Pulmonary Circulation

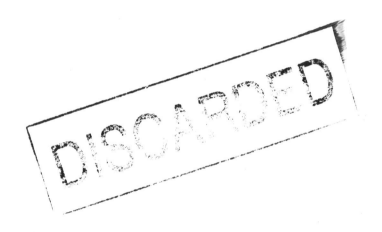

Pulmonary Circulation: Diseases and their Treatment

SECOND EDITION

Edited by

ANDREW J PEACOCK MPhil MD FRCP

Director and Professor of Medicine
Scottish Pulmonary Vascular Unit
Western Infirmary, Glasgow, UK

and

LEWIS J RUBIN MD

Professor of Medicine and Director
Pulmonary Vascular Center at the University of
California, San Diego School of Medicine
La Jolla CA, USA

ARNOLD

A member of the Hodder Headline Group
LONDON

First published in Great Britain in 2004 by
Arnold, a member of the Hodder Headline Group,
338 Euston Road, London NW1 3BH

http://www.hoddereducation.com

Distributed in the United States of America by
Oxford University Press Inc.,
198 Madison Avenue, New York, NY10016
Oxford is a registered trademark of Oxford University Press

Whilst the advice and information in this book are believed to be true and
accurate at the date of going to press, neither the author[s] nor the publisher
can accept any legal responsibility or liability for any errors or omissions
that may be made. In particular (but without limiting the generality of the
preceding disclaimer) every effort has been made to check drug dosages;
however, it is still possible that errors have been missed. Furthermore,
dosage schedules are constantly being revised and new side-effects
recognized. For these reasons the reader is strongly urged to consult the
drug companies' printed instructions before administering any of the drugs
recommended in this book.

British Library Cataloguing in Publication Data
A catalogue record for this book is available from the British Library

Library of Congress Cataloging-in-Publication Data
A catalog record for this book is available from the Library of Congress

ISBN -10: 0 340 80782 2
ISBN -13: 978 0 340 80782 8

2 3 4 5 6 7 8 9 10

Commissioning Editor: Joanna Koster
Development Editor: Sarah Burrows
Project Editor: Zelah Pengilley
Production Controller: Lindsay Smith
Cover Design: Lee-May Lim

Typeset in 10/12 pt Minion by Charon Tec Pvt. Ltd, Chennai, India
Printed and bound in Great Britain by Butler & Tanner Ltd

What do you think about this book? Or any other Arnold title?
Please visit our website: www.hoddereducation.com

To my wife Jila and my children Leila, Johnnie and Vita who have put up with so much over the years. They have tolerated my love for science and medicine even though their own interests lie elsewhere.

AP

To my family for their support, and to our patients, who serve as a constant reminder of the importance of our commitment.

LR

We would like to thank our colleagues from around the world who have been an inspiration to this book and in many cases contributors to it. Whether we work in Respiratory Medicine or Cardiology, we all share the view that the connection between the heart and lungs is important.

Contents

Contributors

Steven H Abman MD
Professor of Pediatrics
Director, Pediatric Heart Lung Center
Department of Pediatrics
University of Colorado Health Sciences Center and
The Children's Hospital
Denver, CO, USA

William R Auger MD
Professor of Clinical Medicine
Division of Pulmonary and Critical Care Medicine
University of California at San Diego
School of Medicine
La Jolla, CA, USA

David B Badesch MD
Professor of Medicine
Division of Pulmonary Sciences and Critical Care
Medicine
Medical Director, Pulmonary Hypertension Center
University of Colorado Health Sciences Center
Denver, CO, USA

Robyn J Barst MD
Professor of Pediatrics
Columbia University College of Physicians and
Surgeons, New York
Director, New York Presbyterian Pulmonary
Hypertension Center
New York, NY, USA

Peter Bärtsch
Medizinische Klinik und Poliklinik
Abteilung Innere Medizin VII: Sportmedizin
Universitätsklinikum, Heidelberg
Germany

Henri Bounameaux MD
Professor of Medicine and Chairman
Department of Internal Medicine
Director, Division of Angiology and Haemostasis
University Hospital of Geneva
Geneva, Switzerland

Angelo Branzi MD
Professor of Cardiology;
Chief Cardiovascular Department and
Director, Institute of Cardiology
University of Bologna, Italy

Oswaldo Castro MD
Professor Emeritus of Medicine
Acting Director, Center for Sickle Cell Disease
Howard University College of Medicine
Washington, DC, USA

Richard N Channick, MD
Associate Professor of Medicine
Division of Pulmonary and Critical Care Medicine
University of California at San Diego
School of Medicine,
La Jolla, CA, USA

Ari Chaouat MD
Department of Pulmonology
Hôpital de Hautepierre
Strasbourg, France

Doina Ciurea DVM
Formerly Assistant Professor of
Comparative Medicine
Center for Laboratory Animal Sciences
Mt Sinai School of Medicine
New York, NY, USA

Barbara A Cockrill MD
Assistant Professor of Medicine
Pulmonary and Critical Care Unit
Massachusetts General Hospital
Harvard Medical School
Boston, MA, USA

Carlyne D Cool MD
Pulmonary Hypertension Center and Department of
Pathology
University of Colorado Health Sciences Center
Denver, CO, USA

Paul A Corris MB FRCP (London) FRCP (Edinburgh)
Professor of Thoracic Medicine
University of Newcastle and Freeman Hospital
Newcastle upon Tyne, UK.

Richard Coulden FRCR FRCP
Consultant Cardiothoracic Radiologist
Papworth and Addenbrooke's Hospitals
Cambridge, UK

Julius H Cranshaw MD BSc MRCP FRCA
Wellcome Trust Training Fellow
Unit of Critical Care, Imperial College of Science,
Technology and Medicine
Royal Brompton Hospital
London, UK

Timothy W Evans MD PhD DSc FRCP FRCA FMedSci
Professor of Intensive Care Medicine
Unit of Critical Care, Imperial College of Science,
Technology and Medicine
Royal Brompton Hospital
London, UK

Karen A Fagan MD
Assistant Professor of Medicine
Division of Pulmonary Sciences and Critical Care
Medicine
Pulmonary Hypertension Center
University of Colorado Health Sciences Center
Denver, CO, USA

Peter F Fedullo MD
Professor of Medicine
Division of Pulmonary and Critical Care Medicine
University of California at San Diego
School of Medicine
San Diego, CA, USA

Terry A Fortin MD
Fellow, Division of Cardiology
Duke University Medical Center
Durham, NC, USA

Sean P Gaine MD PhD FRCPI
Consultant Respiratory Physician
Department of Respiratory Medicine
Mater Misericordiae Hospital
University College Dublin, Ireland

Nazzareno Galiè MD
Associate Professor of Cardiology
Head, Pulmonary Hypertension Center
Institute of Cardiology
University of Bologna, Italy

Jorge Gaspar MD FACC
Head of Interventional Cardiology
Instituto Nacional de Cardiología Ignacio Chávez
Departamento de Hemodinámica, México

J Simon R Gibbs MD FRCP
Senior Lecturer, National Heart and Lung Institute
Imperial College London
Honorary Consultant Cardiologist
Hammersmith Hospital and Royal Brompton Hospital
London, UK

Joan Gil MD
Professor of Pathology
Mount Sinai School of Medicine
New York, NY, USA

Samuel Z Goldhaber MD
Associate Professor of Medicine
Harvard Medical School and
Staff Cardiologist, Director, Venous Thromboembolism
Research Group
Director, Anticoagulation Service
Brigham and Women's Hospital
Boston, MA, USA

Bertron M Groves MD
Professor of Medicine, Division of Cardiology
University of Colorado Health Sciences Center
Denver, CO, USA

Charles A Hales MD
Professor of Medicine
Chief, Pulmonary and Critical Care Unit
Massachusetts General Hospital
Harvard Medical School
Boston, MA, USA

Sheila G Haworth FRCP FRCPath FRCPCH FACC FMedSci
British Heart Foundation, Professor of
Developmental Cardiology
Unit of Vascular Biology and Pharmacology
Institute of Child Health, University College London and
Consultant in Paediatric Cardiology
Great Ormond Street Hospital for Children
London, UK

Douglas Helmerson MD, FRCPC
Clincal Assistant Professor, Medicine
University of Calgary
Calgary, Alberta, Canada

Michael Henein MSc PhD
Senior Lecturer
National Heart and Lung Institute
Imperial College London and
Royal Brompton Hospital
London, UK

Philippe Hervé MD PhD
Pulmonary Vascular Center
Service de Pneumologie et Réanimation Respiratoire
Hôpital Antoine Béclère
Assistance Publique Hôpitaux de Paris
Université Paris Sud
Clamart, France

Marc Humbert MD PhD
Professor of Medicine, Pulmonary Vascular Center
Service de Pneumologie et Réanimation Respiratoire,
Hôpital Antoine Béclère
Assistance Publique Hôpitaux de Paris
Université Paris-Sud
Clamart, France

James E Jackson MB BS MRCP FRCR
Consultant Radiologist and Senior Lecturer
Department of Imaging
Hammersmith Hospital
London, UK

Stuart W Jamieson MB FRCS
Professor of Surgery
Chief of Cardiothoracic Surgery
UCSD Medical Center
San Diego, CA, USA

Trina K Jeffery PhD
CJ Martin Post-Doctoral Fellow, NHMRC(Aus)
University of Cambridge School of Clinical Medicine
Addenbrooke's Hospital
Cambridge, UK

Karina Keogh MD
Division of Pulmonary and Critical Care Medicine
Mayo Clinic College of Medicine
Rochester, MN, USA

Kim M Kerr MD
Associate Clinical Professor of Medicine
Division of Pulmonary and Critical Care Medicine
University of California at San Diego School of Medicine
La Jolla, CA, USA

John P Kinsella MD
Director, ECMO Service
Director, Medical Advisory Group and
Emergency Medical Transport Service
Professor of Neonatology
Department of Pediatrics
University of Colorado School of Medicine and
The Children's Hospital
Denver, CO, USA

Michael J Krowka MD
Professor of Medicine
Mayo Clinic College of Medicine
Division of Pulmonary and Critical Care Medicine
Division of Gastroenterology and Hepatology
Rochester, MN, USA

Marcin Kurzyna MD PhD
Department of Chest Medicine
National Institute of Tuberculosis and Lung Diseases
Warsaw, Poland

David Langleben MD FRCP
Professor of Medicine (Cardiology)
McGill University
Director, Center for Pulmonary Vascular Disease
The Sir Mortimer B Davis-Jewish General Hospital
Montreal, Quebec, Canada

James E Loyd MD
Professor of Medicine
Division of Allergy, Pulmonary and Critical Care Medicine
Vanderbilt University Medical Center
Nashville, TN, USA

William MacNee MB ChB MD FRCP(G) FRCP(E)
Professor of Respiratory and Environmental Medicine
ELEGI, Colt Research Laboratories
Medical School, University of Edinburgh
Edinburgh, UK

Alessandra Manes MD
Coordinator, Pulmonary Hypertension Center
Institute of Cardiology
University of Bologna, Italy

Marco Maggiorini MD
Head of Medical ICU
Department of Internal Medicine
University Hospital
Zurich, Switzerland

Michael D McGoon MD
Consultant, Division of Cardiovascular Diseases
Mayo Clinic
Professor of Medicine
Mayo Medical School
Rochester, MN, USA

Vallerie V McLaughlin MD
Associate Professor of Medicine
Director, Pulmonary Hypertension Program
University of Michigan
Ann Arbor, MI, USA

Keith McNeil MBBS FRACP
Associate Professor of Medicine
University of Queensland
Consultant Respiratory Physician and Head
Transplant and Pulmonary Vascular Diseases Units
Prince Charles Hospital
Brisbane, Australia

Nicholas W Morrell MD FRCP
Director, Pulmonary Vascular Diseases Unit
Addenbrooke's and Papworth Hospitals
University of Cambridge School of Clinical Medicine
Addenbrooke's Hospital
Cambridge, UK

Jane H Morse MD
Professor Emerita of Clinical Medicine
Special Lecturer, Department of Medicine
Columbia University College of Physicians and
Surgeons and Consultant, The Presbyterian Hospital
New York, NY, USA

Heather Mortimer MPhil MRCP
Pulmonary Vascular Fellow and Specialist Registrar
Scottish Pulmonary Vascular Unit
Western Infirmary
Glasgow, UK

Robert Naeije MD PhD
Department of Cardiology
Erasme University Hospital and
Department of Physiology
Erasme Campus of the Free
University of Brussels
Belgium

John H Newman MD
Professor of Medicine
Division of Allergy, Pulmonary and Critical Care Medicine
Vanderbilt University Medical Center
Nashville, TN, USA

Andrea Olschewski MD
Staff Anesthesiologist
Department of Anesthesiology, Intensive Care Medicine
Pain Therapy
University of Giessen School of Medicine
Giessen, Germany

Horst Olschewski MD
Medical Clinic II, Internal Medicine
Critical Care Medicine and Pulmonology
University of Giessen School of Medicine
Giessen, Germany

Andrew J Peacock MPhil MD FRCP
Director and Professor of Medicine
Scottish Pulmonary Vascular Unit
Western Infirmary
Glasgow, UK

Joanna Pepke-Zaba PhD
Consultant Physician
Pulmonary Vascular Diseases Unit
Papworth Hospital
Cambridge, UK

Arnaud Perrier MD FCCP
Senior Lecturer, Medical Clinic
Department of Internal Medicine
Geneva University Hospital
Geneva, Switzerland

Michael R Pinsky MD CM Dr hc FCCP FCCM
Professor of Critical Care Medicine
Bioengineering and Anesthesiology
University of Pittsburgh School of Medicine
Pittsburgh, PA, USA

Marlene Rabinovitch MD
Dwight and Vera Dunlevie Professor of Pediatric
Cardiology and (by courtesy) Developmental Biology,
Research Director of the Wall Center for
Pulmonary Vascular Diseases
Stanford University School of Medicine
Stanford, CA, USA

John T Reeves MD
Professor Emeritus,
Departments of Pediatrics, Medicine and Family Medicine
University of Colorado Health Sciences Center
Denver, CO, USA

Stuart Rich MD
The John H and Margaret V Krehbiel, Professor of
Cardiology, Rush Medical College
Director, Rush Heart Institute Center for
Pulmonary Heart Disease
The Rush University Medical Center
Chicago, IL, USA

Lewis J Rubin MD
Professor of Medicine and Director
Pulmonary Vascular Center
University of California, San Diego School of Medicine
La Jolla, CA, USA

James R Runo MD
Pulmonary Fellow, Division of Allergy, Pulmonary and
Critical Care Medicine
Vanderbilt University Medical Center
Nashville, TN, USA

Julio Sandoval MD FACC
Chief, Cardiopulmonary Department
Instituto Nacional de Cardiología Ignacio Chávez
Mexico

Werner Seeger MD
Professor of Medicine
Chief of the Department of Internal Medicine
Section Head of Respiratory and Critical Care Medicine
University of Giessen School of Medicine
Giessen, Germany

Claire L Shovlin PhD MA FRCP
Senior Lecturer and Honorary Consultant
Respiratory Medicine
Imperial College Faculty of Medicine
National Heart and Lung Institute
Hammersmith Hospital
London, UK

Gérald Simonneau MD
Professor of Medicine
Director, Pulmonary Vascular Center
Service de Pneumologie et Réanimation
Respiratoire
Hôpital Antoine Béclère
Assistance Publique Hôpitaux de Paris
Université Paris-Sud
Clamart, France

Olivier Sitbon MD
Consultant Respiratory Physician
Pulmonary Vascular Center
Service de Pneumologie et Réanimation Respiratoire
Hôpital Antoine Béclère
Assistance Publique Hôpitaux de Paris
Université Paris-Sud
Clamart, France

Rudolf Speich MD FCCP
Professor of Medicine
Department of Internal Medicine
University Hospital
Zurich, Switzerland

Kurt R Stenmark MD
Professor, Pediatric Critical Care Medicine
Director, Developmental Lung Biology
Professor and Section Head
Pediatric Critical Care Medicine
University of Colorado Health Sciences Center
Denver, CO, USA

John Stradling MD FRCP
Professor, Oxford Centre for Respiratory Medicine
Osler Chest Unit, Churchill Hospital
Oxford, UK

Victor F Tapson MD
Associate Professor of Medicine
Director, Pulmonary Hypertension Center
Duke University Medical Center
Durham, NC, USA

Adam Torbicki MD PhD
Professor of Medicine and Head
Department of Chest Medicine
National Institute of Tuberculosis and Lung Diseases
Warsaw, Poland

Rubin M. Tuder MD
Professor of Pathology and Medicine
Divisions of Cardiopulmonary Pathology and
Pulmonary and Critical Care Medicine
Department of Pathology
Johns Hopkins University School of Medicine
Baltimore, MD, USA

Jean-Louis Vincent MD PhD FCCP
Professor, Head, Department of Intensive Care
Erasme University Hospital
University of Brussels
Belgium

Norbert F Voelkel MD
The Hart Family Professor of Emphysema Research
University of Colorado
Health Sciences Center
Denver, CO, USA

Stephen J Watt FRCPEd AFOM
Senior Lecturer, Department of Environmental and
Occupational Medicine
University of Aberdeen
Aberdeen, UK

E Kenneth Weir MD
Chief of Cardiology
VA Medical Center, Minneapolis and
Professor of Medicine and Physiology
University of Minnesota
Minneapolis, MN, USA

Emmanuel Weitzenblum MD
Professor of Medicine and Pulmonology
Head, Department of Pulmonology
Hôpital de Hautepierre
Hôpitaux Universitaires de Strasbourg
Strasbourg, France

Ari L Zaiman MD PhD
Instructor of Medicine
Division of Pulmonary and Critical Care Medicine
Johns Hopkins University School of Medicine
Baltimore, MD, USA

Foreword

Since the first edition of the *Pulmonary Circulation* appeared in 1996, important new information has changed the field. Therefore, a second edition is warranted and timely. It has been necessary to expand the current edition to 52 chapters from 37. Energetic new investigators have brought new concepts and new approaches to the field, including the many authors who are new to this edition. Represented in the current, but not the former, edition is experience from Germany, Ireland, Italy, Mexico, Poland and Switzerland, indicating the increasing global recognition that the lung circulation has a major role to play in health and disease. I have cited below only some of the examples of important new material included in the second edition of *Pulmonary Circulation*.

The description of the human genome and the current genetic revolution has been accompanied by identification of the bone morphogenetic protein and one of its receptors – abnormalities of which may account for 50% of familial and 25% of sporadic cases of primary pulmonary hypertension. Two new chapters indicate not only that these findings will allow screening and early identification of the disease, but also that they hold promise for new therapies. Several etiologies of pulmonary hypertension (PH) not emphasized in the previous edition were considered now to deserve separate chapters.

- One chapter indicates that therapy for PH in connective tissue diseases, and in particular the CREST syndrome of scleroderma, can at least improve the patient's quality of life.
- The chapter on the recently reintroduced appetite suppression drugs implicates serotonin metabolism in the refractory, fatal PH, which can occur in patients taking these drugs.
- Another chapter discusses the frequently unrecognized and highly fatal PH, which occurs in HIV infections.
- Because of the high incidence of pulmonary circulatory disorders in patients with liver cirrhosis and portal vein hypertension, two chapters were included to present the two disparate clinical pictures. Pulmonary

hypertension, which may be severe, occurs in up to 20% of cirrhotic patients and it may respond better to long-term prostacyclin than liver transplant or inhaled NO. At the other end of the spectrum is the pulmonary hypotensive hepatoportal syndrome where shunts through dilated lung arteries cause severe hypoxemia. Here, liver transplantation, although risky, may be effective in the less severely hypoxemic patients.

- Genetic disorders of hemoglobin deserved a chapter in the new edition, because they are worldwide, are not necessarily limited to particular ethnic populations, and have relatively high incidences of PH, which can be rapidly fatal. Because treatment is often unsatisfactory, methods to prevent the development of PH are emphasized.
- Primary pulmonary vascular tumors, mostly sarcomas, are rare but cause rapidly fatal right ventricular failure. Early surgical resection provides the only known potential for cure.
- Particularly when it comes to the lung circulation, children are not just small adults, and primary pulmonary hypertension in the pediatric age group can be rapidly progressive and therapeutically refractory, as discussed in this chapter.
- Veno-occlusive disease, while rare, should be considered, because lung transplantation is the current treatment and initiating arterial dilation risks pulmonary edema.

While individually, each of these varied etiologies of pulmonary vascular disease may be uncommon, together they make up a substantial clinical population. In this second edition, these chapters with detailed presentation of mechanism, incidence, natural history, diagnosis, and management by experts in the field contain important clinical information that has previously not been collected in one volume.

In Western countries, pulmonary thromboembolism is the major cause of death in the puerperium and postoperative period, and is of increasing importance in the aging populations. Therefore, the chapter in the first edition has been replaced by three chapters in the new edition. In the chapter on diagnosis of acute episodes, the authors emphasize for non-massive embolism that combining several tests is needed, while for massive embolism, echocardiography is a good initial screening test. Treatments, in the acute phase, are undergoing substantial evolution away from the use of unfractionated intravenous heparin or inferior vena caval filters to novel anticoagulant strategies. While in chronic PH, thrombectomy has been extremely useful, the challenge remains to prevent, detect, and better treat patients who have small vessel disease.

Some of the most exciting developments detailed in the new version have been in the area of therapy. While there are chapters reviewing and updating conventional therapies for PH, sufficient new drugs or drug strategies have evolved, that a chapter integrating the various approaches is given. The new strategies that are evaluated are the inhalation of a stable analog of prostacyclin (iloprost), the oral and subcutaneous administration of prostacyclin analogs, and the administration of inhaled

nitric oxide, all of which increase adenylcyclase in the pulmonary arteriolar wall. New combinations of these drugs with, for example, phosphodiesterase (to prevent breakdown of cyclic AMP) and inhibitors of endothelin are evaluated. Because right heart failure is the usual precipitating cause of death in PH, one chapter presents the palliation that can be achieved by using atrial septostomy to reduce the load on the right ventricle. Finally, with regard to therapy, the reader is given a glimpse of the future whereby strategies to alter receptor signaling, or to modify the expression of vascular endothelial growth factor, or to reduce the breakdown of matrix have been effective in animal models of pulmonary hypertension.

These new chapters combined with revision of the chapters from the first edition result in a second edition of *Pulmonary Circulation* that upgrades prior and introduces new concepts in an authoritative manner designed to present both a theoretical and clinical review of a rapidly changing field.

John Reeves, 2004

Preface

The consequences of disturbed function of the pulmonary circulation remain an enigma to most clinicians. There is disturbance of pulmonary circulatory function in nearly all cardiac and pulmonary disease, yet this is rarely recognized or treated. The reasons for this relative obscurity when compared, for example, with the systemic circulation, are clear. The pulmonary circulation is difficult to examine clinically and the tools we have for pulmonary circulatory measurement are either crude or invasive, or both. Even when we make invasive measurements with a cardiac catheter we only learn about the circulation in artificial surroundings (the catheter laboratory), in an unrepresentative position (supine on the table) and in a state of artificially restricted activity. Clearly, we need clinical measurement techniques that will allow us to pursue pulmonary circulatory function in all states of human activity both in normal people and those with cardiorespiratory disease. These are coming, but even now we know much about the pulmonary circulation that can help us in looking after patients in the ward and in the intensive care unit. Fortunately, there has been a great deal of research into the structure and function of the pulmonary circulation. We already understand much of its physiology and pathophysiology and, recently, a number of effective therapies have been developed, tested and put into clinical use with great effect. In this book, a distinguished group of authors, most of whom have a clinical background, have presented what is known about the pulmonary circulation in a readable and, more importantly, clinically relevant fashion, so that it can be understood by practising physicians.

This is the second edition, with many completely new sections but a similar though more clinically orientated format. The book has been written especially with the busy clinician in mind, particularly those in respiratory medicine, cardiology, pediatrics and intensive care. It has been deliberately structured so that a subject can be appreciated at any level from the purely clinical right down to the biochemical. This allows the reader to start with a chapter about a particular clinical issue but, if interested, to pursue that subject from clinical to physiological to biochemical level as he or she desires. Each chapter stands alone, so some repetition is inevitable, for which we make no apology, but this hierarchy of structure will, we hope, make the book accessible without diminishing the quality of the information that is presented.

Andrew J Peacock and Lewis J Rubin, 2004

Abbreviations

5-HETE	5-hydroxyeicosotetraenoic acid		CGD	chronic granulomatous disease
5-HT	5-hydroxytryptamine; serotonin		cGMP	cyclic guanosine monophosphate
5-HTT	5-HT transporter		CI	cardiac index; confidence interval
5-LO	5-lipoxygenase		C_K	coefficient of kinship
6MWT	6-minute walk test		CK-MB	creative kinase-myocardial band
8-Br-GMP	8-bromo-guanosine monophosphate		CMS	chronic mountain sickness
^{99m}TcMAA	technetium-99 macroaggregated albumin		CMV	cytomegalovirus
ACE	angiotensin converting enzyme		CNS	central nervous system
ACS	acute chest syndrome		CO	cardiac output
AcT	acceleration time		COPD	chronic obstructive pulmonary disease
AEC	American-European Consensus		CPAP	continuous positive airway pressure
aECA	anti-endothelial antibodies		CPS	carbamoyl-phosphate synthetase
aFGF	acidic fibroblast growth factor		CREB	cAMP response element-binding protein
AIDS	acquired immunodeficiency syndrome		CREST	calcinosis, Raynaud's, sclerodactyly and telangectasia
ALI	acute lung injury			
ALK1	activin receptor-like kinase 1		CSS	Churg–Strauss syndrome
ALT	alanine aminotransferase		CT	computed tomography
AMS	acute mountain sickness		CTD	connective tissue disease
ANA	antinuclear antibody		CTE	chronic thromboembolic
ANCA	antineutrophil cytoplasmic antibody		CTEPH	chronic thromboembolic pulmonary hypertension
ARDS	acute respiratory distress syndrome			
ARNT	aryl hydrocarbon receptor nuclear translocator		CTPA	computed tomography pulmonary angiography
AS	atrial septostomy			
ASD	atrial septal defect		CTR	cardiothoracic ratio
AST	aspartate aminotransferase		CVA	cerebrovascular accident
AVF	atrioventricular fibrillation		CvO_2	mixed venous oxygen content
AVM	arteriovenous malformation		CVP	central venous pressure
AVP	arginine vasopressin		DA	ductus arteriosus
AVSD	atrioventricular septal defect		DCO	diffusing capacity for carbon monoxide
BAL	bronchoalveolar lavage		DLCO	diffusing capacity for carbon monoxide
BBAS	blade balloon atrial septostomy		DLT	double lung transplant
BCPA	bidirectional cavopulmonary anastomosis		DPI	diphenylene iodonium
BDAS	balloon dilation atrial septostomy		DTPA	ethylenediaminepentaacetic acid
bFGF	basic fibroblast growth factor		DVT	deep venous (vein) thrombus (thrombosis)
BLT	bilateral sequential single lung transplant		EBCT	electron beam computed tomography
BMI	body mass index		ECE-1	endothelin-1 converting enzyme
BMP	bone morphogenetic protein		ECG	electrocardiogram
BMPR2	bone morphogenetic protein receptor 2		ECHO	echocardiography
BNP	brain natriuretic protein		ECMO	extracorporeal membrane oxygenation
BPI	bactericidal permeability-increasing protein		EGF	endothelial growth factor; epidermal growth factor
CADD	continuous ambulatory drug delivery			
cAMP	cyclic adenine monophosphate		EGTA	ethyleneglycotetraacetic acid
cANCA	cytoplasmic ANCA		EI	eccentricity index
CcO_2	oxygen content of end-capillary blood		ELISA	enzyme-linked immunoadsorbent assay
CDH	congenital diaphragmatic hernia		ENG	endoglin
CDMP1	cartilage-derived morphogenetic protein-1		eNOS	endothelial nitric oxide synthase
CEMRA	contrast-enhanced magnetic resonance angiography		ENT	ear, nose and throat
			ERK1	extracellular regulated kinase-1

ET	endothelin
ET-1 (2) (3)	endothelin-1 (-2) (-3)
ET_A receptor	endothelin receptor A
ET_B receptor	endothelin receptor B
EVE	endogenous vascular elastase
FAK	focal adhesion kinase
FDA	Federal Drug Administration
FDG-PET	fluorine-18-2-fluoro-2-deoxy-D-glucose positron emission tomography
FDP	fibrin degradation products
FEF	forced expiratory flow
FEV_1	forced expiratory volume in 1 second
FGN	fibrinogen
FIO_2	fraction of inspired oxygen
FLAP	5-lipoxygenase-activating protein
FO	foramen ovale
FPPH	familial primary pulmonary hypertension
FRC	functional residual capacity
FVC	forced vital capacity
G protein	guanine-nucleotide-binding protein
Gd-DTPA	gadolinium-diethylenetriamine pentaacetic acid
GDF	growth and differentiation factor
GI	gastrointestinal
GRE	gradient refocused echo
HAART	highly active antiretroviral therapy
HACE	high-altitude cerebral edema
HAPE	high-altitude pulmonary edema
HFOV	high-frequency oscillatory ventilation
HHT	hereditary hemorrhagic telangiectasia
HHV-8	human herpes virus
HIF	hypoxia-inducible factor
HIV	human immunodeficiency virus
HLT	heart/lung transplant
HOX	homeobox
HPS	hepatopulmonary syndrome
HPV	hypoxic pulmonary vasoconstriction
HPVR	hypoxic pulmonary vascular response
HRCT	high-resolution computed tomography
HSP	Henoch–Schönlein purpura
HVOD	hepatic veno-occlusive disease
HVR	hypoxic ventilatory response
ICAM	intracellular adhesion molecule
ICU	intensive care unit
IGF-1	insulin-like growth factor
IL	interleukin
IMV	intermittent mandatory ventilation
iNO	inhaled nitric oxide
INR	international normalized ratio
IP_3	inositol triphosphate; 1,4,5-inositol triphosphate
IPF	idiopathic pulmonary fibrosis
IPPHS	international primary pulmonary hypertension study
ITP	intrathoracic pressure
IVC	inferior vena cava
IVCCI	inferior vena cava collapsibility index
IVS	interventricular septal
IVUS	intravascular ultrasound

JVP	jugular venous pressure
K_{Ca}	calcium-sensitive potassium channel
KCO	specific gas transfer
KDR	VEGF receptor II
KSV	Kaposi's sarcoma virus
L-Arg	L-arginine
LA	left atrium
LAO	left anterior oblique
LAP	latency-associated protein; left atrial pressure
L-LAMMA	L-monomethylargine
LMWH	low molecular weight heparin
L-NNA	N-nitro-L-arginine
LPA	left pulmonary artery
LTOT	long-term oxygen therapy
LV	left ventricle; left ventricular
LVEDP	left ventricular end-diastolic pressure
LVEF	left ventricular ejection fraction
LVRS	lung volume reduction surgery
MAA	macroaggregates of human serum albumin
MAP	mitogen-activated protein
MCT	monocrotaline
MCTD	mixed connective tissue disease
MIGET	multiple inert gas elimination technique
mLAP	mean left atrial pressure
MMP	matrix metalloproteinase
MPA	microscopic polyangiitis
mPAP	mean pulmonary artery pressure
MRA	magnetic resonance angiography
mRAP	mean right atrial pressure
MRI	magnetic resonance imaging
mRNA	messenger ribonucleic acid
MSI	microsatellite instability
NANC	non-adrenergic, non-cholinergic
NEB	neuroepithelial body
NIH	National Institutes of Health
NMPG	N-mercaptopropionylglycine
NO	nitric oxide
NOS	nitric oxide synthase
NPR-A	atrial natriuretic peptide type A receptor
NYHA	New York Heart Association
OB	obliterative bronchiolitis
OI	oxygenation index
OLT	orthotopic liver transplantation
OSA	obstructive sleep apnea
OSAS	obstructive sleep apnea syndrome
P_A	alveolar pressure
PA	pulmonary artery
$PaCO_2$	arterial PCO_2
PADP	pulmonary artery diastolic pressure
PAH	pulmonary arterial hypertension
PAHRH	pulmonary arterial hypertension related to HIV infection
PAI	protein accumulation index
PAN	polyarteritis nodosa
pANCA	perinuclear ANCA
$P_{A}O_2$	alveolar PO_2
PaO_2	arterial partial pressure of oxygen
PAOP	pulmonary artery occlusion pressure
PAP	pulmonary artery pressure

PAR	pulmonary arterial resistance	RV	right ventricle; right ventricular
PASP	pulmonary artery systolic pressure	RVD	right ventricular dysfunction
PAVM	pulmonary arteriovenous malformation	RVEDP	right ventricular end-diastolic pressure
Paw	airway pressure	RVEF	right ventricular ejection fraction
PAWP	pulmonary artery wedge pressure	RVF	right ventricular failure
PC	phase contrast	RVH	right ventricular hypertrophy
Pc	pulmonary capillary pressure	RVP	right ventricular pressure
PCH	pulmonary capillary hemangiomatosis	RVSP	right ventricular systolic pressure
PCO_2	partial pressure of carbon dioxide	SAC	stretch-activated cation channel
PCP	pulmonary capillary pressure	SaO_2	arterial oxygen saturation
PCWP	pulmonary capillary wedge pressure	SAP	systemic artery pressure
PDA	patent ductus arteriosus	SD	standard deviation
PDE5	phosphodiesterase type 5	SE	spin echo
PDGF	platelet-derived growth factor	SEE	standard error of estimate
PE	pulmonary embolism	SEM	standard error of mean
PEEP	positive end-expiratory pressure	SIRS	systemic inflammatory response syndrome
PG	pressure gradient	SIV	simian immunodeficiency virus
PG	prostaglandin	SLE	systemic lupus erythematosus
PGI_2	prostacyclin	SLT	single lung transplant
PGI_2-R	prostacyclin receptor	SM	smooth muscle
PGI_2-S	prostacyclin synthase	SMC	smooth muscle cell
PH	pulmonary hypertension	SO_2T	systemic oxygen transport
pHi	intramucosal pH	SOD	superoxide dismutase
PKC	protein kinase C	SPH	scleroderma-associated pulmonary
PKG	protein kinase G		hypertension; secondary/severe pulmonary
PO_2	partial pressure of oxygen		hypertension
POPH	portopulmonary hypertension	SSLT	single sequential lung transplantation
PPARγ	nuclear peroxisome proliferator activator	SVC	superior vena cava
	receptor γ	SvO_2	mixed venous O_2 saturation
Ppc	pericardial pressure	SVR	systemic vascular resistance
PPET-1	preproendothelin-1	SVT	supraventricular tachycardia
PPH	primary pulmonary hypertension	TEE	transesophageal echocardiography
PPHN	persistent pulmonary hypertension of the	TF	tissue factor
	newborn	TGA	transposition of the great arteries
Ppl	pleural pressure	TGF-β	transforming growth factor-β
PTCER	pulmonary transcapillary escape route	TIA	transient ischemic attack
PTE	pulmonary thromboendarterectomy	TIMP	tissue inhibitor of matrix metalloproteinases
PVOD	pulmonary vascular obstructive disease	TIPG	tricuspid insufficiency pressure gradient
PVP	pulmonary venous pressure	TIPS	transjugular intrahepatic portosystemic
PVR	pulmonary vascular resistance		shunting
PVZ	pulmonary vascular impedance	TLC	total lung capacity
$\dot{Q}$	blood flow	tPA	tissue-type plasminogen activator
$\dot{Q}P$	pulmonary blood flow	TPR	total pulmonary vascular resistance
$\dot{Q}S$	systemic blood flow	TUNEL	terminal deoxynucleotidyl transferase (TdT)
RA	rheumatoid arthritis; right atrium		mediated dUTP nick end labeling
RANTES	regulated upon activation normal T-expressed	US	lower limb venous compression
	and secreted		ultrasonography
RAP	right atrial pressure	$\dot{V}/\dot{Q}$	ventilation/perfusion
RDS	respiratory distress syndrome	V_A	alveolar ventilation
REM	rapid eye movement	VC	vital capacity
RHC	right heart catheterization	VEGF	vascular endothelial growth factor
RHF	right heart failure	VILI	ventilator-induced lung injury
RIJ	right internal jugular	VO_2	oxygen consumption
RNS	reactive nitrogen species	VSD	ventricular septal defect
ROC	receptor-operated non-selective cation	Vt	tidal volume
	channel	VTE	venous thromboembolism
ROS	reactive oxygen species	WG	Wegener's granulomatosis
RP	Raynaud's phenomenon	Z_0	pulmonary vascular impedance at zero Hz
RSV	respiratory syncytial virus	Z_c	pulmonary vascular characteristic impedance

A note on references

The reference lists are annotated, where appropriate, to guide readers to key primary papers and major review articles as follows:

Key primary papers are indicated by a bullet (•)
Major review articles are indicated by a diamond (◆)

Papers that represent the first formal publication of a management guideline are indicated by an asterisk (∗).

We hope that this feature will render extensive lists of references more useful to the reader and will help to encourage self-directed learning among both trainees and practicing physicians.

PART 1

The structure and function of the normal pulmonary circulation

Pulmonary vascular function

ROBERT NAEIJE

INTRODUCTION

The pulmonary circulation is a high-flow and low-pressure circuit, which favors pulmonary gas exchange by preventing fluid moving out of the pulmonary vessels into the interstitial space, and allows the right ventricle to operate at a low energy cost. However, because of the low pressures, the pulmonary circulation is very sensitive to mechanical influences, and the 'flow generator' right ventricle is thin walled, poorly prepared for rapid changes in loading conditions. In addition, the pulsatility of the pulmonary circulation is more important than that of the systemic circulation, which affects the energy transmission from the right ventricle to the pulmonary arteries.

The gold standard for the functional evaluation of the pulmonary circulation still remains a right heart catheterization with the complex pulmonary artery pressure and flow waves summarized by mean values used for pulmonary vascular resistance (PVR) calculations. Progress in technology now allows refined beat-by-beat non-invasive approaches, which improves the understanding of the coupling of the right ventricle to normal and abnormal pulmonary hemodynamic conditions.

Many cardiac and pulmonary diseases are associated with an abnormal increase in pulmonary artery pressures. The most common causes of pulmonary hypertension are left heart failure and chronic hypoxemic lung diseases. Pulmonary hypertension is the third most common cardiovascular condition, after coronary heart disease and systemic hypertension. As the pulmonary circulation is entirely within the thorax, relatively hidden from clinical examination, and symptoms appear only after pulmonary artery pressures have more than doubled from baseline, a sound physiological approach is essential for the diagnosis and treatment of pulmonary hypertension.

NORMAL PULMONARY VASCULAR PRESSURES AND FLOWS

The interpretation of measurements to evaluate organ function is methodology dependent. The exploration of the pulmonary circulation is normally done with a triple lumen balloon-tipped thermodilution catheter inserted into a central vein and floated through the right heart chambers into the pulmonary artery under constant pressure wave monitoring.[1] The advantage of the small 1 ml balloon at the tip of the catheter is in the ease of placement into the pulmonary artery without fluoroscopic control, and the estimation of **left** ventricular filling pressures while catheterizing the **right** side of the heart. Thus, the pulmonary artery catheter allows successive measurements of a right atrial pressure (RAP), a right ventricular pressure (RVP), a pulmonary artery pressure (PAP), and an occluded PAP (PAOP).

A PAOP gives a satisfactory estimate of left atrial pressure (LAP) provided that the pulmonary vessels are fully recruited with a pulmonary capillary pressure (PCP) higher than surrounding alveolar pressure (P_A). A PCP higher than P_A defines a zone 3 condition according

West's terminology.[2] Lungs of a recumbent normovolemic healthy subject are normally completely in a zone 3 condition.

With the catheter in place, a proximal lumen located 30 cm from the tip serves the measurement of RAP, a distal lumen at the tip the measurement of PAP, and an air-filled lumen serves to inflate the balloon. A thermistor located 4 cm from the catheter tip records small temperature changes in the pulmonary artery induced by the injection of a bolus of cold saline into the right atrium, allowing calculation of a mean pulmonary blood flow ($\dot{Q}$) from a thermodilution curve.

To minimize the influence of intrathoracic pressure changes associated with respiratory movements, pulmonary vascular pressures are measured at end-expiration, when the lungs are at functional residual capacity.

In a streamlined steady-flow hemodynamic system, it is possible to calculate resistance as a pressure drop versus flow ratio. The pulmonary circulation is markedly pulsatile, but a PVR can be estimated as the difference between mean PAP taken as the inflow pressure, and mean LAP taken as the outflow pressure, divided by $\dot{Q}$:

$$PVR = \frac{(PAP - LAP)}{\dot{Q}}$$

A resistance calculation derives from a simple physical law that governs laminar flows of Newtonian fluids through thin, non-distensible circular tubes. This law, initially enunciated by the French physicist Poiseuille, states that resistance R to flow, defined as a pressure drop ΔP to flow $\dot{Q}$ ratio, is equal to the product of the length l of the tube by a viscosity constant η divided by the product of fourth power of the internal radius r by π:

$$R = \frac{\Delta P}{\dot{Q}} = \frac{8l\eta}{\pi r^4}$$

The fact that r in the equation is at the fourth power explains why R is exquisitely sensitive to small changes in caliber radius. Accordingly, PVR is a good indicator of the state of constriction or dilatation of pulmonary resistive vessels, and helpful to monitor disease-induced pulmonary vascular remodeling and/or changes in tone.

The limits of normal of resting pulmonary vascular pressures and flows as derived from measurements obtained in a total of 55 healthy resting supine young adult healthy volunteers[3–5] are shown in Table 1.1. From that study population it is apparent that there are no gender differences in pulmonary hemodynamics after a correction of flow for body dimensions (Table 1.2).

Earlier studies have shown that ageing is associated with an increase in PAP and a decrease in $\dot{Q}$, leading to a doubling of PVR over a life span of five decades (Table 1.3).[6–9]

Table 1.1 *Limits of normal of pulmonary blood flow and vascular pressures*

Variables	Mean	Limits of normal
$\dot{Q}$ (L/min)	6.4	4.4–8.4
Heart rate (bpm)	67	41–93
PAP systolic (mmHg)	19	13–26
PAP diastolic (mmHg)	10	6–16
PAP mean (mmHg)	13	7–19
PAOP (mmHg)	9	5–13
PCP (mmHg)	10	8–12
RAP (mmHg)	5	1–9
PVR (dyn s/cm^5)	55	11–99
SAP mean (mmHg)	91	71–110

PAOP, occluded PAP; PAP, pulmonary artery pressure; PCP, pulmonary capillary pressure; PVR, pulmonary vascular resistance; $\dot{Q}$, cardiac output; RAP, right atrial pressure; SAP, systemic arterial pressure. Limits of normal: from mean -2 SD to mean $+2$ SD; n = 55 healthy resting volunteers (n = 14 for the measurement of PCP). From references 3–5.

Table 1.2 *Influence of gender on pulmonary blood flow and vascular pressures*

Variables (mean + SE)	Men (n = 34)	Women (n = 21)
$\dot{Q}$ (L/min)	6.7 ± 0.9	6.0 ± 1.2*
$\dot{Q}$ (L/min/m^2)	3.5 ± 0.5	3.6 ± 0.6
PAP (mmHg)	13 ± 3	13 ± 3
PAOP (mmHg)	9 ± 2	9 ± 2
RAP (mmHg)	5 ± 2	5 ± 1

CI, cardiac index; PAOP, occluded PAP; PAP, pulmonary artery pressure; $\dot{Q}$, cardiac output; RAP, right atrial pressure. Values are means ± SD. *P < 0.05. From references 3–5.

Table 1.3 *Influence of age on pulmonary blood flow and vascular pressures*

	Age (years)	
	16–28	61–83
Variables (mean + SE)	n = 22	n = 16
$\dot{Q}$ (L/min)	7.6 ± 0.3	5.6 ± 0.3
PAP (mmHg)	13 ± 1	16 ± 1
PAOP (mmHg)	8 ± 1	9 ± 1
PVR (dyn s/cm^5)	54 ± 6	96 ± 7

PAOP, occluded PAP; PAP, pulmonary artery pressure; PVR, pulmonary vascular resistance; $\dot{Q}$, cardiac output. From references 6–9.

EFFECTS OF EXERCISE

Mild to moderate levels of exercise do not normally much increase PAP, which reaches no more than the upper limit of normal of 20 mmHg, while PAOP (or LAP) remains unchanged.[10] Exercise increases cardiac output proportionally more than the pulmonary vascular pressure gradient, and therefore PVR is calculated to decrease.[10,11]

However, high levels of exercise may markedly increase pulmonary vascular pressures. In athletes able to increase their cardiac output to values in the range of 25–35 L/min, PAP may increase to 40–45 mmHg, together with PAOP in the range of 25–35 mmHg.[11] This is illustrated in Figure 1.1, which reports pulmonary hemodynamic measurements in six triathletes at rest and at two levels of exercise.[12]

As pulmonary hypertension is defined by a PAP >25 mmHg at rest and >30 mmHg at exercise,[13] it may thus be stated that well-trained athletes may present with exercise-induced pulmonary hypertension. As also illustrated in Figure 1.2, strenuous exercise-induced pulmonary hypertension appears essentially to be explained by an upstream transmission of increased LAP.[11] Exercise-induced pulmonary hypertension is not accounted for by an increase in PVR.

There may be a question that, for understandable ethical reasons, none of the above-reported pulmonary hemodynamic measurements at high levels of exercise included direct measurements of LAP. However, PAOP at exercise would be unlikely to overestimate LAP. High levels of cardiac output are associated with a complete recruitment of the pulmonary capillary network, which is the prerequisite for the valid estimation of LAP by a PAOP (Figure 1.2). On the other hand, both filling pressures of both ventricles, as assessed by directly measured RAP and indirectly measured LAP, rise at exercise and are related to stroke volume and exercise capacity.[14] Thus, there is strong indirect evidence suggesting that the left ventricle tends to over-use the Frank–Starling mechanism (increase stroke volume by an increased preload, or end-diastolic ventricular volume/pressure) to maximize cardiac output, and thereby increase maximum oxygen consumption by an increase in oxygen delivery to the tissues.[14] On the other hand, PCP is necessarily somewhere between PAP and LAP or PAOP. A PCP >20–25 mmHg is associated with an increased extravascular lung water content because of an increased capillary filtration.[15,16] Strenuous exercise is associated with variable decreases in arterial oxygen pressure (arterial PO_2) and an increase in the alveolar to arterial PO_2 gradient, which may be a cause of maximum oxygen consumption limitation.[17] Exercise-induced hypoxemia may be at least in part explained by exercise-induced pulmonary hypertension.

As mentioned above, PVR increases with ageing, so that the slope of PAP/$\dot{Q}$ plots during exercise averages 1 mmHg/L·min in young adults, but more than doubles, up to 2.5 mmHg/L·min in old subjects, who also present with an earlier and more important increase in PAOP (or LAP).[7,8,11] Earlier increase in LAP in older subjects at exercise could be explained by age-related decreased diastolic compliance of the left ventricle.[8]

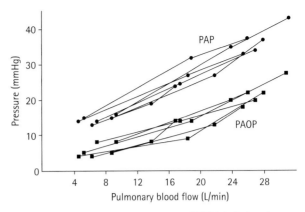

Figure 1.1 *Pulmonary artery pressures (PAP) (circles) and occluded PAP (PAOP) (squares) as a function of pulmonary blood flow in athletes at rest and at two levels of exercise. High levels of exercise are associated with marked increases in PAP and PAOP. (After reference 12).*

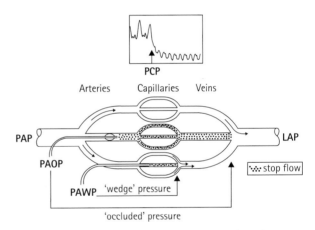

Figure 1.2 *Occluded pulmonary artery pressure (PAOP) is not pulmonary artery wedge pressure (PAWP) or pulmonary capillary pressure (PCP). Stippled areas indicate stop flow.*

PULMONARY CAPILLARY PRESSURE

Pulmonary artery occluded pressure (PAOP) is not the same as pulmonary artery wedge pressure (PAWP) obtained by wedging a pulmonary catheter with a deflated balloon into a small pulmonary arterial branch. As illustrated in Figure 1.2, arterial occlusion creates a stop-flow condition that extends the catheter lumen down to same diameter veins, so that an increase in small vein resistance can conceivably increase PAWP but not PAOP.[18] While in normal subjects PAWP is indistinguishable from PAOP, it has been shown that PAWP may exceed PAOP by an average of 3–4 mmHg in patients with various lung diseases.[19] This can only be explained by an increase in medium to large vein resistances.[19]

Because of the resistance of the smallest veins, which do not contribute to PAWP as being of smaller diameter than the pulmonary artery catheter, and a low but significant capillary resistance, pulmonary capillary pressure (PCP) is necessarily higher than PAWP. A measurement of PCP can be obtained by the analysis of a PAP decay curve after balloon occlusion.[16] As shown in Figure 1.3, such a pressure decay curve is made of a first fast component, which corresponds to the stop of flow through an arterial resistance, and a slower component, which corresponds to the emptying of the compliant capillaries through a venous resistance.[20] The intersection between the two components of the PAP decay curve offers an estimate of PCP that is in good agreement with the reference isogravimetric method.[16]

Measurements of PCP from the analysis of the PAP decay curve after balloon occlusion have recently been reported in young adult volunteers, yielding a mean value of 10 (range 6–14 mmHg).[5] Based on a normal longitudinal distribution of resistances within the pulmonary circulation, ascribing 60% PVR to the arterial segment and 40% to the capillary-venous segment, the normal PCP can also be calculated as proposed by Gaar et al.[16] as

$$PCP = PAOP + 0.4(PAP - PAOP)$$

The Gaar equation becomes obviously invalid in disease states associated with increases in the arterial or the venous components of PVR.

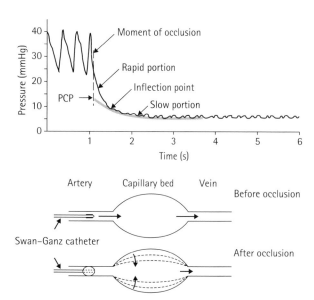

Figure 1.3 *Analysis of the pressure transient after pulmonary arterial occlusion for the estimation of pulmonary capillary pressure (PCP) either by the intersection of the fast and the slow components of the pressure decay curve, or by the extrapolation of the exponential fitting of the slow component of the pressure decay curve to the moment of occlusion. (After reference 20).*

Pulmonary capillary pressure increases with cardiac output and pulmonary venous pressure. Changes in lung volume affect PVR[21] but associated changes in PCP are not known. Hypoxia increases PCP, albeit normally slightly,[5] because of a small venous participation in hypoxic pulmonary vasoconstriction.[22] In a study on 14 healthy volunteers at rest, inspiratory hypoxia increased PAP from 13 ± 3 to 22 ± 3 and PCP from 10 ± 2 to 12 ± 2 mmHg.[5]

Variable increases in PCP have been reported in adult respiratory distress syndrome (ARDS), with recorded values eventually higher than around 20 mmHg, which are known to be associated with hydrostatic edema in normal lungs.[23,24] According to one study, PCP is higher than normal in primary pulmonary hypertension, and may be in relation to a more important venous involvement than previously appreciated in these patients.[25] In the early stages of high altitude pulmonary edema, PCP is higher than 20 mmHg, suggesting a hydrostatic mechanism explaining this, until recently, mysterious entity.[5]

PULMONARY VASCULAR PRESSURE/FLOW RELATIONSHIPS

The inherent assumption of a PVR calculation is that the PAP/Q̇ relationship is linear and crosses the pressure axis at a value equal to PAOP, allowing PVR to be constant whatever the absolute level of pressure of flow. While the (PAP − PAOP)/Q̇ relationship has indeed been shown to be reasonably well described by a linear approximation over a limited range of physiological flows, the zero crossing assumption is true only in the case of well-oxygenated lungs in supine resting subjects, suggesting complete recruitment and minimal distension. Hypoxia and a number of cardiac and respiratory diseases increase both the slope and the extrapolated intercepts of multipoint (PAP − PAOP)/Q̇ plots.[26]

While an increase in the slope of a PAP/Q̇ plot is easily understood as being caused by a decreased cumulative surface section area of pulmonary resistive vessels, the positive extrapolated pressure intercept has inspired various explanatory models. Permutt et al.[27] conceived a vascular waterfall model made of parallel collapsible vessels with a distribution of closing pressures. At low flow, these vessels would be progressively derecruited, accounting for a low flow PAP/Q̇ curve that is concave to the flow axis, and intercepts the pressure axis at the lowest closing pressure to be overcome to generate a flow. At higher flow, completed recruitment and negligible distension account for a linear PAP/Q̇ curve with an extrapolated pressure intercept representing a weighted mean of closing pressures. In this model, the mean closing pressure is the effective outflow pressure of the pulmonary circulation.

A left atrial pressure lower than the mean closing pressure is then an only apparent downstream pressure, and is as irrelevant to flow as is the height of a waterfall. Resistance calculations remain applicable to evaluate the functional state of the pulmonary circulation, provided the apparent downstream pressure is replaced by the effective one.[27]

However, distensible vessel models have been developed which explain the shape of PAP/Q̇ curves by changes in resistance and compliance.[28–30] In fact, as illustrated in Figure 1.4, PAP/Q̇ curves can always be shown to be curvilinear with concavity to flow axis, provided that a large enough number of PAP/Q̇ coordinates are generated and submitted to adequate fitting procedure. On the other hand, derecruitment can be directly observed at low pressures and flows.[31] Both recruitment and distension probably explain most PAP/Q̇ curves. According to this integrated view, at low inflow pressure, many pulmonary vessels are closed as an effect of their intrinsic tone and surrounding alveolar pressure, and those that are open are relatively narrow. As inflow pressure increases, previously closed vessels progressively open (recruitment), and previously narrow vessels progressively dilate (distension). Both mechanisms explain a progressive decrease in the slope of pulmonary vascular pressure/flow relationships with increasing flow or pressure.

The practical consequence is that single PVR determinations cannot be reliable for the evaluation of the functional state of the pulmonary circulation at variable flow (Figure 1.4). A better description of the resistive properties of the pulmonary circulation requires measurements of pulmonary vascular pressure at several levels of flow. The problem is to alter flow without affecting vascular tone. This could be achieved with low-dose dobutamine.[25] Exercise to alter flow may lead to spuriously increased slopes with of PAP/Q̇ plots in patients with cardiac or pulmonary diseases, probably because of exercise-induced pulmonary vasoconstriction, due to a decrease in mixed venous PO_2, sympathetic nervous system activation, and exercise-associated increase in left atrial pressure.[25,32]

PASSIVE REGULATION OF THE PULMONARY CIRCULATION

Left atrial pressure and cardiac output

At a given Q̇, an increase in LAP is transmitted upstream to PAP in a less than one-for-one proportion, depending on the state of arterial distension and the presence, or not, of a closing pressure higher than LAP.[30] As discussed above, an increase in Q̇ at a given LAP increases PAP but decreases PVR because of variable combination of pulmonary vascular recruitment and distension.

Lung volume

An increase in lung volume above functional residual capacity increases the resistance of alveolar vessels, which are the vessels exposed to alveolar pressure, but decreases the resistance of extra-alveolar vessels, which are the vessels exposed to interstitial pressure. A decrease in lung volume below functional residual capacity has the opposite effects. It has been shown that the combination of alveolar and extra-alveolar vessel resistance that gives the lowest resultant PVR is observed at functional residual capacity.[21,33]

Gravity

Pulmonary blood flow increases almost linearly from non-dependent to dependent lung regions. This inequality of pulmonary perfusion is best demonstrated in an upright lung.[2] The vertical height of a lung is, on average, about 30 cm. The difference in pressure between the

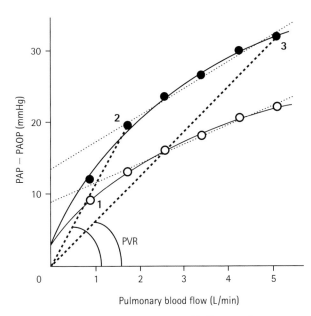

Figure 1.4 *Pulmonary artery pressure (PAP) versus flow coordinates at two levels of pulmonary hypertension are correctly described by a linear approximation over a physiological range of flows. The extrapolated pressure intercepts of these linearized pressure/flow relationships are positive, suggesting a closing pressure higher than left atrial pressure. However, the pressure/flow coordinates are better described by a curvilinear fitting, which takes more adequately into account the natural distensibility of the pulmonary vessels. In both situations, pulmonary vascular resistance (PVR) calculations are misleading: from A to B, PVR does not change, and from A to C, PVR decreases in the presence of aggravated pulmonary hypertension, as assessed by higher pressures at a given flow. PAOP, pulmonary artery occlusion pressure.*

extremities of a vertical column of blood of the same size amounts to 23 mmHg, which is quite large compared to the mean perfusion pressure of the pulmonary circulation. Accordingly, the physiological inequality of the distribution of perfusion of a normal lung can be explained by a gravity-dependent interplay between arterial, venous and alveolar pressures.[2] At the top of the lung, alveolar pressure (P_A) is higher than mean PAP and pulmonary venous pressure (PVP). In this **zone 1**, flow may be present only during systole, or not at all. Zone 1 is extended in clinical situations of low flow, such as hypovolemic shock, or increased P_A such as during ventilation with a positive end-expiratory pressure (PEEP). Further down the lung there is a **zone 2** where PAP $> P_A >$ PVP. In this zone 2, P_A is an effective closing pressure, and the driving pressure for flow is the gradient between mean PAP and P_A. As mentioned above, such a flow condition can be likened to a waterfall since PVP, the apparent outflow pressure, is irrelevant to flow, as is the height of a waterfall. In **zone 3**, PVP is higher than P_A, so that the driving pressure for flow is PAP $-$ PVP.

At the most dependent regions of upright lung, there is an additional region where flow decreases.[33] This **zone 4** has been attributed to an increase in the resistance of extra-alveolar vessels because it expands when lung volume is reduced or in the presence of lung edema. Active tone may be an additional explanation for zone 4 as it is also reduced by the administration of vasodilators.

The vertical height of lung tissue in a supine subject is of course much reduced compared to the upright position and, accordingly, the lung is then normally almost completely in zone 3, with, however, persistence of a still measurable increase in flow from non-dependent to dependent lung regions.

While gravity is the major determinant of regional changes in blood flow in the normal pulmonary circulation, three-dimensional reconstructions using single-photon-emission computed tomography have shown that there is also a decrease in blood flow from the center of the lung to the periphery.[34] This may reflect an intrinsic effect of pulmonary vascular geometry, and has not been shown to be relevant to gas exchange.

ACTIVE HYPOXIC REGULATION OF THE PULMONARY CIRCULATION

There is an active intrapulmonary control mechanism able to some extent correct the passive gravity-dependent distribution of pulmonary blood flow: a decrease in PO_2 increases pulmonary vascular tone. Hypoxic pulmonary vasoconstriction was first reported by von Euler and Liljestrand,[35] who proposed a functional interpretation that can still be considered valid. In lung tissue, PO_2 is determined by a ratio between O_2 carried to the lung by alveolar ventilation (V_A) and O_2 carried away from the lung by blood flow ($\dot{Q}$):

$$PO_2 = \frac{V_A}{\dot{Q}}$$

in contrast to hypoxic vasodilation in systemic tissue, where local PO_2 is accordingly determined by a ratio flow of O_2 carried to the tissues ($\dot{Q}$) and local O_2 consumption (VO_2):

$$PO_2 = \frac{\dot{Q}}{VO_2}$$

The hypoxic pulmonary pressor response is universal in mammals and in birds, but with considerable interspecies and inter-individual variability.[10,36] The attributes of hypoxic pulmonary vasoconstriction can be summarized as follows.[10,36,37] The response is vigorous in cattle and in pigs, moderate in humans, dogs and camelids (including the llama), and almost absent in guinea pigs and rabbits. It is turned on in a few seconds, fully developed after 1–3 minutes, and more or less stable thereafter according to the experimental conditions. It is reversed in less than a minute. It is observed in lungs devoid of nervous connections, and indeed also in isolated pulmonary arterial smooth muscle cells. Hypoxic pulmonary vasoconstriction is enhanced by acidosis, a decrease in mixed venous PO_2, repeated hypoxic exposure (in some experimental models), perinatal hypoxia, decreased lung segment size, cyclooxygenase inhibition, nitric oxide inhibition, and certain drugs or mediators which include almitrine and low-dose serotonin. Hypoxic pulmonary vasoconstriction is inhibited by alkalosis, hypercapnia, an increase in pulmonary vascular or alveolar pressures, vasodilating prostaglandins, nitric oxide, complement activation, low-dose endotoxin, calcium channel blockers, β_2-stimulants, nitroprusside and, paradoxically, by peripheral chemoreceptor stimulation. The hypoxic pressor response is biphasic, with a progressive increase as PO_2 is progressively decreased to approximately 35–40 mmHg, followed by a decrease ('hypoxic vasodilatation') in more profound hypoxia.

The hypoxia-induced increase in PVR is mainly caused by a constriction of precapillary small arterioles.[10,36] Small pulmonary veins also constrict in response to hypoxia, but this should not normally contribute to more than 20–30% of the total change in PVR.[5,22] An exaggerated hypoxic constriction of small pulmonary veins could explain high altitude pulmonary edema.[5]

While hypoxic pulmonary vasoconstriction has been shown by sophisticated modeling to be an only moderately efficient feedback mechanism,[4,38] it may still produce substantial improvements in arterial oxygenation of patients with inhomogeneous lungs such as in chronic obstructive pulmonary disease (hypoxemia mainly explained by low ventilation/perfusion ratios) or in the acute respiratory distress syndrome (hypoxemia mainly explained by ventilation/perfusion ratios equal to zero, or shunt).[39] Topographical blood flow distribution [positron emission tomography (PET) scan] and arterial PO_2 can be shown to conform to the expected functional effects of hypoxic pulmonary vasoconstriction in experimental acute lung injury models, as an inhibition of the response prevents redistribution of blood flow to non-dependent lung regions and markedly aggravates shunt and arterial hypoxemia.[40,41]

The biochemical mechanism of hypoxic pulmonary vasoconstriction remains incompletely understood. Current thought is that a decrease in PO_2 inhibits smooth muscle cell voltage-dependent potassium channels, resulting in membrane depolarization, influx of calcium, and cell shortening.[37] Two such channels, $Kv_{2.1}$ and $Kv_{1.5}$, have been identified in rat pulmonary arteries.[42] However, the nature of the low PO_2 sensing mechanism remains elusive.[37] Inhibition of voltage-dependent potassium channels has been observed in isolated pulmonary artery smooth muscle cells of patients with primary pulmonary hypertension, and might thus be a universal pathway to enhanced pulmonary vascular reactivity and subsequent remodeling.[43] The reversal of hypoxic vasoconstriction by profound hypoxia is caused by activation of ATP-dependent potassium channels.[37]

The normal as well as the abnormal pulmonary vascular tone has been shown to be modulated by a series of endothelium-derived and circulating mediators.[44] Endothelium-derived relaxing factors include nitric oxide, prostacyclin and the endothelium-derived hyperpolarizing factor. The major endothelium-derived contracting factor is endothelin. These observations are at the basis of current attempts at treating pulmonary hypertension with inhaled nitric oxide, intravenous prostacyclin, or oral anti-endothelins. It is of interest to note that the pulmonary vasodilating effects of nitric oxide and prostacyclin are mediated by the cyclic-GMP and the cyclic-AMP pathways, respectively, suggesting the possibility of additive effects.

The pulmonary circulation is richly innervated by the autonomic nervous system, which includes adrenergic, cholinergic, and non-adrenergic non-cholinergic (NANC) pathways.[10,36,45] However, the role played by the autonomic nervous system in the control of pulmonary vascular tone appears to be minor. In fact, autonomic innervation of the pulmonary arterial tree is predominantly proximal, suggesting a more important effect in the modulation of proximal compliance.[45]

PULSATILE FLOW PULMONARY HEMODYNAMICS

The study of the pulmonary circulation as a steady flow system is a simplification, since pulmonary arterial pulse pressure, or the difference between systolic and diastolic PAP, is in the order of 40–50% of mean pressure, and instantaneous flow varies from a maximum at mid-systole to around zero in diastole.[10,36,46] While PAP and flow waves are superimposable in normal subjects, they become markedly different in aspect and desynchronized in patients with pulmonary hypertension.[46]

In patients with severe pulmonary hypertension, the right ventricular pressure wave is characterized by a sharp initial upstroke, followed by a short plateau, and by a late systolic peaking, and the PAP wave is characterized by a huge pulse pressure and a late systolic peaking. In the most severe forms of pulmonary hypertension the PAP wave looks 'ventricularized'. On the other hand, the pulmonary blood flow wave presents with a late systolic deceleration, or even a mid-systolic deceleration.

These morphological aspects of pulmonary artery pressure and flow waves in pulmonary hypertension are completely explained by decreases in pulmonary arterial compliance and by earlier return of reflected waves on forward waves. It can be shown experimentally that right ventricular output decreases because of an increased afterload if, at a given resistance, pulmonary arterial compliance decreases and/or wave reflection increases.[47,48]

Pulmonary artery pressure and flow waves can be decomposed into their constituent harmonic oscillations by an application of the Fourier theorem.[10,46] This analysis is possible because the pulmonary circulation acts as a linear system, that is, that a purely sinusoidal flow oscillation produces a purely sinusoidal pressure oscillation of the same frequency. From the spectral analysis of the pulmonary arterial pressure and flow waves, one calculates pulmonary vascular impedance (PVZ).[10,46] Pulmonary vascular impedance is the ratio of pressure oscillations to flow oscillations. It is graphically represented as a pressure/flow ratio and a phase angle, both as a function of frequency. Typical PVZ spectra are illustrated in Figure 1.5.

Pulmonary vascular impedance at zero Hz (Z_0) corresponds to PVR calculated as PAP/$\dot{Q}$. Normally, the ratio of pressure and flow decreases rapidly to a first minimum at 2–3 Hz and increases again to a first maximum at 5–6 Hz. At low frequencies, the phase angle is negative, indicating that flow leads pressure.

An increase in the pressure/flow ratio at all frequencies indicates a decreased pulmonary arterial distensibility. A shift of the first minimum and maximum to higher frequencies indicates an increased wave velocity or a change in the dominant reflection site.

The PVZ spectrum allows the quantification of characteristic impedance (Z_c) defined as PVZ without wave reflection. Characteristic impedance is measured as the average pressure/flow ratio at the highest frequencies. It can also be measured as the linearized slope of the early systolic pulmonary artery pressure/flow relationship.

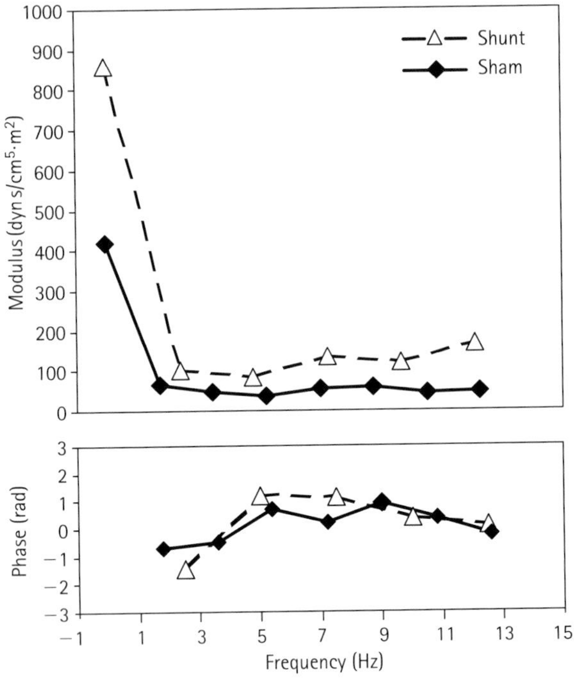

It is thus apparent that a PVZ calculation allows the quantification of the forces that oppose right ventricular ejection, or afterload, as a dynamic interplay between resistance, compliance and wave reflection.

The pulsatile hydraulic power is most important in the proximal pulmonary arterial tree[10,46] and, accordingly, PVZ calculations are relatively insensitive to peripheral physiological or pathological changes. The spectrum of PVZ is little affected by normal breathing,[49] or by disease processes limited to alveolar or juxta-alveolar vessels.[48,50] By contrast, proximal pulmonary arterial obstruction markedly affects pressure and flow wave morphology, the PVZ spectrum and, at any given PVR, has a more important depressant effect on right ventricular output.[47,51]

NON–INVASIVE EVALUATION OF THE PULMONARY CIRCULATION

Non-invasive methods to evaluate the pulmonary circulation have made a lot of progress in recent years. Doppler echocardiography, introduced in the early 1980s[52,53] has already entered routine cardiology practice, allowing for easy measurement of instantaneous pulmonary arterial flow velocity and satisfactory recalculation of instantaneous PAPs.[54]

Pulmonary flow velocity measured by the pulsed Doppler technique normally exhibits a dome-like contour, with a peak in the middle of systole.[52,54] Pulmonary hypertension is associated with a decrease in the acceleration time (from start to peak velocity of flow) and with late systolic deceleration of flow. Severe pulmonary hypertension is associated with extreme shortening of acceleration time and a mid-systolic deceleration of flow, eventually with a late systolic reversal of flow.[52,54] These aspects had been previously observed using electromagnetic volume flow measurements.[46] Acceleration time is affected by heart rate, and it is therefore reasonable to correct the measurement for the ejection time.[54] Acceleration time normally exceeds 100 ms. The limits of normal of acceleration time corrected for ejection time vary from 0.35 to 0.47. Acceleration time is inversely correlated to invasively measured PAP and PVR, but, in spite of correlation coefficients reported in the range of 0.8–0.9 in many studies, the predictive value of PAP or PVR from the acceleration time on an individual basis is usually poor.[52,54] This is explained by operator-dependent variability of the measurement, insufficient frequency response of fluid-filled pulmonary catheters, and the fact that, as developed above, a flow cannot be considered physiologically identical to a pressure or to a resistance calculation.[54]

The detection of a tricuspid regurgitation as measured by continuous Doppler allows the calculation of a trans-tricuspid pressure gradient using the simplified

Figure 1.5 *Pulmonary vascular impedance (PVZ) spectra in a piglet at baseline (black diamonds) and after a high pulmonary blood flow (by a surgical aortopulmonary shunt) during 3 months (white traingles). The PVZ spectrum at baseline is characterized by a relatively high value of the ratio of pulmonary artery pressure and flow moduli (modulus) at 0 Hz, corresponding to a 'total' PVR (PVR without inclusion of left atrial pressure), that rapidly decreases at low frequency, to oscillate around a low characteristic impedance (Z_c) estimated by the ratio of pressure and flow moduli at the highest frequencies. At low flow, phase is slightly negative, indicating that flow normally slightly leads pressure. Prolonged increase in pulmonary blood flow (as seen in persistent ductus arteriosus) increases both PVR and Z_c with a more negative low frequency phase angle, indicating increased resistance, elastance and wave reflection (B Rondelet, personal communication).*

Characteristic impedance is dependent on the ratio of inertia and compliance of the pulmonary circulation, and can be approximated by the equation:

$$Z_c = \frac{(\rho / \pi r^4)}{\Delta \pi r^2 / \Delta P}$$

where ρ is the density of blood, r the mean internal radius, $\rho/\pi r^4$ the inertance and $\Delta \pi r^2 / \Delta P$ the compliance of the pulmonary arterial tree.

The extent of the difference between Z_0 and Z_c can be used to calculate and index of wave reflection as:

$$Rc = \frac{(1 - Z_c / Z_0)}{(1 + Z_c / Z_0)}$$

where Rc is reflection coefficient and Z_0 is vascular impedence at 0 Hz.

form of the Bernouilli equation:

$$\Delta P = 4 \times v^2$$

where ΔP is the pressure gradient and v is the velocity of flow. In general, a systolic pulmonary artery pressure is calculated from the maximum velocity of the regurgitant flow and an estimated or a measured right atrial pressure.[53,54] Tricuspid regurgitant flows can be recorded in about 60% of normal subjects, and in most patients with pulmonary hypertension. There is a good correlation between systolic pulmonary artery pressures directly measured during a right heart catheterization and predicted from the tricuspid regurgitant jets.[53,54] However, the prediction of invasive from non-invasive measurements can be disappointing on an individual basis because of the assumptions of the pressure gradient calculation, and also because of the limited frequency response of fluid-filled catheters to measure right ventricular pressures.[54] The shape of the tricuspid regurgitant jet is interesting to analyze as it shows a late systolic peaking in patients with severe pulmonary hypertension, like the directly measured pulmonary artery pressure curve.[48]

It is possible to apply the Bernouilli equation to the tricuspid and pulmonary regurgitant jets to recalculate complete PAP curves.[55] This method has been reported to be as accurate as direct invasive measurements to show significant differences in morphology of pulmonary artery pressure curves in patients with primary pulmonary hypertension, a disease process which mainly involves small peripheral arterioles compared to patients with proximal thromboembolic obstruction of the pulmonary arteries.

KEY POINTS

- Pulmonary artery pressures are normally low, but increase passively with left atrial pressure and with pulmonary blood flow.
- There are no gender differences in pulmonary hemodynamics, provided that pulmonary blood flow is corrected for body size.
- Pulmonary vascular resistance increases at high and at low pulmonary volumes, is minimal at functional residual capacity, and approximately doubles with ageing.
- Pulmonary hypertension may be associated with an increase in pulmonary capillary filtration pressure, which is estimated from the analysis of the pulmonary arterial pressure decay curve after balloon occlusion, or by adding to left atrial pressure 40% of the difference between mean pulmonary artery pressure and left atrial pressure.

- Gravity determines an increase in pulmonary blood flow from non-dependent to dependent lung regions.
- Hypoxic pulmonary vasoconstriction redistributes blood flow to better aerated lung areas, thereby limiting the hypoxemic effects of local decreases in ventilation/perfusion relationships. Right ventricular afterload is determined by a complex interplay between pulmonary arterial resistance, compliance and wave reflection.
- The determinants of right ventricular afterload can be quantified from invasive or non-invasive pressure and waveform morphology analysis.

REFERENCES

●1 Swan HJC, Ganz W, Forrester JS et al. Catheterization of the heart in man with use of a flow-directed catheter. N Engl J Med 1970;**283**:447–51.
●2 West JB, Dollery CT, Naimark A. Distribution of blood flow in isolated lung: relation to vascular and alveolar pressures. J Appl Physiol 1964;**19**:713–24.
3 Naeije R, Mélot C, Mols P et al. Effects of vasodilators on hypoxic pulmonary vasoconstriction in normal man. Chest 1982;**82**:404–10.
4 Mélot C, Naeije R, Hallemans R et al. Hypoxic pulmonary vasoconstriction and pulmonary gas exchange in normal man. Respir Physiol 1987;**68**:11–27.
5 Maggiorini M, Mélot C, Pierre S et al. High altitude pulmonary edema is initially caused by an increased capillary pressure. Circulation 2001;**103**:2078–83.
6 Holmgren A, Jonsson B, Sjostrand T. Circulatory data in normal subjects at rest and during exercise in the recumbent position, with special reference to the stroke volume at different working intensities. Acta Physiol Scand 1960;**49**:343–63.
7 Granath A, Strandell T. Relationships between cardiac output, stroke volume, and intracardiac pressures at rest and during exercise in supine position and some anthropometric data in healthy old men. Acta Med Scand 1964;**176**:447–66.
8 Granath A, Jonsson B, Strandell T. Circulation in healthy old men, studied by right heart catheterization at rest and during exercise in supine and sitting position. Acta Med Scand 1964;**176**: 425–46.
9 Bevegaard S, Holmgren A, Jonsson B. Circulatory studies in well trained athletes at rest and during heavy exercise, with special reference to stroke volume and the influence of body position. Acta Physiol Scand 1963;**57**:26–50.
◆10 Fishman AP. Pulmonary circulation. In: Handbook of physiology. The respiratory system. Circulation and nonrespiratory functions, sect 3, vol 1, chap f3. Bethesda: Am Physiol Soc, 1985; 93–166.
◆11 Reeves JT, Dempsey JA, Grover RF. Pulmonary circulation during exercise. In: Weir EK, Reeves JT (eds), Pulmonary vascular physiology and physiopathology, chap 4. New York: Marcel Dekker, 1989; 107–33.

12 Naeije R, Mélot C, Niset G *et al.* Improved arterial oxygenation by a pharmacological increase in chemosensitivity during hypoxic exercise in normal subjects. *J Appl Physiol* 1993;**74**:1666–71.

13 Rubin LJ. Primary pulmonary hypertension. *N Engl J Med* 1997;**336**:111–17.

14 Reeves JT, Groves BM, Cymerman A *et al.* Operation Everest II: cardiac filling pressures during cycle exercise at sea level. *Respir Physiol* 1990;**80**:147–54.

◆15 Dempsey JA, Wagner PD. Exercise-induced arterial hypoxemia. *J Appl Physiol* 1999;**87**:1997–2006.

●16 Gaar KA Jr, Taylor AE, Owens LJ *et al.* Pulmonary capillary pressure and filtration coefficient in the isolated perfused lung. *Am J Physiol* 1967;**213**:910–14.

◆17 Cope DK, Grimbert F, Downey JM *et al.* Pulmonary capillary pressure: a review. *Crit Care Med* 1992;**20**:1043–56.

●18 Zidulka A, Hakim TS. Wedge pressure in large vs small pulmonary arteries to detect pulmonary venoconstriction. *J Appl Physiol* 1985;**59**:1329–32.

19 Teboul JL, Andrivet P, Ansquer M *et al.* Bedside evaluation of the resistance of large and medium pulmonary veins in various lung diseases. *J Appl Physiol* 1992;**72**:998–1003.

20 Perret C, Tagan D, Feihl F *et al. The pulmonary artery catheter in critical care.* Oxford: Blackwell Science, 1996.

21 Howell JBL, Permutt S, Proctor DF *et al.* Effect of inflation of the lung on different parts of the pulmonary vascular bed. *J Appl Physiol* 1961;**16**:71–6.

22 Hillier SC, Graham JA, Hanger CC *et al.* Hypoxic vasoconstriction in pulmonary arterioles and venules. *J Appl Physiol* 1997;**82**:1084–90.

23 Collee CG, Lynch KE, Hill D *et al.* Bedside measurements of pulmonary capillary pressure in patients with acute respiratory failure. *Anesthesiology* 1987;**66**:614–20.

24 Rossetti M, Guenard H, Gabinski C. Effects of nitric oxide on pulmonary serial resistances in ARDS. *Am J Respir Crit Care Med* 1996;**154**:1375–81.

25 Abdel Kafi S, Mélot C, Vachiéry JL *et al.* Partitioning of pulmonary vascular resistance in primary pulmonary hypertension. *J Am Coll Cardiol* 1998;**31**:1372–6.

◆26 McGregor M, Sniderman A. On pulmonary vascular resistance: the need for more precise definition. *Am J Cardiol* 1985;**55**:217–21.

●27 Permutt S, Bromberger-Barnea B, Bane HN. Alveolar pressure, pulmonary venous pressure and the vascular waterfall. *Med Thorac* 1962;**19**:239–60.

●28 Zhuang FY, Fung YC, Yen RT. Analysis of blood flow in cat's lung with detailed anatomical and elasticity data. *J Appl Physiol* 1983;**55**:1341–8.

29 Nelin LD, Krenz GS, Rickaby DA *et al.* A distensible vessel model applied to hypoxic vasoconstriction in the neonatal pig. *J Appl Physiol* 1992;**73**:987–94.

30 Mélot C, Delcroix M, Lejeune P *et al.* Starling resistor versus viscoelastic models for embolic pulmonary hypertension. *Am J Physiol* 1995;**267**(*Heart Circ Physiol* **36**):H817–27.

31 Glazier JB, Hughes JMB, Maloney JE *et al.* Measurements of capillary dimensions and blood volume in rapidly frozen lungs. *J Appl Physiol* 1969;**26**:65–76.

32 Janicki JS, Weber KT, Likoff MJ *et al.* The pressure-flow response of the pulmonary circulation in patients with heart failure and pulmonary vascular disease. *Circulation* 1985;**72**:1270–8.

●33 Hughes JM, Glazier JB, Maloney JR *et al.* Effect of lung volume on the distribution of pulmonary blood flow in man. *Respir Physiol* 1968;**4**:58–72.

34 Hakim TS, Lisbona R, Michel RP *et al.* Role of vasoconstriction in gravity-nondependent central-peripheral gradient in pulmonary blood flow. *J Appl Physiol* 1993;**63**:1114–21.

●35 von Euler US, Liljestrand G. Observations on the pulmonary arterial blood pressure in the cat. *Acta Physiol Scand* 1946;**12**:301–20.

◆36 Grover RF, Wagner WW, McMurtry IF *et al.* Pulmonary circulation. In: *Handbook of physiology. The cardiovascular system. Peripheral circulation and organ blood flow*, sect 2, vol III, part 1, chap 4. Bethesda: Am Physiol Soc, 1983; 103–36.

◆37 Weir EK, Archer SL. The mechanism of acute hypoxic pulmonary vasoconstriction: the tale of two channels. *FASEB J* 1995;**9**:183–9.

38 Grant BJB. Effect of local pulmonary blood flow control on gas exchange: theory. *J Appl Physiol Respir Environ Exercise Physiol* 1982;**53**:1100–9.

39 Brimioulle S, Lejeune P, Naeije R. Effects of hypoxic pulmonary vasoconstriction on gas exchange. *J Appl Physiol* 1996;**81**:1535–43.

40 Gust R, Kozlowski J, Stephenson AH *et al.* Synergistic hemodynamic effects of low-dose endotoxin in acute lung injury. *Am J Respir Crit Care Med* 1998;**157**:1919–26.

◆41 Naeije R, Brimioulle S. Physiology in medicine: the importance of hypoxic pulmonary vasoconstriction in maintaining arterial oxygenation during acute lung injury. *Crit Care* 2001;**5**:67–71.

42 Archer SL, Souil E, Dinh-Xuan AT *et al.* Molecular identification of the role of voltage-gated K^+ channels, Kv1.5 and Kv2.1, in hypoxic pulmonary vasoconstriction and control of resting membrane potential in rat pulmonary artery myocytes. *J Clin Invest* 1998;**101**:2319–30.

43 Yuan XJ, Aldinger AM, Juhaszova M *et al.* Dysfunctional voltage-gated K^+ channels in pulmonary artery smooth cells of patients with primary pulmonary hypertension. *Circulation* 1998;**98**:1400–6.

◆44 Barnes PJ, Liu SF. Regulation of pulmonary vascular tone. *Pharmacol Rev* 1995;**47**:87–131.

◆45 Downing SE, Lee JC. Nervous control of the pulmonary circulation. *Annu Rev Physiol* 1980;**42**:199–210.

◆46 Nichols WW, O'Rourke MF. *McDonald's blood flow in arteries*, 4th edn. London: Edward Arnold, 1998.

●47 Elzinga G, Piene H, de Jong J.P. Left and right ventricular pump function and consequences of having two pumps in one heart. *Circ Res* 1980;**46**:564–74.

48 Furuno Y, Nagamoto Y, Fujita M *et al.* Reflection as a cause of mid-systolic deceleration of pulmonary flow wave in dogs with acute pulmonary hypertension: comparison of pulmonary artery constriction with pulmonary embolisation. *Cardiovasc Res* 1991;**25**:118–24.

49 Murgo JP, Westerhof N. Input impedance of the pulmonary arterial system in normal man: effects of respiration and comparison to systemic impedance. *Circ Res* 1984;**54**:666–73.

50 Pagnamenta A, Bouckaert Y, Wauthy P *et al.* Continuous versus pulsatile pulmonary hemodynamics in oleic acid lung injury. *Am J Respir Crit Care Med* 2000;**162**:936–40.

51 Fitzpatrick JM, Grant BJB. Effects of pulmonary vascular obstruction on right ventricular afterload. *Am Rev Respir Dis* 1990;**141**:944–52.

●52 Kitabatake A, Inoue M, Asao M *et al*. Noninvasive evaluation of pulmonary hypertension by a pulsed Doppler technique. *Circulation* 1983;**68**:302–9.

●53 Yock P, Popp R. Noninvasive estimation of right ventricular systolic pressure by Doppler ultrasound in patients with tricuspid regurgitation. *Circulation* 1984;**70**:657–62.

◆54 Naeije R, Torbicki A. More on the noninvasive diagnosis of pulmonary hypertension: Doppler echocardiography revisited. *Eur Respir J* 1995;**8**:1445–9.

55 Nakayama Y, Sugimachi M, Nakanishi N *et al*. Noninvasive differential diagnosis between chronic pulmonary thromboembolism and primary pulmonary hypertension by means of Doppler ultrasound measurement. *J Am Coll Cardiol* 1998;**31**:1367–71.

Functional anatomy of the pulmonary microcirculation

JOAN GIL AND DOINA CIUREA

INTRODUCTION

The circulation in the lung is more complex than in any other organ. This is true both in terms of anatomy and of physiology. Nomenclature, unique characteristics and functional responses are so diverse as to confuse the non-specialist. The emphasis in this chapter is on the organization of the alveolar wall capillaries (the so-called 'microcirculation') and their potential for continuous adaptation to the prevailing vascular and air pressures. In general, when referring to the anatomy of body organs, most people think of rigid, stable structures where changes, physiological or pathological, develop only slowly over a long period of time. Histology is mostly stable and unlikely to change suddenly. This is not true of the air-filled lung, where both alveolar and capillary configurations and dimensions change rapidly in response to a new set of transmural pressures (air, arterial or venous pressures).[1–7] A practical consequence, for instance, is that the configuration of the gas-exchanging apparatus of a patient being ventilated using positive end-expiratory pressure (PEEP) differs from that of a patient walking the street.

Before reaching the main topic, the alveolar wall circulation, the structure of the conducting vessels (arteries and veins) that lead the blood into the alveolar walls is reviewed; it is in their walls where most recognizable hypertensive changes take place, including those occurring due to hypoxic vasoconstriction.

THE EXTRA-ALVEOLAR AND CORNER VESSELS: CONNECTIONS AND FUNCTIONAL DIFFERENCES BETWEEN LARGE CONDUCTING VESSELS AND ALVEOLAR CAPILLARIES

In the systemic circulation, vessels can be classified into large conducting arteries and veins that differ from each other in diameter, wall structure and wall thickness, arterioles and venules (with a minimal medial layer) and capillaries. In the lung, however, the situation is different. One major difference between systemic and pulmonary circulation is that for a given caliber, the medial layer of muscle is comparatively much thinner, which reflects the lower pressures prevailing in the pulmonary circulation. A second difference, arterioles and venules similar to those in the systemic circulation are not present. This is important because systemic arterioles are the site of most peripheral resistance to flow and their absence results in the transmission of much of the pulmonary arterial pressure to the alveolar capillaries and probably in a highly pulsatile flow. Structurally, there are transitional equivalents between arteries and capillaries, which in the lung are often called 'precapillary arteries' and 'postcapillary veins'.

But even beyond these two differences, which are already substantial, two new elements exist that are unique to the lungs: first, the so-called **extra-alveolar vessels**, both arteries and veins, first defined by Howell *et al.*[8] on the basis of functional criteria but which have an anatomic counterpart and can be structurally identified. The most significant anatomic characteristic of extra-alveolar vessels is that they are surrounded by a sheath of loose connective tissue, which contains the origin of the pulmonary lymphatics, and that the alveolar septa insert radially in their periphery. The effect of this arrangement is that the radial pull exerted by the alveolar walls during inflation results in the creation of a perivascular subatmospheric pressure leading to their increase in diameter during inspiration. The second element unique to pulmonary circulation is the **corner vessels**. The latter are inside the alveolar parenchyma, and they are therefore not surrounded by a connective sheath of their own. They differ functionally from other alveolar wall capillaries in that they are protected against high alveolar air pressures and therefore stay open even when air pressures (during the use of the abdominal press for instance) cause the closure of most alveolar septal capillaries. These two types of blood vessels are often confused with each other; it is therefore warranted to describe them in some detail.

Figure 2.1 shows the position of large conducting arteries between the hilum and the point where they enter the gas exchange parenchyma. Arteries that accompany the bronchi are called 'axial' because the companion bronchus is always located in the axis of all wedge-shaped units (such as lobules or acini) that make up the lung. There are many more arteries than bronchi; this is due to the existence of the **supernumerary** arteries described by Hislop and Reid[9] that often sharply bend off the bronchial artery, leave the axis and head straight for the alveolar parenchyma where they break down into smaller vessels entering finally the alveolar parenchyma and opening to the alveolar capillary network at locations that are difficult to characterize. This means that an acinus (or a lobule) does not get a straightforward perfusion from its axis toward the pleura and the periphery (where the collecting veins are located). It instead receives arterial blood supply at different points which must result in complex directional patterns in the alveolar wall, turbulence and possibly even anastomosis between neighboring acini or lobules. A recognizable artery, whether axial or supernumerary, is never immediately exposed to the alveolar air; instead, as described above, it is always surrounded by a loose connective tissue sheath (Figure 2.2), an arrangement of great functional significance. The sheath is outwardly lined by epithelium and numerous alveolar septa are radially inserted. Large axial arteries share this sheath with a bronchus (Figures 2.1 and 2.2), but supernumerary arteries have an independent sheath from the beginning.

In summary, we call 'extra-alveolar' all arteries or veins surrounded by a connective tissue sheath which are seen isolated in the lung parenchyma and surrounded by

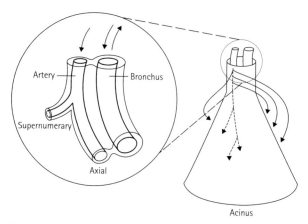

Figure 2.1 *Diagram showing the arrangement of arteries and bronchi with respect to the acinus. Originally, both appear in the hilum of the acinus. Bronchi and bronchioles always remain in an axial (central) position for as long as they exist and are followed by the lumen of alveolar ducts throughout the distal lung parenchyma. Arterial branches accompanying the bronchi are also called axial. Other arterial branches, however, leave the axis, penetrate into the surrounding parenchyma and are called supernumerary. This model shows the supernumeraries returning peripherally to the acinus and supplying it with blood. The possibility that they also perfuse adjoining acini cannot be ruled out. There are many more supernumerary than axial arteries.*

insertions of alveolar septa. Their connective tissue cuff is of crucial importance to our understanding of pulmonary function, circulation and edema development. It is held that a fibrous continuum[10] exists in the lung, that is, that all connective tissue compartments of the lung are connected with each other. This fibrous compartment forms a three-dimensional mesh that extends from the hilum to the pleura and includes the connective tissue sheath surrounding both blood vessels and bronchi. It has been established that the interstitial pressure in this connective tissue is negative and different in each compartment.[11] The cause of this is the pull originating from the pleural expansion transmitted by mechanical interdependence throughout the lung and exerted by the perpendicularly inserted alveolar walls in the periphery of the connective tissue cuff, which is opposed by the intrinsic recoil force of the lung, including the alveolar surface tension.

The practical consequence of this arrangement is that extra-alveolar vessels are surrounded by a subatmospheric pressure that becomes more negative during inflation. This means that while septal capillaries become compressed and empty during positive pressure inflation, the extra-alveolar blood vessels become enlarged (wider and longer) during inspiration and smaller (narrower and shorter) during expiration. Because of this they may temporarily store substantial volumes of blood, in the lung, but outside of the alveolar walls. This was shown to be the case years ago in a classic experiment by Howell et al.[8] and is summarized in Figure 2.3. Functionally, the important characteristic of extra-alveolar vessels is their capability of enlarging whenever lung volume increases.

Corner vessels are alveolar vessels that look like large capillaries (they do not have muscular or adventitial wall layers) and, due to their anatomic location in alveolar corners, are capable of resisting collapse even when alveolar air pressure exceeds arterial pressure (Figure 2.3). In this, they differ functionally from the other alveolar capillaries at non-corner locations, which will collapse during positive air pressure inflation, whenever the air pressure is higher than the vascular pressure. Corner vessels are described in

more detail later. Corner pleats are a particular form of corner vessels present mostly under zone 2 conditions, where a bundle of capillaries is formed in a corner due to a small pleating and infolding of alveolar walls.

ALVEOLAR WALLS AND THE MICROCIRCULATION

At the end of the last conducting bronchiole (ignoring the transitional zone or respiratory bronchioles where conducting and gas-exchanging elements coexist), air

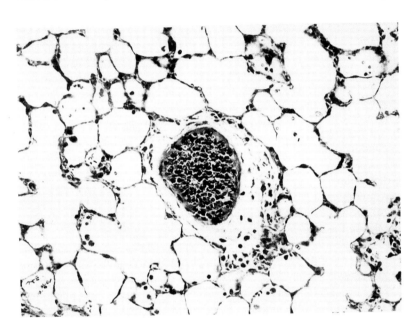

Figure 2.2 *Human lung fixed by instillation of buffered formalin into the airways. Note an extra-alveolar vessel surrounded by a loose connective tissue sheath. Alveolar walls inset radially in the periphery of the sheath. Physiological properties of these vessels are related to the pull exerted by the alveolar septa during lung inflation (×240).*

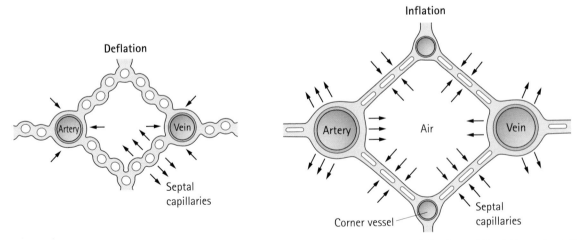

Figure 2.3 *Effects of inflation: alveolar vs. extra-alveolar vessels. The left panel shows a deflated alveolus, and the right panel an inflated alveolus subjected to a higher intra-alveolar air pressure. Note the opposite effect of air pressure on septal capillaries on one side and extra-alveolar arteries and veins on the other. During air inflation with positive pressure, the luminal air pressure may cause the compression and closure of septal capillaries, whereas the radial pull of the septal walls on the periphery of the connective tissue sheaths of extra-alveolar vessels causes these to increase in diameter during inflation. The extrapulmonary expansion will evidently occur even when the inflation is achieved without positive air pressure. Note, however, the difference between extra-alveolar and corner vessels (compare Figure 2.6).*

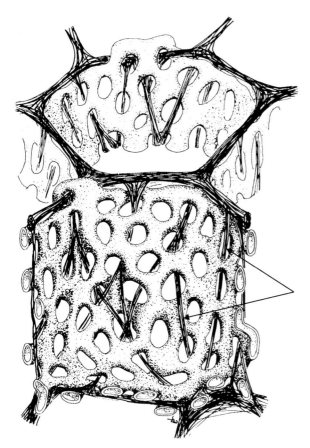

Figure 2.4 *Representation of the dense capillary network present in the alveolar septa (here secondary walls). Previously, Weibel had shown that this unique network can be morphometrically viewed as a hexagonal mesh. Epithelial and connective tissue cells occupy the centers of the hexagons. The sparse fibers (arrows) lend limited support to the network but its capillaries are deformable and distensible. (Reproduced with permission from Weibel and Gil.)[10]*

and blood enter the alveolar gas-exchanging parenchyma. The path of the air leads into the alveolar ducts, whose walls, the alveolar septa, constitute the gas-exchanging parenchyma (Figures 2.3–2.5). The foremost characteristic of the alveolar walls is that over 90% of their substance consists of blood capillaries. Beyond the last bronchiole, the content of the last axial blood vessels also penetrates into the alveolar network where it joins blood from the supernumerary arteries that is already there. While a wedge-shaped lobule or acinus is ventilated by air from a bronchiole from its apex, blood supply is far less regular and may come from the corresponding axial arteries or from neighboring supernumerary units from the same or from another axis, a matter virtually impossible to investigate. Finally, air and blood come within a very close distance from each other but stay separated at all times by an attenuated air–blood barrier, consisting at least of an endothelial and an epithelial cell sharing a fused basement membrane.

The morphology of the capillary network was described by Weibel.[12] The major differences between pulmonary and systemic capillary networks is that in the peripheral organs the arterioles break down into a brush-like bundle of capillaries, which are collected again to reconstruct a venule on the venous side whereas, in the lung, the capillaries are situated in the wall of ventilated cavities for the purpose of enabling gas exchange. Lung capillaries form a dense anastomosing hexagonal network without obvious beginning or end, periodically fed and drained by arteries and veins. Figure 2.4 is a reconstruction of a dense alveolar capillary network shown here devoid of lining epithelium. For modeling purposes, this structure can be regarded as a hexagonal mesh, as shown by Weibel.

It was pointed out[2] that all capillaries cannot be on the same plane. Alveolar septa can be categorized in two

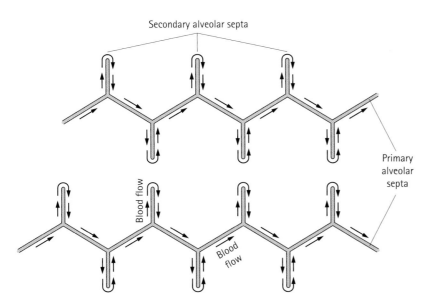

Figure 2.5 *Alveolar parenchyma showing the difference between primary and secondary alveolar walls. Primary septa form the cylindrical outer shell of alveolar ducts and always belong to two different neighboring alveolar ducts. They continuously extend from the most distal respiratory bronchiole to the insertion of the acinus into the pleural connective tissue. Secondary septa grow out of the primary walls to variable lengths into the ductal lumen. Their variable development accounts for the irregular shape and size of most individual alveoli; they are first to be destroyed in emphysema. The capillaries present within secondary septa must necessarily be collateral to those present in primary walls, to which they must return.*

groups: primary walls, which are those separating contiguous alveolar ducts, and secondary walls, perpendicular to the primary, which are placed between contiguous alveoli belonging to the same duct and in the original three-dimensional parenchyma terminate in the so-called 'alveolar entrance rings' but are seen in histological sections as having a free tip (Figure 2.5). In a study of human lungs it was shown that while primary walls are constant features, secondary walls are variably and generally irregularly developed.[13] There is reason to suspect that secondary septa are the first to be lost in pulmonary emphysema. It is evident that primary walls are in the same axis of the axial arteries while capillary networks located inside the secondary septa are blind collaterals that must rejoin the primary septa and can only be perfused if blood flows in two different directions. This is a major complication whose effects on the alveolar circulation have not been studied but it must result in the development of substantial turbulence at the capillary level.

Capillaries in the systemic circulation and in Weibel's hexagonal model are tubular. Flow resistance can be computed in principle following Poiseuille's law. What may well prevent its application is the excessive number of turbulent areas. Fung, Sobin and co-workers[14–17] proposed the notion of the sheet flow, whereby alveolar flow of blood was to be compared to the progression of a lamella (sheet) of blood moving parallel to the alveolar surfaces, interrupted only at regular intervals by the 'posts' (the solid tissue at the center of the capillary hexagon), which the authors compared to the columns of a parking garage. Supporters and detractors of the sheet flow versus capillary theory have clashed bitterly.[17–19] Both groups believe

that the published descriptions or pictures of lung vasculature support or refute their conceptions. Actually, the tissue elements in the alveolar wall are soft and devoid of skeletal or connective tissue support (Figures 2.3–2.5) and acquire a different appearance depending on the fixation method utilized. Therefore, the findings are consistent with both interpretations because alveolar wall anatomy in terms of surface configuration is not rigid. The ultimate determinants of the final appearance of the alveolar septal surface, and of its contained capillaries, are three pressures: arterial inflow pressure, venous return pressure and intra-alveolar air pressure. These pressures occur in three combinations that can be reproduced experimentally in the laboratory.[7,19–24]

THE THREE ZONES: DYNAMIC CHANGES AND ANASTOMOSES

The three zones described by West in the upright lung are the result of the following pressure combinations, which can be ultimately attributed to the effects of gravity on the arterial and venous pressures:

- zone 1: air pressure is higher than both arterial and venous pressures;
- zone 2: arterial pressure is highest, air pressure second and venous pressure is lowest. This is the situation in patients attached to a respirator;
- zone 3: both arterial and venous pressure exceed air pressure.

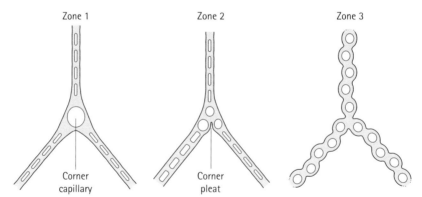

Figure 2.6 *Results of the interplay between arterial, venous and air pressures in the zonal model of the lung. In zone 1, the flow is limited to alveolar corner vessels; whereas most alveolar wall capillaries are compressed and closed by the high air pressure, the corner vessels are protected by the alveolar curvature and accommodate the entire arterio-venous flow. Zone 2 is similar to zone 1 except that alveolar wall perfusion is already increased by patches of open capillaries, which typically have quadrangular profiles and a smoothed-out surface. Corner vessels and pleats are prominent and account for the bulk of perfusion flow. In Zone 3, corner vessels, corner pleats and areas of alveolar septal closure have disappeared: instead, all alveolar wall capillaries are open and have a rounded outlines indicating that the venous pressure exceeds the air pressure. Note in this scheme the difference between corner vessels, capillaries found in corners between alveoli which are highlighted under the pressure conditions of zones 1 or 2 and extra-alveolar vessels (Figure 2.3), arteries or veins surrounded by connective tissue.*

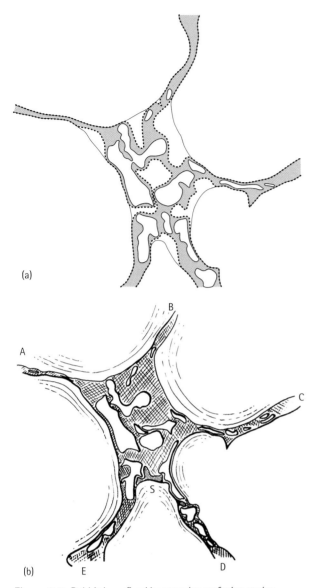

(a)

(b)

Figure 2.7 *Rabbit lung fixed by vascular perfusion under controlled pressure conditions. Part (a) is a micrograph of a septal corner as frequently seen in zone 2 (and less commonly in zone 1). The pleat is formed by folding of small segments of alveolar septa containing capillaries but is devoid of significant numbers of connective tissue fibers. The panel to the left shows, in a broken line, the reversible folding axis of the walls. Surface crevices and irregularities are filled by pools of surfactant and by alveolar macrophages. By serial reconstruction it can be shown that the tufts of capillaries contained within the pleat are fed by an artery and drained by a vein; they therefore are functionally equivalent to the corner vessels and represent arterio-venous shortcuts that stay patent when much of the septal capillary network is closed by high pressure (which is the situation in patients placed on a respirator). These pleats represent high-velocity gas exchangers (note the thinness of the tissue barrier interposed between vascular space and air) (original magnification × 1250).*

Structural studies of rat and rabbit lungs fixed by vascular perfusion in each one of the above conditions have been performed.[7] The observations are summarized in Figure 2.6. Whenever the air pressure exceeds the venous pressure (zones 1 and 2) the alveolar surface is completely smooth. This is because in both cases the 'ironing' force developed by surface tension at the air–tissue interface exceeds the venous pressure.

Blood perfusion in zone 1 is confined mostly to the corners of alveoli, while most septal capillaries appear collapsed. The open corner vessels, which because of their location are protected against intra-alveolar air pressures, are generally larger than common septal capillaries because they are distensible and must accommodate a high flow volume because of the closure of large segments of the capillary network. The existence of corner vessels has been well documented in physiological experiments based on completely different methodologies.[21,22] Zone 2 is similar, except for the additional presence of patches of capillaries with flattened, slit-like (opposite to round) lumen. Sometimes it is possible to see corner vessels in the less common form of 'corner pleats'. These are caused by small inward foldings and pleatings of the alveolar wall that occur where at least three alveolar septa meet and contain round, wide-open capillaries (Figure 2.7). An interesting finding is that crevices and depressions of the wall in such areas are filled with pools of extracelullar surfactant, which originally led to the suggestion that they served as important players in alveolar micromechanics. The therein contained capillary bundles differ little from the corner vessels of zone 1. It has been demonstrated by serial sectioning that the capillaries of septal pleats are fed on one side by a small precapillary vessel (the equivalent of an arteriole) and drained on the other by a postcapillary vein (venule).[7] These therefore represent arteriovenous shortcuts characteristic of zone 2 and which remain patent despite the effects of high intra-alveolar air pressure (Figure 2.8). The reality of circulatory changes has also been independently studied.[19,23,24] In zone 3, the striking alveolar smoothness of zones 1 and 2 has been lost because even venous return pressure exceeds the flattening capabilities of the low surface tension, which has an influence on capillary volume and compliance.[24] Whenever venous pressure exceeds air pressure, capillaries bulge freely into the air spaces. Septal pleats and corner vessels are no longer recognizable as distinct entities. It is in zone 3 that the whole alveolar surface is being perfused and optimally available for gas exchange.

One of the most interesting features of zone 2 comprises the septal pleats described above, which must be regarded as the functional equivalent of the corner vessels seen in zone 1. Put in the perspective of an extensive alveolar capillary continuum with an area of 130 m² fed and drained at intervals by arteries and veins, the pleat in the corner is a shortcut between arteries and veins formed whenever air pressure closes down most of the network.

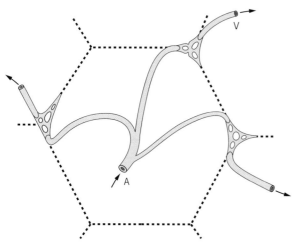

Figure 2.8 *Model representation of the protected, anastomosing role of corner vessels or pleats (triangular shadowed areas) as permanently open communications between arteries and veins regardless of alveolar pressures. Blood flow will continue (and gas exchange will take place) at least at these locations, no matter how high the air pressure and regardless of collapse of the rest of septal vessels. The artery (A) and vein (V) shown are extra-alveolar vessels surrounded by connective tissue which actually dilate with high alveolar air pressures.*

They have the function of maintaining a patent communication between the right and left ventricle. The definition of corner vessel simply implies a blood vessel located in a corner that cannot be closed by high alveolar air pressures. It applies to both a solitary vessel and to a septal pleat as described above. When originally described,[5,6] septal pleats were viewed as adaptive mechanisms in pulmonary mechanics, an opinion enhanced by the finding of pools of surfactant in alveolar epithelial crevices. The understanding was that during respiration alveolar size would change by pleating and unpleating alveolar walls. Experimentally, it is very difficult to separate the effects of inflation from adjustments to serve the needs of pulmonary microcirculation. We now know, however, that septal folds are related solely to zone 2 pressure conditions and are *per se* independent of alveolar inflation. Finally, regarding the controversy between tubular and sheet flow theories mentioned above, it is interesting to note that the morphology of zone 2 appears best to accommodate sheet flow theory (in particular, because of the patches of slit-like capillaries), while zone 3 is most consistent with the tubular flow approach.

GAS EXCHANGE IN THE THREE ZONES

Alveolar and capillary configurations are different in the three zones. Gas exchange naturally depends on lung anatomy. In zone 1, blood appears only in corner vessels and any gas exchange must be limited to such narrow areas. In zone 3, at the other extreme, every single blood capillary is filled with blood. If ventilation is even, there will be maximal utilization of the entire alveolar surface.

It has been convincingly shown by Lamm *et al.*[21] that the corner vessels open in zone 1 are capable of gas exchange. Special attention should be paid to the situation in zone 2, particularly in regard to septal pleats in the corner areas and the collapse of the capillaries present in the flattened walls. The problem has more than theoretical significance as the whole lungs of patients on a respirator with added PEEP are in that condition. The morphological findings indicate that much (perhaps most, depending on the precise pressures) of the capillary network is closed except for small patches of alveolar wall with slit-like capillaries, and that most of the flow is confined to corners and pleated capillaries which function as shortcuts between arteries and veins. Under the circumstances, one might expect that a substantial part of gas-exchanging potential could be lost, at least for the duration of the PEEP. In fact the loss fails to materialize because the septal pleat in itself must function as an excellent gas exchanger. As known from glomerular renal physiology, convoluted capillaries generally do not generate a substantial flow resistance. If parts of the capillary network are closed, the flow velocity in the pleats that stay open must be high. Micrographs always show the existence of very thin air–blood barriers between air and unfolded capillaries, which would allow for optimal gas exchange even at very high flow rates. Therefore, rather than homogeneously distributed gas exchange throughout the whole alveolar surface, what we find under zone 2 is intensive gas exchange concentrated in a few areas with high flow velocity. The above holds true only if the alveolar spaces are dry because alveolar filling results in a dramatic change in capillary morphology leading to the elimination of all corner vessels, alveolar pleats and reopening of all alveolar wall capillaries, thus creating a configuration reminiscent of that under zone 3.[4] The major difference is that an alveolus flooded through edema is incapable of gas exchange but the change in morphology may be advantageous when ventilating the lung with special fluids.

Much of what is reported in this chapter is the result of quantitative morphological studies conducted in lungs fixed by perfusion with osmium under controlled pressure conditions. Rapid freezing studies, which would have the advantage of preserving the intravascular blood, have also been published but their usefulness is technically limited by the formation of freezing artifacts and the generally poor histological quality. Morphological techniques are challenging[3] but the interest in microscopic studies has never waned and intravital studies, for instance through a window on the pleura, have always played a major role in pulmonary physiology. Even today, newer technologies only increase our interest in all forms of optical imaging.[25] *In vivo* studies are of particularly difficult interpretation because they are limited to the subpleural region because the authors view as alveoli the distance between alveolar walls, and because the position of the capillaries in the context of complex alveolar duct anatomy is ambiguous. The study of alveolar microcirculation is difficult but is not closed and newer emerging technologies may well soon enhance our knowledge.

KEY POINTS

- Extra-alveolar vessels are arteries and veins surrounded by connective tissue cuffs into which surrounding alveolar walls radially insert. They increase in volume and length during inflation and decrease during deflation.
- Corner vessels are single alveolar wall capillaries located in corners that cannot be closed by high air pressures. They are characteristic of zone 1.
- Alveolar pleats are bundles of capillaries located in corners characteristic of zone 2 lungs. They are functionally similar to the corner vessels of zone 1.
- Alveolar wall capillaries are unique in that they form large, dense hexagonal networks periodically fed and drained by arteries and veins.
- There are fewer axial arteries (those associated with bronchi) than extranumerary arteries.
- In primary alveolar septa, blood flows in the general direction from the hilum toward the pleura; in secondary alveolar septa, it may have to flow in two directions.
- In zone 1, only corner capillaries are open, maintaining the patency of pulmonary circulation.
- In zone 2, only capillaries in corner pleats and some patches of slit-like septal capillaries are open.
- In zone 3, all septal capillaries are open and the alveolar surface is undulating.
- The corner and pleated vessels of zones 1 and 2 are capable of gas exchange.
- Tubular and sheet flow theories are competing models of alveolar capillary flow. Both are based on anatomic findings which may result from reversible adaptations to pressure.

REFERENCES

1 Gil J. The normal pulmonary circulation. In: Fishman AP (ed.), *The pulmonary circulation, normal and abnormal.* Philadelphia: University of Pennsylvania Press, 1990.

2 Gil J. Morphologic aspects of alveolar microcirculation. *Fed Proc* 1978;**37**:2462-5.

◆3 Gil J. Controlled and reproducible fixation of the lung for correlated studies. In: Gil J (ed.), *Models of lung disease: methods in microscopy.* New York: Marcel Dekker, 1990.

●4 Gil J, Bachofen H, Gehr P *et al.* Alveolar volume–surface area relation in air- and saline-filled lungs fixed by vascular perfusion. *J Appl Physiol* 1979;**47**:990-1001.

●5 Gil J, Weibel ER. Morphological study of pressure–volume hysteresis in rat lungs fixed by vascular perfusion. *Respir Physiol* 1972;**15**:190-213.

6 Gil J. The normal lung circulation. State of the Art. *Chest* 1988;**93**:805-25.

●7 Ciurea D, Gil J. Morphometry of capillaries in three zones of rabbit lungs fixed by vascular perfusion. *Anat Record* 1996;**244**:182-92.

●8 Howell JBL, Permutt S, Proctor DF *et al.* Effect of inflation of the lung on different parts of the pulmonary vascular bed. *J Appl Physiol* 1962;**16**:71-6.

●9 Hislop A, Reid L. Pulmonary arterial development during childhood: branching pattern and structure. *Thorax* 1973;**28**:129-35.

◆10 Weibel ER, Gil J. Structure function relationships of the alveolar level. In: West JB (ed.), *Bioengineering aspects of the lung.* New York: Marcel Dekker, 1977.

11 Lai-Fook JS. Mechanical factors in lung liquid distribution. *Annu Res Physiol* 1992;**55**:155-79.

●12 Weibel ER. *Morphometry of the human lung.* Berlin: Springer Verlag/New York: Academic Press, 1963.

13 Ciurea D, Gill J. (1989) Morphometric study of human alveolar ducts based on serial sections. *J Appl Physiol,* **67,** 2512-21.

14 Sobin SS, Fung YC. Response to challenge to the Sobin–Fung approach to the study of pulmonary microcirculation. *Chest* 1992;**101**:1135-43.

◆15 Fung YC, Sobin SS. Pulmonary alveolar blood flow. In: West JB (ed.), *Bioengineering aspects of the lung.* New York: Marcel Dekker, 1977; 267-359.

16 Fung Y, Yen RT. A new theory of pulmonary blood flow in zone 2 condition. *J Appl Physiol* 1986;**60**:1638-50.

●17 Sobin SS, Fung YC, Tremer HM *et al.* Elasticity of the pulmonary alveolar microvascular sheet in the cat. *Circ Res* 1972;**30**:440-50.

18 Guntheroth WG, Luchtel DL, Kawabori J. Functional implications of the pulmonary microcirculation. An update. *Chest* 1992;**101**:1131-4.

19 Bachofen H, Wagensteen D, Weibel ER. Surfaces and volumes of alveolar tissue under zone II and zone III conditions. *J Appl Physiol* 1982;**53**:879-85.

20 Koyama S, Hildebrandt J. Air interface and elastic recoil affect vascular resistance in three zones of rabbit lungs. *J Appl Physiol* 1991;**70**:2422-31.

21 Lamm WJ, Obermiller T, Hlastala MP *et al.* Perfusion through vessels open in zone 1 contributes to gas exchange in rabbit lungs *in situ. J Appl Physiol* 1995;**79**:1895-9.

22 Lamm WJ, Kirk KR, Hanson WL *et al.* Flow through zone 1 lungs utilizes alveolar corner vessels. *J Appl Physiol* 1991;**70**:1518-23.

23 Conhaim RL, Rodenkirch LA. Functional diameters of alveolar microvessels at high lung volume in zone II. *J Appl Physiol* 1998;**85**:47-52.

24 Topulos GP, Brown ER, Butler JP. Increased surface tension decreases pulmonary capillary volume and compliance. *J Appl Physiol* 2002;**93**:1023-9.

25 Lawler C, Suk WA, Pitt BR *et al.* Multimodal optical imaging. *Am J Physiol Lung Cell Mol Physiol* 2003;**285**:L269-80.

PART 2

Pathophysiology and pathology of pulmonary vascular disease

3

Pathology of pulmonary vascular disease

RUBIN M TUDER AND ARI L ZAIMAN

INTRODUCTION

The uniqueness of clinical and pathological manifestations of pulmonary vascular diseases is a reflection of the specialized cellular and physiological properties of the pulmonary circulatory system. As elegantly outlined by Wagenvoort and Wagenvoort, the pulmonary vascular bed progressively remodels after birth in order to accommodate the low-pressure right ventricular cardiac output.[1] By means of complex and incompletely understood mechanisms, the pulmonary vascular bed can tightly control the blood flow throughout the pulmonary capillaries. A prominent elastic medium usually extends from the larger, extrapulmonary, arterial branches into vessels approximately 500 μm in diameter. Scattered smooth muscle cells are interspersed between a rich mesh of elastic fibers in pulmonary arteries of this size range. In pulmonary arteries ranging from 500 μm to approximately 70 μm in diameter, the smooth muscle cells progressively become more abundant, as compared to the relative amounts of elastic tissue (Plate 3.1). The vascular segments proximal to alveolar capillaries are devoid of smooth muscle cells in the media, and therefore constitute a true precapillary bed with little potential for tone control (Plate 3.1c–e). At the light microscopic level, the intima and the adventitia have similar features in the different pulmonary vascular segments. Remarkable in comparison with the systemic vessels is the lack of a classic (i.e. systemic vessel-like) adventitial vasa vasorum in pulmonary arteries.

This apparently simple cellular structure belies a complex array of phenotypic characteristics that ultimately regulate pulmonary blood flow. Comparison of the diseased lung tissue with the normal pulmonary circulation has given us insight into the phenotypic characteristics of pulmonary vascular cells, and how their functional properties relate to their morphologies. The morphological alterations present in pulmonary vascular diseases have to be appreciated in the context of the pathobiology of these very same diseases. Such an integrated approach between pathology and pathobiology is ever more pertinent in the studies concerning non-neoplastic lung diseases. Using this approach, modern pathological studies of pulmonary vascular diseases have had broad ramifications into studies related to the pathobiology, diagnosis and therapies of pulmonary hypertension.

It is the authors' goal to outline the morphological alterations observed in pulmonary hypertension, an integral part of a pathobiological process known as pulmonary vascular remodeling. The interplay between the alterations of the pulmonary vascular structure and cellular and molecular signaling underlying these alterations are covered in Chapters 5 and 13A. The overall implications of the patterns of pulmonary vascular remodeling in the pathogenesis and prognosis of pulmonary hypertension are emphasized. To illustrate the integrated approach for the assessment of the morphological information in pulmonary hypertension provided in this chapter, the authors include the clinicopathological discussion of five cases of pulmonary hypertension (see cases 1–5; Plates 3.3–3.7).

PULMONARY HYPERTENSION

Pulmonary hypertension, defined as an elevation of the mean pulmonary artery pressures above 25 mmHg, is frequently present in association with a variety of interstitial and chronic obstructive pulmonary diseases. Up to 30% of interstitial lung diseases present with pulmonary hypertension.[2] In a small fraction of patients, the mean pulmonary artery pressure reaches levels above 45 mmHg. We will refer to this form of the disease as severe pulmonary hypertension (SPH). This may present in an idiopathic form, also called primary pulmonary hypertension (PPH), or associated with underlying diseases, which include liver cirrhosis, viral infections (HIV and hepatitis C), congenital heart malformations with left-to-right shunting, and collagen vascular diseases. SPH occurs, albeit infrequently, associated with idiopathic interstitial lung diseases such as sarcoid or eosinophilic granuloma.[3] We will refer to pulmonary hypertension with mean pulmonary artery pressures ranging between 25 and 45 mmHg as mild pulmonary hypertension. This arbitrary classification is more in tune with the clinical presentation, hemodynamics data and outcome.[4]

The discussion on the morphological alterations in pulmonary hypertension is based on the recommendations of the Executive Summary from the World Symposium – Primary Pulmonary Hypertension.[5] This recommendation, which stresses the adoption of a descriptive pathological diagnosis, is a departure from the First international meeting on PPH since the limitations of the pathological assessment of lungs with pulmonary hypertension with regard to the impact on clinical presentation, prognosis, and therapies of pulmonary hypertension became apparent.[6] To a large degree, this different stand resulted from the inability of the pathologists to uncover clinically and physiologically relevant information by observing the lung morphology[6,7] and a delay to incorporate the modern tools of molecular pathology, such as immunohistochemistry, *in situ* hybridization, and lung cell sampling using laser microdissection.

Over the past 20 years, the current standards of care of SPH have been based on the hemodynamic analysis of pulmonary vascular reactivity and have been tailored to the administration of calcium channel blockers or prostacyclin.[8] In fact, pathologists assumed a secondary role in the diagnosis of pulmonary hypertension, usually restricted to postmortem confirmation of clinical data. However, pathology has significantly evolved during this time. The information provided by the 'blue and pink' slides (hematoxylin- and eosin-stained cellular structures, respectively) has been expanded by the incorporation of *in situ* detection of proteins and antigens by immunohistochemistry, mRNA by *in situ* hybridization, and cell- and structure-specific molecular studies using laser microdissection. Novel information concerning molecules that carry out the functional roles of the vascular cells, and modern concepts of cellular and molecular (patho)biology have led to an increased understanding of the relevant pathological alterations in pulmonary hypertension. Indeed, some of the most significant advances of our understanding of the pathogenesis of severe pulmonary hypertension originated from the interrogation of human diseased lung tissue (see Chapter 13A). As will become apparent, the recent introduction of these tools has expanded the role of the pathological assessment of pulmonary vascular remodeling and improved our understanding of the cellular alterations in pulmonary hypertension. Unfortunately, we still lack key information concerning several of the cellular alterations to be discussed herein. In line with the recommendation of the World Symposium in PPH, we describe the pathological features and their diagnostic significance for each layer of the pulmonary vasculature.

Intimal changes

The intima consists of the cellular matrix (basement membrane) and the endothelium interposed between the internal elastic lamina and the vascular lumen. The normal intima (which measures roughly 1–2 μm) can be altered by increased cellularity and/or intercellular matrix. The only cells capable of proliferation within the intima are the resident endothelial cells and smooth muscle cells that migrate from the vascular media. Below, we expand on the characteristics of endothelial cell-, smooth muscle cell-, and intercellular matrix processes.

ENDOTHELIAL CELLS

The pulmonary artery endothelial cells form an obligatory monolayer throughout the entire pulmonary vascular bed. Microscopically, endothelial cells lining the different segments of pulmonary arteries are similar. In pulmonary hypertension, endothelial cells that maintain their monolayer properties are indistinguishable at the microscopic level from those that line normotensive pulmonary arteries. However, several key functional alterations in endothelial cells of lungs with SPH can be demonstrated by immunohistochemistry. The expression of endothelial cells enzymes such as nitric oxide synthase and prostacyclin synthase is decreased in endothelial cells of SPH lungs,[9,10] whereas the expression of 5-lipoxygenase (an enzyme critical in the synthesis of leukotriene A$_4$), and of endothelin is increased.[11,12] The pathobiological relevance of these phenotypic alterations is discussed in detail elsewhere in this book.

In the process of determining other histopathological markers that may aid in the recognition of the altered endothelial cell phenotype in SPH, we have observed increased expression of cellular proliferation markers, such as the proliferating cell nuclear antigen, the cell proliferation-related antigen Ki67, or phosphorylated histone. The pulmonary endothelium, with a predicted doubling time of more than 180 days, is a very stable cell population, which does not normally express proliferation markers (R M Tuder, unpublished observation; Plate 3.1). The use of proliferation markers in the pathological work-up of pulmonary hypertension has been proposed,[13] but prospective studies are needed to validate this approach.

Endothelial cell proliferation is one of the characteristic feature of SPH.[14] Clusters of endothelial cells are present in pulmonary arteries of lungs with SPH. Since these clusters expand the wall of the compromised pulmonary artery,[15] they resemble small tumors or tumorlets.[16] Fully developed lesions form the so-called plexiform lesions. Plexiform lesions consist of an irregular mass of endothelial cells admixed with scanty myofibroblasts. As assessed by three-dimensional reconstruction studies, endothelial cells form a centrally dense syncytial core, with focal intracellular lumen formation, or thin-walled capillaries.[7,15,17,18] In the past, the encounter of plexiform lesions would suffice to warrant a diagnosis of plexogenic pulmonary hypertension.[6] The World Symposium – Primary Pulmonary Hypertension has discouraged the use of such a terminology since plexiform lesions are observed in PPH and in secondary SPH. Plexiform lesions from primary pulmonary hypertension are structurally similar to those present in secondary SPH. The pulmonary arteries with plexiform lesions were significantly smaller (79 μm) in PPH patients compared with secondary pulmonary hypertension due to Eisenmenger's syndrome (210 μm).

More recently, this abnormal growth of endothelial cells has been compared to endothelial cell growth seen in angiogenic processes, since the endothelial cells in plexiform lesions express angiogenic markers such as vascular endothelial growth factor, vascular endothelial growth factor receptor II (KDR/Flk), and the α- and β-subunits of the hypoxia-inducible factor (HIF).[19] Plexiform lesions resemble the glomeruloid angioproliferative vascular lesions induced by subcutaneous overexpression of vascular endothelial growth factor in the rabbit ear.[20,21] Markers of angiogenesis or structural endothelial cell proteins may be used to aid in the identification of endothelial cell tumorlets (Plate 3.2).[13]

Endothelial cell tumorlets are pathognomonic of SPH. Endothelial cell clusters or endothelial cell proliferation have not been seen in milder forms of pulmonary hypertension.[22] While no study has methodically addressed the true frequency of plexiform lesions using morphometric analysis, some studies approximate their occurrence at one lesion per 20 high-power fields.[17] Significantly, only 'classic' plexiform lesions were identified in these studies.

So-called early plexiform lesions, whose recognition cannot be made without the help of endothelial cell immunohistochemistry, were not included.

Angiomatoid lesions, a cluster of dilated capillary-like structures located in alveolar septa, are often seen in proximity of plexiform lesions. Therefore, angiomatoid lesions, as stated for plexiform lesions, are characteristic of SPH. Whether the angiomatoid lesions results from the abnormal angiogenic process in SPH is unknown. Overactive Tie-2 receptor, because of an activating intracellular mutation or overexpression of angiopoietin-2, a natural inhibitor of angiopoietin-1, the ligand for Tie-2, results in a lack of vascular wall maturation by incorporation of smooth muscle cells and pericytes. Whether abnormal Tie-2 signaling is present in SPH with angiomatoid lesions is unknown.[23,24]

Concentric lesions with an onionskin arrangement of intimal cells are also characteristically observed in SPH. The concentric lesions occur in close proximity of plexiform lesions. In three-dimensional reconstruction studies, we observed that concentric lesions occurred proximally to a well-developed plexiform lesions.[15] Furthermore, concentric lesions are composed of endothelial cells.[25] The close proximity between plexiform lesions and concentric lesions, the endothelial cell composition of both lesions, and the lack of evidence of cellular proliferation in the concentric lesion led us to the hypothesis that concentric lesion results from a continuous remodeling of a plexiform lesion at its most proximal site.[19]

SMOOTH MUSCLE CELLS

Eccentric thickening of the intima is characterized by a segmental thickening, composed of myofibroblasts embedded in a mucopolysaccharide matrix and lined with an endothelial monolayer. Although described as the most common intimal lesion in pulmonary hypertension, eccentric thickening of the intima is a common and a relatively non-specific finding in human pulmonary human arteries. In fact, eccentric thickening may be seen associated with peribronchiolar and interstitial inflammatory lung processes, or in localized thromboembolic disease, with or without pulmonary hypertension.

There is no particular feature that categorically distinguishes the eccentric pulmonary artery thickening present in lungs with mild or SPH. However, in collagen vascular disease-associated SPH (particularly the variant CREST – calcinosis, Raynaud's, sclerodactyly and telangectasia), there is marked, almost acellular, intimal thickening, which circumferentially encroaches on the vascular lumen instead of the more frequent localized pattern of eccentric intima thickening. In fact, the low-power view of such a lesion is very similar to a long, cylinder-like, fibrotic core, which takes off from a muscular artery and extends peripherally into the alveolar region. In marked contrast, in thromboembolic disease, the eccentric thickening is more cellular and less restricting than in CREST. Furthermore, the extent of intima thickening relative to the total vessel diameter is significantly increased in lungs with PPH and scleroderma-associated pulmonary hypertension compared with normal and thromboembolic diseased lungs.[26] The cause of intimal scarring by myofibroblasts is unknown. It is possible to cause intima scarring in experimental models by combining increased shear stress with pulmonary artery endothelial cell injury by the alkaloid monocrotaline.[27] The potential for pharmacological regression of these vascular lesions is probably low due to the stable nature of the population of myofibroblasts in the intimal scarring.

A unique type of myofibroblastic remodeling associated with eccentric intima thickening, the 'bridge septation', occurs in the vascular lumen in thromboembolic disease. When focal in the lung, this process may not be associated with pulmonary hypertension. However, multiple and multifocal intima 'bridge' lesions are often associated with significant pulmonary hypertension. Assessment of media hypertrophy in pulmonary artery segments not affected by the intima changes may be of help in the final diagnosis of pulmonary hypertension. The vast majority of cases of thromboembolic pulmonary hypertension lack plexiform lesions or evidence of endothelial cell proliferation. A recent study described the presence of plexiform lesions in a subset of patients with thromboembolic disease.[26] These cases evolved with SPH and the lesions persisted after endoarterectomy, suggesting that these cases might have been PPH with thromboembolic lesions.

Pulmonary vascular media

SMOOTH MUSCLE CELLS

Histological assessment of media thickening is frequently used to diagnose the different forms of pulmonary hypertension; however, it is unknown whether the alterations of vascular smooth muscle cell are the same in different forms of pulmonary hypertension. Morphometric analysis of the extent of media thickening in cases of SPH revealed that the percentage of medial thickening is increased to a similar degree in PPH and pulmonary hypertension associated with Eisenmenger's syndrome. In both settings, the per cent medial thickening was higher than that in normal and chronic thromboembolic disease.[26]

While informative in pulmonary hypertension associated with congenital heart malformation, the extension of the Heath and Edwards classification to all forms of pulmonary hypertension is misleading.[7] Not only does it fail to account for the phenotypic heterogeneity of medial smooth muscle cells, it has led to the misconceptions that

the media thickening occurs because of increased blood flow, it precedes other processes in pulmonary vascular remodeling, and it follows a common and predictable pathway. In reality, we know little about the mechanisms of media thickening, and whether the smooth muscle cell response is unique in the different forms and grades of pulmonary hypertension.

The process of media thickening is characterized by an increase in the overall contribution of the media to the total pulmonary artery diameter and, perhaps more importantly, by a peripheral extension of smooth muscle cells to pulmonary artery branches less than $70\,\mu m$ in diameter. Initially characterized in pulmonary hypertension associated with left-to-right shunts, a uniform peripheral extension was thought to occur in all forms of pulmonary hypertension. In our experience, the peripheral extension of smooth muscle cells into non-muscularized pulmonary arteries occurs in an irregular pattern in PPH and in HIV-associated pulmonary hypertension. In liver cirrhosis and collagen vascular disease-associated pulmonary hypertension, there is more uniform and extensive peripheral extension, which is also associated with marked intimal scarring.

The pathobiological importance of media thickening in pulmonary hypertension has relied on the role of medial smooth muscle cells in the control of pulmonary artery vasomotor tone and the media remodeling that is present in experimental models of pulmonary hypertension. Yet the relevance of these models to the human SPH has only recently been reviewed.[28] In fact, these models of pulmonary hypertension, are of relative short duration (i.e. 3 weeks) and are characterized by smooth muscle cell proliferation (hyperplasia).[29,30] On the other hand, we have recently highlighted that, in established human pulmonary hypertension, one seldom finds any evidence of medial smooth muscle cell proliferation.[31] If smooth muscle cell proliferation does indeed occur in pulmonary hypertension, this proliferation is brief and restricted to a few cell doublings. Furthermore, the current morphometric approach, which relies on the postulated relationship between the levels of pulmonary artery pressures and the degree of pulmonary artery medial thickening, adds limited information to the etiological nature and the extent of pulmonary hypertension. Since medial thickening occurs in mild pulmonary hypertension, the degree of medial hypertrophy alone does not allow one to discriminate mild from severe pulmonary hypertension.

The usefulness of the extent (number and degree of vessel involvement) of medial thickening in the diagnosis and prognosis of pulmonary hypertension is limited. The pathobiological importance of the medial thickening is not understood, and the fine phenotypic characterization of media smooth muscle cells in mild and severe pulmonary hypertension has not been performed. There are no markers that can help us distinguish the distinct vascular smooth muscle cell responses in the different forms of pulmonary hypertension. In summary, the authors advise that a final morphological diagnosis of pulmonary hypertension be made only in the presence of proliferated endothelial cells (in case of SPH) or extensive intima thickening by myofibroblasts (as in collagen vascular disease). Otherwise, when proliferating endothelial cells are not present, the diagnosis should contain descriptive terminology and, if appropriate, the final diagnosis should be rendered only in the context of conclusive clinical evidence of pulmonary hypertension.

Pulmonary vascular adventitia

Adventitial thickening, characterized by increase in numbers of fibroblasts, is a finding in neonatal pulmonary hypertension and in collagen vascular disease-associated pulmonary hypertension. In the vast majority of cases of mild pulmonary hypertension and SPH, there is limited adventitial thickening.

Inflammatory cells

An increase in inflammatory cells has been described in cases of SPH with plexiform lesions.[32] Further expanding this observation using cell-specific antibodies, we noted the perivascular clustering of macrophages and T and B lymphocytes around the most remodeled pulmonary arteries.[25] Importantly, this inflammatory infiltrate did not qualify as a vasculitis since there was no active vascular wall destruction by inflammatory cells.[33] Furthermore, we have not observed necrotizing arteritis as a complication of end-stage SPH, as previously described.[34] In our experience, the perivascular clustering in SPH is more pronounced in PPH when compared with secondary SPH.

CLINICOPATHOLOGICAL DISCUSSION OF CASES OF PULMONARY HYPERTENSION

Case 1

The patient is a 42-year-old man who was diagnosed with PPH 4 years ago after his right heart catheterization revealed a pulmonary artery pressure of 78/30 with a mean of 46 mmHg. He improved markedly after initiating continuous prostacyclin therapy and was removed from the transplant list. Six months ago he began to develop symptoms of severe right heart failure with increasing dyspnea on exertion, decreasing renal function, and increasing ascites. Dopamine was started and resulted in prompt diuresis; however, he continued to decline. Repeat echocardiogram showed a small left ventricle, a dilated right atrium and ventricle, severe tricuspid regurgitation,

and severe pulmonary hypertension with an estimated right ventricular systolic pressure (RVSP) of 63 mmHg. He underwent a bilateral lung transplant.

PATHOLOGY

See Plate 3.3.

DIAGNOSIS

Severe Pulmonary hypertension with endothelial cell proliferation, consistent with primary pulmonary hypertension.

COMMENTS

This is a classic case of SPH, demonstrating all the morphological findings associated with pulmonary vascular remodeling. The large vessel atherosclerotic change seen in Plate 3.3a is a common finding in clinical situations where there is an elevation in pulmonary artery pressures. These atherosclerotic lesions do not impart an increase in pulmonary vascular resistance. The marked intima thickening, with near complete obliteration of the vascular lumen, should impart a major increase in resistance to the blood flow. This thickening is composed of both myofibroblasts and endothelial cell proliferation. The most characteristic features of severe pulmonary hypertension are the plexiform and the angiomatoid lesions.

Case 2

The patient is a 52-year-old woman who was diagnosed 4 years earlier with PPH after a short exposure to the anorexigen phentermine and who symptomatically improved with continuous prostacyclin therapy. However, in recent months, her symptoms have worsened and she complained of dyspnea at rest, increasing ascites and syncope. An echocardiogram revealed a severely dilated right heart, severe tricuspid regurgitation, and an estimated right ventricular pressure of 75 mmHg. Nuclear study estimated the right ventricular ejection fraction at 10%. She underwent bilateral lung transplant.

PATHOLOGY

See Plate 3.4.

DIAGNOSIS

Severe pulmonary hypertension with endothelial cell proliferation consistent with primary pulmonary hypertension.

COMMENTS

The vascular alterations seen in the present case are similar to those shown in case 1. The present case, however, shows vascular occlusion by a recent thrombus. Thrombosis of pulmonary arteries is not a frequent finding in the recent cases examined by the authors, as compared with previous reports of the histological findings in PPH.[17] The myofibroblastic eccentric thickening is not a pathognomonic feature of pulmonary hypertension since it can be seen as a 'bystander' finding in inflammatory lung diseases. However, when the intima thickening by myofibroblasts is pronounced (as seen in the present case), it is strongly suggestive of pulmonary hypertension.

Case 3

The patient is a 38-year-old woman with a history of increasing dyspnea on exertion who presented after a syncopal episode. Echocardiography showed evidence of bidirectional shunting at the atrial septum. Cardiac catheterization revealed severe pulmonary hypertension (PA pressure 85/35, mean 57, PCWP 10, cardiac output 0.9); however, there was no evidence of a significant left-to-right shunt. Based on the elevated pressures, the patient underwent bilateral lung transplantation.

PATHOLOGY

See Plate 3.5.

DIAGNOSIS

Severe pulmonary hypertension with endothelial cell proliferation consistent with secondary pulmonary hypertension due to Eisenmenger's syndrome.

COMMENTS

The morphological alterations in this case are similar to those present in cases 1 and 2. Atherosclerotic lesions are seen in large elastic pulmonary arteries. Evidence of endothelial cell proliferation is also seen in muscular pulmonary arteries in sizes ranging from 100 to 250 μm. The muscularization of pulmonary arteries is more consistently seen in cases of secondary pulmonary hypertension associated with congenital heart malformations. The inflammatory component seen surrounding the vascular lesions is similar in secondary pulmonary hypertension to the lesion seen in PPH.

Case 4

The patient is a 49-year-old woman with a 10-year history of scleroderma, which was diagnosed after presenting with joint pain, Raynaud's phenomenon and esophageal reflux. She remained relatively stable until 2 years prior to presentation when she developed increasing fatigue and shortness of breath. Open lung biopsy revealed non-specific interstitial fibrosis and right heart catheterization revealed marked pulmonary hypertension: RA 12 mmHg, PCWP 12 mmHg, PA 80/30 (mean 50) mmHg, CO 3.61 mmHg. She underwent a vasodilator trial and was started on intravenous prostacyclin. Although she had improvement in some symptoms, her pulmonary artery pressure appeared elevated by echocardiogram and there was increased scarring at the bases. She was referred for transplant.

PATHOLOGY

See Plate 3.6.

DIAGNOSIS

Severe pulmonary hypertension characterized by medial hypertrophy, marked intima thickening (intima fibrosis), and recent thrombosis. Non-specific interstitial pneumonitis, type II, consistent with scleroderma.

COMMENTS

The present case shows an association between interstitial lung disease and marked vascular remodeling. Marked intima thickening and medial hypertrophy characterize the vascular remodeling. The intimal lesions predominate over the extent of the medial thickening with respect to the degree of obliteration of the vascular lumen. These findings are more suggestive of an ongoing pulmonary vascular lesion resulting from damage of the endothelium. Importantly, the vascular alterations are seen in areas where the interstitial process is less evident (better seen in Plate 3.6c). The contribution of the angiogenesis associated with the inflammatory interstitial disease (as seen in Plate 3.6b) has unknown significance on pulmonary vascular resistance and pulmonary hypertension. The SPH in the present case is probably the result of pulmonary vascular remodeling and the interstitial lung disease. Interstitial inflammatory diseases may be associated with mild pulmonary hypertension; in this circumstance, the vascular remodeling, with medial hypertrophy and intima thickening, is restricted to the scarred areas, and it does not involve pulmonary arteries of normal lung parenchyma.

Case 5

The patient is a 30-year-old man who initially presented with watery diarrhea. During his work-up, he noted decreasing vision bilaterally and was found to have occlusive retinal disease with some revascularization. He was referred to pulmonary clinic after developing dyspnea on exertion that rapidly progressed to dyspnea at rest. He was given a trial of empiric steroids without relief. After a low-probability V/Q scan, a thoracic CT revealed upper apical bullae and a diffuse alveolar filling process. Right heart catheterization revealed moderate pulmonary hypertension with PAP 56/20, mean of 33, PCWP of 17 and CO of 6.5.

PATHOLOGY

See Plate 3.7.

DIAGNOSIS

Pulmonary capillary hemangiomatosis.

COMMENT

This is an invasive aggressive infiltration of vascular structures in the lung by capillary-like structures. The primary involvement occurs within pulmonary veins, and extends into alveolar septa. Pulmonary hypertension due to venous abnormalities in the lung eventually compromises pulmonary arteries. Pulmonary medial thickening and variable degrees of intima thickening may be seen associated with venous pulmonary hypertension. Whether the vascular proliferation is neoplastic remains undetermined. As a group, pulmonary hypertension of venous origin is remarkable for pulmonary vascular medial thickening with smooth muscle cell hypertrophy. Careful examination may, however, reveal diffuse prominence of alveolar capillaries and presence of hemosiderin deposits in alveolar macrophages, strongly suggestive of left-sided heart failure and eventual venous pulmonary hypertension. Infrequently, one may observe prominence of peri-interlobular septal capillaries, somewhat reminiscent of a pattern resembling superficially lung fibrosis. This case warrants close examination of pulmonary veins, which run along the interlobular septa. Finding of intimal thickening or intraluminal fibrotic bridges may be indicative of pulmonary veno-occlusive disease. Characteristic lesions consist of identification of occlusive or partially recanalized thrombi.

KEY POINTS

- The pulmonary arteries are structurally organized in order to accommodate the equivalent of the systemic cardiac output under low perfusion pressures.
- In the 500 to 70 μm diameter range of arteries, the medial smooth muscle coat predominates, with progressive loss of a classic medial layer in the precapillary pulmonary arteries.

- In broad clinical and pathological terms, one may divide the cases of pulmonary hypertension as mild/moderate and severe pulmonary hypertension.
- A purely descriptive pathological approach to the pulmonary artery alterations in pulmonary hypertension, as proposed in the Evian World Symposium on PPH, is more in tune the standards of care and pathobiological understanding of pulmonary hypertension.
- Intima alterations in pulmonary hypertension involve endothelial cell proliferation or expansion of myofibroblasts originated from the medial smooth muscle cells.
- The proliferation of endothelial cells can manifest as a small cluster of cells or as plexiform lesions, as angiomatoid or as concentric lesions, and is the only finding that accurately discriminates between severe versus mild/moderate pulmonary hypertension.
- Smooth muscle cell hypertrophy and hyperplasia occur to a variable degree in pulmonary hypertension; however, there are no data on the correlation of the extent of media thickening or smooth muscle cell phenotype in discriminating mild/moderate versus severe pulmonary hypertension.
- The presence of intima fibrotic bridges associated with medial hypertrophy is suggestive of thromboembolic disease.
- A case with medial hypertrophy with absence of endothelial cell proliferation or extensive intima scarring should be interpreted with care, and a final diagnosis of pulmonary hypertension should be rendered only after careful clinico-pathological correlation.

REFERENCES

♦1 Wagenvoort CA, Wagenvoort N. Normal pulmonary and bronchial vasculature. In: Wagenvoort CA, Wagenvoort N (eds), *Pathology of pulmonary hypertension*. New York: John Wiley & Sons, 1977;17–55.

2 Tuder RM, Cool CD, Jennings C *et al*. Pulmonary vascular involvement in interstitial lung disease. In: Schwartz SM, King TEJ (eds), *Interstitial lung disease*. Hamilton: BC Decker, 1998;251–63.

3 Fartoukh M, Humbert M, Capron F *et al*. Severe pulmonary hypertension in histiocytosis X. *Am J Respir Crit Care Med* 2000;**161**:216–23.

♦4 Voelkel NF, Tuder RM. Severe pulmonary hypertensive diseases: a perspective. *Eur Respir J* 1999;**14**:1246–50.

◆5 Haworth SG, Rabinovitch M, Meyrick B *et al*. Primary pulmonary hypertension: executive summary. In: Rich S (ed.), *World Symposium – Primary pulmonary hypertension*. Geneva: World Health Organization, 1988;2–5.

6 Heath D, Wagenvoort CA. Classification and nomenclature. In: Hatano S, Strasser T (eds), *Primary pulmonary hypertension: report on a WHO meeting, October 15–17, 1973*. Geneva: World Health Organization, 1975;7–45.

◆7 Heath D, Edwards JE. The pathology of pulmonary hypertensive disease. A description of six grades of structural changes in the pulmonary arteries with special reference to congenital cardiac septal changes. *Circulation* 1958;**18**:533–47.

8 Higenbottam T, Wheeldon D, Wells F *et al*. Long-term treatment of primary pulmonary hypertension with continuous intravenous epoprostenol (prostacyclin). *Lancet* 1984;**i**:1046–7.

9 Giaid A, Saleh D. Reduced expression of endothelial nitric oxide synthase in the lungs of patients with pulmonary hypertension. *N Engl J Med* 1995;**333**:214–21.

10 Tuder RM, Cool CD, Geraci MW *et al*. Prostacyclin synthase expression is decreased in lungs from patients with severe pulmonary hypertension. *Am J Respir Crit Care Med* 1999;**159**:1925–32.

11 Giaid A, Yanagisawa M, Langleben D *et al*. Expression of endothelin-1 in the lungs of patients with pulmonary hypertension. *N Engl J Med* 1993;**328**:1732–9.

12 Wright L, Tuder RM, Cool CD *et al*. 5-Lipoxygenase and 5-lipoxygenase activating protein (FLAP) immunoreactivity in lungs from patients with primary pulmonary hypertension. *Am J Respir Crit Care Med* 1998;**157**:219–29.

13 Voelkel NF, Tuder RM, Cool CD *et al*. Severe chronic pulmonary hypertension and the pressure-overloaded right ventricle. In: Banner NR, Polak JM, Yacoub MH (eds), *Lung transplantation*. Cambridge: Cambridge University Press, 2002;Chapter 29:29–38.

14 Cool CD, Kennedy D, Voelkel NF *et al*. Pathogenesis and evolution of plexiform lesions in pulmonary hypertension associated with scleroderma and human immunodeficiency virus infection. *Hum Pathol* 1997;**28**:434–42.

15 Cool CD, Stewart JS, Werahera P *et al*. Three-dimensional reconstruction of pulmonary arteries in plexiform pulmonary hypertension using cell specific markers: evidence for a dynamic and heterogeneous process of pulmonary endothelial cell growth. *Am J Pathol* 1999;**155**:411–19.

◆16 Voelkel NF, Cool CD, Lee SD *et al*. Primary pulmonary hypertension between inflammation and cancer. *Chest* 1999;**114**:225S–30S.

●17 Wagenvoort CA, Wagenvoort N. Primary pulmonary hypertension. A pathologic study of the lung vessels in 156 clinically diagnosed cases. *Circulation* 1970;**42**:1163–84.

●18 Tuder RM, Groves BM, Badesch DB *et al*. Exuberant endothelial cell growth and elements of inflammation are present in plexiform lesions of pulmonary hypertension. *Am J Pathol* 1994;**144**:275–85.

19 Tuder RM, Chacon M, Alger LA *et al*. Expression of angiogenesis-related molecules in plexiform lesions in severe pulmonary hypertension: evidence for a process of disordered angiogenesis. *J Pathol* 2001;**195**:367–74.

20 Sundberg C, Nagy JA, Brown LA *et al*. Glomeruloid microvascular proliferation follows adenoviral vascular permeability factor/vascular endothelial growth factor-164 gene delivery. *Am J Pathol* 2001;**168**:1145–60.

21 Tuder RM, Voelkel NF. Plexiform lesion in severe pulmonary hypertension: association with glomeruloid lesion. *Am J Pathol* 2001;**159**:382–3.

◆22 Tuder RM, Cool CD, Yeager ME *et al*. The pathobiology of pulmonary hypertension. Endothelium. *Clin Chest Med* 2001;**22**:405–18.

23 Maisonpierre PC, Suri C, Jones PF *et al*. Angiopoietin-2, a natural antagonist for Tie2 that disrupts *in vivo* angiogenesis. *Science* 1997;**277**:55–60.

24 Vikkula M, Boon LM, Carraway KL *et al*. Vascular dysmorphogenesis caused by an activating mutation in the receptor tyrosine kinase TIE2. *Cell* 1996;**87**:1181–90.

25 Badesch DB, Zamora M, Fullerton D *et al*. Pulmonary capillaritis: a possible histologic form of acute pulmonary allograft rejection. *J Heart Lung Transplant* 1998;**17**:415–22.

26 Yi ES, Kim H, Ahn H *et al*. Distribution of obstructive intimal lesions and their cellular phenotypes in chronic pulmonary hypertension. A morphometric and immunohistochemical study. *Am J Respir Crit Care Med* 2000;**162**(4 Pt 1):1577–86.

27 Schuster JM, Nelson PS. Toll receptors: an expanding role in our understanding of human disease. *J Leukoc Biol* 2000;**67**:767–73.

◆28 Voelkel NF, Tuder RM. Hypoxia-induced pulmonary vascular remodeling – a model for what human disease? *J Clin Invest* 2000;**106**:733–8.

29 Meyrick B, Reid L. Hypoxia and incorporation of ^{3}H-thymidine by cells of the rat pulmonary arteries and alveolar wall. *Am J Pathol* 1979;**96**:51–70.

30 Meyrick B, Reid L. Development of pulmonary arterial changes in rats fed *Crotalaria spectabilis*. *Am J Pathol* 1979;**94**:37–51.

31 Tuder RM, Zaiman AL. Prostacyclin analogs as the brakes for pulmonary artery smooth muscle cell proliferation. Is it sufficient to treat severe pulmonary hypertension? *Am J Respir Cell Mol Biol* 2002;**26**:171–4.

32 Caslin AW, Heath D, Madden B *et al*. The histopathology of 36 cases of plexogenic pulmonary arteriopathy. *Histopathology* 1990;**16**:9–19.

33 Tuder RM, Voelkel NF. Pulmonary hypertension and inflammation. *J Lab Clin Med* 1998;**132**:16–24.

◆34 Wagenvoort CA, Wagenvoort N. Unexplained plexogenic pulmonary arteriopathy: primary pulmonary hypertension. In: Wagenvoort CA, Wagenvoort N (eds), *Pathology of pulmonary hypertension*. New York: John Wiley & Sons, 1977;119–42.

4

Hypoxic pulmonary vasoconstriction and hypertension

ANDREA OLSCHEWSKI AND E KENNETH WEIR

INTRODUCTION

Hypoxic pulmonary vasoconstriction (HPV) is a physiological response of small pulmonary arteries that diverts mixed venous blood away from hypoxic alveoli, thus optimizing the matching of perfusion and ventilation and preventing arterial hypoxemia. HPV has been an area of intensive investigation since it was reported more than 100 years ago[1] and was more precisely described in 1946 by von Euler and Liljestrand.[2] Although the responses to hypoxia are relatively well characterized, the molecular mechanisms of O_2 signaling and how changes in environmental O_2 are translated into signals recognizable by the cell are just beginning to be understood.

HYPOXIC PULMONARY VASOCONSTRICTION

The pulmonary vascular bed is unique compared with most studied systemic vascular beds. During normoxic conditions, the pulmonary circulation is at low pressure – that is, vasodilated – compared with the high-pressure systemic circulation. In the systemic circulation, hypoxemia elicits vasodilatation that increases O_2 delivery to the tissues. In contrast, small resistance arteries in the pulmonary circulation constrict in response to hypoxia. In the developing fetus, gas exchange occurs via the placenta. HPV helps to maintain the high pulmonary vascular resistance that diverts blood flow away from the fetal lung through the ductus arteriosus (DA). Postpartum, in concert with inflation of the lungs, the pulmonary vasculature relaxes and promotes better perfusion of the lung vessels. HPV can be defined as the rapid, reversible increase in pulmonary vascular resistance, caused by contraction of the small muscular pulmonary arteries with an internal diameter of about 200–600 μm, in response to physiological levels of hypoxia.[3] Hypoxic vasoconstriction depends largely on the alveolar and not on the mixed venous PO_2,[4,5] and starts within seconds of the onset of airway hypoxia by a decrease in alveolar O_2 tension below a threshold fractional inspired O_2 concentration of approximately 10%.[5,6] The response to alveolar hypoxia shows a biphasic character, with an early pulmonary arterial pressure peak and a more protracted secondary pressure elevation, as observed in intact dogs[7] and rabbits,[8] and in isolated ferret[9] and rabbit lungs.[5] The acute, initial transient vasoconstrictor phase one is independent of the endothelium. The slowly developing increase in vascular tone (second phase) appears to be dependent on the presence of endothelium and extracellular Ca^{2+}. When only a small region of the lung is hypoxic, HPV can occur without significant effect on pulmonary arterial pressure.[10] However, when hypoxia is generalized, as seen with many lung diseases and in high-altitude exposure, the subsequent pulmonary vasoconstriction contributes to pulmonary hypertension, heart failure and death.

Superimposed effects of acidosis, alkalosis and hyperventilation

Hypoxia stimulates ventilation and ventilation *per se* can affect pulmonary vascular tone. The mechanisms of the alkalosis- and hypocapnia-dependent vasodilatory responses are not fully understood. Hyperventilation has been demonstrated to reduce elevated pulmonary arterial pressure in different animal models, and is employed during anesthesia for the treatment of children with pulmonary hypertensive disorders. The induction of hypocapnic alkalosis is believed to play an important role in these vasodilatory effects,[11,12] with alkalosis but not hypocapnia being the crucial factor.[13] Although the results generally indicate that extracellular alkalosis inhibits, and hypercapnia or acidosis potentiates, the hypoxic pressor response, there are discordant findings. Raffestin and McMurtry have reported that intracellular alkalosis increases and acidosis attenuates HPV by unknown mechanisms.[14] During respiratory alkalosis, exhalation of the potent vasodilator nitric oxide (NO) is increased in rabbit lungs.[15,16] However, there is also evidence that alkalosis-induced pulmonary vasodilation is independent of both NO[11] and prostacyclin synthesis.[17]

Hyperventilation is itself capable of inducing the release of vasoactive mediators via mechanical forces. In human volunteers, hyperventilation stimulates the release of the vasodilator prostaglandins PGE_1 and PGI_2, independent of respiratory alkalosis.[18] Moreover, the production of PGI_2 in lung cells is significantly affected by the frequency and magnitude of pulsatile stretch in the rat[19] and hyperventilation augments the release of PGI_2 in isolated mouse lungs.[20] In addition, the exhalation of NO increases with lung distension induced by different ventilation strategies in rabbits.[16] The intracellular signaling events in response to these mechanical forces may include activation of stretch-sensitive ion channels and cascades of protein kinases. Due to the complexity of pulmonary tissue and the variety of cells capable of perceiving mechanical forces, the origin of these vasoactive mediators is not exactly known, but airway epithelial and vascular endothelial cells, as well as pulmonary nerves (for generation of NO), must be considered.

Effector mechanism (intracellular and extracellular sources of Ca^{2+})

Hypoxia appears to activate mechanisms intrinsic to the pulmonary vasculature, which are independent of blood-borne factors or influences requiring the central nervous system, as HPV can be demonstrated in isolated perfused lungs and isolated pulmonary arteries.[5,21,22] According to current knowledge, neither angiotensin, prostaglandins, thromboxane nor arachidonic acid lipoxygenase products directly mediate the mechanism of acute HPV. In contrast, hypoxic vasoconstriction is blocked by calcium antagonists and reduced by endothelin antagonists and α-adrenergic antagonists, suggesting not only involvement of voltage-dependent calcium channels and extracellular calcium but also of the endothelin pathway and possibly of catecholamines. Vasodilatators such as NO and prostacyclin are able to override HPV, but this does not necessarily suggest an endogenous role of these substances in the mechanism.

Acute exposure to hypoxia increases the pulmonary arterial pressure in whole animals and in isolated lungs, as already described. Hypoxia also causes contraction in isolated pulmonary arteries[23–25] as well as in pulmonary artery rings denuded of endothelium[26,27] and in single isolated smooth muscle cells from resistance pulmonary arteries,[28] indicating that the basic mechanism of HPV is intrinsic to the vascular wall of pulmonary arteries. An increase of the cytosolic Ca^{2+} concentration ($[Ca^{2+}]_i$) is necessary to elicit constriction of the vessels. In excitable cells, $[Ca^{2+}]_i$ is increased by Ca^{2+} influx through Ca^{2+}-permeable channels and/or by Ca^{2+} mobilization from intracellular Ca^{2+} stores (e.g. endoplasmic/sarcoplasmic reticulum). There are three main pathways by which extracellular Ca^{2+} can enter into the PA smooth muscle cells:

- voltage-dependent Ca^{2+} channels
- receptor-activated Ca^{2+} channels and
- store-operated Ca^{2+} channels.

However, store-operated Ca^{2+} channels are frequently defined as a major subfamily of receptor-activated Ca^{2+} channels. Voltage-dependent Ca^{2+}-channel blockers such as verapamil or SFK-525 significantly reduce HPV in isolated perfused lungs[29] and BAY K 8644, a voltage-dependent Ca^{2+}-channel agonist, enhances it.[30,31] The increase in $[Ca^{2+}]_i$ is smaller in the absence of extracellular calcium,[32] indicating significant contributions from calcium entry through calcium channels. Our own experiments using fura-2 loaded myocytes from resistance pulmonary arteries shows that the hypoxia-induced increase in $[Ca^{2+}]_i$ is approximately 70% reduced by removal of extracellular Ca^{2+} (Figure 4.1). Hypoxia-induced increase in $[Ca^{2+}]_i$ is entirely inhibited in type I cells in the absence of extracellular Ca^{2+}.[33] Robertson *et al.* found that a low concentration of La^{3+} ($<3\,\mu M$), which is a non-selective blocker of Ca^{2+} entry almost abolished vasoconstriction in isolated pulmonary artery rings and increase of $[Ca^{2+}]_i$.[34] These observations suggest that both sources of Ca^{2+} may be important. Calcium influx via voltage-dependent Ca^{2+} channels in vascular smooth muscle cells is controlled by

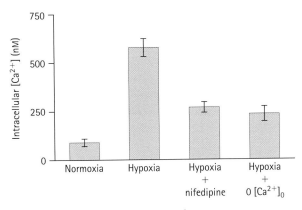

Figure 4.1 *The hypoxic increase in [Ca^{2+}]$_i$ of pulmonary artery smooth muscle cells comes from both inside and outside the cell. The data are given as mean ± SEM (n = 10).*

the resting membrane potential (E$_m$) of these cells. E$_m$ is controlled by potassium permeability, which is determined by sarcolemmal potassium (K$^+$) channel conductance. Hypoxia causes both an inhibition of whole cell K$^+$ current and membrane depolarization in isolated PA smooth muscle cells,[35,36] leading to opening of voltage-gated calcium channels and entry of calcium into the cells.

Stores of Ca^{2+} in the cell also provide the potential for release of Ca^{2+} during physiological signaling of hypoxia. The main storage compartment is the sarcoplasmic reticulum, and this organelle has a major role in maintaining low [Ca^{2+}]$_i$. Hypoxia still increases [Ca^{2+}]$_i$ in isolated PA smooth muscle cells in the absence of external calcium[37] and the hypoxia-induced change in [Ca^{2+}]$_i$ is inhibited by the use of thapsigargin, ryanodine or cyclopiazonic acid, that reduce Ca^{2+} release from the sarcoplasmic reticulum, suggesting that hypoxia may alter Ca^{2+} handling by the sarcoplasmic reticulum.[38] Pretreatment with cyclopiazonic acid also inhibits the acute, initial transient vasoconstrictor phase of hypoxic vasoconstriction in intrapulmonary arteries, at least in rats.[34] These findings suggest that the mechanisms that are necessary for sensing and responding acutely to hypoxia are intrinsic to the PA smooth muscle cells and that both intracellular and extracellular Ca^{2+} are important.

MECHANISM OF ACUTE HYPOXIC VASOCONSTRICTION: HYPOXIC SIGNALING

Knowledge of the mechanism of O$_2$ sensing and the signaling pathways that mediate the cellular response to hypoxia has developed rapidly in the last decade. The most widely distributed structures mediating the effect of changes in PO$_2$ are ion channels. Several studies have provided direct evidence that hypoxic vasoconstriction of PA smooth muscle cells is mediated, at least in part, by

the inhibition of one or several K$^+$ channels leading to cell depolarization, opening of voltage-gated Ca^{2+} channels and myocyte contraction.[22,35,39–41] In addition, hypoxia potentiates Ca^{2+} entry through L-type Ca^{2+} channels in a subset of resistance vessel myocytes.[33,42,43] Ca^{2+} released from ryanodine-sensitive stores in hypoxia could also contribute to constriction either directly or through blockade of K$^+$ channels.[44,45]

Potassium channels

The potassium current in PA smooth muscle cells is an ensemble, reflecting activity of many different channels. At least three classes of potassium channels have been identified in PA smooth muscle cells: voltage-dependent potassium channels (Kv),[39,45,46] calcium-activated potassium channels (K$_{Ca}$)[47,48] and ATP-sensitive potassium channels (K$_{ATP}$).[49] The potassium channels which control E$_m$ in PA smooth muscle cells, and inhibition of which initiates HPV, conduct an outward current which is slowly inactivating and blocked by the Kv channel blocker 4-aminopyridine (4-AP) but not by inhibitors of K$_{Ca}$ or K$_{ATP}$, at least in the rat.[39,40,50] At the molecular level, Kv channels are homo- or heteromultimeric tetramers that are composed of two structurally distinct subunits: the pore-forming α-subunits and the regulatory β-subunits.[51] Nine families of Kv channel α-subunits are recognized from cloning studies (Kv1–9),[51,52] each with subtypes (e.g. Kv1.1–1.6). The molecular identification of the specific Kv channels that control E$_m$ is difficult, even with advanced electrophysiological techniques, mainly because of the lack of specific blockers. However, the intracellular dialysis of specific Kv antibodies combined with patch-clamp recording, studies in expression systems, or the use of reverse transcription polymerase chain reaction may throw light on the involvement of K$^+$ channels in the mechanism of HPV. The potential candidate Kv channel α-subunits that could form O$_2$-sensitive channels in PA smooth muscle cells are Kv1.2,[53,54] Kv1.5,[50,53] Kv2.1,[50,54,55] Kv3.1,[56] and Kv9.3.[54,55]

The O$_2$ sensitivity of Kv1.2 channels was recently examined by Hulme *et al.*,[54] who found that, when expressed in mouse L cells, the Kv1.2 was significantly inhibited by hypoxia. Low O$_2$ tension also inhibited Kv1.2 channels expressed in PC 12 cells.[57] Conversely hypoxia failed to inhibit Kv1.2 channels.[56] It has been reported that hypoxia initiates HPV by inhibiting Kv1.5 and perhaps Kv2.1.[50] In addition, HPV is markedly suppressed in Kv1.5 knockout mice compared with the wild type.[58] However, Kv1.5 is not sensitive to hypoxia when expressed as a homotetramer in L cells,[54] or COS-7 cells.[54] When coexpressed, Kv1.2 and Kv1.5 α-subunits in L cells produced currents that displayed kinetic and pharmacological properties distinct from Kv1.2 and

Kv1.5 alone and this current was significantly inhibited by hypoxia in the voltage range of the PA smooth muscle cells' resting membrane potential.[54]

Hypoxia was found to inhibit recombinant rat Kv2.1 channels expressed in COS cells[55] and mouse L cells.[54] In contrast, Conforti et al. found the Kv2.1 current to be insensitive when expressed in Xenopus oocytes.[57] Patel et al. have provided support for the role of Kv2.1 in O_2 sensing.[55] When Kv2.1 was coexpressed with the 'silent' Kv9.3 α-subunit, cloned from myocytes of the pulmonary artery, effect of hypoxia was enhanced.[55] More importantly, Kv9.3 shifted the voltage-dependent activation of the heteromeric Kv2.1/Kv9.3 channel into the voltage range of the resting membrane potential of PA smooth muscle cells, supporting the role of the Kv2.1/Kv9.3 current in the physiological response of PA smooth muscle cells to hypoxia.[54,55]

The β-subunit could also confer O_2 sensitivity on a K^+ channel. It has been reported that expression of Kv4.2 channels plus Kvβ1.2 subunit in HEK293 cells conferred sensitivity to redox modulation and O_2 sensitivity.[59]

Redox modulation of channels

Multiple pathways may exist for hypoxia-induced Kv channel inhibition. Hypoxic signaling may be related to:

- a conformational change of a membrane-bound heme-linked protein closely associated with the channel, secondary to the binding of O_2;
- a change in cellular (sarcoplasmic or cytoplasmic) redox status, secondary to altered NAD(P)H oxidase- and/or mitochondrial-dependent oxygen radical formation; or
- an increase in the ratios of the cytosolic redox couples (NADH/NAD; NADPH/NADP; GSH/GSSG), secondary to slowing of mitochondrial electron transfer; or
- release of intracellularly stored Ca^{2+}.

CONFORMATIONAL CHANGE ALTERING CHANNEL FUNCTION

Iron-containing heme proteins, including cytochromes and NAD(P)H oxidases, were proposed some time ago as potential O_2 sensors in a variety of cellular systems. The heme protein in the deoxy conformation could activate effectors either directly or through a signaling cascade. Some native[60,61] and recombinant channels[56,59] have been reported to retain O_2 sensitivity in excised membrane patches in the absence of intracellular mediators, which could suggest a direct interaction between channels and O_2 sensors, or between channels and oxygen itself. The existence of a putative sensor is also supported by the observation that carbon monoxide, which has a high binding affinity to the heme protein, significantly reverses

the hypoxic inhibition of the O_2-sensitive K channel of rabbit carotid body type I cells[62] and of the Kv channels expressed in HEK cells.[59] However, the major problem of the heme model is a lack of direct experimental support. In addition, recent data have shown that CO can interact directly with hypoxia-inducible factor (HIF)-1α and the inhibition of heme synthesis fails to show any effect on hypoxia responsiveness, suggesting that heme proteins are not involved in the more chronic sensing of hypoxia.[63]

POTENTIAL ROLE OF REACTIVE OXYGEN SPECIES

O_2 sensing could be achieved through production of reactive oxygen species (ROS), thus altering the redox status of signaling molecules and the function of effectors. ROS, including superoxide anion (O_2^-), hydroxyl radical (OH$\cdot$) and hydrogen peroxide (H_2O_2), are produced in the lung in proportion to the ambient O_2 tension. The superoxide anion is formed by the one electron reduction of molecular oxygen (O_2), mediated by enzymes such as NAD(P)H oxidases and xanthine oxidases, or non-enzymatically by redox reactive compounds such as the semi-ubiquinone compound of the mitochondrial electron transport chain. SOD converts superoxide enzymatically into hydrogen peroxide. In the presence of reduced transition metals, hydrogen peroxide can be converted into the highly reactive hydroxyl radical or alternatively into water by the enzymes catalase or glutathione peroxidase. Several studies have shown that hypoxia decreases production and tissue levels of ROS,[64–70] although this is still disputed[71–76] (Table 4.1).

Extracellularly applied H_2O_2 enhances the O_2-sensitive outward K^+ current[77–79] and hypoxia inhibits this K^+ current in lung neuroepithelial body (NEB) cells.[78,79] Therefore, if ROS are involved in O_2 sensing, hypoxia must reduce ROS. Direct effects of ROS on voltage-gated K^+ channels have also been demonstrated in the HERG channel,[80] in the small cell lung carcinoma (H-146) cell line[69] and in smooth muscle cells of the ductus arteriosus.[70]

Regardless of the direction of the change in the level of ROS, the redox couples within the cytosol could be affected and modify channel activity, or alternatively the ROS could directly alter ion channel activity. Under normoxic levels of O_2, glycolysis results in the production of reducing equivalents such as NADH. Hypoxia increases the ratios of the reduced to the oxidized form of the cytosolic redox pairs such as NADH/NAD, NADPH/ NADP and/or glutathione (GSH/GSSG)[81–83] and thus shifts the cells to a more reduced state. Exogenous reducing agents mimic the effect of hypoxia on several types of O_2-sensitive K^+ channels, membrane potential or $[Ca^{2+}]_i$[84,85] (Figure 4.2). Reduced glutathione (GSH) in cultured PA smooth muscle cells causes an inhibition in the whole-cell K^+ current and significant membrane depolarization. In the presence of GSH in these cells, hypoxia has

Table 4.1 *Effect of acute hypoxia on reactive oxygen species (ROS) production*

Tissue	ROS	Technique	Reference
Human neutrophils	↓	Superoxide-mediated cytochrome c reduction	Gabig et al. (1979)[64]
Lung tissue slices (rat)	↓	CN⁻-resistant respiration	Freeman and Crapo (1981)[65]
Lung (rat)	↓	Lucigenin-enhanced chemiluminescence Luminol-enhanced chemiluminescence	Archer et al. (1989)[66]
Lung (rabbit)	↓	Lucigenin-enhanced chemiluminescence	Paky et al. (1993)[67]
Pulmonary artery (PA) ring (rat)	↓	Lucigenin-enhanced chemiluminescence	Archer et al. (1999)[68]
Small cell lung carcinoma cell line (H-146)	↓	2′,7′-dichlorodihydrofluorescein diacetate (H_2DCFDA) fluorescence	O'Kelly et al. (2000)[69]
Ductus arteriosus rings (rabbit)	↓	Lucigenin-enhanced chemiluminescence Luminol-enhanced chemiluminescence	Reeve et al. (2000)[70]
PA smooth muscle cells (calf)	↑	Lucigenin-enhanced chemiluminescence	Marshall et al. (1996)[71]
Cardiomyocytes (chick)	↑	2′,7′-dichlorofluorescein diacetate (DCFH-DA) fluorescence	Duranteau et al. (1998)[72]
PA smooth muscle cells	↑	DCFH-DA fluorescence	Killilea et al. (2000)[73]
PA smooth muscle cells (rat)	↑	DCFH-DA fluorescence	Waypa et al. (2001)[75]

no further effect on K^+ current or resting membrane potential, suggesting that both hypoxia and GSH block the same K^+ channels.[84] Oxidized gluthatione (GSSG), co-enzyme Q_{10} and duroquinone, on the other hand, increase whole-cell K^+ current and hyperpolarize the resting membrane potential.[22,86] Complementary to these findings, in the ductus arteriosus the reducing agent *N*-mercaptopropionylglycine (NMPG) both increases K^+ current and dilates normoxic-constricted rings.[70] These data suggest that changes in the redox status of the cytoplasm might alter the gating of K^+ channels, such that hypoxia closes channels in pulmonary artery and opens them in ductus arteriosus smooth muscle cells.

SOURCES OF ROS PRODUCTION

Two principal systems produce ROS: the NAD(P)H oxidases and the mitochondria. NAD(P)H oxidase, a flavocytochrome, is expressed in a variety of O_2-sensitive tissues, including NEBs,[87] pulmonary artery smooth muscle cells,[71,88,89] endothelial cells[90] and carotid bodies.[91] The NAD(P)H oxidase isoforms of the cardiovascular system are membrane-associated enzymes and the rate of superoxide production in these cells is only about one-third of that of neutrophils. The classical form of this enzyme is comprised of a membrane-bound flavocytochrome containing two subunits, gp91[phox] and p22[phox], and the cytosolic proteins p47[phox] and p67[phox].[92,93] There is support for the central role of an NAD(P)H oxidase in O_2 sensing in lung NEBs and the H-146 cell line.[69,77] In these cells, the hypoxia-sensitive K^+ current is potentiated by H_2O_2 or by the activation of the oxidase with phorbol esters.[69,77] The involvement of this oxidase has received further reinforcement by the observation that K^+

channels of NEB cells recorded from gp91[phox] knockout mouse lung slices were insensitive to acute hypoxia.[79] Recently, a microsomal NAD(P)H oxidase has also been implicated as an oxygen sensor in bovine pulmonary arteries, where changes in oxygen tension regulate vascular relaxation through changes in ROS production and cGMP formation.[94]

Several studies report evidence against the involvement of an NAD(P)H oxidase on O_2 sensing. In isolated and cultured NEB cells, the hypoxia-induced inhibition of K^+ channels was found to be suppressed by the relatively non-selective NAD(P)H oxidase inhibitor, diphenylene iodonium (DPI)[77] but DPI did not mimic the hypoxia response when given during normoxia. Similarly, the involvement of the neutrophil NAD(P)H oxidase as an O_2 sensor in the pulmonary circulation has been discounted by the recent observation that the gp91[phox] knockout mouse has normal HPV and hypoxia still inhibits K^+ channels in their PA smooth muscle cells. Moreover, patients with genetic subtypes of chronic granulomatous disease (CGD), characterized by absence or abnormality of each of the NAD(P)H subunits, have a very restricted clinical phenotype with no apparent evidence of disordered O_2 sensing. Finally, Wenger et al. showed that CGD-derived lymphoid cell lines, deficient in either the gp91[phox] or p22[phox] subunits, were still able to express vascular endothelial growth factor and aldolase mRNA in response to hypoxia, similar to the wild-type controls.[95]

Because the lion's share of oxygen metabolism takes place in the mitochondria, this organelle might seem to be critical for the sensing of hypoxia. Depletion of high-energy phosphates, a shift toward the reduced form of redox couples, or cytochromes with an unusually low

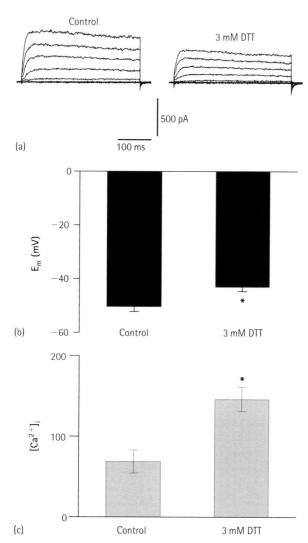

Figure 4.2 *Effect of the reducing agent dithiothreitol (DTT) on whole-cell outward potassium current, resting membrane potential and intracellular $[Ca^{2+}]$ of adult rabbit pulmonary artery (PA) smooth muscle cells. (a) Representative traces demonstrate whole-cell potassium currents from adult rabbit PA smooth muscle cells under normoxic conditions (left) and after 3 mM DTT (right). Currents were evoked from a holding potential of -70 mV to $+50$ mV in 20 mV steps. (b) DTT depolarizes the resting membrane potential (E_m) (n = 5). (c) DTT increases the $[Ca^{2+}]_i$ of PA smooth muscle cells (n = 14). The data are given as mean $\pm$ SEM. *P $<$ 0.05 for difference from control.*

affinity for PO_2 could act as a sensor for hypoxia. A model of O_2 sensing based on the mitochondria comes from observations on the carotid body. A cytochrome with an unusually low affinity for O_2 was reported 30 years ago in carotid body mitochondria.[96] Duchen and Biscoe have described a graded increase in NAD(P)H autofluorescence in type I cells in response to decreasing levels of PO_2 over a physiologically significant range (below a PO_2 of about 60 mmHg), reflecting a rise in

NAD(P)H/NAD(P) ratio.[97,98] In similarly isolated chromaffin cells and dorsal root ganglion neurons no measurable change in autofluorescence was seen until the PO_2 fell close to zero. They interpreted these results to suggest that specialized mitochondrial electron transport might confer the unusual oxygen sensitivity in type I cells.

Further support for involvement of mitochondria has come from observations on Hep 3B cells[99–101] and cardiomyocytes.[75,101–103] These observations suggest that hypoxia reversibly decreases the V_{max} of the cytochrome oxidase. The decrease in V_{max} results in accumulation of electrons and an increase in NADH concentration of the cell during moderate hypoxia (20–50 mmHg).[104] This adaptation in enzyme function appears to develop over 1–2 hours in some cell types,[105] whereas other cells undergo the change more rapidly.[103] So again, if mitochondrial production of ROS were to be important, a cytochrome with a low affinity for O_2 could be essential.

Primary role of $[Ca^{2+}]_i$ on potassium channel function

One mechanism proposed to explain K^+ channel modulation during hypoxia is the direct influence of increased cytosolic $[Ca^{2+}]$ on K^+ channels. Exposure to hypoxia of PA smooth muscle cells may cause rapid mobilization of Ca^{2+} from intracellular stores.[32] It is possible that the first effect of hypoxia is the release of intracellular calcium, which could in turn lead to inhibition of K^+ channels and influx of external calcium.[37,45] However, this mechanism seems less likely given the observation that hypoxic inhibition of potassium current can be demonstrated in type I cells using the whole-cell patch-clamp technique with EGTA in the patch pipette to maintain a low intracellular Ca^{2+} concentration.[106]

CHRONIC HYPOXIC VASOCONSTRICTION: HYPOXIC PULMONARY HYPERTENSION

Chronic hypoxia, for example related to chronic obstructive lung disease, or a prolonged stay at high altitude, results in both structural changes in the PA and a sustained increase in pulmonary vascular tone. The increase in vascular tone may be due to depolarization through inactivation or lack of expression of K^+ channels[107] and decreased levels of cGMP and cAMP caused by increased phosphodiesterase activity,[108] in addition to increased levels of endogenous vasoconstrictors, such as angiotensin II,[109–111] thromboxane A_2,[112] endothelin-1 (ET-1),[113] and 5-hydroxytryptamine (5-HT).[114,115]

Each cell type in the small pulmonary arteries less than 500 μm in diameter – endothelial cells, smooth muscle cells and adventitial fibroblasts – is involved in

Color plates

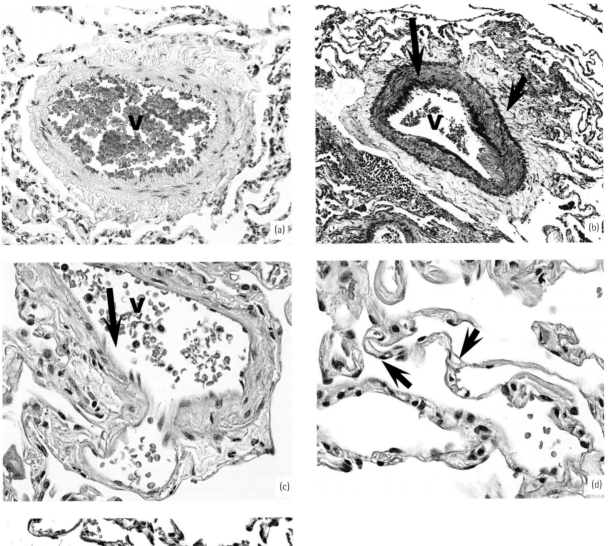

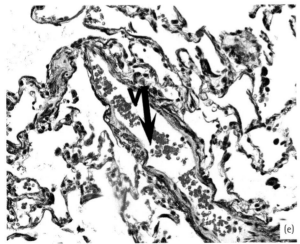

Plate 3.1 *Morphology of normal pulmonary arteries. (a) Muscular pulmonary artery (V) (hematoxylin and eosin, ×200 original magnification). (b) Movat-stained pulmonary artery (V) with internal (arrow) and external elastic lamina (arrowhead). Note, in yellow, the delicate collagenous adventitia. Although this is a normal pulmonary artery, there is a focal intima thickening (thin arrow) (×100 original magnification). (c) Muscular pulmonary artery (V) merging into a thin-walled, amuscular precapillary artery. Normal pulmonary arteries lose the muscular layer in the range of 70 μm vessel diameter. (d) Alveolar septa with thin capillary units (arrowheads) (hematoxylin and eosin, ×400 original magnification). (e) Movat-stained pulmonary artery (V) showing lack of muscular media and single elastic tissue (arrow).*

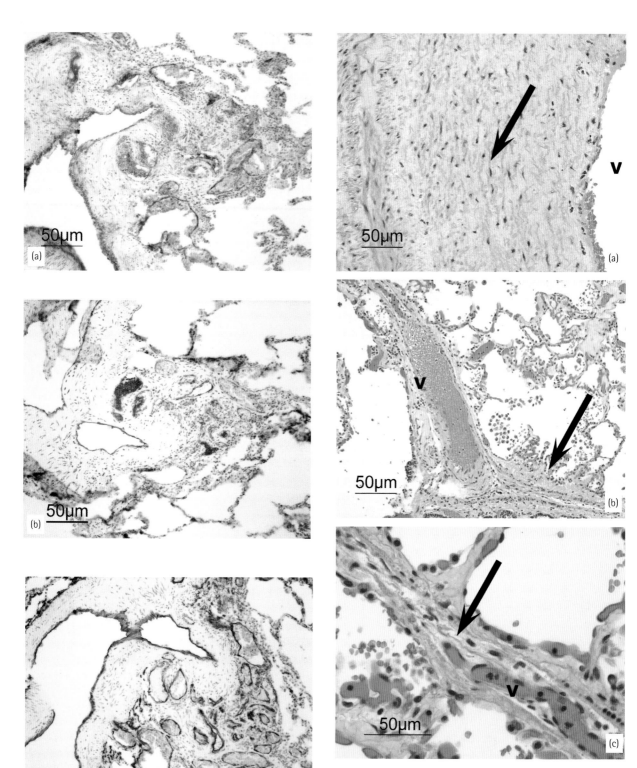

Plate 3.2 *Immunohistochemical detection of the endothelial cell antigens Factor VIII-related antigen (a), CD-31 (b) and CD-34 (c) in serial sections of a plexiform lesions (bar = 50 μm).*

Plate 3.3 *(a) Large pulmonary artery composed mostly of elastic media showing an increase of the intima thickness due to myxoid tissue admixed with myofibroblasts. This lesion is similar to atherosclerotic lesions seen in the aorta and large systemic vessels. This is a non-specific reaction due to the elevation of pulmonary artery pressures (hematoxylin and eosin, ×50 original magnification). (b) Muscularized pulmonary artery, showing an increase in medial thickness. The branch, which takes off to the right of the microscopic field, shows intima obliteration (arrow) (hematoxylin and eosin, bar = 50 μm). (c) Close-up of the vascular segment highlighted by an arrow in (b), showing intima thickening due to myxoid tissue admixed with myofibroblasts (arrow) (hematoxylin and eosin, bar = 50 μm).*

(Continued opposite)

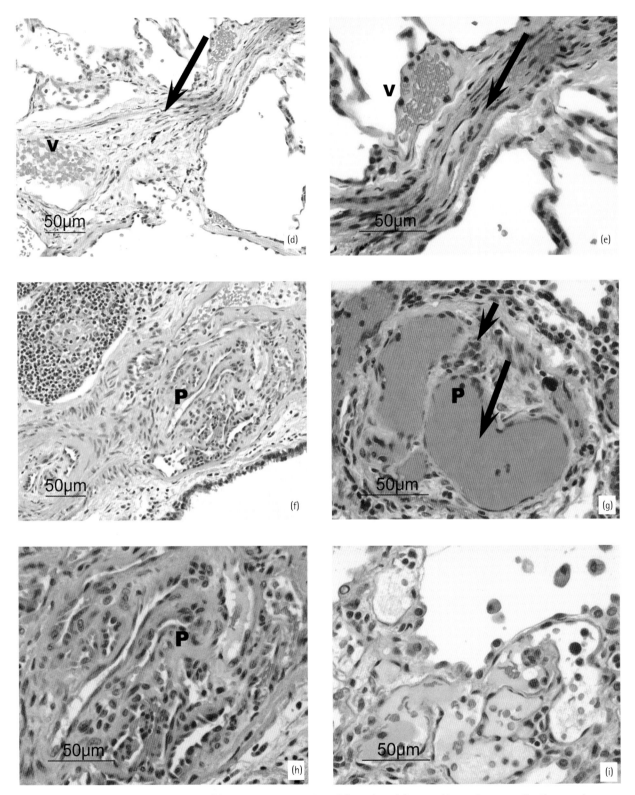

Plate 3.3 *(d) Small size pulmonary artery (V) showing near complete obliteration of the vessel lumen by connective tissue and myofibroblasts (arrow) (hematoxylin and eosin, bar = 50 μm). (e) Close-up of pulmonary arteries shown in (d). Note the obliteration of the vascular lumen by elongated myofibroblastic cells (arrow) (hematoxylin and eosin, bar = 50 μm). (f) Plexiform lesion (P) compromising medium-sized pulmonary artery. Note near-complete obliteration of vascular lumen by the lesion (hematoxylin and eosin, bar = 50 μm). (g, h) Close-up of two plexiform lesions (P). Note the core of endothelial cells (arrow) in variable stages of blood vessel formation The endothelial cells appear more rounded and disorganized than intima myofibroblasts. Often, they are seen in continuity with endothelial cells lining the lumen of incipient blood vessels (arrowheads). Lesion in (c) is shown in a cross-section (hematoxylin and eosin, bar = 50 μm).*

(Continued over)

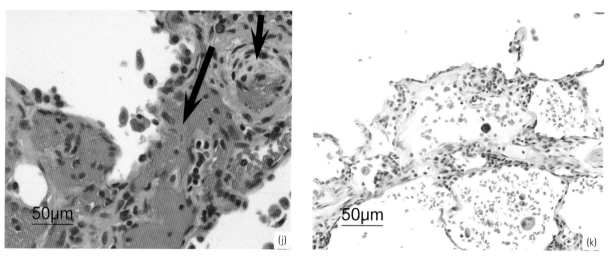

Plate 3.3 *(i–k) Angiomatoid lesion, characterized by the formation of conglomerates of thin-walled vessels, devoid of smooth muscle cells, and lined by single layer endothelium. In (j), the angiomatoid lesion is seen distally to a concentric lesion possibly representing an early plexiform lesion. Angiomatoid vessels are highlighted by the arrow (hematoxylin and eosin, bar = 50 μm).*

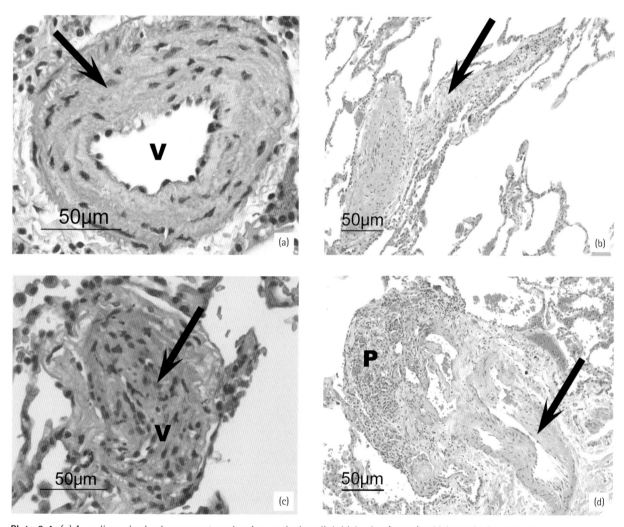

Plate 3.4 *(a) A medium-sized pulmonary artery showing marked medial thickening (arrow), which results in minimal reduction of vascular lumen. Note the presence of a monolayer of endothelial cells lining the vascular lumen (hematoxylin and eosin, bar = 50 μm). (b) Medium-sized pulmonary artery, the proximal segment is in the left-lower corner of the figure and progresses distally (right-upper corner) with marked intimal thickening, leading to the effacement of the vascular lumen (arrow) (hematoxylin and eosin, bar = 50 μm). (c) Close-up of small precapillary pulmonary artery (V) showing complete effacement of the vascular lumen due to proliferation of myofibroblastic-like cells (arrows) (hematoxylin and eosin, bar = 50 μm). (d) Plexiform lesion (P), which distally drains into an angiomatoid-like process highlighted by the arrow (hematoxylin and eosin, bar = 50 μm).*

(Continued opposite)

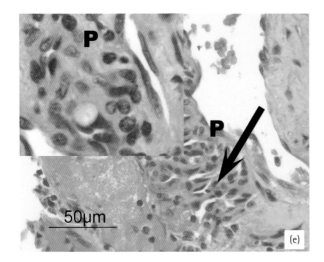

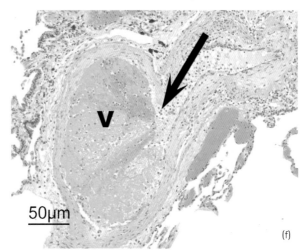

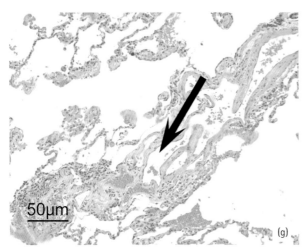

Plate 3.4 *(e) High magnification of plexiform lesion (P). The feeding vessel is shown on the right side of the picture. Note the proliferating endothelial cells, which form on a regular mass of cells (arrow). The cellular nature of the endothelial cell mass is better illustrated in the close-up (insert) where the endothelial cells are distributed in a haphazard distribution, with intracytoplasmic lumina and progressive formation of thin-walled blood vessels (hematoxylin and eosin, bar = 50 μm). (f) Pulmonary artery (V) showing complete obliteration of the feeding portion with a recent thrombus (arrow) (hematoxylin and eosin, bar = 50 μm). (g) Plexiform lesion followed by angiomatoid lesion (arrow). Note the clustering of muscularized small pulmonary arteries within the alveolar septum surrounding the lesion (hematoxylin and eosin, bar = 50 μm).*

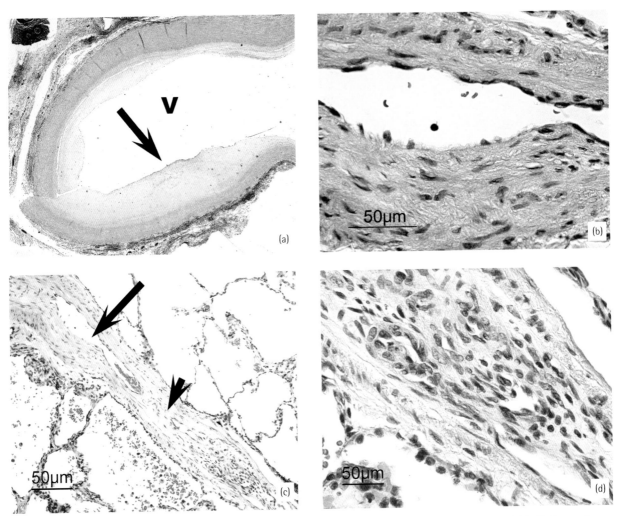

Plate 3.5 *(a) Elastic pulmonary artery (V) showing marked intima thickening due to myxoid connective tissue rich in lipid vacuoles. This lesion is morphologically similar to the atherosclerotic lesions present in the systemic circulation (bar = 50 μm).*
(b) Pulmonary artery showing a marked intima thickening due to infiltration by abundant myofibroblasts (bar = 50 μm).
(c) Pulmonary artery profile showing a uniform thickening of the intima (arrow), which shows partial obliteration of the vessel lumen (arrowhead). In the bottom right segment, there is evidence of proliferating endothelial cells (hematoxylin and eosin, bar = 50 μm).
(d) Close-up of proliferating endothelial cells shown in Figure 3.1c. Note the regular clustering of slightly hyperchromatic endothelial cells, in different variable stages of blood vessel formation (hematoxylin and eosin, bar = 50 μm).

(Continued opposite)

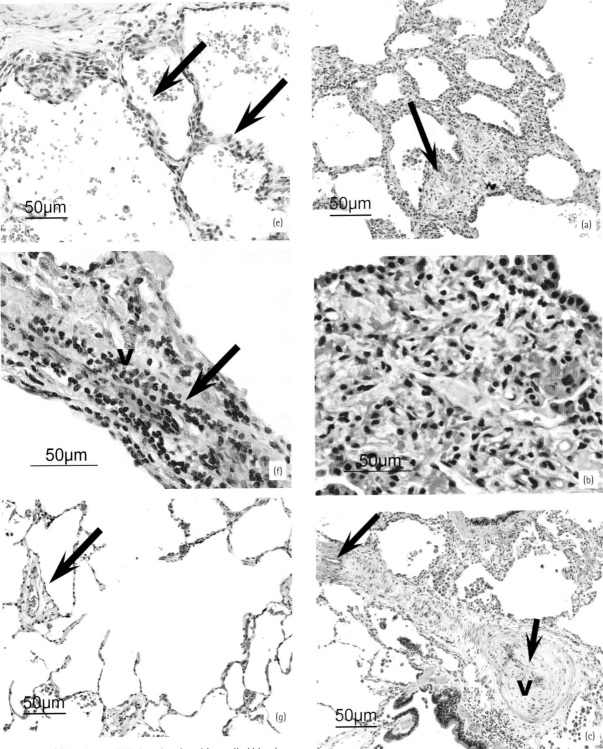

Plate 3.5 *(e) Angiomatoid lesion showing thin-walled blood vessels (arrow). In the upper-left corner, protruding into one of the vascular lakes, is a cluster of endothelial cells in a whorl-like arrangement (hematoxylin and eosin, bar = 50 μm). (f) Small-sized pulmonary artery (V) showing infiltration by lymphomononuclear cells (arrow). Note a marked reduction of the vascular lumen by connective tissue and inflammatory cells (hematoxylin and eosin, bar = 50 μm). (g) Alveolated parenchyma showing progressive muscularization and thickening of precapillary pulmonary arteries (arrow). Note that other alveoli septa do not show thickening by smooth muscle cells (lower-right corner) (hematoxylin and eosin, bar = 50 μm).*

Plate 3.6 *(a) Interstitial lung disease with homogeneous thickening of alveolar septa (arrowhead). The thickened small pulmonary arteries appear in clusters (hematoxylin and eosin, bar = 50 μm). (b) High magnification of interstitial inflammatory process showing marked increase in capillaries (hematoxylin and eosin, bar = 50 μm). (c) Muscular pulmonary artery showing marked intima thickening (arrowhead), which extends into the segment present in the alveolated lung parenchyma (arrowhead). The boxed areas are shown in close-up in (d) and (e) (hematoxylin and eosin, bar = 50 μm).*

(Continued over)

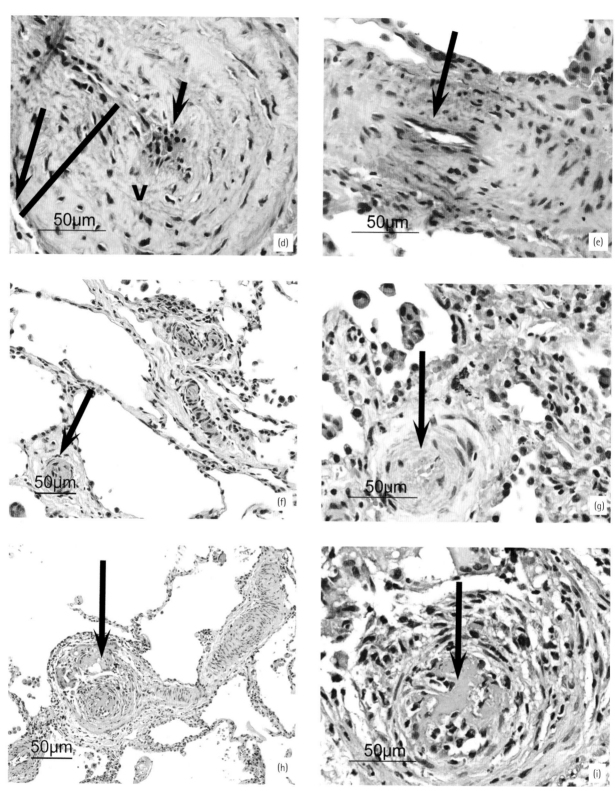

Plate 3.6 *(d) Marked intima thickening of small pulmonary artery shown in (c) (V). The intima thickening probably results from an almost concentric growth of myofibroblasts embedded in a collagenous, somewhat myxoid background. The outside boundary (i.e. smooth muscle cell media, arrow) is delineated by bracketed line (hematoxylin and eosin, bar = 50 μm). (e) Precapillary segment of pulmonary artery shown in (c). The internal thickening, shown in (d), extends to the prealveolar segment of pulmonary artery (hematoxylin and eosin, bar = 50 μm). (f) In areas relatively spared of interstitial involvement, precapillary pulmonary arteries show marked media and intima thickening. Note the increase in perivascular adventitia (arrow) (hematoxylin and eosin, bar = 50 μm). (g) In detail, the intima concentric thickening of a vessel similar to those shown in (f) is better appreciated. There is a concomitant component of interstitial lung disease (hematoxylin and eosin, bar = 50 μm). (h) Pulmonary artery thrombosis in medium-sized pulmonary artery (arrow). (i) Close-up of artery (V) with inflammation of intima (arrowheads) and superimposed thrombosis (arrow) (hematoxylin and eosin, bar = 50 μm).*

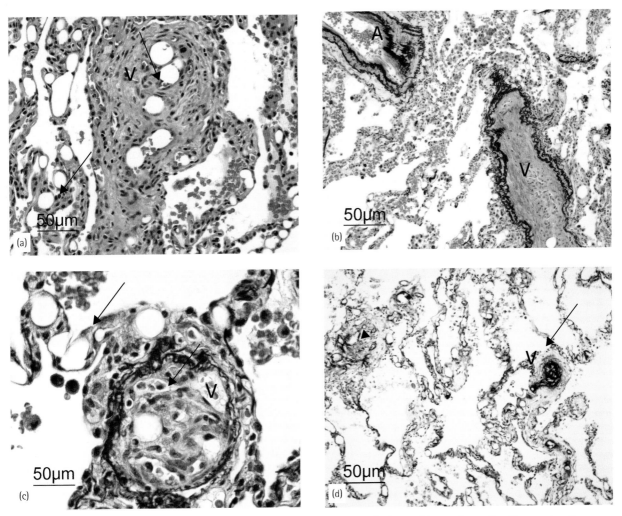

Plate 3.7 *(a) A large number of capillaries are seen infiltrating pulmonary vascular lumen (V, arrow) as well as the vessel wall. Note the extension into the adjacent alveolar septae (arrow) (hematoxylin and eosin, bar = 50 μm). (b) Pulmonary artery (A) and pulmonary vein (V) shown, with obliteration of the vein lumen by infiltrating capillaries (hematoxylin and eosin, bar = 50 μm). (c) High magnification of pulmonary vessel (V) showing extensive infiltration of the vascular lumen, the vascular wall and alveolar septa by capillaries (arrows) (hematoxylin and eosin, bar = 50 μm). (d) Factor VIII Ag immunostaining highlighting the proliferated endothelial cells, forming the invasive capillaries both in the vascular lumen (V, arrow) as well as within alveolar septae (arrowheads) (hematoxylin and eosin, bar = 50 μm).*

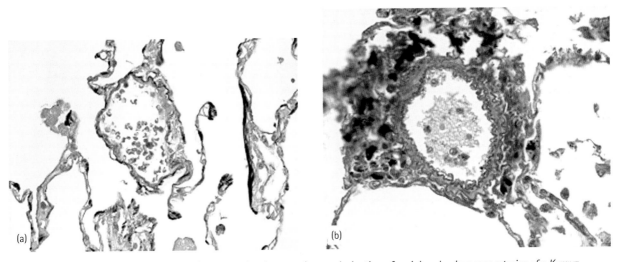

Plate 5.1 *Histological sections of lungs demonstrating increased muscularization of peripheral pulmonary arteries of a Kyrgyz highlander living at an altitude greater than 3000 m (b) compared with a normal artery (a).*

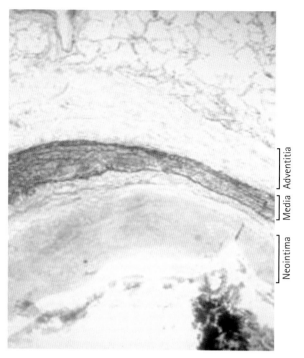

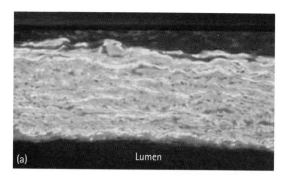

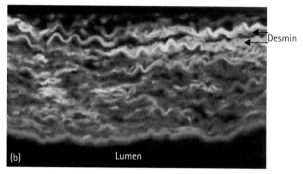

Plate 5.2 *Histological section of a segmental pulmonary artery from a patient with primary pulmonary hypertension stained to demonstrate elastin and showing thickening of the adventitia and media and formation of neointima.*

Plate 5.4 *Fluorescent immunohistochemical staining of a normal proximal human pulmonary artery showing a homogeneous pattern of staining for smooth muscle actin (a) but heterogeneity in desmin immunostaining (b), suggesting the existence of a phenotypically distinct smooth muscle cells within the vessel wall.*

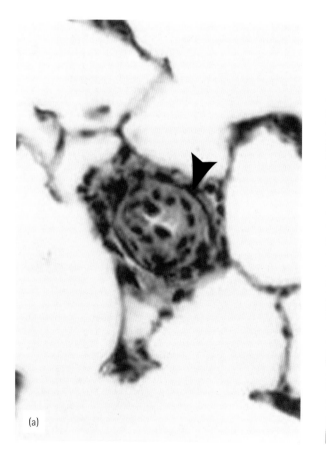

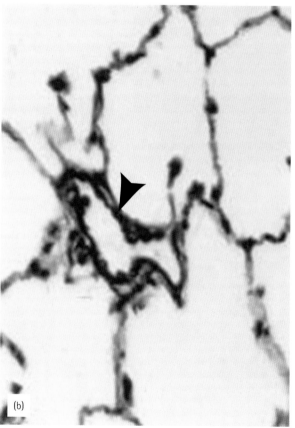

Plate 5.3 *Histological sections of lungs from rats treated with monocrotaline and pneumonectomy (a) and normal rats (b). Arrows indicate the position of the internal elastic laminae. The formation of the neointima is seen in (a).*

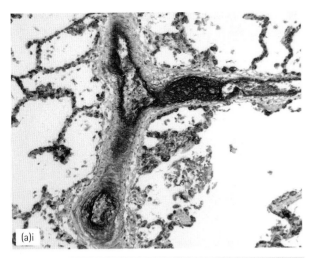

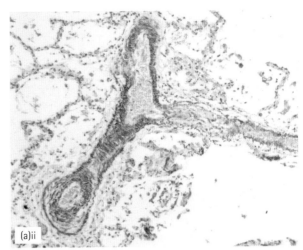

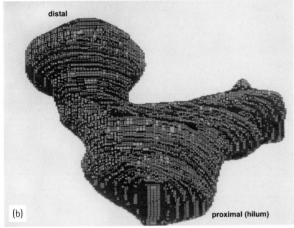

Plate 13A.1 *(a) Factor VIII-related antigen and smooth muscle specific antigen staining. (b) Three-dimensional reconstruction of a plexiform lesion at precapillary arteriolar branch point in primary pulmonary hypertension.*

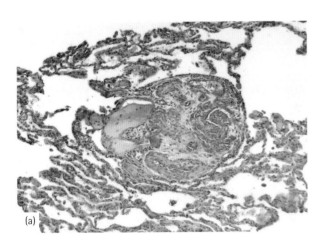

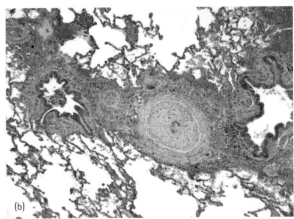

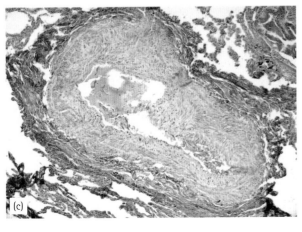

Plate 13A.2 *Lack or decrease of expression of the prostacyclin receptor protein in vascular smooth muscle cells in a plexiform lesion of a patient with primary pulmonary hypertension. (a) Complex vascular lesion, (b) concentric lesions, and (c) heavily muscularized artery. Brown staining indicates intact, normal expression.*

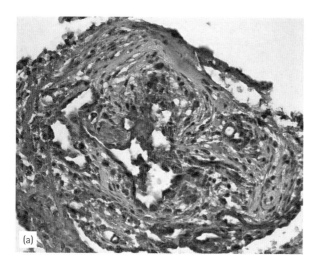

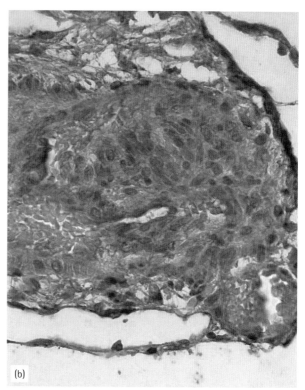

Plate 13A.3 *Immunohistochemical staining (brown) for nitrotyrosine of lung sections from patients with severe primary pulmonary hypertension. (a) Plexiform lesion demonstrating positive staining in many of the cells that comprise the abnormal vascular structure. (b) Plexiform lesion with intense positive nitrotyrosine expression in all of the cells.*

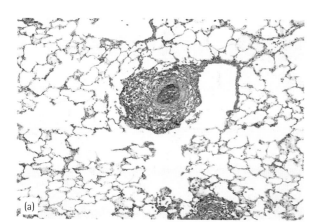

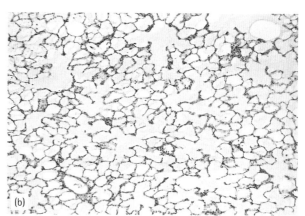

Plate 13A.4 *(a) Vascular lesions in lung from a rat treated with the vascular endothelial growth factor (VEGF) receptor blocker SU5416 and kept chronically hypoxic for 3 weeks, staining for the VEGF receptor II (KDR). (b) Treatment of a rat with simvastatin following the combined treatment with SU5416 plus chronic hypoxic for 3 weeks reduces the severity of pulmonary arteriolar lesions and renders patent the lumen of most of the vessels obliterated as a consequence of SU5416 + hypoxia treatment.*

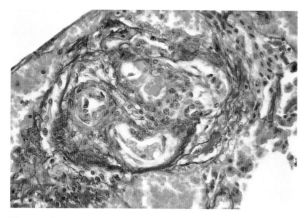

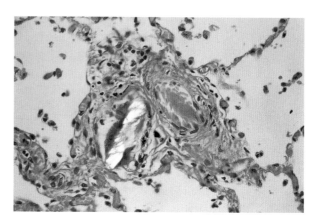

Plate 13G.1 *Plexiform lesions in a HIV-infected intravenous drug user with pulmonary arterial hypertension related to HIV infection (PAHRH).*

Plate 13G.2 *Occasional birefringent talc particles that usually were located adjacent to and not within the plexiform lesions.*

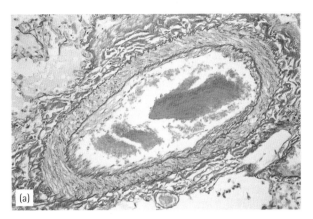

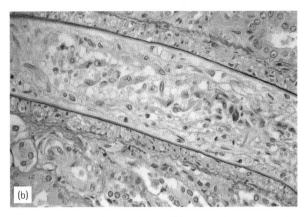

Plate 13G.3 *Autopsy findings of a patient with PAHRH showing microangiopathic changes in a renal artery (a) and a pulmonary vessel with concurrent intimal fibrosis and medial hypertrophy (b).*

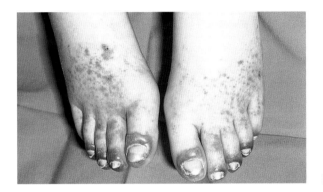

Plate 13G.4 *Purpura fulminans in a patient with PAHRH.*

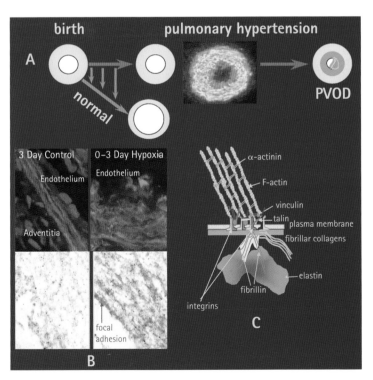

Plate 13H.1 *The upper figure (A) illustrates the rapid reduction in pulmonary arterial wall thickness occurring immediately after birth in the normal lung. This process is profoundly disturbed in neonatal pulmonary hypertension and an increase in medial thickness eventually leads to pulmonary vascular obstructive disease (PVOD) if the pressure remains high. Insert shows abnormal, hypertensive human peripheral pulmonary artery at 3 days, stained for γ-actin. Mechanisms are illustrated in (B) and (C). In (B), confocal and transmission electron microscopy shows, in the left-hand panel, the normal porcine peripheral pulmonary artery and in the right-hand panel, the pulmonary hypertensive vessel at 3 days. Normal remodeling entails reorganization of the smooth muscle cell actin cytoskeleton which undergoes transient disassembly as the cells thin and elongate to spread around an enlarging lumen. In pulmonary hypertension, larger cells are packed with red actin myofilaments (phalloidin stained) while immunoelectron-microscopy reveals sheets of actin bundles labeled with gold particles rather than actin being diffusely distributed in the cytosol. (C) All aspects of vessel wall remodeling are disturbed in pulmonary hypertension, from the excessive myofilament assembly within the cell, focal adhesion remodeling at the membrane and excessive connective tissue deposition in the matrix. Gene expression of tropoelastin and type I procollagen is abnormally high and steady-state protein levels are increased.[48,49] Vessels appear to become fixed in an incompletely dilated state. This is the beginning of PVOD in the young if the process cannot be arrested therapeutically.*

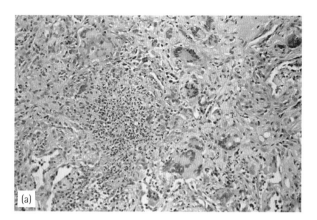 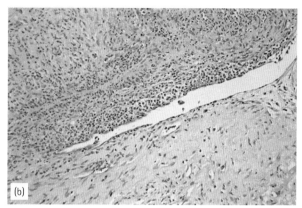

Plate 13I.1 *Pathology of Wegener's granulomatosis. (a) Granuloma with multiple giant cells in lung. (b) Small artery demonstrating thickened wall infiltrated with leukocytes and perivascular inflammation. (Photomicrographs provided courtesy of the Mayo Foundation.)*

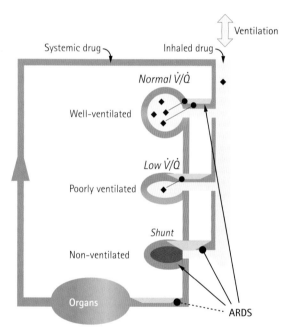

Plate 13M.1 *Scheme of the pulmonary ventilation and perfusion distribution. Green blocks: precapillary vascular resistance. In normals, most of the lung represents well-ventilated areas with high alveolar partial pressure of oxygen (PO_2) and hardly any vasoconstriction of the pulmonary arteries. In acute respiratory distress syndrome (ARDS) there are many low ventilation/perfusion ($\dot{V}/\dot{Q}$) and shunt areas with alveolar hypoxia resulting in hypoxic pulmonary vasoconstriction (HPV), contributing to pulmonary hypertension. Systemic vasodilators will block HPV and worsen the $\dot{V}/\dot{Q}$ mismatch, while inhaled vasodilators will preferentially vasodilate the well-ventilated areas.*

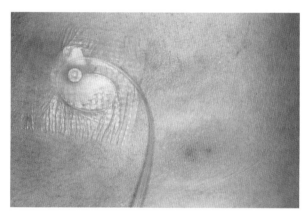

Plate 13N.1 *Site reaction.*

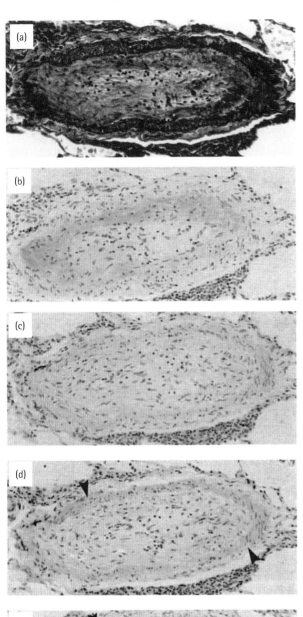

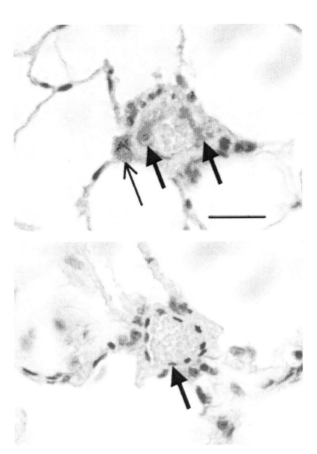

Plate 13Q.2 *Representative examples of active caspase-3 immunostaining of lung sections harvested 2 weeks after monocrotaline (MCT) alone or together with cell-based gene transfer of vascular endothelial growth factor (VEGF). In animals treated with MCT alone (top), immunostaining was seen largely localized to endothelial cells of small arterioles (thick arrows), with occasional positivity of surrounding pericytes (thin arrow), whereas in sections from animals treated with MCT and VEGF gene transfer (bottom), endothelial staining for active caspase-3 was infrequent. (Reproduced with permission from Campbell AI, Zhao Y, Sandhu R et al. Cell-based gene transfer of vascular endothelial growth factor attenuates monocrotaline-induced pulmonary hypertension.* Circulation *2001;104:2242–8.)*

Plate 13Q.1 *Procollagen and transforming growth factor (TGF)-β immunohistochemistry do not co-localize in occluded hypertensive pulmonary artery. Immunohistochemistry was performed on lung parenchyma from a second patient undergoing single-lung transplantation for primary pulmonary hypertension. Procollagen immunoreactivity (b) is present only within the neointima of this occluded artery. TGF-β3 (e) and TGF-β2 (d) immunoreactivity is most intense in the medial layer (arrowhead), although faint staining for TGF-β3 is observed within the neointima. TGF-β1 (c) is not detected. An elastin–van Gieson stain demonstrates vascular structures (a). (Reproduced with permission from Botney MD, Bahadori L, Gold LI. Vascular remodelling in primary pulmonary hypertension. Potential role for transforming growth factor-beta.* Am J Pathol *1994;144:286–95.)*

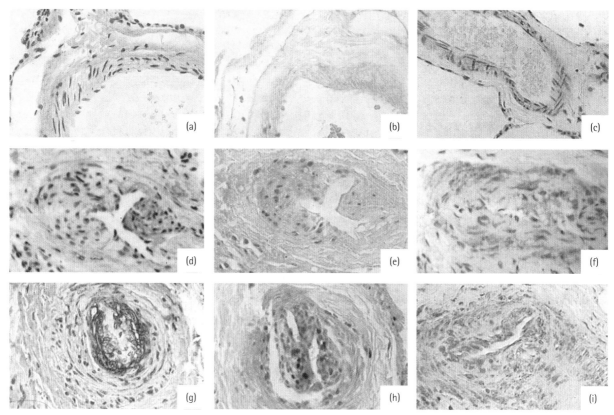

Plate 13Q.3 *Representative photomicrographs showing immunoperoxidase staining for tenascin-C (TN) (a, d and g), proliferating cell nuclear antigen (PCNA) (b, e and h) and epidermal growth factor (EGF) (c, f and i) in graded lung biopsy tissue sections. (a–c) Vessel showing a typical grade I^A lesion. (d–f) Vessel showing a typical grade I^C lesion. (g–i) Vessel showing a typical grade III^C lesion. In low-grade lesions (a), modest TN immunostaining was evident in the adventitia. With medial hypertrophy, TN immunoreactivity became more prominent in the periendothelium (d), with the most intense immunostaining being apparent within the neointima of high-grade lesions showing occlusive neointimal formation (g). In the lowest grade of lesion, PCNA was negative (b), despite foci of EGF in the media. With medial hypertrophy, PCNA was expressed in the media (e), together with foci of EGF (f). With the development of higher-grade occlusive lesions, TN (g), PCNA (h) and EGF (i) co-localized to the neointimal cell layers. Note that TN and PCNA staining was performed on serial sections, whereas EGF detection was carried out on similar vessels within the same biopsy. Original magnification × 40. (Reproduced with permission from Jones PL, Cowan KN, Rabinovitch M. Progressive pulmonary vascular disease is characterized by a proliferative response related to deposition of tenascin-C and is preceded by subendothelial accumulation of fibronectin. Am J Pathol 1997;150:1349–60.)*

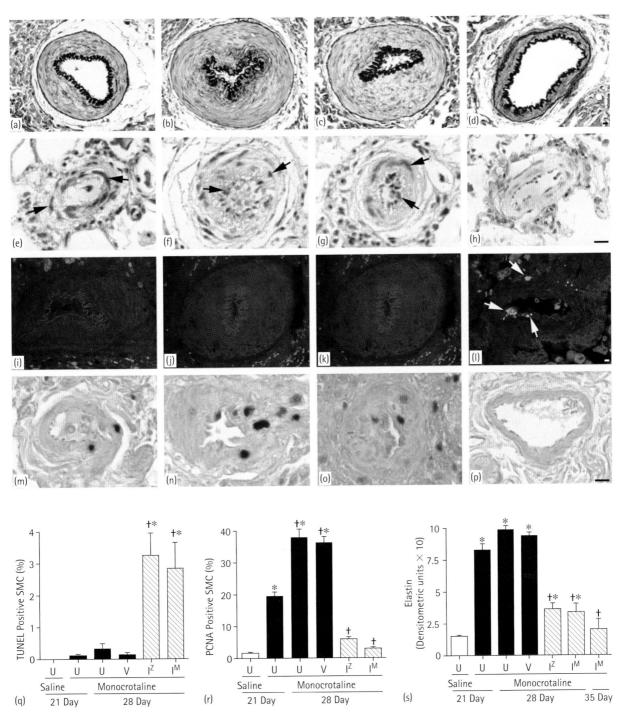

Plate 13Q.4 *Cellular mechanism responsible for reversal of pulmonary artery muscularity. Elastase inhibition arrests tenascin-C accumulation and proliferation and induces apoptosis and loss of extracellular matrix (such as elastin). For (a–p) (days refer to time after injection of monocrotaline): first row, day 21; second row, day 28; third row, day 28; last row, day 28. (a–d) Saline-perfused pulmonary arteries stained with Movat pentachrome stain. (e, h) Pulmonary arteries after tenascin-C immunohistochemistry. Arrows, positive brown peroxidase staining. (i, j) In situ terminal deoxynucleotidyl transferase (TdT) mediated dUTP nick end labeling (TUNEL) assays identifying apoptosis. White arrows, TUNEL-positive vascular cells. (m–p) Proliferating vascular cells, shown by immunohistochemistry or proliferating cell nuclear antigen (PCNA); dark nuclei are PCNA-positive cells. (q, r) Percentage of smooth muscle cells (SMC) that are TUNEL-positive (q) or PCNA-positive (r). (s) Densitometric quantification of elsatin. U, untreated; V, vehicle-treated; I, inhibitor-treated (I^Z, ZD08921; I^M, M249314). Graphed data represent mean + SEM of n = 4. Scale bars represent 5 μm. *P < 0.05, compared with †P < 0.05, compared with results on day 21 in rates treated with monocrotaline. (Reproduced with permission from Cowan KN, Heilbot A, Lam C. Reversal of severe pulmonary hypertension by a serine elastase inhibitor. Nat Med 2000;6:698–702.)*

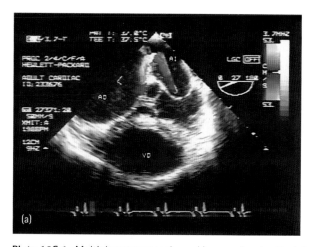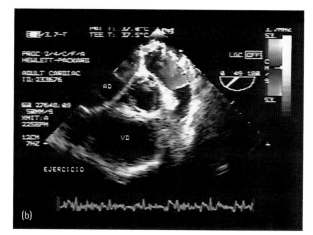

Plate 13S.1 *Multiplane transesophageal images showing the inter-atrial shunt by color-flow at rest (a), and during exercise (b). AD, right atrium; AI, left atrium; VD, right ventricle; EJERCICIO, exercise (supine).*

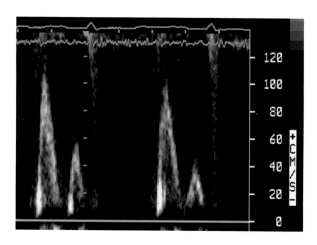

Plate 14A.1 *Transmitral Doppler flow velocities from a patient with severe left ventricular disease and restrictive filling showing fast acceleration and deceleration of early diastolic component.*

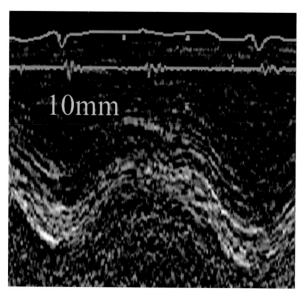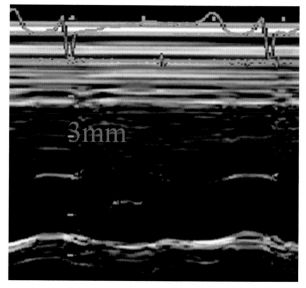

Plate 14A.2 *Right ventricular free wall long axis excursion from a patient with pulmonary hypertension (left) and after developing severe ventricular disease (right). Note the marked drop in the extent of free wall movement.*

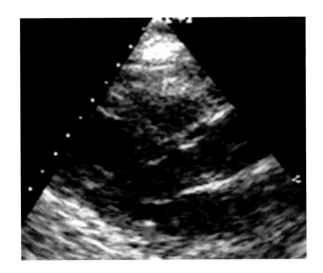

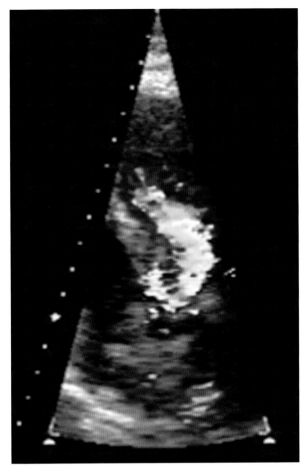

Plate 14A.3 *Parasternal long axis view from an elderly patient with exertional breathlessness demonstrating basal septal hypertrophy (above) and raised velocities shown by the aliasing colour Doppler (right).*

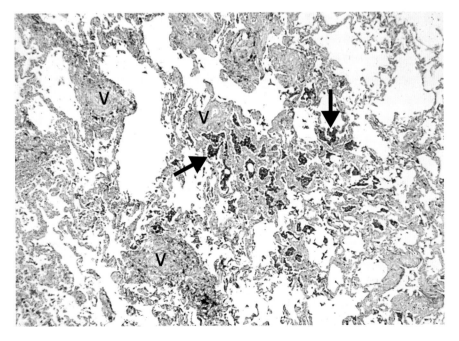

Plate 14B.1 *Low-power photomicrograph showing multiple small veins (V) with sclerosis, interstitial fibrosis (center right) and hemosiderin (arrows).*

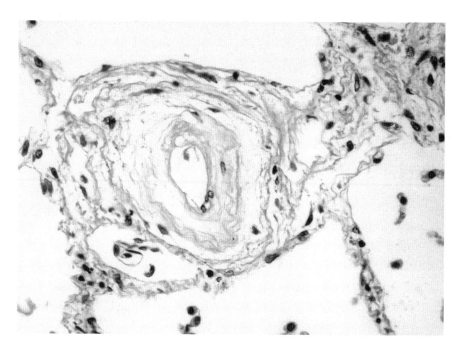

Plate 14B.2 *High-power photomicrograph showing a small vein with both intimal and medial thickening resulting in marked luminal narrowing.*

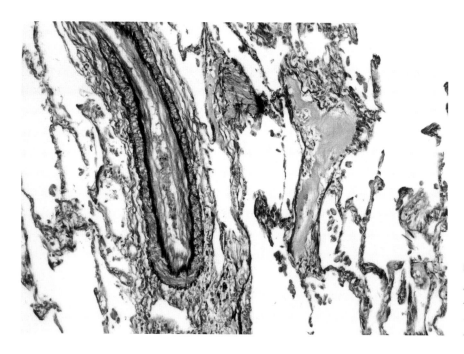

Plate 14B.3 *Medium-power photomicrograph elastin tissue stain showing a sclerotic vein (right) and an arteriole with intimal hypertensive changes (left).*

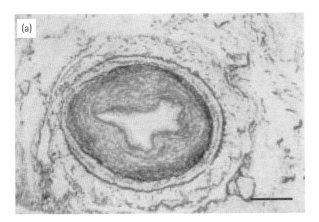

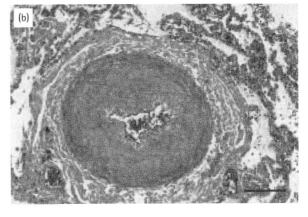

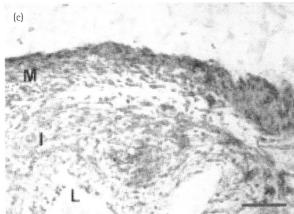

Plate 15C.1 *Serial sections of a muscular pulmonary artery from a patients with chronic obstructive pulmonary disease (COPD) showing prominent internal thickening and luminal narrowing. (a) Orcein stain showing abundant elastin and (b) Masson's trichrome stain showing collagen within the intima (c) section of artery wall showing intimal thickening and luminal narrowing. The section is stained for α-smooth muscle actin which is prominent in both the intimal and medial layers. A, adventitia; M, medial layer; I, intimal layer; L, lumen. (Reproduced with permission from Sontas S, Peinado VI, Ramirez J et al. Characterization of pulmonary vascular remodeling in smokers and patients with mild COPD.* Eur Respir J *2002;19:632–8.)*

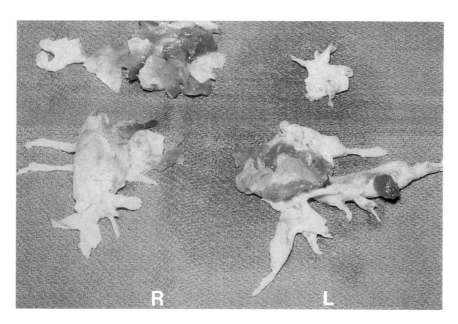

Plate 17.1 *Chronic thromboembolic material removed at the time of thrombo-endarterectomy from the patient featured in Figures 17.1 and 17.3.*

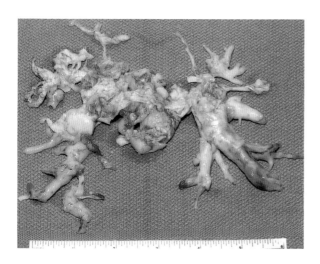

Plate 18.1 *Gross photograph of a large sarcoma resected via endarterectomy from the right and left pulmonary arteries of a 77-year-old female.*

effecting the response to chronic hypoxia. Morphometric data have shown proliferative and obliterative changes in these small pulmonary arteries. The lesions are influenced by cytokines and growth factors. In the precapillary vessel wall a variety of cellular phenotypic changes develop at the same time. An extension of muscle into peripheral arteries has been described as an early event during hypoxic remodeling.[116] This extension is followed by an increase in medial thickness of the muscular arteries, caused by hypertrophy and hyperplasia of pre-existing smooth muscle cells and by an increase in the extracellular matrix, including connective tissue proteins, which leads to both stiffening and vasoconstriction of the vessels.[117]

Because K^+ channels are important determinants of vascular tone control and the proliferative status of vascular smooth muscle cells, the role of K^+ channels and membrane potential have been investigated in several animal models of chronic pulmonary hypertension. Shortly after the first reports about the effect of acute hypoxia on K^+ channels, Smirnov et al. demonstrated that PA smooth muscle cells of rats raised for 4 weeks in an hypoxic environment have reduced Kv current compared with normoxic rats.[107] The resting potential of PA smooth muscle cells from chronically hypoxic animals was significantly more positive.[107] It was proposed that the observed reduction in K^+-current amplitudes was as a result of decreased channel expression. The first evidence for a down-regulation of Kv-channel α-subunits (Kv1.2 and Kv1.5) in cultured rat PA smooth muscle cells under chronic hypoxia was provided by Wang et al.[53] More recently, it was reported that chronic hypoxia also decreases the mRNA expression of Kv1.1, Kv1.5, Kv2.1, Kv4.3 and Kv9.3 α-subunits in cultured rat PA smooth muscle cells.[118,119] Similar results have been observed in freshly isolated PA smooth muscle cells from chronically hypoxic animals.[120–123] In contrast, chronic hypoxia fails to inhibit the expression of Kv-channel α- or β-subunits examined in mesenteric arterial smooth muscle cells.[118,119] As discussed above, a reduction of the Kv-channel activity and the consequent membrane depolarization appears to be involved in the development of chronic hypoxia-mediated pulmonary hypertension by mediating pulmonary vasoconstriction and vascular remodeling through increased $[Ca^{2+}]_i$ in PA smooth muscle cells.

If the decreased acute HPV found in chronic hypoxia[124] is due to loss of hypoxia-sensitive Kv channels, what is the mechanism of that loss? Chronic hypoxia has been reported to increase the reduced glutathione levels before the Kv1.5- and Kv2.1-channel protein is decreased.[123] These data suggest that the cytosol is reduced before changes in K^+-channel expression occurs in hypoxia. In addition, it has been recently reported that overexpression of c-jun gene significantly decreases whole-cell Kv current, down-regulates the mRNA expression of the Kv1.5-channel α-subunit and accelerates Kv-current inactivation in cultured PA smooth muscle cells.[125] A significant membrane depolarization and stimulated smooth muscle cell proliferation in these cells has also been demonstrated caused by overexpression of the gene and Kv-channel inhibition.[125] There is a large body of data indicating that the c-jun family of genes is inducible by hypoxia.[126–128] Yu et al. interpreted their results to suggest that c-jun may indirectly down-regulate transcription of the Kv1.5 gene and decrease Kv current.[125] The resultant membrane depolarization could increase $[Ca^{2+}]_i$ and induce cell growth.

There is accumulating evidence that chronic hypoxic exposure is associated with protein phosphorylation and/or redox modulation of transcription factors, including hypoxia-inducible factor-1 (HIF-1). HIF-1 is a heterodimeric basic helix–loop–helix–Per/ARNT/Sim (PAS)-domain transcription factor composed of HIF-1α and HIF-1β subunits.[129,130] HIF-1β is expressed constitutively in many cells, but HIF-1α, almost absent in normoxia, is induced by hypoxia. The expression of HIF-1α in the lung, regulated by the inspired O_2 concentration, has been demonstrated recently.[131] The role of HIF-1α in hypoxia-induced pulmonary vascular remodeling has been reported by Yu et al.[132] They found that in comparison with wild-type mice, the muscularization of pulmonary arterioles was significantly decreased in heterozygous HIF-1α± mice exposed to hypoxia for 3 weeks. HIF-1 has been implicated in the regulation of an ever-growing number of genes, the products of which include vascular endothelial growth factor (VEGF), endothelin-1 (ET-1), and nitric oxide synthase-2. VEGF is expressed in nearly all cells and tissues and is important in the regulation of new blood vessel formation. The expression of VEGF has been shown to be markedly increased by hypoxia.[133] The role of ET-1 in the development of chronic hypoxic pulmonary hypertension has been shown in several animal models.[134] ET-1 is increased in plasma and in lungs of rats following exposure to hypoxia,[113,135], in fawn-hooded rats that develop severe pulmonary hypertension when raised under mild hypoxia,[136] and in monocrotaline-treated rats.[137] Aguirre et al. demonstrated recently the importance of ET-1 in the vascular remodeling associated with chronic hypoxia through its mitogenic effect on vascular smooth muscle cells.[138] It has been supposed that hypoxia also increases the transcription rate of 5-hydroxytriptamine (5-HT) transporter gene through HIF-1.[139] The serotonin (5-HT) transporter in pulmonary vascular smooth muscle cells isolated from rat and bovine pulmonary arteries has many attributes, suggesting that it may be a key determinant of pulmonary vessel remodeling.[140,141] Moreover, in mice lacking the 5-HT transporter gene, where platelets are depleted of serotonin and exposed to chronic hypoxia, the number and the wall thickness of muscularized pulmonary arteries were already decreased after 2 weeks of

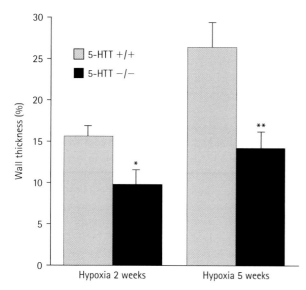

Figure 4.3 *The normalized wall thickness of muscular arteries is less in mice lacking the 5-hydroxytryptamine transporter (5-HTT) gene after exposure to chronic hypoxia. Normalized wall thickness measured in fully muscular arteries in lungs from control (5-HTT+/+) and mice lacking the 5-HTT gene (5-HTT−/−) exposed to chronic hypoxia over 2 weeks (n = 9 mice of each genotype) or 5 weeks (n = 8 mice of each genotype). *P< 0.05, **P< 0.01 compared with values in 5-HTT+/+ mice exposed to hypoxia after the same durations. (Reproduced with permission from Eddahibi et al.)[142]*

hypoxia compared with wild-type controls[142] (Figure 4.3). In addition, pulmonary artery pressure was lower and the right ventricle hypertrophy less marked in the mutant mice, providing further evidence that 5-HT plays a major role in hypoxia-induced pulmonary vascular remodeling.[139,142]

SUMMARY

A variety of cells in the body have been demonstrated to have great sensitivity to acute changes in oxygen tension. These include the type I cell of the carotid body, NEB cells and the associated small cell lung carcinoma cell line, phaeochromocytoma (PC12) cells and vascular smooth muscle cells, especially those of the ductus arteriosus and small pulmonary arteries.

It is striking that all of these cells have been found to have changes in K^+-channel gating, membrane potential and cytosolic $[Ca^{2+}]$ in response to alteration in oxygen tension. It is also remarkable that chronic changes in oxygen levels alter K^+-channel expression. There is evidence that both the acute and chronic effects of oxygen on K^+ channel are achieved by changes in intracellular redox status. This change in redox status may well also control calcium release from the sarcoplasmic reticulum.

KEY POINTS

- Hypoxic pulmonary vasoconstriction (HPV) involves both influx of calcium and intracellular release of calcium in pulmonary artery smooth muscle cells.
- Hypoxia inhibits one or more sarcolemmal K^+ channels leading to membrane depolarization and calcium entry through voltage-gated Ca^{2+} channels.
- Hypoxia likely inhibits K^+ channels and releases Ca^{2+} from the sarcoplasmic reticulum by changing production of reactive oxygen species and/or levels of redox couples such as GSH/GSSG and NADPH/NADP.
- Chronic hypoxia leads to inactivation, or lack of expression, of specific K^+ channels, probably through modulation of HIF-1α.
- Serotonin and endothelin-1 play a part in remodeling of the pulmonary vasculature caused by chronic hypoxia.

ACKNOWLEDGMENTS

The authors are grateful for the many contributions of Dr SL Archer to the development of the 'redox' hypothesis.

Andrea Olschewski is supported by the Deutsche Forschungsgemeinschaft (DFG: Ol 127/1-1 and SFB 547). E Kenneth Weir is supported by VA Merit Review Funding and NIH (RO1-HL 65322-01A1).

REFERENCES

● 1 Bradford JR, Dean HP. The pulmonary circulation. *J Physiol* 1894;16:34–96.
● 2 Euler v US, Liljestrand G. Observations on the pulmonary arterial blood pressure in the cat. *Acta Physiol Scand* 1946;**12**:301–20.
3 Shirai M, Sada K, Ninomiya I. Effects of regional alveolar hypoxia and hypercapnia on small pulmonary vessels in cats. *J Appl Physiol* 1986;**61**:440–8.
4 Marshall C, Marshall BE. Influence of perfusate pO₂ on hypoxic pulmonary vasoconstriction in rats. *Circ Res* 1983;**52**:691–6.
5 Weissmann N, Grimminger F, Walmrath D *et al.* Hypoxic vasoconstriction in buffer-perfused rabbit lungs. *Respir Physiol* 1995;**100**:159–69.
6 Jensen KS, Micco AJ, Czartolomna J *et al.* Rapid onset of hypoxic vasoconstriction in isolated lungs. *J Appl Physiol* 1992;**72**:2018–23.
7 Welling KL, Sanchez R, Ravn JB *et al.* Effect of prolonged alveolar hypoxia on pulmonary arterial pressure and segmental vascular resistance. *J Appl Physiol* 1993;**75**:1194–200.

8 Vejlstrup NG, Dorrington KL. Intense slow hypoxic pulmonary vasoconstriction in gas-filled and liquid-filled lungs: an *in vivo* study in the rabbit. *Acta Physiol Scand* 1993;**148**:305–13.

9 Wiener CM, Sylvester JT. Effects of glucose on hypoxic vasoconstriction in isolated ferret lungs. *J Appl Physiol* 1991;**70**:439–46.

10 Nakanishi K, Tajima F, Osada H *et al.* Pulmonary, vascular responses in rats exposed to chronic hypobaric hypoxia at two different altitude levels. *Pathol Res Pract* 1996;**192**:1057–67.

11 Fineman JR, Wong J, Soifer SJ. Hyperoxia and alkalosis produce pulmonary vasodilation independent of endothelium-derived nitric oxide in newborn lambs. *Pediatr Res* 1993;**33**:341–6.

12 Yamaguchi K, Takasugi T, Fujita H *et al.* Endothelial modulation of pH-dependent pressor response in isolated perfused rabbit lungs. *Am J Physiol* 1996;**270**:H252–8.

13 Schreiber MD, Heymann MA, Soifer SJ. Increased arterial pH, not decreased $PaCO_2$, attenuates hypoxia-induced pulmonary vasoconstriction in newborn lambs. *Pediatr Res* 1986;**20**:113–17.

14 Raffestin B, McMurtry IF. Effects of intracellular pH on hypoxic vasoconstriction in rat lungs. *J Appl Physiol* 1987;**63**:2524–31.

15 Carlin RE, Ferrario L, Boyd JT *et al.* Determinants of nitric oxide in exhaled gas in the isolated rabbit lung. *Am J Respir Crit Care Med* 1997;**155**:922–7.

16 Stromberg S, Lonnqvist PA, Persson MG *et al.* Lung distension and carbon dioxide affect pulmonary nitric oxide formation in the anaesthetized rabbit. *Acta Physiol Scand* 1997;**159**:59–67.

17 Morin FC, III. Hyperventilation, alkalosis, prostaglandins, and pulmonary circulation of the newborn. *J Appl Physiol* 1986;**61**:2088–94.

18 Ishii Y, Kitamura S. Hyperventilation stimulates the release of prostaglandin I2 and E2 from lung in humans. *Prostaglandins* 1990;**39**:685–91.

19 Skinner SJ, Somervell CE, Olson DM. The effects of mechanical stretching on fetal rat lung cell prostacyclin production. *Prostaglandins* 1992;**43**:413–33.

20 von Bethmann AN, Brasch F, Nusing R *et al.* Hyperventilation induces release of cytokines from perfused mouse lung. *Am J Respir Crit Care Med* 1998;**157**:263–72.

21 Barnes PJ, Liu SF. Regulation of pulmonary vascular tone. *Pharmacol Rev* 1995;**47**:87–131.

♦22 Weir EK, Archer SL. The mechanism of acute hypoxic pulmonary vasoconstriction: the tale of two channels. *FASEB J* 1995;**9**:183–9.

●23 Kato M, Staub NC. Response of small pulmonary arteries to unilobar hypoxia and hypercapnia. *Circ Res* 1966;**19**:426–40.

●24 Harder DR, Madden JA, Dawson C. Hypoxic induction of Ca^{2+}-dependent action potentials in small pulmonary arteries of the cat. *J Appl Physiol* 1985;**59**:1389–93.

●25 Madden JA, Dawson CA, Harder DR. Hypoxia-induced activation in small isolated pulmonary arteries from the cat. *J Appl Physiol* 1985;**59**:113–18.

26 Yuan XJ, Tod ML, Rubin LJ *et al.* Contrasting effects of hypoxia on tension in rat pulmonary and mesenteric arteries. *Am J Physiol* 1990;**259**:H281–9.

27 Jin N, Packer CS, Rhoades RA. Pulmonary arterial hypoxic contraction: signal transduction. *Am J Physiol* 1992;**263**:L73–8.

28 Madden JA, Vadula MS, Kurup VP. Effects of hypoxia and other vasoactive agents on pulmonary and cerebral artery smooth muscle cells. *Am J Physiol* 1992;**263**:L384–93.

●29 McMurtry IF, Davidson AB, Reeves JT *et al.* Inhibition of hypoxic pulmonary vasoconstriction by calcium antagonists in isolated rat lungs. *Circ Res* 1976;**38**:99–104.

●30 McMurtry IF. BAY K 8644 potentiates and A23187 inhibits hypoxic vasoconstriction in rat lungs. *Am J Physiol* 1985;**249**:H741–6.

31 Tolins M, Weir EK, Chesler E *et al.* Pulmonary vascular tone is increased by a voltage-dependent calcium channel potentiator. *J Appl Physiol* 1986;**60**:942–8.

●32 Salvaterra CG, Goldman WF. Acute hypoxia increases cytosolic calcium in cultured pulmonary arterial myocytes. *Am J Physiol* 1993;**264**:L323–8.

33 Urena J, Franco-Obregon A, Lopez-Barneo J. Contrasting effects of hypoxia on cytosolic Ca^{2+} spikes in conduit and resistance myocytes of the rabbit pulmonary artery. *J Physiol* 1996;**496**:103–9.

34 Robertson TP, Hague D, Aaronson PI *et al.* Voltage-independent calcium entry in hypoxic pulmonary vasoconstriction of intrapulmonary arteries of the rat. *J Physiol* 2000;**525**:669–80.

●35 Post JM, Hume JR, Archer SL *et al.* Direct role for potassium channel inhibition in hypoxic pulmonary vasoconstriction. *Am J Physiol* 1992;**262**:C882–90.

36 Yuan XJ, Goldman WF, Tod ML *et al.* Hypoxia reduces potassium currents in cultured rat pulmonary but not mesenteric arterial myocytes. *Am J Physiol* 1993;**264**:L116–23.

37 Gelband CH, Gelband H. Ca^{2+} release from intracellular stores is an initial step in hypoxic pulmonary vasoconstriction of rat pulmonary artery resistance vessels. *Circulation* 1997;**96**:3647–54.

38 Dipp M, Nye PC, Evans AM. Hypoxic release of calcium from the sarcoplasmic reticulum of pulmonary artery smooth muscle. *Am J Physiol* 2001;**281**:L318–25.

39 Yuan XJ. Voltage-gated K^+ currents regulate resting membrane potential and $[Ca^{2+}]_i$ in pulmonary arterial myocytes. *Circ Res* 1995;**77**:370–8.

40 Archer SL, Huang JM, Reeve HL *et al.* Differential distribution of electrophysiologically distinct myocytes in conduit and resistance arteries determines their response to nitric oxide and hypoxia. *Circ Res* 1996;**78**:431–42.

41 Osipenko ON, Evans AM, Gurney AM. Regulation of the resting potential of rabbit pulmonary artery myocytes by a low threshold, O_2-sensing potassium current. *Br J Pharmacol* 1997;**120**:1461–70.

●42 Franco-Obregon A, Lopez-Barneo J. Differential oxygen sensitivity of calcium channels in rabbit smooth muscle cells of conduit and resistance pulmonary arteries. *J Physiol* 1996;**491**:511–18.

43 Bakhramov A, Evans AM, Kozlowski RZ. Differential effects of hypoxia on the intracellular Ca^{2+} concentration of myocytes isolated from different regions of the rat pulmonary arterial tree. *Exp Physiol* 1998;**83**:337–47.

44 Vadula MS, Kleinman JG, Madden JA. Effect of hypoxia and norepinephrine on cytoplasmic free Ca^{2+} in pulmonary and cerebral arterial myocytes. *Am J Physiol* 1993;**265**:L591–7.

45 Post JM, Gelband CH, Hume JR. $[Ca^{2+}]_i$ inhibition of K^+ channels in canine pulmonary artery. Novel mechanism for hypoxia-induced membrane depolarization. *Circ Res* 1995;**77**:131–9.

46 Evans AM, Osipenko ON, Gurney AM. Properties of a novel K^+ current that is active at resting potential in rabbit pulmonary artery smooth muscle cells. *J Physiol* 1996;**496**:407–20.

47 Albarwani S, Robertson BE, Nye PC et al. Biophysical properties of Ca^{2+}- and Mg-ATP-activated K^+ channels in pulmonary arterial smooth muscle cells isolated from the rat. *Pflügers Arch* 1994;**428**:446–54.

48 Peng W, Hoidal JR, Farrukh IS. Role of a novel KCa opener in regulating K^+ channels of hypoxic human pulmonary vascular cells. *Am J Respir Cell Mol Biol* 1999;**20**:737–45.

♦49 Nelson MT, Quayle JM. Physiological roles and properties of potassium channels in arterial smooth muscle. *Am J Physiol* 1995;**268**:C799–822.

●50 Archer SL, Souil E, Dinh-Xuan AT et al. Molecular identification of the role of voltage-gated K^+ channels, Kv1.5 and Kv2.1, in hypoxic pulmonary vasoconstriction and control of resting membrane potential in rat pulmonary artery myocytes. *J Clin Invest* 1998;**101**:2319–30.

51 Hille B. Potassium channels and chloride channels. In: Hille B (ed.), *Ion channels of excitable membranes*. Sunderland: Sinauer Associates Inc., 2001;131–67.

♦52 Pongs O. Molecular biology of voltage-dependent potassium channels. *Physiol Rev* 1992;**72**:S69–88.

●53 Wang J, Juhaszova M, Rubin LJ et al. Hypoxia inhibits gene expression of voltage-gated K^+ channel alpha subunits in pulmonary artery smooth muscle cells. *J Clin Invest* 1997;**100**:2347–53.

●54 Hulme JT, Coppock EA, Felipe A et al. Oxygen sensitivity of cloned voltage-gated $K^{(+)}$ channels expressed in the pulmonary vasculature. *Circ Res* 1999;**85**:489–97.

55 Patel AJ, Lazdunski M, Honore E. Kv2.1/Kv9.3, a novel ATP-dependent delayed-rectifier K^+ channel in oxygen-sensitive pulmonary artery myocytes. *EMBO J* 1997;**16**:6615–25.

●56 Osipenko ON, Tate RJ, Gurney AM. Potential role for kv3.1b channels as oxygen sensors. *Circ Res* 2000;**86**:534–40.

57 Conforti L, Bodi I, Nisbet JW et al. O_2-sensitive K^+ channels: role of the Kv1.2 -subunit in mediating the hypoxic response. *J Physiol* 2000;**524**:783–93.

●58 Archer SL, London B, Hampl V et al. Impairment of hypoxic pulmonary vasoconstriction in mice lacking the voltage-gated potassium channel Kv1.5. *FASEB J* 2001;**15**:1801–3.

59 Perez-Garcia MT, Lopez-Lopez JR, Gonzalez C. Kvbeta1.2 subunit coexpression in HEK293 cells confers O_2 sensitivity to kv4.2 but not to Shaker channels. *J Gen Physiol* 1999;**113**:897–907.

●60 Ganfornina MD, Lopez-Barneo J. Single K^+ channels in membrane patches of arterial chemoreceptor cells are modulated by O_2 tension. *Proc Natl Acad Sci USA* 1991;**88**:2927–30.

●61 Jiang C, Haddad GG. A direct mechanism for sensing low oxygen levels by central neurons. *Proc Natl Acad Sci USA* 1994;**91**:7198–201.

62 Lahiri S, Acker H. Redox-dependent binding of CO to heme protein controls $P(O_2)$-sensitive chemoreceptor discharge of the rat carotid body. *Respir Physiol* 1999;**115**:169–77.

63 Srinivas V, Zhu X, Salceda S et al. Hypoxia-inducible factor 1alpha (HIF-1alpha) is a non-heme iron protein. Implications for oxygen sensing. *J Biol Chem* 1998;**273**:18019–22.

64 Gabig TG, Bearman SI, Babior BM. Effects of oxygen tension and pH on the respiratory burst of human neutrophils. *Blood* 1979;**53**:1133–9.

●65 Freeman BA, Crapo JD. Hyperoxia increases oxygen radical production in rat lungs and lung mitochondria. *J Biol Chem* 1981;**256**:10986–92.

66 Archer SL, Nelson DP, Weir EK. Detection of activated O_2 species *in vitro* and in rat lungs by chemiluminescence. *J Appl Physiol* 1989;**67**:1912–21.

67 Paky A, Michael JR, Burke-Wolin TM et al. Endogenous production of superoxide by rabbit lungs: effects of hypoxia or metabolic inhibitors. *J Appl Physiol* 1993;**74**:2868–74.

68 Archer SL, Reeve HL, Michelakis E et al. O_2 sensing is preserved in mice lacking the gp91 phox subunit of NADPH oxidase. *Proc Natl Acad Sci USA* 1999;**96**:7944–9.

69 O'Kelly I, Lewis A, Peers C et al. O_2 sensing by airway chemoreceptor-derived cells. Protein kinase c activation reveals functional evidence for involvement of NADPH oxidase. *J Biol Chem* 2000;**275**:7684–92.

●70 Reeve HL, Tolarova S, Nelson DP et al. Redox control of oxygen sensing in the rabbit ductus arteriosus. *J Physiol* 2001;**533**:253–61.

71 Marshall C, Mamary AJ, Verhoeven AJ et al. Pulmonary artery NADPH-oxidase is activated in hypoxic pulmonary vasoconstriction. *Am J Respir Cell Mol Biol* 1996;**15**:633–44.

72 Duranteau J, Chandel NS, Kulisz A et al. Intracellular signaling by reactive oxygen species during hypoxia in cardiomyocytes. *J Biol Chem* 1998;**273**:11619–24.

73 Killilea DW, Hester R, Balczon R et al. Free radical production in hypoxic pulmonary artery smooth muscle cells. *Am J Physiol* 2000;**279**:L408–12.

74 Weissmann N, Tadic A, Hanze J et al. Hypoxic vasoconstriction in intact lungs: a role for NADPH oxidase-derived H_2O_2? *Am J Physiol* 2000;**279**:L683–90.

75 Waypa GB, Chandel NS, Schumacker PT. Model for hypoxic pulmonary vasoconstriction involving mitochondrial oxygen sensing. *Circ Res* 2001;**88**:1259–66.

76 Weissmann N, Winterhalder S, Nollen M et al. NO and reactive oxygen species are involved in biphasic hypoxic vasoconstriction of isolated rabbit lungs. *Am J Physiol* 2001;**280**:L638–45.

●77 Wang D, Youngson C, Wong V et al. NADPH-oxidase and a hydrogen peroxide-sensitive K^+ channel may function as an oxygen sensor complex in airway chemoreceptors and small cell lung carcinoma cell lines. *Proc Natl Acad Sci USA* 1996;**93**:13182–7.

78 Fu XW, Nurse C, Wang YT et al. Selective modulation of membrane currents by hypoxia in intact airway chemoreceptors from neonatal rabbit. *J Physiol* 1999;**514**:139–50.

79 Fu XW, Wang D, Nurse CA et al. NADPH oxidase is an O_2 sensor in airway chemoreceptors: evidence from K^+ current modulation in wild-type and oxidase-deficient mice. *Proc Natl Acad Sci USA* 2000;**97**:4374–9.

80 Berube J, Caouette D, Daleau P. Hydrogen peroxide modifies the kinetics of HERG channel expressed in a mammalian cell line. *J Pharmacol Exp Ther* 2001;**297**:96–102.

81 Chander A, Dhariwal KR, Viswanathan R *et al.* Pyridine nucleotides in lung and liver of hypoxic rats. *Life Sci* 1980;**26**:1935–45.

82 Archer SL, Huang J, Henry T *et al.* A redox-based O_2 sensor in rat pulmonary vasculature. *Circ Res* 1993;**73**:1100–12.

83 Shigemori K, Ishizaki T, Matsukawa S *et al.* Adenine nucleotides via activation of ATP-sensitive K^+ channels modulate hypoxic response in rat pulmonary arteries. *Am J Physiol* 1996;**270**:L803–9.

84 Yuan XJ, Tod ML, Rubin LJ *et al.* Deoxyglucose and reduced glutathione mimic effects of hypoxia on K^+ and Ca^{2+} conductances in pulmonary artery cells. *Am J Physiol* 1994;**267**:L52–63.

85 Park MK, Bae YM, Lee SH *et al.* Modulation of voltage-dependent K^+ channel by redox potential in pulmonary and ear arterial smooth muscle cells of the rabbit. *Pflügers Arch* 1997;**434**:764–71.

86. Reeve HL, Weir EK, Nelson DP *et al.* Opposing effects of oxidants and antioxidants on K^+ channel activity and tone in rat vascular tissue. *Exp Physiol* 1995;**80**:825–34.

●87 Youngson C, Nurse C, Yeger H *et al.* Oxygen sensing in airway chemoreceptors. *Nature* 1993;**365**:153–5.

88 Mohazzab KM, Wolin MS. Properties of a superoxide anion-generating microsomal NADH oxidoreductase, a potential pulmonary artery PO_2 sensor. *Am J Physiol* 1994;**267**:L823–31.

89 Mohazzab KM, Fayngersh RP, Kaminski PM *et al.* Potential role of NADH oxidoreductase-derived reactive O_2 species in calf pulmonary arterial PO_2-elicited responses. *Am J Physiol* 1995;**269**:L637–44.

90 Zulueta JJ, Yu FS, Hertig IA *et al.* Release of hydrogen peroxide in response to hypoxia-reoxygenation: role of an NAD(P)H oxidase-like enzyme in endothelial cell plasma membrane. *Am J Respir Cell Mol Biol* 1995;**12**:41–9.

●91 Kummer W, Acker H. Immunohistochemical demonstration of four subunits of neutrophil NAD(P)H oxidase in type I cells of carotid body. *J Appl Physiol* 1995;**78**:1904–9.

92 Jones SA, Hancock JT, Jones OT *et al.* The expression of NADPH oxidase components in human glomerular mesangial cells: detection of protein and mRNA for p47phox, p67phox, and p22phox. *J Am Soc Nephrol* 1995;**5**:1483–91.

93 Umeki S. Activation factors of neutrophil NADPH oxidase complex. *Life Sci* 1994;**55**:1–13.

94 Wolin MS, Burke-Wolin TM, Mohazzab H. Roles for NAD(P)H oxidases and reactive oxygen species in vascular oxygen sensing mechanisms. *Respir Physiol* 1999;**115**:229–38.

95 Wenger RH, Marti HH, Schuerer-Maly CC *et al.* Hypoxic induction of gene expression in chronic granulomatous disease-derived B-cell lines: oxygen sensing is independent of the cytochrome b_{558}-containing nicotinamide adenine dinucleotide phosphate oxidase. *Blood* 1996;**87**:756–61.

●96 Mills E, Jobsis FF. Mitochondrial respiratory chain of carotid body and chemoreceptor response to changes in oxygen tension. *J Neurophysiol* 1972;**35**:405–28.

97 Duchen MR, Biscoe TJ. Mitochondrial function in type I cells isolated from rabbit arterial chemoreceptors. *J Physiol* 1992;**450**:13–31.

98 Duchen MR, Biscoe TJ. Relative mitochondrial membrane potential and $[Ca^{2+}]_i$ in type I cells isolated from the rabbit carotid body. *J Physiol* 1992;**450**:33–61.

99 Chandel NS, Maltepe E, Goldwasser E *et al.* Mitochondrial reactive oxygen species trigger hypoxia-induced transcription. *Proc Natl Acad Sci USA* 1998;**95**:11715–20.

100 Chandel NS, McClintock DS, Feliciano CE *et al.* Reactive oxygen species generated at mitochondrial complex III stabilize hypoxia-inducible factor-1alpha during hypoxia: a mechanism of O_2 sensing. *J Biol Chem* 2000;**275**:25130–8.

101 Chandel NS, Schumacker PT. Cellular oxygen sensing by mitochondria: old questions, new insight. *J Appl Physiol* 2000;**88**:1880–9.

102 Budinger GR, Chandel NS, Shao ZH *et al.* Cellular energy utilization and supply during hypoxia in embryonic cardiac myocytes. *Am J Physiol* 1996;**270**:L44–53.

103 Budinger GR, Duranteau J, Chandel NS *et al.* Hibernation during hypoxia in cardiomyocytes. Role of mitochondria as the O_2 sensor. *J Biol Chem* 1998;**273**:3330–6.

104 Chandel NS, Budinger GR, Choe SH *et al.* Cellular respiration during hypoxia: role of cytochrome oxidase as the oxygen sensor in hepatocytes. *J Biol Chem* 1997;**272**:111–12.

105 Chandel NS, Budinger GR, Kemp RA *et al.* Inhibition of cytochrome-c oxidase activity during prolonged hypoxia. *Am J Physiol* 1995;**268**:L918–25.

●106 Lopez-Barneo J, Lopez-Lopez JR, Urena J *et al.* Chemo-transduction in the carotid body: K^+ current modulated by pO_2 in type I chemoreceptor cells. *Science* 1988;**241**:580–2.

●107 Smirnov SV, Robertson TP, Ward JP *et al.* Chronic hypoxia is associated with reduced delayed rectifier K^+ current in rat pulmonary artery muscle cells. *Am J Physiol* 1994;**266**:H365–70.

108 MacLean MR, Johnston ED, Mcculloch KM *et al.* Phosphodiesterase isoforms in the pulmonary arterial circulation of the rat: changes in pulmonary hypertension. *J Pharmacol Exp Ther* 1997;**283**:619–24.

109 Morrel NW, Atochina EN, Morris KG *et al.* Angiotensin converting enzyme expression is increased in small pulmonary arteries of rats with hypoxia-induced pulmonary hypertension. *J Clin Invest* 1995;**96**:1823–33.

110 Zhao L, al-Tubuly R, Sebhki A *et al.* Angiotensin II receptor expression and inhibition in the chronically hypoxic rat lung. *Br J Pharmacol* 1996;**119**:1217–22.

111 Chassagne C, Eddahibi S, Adamy C *et al.* Modulation of angiotensin II receptor expression during development and regression of hypoxic pulmonary hypertension. *Am J Respir Cell Mol Biol* 2000;**22**:323–32.

112 Christman BW, McPherson CD, Newman JH *et al.* An imbalance between the excretion of thromboxane and prostacyclin metabolites in pulmonary hypertension. *N Engl J Med* 1992;**327**:70–5.

113 Li H, Chen SJ, Chen YF *et al.* Enhanced endothelin-1 and endothelin receptor gene expression in chronic hypoxia. *J Appl Physiol* 1994;**77**:1451–9.

114 Lee SL, Dunn J, Yu FS *et al.* Serotonin uptake and configurational change of bovine pulmonary artery smooth muscle cells in culture. *J Cell Physiol* 1989;**138**:145–53.

●115 Eddahibi S, Fabre V, Boni C *et al.* Induction of serotonin transporter by hypoxia in pulmonary vascular smooth muscle cells. Relationship with the mitogenic action of serotonin. *Circ Res* 1999;**84**:329–36.

●116 Meyrick B, Reid L. Hypoxia and incorporation of ^{3}H-thymidine by cells of the rat pulmonary arteries and alveolar wall. *Am J Pathol* 1979;**96**:51–70.

117 Rabinovitch M. Pathobiology of pulmonary hypertension. Extracellular matrix. *Clin Chest Med* 2001;**22**:433–49.

118 Sweeney M, Yuan JX. Hypoxic pulmonary vasoconstriction: role of voltage-gated potassium channels. *Respir Res* 2000;**1**:40–8.

119 Platoshyn O, Yu Y, Golovina VA *et al.* Chronic hypoxia decreases K(v) channel expression and function in pulmonary artery myocytes. *Am J Physiol* 2001;**280**:L801–12.

●120 Osipenko ON, Alexander D, MacLean MR *et al.* Influence of chronic hypoxia on the contributions of non-inactivating and delayed rectifier K currents to the resting potential and tone of rat pulmonary artery smooth muscle. *Br J Pharmacol* 1998;**124**:1335–7.

121 Li K-X, Fouty B, McMurtry IF *et al.* Enhanced ETA-receptor-mediated inhibition of Kv channels in hypoxic hypertensive rat pulmonary artery myocytes. *Am J Physiol* 1999;**277**:H363–70.

122 Shimoda LA, Sylvester JT, Sham JS. Chronic hypoxia alters effects of endothelin and angiotensin on K$^+$ currents in pulmonary arterial myocytes. *Am J Physiol* 1999;**277**:L431–9.

123 Reeve HL, Michelakis E, Nelson D *et al.* Alterations in a redox oxygen sensing mechanism in chronic hypoxia. *J Appl Physiol* 2001;**90**:2249–56.

●124 McMurtry IF, Petrun MD, Reeves JT. Lungs from chronic hypoxic rats have decreased pressor response to acute hypoxia. *Am J Physiol* 1978;**235**:H104–9.

●125 Yu Y, Platoshyn O, Zhang J *et al.* c-Jun decreases voltage-gated K$^+$ channel activity in pulmonary artery smooth muscle cells. *Circulation* 2001;**104**:1557–63.

126 Webster KA, Discher DJ, Bishopric NH. Induction and nuclear accumulation of Fos and Jun proto-oncogenes in hypoxic cardiac myocytes. *J Biol Chem* 1993;**268**:16852–8.

127 Munell F, Burke RE, Bandele A *et al.* Localisation of c-*fos*, c-*jun*, and *hsp70* mRNA expression in brain after neonatal hypoxia-ischemia. *Dev Brain Res* 1994;**77**:111–21.

◆128 Bunn HF, Poyton RO. Oxygen sensing and molecular adaptation to hypoxia. *Physiol Rev* 1996;**76**:839–85.

129 Semenza GL. HIF-1: mediator of physiological and pathophysiological responses to hypoxia. *J Appl Physiol* 2000;**88**:1474–80.

◆130 Semenza GL. Oxygen-regulated transcription factors and their role in pulmonary disease. *Respir Res* 2000;**1**:159–62.

131 Yu AY, Frid MG, Shimoda LA *et al.* Temporal, spatial, and oxygen-regulated expression of hypoxia-inducible factor 1 in the lung. *Am J Physiol* 1998;**275**:L818–26.

●132 Yu AY, Shimoda LA, Iyer NV *et al.* Impaired physiological response to chronic hypoxia in mice partially deficient for hypoxia-inducible factor 1alpha. *J Clin Invest* 1999;**103**:691–6.

133 Shweiki D, Itin A, Soffer D *et al.* Vascular endothelial growth factor induced by hypoxia may mediate hypoxia-initiated angiogenesis. *Nature* 1992;**359**:843–5.

134 Fagan KA, McMurtry IF, Rodman DM. Role of endothelin-1 in lung disease. *Respir Res* 2001;**2**:90–101.

●135 Li H, Elton TS, Chen YF *et al.* Increased endothelin receptor gene expression in hypoxic rat lung. *Am J Physiol* 1994;**266**:L553–60.

136 Stelzner TJ, O'Brien RF, Yanagisawa M *et al.* Increased lung endothelin-1 production in rats with idiopathic pulmonary hypertension. *Am J Physiol* 1992;**262**:L614–20.

137 Frasch HF, Marshall C, Marshall BE. Endothelin-1 is elevated in monocrotaline pulmonary hypertension. *Am J Physiol* 1999;**276**:L304–10.

138 Aguirre JI, Morrel NW, Long L *et al.* Vascular remodeling and ET-1 expression in rat strains with different responses to chronic hypoxia. *Am J Physiol* 2000;**278**:L981–7.

139 MacLean MR, Herve P, Eddahibi S *et al.* 5-Hydroxytriptamine and the pulmonary circulation: receptors, transporters and relevance to pulmonary arterial hypertension. *Br J Pharmacol* 2000;**131**:161–8.

140 Lee SL, Wang WW, Moore BJ *et al.* Dual effect of serotonin in growth of bovine pulmonary artery smooth muscle cells in culture. *Circulation* 1991;**68**:1362–8.

141 Pitt BR, Weng W, Steve AR *et al.* Serotonin increase DNA synthesis in rat proximal and distal pulmonary vascular smooth muscle cells in culture. *Am J Physiol* 1994;**266**:L178–86.

●142 Eddahibi S, Hanoun N, Lanfumey L *et al.* Attenuated hypoxic pulmonary hypertension in mice lacking the 5-hydroxytryptamine transporter gene. *J Clin Invest* 2000;**105**:1555–62.

5

Pulmonary vascular remodeling

NICHOLAS W MORRELL AND TRINA K JEFFERY

DEFINITION

Pulmonary vascular remodeling involves structural and functional changes to the normal architecture of the walls of pulmonary arteries. The process of vascular remodeling can occur as a primary response to injury, or stimulus such as hypoxia, within the resistance vessels of the lung. Alternatively, the changes seen in more proximal vessels are probably the result of a sustained rise in intravascular pressure. In order to withstand the chronic increase in intraluminal pressure, the vessel wall becomes thickened and stronger. This arises from Laplace's law, i.e. $P = T/r$, where T is tangential tension, P is pressure difference across the wall of the vessel and r is the radius. Thus tension within the vessel wall rises as a consequence of increased pressure. This 'armoring' of the vessel wall with extra smooth muscle and extracellular matrix leads to a decrease in lumen diameter and reduced capacity for vasodilatation. This maladaptive response results in increased pulmonary vascular resistance and, consequently, sustained pulmonary hypertension.

PHYSIOLOGICAL CONSEQUENCES OF PULMONARY VASCULAR REMODELING

The normal adult pulmonary circulation is a high-flow, low-resistance vascular bed with little or no resting tone.

The capacity for recruitment and vasodilatation in the normal pulmonary circulation is such that large increases in cardiac output cause little elevation of pulmonary arterial pressure (Figure 5.1). Thus, pulmonary vascular

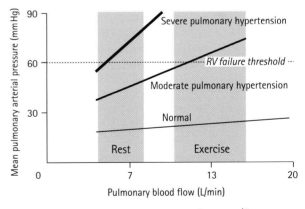

Figure 5.1 *Diagramatic representation of pressure/flow curves, at rest and on exercise, in the normal pulmonary circulation and in pulmonary hypertension, in the face of increasing remodeling. The slope of the lines is equivalent to the pulmonary vascular resistance (PVR). Thus, an increase in remodeling leads to increases in PVR and thus pressure. Note that an increase in resting PVR is accompanied by truncation of the pressure/flow curve on exercise and a marked increase in exercise PVR in pulmonary hypertension. RV, right ventricle.*

resistance (PVR) decreases as pulmonary blood flow increases. However, when the pulmonary circulation is remodeled, there is a reduced capacity for vasodilatation and a decrease in the cross-sectional area of the pulmonary vascular bed. Therefore, pulmonary arterial pressure may be elevated at rest and rise further on exercise. The greater the degree of remodeling, the greater the rise in pressure for a given cardiac output. So, for example, in patients with idiopathic pulmonary hypertension in whom florid vascular remodeling is observed, severe pulmonary hypertension can lead to right ventricular failure at rest. At a mean right ventricular pressure of >60 mmHg, right ventricular overload occurs and the capacity to further increase cardiac output is compromised (see Chapter 2).

MORPHOLOGICAL FEATURES

Normal pulmonary arteries

The anatomy of pulmonary arteries alters in a systematic way from the central 'conduit' arteries to the peripheral 'resistance' vessels (see Chapter 1). Proximal arteries are thin walled relative to their luminal diameter. The muscular media is composed of many elastic laminae separated by layers of smooth muscle. As the diameter of the arterial lumen decreases, the elastic laminae become less prominent and are replaced by smooth muscle. Beyond the terminal bronchioles, within the respiratory acinus, the arteries become only partially muscularized as the smooth muscle layer tails off in a spiral, with no smooth muscle found within the smaller intra-acinar arteries.[1,2] This precapillary segment of the pulmonary vascular bed is the site of the greatest pressure drop along the pulmonary circulation. As this site contributes to the majority of pulmonary vascular resistance, it follows that small changes in tone or wall structure at this level can lead to large elevations of pulmonary arterial pressure. For example, from Poiseuille's law for steady flow:

$$PVR \propto 8\,\mu L/\pi D^4$$

where L is vascular length, μ is the viscosity of blood, and D is vessel diameter; it can be seen that at constant length, the resistance in a tube doubles if D is decreased by 16%. The most distal segments of the precapillary arterioles contain an endothelial layer underlined by a single elastic lamina. Two smooth muscle-like cell types are found in the more distal segments:

- intermediate cells that, unlike smooth muscle cells, lie inside the internal elastic lamina and
- pericytes that lie beneath the endothelium in small precapillary vessels that do not possess an elastic lamina.

Distal muscularization of normally non-muscular arteries

A feature common to all forms of pulmonary hypertensive remodeling is the appearance of a layer of smooth muscle in small peripheral, normally non-muscular, pulmonary arteries within the respiratory acinus. The cellular processes underlying muscularization of this distal segment of the pulmonary arterial tree are incompletely understood. In precapillary vessels, intermediate cells, inside the internal elastic lamina, proliferate and differentiate into smooth muscle cells.[3] In the most distal vessels, which lack an elastic lamina (20–30 μm diameter), differentiation of pericytes and recruitment of interstitial fibroblasts from the surrounding lung parenchyma contribute to the process of muscularization.[4] These cells subsequently take on a smooth muscle-like phenotype.

It has been emphasized, particularly by the late Donald Heath, that when pulmonary hypertension occurs associated with alveolar hypoxia, such as hypoxic lung disease or from residence at high altitude, the remodeling observed in small pulmonary arteries is rather different from that seen in other forms of pulmonary hypertension. Although distal neomuscularization still occurs, laying down of longitudinally orientated layer of smooth muscle within the intima of small (80–500 μm) pulmonary arteries (Plate 5.1), and formation of 'inner muscular tubes' is characteristic of hypoxia-induced pulmonary hypertension in man.[5]

Increased muscularization of muscular pulmonary arteries

In the more proximal muscular arteries, subjected to a higher intraluminal pressure secondary to vasoconstriction and remodeling in the small peripheral arteries, proliferation and hypertrophy of medial smooth muscle occurs, leading to a 'fixed' reduction in the diameter of the vessel lumen.[6,7] New elastic laminae are deposited between the muscle layers, and increased type I collagen deposition serves to stiffen the vessel wall.[7] In addition to the changes in the media, there is proliferation of fibroblasts in the adventitial layer along with collagen deposition.[7] In pulmonary hypertension due to raised left atrial pressure, similar though less marked changes may be observed in the pulmonary veins.[8] The mechanism leading to excess vascular muscularization in the proximal pulmonary arteries includes endothelial damage/activation leading to increased permeability to factors in the serum (see below). For example, activation of elastases disrupts the elastic laminae of the vessel and promotes proliferation and hypertrophy of activated smooth muscle cells and deposition of extracellular matrix.[9,10]

Neointima formation

A hallmark of severe pulmonary hypertension (e.g. primary pulmonary hypertension, or congenital heart disease) is the formation of a layer of cells and extracellular matrix between the endothelium and the internal elastic lamina, termed the neointima (Plate 5.2).[11,12] This important lesion occurs in small and large arteries and contributes significantly to the increased vascular resistance. Neointima formation appears to be a frequent non-specific response to vascular injury and is also found in restenosis following angioplasty, and the atherosclerosis of coronary arteries in transplanted hearts. The commonly used animal models of pulmonary hypertension (e.g. chronically hypoxic rat, or monocrotaline) do not recapitulate this important feature. However, when vascular injury (monocrotaline) is combined with high flow (induced by pneumonectomy), the rat also develops a neointima (Plate 5.3).[13,14] These observations suggest that increased blood flow, such as that seen in congenital left-to-right shunts, is an important stimulus to neointima formation and disease progression.

The cells comprising the neointima are myofibroblasts. These cells express smooth muscle markers such as α-smooth muscle (α-SM) actin and vimentin, but are distinguished from mature smooth muscle cells by their lack of expression of markers characteristic of highly differentiated smooth muscle cells, such as smooth muscle myosin. Neointimal cells do not express endothelial cell markers such as CD31, CD34 or factor VIII.[12] *In vitro*, myofibroblasts derived from the neointima, exhibit different responses to growth factors than cells derived from the media.[15] The origin of neointimal cells in severe pulmonary hypertension is unknown. It is possible that these cells arise by transdifferentiation of endothelial cells, by migration of 'smooth muscle cell-like cells' from the media, or by migration of adventitial fibroblasts. In the systemic circulation, using pulse-labeling of dividing cells with bromodeoxyuridine, the available evidence suggests that proliferating cells arising in the media and adventitia of injured arteries migrate to the subendothelial space.[16,17] Furthermore, labeled adventitial fibroblasts stably transfected with a *lacZ* retrovirus were found capable of migrating from the adventitia to the media and neointima.[18] Study of the relative contribution from adventitial fibroblasts and poorly differentiated medial smooth muscle cells to neointima formation is hampered by the lack of specific markers to differentiate between these cells.

Formation of plexiform lesions

Another important form of vascular remodeling in severe pulmonary hypertension is the disorganized proliferation of endothelial cells leading to formation of the so-called plexiform lesion. This disorganized growth of new vessels is seen in 80% of cases of idiopathic pulmonary hypertension and in severe cases of secondary pulmonary hypertension. They are typically seen arising from arteries of diameter 200–400 μm and subtle differences have been reported in the site of lesions. Therefore, lesions occur in smaller arteries in primary pulmonary hypertension compared with pulmonary hypertension secondary to congenital heart disease.[12] The cells comprising these lesions are endothelial channels supported by a stroma containing matrix proteins and α-SM actin expressing myofibroblasts.[12] The endothelial cells within these lesions express markers of angiogenesis, such as VEGF and its receptors.[19,20] Recent studies have shown that the cells comprising plexiform lesions in cases of primary pulmonary hypertension are monoclonal in origin, whereas cells in cases of secondary pulmonary hypertension are polyclonal in origin.[21,22] Therefore, although the lesions themselves may be hemodynamically irrelevant, they may represent more than simply the result of severe elevation of intravascular pressures. Rather, the endothelial proliferation seen in these lesions may be a marker of a fundamental endothelial abnormality in primary pulmonary hypertension, possibly playing a key role in the pathogenesis of the condition (see Chapter 7).[23]

PULMONARY VASCULAR REMODELING IN ANIMAL MODELS

A number of different animal models have been used to investigate the mechanisms underlying pulmonary vascular remodeling. Each model imitates human disease to a greater or lesser extent, with, to date, no good model that mimics primary pulmonary hypertension in humans. Nevertheless, these models have been invaluable in the preclinical assessment of many of the emerging new treatments for clinical pulmonary hypertension, and in advancing our understanding of disease mechanisms *in vivo*.

Hypoxia

In the most commonly used model, rats are exposed to normobaric (10% oxygen) or hypobaric (320 mmHg) hypoxia for 2–3 weeks, leading to a 50% increase in mean pulmonary arterial pressure, and a doubling in weight of the right ventricle.[24] Muscular arteries undergo a doubling in their wall thickness and there is distal extension of smooth muscle into normally non-muscular arteries.[6,24] On return to room air, the hemodynamic changes largely resolve within 10 days, but the muscularization of small pulmonary arteries reverses more slowly (1 month). In larger vessels the regression is only partial.[7,25,26] This model has been criticized for not being particularly representative of any human disease, though most closely paralleling prolonged residence at high altitude.[27] Nevertheless, it is a convenient model and the key process of distal muscularization is a prominent feature. Different strains of rat respond with differing severity to chronic hypoxia. For example the Fisher (F344) strain is relatively resistant, whereas the Wistar–Kyoto strain is relatively susceptible to hypoxia-induced pulmonary hypertension, a feature that can be exploited in genetic studies.[28]

The rodent model has been successfully adapted to allow physiological and morphometric studies in the mouse, which responds similarly, if a little less obviously, to chronic hypoxia as the rat. This advance has meant that genetically engineered mice can readily be studied. Recently, many key observations have been possible using this approach, which allows measurement of the effect of disrupting specific pathways when pharmacological inhibitors may either be unavailable or lacking in specificity. For example, mice lacking the genes for endothelial nitric oxide synthase (eNOS),[29] prostacyclin receptor[30] and atrial natriuretic peptide type A receptor (NPR-A)[31] develop more severe pulmonary hypertension after exposure to hypoxia than wild-type littermates. The role of individual transcription factors can also be dissected; for example, mice deficient in hypoxia-inducible factor-1 (HIF-1) develop less severe pulmonary hypertension than controls.[32] A further well-characterized model of hypoxia-induced pulmonary hypertension is the chronically hypoxic newborn calf.[33] This model develops suprasystemic pulmonary hypertension with exuberant medial and adventitial thickening. The newborn pulmonary circulation seems particularly susceptible to hypoxic injury with profound remodeling. Similar lesions are seen in patients with persistent pulmonary hypertension of the newborn.

Hyperoxia

This model is less widely used than the hypoxic model, though is a useful model of hyperoxic or oxidant lung injury. Rats are exposed to normobaric 89% oxygen for 2–3 weeks, leading to the development of pulmonary hypertension.[34]

Monocrotaline

The pyrrolizidine alkaloids, such as monocrotaline, usually given as a single intraperitoneal dose, cause widespread vascular injury and inflammation, particularly endothelial cell injury. Pulmonary hypertension and vascular remodeling occur in rats 2–3 weeks following administration of monocrotaline.[35,36] Species differ in their susceptibility to monocrotaline, which is partly dependent on the activity of cytochrome P450 isoenzymes, which metabolize the toxin. Mice, in particular, are more resistant to the pulmonary vascular effects of monocrotaline.

High flow

Systemic-to-pulmonary artery shunts can be created in rats by surgical anastomosis, or alternatively, removal of one lung increases flow. Interestingly, the combination of monocrotaline and pneumonectomy has been used recently to induce vascular remodeling characterized by neointimal proliferation (a feature of severe pulmonary hypertension in man), not found in other animal models of pulmonary hypertension.[14] This observation has given rise to the hypothesis that the formation of the neointima requires 'two hits', that is, both endothelial injury and changes in pulmonary artery hemodynamics must occur for this lesion to develop.[13]

CELLULAR CHANGES IN PULMONARY VASCULAR REMODELING

Endothelium

The endothelium is the interface between hemodynamics and the underlying vascular wall. In addition, the endothelium provides an antithrombogenic, semipermeable barrier between the vascular and extravascular fluid compartments. The endothelium fulfils a variety of metabolic functions as well as exerting profound effects on vascular tone, growth and differentiation, and response to injury. The initiating injury in the context of pulmonary hypertension may be hypoxia, increased flow (shear stress), inflammation, or the response to drugs (e.g. dexfenfluramine) or toxins (e.g. adulterated rape seed oil, monocrotaline) on a background of genetic susceptibility. The endothelial cell may respond to specific forms of injury in various ways that can affect the process of vascular remodeling. As well as influencing cell growth and differentiation, injury may directly damage the normal homeostatic functions of the endothelium by altering endothelial permeability, metabolism, production of growth factors, and coagulation pathways.

In the chronically hypoxic rat model of pulmonary hypertension, a threefold increase in the number of endothelial cells replicating (measured by ^{3}H-thymidine uptake *in vivo*) in main pulmonary arteries is observed within 24 hours, and an increase in the number of replicating endothelial cells is seen in small muscular arteries at 7 and 10 days.[37] In hypoxic neonatal calves, the endothelial proliferative response to hypoxia is complex. In normal calves the endothelial proliferative index (measured by bromodeoxyuridine uptake *in vivo*) in small arteries (<1500 μm diameter) falls from 27% at day 1 to 2% by

14 days. Under conditions of hypoxia, the index at day 1 is suppressed (14%) but at day 14 enhanced proliferation is observed (8%).[38] Thus, endothelial cell hypertrophy and hyperplasia appear to contribute to intimal thickening, as does edema, thickening of the endothelial basement membrane and increased elastin synthesis.[39–41] At the ultrastructural level, the number/size of lamellar structures and organelles are increased, contributing to the swollen appearance of endothelial cells.[3,40]

A shear stress is imposed upon the endothelium exposed to the flowing blood (in systemic vessels, 15 dyn/cm^2). Increases in shear stress are caused by increases in blood flow, seen most notably in the presence of left-to-right shunts (e.g. congenital heart disease). Shear stress is transduced by the endothelium, which produces vasoactive mediators [e.g. endothelin-1 (ET-1), angiotensin II, thromboxane, nitric oxide, prostacyclin] and growth factors [e.g. platelet-derived growth factor (PDGF), transforming growth factor-β (TGF-β)] to maintain vascular homeostasis by reducing or increasing the vessel diameter. Transduction of the shear stress signal is probably achieved via alterations in the extracellular matrix/integrin/cytoskeleton structure, particularly at the focal adhesion complexes, where cytoskeletal components are tethered at the cell membrane.[42] Protein kinases are activated at these sites, which phosphorylate and activate downstream signals. Changes in shear stress can induce patterns of gene expression that can alter endothelial function, or the release of mediators that influence the biology of underlying smooth muscle cells.

A feature common to patients with severe pulmonary hypertension secondary to congenital heart disease and pulmonary hypertension in rats induced by the toxin, monocrotaline, is fragmentation of the internal elastic lamina.[43,44] This observation, together with the increased pulmonary transvascular protein leak observed in hypoxic rats, suggests that increased permeability of the intima may allow increased access of circulating growth mediators to the subendothelial compartment in pulmonary hypertension.

One of the major functions of the pulmonary endothelium under normal conditions is to prevent the formation of thrombus. In addition, small thrombi from the systemic veins will be continuously filtered by the lungs and presumably undergo fibrinolysis in the small pulmonary vessels. Alterations in endothelial coagulation and fibrinolytic factors may therefore contribute to the pathogenesis of idiopathic and thromboembolic pulmonary hypertension. *In situ* thrombosis in small pulmonary arteries is a feature of patients with idiopathic pulmonary hypertension.[45] In addition, anticoagulant therapy with warfarin improves the survival of these patients. Thrombin disrupts the endothelial barrier, causing leakage of proteins and interstitial edema, and promotes growth of fibroblasts and stimulates deposition of collagen in the interstitium.

Thrombin also promotes neutrophil adherence to the endothelium. Fibrin degradation products (FDPs), formed during fibrinolysis, also contribute to microvascular injury and can stimulate proliferation of lung interstitial fibroblasts.[46] Recent studies have shown that there are marked elevations of circulating plasminogen activator inhibitor and von Willebrand factor in severe idiopathic pulmonary hypertension, as well as reduced soluble thrombomodulin, indicating impaired local fibrinolysis.[47] Whether these changes are involved in the pathogenesis of this condition or are secondary to endothelial injury are not yet known. For example, alterations in blood flow and shear stress can alter the expression of regulators of the coagulation and fibrinolytic pathways (reviewed in reference 48). In addition to changes in shear stress, hypoxia itself exerts profound effects on endothelial cell function leading to increased endothelial permeability, expression of procoagulant factors (e.g. thrombomodulin), and induction of inflammatory molecules [e.g. interleukin-1 (IL-1), intracellular adhesion molecule-1 (ICAM-1)].

In response to these stimuli (hypoxia, increased shear stress, injury), endothelial cells in the hypertensive pulmonary circulation produce more vasoconstricting, proproliferative factors (ET-1, angiotensin II, thromboxane A_2), and less vasodilating, antiproliferative mediators (NO, PGI$_2$), which may serve to maintain the vessel wall in the remodeled hypertensive state.

Smooth muscle

During the development of pulmonary hypertension, smooth muscle cells undergo hypertrophy and proliferation, migration and changes in matrix deposition. Hypertrophy of smooth muscle cells makes a greater contribution than hyperplasia in the larger, more proximal arteries, whereas hyperplasia is more prevalent in the smaller resistance arteries.[7,37,39] In large hilar arteries, cells take on a more 'synthetic' as opposed to the usual 'contractile' smooth muscle cell phenotype. They show prominent rough endoplasmic reticulum and Golgi apparatus.[7] Cells from hypertensive arteries produce more collagen (types I and IV) and elastin in culture.[49]

Under normal conditions, the smooth muscle cells comprising the adult pulmonary arterial media display minimal basal cell division. In contrast, during the development of pulmonary hypertension this suppression of cell proliferation is perturbed by the up-regulation of stimulatory pathways (changes in ion channel activity, altered balance of vasoactive mediators, and growth factor expression – see below). Similar to the manner in which endothelial cells respond to changes in shear stress, smooth muscle cells are affected by mechanical stimuli, such as increased transmural pressures imposing circumferential stretch to the vessel wall. For example, mechanical stretch increases

DNA synthesis in pulmonary artery smooth muscle cells, and increases collagen expression in pulmonary artery fibroblasts exposed to cyclical mechanical loading.[50,51]

The process of extension of smooth muscle into normally non-muscular arteries is probably brought about by differentiation and hypertrophy of intermediate cells and pericytes already present in the wall. Indeed, pericytes have been shown to exhibit great plasticity in culture, being capable of differentiation into phagocytes, osteoblasts and adipocytes.[52] In addition, in hyperoxia-induced pulmonary hypertension, recruitment of interstitial fibroblasts from alveolar walls contributes to the formation of muscularized microvessels in the rat lung.[4]

It has become apparent that heterogeneity of pulmonary artery smooth muscle cells exists within the medial layer. This has been most elegantly demonstrated in the media of the bovine main pulmonary artery, where differently oriented cell populations, which differentially express mRNA for procollagen and tropoelastin, are visible by light microscopy.[53] By utilizing a panel of antibodies to contractile and cytoskeletal proteins at least four cell phenotypes can be discerned, which arise early during development of the arterial media (Plate 5.4).[54] These subpopulations are distinct with regard to their state of differentiation, expression of smooth muscle markers, proliferative response to growth factors, and to hypoxia.[55] When isolated in tissue culture, these subpopulations display markedly different rates of proliferation, and matrix protein expression. Thus, at any given level of the vessel wall there may be distinct smooth muscle cell subpopulations that may play diverse roles in vascular homeostatis and can respond in an injury-specific manner during the development of pulmonary hypertension.[55–58] Although the media of the human pulmonary artery appears homogeneous by conventional histochemical staining techniques and light microscopy, heterogeneity is apparent using antibodies directed against contractile proteins (Plate 5.3). In addition, heterogeneity in medial cell function is apparent *in vitro*, for example the release of adrenomedullin[59] and expression of binding sites for angiotensin II.[60] Furthermore, heterogeneity in smooth muscle cells is also observed in cells isolated from different anatomic locations in the lung, i.e. proximal versus peripheral arteries. For example, human pulmonary artery smooth muscle cells from the peripheral pulmonary circulation (arteries 1–2 mm diameter) proliferate more rapidly and are more sensitive to the antiproliferative effects of prostacyclin analogs than cells isolated from the main pulmonary artery.[61] Further elucidation of which cells respond to which stimuli will help our understanding of the process of vascular remodeling.

Fibroblasts

Early studies demonstrated that in rats exposed to hypoxia there is an early peak (2–3 days) in fibroblast proliferation

and hypertrophy in the adventitia of hilar arteries.[7,39] This coincides with increased deposition of type I collagen and elastin. In small peripheral muscular arteries, fibroblast hyperplasia and increased production of extracellular matrix protein is also prominent.[62] Type I collagen deposition and elastin synthesis in the adventitia contribute to the narrowing of the vascular lumen and probably to the reduced capacity for vasodilatation in advanced pulmonary hypertension.[63,64]

Recent evidence supports an active role for the adventitial fibroblast in the remodeling of the pulmonary circulation during the development of pulmonary hypertension. Adventitial fibroblasts undergo a transition in phenotype during the development of pulmonary hypertension, as evidenced by the expression of smooth muscle contractile proteins such as α-SM actin.[65] These α-SM actin-expressing fibroblasts are often referred to as myofibroblasts, and are thought to represent a response to injury. As such, they are found in the adventitial layer of systemic arteries following balloon injury and in the injured dermis contribute to wound healing and scar contraction.[66] Although adventitial remodeling occurs in primary pulmonary hypertension,[67] it occurs most dramatically in neonatal forms of pulmonary hypertension.[33] The heightened proliferative response of the neonatal fibroblast may be due to developmental differences in protein kinase C signaling.[68,69]

Similar to smooth muscle cells, phenotypically distinct subpopulations of fibroblasts exist within the adventitia.[70] In addition, fibroblasts are also heterogeneous in their responses to hypertensive stimuli. For example, in response to hypoxia some pulmonary artery fibroblasts proliferate, with increased activity of mitogen-activated protein (MAP) kinases,[71,72] whereas in others no response is observed.[70] It has been proposed that in pulmonary hypertension there is selective expansion of subpopulations of fibroblasts within the adventitia.[71] In fetal cells, the hypoxia-induced proliferation is related to the to the activity of specific isoforms of protein kinase C.[73]

In arterial remodeling, the adventitial layer is now seen as an important modulator of remodeling through its interactions with other layers of the vessel wall. Much of what is known originates from observations in the systemic circulation in the context of vascular injury following balloon angioplasty. The adventitial fibroblast may contribute to remodeling by transition of fibroblasts to myofibroblasts (expressing contractile proteins, e.g. α-SM actin), myofibroblast migration into the intima, adventitial fibrosis and expression of MMPs (see below).

MATRIX DEPOSITION

Although the deposition of collagen is often thought of as an irreversible process, the fractional synthesis rate of collagen is about 3% per day in the rabbit pulmonary artery.[74] Small changes in the rate of collagen synthesis and metabolism therefore cause a marked alteration in collagen content. Elastin and collagen deposition is increased during the development of pulmonary hypertension.[39] Endothelial cells in the microvasculature secrete type IV collagen and elastin. In larger arteries, smooth muscle cells and fibroblasts produce collagen and elastin within the media and adventitia, respectively. This appears to be in response to increased wall tension, since isolated stretched vessels also do this.[75] In the hypoxic model, the increased connective tissue maintains its normal relationship to muscle mass. In other models (e.g. neonatal hypoxic calves) there is greatly increased collagen deposition in the adventitia.[33,63] Connective tissue turnover is regulated in the vessel wall by the production of collagen and elastin on the one hand and its breakdown on the other. The degradation of matrix proteins is in large part due to the activity of matrix metalloproteinases (collagenases and elastases), the activity of which is in turn regulated by tissue inhibitors of matrix metalloproteinases (TIMPs) (see below).

ROLE OF ENDOGENOUS VASCULAR ELASTASES AND PROTEASES

One of the earliest features of pulmonary vascular remodeling is fragmentation of the internal elastic lamina, implying that elastases are activated in the vessel wall.[76] Inhibition of serine elastase activity with serine protease inhibitors (e.g. α_1-antitrypsin) during the early stages of monocrotaline or hypoxia-induced pulmonary hypertension prevents disruption of the internal elastic lamina and reduces vascular remodeling.[9,10,77] Elastase activation is related to serum factors leaking into the arterial wall because of damage to the endothelium. Within the media, elastase also degrades proteoglycans that serve as storage sites for growth factors, releasing biologically active forms of basic fibroblast growth factors (bFGF) and transforming growth factor-β (TGF-β).[78] In addition, elastase and the matrix metalloproteinases, as well as FGF-2, can induce production of the matrix glycoprotein tenascin-C.[79]

Tenascin-C is localized to sites of active vascular remodeling within the neointima in pulmonary hypertension secondary to congenital heart disease, where it co-localizes with proliferating cells and epidermal growth factor.[79] Tenascin augments the proliferative response to growth factors by a mechanism that involves binding of its cell surface integrin ($\alpha_v\beta_3$), leading to a rearrangement of the cytoskeleton and clustering and priming of growth factor receptors (e.g. epidermal growth factor receptors).[80] Furthermore, continued activity of elastase releases elastin peptides that stimulate the production of the matrix protein fibronectin, which changes smooth muscle cells from a contractile to a migratory phenotype.

Matrix metalloproteinases are a family of degradative enzymes that have important functions in cellular migration, and regulating the composition and amount of extracellular matrix. Members of this family are secreted in a latent form and are cleaved by other proteases to active forms. Several MMPs (including MMP-1, 2, 3 and 9) are produced by vascular smooth muscle cells in the arterial wall. The counteracting TIMP modulates MMP activities and the balance between MMP and TIMP is thought to determine the turnover of matrix proteins. Studies in the pulmonary circulation suggest that MMP activity is increased in rat pulmonary artery after removal from a hypoxic environment, accompanying active resorption of collagen, and resolution of remodeling, suggesting that MMPs may mediate the breakdown of excess collagen during recovery.[81] Futhermore, inhibition of MMP by TIMP-1 gene transfer or adminstration of doxycyline (MMP inhibitor) worsened the development of pulmonary hypertension, including increased muscularization and peradventitial collagen accumulation, in rats exposed to hypoxia.[82] In addition, inhibition of MMP activity suppresses tenascin-C expression.[83,84]

APOPTOSIS

Tissue remodeling also involves apoptosis, or programmed cell death. Either excessive or limited apoptosis can lead to the development of a variety of diseases, including pulmonary hypertension. In contrast to cell necrosis, apoptosis is a tightly regulated process that requires energy from ATP, gene transcription and protein synthesis. The role of apoptosis in pulmonary vascular remodeling is under investigation. In the monocrotaline model, apoptosis was only seen in the endothelial cells of the pulmonary artery, suggesting a mechanism for access of serum factors to the subendothelial space.[85] In patients with primary pulmonary hypertension, cells within plexiform lesions exhibit somatic mutations in genes regulating apoptosis (Bax) as well as cell proliferation (MutS homolog 2 gene and TGF-β type II receptor).[86] It is hypothesized that acquisition of somatic mutations in these genes allows clonal expansion of endothelial cells in PPH.[86]

Interestingly, hypoxia is a powerful promoter of apoptosis in many cell systems, and resistance to hypoxia-induced apoptosis allows clonal expansion of cells in some tumors. Little or no increase in the number of apoptotic cells is observed within the media of the chronically hypoxic rat. However, on return to room air apoptosis is maximal after 3 days and is likely to be involved in the involution of vascular remodeling during recovery from chronic hypoxic exposure.[87] The potential importance of targeting apoptosis in the therapeutic reversal of established pulmonary vascular remodeling was shown in monocrotaline-induced pulmonary hypertensive rats. Treatment of rats with serine elastase inhibitors led to myocyte apoptosis and loss of extracellular matrix, and normalized pulmonary artery structure and pressure.[75]

GROWTH FACTORS AND OTHER MEDIATORS INVOLVED IN VASCULAR REMODELING

Numerous cell-derived growth factors, vasoactive peptides and cytokines are involved in modulation of the vascular remodeling process. In addition, small molecules such as nitric oxide and reactive oxygen species play important roles. Table 5.1 lists the factors thought to be involved in smooth muscle cell growth and collagen synthesis in the vascular wall.

The cell surface receptors for most growth factors are transmembrane tyrosine-specific protein kinases, also known as receptor tyrosine kinases. These include receptors for PDGF, FGFs, insulin-like growth factor-1 (IGF-1), epidermal growth factor (EGF) and VEGF. Ligand binding leads to phosphorylation of the intracellular part of the receptor and initiation of intracellular signaling cascades. The TGF-β and bone morphogenetic protein family of growth factors signal via receptor serine/threonine kinases. The intracellular signaling pathways downstream of these receptors are complex and depend upon the tissue and cell type under investigation, which lends specificity to the responses.[88] However, many of the factors involved in vascular remodeling converge on common key signaling pathways within the cell. For example, a number of antiproliferative molecules in vascular smooth muscle stimulate production of the important intracellular second messengers, cyclic nucleotides (cAMP and cGMP). Vasoconstrictors and growth factors tend to converge to stimulate phosphorylation of MAP kinases. Different growth factors tend to operate at different stages of the cell cycle (the process of cell division), underlining the importance of multiple signals operating in concert *in vivo*.

MECHANISMS OF VASCULAR REMODELING IN PRIMARY PULMONARY HYPERTENSION

Although many factors act in concert to orchestrate pulmonary vascular remodeling, recent advances in our understanding of the pathogenesis of primary pulmonary hypertension have demonstrated that alterations in certain key pathways may play a central role in initiating disease, or causing disease progression (Figure 5.2).

TGF-β/bone morphogenetic proteins

Mutations in the gene encoding the bone morphogenetic protein (BMP) type II receptor (BMPR-II) were recently identified in familial and some apparently sporadic cases of primary pulmonary hypertension (see Chapter 6). BMPR-II is a constitutively active serine/threonine kinase receptor, signaling via formation of heterocomplexes with one of

Table 5.1 *Factors involved in the stimulation and inhibition of cell proliferation and collagen synthesis*

Smooth muscle cell growth		Type I collagen synthesis	
Stimulate	**Inhibit**	**Stimulate**	**Inhibit**
IGF-1	TGF-βBMPs	IGF-1	Prostaglandins
IGF-2	IL-1	IGF-2	Interferons
PDGF	Prostaglandins	TGF-β	Nitric oxide
EGF	Interferons	PDGF	ANP
bFGF	TNF-α	Angiotensin II	
aFGF	Heparin sulphates	Tenascin	
Insulin	Nitric oxide		
Heparin	Carbon monoxide		
Thromboxane A$_2$	Adrenomedullin		
Endothelin-1	ANP		
Angiotensin II	Isoproterenol		
Serotonin			
Tenascin			
Leukotrienes			
ROS			

aFGF, acidic fibroblast growth factor; ANP, atrial natriuretic peptide; bFGF, basic fibroblast growth factor; BMPs, bone morphogenetic proteins; EGF, epidermal growth factor; FGF, fibroblast growth factor (prefix a or b indicates acidic or basic, respectively); IGF, insulin-like growth factor; IL, interleukin; PDGF, platelet-derived growth factor; ROS, reactive oxygen species; TGF, transforming growth factor; TNF, tumour necrosis factor.

three type I receptors (ALK-3/BMPR-IA, ALK-6/BMPR-IB or ALK-2) in response to ligand (BMP2, BMP4 and BMP7). BMPR-II phosphorylates the associated type I receptor, thereby activating intracellular signaling via the Smad family of proteins (reviewed in reference 89), though alternative pathways involving MAP kinases, including $p38^{MAPK}$ and JNK kinases, are now recognized.[90] BMPR-II is present predominantly on the pulmonary vascular endothelium, and to a lesser extent on medial smooth muscle cells.[91] Endothelial expression of BMPR-II mRNA and protein is reduced in cases of primary pulmonary hypertension, whether or not an identified mutation exists in BMPR-II gene coding sequence (Figure 5.3).[91] Furthermore, immunohistochemical and *in situ* hybridization studies have demonstrated that BMPR-II is expressed in endothelial cells of plexiform lesions and myofibroblast cells within concentric and obliterative lesions.[91]

The role of BMPs in pulmonary vascular remodeling is not easy to predict, because the TGF-β family exerts complex effects on vascular cell function, which vary depending on the cell phenotype and the context. However, in general, TGF-β exerts antiproliferative effects on smooth muscle cells and promotes cell differentiation. Similarly, BMPs tend to suppress proliferation of smooth muscle

cells from normal proximal pulmonary arteries and from patients with secondary pulmonary hypertension.[58] In contrast, BMPs fail to suppress proliferation of smooth muscle cells from patients with primary pulmonary hypertension.[58] Thus, at least one mechanism for the abnormal proliferation of cells in the lesions of primary pulmonary hypertension may be a failure to respond to the growth suppressive effects of BMPs.

Since clinical pulmonary hypertension manifests in only a minority of disease gene carriers within families (10–20%) harboring *BMPR2* mutations, *BMPR2* mutation is necessary but not alone sufficient to cause disease. Thus, it has been proposed that a 'second hit' is necessary to bring about manifestation of the disease. This second hit could take the form of an environmental insult such as exposure to dexfenfluramine or a further genetic insult such as a somatic mutation in the normal *BMPR2* allele or related/interacting gene. Although individuals harboring *BMPR2* mutations may not manifest disease clinically, it is possible that these individuals have an abnormal pulmonary circulation. Indeed it is interesting to note that relatives of primary pulmonary hypertensive patients have an elevated pulmonary vascular resistance.[92] These various interacting factors are summarized in Figure 5.4.

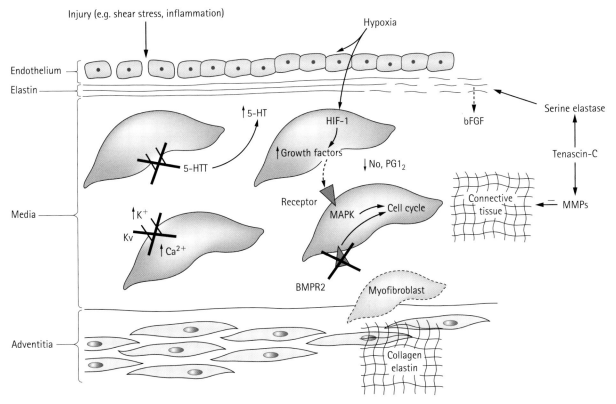

Figure 5.2 *Diagramatic representation of the various mechanisms involved in pulmonary vascular remodeling. 5HT, 5-hydroxytryptamine (serotonin); 5HTT, 5-HT transporter; bFGF, basic fibroblast growth factor; BMPR2, bone morphogenetic protein receptor 2; HIF-1, hypoxia inducible factor-1; Kv voltage-gated K⁺ channels; MMP, matrix metalloprotein; PGI₂, prostacyclin.*

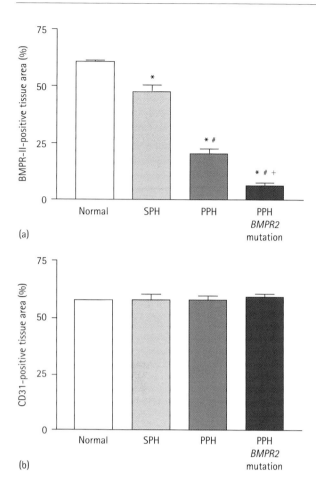

(a)

(b)

Figure 5.3 *(a) Pulmonary endothelial expression of* BMPRII *in lung tissue from normal, secondary (SPH) and primary pulmonary hypertensive (PPH) patients (with or without mutations in* BMPR2*). (b) The amount of endothelial positive tissue was determined by staining with the endothelial marker CD31. Image analysis confirmed that expression of* BMPRII *was markedly reduced in the peripheral lung of primary pulmonary hypertensive patients especially in those harboring* BMPR2 *mutations.*

A further defect in the TGF-β signaling pathway has been demonstrated in primary pulmonary hypertension. In approximately 30% of primary pulmonary hypertensive plexiform lesions there is a frameshift mutation in the TGF-βR2 gene encoding a premature stop codon.[86] Furthermore, in 90% of plexiform lesions, TGF-βR2 protein is not expressed, in contrast to the abundant expression in endothelial cells outside these lesions. It has been proposed that the monoclonal cell expansion of endothelial cells within plexiform lesions may thus result from somatic mutations in growth regulatory genes. In primary pulmonary hypertension patients the expression of the ligands for this receptor, namely TGF-β2 and TGF-β3, is reduced although no difference in TGF-β1 expression has been reported.[93] TGF-β is also known to increase production of extracellular matrix. For example, in human lung fibroblasts, TGF-β increases elastin expression by stabilization of elastin mRNA[94] and thus it is possible that increased elastin expression observed in primary pulmonary hypertension may be also due to alterations in this pathway.

Serotonin

In clinical pulmonary hypertension, platelet and plasma 5-hydroxytryptamine (5-HT; serotonin) levels are increased[95,96] and in addition, fawn-hooded rats, which have a deficiency in the storage of 5-HT by platelets, have a genetic predisposition to the development of pulmonary hypertension.[97,98]

5-HT induces hyperplasia and hypertrophy of human pulmonary artery smooth muscle cells,[99–101] although no mitogenic effect has been observed in endothelial cells or fibroblasts.[99,102,103] 5-HT also acts as a co-mitogen since in combination with other growth factors, including PDGF, EGF and FGF, the proliferative response is greater in magnitude than either mitogen alone.[99,102] Pulmonary cells from arteries of primary pulmonary hypertensive patients display a greater proliferative response to 5-HT compared with normal cells.[104] It appears that the 5-HT transporter (5-HTT), rather than its cell surface receptors, plays a pivotal role in 5-HT-induced cell proliferation.[101] In primary pulmonary hypertensive patients, 5-HT uptake and binding of the 5-HTT inhibitor, citalopram, is increased and this is due to increased expression of 5-HTT in these lungs.[104] The importance that the 5-HTT plays in vascular remodeling is further illustrated by the fact that when 5-HTT knockout mice are exposed to hypoxia, medial thickening and neomuscularization are significantly less than in wild-type mice.[105] These findings raise the possibility that 5-HTT inhibitors, such as fluoxetine, could be useful in the treatment of pulmonary hypertension.

Potassium channels

Potassium currents through voltage-gated K^+ (Kv) channels regulate the resting membrane potential within pulmonary artery smooth muscle cells with inhibition of these Kv channels leading to cell depolarization and a corresponding increase in intracellular calcium.[106] It is the intracellular calcium levels that influence not only the contractile but also the proliferative status of pulmonary smooth muscle cells.[107] In primary pulmonary hypertension, basal intracellular calcium levels and resting membrane potential are significantly greater in pulmonary smooth muscle cells than in cells from control and secondary pulmonary hypertensive patients.[108] This is due to both a decrease in Kv channel expression and impaired function since both the amplitude of current through the I_{KV}-type K^+ channels and the response of intracellular calcium levels to a Kv channel blocker is reduced.[106,107]

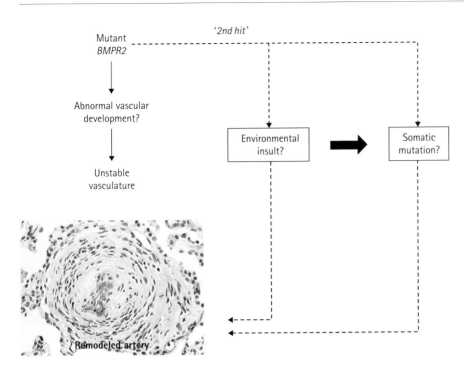

Figure 5.4 *Hypothetical mechanisms underlying the pathogenesis of primary pulmonary hypertension associated with BMPR2 mutation.*

Kv channels are also oxygen sensitive and in response to *in vitro* and *in vivo* hypoxia the expression and activity of these channels, is reduced.[109–113]

K$^+$ channels also appear to play an important role in apoptosis since activation of K$^+$ channels and hence the subsequent reduction in intracellular potassium leads to pulmonary artery cell apoptosis.[114,115] Thus, it has been proposed that the dysfunction in Kv channels seen in primary pulmonary hypertension may also contribute to a reduction in apoptosis and thus contribute to remodeling.[115]

MECHANISMS OF REMODELING IN HYPOXIA–INDUCED PULMONARY HYPERTENSION

The mechanism by which hypoxia leads to remodeling and hence pulmonary hypertension remains unclear. *In vitro* studies have demonstrated that hypoxia has direct effects on cell growth, with proliferation of pulmonary fibroblasts,[70,116] inhibition of endothelial cell growth[117] and either stimulation or inhibition of pulmonary artery smooth muscle cell growth.[118] This differential effect appears, at least for smooth muscle cells and fibroblasts, to be related to protein kinase C activation and cell population subtype examined.[70,56,118] Components of the extracellular matrix are also affected with less accumulation of one or more proteoglycans/glycosaminoglycans (e.g. heparan sulfates and hyaluronic acid) in hypoxic exposed pulmonary endothelial and smooth muscle cells.[119,120]

However, in contrast, in pulmonary fibroblasts hypoxia stimulates the production of heparan sulfate.[120] The proteoglycans have effects on cell proliferation and in rat lung pericytes and endothelial cells heparin, heparan sulfate, chondroitin sulfate and dermatan sulfate inhibit proliferation.[121]

Hypoxia is able to influence cell proliferation by exerting effects on a wide of variety of mediators. For example, hypoxia inhibits the production and/or release of antimitogenic factors (e.g. NO, prostacyclin),[122] whilst increasing the production and/or release of mitogenic stimuli from smooth muscle cells and endothelial cells (e.g. ET-1, angiotensin II, 5-HT, PDGF, IL-1, VEGF and bFGF).[123–126] Various inflammatory mediators, including IL-1β, IL-6, IL-8, PAF, monocyte chemoattractant factor-1 and macrophage inflammatory protein-2, which have been proposed to have mitogenic properties, also appear to be regulated by hypoxia.[127,128]

Hypoxic induction of the numerous mitogenic factors has been proposed to occur via the activation of a specific, as yet unknown, oxygen sensor leading to the induction or down-regulation of various transcription factors [e.g. HIF-1, activating protein-1, NFκB and cAMP response element-binding protein (CREB)] controlling the transcriptional activation of the genes. Of the transcription factors stimulated by hypoxia, HIF-1 appears to be one of the most potent inducers of gene expression. HIF-1, a heterodimer composed of HIF-1α and HIF-1β subunits, was first identified as a requirement for the induction of the erythropoietin gene by hypoxia.[130–132] Both *in vitro* and *in vivo* studies have demonstrated that it is the HIF-1α subunit that is regulated by hypoxia in the pulmonary vasculature.[32,133,134] The genes induced by HIF-1 include type II NOS,[132] heme oxygenase-1[134] and VEGF.[135] In contrast to HIF-1, the transcription factor CREB is down-regulated in response to hypoxia. Under normal physiological conditions, CREB expression maintains cells in a state of quiescence, which is proposed to involve the down-regulation of various cell cycle proteins (e.g. cdk4 and cyclin G and D2) as well as growth factors and cytokines including VEGF, ET-1 and IL-6.[136] Thus down-regulation of CREB by hypoxia is likely to play a pivotal role in cases of hypoxia-induced cell proliferation.

THERAPEUTIC REVERSAL OF PULMONARY VASCULAR REMODELING

Most of the current therapies available for the treatment of severe pulmonary hypertension were designed to target the process of vasoconstriction rather than the remodeling process. The relationship between vasoconstriction and remodeling has not been clearly established. It is probably not correct to assume that all vasodilators will inhibit or reverse the process of remodeling, though the mechanisms of action of many vasodilators (e.g. calcium channel blockers, activation of cyclic nucleotides) have an impact on known growth pathways. Nevertheless, since vessel remodeling is critical in the pathogenesis of pulmonary hypertension, it would seem advantageous to design treatments that specifically target this process (see Chapter 13).

Prostacyclin therapy (intravenous, inhaled or oral administration) has been a significant advance in the treatment of primary pulmonary hypertension. Many trials have found prostacyclin or its analogues to not only reduce pulmonary artery pressure but, more importantly, improve long-term survival (reviewed in reference 137). Although primarily used for its vasodilator properties, there is the suggestion that prostacyclin has antiproliferative effects.[138] Indirect evidence for this comes from the observation that patients who do not show an initial acute vasodilator response to prostacyclin still demonstrate a reduction in pulmonary vascular resistance during long-term administration,[139,140] though effects on cardiac function have yet to be excluded. Direct evidence for the antiproliferative effects of PGI_2 is derived from both in vitro cell culture studies[141] and from animal models of the disease.[61,142]

Endothelin, a potent smooth muscle mitogen, is thought to play an important role in pulmonary hypertension since there are various alterations in the endothelin pathway in pulmonary hypertension (reviewed in reference 143). The endothelin receptor antagonists, BQ-123 and bosentan, have been subjected to clinical trials in pulmonary hypertension.[144–146] In the two double-blind, placebo-controlled studies, bosentan (ET_A/ET_B receptor antagonist) significantly increased exercise capacity and improved hemodynamics in both primary and secondary pulmonary hypertensive patients.[145,146] The mechanism of action of endothelin receptor antagonists may relate to its vasodilatory properties although antimitogenic effects cannot be ruled out since numerous studies in animal models of the disease have found that endothelin antagonists can not only prevent the development of, but also completely reverse, remodeling.[147–149]

The importance of elastase in the development of vascular remodeling in pulmonary hypertension has already been discussed (see above). Serine elastase inhibitors and even gene therapy targeting serine elastase may in the future prove to be beneficial in treating pulmonary vascular remodeling associated with pulmonary hypertension. In animal models of pulmonary hypertension, various serine elastase inhibitors have been demonstrated to inhibit, and for some even completely reverse, existing remodeling.[9,10,77,150] Targeted overexpression of the serine elastase inhibitor elafin, in mice, has been found to not only suppress the up-regulation of MMP-9 seen in non-transgenic mice exposed to hypoxia but also to reduce remodeling.[151] Future developments are likely to include targeting the serotonin system and the BMP/TGF-β signaling pathways.

KEY POINTS

- The structure of the pulmonary arterial wall varies systematically from the large (proximal) vessels to the small (distal) pre-acinar vessels.
- Vascular remodeling involves thickening of the vessel wall to withstand any increase in intravascular pressure or flow, but also lumen narrowing and reduced capacity for vasodilatation.
- Smooth muscle cells, fibroblasts and endothelial cells contribute to remodeling by a combination of migration, hypertrophy and proliferation.
- Increased synthesis of collagen and elastin serves to reduce vascular wall compliance.
- Animal models mimic some, but not all of the features of human pulmonary vascular remodeling.
- Vascular wall elastases and matrix metalloproteinases (and their inhibitors – TIMPs) regulate matrix protein deposition and smooth muscle during remodeling.
- Disruption of the elastic lamina is an early feature of remodeling, resulting from leakage of serum proteins through a damaged endothelium and activation of endogenous vascular elastases.

- Receptor tyrosine kinase growth factors (e.g. EGF, PDGF, IGF, FGF, VEGF), receptor serine/threonine kinases (BMPs/TGF-β), hypoxia and potassium channels are involved in cell differentiation and proliferation.
- Activation of mitogen-activated protein kinases is a common feature of growth signals acting via G-protein coupled receptors and receptor tyrosine kinases.
- Specific targeting of the pathways regulating pulmonary vascular remodeling may lead to new treatments aimed at preventing or reversing pulmonary hypertension.

REFERENCES

1 deMello DE, Sawyer D, Galvin N et al. Early fetal development of lung vasculature. Am J Respir Cell Mol Biol 1997;16:568–71.
2 Davies P, Maddalo F, Reid L. Effects of chronic hypoxia on structure and reactivity of rat lung microvessels. J Appl Physiol 1985;58:795–801.
3 Meyrick B, Reid L. The effect of continued hypoxia on rat pulmonary arterial circulation. Lab Invest 1978;38:188–200.
4 Jones R, Jacobson M, Steudel W. α-Smooth muscle actin and microvascular precursor smooth-muscle cells in pulmonary hypertension. Am J Respir Cell Mol Biol 1999;20:582–94.
5 Heath D. Pulmonary vascular disease. Pathology of the lung, 5 edn. London: McGraw-Hill, 1996.
•6 Hislop A, Reid L. New findings in pulmonary arteries of rats with hypoxia-induced pulmonary hypertension. Br J Exp Pathol 1976;57:542–54.
7 Meyrick B, Reid L. Hypoxia-induced structural changes in the media and adventitia of the rat hilar pulmonary artery and their regression. Am J Pathol 1980;100:151–78.
8 Wagenvoort CA, Wagenvoort N. Primary pulmonary hypertension. A pathological study of the lung vessels in 156 clinically diagnosed cases. Circulation 1970;42:1163–84.
9 Ilkiw R, Todorovich-Hunter L, Maruyama K et al. SC-39026, a serine elastase inhibitor, prevents muscularization of peripheral arteries, suggesting a mechanism of monocrotaline-induced pulmonary hypertension in rats. Circ Res 1989;64:814–25.
10 Maruyama K, Ye CL, Woo M et al. Chronic hypoxic pulmonary hypertension in rats and increased elastolytic activity. Am J Physiol 1991;261:H1716–26.
11 Botney MD, Kaiser LR, Cooper JD et al. Extracellular matrix protein gene expression in atherosclerotic hypertensive pulmonary arteries. Am J Pathol 1992;151:1019–25.
•12 Yi ES, Kim H, Ahn H et al. Distribution of obstructive intimal lesions and their cellular phenotypes in chronic pulmonary hypertension. Am J Respir Crit Care Med 2000;162:1577–86.
13 Botney MD. Role of hemodynamics in pulmonary vascular remodeling. Am J Respir Crit Care Med 1999;159:361–4.

14 Okada K, Tanaka Y, Bernstein M et al. Pulmonary hemodynamics modify the rat pulmonary artery response to injury. A neointimal model of pulmonary hypertension. Am J Pathol 1997;151:1019–25.
15 Morrell NW, Yang X, Upton PD et al. Altered growth responses of human pulmonary artery smooth muscle and neointimal cells from patients with pulmonary hypertension. Am J Respir Crit Care Med 1999;159:A696.
16 Shi Y, O'Brien JE, Fard A et al. Adventitial myofibroblasts contribute to neointimal formation in injured porcine coronary arteries. Circulation 1996;94:1655–64.
17 Scott NA, Cipolla GD, Ross CE et al. Identification of a potential role for the adventitia in vascular lesion formation after balloon overstretch injury of porcine coronary arteries. Circulation 1996;93:2178–87.
18 Li G, Chen SJ, Oparil S et al. Direct in vivo evidence demonstrating neointimal migration of adventitial fibroblasts after balloon injury of rat carotid arteries. Circulation 2000;101:1362–5.
•19 Hirose S, Hosoda Y, Furuya S et al. Expression of vascular endothelial growth factor and its receptors correlates closely with formation of the plexiform lesion in human pulmonary hypertension. Pathol Int 2000;50:472–9.
•20 Tuder RM, Chacon M, Alger L et al. Expression of angiogenesis-related molecules in plexiform lesions in severe pulmonary hypertension: evidence for a process of disordered angiogenesis. J Pathol 2001;195:367–74.
•21 Cool CD, Stewart JS, Werahera P et al. Three-dimensional reconstruction of pulmonary arteries in plexiform pulmonary hypertension using cell-specific markers. Am J Pathol 1999;155:411–19.
•22 Lee SD, Shroyer KR, Markham NE et al. Monoclonal endothelial cell proliferation is present in primary but not secondary pulmonary hypertension. J Clin Invest 2002;101:927–34.
23 Voelkel NF, Tuder RM, Weir EK. Pathophysiology of primary pulmonary hypertension: from physiology to molecular mechanisms. In: Rubin LJ, Rich S (eds), Primary pulmonary hypertension, vol. 99. New York: Marcel Dekker Inc., 1997;83–129.
•24 Rabinovitch M, Gamble W, Nadas AS et al. Rat pulmonary circulation after chronic hypoxia: hemodynamic and structural features. Am J Physiol 1979;236:H818–27.
25 Hislop A, Reid L. Changes in the pulmonary arteries of the rat during recovery from hypoxia-induced pulmonary hypertension. Br J Exp Pathol 1977;58:653–62.
26 Fried R, Reid L. Early recovery from hypoxic pulmonary hypertension: a structural and functional study. J Appl Physiol 1984;57:1247–53.
27 Heath D. The rat is a poor animal model for the study of human pulmonary hypertension. Cardioscience 1992;3:1–6.
28 Aguirre JI, Morrell NW, Long L et al. Vascular remodeling and ET-1 expression in rat strains with different responses to chronic hypoxia. Am J Physiol 2000;278:L981–7.
29 Fagan KA, Fouty BW, Tyler RC et al. The pulmonary circulation of homozygous or heterozygous eNOS-null mice is hyperresponsive to mild hypoxia. J Clin Invest 1999;103:291–99.

30 Hoshikawa Y, Voelkel NF, Gesell TL *et al*. Prostacyclin receptor-dependent modulation of pulmonary vascular remodeling. *Am J Respir Crit Care Med* 2001;**164**:314–18.

31 Zhao L, Long L, Morrell NW *et al*. NPR-A deficient mice show increased susceptibility to hypoxia-induced pulmonary hypertension. *Circulation* 1999;**99**:605–7.

32 Yu AY, Shimoda LA, Iyer NV *et al*. Impaired physiological responses to chronic hypoxia in mice partially deficient for hypoxia-inducible factor 1α. *J Clin Invest* 1999;**103**:691–6.

33 Stenmark KR, Fasules J, Hyde DM *et al*. Severe pulmonary hypertension and arterial adventitial changes in newborn calves at 4,300 m. *J Appl Physiol* 1987;**62**:821–30.

34 Jones R, Reid L. Vascular remodelling in clinical and experimental pulmonary hypertensions, In: Bishop JE, Reeves JT, Laurent GJ (eds), *Pulmonary vascular remodelling*. London: Portland Press, 1995;47–115.

35 Meyrick B, Gamble W, Reid LM. Development of *Crotalaria* pulmonary hypertension: hemodynamic and structural study. *Am J Physiol* 1980;**239**:692–702.

36 van Suylen RJ, Smits JF, Daemen MJ. Pulmonary artery remodeling differs in hypoxia- and monocrotaline-induced pulmonary hypertension. *Am J Respir Crit Care Med* 1998;**157**:1423–8.

37 Meyrick B, Reid L. Hypoxia and incorporation of ³H-thymidine by cells of the rat pulmonary arteries and alveolar wall. *Am J Pathol* 1979;**96**:51–70.

38 Stiebellehner L, Belknap JK, Ensley B *et al*. Lung endothelial cell proliferation in normal and pulmonary hypertensive neonatal calves. *Am J Physiol* 1998;**275**:L593–600.

39 McKenzie JC, Clancy J, Klein RM. Autoradiographic analysis of cell proliferation and protein synthesis in the pulmonary trunk of rats during the early development of hypoxia-induced pulmonary hypertension. *Blood Vessels* 1984;**21**:80–9.

40 Meyrick B, Reid L. Endothelial and subintimal changes in rat hilar pulmonary artery during recovery from hypoxia. A quantitative ultrastructural study. *Lab Invest* 1980; **42**:603–15.

41 Vyas-Somani AC, Aziz S, Arcot SA *et al*. Temporal alterations in basement membrane components in the pulmonary vasculature of the chronically hypoxic rat: impact of hypoxia and recovery. *Am J Med Sci* 1996;**312**:54–67.

42 Fisher AB, Chien S, Barakat AI *et al*. Endothelial cellular responses to altered shear stress. *Am J Physiol* 2001;**281**:L529–33.

43 Rabinovitch M, Bothwell T, Hayakawa BN *et al*. Pulmonary artery endothelial abnormalities in patients with congenital heart defects and pulmonary hypertension. A correlation of light with scanning electron microscopy and transmission electron microscopy. *Lab Invest* 1986;**55**:632–53.

44 Todorovich-Hunter L, Johnson DJ, Ranger P *et al*. Altered elastin and collagen synthesis associated with progressive pulmonary hypertension induced by monocrotaline. A biochemical and ultrastructural study. *Lab Invest* 1988;**58**:184–95.

45 Hassell KL. Altered hemostasis in pulmonary hypertension. *Blood Coagul Fibrinolysis* 1998;**9**:107–17.

46 Gray AJ, Bishop JE, Reeves JT *et al*. Partially degraded fibrin(ogen) stimulates fibroblast proliferation *in vitro*. *Am J Respir Cell Mol Biol* 1995;**12**:684–90.

47 Welsh CH, Hassell KL, Badesch DB *et al*. Coagulation and fibrinolytic profiles in patients with severe pulmonary hypertension. *Chest* 1996;**110**:710–17.

48 Turitto VT, Hall CL. Mechanical factors affecting hemostasis and thrombosis. *Thromb Res* 1998;**92**:S25–31.

49 Crouch EC, Parks WC, Rosenbaum JL *et al*. Regulation of collagen production by medial smooth muscle cells in hypoxic pulmonary hypertension. *Am Rev Respir Dis* 1989;**140**:1045.

●50 Weiser MC, Majack RA, Tucker A *et al*. Static tension is associated with increased smooth muscle cell DNA synthesis in rat pulmonary arteries. *Am J Physiol* 1995;**268**:H1133–8.

51 Bishop JE, Butt RP, Low RB. The effect of mechanical forces on cell function: implications for pulmonary vascular remodelling due to hypertension. In: Bishop JE, Reeves JT, Laurent GJ (eds), *Pulmonary vascular remodelling*. London: Portland Press, 1995;213–39.

52 Hirschi KK, D'Amore PA. Pericytes in the microvasculature. *Cardiovasc Res* 1996;**32**:687–98.

53 Prosser IW, Stenmark KR, Suthar M *et al*. Regional heterogeneity of elastin and collagen gene expression in intralobar arteries in response to hypoxic pulmonary hypertension as demonstrated by *in situ* hybridization. *Am J Pathol* 1989;**135**:1073–88.

●54 Frid MG, Moiseeva EP, Stenmark KR. Multiple phenotypically distinct smooth muscle cell populations exist in the adult and developing bovine pulmonary arterial media *in vivo*. *Circ Res* 1994;**75**:669–81.

55 Frid MG, Aldashev AA, Dempsey EC *et al*. Smooth muscle cells isolated from discrete compartments of the mature vascular media exhibit unique phenotypes and distinct growth capabilities. *Circ Res* 1997;**81**:940–52.

56 Dempsey EC, Frid MG, Aldashev AA *et al*. Heterogeneity in the proliferative response of bovine pulmonary artery smooth muscle cells to mitogens and hypoxia: importance of protein kinase C. *Can J Physiol Pharmacol* 1997;**75**:936–44.

●57 Wohrley JD, Frid MG, Moiseeva EP *et al*. Hypoxia selectively induces proliferation in a specific subpopulation of smooth muscle cells in the bovine neonatal pulmonary arterial media. *J Clin Invest* 1995;**96**:273–81.

●58 Morrell NW, Yang X, Upton PD *et al*. Altered growth responses of pulmonary artery smooth muscle cells from patients with primary pulmonary hypertension to transforming growth factor-β₁ and bone morphogenetic proteins. *Circulation* 2001;**104**:790–5.

59 Upton PD, Wharton J, Davie N *et al*. Differential adrenomedullin release and endothelin receptor expression in distinct subpopulations of human airway smooth-muscle cells. *Am J Respir Cell Mol Biol* 2001;**25**:316–25.

60 Morrell NW, Upton PD, Kotecha S *et al*. Angiotensin II activates MAPK and stimulates growth of human pulmonary artery smooth muscle via AT₁ receptors. *Am J Physiol* 1999;**277**:L440–8.

61 Wharton J, Davie N, Upton PD *et al*. Prostacyclin analogues differentially inhibit growth of distal and proximal human pulmonary artery smooth muscle cells. *Circulation* 2000;**102**:3130–6.

62 Riley DJ, Poiani GJ, Tozzi CA *et al*. Collagen and elastin gene expression in the hypertensive pulmonary artery of the rat. *Trans Assoc Am Phys* 1986;**99**:180–8.

63 Mecham RP, Whitehouse LA, Wrenn DS *et al*. Smooth muscle mediated-connective tissue remodelling in pulmonary hypertension. *Science* 1987;**237**:423–6.

64 Tozzi CA, Christiansen DL, Poiani GJ *et al*. Excess collagen in hypertensive pulmonary arteries decreases vascular distensibility. *Am J Respir Crit Care Med* 1994;**149**:1317–26.

◆65 Stenmark KR, Mecham RP. Cellular and molecular mechanisms of pulmonary vascular remodeling. *Annu Rev Physiol* 1997;**59**:89–144.

◆66 Straus BH, Rabinovitch M. Adventitial fibroblasts. Defining a role in vessel wall remodeling. *Am J Respir Cell Mol Biol* 2000;**22**:1–3.

◆67 Chazova I, Loyd JE, Zhdanov VS *et al*. Pulmonary artery adventitial changes and venous involvement in primary pulmonary hypertension. *Am J Pathol* 1995;**146**:389–97.

68 Das M, Stenmark KR, Ruff LJ *et al*. Selected isozymes of PKC contribute to augmented growth of fetal and neonatal bovine PA adventitial fibroblasts. *Am J Physiol* 1997;**273**:L1276–84.

69 Das M, Stenmark KR, Dempsey EC. Enhanced growth of fetal and neonatal pulmonary artery adventitial fibroblasts is dependent on protein kinase C. *Am J Physiol* 1995;**269**:L660–7.

●70 Das M, Dempsey EC, Reeves JT *et al*. Selective expansion of fibroblast subpopulations from pulmonary artery adventitia in response to hypoxia. *Am J Physiol* 2002;**282**:L986.

71 Das M, Bouchey DM, Moore MJ *et al*. Hypoxia-induced proliferative response of vascular adventitial fibroblasts is dependent on G protein-mediated activation of mitogen-activated protein kinases. *J Biol Chem* 2001;**276**:15631–40.

72 Welsh DJ, Peacock AJ, MacLean M *et al*. Chronic hypoxia induces constitutive p38 mitogen-activated protein kinase activity that correlates with enhanced cellular proliferation in fibroblasts from rat pulmonary but not systemic arteries. *Am J Respir Crit Care Med* 2001;**164**:282–9.

◆73 Das M, Dempsey EC, Bouchey D *et al*. Chronic hypoxia induces exaggerated growth responses in pulmonary artery adventitial fibroblasts. *Am J Respir Cell Mol Biol* 2000;**22**:15–25.

74 Reeves JT, Bishop JE, Laurent GJ. Functional basis for the structure of the pulmonary arterial tree. In: Bishop JE, Reeves JT, Laurent GJ (eds), *Pulmonary vascular remodelling*. London: Portland Press, 1995;1–19.

75 Tozzi CA, Poiani GJ, Harangozo AM *et al*. Pressure-induced connective tissue synthesis in pulmonary artery segments is dependent on intact endothelium. *J Clin Invest* 1989;**84**:1005–12.

●76 Todorovich-Hunter L, Dodo H, Ye C *et al*. Increased pulmonary artery elastolytic activity in adult rats with monocrotaline-induced progressive hypertensive pulmonary vascular disease compared with infant rats with nonprogressive disease. *Am Rev Respir Dis* 1992;**146**:213–23.

77 Cowan KN, Heilbut A, Humpl T *et al*. Complete reversal of fatal pulmonary hypertension in rats by a serine elastase inhibitor. *Nat Med* 2000;**6**:698–702.

●78 Thompson K, Rabinovitch M. Exogenous leukocyte and endogenous elastases can mediate mitogenic activity in pulmonary artery smooth muscle cells by release of extracellular-matrix bound basic fibroblast growth factor. *J Cell Physiol* 1996;**166**:495–505.

79 Lloyd Jones P, Cowan KN, Rabinovitch M. Tenascin-C, proliferation and subendothelial fibronectin in progressive pulmonary vascular disease. *Am J Pathol* 1997;**150**:1349–60.

80 Lloyd Jones P, Crack J, Rabinovitch M. Regulation of tenascin-C, a vascular smooth muscle cell survival factor that interacts with the $\alpha_v\beta_3$ integrin to promote epidermal growth factor receptor phosphorylation and growth. *J Cell Biol* 1997;**139**:279–93.

81 Thakker-Varia S, Tozzi CA, Poiani GJ *et al*. Expression of matrix-degrading enzymes in pulmonary vascular remodeling in the rat. *Am J Physiol* 1998;**275**:L398–406.

82 Vieillard-Baron A, Frisdal E, Eddahibi S *et al*. Inhibition of matrix metalloproteinases by lung TIMP-1 gene transfer or doxycycline aggravates pulmonary hypertension in rats. *Circ Res* 2000;**87**:418–25.

83 Cowan KN, Jones PL, Rabinovitch M. Regression of hypertrophied rat pulmonary arteries in organ culture is associated with suppression of proteolytic activity, inhibition of tenascin-C, and smooth muscle cell apoptosis. *Circ Res* 1999;**84**:1223–33.

84 Cowan KN, Jones PL, Rabinovitch M. Elastase and matrix metalloproteinase inhibitors induce regression, and tenascin-C antisense prevents progression, of vascular disease. *J Clin Invest* 2000;**105**:21–34.

85 Thomas HC, Lame MW, Dunston SK *et al*. Monocrotaline pyrrole induces apoptosis in pulmonary artery endothelial cells. *Toxicol Appl Pharmacol* 1998;**151**:236–44.

●86 Yeager ME, Halley GR, Golpon HA *et al*. Microsatellite instability of endothelial cell growth and apoptosis genes within plexiform lesions in primary pulmonary hypertension. *Circ Res* 2001;**88**:e2–11.

◆87 Riley DJ, Thakker-Varia S, Wilson FJ *et al*. Role of proteolysis and apoptosis in regression of pulmonary vascular remodelling. *Physiol Res* 2000;**49**:577–85.

88 Alberts B, Bray D, Lewis J *et al*. *Molecular biology of the cell*, 3rd edn. New York: Garland Publishing, 1994.

◆89 Kawabata M, Imamura T, Miyazono K. Signal transduction by bone morphogenetic proteins. *Cytokine Growth Factor Rev* 1998;**9**:49–61.

90 Roberts AB. The ever-increasing complexity of TGF-beta signaling. *Cytokine Growth Factor Rev* 2002;**13**:3–5.

●91 Atkinson C, Stewart S, Upton PD *et al*. Primary pulmonary hypertension is associated with reduced pulmonary vascular expression of type II bone morphogenetic protein receptor. *Circulation* 2002;**105**:1672–8.

92 Grunig E, Janssen B, Mereles D *et al*. Abnormal pulmonary artery pressure response in asymptomatic carriers of primary pulmonary hypertension gene. *Circulation* 2000;**102**:1145–50.

93 Botney MD, Bahadori L, Gold LI. Vascular remodelling in primary pulmonary hypertension. Potential role for transforming growth factor-β. *Am J Pathol* 1994;**144**:286–95.

94 Kucich U, Rosenbloom JC, Abrams WR *et al*. Transforming growth factor-β stabilizes elastin mRNA by a pathway requiring active smads, protein kinase C-delta, and p38. *Am J Respir Cell Mol Biol* 2002;**26**:183–8.

95 Herve P, Drouet L, Dosquet C *et al*. Primary pulmonary hypertension in a patient with familial storage pool disease: role of serotonin. *Am J Med* 1990;**89**:117–20.

96 Herve P, Launay JM, Scrobahaci M-L *et al.* Increased plasma serotonin in primary pulmonary hypertension. *Am J Med* 1995;**99**:249–54.

97 Gonzalez AM, Smith AP, Emery CJ *et al.* The pulmonary hypertensive fawn-hooded rat has a normal serotonin transporter coding sequence. *Am J Respir Cell Mol Biol* 1998;**19**:245–9.

98 Sato K, Webb S, Tucker A *et al.* Factors influencing the idiopathic development of pulmonary hypertension in the fawn hooded rat. *Am Rev Respir Dis* 1992;**145**:793–7.

●99 Lee SL, Wang WW, Lanzillo JJ *et al.* Serotonin produces both hyperplasia and hypertrophy of bovine pulmonary artery smooth muscle cells in culture. *Am J Physiol* 1994; **266**:L46–52.

◆100 Fanburg BL, Lee SL. A new role for an old molecule: serotonin as a mitogen. *Am J Physiol* 1997;**272**:L795–806.

●101 Eddahibi S, Fabre V, Boni C *et al.* Induction of serotonin transporter by hypoxia in pulmonary vascular smooth muscle cells. Relationship with the mitogenic action of serotonin. *Circ Res* 1999;**84**:329–36.

102 Lee SL, Wang WW, Moore BJ *et al.* Dual effect of serotonin on growth of bovine pulmonary artery smooth muscle cells in culture. *Circ Res* 1991;**68**:1362–8.

103 Pitt BR, Weng W, Steve AR *et al.* Serotonin increases DNA synthesis in rat proximal and distal pulmonary vascular smooth muscle cells in culture. *Am J Physiol* 1994;**266**:L178–86.

●104 Eddahibi S, Humbert M, Fadel E *et al.* Serotonin transporter overexpression is responsible for pulmonary artery smooth muscle hyperplasia in primary pulmonary hypertension. *J Clin Invest* 2001;**108**:1141–50.

105 Eddahibi S, Hanoun N, Lanfumey L *et al.* Attenuated hypoxic pulmonary hypertension in mice lacking the 5-hydroxytryptamine transporter gene. *J Clin Invest* 2000;**105**:1555–62.

106 Yuan XJ. Voltage-gated K⁺ currents regulate resting membrane potential and [Ca²⁺]ᵢ in pulmonary arterial myocytes. *Circ Res* 1995;**77**:370–8.

107 Platoshyn O, Golovina VA, Bailey CA *et al.* Sustained membrane depolarization and pulmonary artery smooth muscle cell proliferation. *Am J Physiol* 2000;**279**:C1540–9.

●108 Yuan JX-J, Aldinger AM, Juhaszova M *et al.* Dysfunctional voltage-gated K⁺ channels in pulmonary artery smooth muscle cells of patients with primary pulmonary hypertension. *Circulation* 1998;**98**:1400–6.

●109 Yuan JX-J, Wang J, Juhaszova M *et al.* Attenuated K⁺ channel gene transcription in primary pulmonary hypertension. *Lancet* 1998;**351**:726–7.

110 Smirnov SV, Robertson TP, Ward JP *et al.* Chronic hypoxia is associated with reduced delayed rectifier K⁺ current in rat pulmonary artery muscle cells. *Am J Physiol* 1994;**266**:H365–70.

111 Wang J, Juhaszova M, Rubin LJ *et al.* Hypoxia inhibits gene expression of voltage-gated K⁺ channel alpha subunits in pulmonary artery smooth muscle cells. *J Clin Invest* 1997;**100**:2347–53.

112 Yuan JX-J, Goldman WF, Tod ML *et al.* Hypoxia reduces potassium currents in cultured rat pulmonary but not mesenteric arterial myocytes. *Am J Physiol* 1993; **264**:L116–23.

113 Platoshyn O, Lu Y, Golovina VA *et al.* Chronic hypoxia decreases Kᵥ channel expression and function in pulmonary artery myocytes. *Am J Physiol* 2001;**280**:L801–12.

114 Krick S, Platoshyn O, Sweeney M *et al.* Activation of K⁺ channels induces apoptosis in vascular smooth muscle cells. *Am J Physiol* 2001;**280**:C970–9.

115 Ekhterae D, Platoshyn O, Krick S *et al.* Bcl-1 decreases voltage-gated K⁺ channel activity and enhances survival in vascular smooth muscle cells. *Am J Physiol* 2001;**281**:C157–65.

●116 Welsh DJ, Scott P, Plevin R *et al.* Hypoxia enhances cellular proliferation and inositol 1,4,5-triphosphate generation in fibroblasts from bovine pulmonary artery but not from mesenteric artery. *Am J Respir Crit Care Med* 1998; **158**:1757–62.

117 Tucci M, Hammerman SI, Furfaro S *et al.* Distinct effect of hypoxia on endothelial cell proliferation and cycling. *Am J Physiol* 1997;**272**:C1700–8.

118 Dempsey EC, McMurtry IF, O'Brien RF. Protein kinase C activation allows pulmonary artery smooth muscle cells to proliferate to hypoxia. *Am J Physiol* 1991;**260**:L136–45.

119 Humphries DE, Lee SL, Fanburg BL *et al.* Effects of hypoxia and hyperoxia on proteoglycan production by bovine pulmonary artery endothelial cells. *J Cell Physiol* 1986;**126**:249–53.

120 Papakonstantinou E, Karakiulakis G, Tamm M *et al.* Hypoxia modifies the effect of PDGF on glycosaminoglycan synthesis by primary human lung cells. *Am J Physiol* 2000;**279**:L825–34.

121 Khoury J, Langleben D. Heparin-like molecules inhibit pulmonary vascular pericyte proliferation *in vitro*. *Am J Physiol Lung Cell Mol Physiol* 2000;**279**:L252–61.

122 Madden MC, Vender RL, Friedman M. Effect of hypoxia on prostacyclin production in cultured pulmonary artery endothelium. *Prostaglandins* 1986;**31**:1049–62.

123 Cooper AL, Beasley D. Hypoxia stimulates proliferation and interleukin-1α production in human vascular smooth muscle cells. *Am J Physiol* 1999;**277**:H1326–37.

124 Ambalavanan N, Bulger A, Philips JB. Hypoxia-induced release of peptide growth factors from neonatal porcine pulmonary artery smooth muscle cells. *Biol Neonate* 1999;**76**:311–19.

125 Klekamp JG, Jarzecka K, Hoover RL *et al.* Vascular endothelial growth factor is expressed in ovine pulmonary vascular smooth muscle cells *in vitro* and regulated by hypoxia and dexamethasone. *Pediatr Res* 1997;**42**:744–9.

126 Dawes KE, Peacock AJ, Gray AJ *et al.* Characterization of fibroblast mitogens and chemoattractants produced by endothelial cells exposed to hypoxia. *Am J Respir Cell Mol Biol* 1994;**10**:552–9.

127 Tamm M, Bihl M, Eickelberg O *et al.* Hypoxia-induced interleukin-6 and interleukin-8 production is mediated by platelet-activating factor and platelet-derived growth factor in primary human lung cells. *Am J Respir Cell Mol Biol* 1998;**19**:653–61.

●128 Minamino T, Christou H, Hsieh C *et al.* Targeted expression of heme oxygenase-1 prevents the pulmonary inflammatory and vascular responses to hypoxia. *Proc Natl Acad Sci USA* 2001;**98**:8798–803.

129 Semenza GL, Wang GL. A nuclear factor induced by hypoxia via de novo protein synthesis binds to human erythropoietin gene enhancer at a site required for transcriptional activation. *Mol Cell Biol* 1992;**12**:5447–54.

130 Semenza GL, Nejfelt MK, Chi SM *et al*. Hypoxia inducible factors bind to an enhancer element located 3′ to the human erythropoietin gene. *Proc Natl Acad Sci USA* 1991;**88**:5680–4.

●131 Wang GL, Semenza GL. Characterization of hypoxia-inducible factor 1 and regulation of DNA binding activity by hypoxia. *J Biol Chem* 1993;**268**:21513–18.

●132 Palmer LA, Semenza GL, Stoler MH *et al*. Hypoxia induces type II NOS gene expression in pulmonary artery endothelial cells via HIF-1. *Am J Physiol* 1998;**274**:L212–19.

133 Wiener CM, Booth G, Semenza GL. *In vivo* expression of mRNAs encoding hypoxia-inducible factor 1. *Biochem Biophys Res Commun* 1996;**225**:485–8.

134 Lee PJ, Jiang B, Chin BY *et al*. Hypoxia inducible factor-1 mediates transcriptional activation of the heme-oxygenase-1 gene in response to hypoxia. *J Biol Chem* 1997;**272**:5375–81.

135 Liu Y, Cox SR, Morita T *et al*. Hypoxia regulates vascular endothelial growth factor gene expression in endothelial cells. *Circ Res* 1995;**77**:638–43.

136 Klemm DJ, Watson PA, Frid MG *et al*. cAMP response element-binding protein content is a molecular determinant of smooth muscle cell proliferation and migration. *J Biol Chem* 2001;**276**:46132–41.

♦137 Galie N, Manes A, Branzi A. Medical therapy of pulmonary hypertension. The prostacyclins. *Clin Chest Med* 2001; **22**:529–37.

138 McLaughlin VV, Gentthner DE, Panella MM *et al*. Reduction in pulmonary vascular resistance with long-term epoprostenol (prostacyclin) therapy in primary pulmonary hypertension. *N Engl J Med* 1998;**338**:273–7.

139 Barst RJ, Rubin LJ, McGoon MD *et al*. Survival in primary pulmonary hypertension with long-term continuous intravenous prostacyclin. *Ann Intern Med* 1994;**121**:409–15.

140 Barst RJ. A comparison of continuous intravenous epoprostenol (prostacyclin) with conventional therapy for primary pulmonary hypertension. *N Engl J Med* 1996;**334**:296–301.

141 Clapp LH, Finney P, Turcato S *et al*. Differential effects of stable prostacyclin analogs on smooth muscle proliferation and cyclic AMP generation in human pulmonary artery. *Am J Respir Cell Mol Biol* 2002;**26**:194–201.

142 Nagaya N, Yokoyama C, Kyotani S *et al*. Gene transfer of human prostacyclin synthase ameliorates monocrotaline-induced pulmonary hypertension in rats. *Circulation* 2000;**102**:2005–10.

♦143 MacLean MR. Endothelin-1 and serotonin: mediators of primary and secondary pulmonary hypertension? *J Lab Clin Med* 1999;**134**:105–14.

144 Prendergast B, Newby DE, Wilson DE *et al*. Early therapeutic experience with the endothelin antagonist BQ-123 in pulmonary hypertension after congenital heart surgery. *Heart* 1999;**82**:505–8.

●145 Channick RN, Simonneau G, Sitbon O *et al*. Effects of dual endothelin-receptor antagonist bosentan in patients with pulmonary hypertension: a randomised placebo-controlled study. *Lancet* 2001;**358**:1119–23.

146 Rubin LJ, Badesch DB, Barst RJ *et al*. Bosentan therapy for pulmonary arterial hypertension. *N Engl J Med* 2002;**346**:933–5.

147 Chen S, Chen Y, Meng QC *et al*. Endothelin-receptor antagonist bosentan prevents and reverses hypoxic pulmonary hypertension in rats. *J Appl Physiol* 1995;**79**:2122–31.

148 Chen S, Chen Y, Opgenorth TJ *et al*. The orally active nonpeptide endothelin A-receptor antagonist A-127722 prevents and reverses hypoxia-induced pulmonary hypertension and pulmonary vascular remodelling in Sprague–Dawley rats. *J Cardiovasc Pharmacol* 1997;**29**:713–25.

149 Tilton RG, Munsch CL, Sherwood SJ *et al*. Attenuation of pulmonary vascular hypertension and cardiac hypertrophy with sitaxsentan sodium, an orally active ET(A) receptor antagonist. *Pulm Pharmacol Ther* 2000;**13**:87–97.

150 Ye CL, Rabinovitch M. Inhibition of elastolysis by SC-37698 reduces development and progression of monocrotaline pulmonary hypertension. *Am J Physiol* 1991;**261**:H1255–67.

151 Zaidi SH, You XM, Ciura S *et al*. Overexpression of the serine elastase inhibitor elafin protects transgenic mice from hypoxic pulmonary hypertension. *Circulation* 2002;**105**:516–21.

6

The genetics of pulmonary hypertension

HEATHER MORTIMER, JANE H MORSE* AND ANDREW J PEACOCK[†]

PULMONARY HYPERTENSION

Pulmonary hypertension is a rare condition characterized by a resting mean pulmonary artery pressure $>25\,mmHg$ or $>30\,mmHg$ on exercise with a normal pulmonary artery wedge pressure. Untreated survival following diagnosis rarely exceeds 3 years.[1] Current treatments aim to decrease peripheral vascular resistance and increase exercise tolerance. It is likely, however, that cure will only be possible when we have determined the molecular mechanisms of the disease.

Disease classification

Pulmonary hypertension can occur as a primary disease process so-called primary pulmonary hypertension (PPH), i.e. when no cause can be discovered, or secondary to other conditions. In 1998, the World Health Organization reclassified pulmonary arterial hypertension (PAH) into four main groups (for review see Chapter 12).[2] Interestingly, the patients who have disease localized to the pulmonary arteries often show similar histology despite differing etiologies.

Histology

Despite the many causes of PAH, the underlying pathology of the condition remains remarkably consistent with expansion and remodeling of all three compartments of the vascular wall, specifically: intimal proliferation, smooth muscle cell hypertrophy, and *in situ* thrombosis and fibrosis, which result in the classical plexiform lesions (for review see Chapter 5).[3] The primary form of the disease (PPH) has been studied most in order to gain a more detailed understanding of why such apparently disparate agents – for example anorexigens, thyroid dysfunction and HIV infection – should all result in the same pathological process.

This chapter considers the various pulmonary vascular diseases known to have a genetic basis.

PRIMARY PULMONARY HYPERTENSION

Primary pulmonary hypertension (PPH) is a rare condition with an incidence of approximately 1–2 per million. The National Institutes of Health Prospective Trial, which looked at 187 patients with a diagnosis of PPH in the USA, found that more than 90% of cases were sporadic, and only 6% were familial.[2] Clarke is credited for being the first investigator to appreciate the familial form of the disease.[4]

---

*JHM has contributed sections on the genetics of PPH. [†] AJP has contributed sections on the genetics of hypoxic lung disease.

Pattern of inheritance

The largest study to investigate the pattern of inheritance of PPH looked at 429 family members of 124 patients with this disease.[5] Using retrospective pedigree analysis, Loyd et al.[5] demonstrated vertical transmission of PPH over at least five generations, which is highly suggestive of a dominant gene. They also demonstrated male-to-male transmission, effectively ruling out an X-linked condition. More women than men were found to carry the gene – defined as either having the disease or progeny with the disease (female:male, 84:40) – and more women with the gene went on to develop PPH (72 of 84 compared with 27 of 40). The pattern of disease was identical between the sexes. Penetrance was highly variable across different families with only 20% of those carrying the gene being affected by the disease process.[5] More female children were born to those with PPH, suggesting perhaps selective loss of male fetuses in utero. Inheritance of PPH also appears to exhibit genetic anticipation, i.e. it becomes clinically evident at earlier ages and in a more severe form in subsequent generations.[6]

Chromosomal locus of PPH1 gene

Two groups independently mapped the gene for PPH1 to chromosome 2q31,32 by using the technique of genome scanning across the autosomes with microsatellite markers followed by linkage analysis.[7,8] Nichols and colleagues[8] reported a multipoint lod score of 8.86 at D2S311 in six families and Morse and colleagues[7] a lod score of 3.87 between markers D2S350 and D2S364 in two families. The locus initially mapped to an ≈25–27 centimorgan (cM) region using a single family shared by both groups, was later refined to a more telomeric 3 cM region at 2q33.[9,10] The microsatellite haplotypes were exclusive to each family, making the possibility of a single founder unlikely. All of these families appeared to be linked to this locus, but families with only a few affected individuals did not have sufficient statistical power to rule out linkage to other chromosomes.

Identification of PPH1 gene as BMPR2

Nucleic acid sequencing identified the PPH1 gene as the gene for a previously known molecule, bone morphogenetic protein receptor 2 (BMPR2),[11,12] a member of the transforming growth factor-β (TGF-β) superfamily of receptors. Prior to sequencing BMPR2, both groups independently sequenced two immunological molecules, CTLA4 and CD28, which failed to segregate with PPH. The TGF-β superfamily exerts a major controlling influence on the cell cycle affecting cell proliferation, apoptosis, cell adhesion and migration.[13] Disordered TGF-β

signaling has been implicated in various pathological processes, for example, malignancies, atherosclerosis and fibrogenesis.[14] The role of BMP, originally thought to be confined to osteo- and chondrogenesis during early development, now appears to function variably throughout the life cycle and in a tissue-specific manner. New data are emerging on the role of BMP in adult lung physiology and how BMPR2 mutations might result in the development of pulmonary hypertension.[15,16]

Initially, heterozygous germline missense, nonsense and frameshift mutations in BMPR2 were found in 7 of 8,[11] 9 of 19,[12] and later in 23 of 47 (≈50%) of FPPH families.[17] One family had a proband whose new mutation not found in either parent.[12] These mutations have not been found in 196 and 150 normal chromosomes. The BMPRII molecule, a serine threonine kinase, has 13 exons: exons 1–3 code for extracellular components, exon 4 transmembrane components, exons 5–10 make the kinase domain, and exon 12 the large cytoplasmic intracellular tail of unknown function. It was noted that each of the amino acid substitutions occurred in highly conserved or a functionally important site of the BMPR2 molecule, and speculated that these mutations would interrupt the BMPR2 signaling pathway by hindering ligand binding, eliminating kinase activity or reducing the heterodimer formation. So far, 46 different mutations in the BMPR2 gene have been identified, which occur throughout the gene with the exception of exons 10 and 13.[12,17,18] There have been no mutational 'hot spots'.

Where are the other mutations?

BMPR2 mutations have been reported in only 55% of all FPPH families, suggesting either a technical problem or the potential involvement of other genes. Janssen et al.[19] have reported a second locus of interest at D2S1238: PPH2 located within the original 27 cM locus identified by Nichols and Morse but more centromeric to BMPR2.[19] The problem may still be a technical one since mutations within the regulatory regions and introns of BMPR2 have not yet been sequenced. Extensive genome screening across the autosomes to look for other causative or modifying genes has not been reported.

BMPR2 mutations function via haploinsufficiency and a dominant negative effect

Both the Columbia group and the PPH Consortium identified a single mutated copy of BMPR2.[11,12] This suggests that the abnormal receptor functions either by haploinsufficiency or by exerting a dominant negative effect. Haploinsufficiency would produce approximately 25–75% of expected functioning receptors. Machado *et al.*[17] found loss of function using the *in vitro* expression of two recombinant *BMPR2* mutants, either the D485G or I860fs(+0), predicted to encode 83% of the normal protein, consistent with a model of haploinsufficiency.

Two recent functional analyses of *BMPR2* mutants are consistent with a dominant negative effect and with the requirement of additional factors for certain types of mutations.[15,16] Some *BMPRII* mutants demonstrated loss of most of their signal-transcriptional activity and ability to phosphorylate Smad proteins, whereas others retained the majority of their function. Missense mutations within the extracellular and kinase domains abrogated *BMPR* signal transduction abilities. Mutations in conserved cysteine residues in the extracellular and kinase domains were found in the cytoplasm, suggesting that the loss of signaling ability associated with these mutations was due to altered subcellular localization. Constructs with mutations causing truncation of the cytoplasmic tail retained their ability to transduce BMP signals and trafficked to the cell surface. Signalling by normal *BMPRII* was reduced by the addition of certain extracellular and kinase mutant constructs, consistent with a dominant negative effect.[15] A second functional analysis of *BMPRII* mutants[16] found similar results but noted that the transfection of mutant but not wild-type constructs into a mouse epithelial cell line led to activation of p38MAPK and increased serum-induced proliferation. They concluded that *BMPRII* mutations heterogeneously inhibit BMP/Smad-mediated signaling by diverse molecular mechanisms but that all mutants demonstrated a gain of function involving up-regulation of p38MAPK-dependent proproliferative pathways.

In addition, *BMPR* complexes on the surface of live cells provide different oligomerization modes.[20] Signals induced by binding *BMP2* to preformed receptor complexes activate the Smad pathway whereas *BMP2*-induced recruitment of receptors activate a different Smad-independent pathway, resulting in the induction of alkaline phosphatase activation via p38MAPK.[21] Deng *et al.*[12] had speculated initially that the MAPK pathway might be involved. Interestingly, Du *et al.*[22] have reported that angiopoietin-1 shuts off the expression of *BMPRIa*, providing a mechanistic link between FPPH and non-familial PPH via the BMP/TGF-β pathway. There may be other unrecognized and uninvestigated pathways as well.

The *BMPR2* mutation confers a pathological disadvantage

Grunig *et al.*[23] reported that asymptomatic carriers of the gene in FPPH families had elevated systolic PAP on stress echoes. This suggests that either there is an increased risk of developing PPH in this group or that elevated mPAP on exercise represents a *forme fruste* of the condition.

If substantiated, this would suggest that a reduction in numbers of functioning receptors does confer a pathological disadvantage regardless of the absence of symptoms. Furthermore, the fact that only 20% of those carrying the gene go on to develop overt PPH suggests that a single mutation alone is insufficient to cause PAH and that additional factors are required.

FAMILIAL PPH: TWO–HIT HYPOTHESIS AND RELATIONSHIP TO CANCER

The discovery of endothelial cell microsatellite instability in patients with FPPH and sporadic PPH (SPPH) supports the theory that PPH develops as a result of an additional insult in a susceptible individual.[24,25] The requirement of two signals, whether genetic or environmental, had originally been proposed by the same investigators[26] in their comparison of PPH to cancer, even prior to the *BMPR2* discovery. Microsatellite instability is caused by either the insertion or deletion of base pairs in DNA during faulty repair mechanisms and is frequently seen in malignancy.[13] Yeager *et al.*[25] demonstrated instability in up to 50% of plexogenic lesions in tissue taken from PPH patients. Somatic mutations could be acquired under such circumstances following an additional environmental or genetic stimulus.

BMPR2 MUTATIONS IN SPORADIC PPH: A FORM OF FAMILIAL PPH?

The low incidence of PPH and the presence of *BMPR2* mutations in FPPH led to the hypothesis that sporadic cases of PPH were in fact unrecognized FPPH and that *BMPR2* mutations could provide a single explanation for the disease process.[18,27] Thomson *et al.*[18] estimated that the frequency of the *BMPR2* mutations was in excess of 26% in their sample of sporadic PPH patients. Newer evidence suggests that their estimate is too high. Complete parental samples were lacking for at least five of the other *BMPR2* mutation-positive patients. In another study, three of 33 unrelated French patients (9%) who developed PPH following fenfluramine exposure had *BMPR2* mutations,[28] suggesting a frequency closer to the original NIH registry.

In contrast, support for sporadic PPH as a separate disease process has been demonstrated by microarray analysis of lung tissue from PPH, sporadic PPH and normal lung.[29] Geraci *et al.*[29] looked at the relative patterns of gene expression in normal, PPH and SPPH lung and found that only 307 genes were significantly different in their patterns of expression. There was a substantial imbalance in the expression of genes that control cell replication and apoptosis between normal and pulmonary hypertensive lung.[30] The most surprising finding was that patterns of gene expression seen in FPPH lung bore greater similarities to that of normal than that of sporadic PPH lung. In particular, there was up-regulation of a mutated TGF-β receptor and Bax in sporadic PPH, both of which have been implicated in neoplasia.[31,32] These mutations were not seen in FPPH, suggesting that sporadic and familial PPH are separate entities. Unfortunately, *BMPR2* mutations were not determined in either of the two studies by Geraci *et al.*

BMPR2 MUTATION AND ANOREXIGEN-INDUCED PULMONARY HYPERTENSION

The introduction of aminorex in the 1960s and fenfluramine and dexfenfluramine in the 1980s caused two distinct epidemics of pulmonary hypertension (for review see Chapter 13E). The fenfluramine studies suggested that a 3-month exposure increased the risk of developing pulmonary hypertension by a factor of 30.[33] However, case studies suggest the existence of a subgroup within this population that is at a further increased risk of rapid-onset pulmonary hypertension: Mark *et al.*[34] document the development of pulmonary hypertension following a 23-day history of exposure, whilst Douglas *et al.*[35] detail a family history of pulmonary hypertension following exposure to dexfenfluramine. There appears to be a subgroup further predisposed to developing the condition at an even earlier stage, possibly as a result of an inherited *BMPR2* mutation.[28]

Anorexigen-associated PPH and serotonin (5-HT) genetics

Aminorex, fenfluramine and dexfenfluramine are structurally related to amphetamines. They are thought to function as appetite suppressants via suppression of neuronal reuptake of serotonin (5-HT) in the hypothalamus. Several observations have implicated 5-HT as an etiological agent in the development of PPH. Plasma serotonin levels are elevated in PPH,[36] in PAH associated with platelet storage disease[37] and are up-regulated in von Gierke's (Ia) and (Ib) forms of glycogen storage disease.[38] The highest levels of 5-HT were found in a patient with type-1a glycogen storage disease and PAH.[39] Serotonin is a known mitogen for pulmonary vascular smooth muscle cells and is a potent vasoconstrictor.[40]

In animal studies, Eddahibi *et al.*[41] have shown that 5-HT is up-regulated in the lung following fenfluramine infusion in rats. They also demonstrated a significant increase in the number of 5-HT transporters (5-HTTs) expressed on rat pulmonary artery smooth muscle cells

in the same study. Both 5-HT and 5-HTT up-regulation are further augmented by hypoxic exposure. This has led to the speculation that 5-HTT overexpression may promote the development of PAH and may be involved in the genesis of hypoxic PAH. Fluoxetine and paroxetine, both 5-HTT inhibitors, have been shown to attenuate this response reducing pulmonary artery smooth muscle cell proliferation and pulmonary artery pressure.[40]

The discovery of 5-HTT polymorphisms affecting the numbers of expressed receptors has lent further support for the hypothesis that 5-HTT expression may be involved in the etiology of PPH.[42] The polymorphism involves either an insertion (long/L) or deletion (short/S) on the 5-HTT gene located at chromosome 17q11.2.[43] The L/L genotype results in a threefold increase in 5-HTT expression. This increase in 5-HTT expression has also been demonstrated in platelets as well as pulmonary artery smooth muscle cells and suggests that this polymorphism results in up-regulation of 5-HTT throughout the organism rather than in the pulmonary circulation alone.

Eddahibi *et al.*[44] found that 5-HTT mRNA and protein expression was significantly increased in pulmonary artery smooth muscle cells of PPH patients compared with controls. The frequency of the L/L genotype was 65% in PPH patients and only 27% in controls, but 5-HTT expression was significantly greater in L/L-positive PPH patients than in L/L-positive controls. This also suggests that further environmental factors are required for the development of overt PPH.

PULMONARY VENO-OCCLUSIVE DISEASE AND *BMPR2* MUTATIONS

Pulmonary veno-occlusive disease has also been linked to *BMPR2* mutation in one recently published case history.[45] The mutation was present in both the patient and her asymptomatic sibling, implying that it had been inherited from their mother rather than occurring as a spontaneous somatic mutation (for review see Chapter 14B).

HIV AND *BMPR2* MUTATIONS

No *BMPR2* mutations were found in 19 French patients with HIV-associated PAH, 11 via intravenous drug abuse and 8 via sexual or blood transmission.[46] The PAH response has been postulated to be immunologically mediated because the HIV virus was not detected in the lung lesions.[47] It is anticipated that frequency of PAH will continue to decline with the introduction of antiprotease therapies (for review see Chapter 13G).

HEREDITARY HEMORRHAGIC TELANGIECTASIA (HHT) AND DYSFUNCTION OF TGF-β SIGNALING

Hereditary hemorrhagic telangiectasia (HHT) or Osler–Weber–Rendu syndrome, an autosomal dominant condition, is associated with the development of angioid lesions in the lungs, brain and skin, leading to the development of arteriovenous malformations in affected tissues (for review see Chapter 13D). *HHT1* is identified with mutations in endoglin (ENG), an accessory receptor similar to TGF-β type 3 on chromosome 9 and *HHT2* with mutations in activin-like kinase 1 (ALK-1), a TGF-β type 1 receptor located on chromosome 12q13.[48,49] Arteriovenous malformations are more often associated with ENG mutations so it was a surprise when Trembath et al.[50] described six HHT type 2 families with ALK-1 mutations who had family members with PPH. The mutations in exons 2, 3, 6, 8 and 10 consisted of missense, nonsense and deletions. The newly appreciated mutations in exons 2 and 10 were in the extracellular and serine/threonine kinase domains, respectively. PAH associated with HHT re-emphasizes the importance of the TGF-β signaling pathway in the genesis of PAH from a variety of causes and its relation to cancer.

HYPOXIA–INDUCED PULMONARY HYPERTENSION

Hypoxic exposure results in pulmonary vasoconstriction,[51] which if maintained results in vascular wall remodeling[52] and histological changes similar to those seen in PPH.[3] There is evidence that these changes can be partially reversed with reoxygenation,[53] but if hypoxia is chronic, established pulmonary hypertension occurs with eventual right ventricular failure. In humans the effects of chronic hypoxic exposure can be seen in the development of conditions such as chronic mountain sickness (CMS) or in the right heart failure developed in association with hypoxic lung diseases such as chronic obstructive pulmonary disease (COPD) or fibrotic lung disease associated with connective tissue diseases (for reviews see Chapters 15A and 13D).

Animal studies have demonstrated a genetic component to hypoxia-related pulmonary hypertension. Weir et al.[54] demonstrated that cattle bred exclusively from susceptible animals at sea level developed signs of right heart failure when relocated to 2100 m. Cruz et al.[55] showed that intrauterine transfer of embryos from susceptible cattle into resistant surrogates demonstrated elevated mean pulmonary artery pressures when raised at altitude.

In man, Niermeyer et al.[56] demonstrated that Tibetan infants had consistently higher oxygen saturations over the first 4 months of life than infants of the Han Chinese. Native Tibetans have been resident on the Himalayan Plateau for approximately 25 000 years, the Han Chinese since the Chinese occupation in 1951. Niermeyer and colleagues theorized that genetic adaptation in the Tibetans had led to an improved ability to withstand the effects of a chronically hypoxic environment. In support of this theory Groves et al.[57] found that in adult Tibetan males the mPAP was similar to that expected at sea level. Also, all bar one of the subjects who underwent right heart catheterization were able to significantly increase their cardiac output on exertion.[57] Morrell and colleagues demonstrated that 6% of Kyrghyz highlanders, a population resident at 3000 m, go on to develop right heart failure in association with CMS. This figure was later estimated as 14% on the basis of electrocardiogram (ECG) changes indicative of cor pulmonale.[58,59]

Possible candidate genes associated with hypoxia related pulmonary hypertension

SEROTONIN TRANSPORTERS AND HYPOXIC LUNG DISEASE

See '*BMPR2* mutation and anorexigen-induced pulmonary hypertension'.

ANGIOTENSIN CONVERTING ENZYME (ACE) GENETICS AND HYPOXIC LUNG DISEASE

There has been a considerable body of work that looks at the role of ACE in the genesis of hypoxia-mediated pulmonary hypertension. Rigat et al.[60] identified two distinct ACE genotypes characterized either by the insertion (I) or deletion (D) of part of the genome located on chromosome 17q23. The I/I genotype producing the lowest, D/D the highest and I/D an intermediate level of ACE. It has been suggested that high circulating levels of ACE would have a negative effect in hypoxic pulmonary artery hypertension.[60] Morrell et al.[61] demonstrated that ACE was up-regulated in the muscular arteries of hypoxic rats although total lung ACE levels were reduced. They also demonstrated that ACE inhibitors partially attenuated hypoxic pulmonary artery hypertension in rats.[62]

Several studies examine a potential association of the ACE genotype with hypoxic lung diseases such as COPD. The results have been confusing. Abraham et al.[63] identified an association between hypoxic pulmonary artery hypertension and the D/D genotype. Paradoxically the D/D genotype was identified with lower mPAP and PVR than either the I/I or I/D genotype, suggesting that the D/D genotype is an adaptive phenomenon.[63] However, Kanazawa et al.[64] found that COPD patients with the D/D genotype had worse pulmonary hypertension than the other allelic combinations. Van Suylen et al.[65] found a negative association between D/D genotype and ECG evidence of right heart hypertrophy in male patients only. Surprisingly, Morrell and colleagues found that the I/I genotype was associated with an increased tendency to develop chronic mountain sickness.[59] A further study by the same group demonstrated that the I/I genotype was associated with a threefold increase in frequency of high-altitude pulmonary hypertension and that the mPAP was higher in asymptomatic carriers of the I/I genotype.[58] The I/I genotype may be linked to another causative gene. The functional role of ACE genotype in the etiology of hypoxic pulmonary hypertension in man is still unknown.

ENDOTHELIAL NITRIC OXIDE SYNTHASE (eNOS) GENETICS AND HYPOXIA–INDUCED PULMONARY HYPERTENSION IN ANIMALS

Nitric oxide (NO) is produced by endothelial cells by the action of endothelial nitric oxide sythase (eNOS) on L-arginine. It has a short half-life and acts as a local vasodilator modulating basal vascular tone. As with the data on ACE genetics, the studies on the influence of eNOS and NO are conflicting. In animal studies, mice null for eNOS have a greater rise in mPAP on exposure to hypoxia than similar animals maintained under normoxic conditions.[66] Interestingly, Fagan and co-workers also demonstrated that mice +/− for eNOS also developed a similar degree of PAH on exposure to hypoxia, suggesting that eNOS activity 50% of normal is inadequate to maintain basal pulmonary artery tone. However Quinlan et al.[67] demonstrated that mice deficient in eNOS showed less pulmonary vascular proliferation and remodeling to chronic hypoxia. Champion and colleagues[68] demonstrated that hypoxic pulmonary artery hypertension in mice null for eNOS could be ameliorated by endotracheal administration of eNOS attached to an adenoviral vector. Tyler et al.[69] demonstrated that eNOS protein and mRNA were up-regulated in the endothelium and neomuscularized pulmonary arteries of chronically hypoxic rats. It was suggested that this might be as a result of increased shear stress as only the hypertensive arteries appeared to be affected. Again the data are conflicting: Resta et al.[70] suggested that eNOS mRNA remained up-regulated following hypoxic exposure as a result of shear stress, but Everett et al.[71] found that eNOS mRNA and protein were not elevated as a result of iatrogenic left-to-right shunt in Sprague–Dawley rats.

NO GENETICS IN MAN

So far NO genetics have only been implicated in the development of high-altitude pulmonary edema (HAPE): the association of pulmonary hypertension, hypoxemia and pulmonary edema following acute exposure to altitude (for review see Chapter 24)[72,73] and not with pulmonary hypertension associated with chronic hypoxic exposure. HAPE occurs in susceptible individuals following rapid ascent to altitude combined with exertion. The pulmonary edema is thought to result from a combination of hypoxia-mediated vasoconstriction and endothelial incompetence. As a fulminant condition it is comparatively rare and is associated with reduced exhaled NO. Susceptible individuals improve on treatment with NO, acetazolamide and steroids.[74]

Droma et al.[75] found an association between the Glu298Asp polymorphism and the eNOS4b/a alleles localized to chromosome 7q35–6 and an increased risk of developing HAPE in a Japanese population. If both polymorphisms were present, then the risk of HAPE was significantly increased. The frequency of these genes varies between populations: Droma and colleagues found an incidence of 90.2% for the Glu298Asp allele in the indigenous Japanese population whilst Lacolley et al.[76] found a frequency of 56% in France. Similar variations in the eNOS4b/a allele frequency were demonstrated in Australian and Japanese populations. However, other work in a European population has not confirmed the Japanese group's conclusions.[77]

KEY POINTS

- PPH is a rare condition with an incidence of 1–2 per million. Of these, 6% represent familial, or FPPH, and the remainder are sporadic, or SPPH.
- Inheritance of FPPH appears to be autosomal dominant with variable penetrance of approximately 20%, suggesting that the mutation alone is insufficient to result in expression of the disease phenotype.
- *PPH1* was identified in 1987 to chromosome 2q31,33 but was later narrowed to 2q33.
- BMPRII was identified as the mutated gene product of 2q33. BMPRII is a member of the TGF-β superfamily, a group of serine kinase transmembrane signals which have also been implicated in other pathologies such as neoplasia and atherosclerosis.
- The *BMPR2* mutation is present in 55% of FPPH. *PPH2* has been located at a more centromeric region of the original 27 cM area identified in 1987. Further mutations may be identified following analysis of intronic portions of the gene and those located near the control region of the gene.
- Mutations have been identified throughout the *BMPR2* gene (except in exons 5,10 and 13) and take the form of missense, nonsense and frameshift mutations resulting in a non-functioning receptor. The mutations function by

both haploinsufficiency and dominant negative effects.
- SPPH appears to be a different pathological process from FPPH (on the basis of microarray analysis of SPPH, FPPH and normal lung tissue). It does not seem to represent unidentified FPPH.
- No evidence of *BMPR2* mutations have been discovered in PPH related to HIV infection. A single case study makes the association between pulmonary veno-occlusive disease (PVOD) and *BMPR2* mutation. There may be a subgroup in those with anorexigen-associated PPH who carry the *BMPR2* mutation and are at a higher risk of developing early-onset PPH in addition to the established risk associated with anorexigen use.
- HHT-associated PPH is linked with mutations in activin-like kinase-1 (ALK-1), a TGF-β type 1 receptor located on chromosome12q13.
- Hypoxia-associated PPH may be linked to the serotonin transporter (5-HTT) L/L genotype, the ACE I/I genotype and HAPE may be linked to the Glu298Asp polymorphism and eNOS4b/a alleles localized to chromosome 7q35–6.

REFERENCES

1 D'Alonzo GE, Barst RJ, Ayres SM et al. Survival in patients with primary pulmonary hypertension. Results from a national prospective registry. Ann Intern Med 1991; 115:343–9.
●2 Rich S, Dantzker DR, Ayres SM et al. Primary pulmonary hypertension: a national prospective study. Ann Intern Med 1987;107:216–23.
3 Stenmark KR, Meecham RP. Cellular and molecular mechanisms of pulmonary vascular remodelling. Annu Rev Physiol 1997;59:98–144.
4 Clarke RC, Coombs CF, Hadfield G et al. On certain abnormalities, congenital and acquired, of the pulmonary artery. Q J Med 1927;21:51–68.
●5 Loyd JE, Butler MG, Ford TM et al. Genetic anticipation and abnormal gender ratio at birth in familial primary pulmonary hypertension. Am J Respir Crit Care Med 1995;152:93–7.
●6 Loyd JE, Primm RK, Newman JH. Familial primary pulmonary hypertension: clinical patterns. Am Rev Respir Dis 1984; 129:194–7.
●7 Morse JH, Jones AC, Barts RJ et al. Mapping of familial primary pulmonary hypertension locus (PPH1) to chromosome 2q31-32. Circulation 1997;95:2603–6.
●8 Nichols WC, Koller DL, Slovis B et al. Localization of the gene for familial primary pulmonary hypertension to chromosome 2q31-32. Nat Genet 1997;15:277–80.
●9 Deng Z, Haghighi F, Helleby L et al. Fine mapping of PPH1, a gene for familial primary pulmonary hypertension, to a 3 cM region on chromosome 2q22. Am J Respir Crit Care Med 2000;161:1055–9.
●10 Machado RD, Pauciulo MW, Fretwell N et al. A physical and transcript map bases upon refinement of the critical interval for PPH1, a gene for familial primary pulmonary hypertension. Genomics 2000;68:220–8.
●11 Lane KB, Machada RD, Pauciulo MW et al. Heterozygous germline mutations in BMPR2, encoding a TGF-beta receptor, cause familial primary pulmonary hypertension. The International PPH Consortium. Nat Genet 2000;26:81–4.
●12 Deng Z, Morse JH, Slager SL et al. Familial primary pulmonary hypertension (gene PPH1) is caused by mutations in the bone morphogenetic protein receptor-II gene. Am J Hum Genet 2000;67:737–44.
♦13 Massague J, Wotton D. Transcriptional control by the TGF-beta/Smad signalling system. EMBO J 2000;19:1745–54.
♦14 Blobe GC, Schiemann WP, Lodish HF. Mechanisms of disease: role of transforming growth factor (beta) in human disease. N Engl J Med 2000; 342:1350–8.
15 Nishihara A, Watabe T, Imamura T et al. Functional heterogeneity of bone morphogenetic protein receptor II mutants found in patients with primary pulmonary hypertension. Mol Biol Cell 2002;13:3055–63.
16 Rudarakanchana N, Flanagan JA, Chen H et al. Functional analysis of bone morphogenetic protein type II receptor mutations underlying primary pulmonary hypertension. Hum Mol Genet 2002;11:1517–25.
●17 Machado RD, Pauciulo NW, Thomson JR et al. BMPR2 haplo-insufficiency as the inherited molecular mechanism for primary pulmonary hypertension. Am J Hum Genet 2001; 68:92–102.
18 Thomson JR, Machada RD, Pauciulo NW et al. Sporadic primary pulmonary hypertension is associated with germline mutations of the gene encoding BMPR-II, a receptor member of the TGF beta family. J Med Genet 2000;37:741–5.
●19 Janssen B, Rinderman M, Barth U et al. Linkage analysis in a large family with primary pulmonary hypertension: genetic heterogeneity and a second primary pulmonary hypertension locus on 2q31-32. Chest 2002;121(3 Suppl):54s–6s.
20 Gilboa L, Nohe A, Geisendorfer T et al. Bone morphogenetic protein receptor complexes on the surface of live cells: a new oligomerization mode for serine/threonine kinase receptors. Mol Biol Cell 2000;11:1023–35.
21 Nohe A, Hassel S, Ehrlich M et al. The mode of bone morphogenetic protein (BMP) receptor oligomerization determines different BMP-2 signalling pathways. J Biol Chem 2001;277:5330–8.
22 Du L, Sullivan CD, Chu D et al. Signalling molecules in nonfamilial pulmonary hypertension. N Engl J Med 2003; 348:500–9.
●23 Grunig E, Janssen B, Mereles D et al. Abnormal pulmonary artery pressure response in asymptomatic carriers of primary pulmonary hypertension gene. Circulation 2000;102: 1145–50.
●24 Yeager ME, Golpon H, Voelkel NF et al. Microsatellite mutational analysis of endothelial cells within plexiform lesions from patients with familial, pediatric, and sporadic pulmonary hypertension. Chest 2002;121:61S.
25 Yeager ME, Halley GR, Golpon HA et al. Microsatellite instability of endothelial cell growth and apoptosis genes within plexiform lesions in primary pulmonary hypertension. Circ Res 2001;88:e2–11.

26 Voelkel NF, Cool C, Lee SD *et al*. Primary pulmonary hypertension between inflammation and cancer. *Chest* 1998;**114**(3 Suppl):225s–30s.

27 Newman JH, Wheeler L, Lane KB *et al*. Mutation in the gene for bone morphogenetic protein receptor II as a cause of primary pulmonary hypertension in a large kindred. *N Engl J Med* 2001;**345**:319–24.

28 Humbert M, Deng Z, Simmoneau G *et al*. BMPR2 germline mutations in pulmonary hypertension associated with fenfluramine derivatives. *Eur Respir J* 2002;**20**:518–23.

29 Geraci MW, Hoshikawa Y, Yeager M *et al*. Gene expression profiles in pulmonary hypertension. *Chest* 2002;**121**:104s–5s.

●30 Geraci MW, Moore M, Gessell R *et al*. Gene expression patterns in the lungs of patients with primary pulmonary hypertension: a gene microarray analysis. *Circ Res* 2001; **88**:555–62.

31 Rampino N, Yamamoto H, Ionor Y *et al*. Somatic frameshift mutations in the Bax gene in colon cancers of the microsatelite mutator phenotype. *Science* 1997;**275**:967–9.

32 Meyeroff LL, Parsons R, Kum SJ *et al*. A transforming growth factor beta type II mutation common in colon and gastric but rare in endometrial cancers with microsatellite instability. *Cancer Res* 1995;**55**:5545–7.

33 Abenheim L, Moride Y, Brenot F. Appetite suppressant drugs and the risk of primary pulmonary hypertension. *N Engl J Med* 1996;**335**:609–16.

34 Mark EJ, Patalas E, Chang HT *et al*. Fatal pulmonary hypertension associated with short-term use of fenfluramine and phentermine. *N Engl J Med* 1997;**337**:602–6.

35 Douglas JG, Monro JF, Kitchin AH *et al*. Pulmonary hypertension and fenfluramine. *Br Med J (Clin Res Edn)* 1981;**283**:881–3.

36 Herve P, Launay JM, Scrobahaci ML *et al*. Increased plasma serotonin in primary pulmonary hypertension. *Am J Med* 1995;**99**:249–54.

37 Herve P, Drouet L, Dosquet C *et al*. Primary pulmonary hypertension in a patient with a familial platelet storage pool disease: role of serotonin. *Am J Med* 1990;**89**:117–20.

38 Pizzo CJ. Type I glycogen storage disease with focal nodular hyperplasia of the liver and vasoconstrictive pulmonary hypertension. *Paediatrics* 1980;**65**:341–3.

39 Humbert M, Labrune P, Sitbon O *et al*. Pulmonary arterial hypertension and type-1 glycogen-storage disease: the serotonin hypothesis. *Eur Respir J* 2002;**20**:59–65.

40 Eddahibbi S, Fabre V, Boni C *et al*. Induction of serotonin transporter by hypoxia in pulmonary vascular smooth muscle cells. Relationship with the mitogenic action of serotonin. *Circ Res* 1999;**84**:329–36.

41 Eddahibi S, Adnot S, Frisdal E *et al*. Dexfenfluramine-associated changes in 5-hydroxytryptamine transporter expression and development of hypoxic pulmonary hypertension in rats. *J Pharmacol Exp Ther* 2000;**148**:148–54.

42 Lesch KP, Bengel D, Heils A *et al*. Association of anxiety-related traits with a polymorphism in the serotonin transporter gene regulatory region. *Science* 1996;**274**: 1527–31.

43 Ramamoorthy S. Antidepressant and cocaine-sensitive human serotonin transporter: molecular cloning, expression, and chromosomal localization. *Proc Natl Acad Sci USA* 1993;**90**:2542–6.

44 Eddahibi S, Humbert M, Fadel E *et al*. Serotonin transporter overexpression is responsible for pulmonary artery smooth muscle hyperplasia in primary pulmonary hypertension. *J Clin Invest* 2001;**108**:1141–50.

45 Runo JR, Vnencak-Jones CL, Prince M *et al*. Pulmonary veno-occlusive disease caused by an inherited mutation in bone morphogenetic protein receptor II. *Am J Respir Crit Care Med* 2003;**167**:889–94.

46 Nunes H, Humbert M, Sitbon O *et al*. Prognostic factors for survival in human immunodeficiency virus-associated pulmonary arterial hypertension. *Am J Respir Crit Care Med* 2003;**167**:1433–9.

47 Mette SA, Palevsky HI, Peitra GG *et al*. Primary pulmonary hypertension in association with human immunodeficiency virus infection. A possible viral etiology for some forms of hypertensive pulmonary arteriopathy. *Am Rev Respir Dis* 1992;**145**:1196–200.

48 Burg JN, Uttmacher AE, Marchuk DA *et al*. Clinical heterogeneity in hereditary haemorrhagic telangiectasia: are pulmonary arteriovenous malformations more common in families linked to endoglin? *J Med Genet* 1996;**33**:256–7.

49 Johnson DW, Berg JN, Baldwin MA *et al*. Mutations in the activin receptor-like kinase 1 gene in hereditary haemorrhagic telangiectasia type 2. *Nat Genet* 1996; **13**:189–95.

50 Trembath RC, Thomson JR, Machado RD *et al*. Clinical and molecular genetic features of pulmonary hypertension in patients with hereditary hemorrhagic telangiectasia. *N Engl J Med* 2001;**345**:325–34.

51 Euler v US, Liljestrand J. Observations on the pulmonary arterial blood pressure in the cat. *Acta Physiol Scand* 1946;**12**:301–20.

52 Meyrick B, Reid L. Hypoxia and the incorporation of ^{3}H-thymidine by cells of the rat pulmonary arteries and alveolar wall. *Am J Pathol* 1979;**96**:51–69.

53 Meyrick B, Reid L. Hypoxia-induced structural changes in the media and adventitia of the rat hilar pulmonary artery and their regression. *Am J Pathol* 1980;**100**:151–69.

54 Weir EK, Tucker A, Reeves JT *et al*. The genetic factor influencing pulmonary hypertension in cattle at high altitude. *Cardiovasc Res* 1974;**8**:745–9.

55 Cruz JC, Reeves JT, Russell BE *et al*. Embryo transplanted calves: the pulmonary hypertensive trait is genetically transmitted. *Proc Soc Exp Biol Med* 1980;**164**:142–5.

56 Niermeyer S, Yang P, Shanmina *et al*. Arterial oxygen saturation in Tibetan and Han infants born in Lhasa, Tibet. *N Engl J Med* 1995;**333**:1248–52.

57 Groves BM, Droma T, Sutton JR *et al*. Minimal hypoxic pulmonary hypertension in normal Tibetans at 3,658 m. *J Appl Physiol* 1993;**74**:312–18.

58 Aldashev AA, Sarybaev AS, Sydykov AS *et al*. Characterization of high-altitude pulmonary hypertension in the Kyrgyz: association with angiotensin-converting enzyme genotype. *Am J Respir Crit Care Med* 2002;**166**:1396–402.

59 Morrell NW, Sarybaev AS, Alikhan A *et al*. Ace genotype and risk of high altitude pulmonary hypertension in Kyrghyz highlanders. *Lancet* 1999;**353**:814.

60 Rigat B, Humbert H, Alhenc-Gelas F *et al*. An insertion/deletion polymorphism in the angiotensin I converting

enzyme gene accounting for half the variance of serum enzyme levels. *J Clin Invest* 1990;**86**:1343–6.

61 Morrell NW, Morris KG, Stenmark KR. Role of angiotensin-converting enzyme and angiotensin II in development of hypoxic pulmonary hypertension. *Am J Physiol* 1995; **269**(4 Pt 2):H1186–94.

62 Morrell NW, Atochina EN, Morris KG *et al.* Angiotensin converting enzyme expression is increased in small pulmonary arteries of rats with hypoxia-induced pulmonary hypertension. *J Clin Invest* 1995;**96**:1823–33.

63 Abraham WT, Reynolds MV, Gottschall B *et al.* Importance of angiotensin converting enzyme in pulmonary hypertension. *Cardiology* 1995;**86**(Suppl 1):9–15.

64 Kanazawa H, Otsuka T, Hirata K *et al.* Association between the angiotensin-converting enzyme gene polymorphisms and tissue oxygenation during exercise in patients with COPD. *Chest* 2002;**121**:697–701.

65 van Suylen RJ, Wouters EF, Pennings HJ *et al.* The DD genotype of the angiotensin converting enzyme gene is negatively associated with right ventricular hypertrophy in male patients with chronic obstructive pulmonary disease. *Am J Respir Crit Care Med* 1999;**159**:1791–5.

66 Fagan KA, Fouty BW, Tyler RC *et al.* The pulmonary circulation of homozygous or heterozygous eNOS-null mice is hyperresponsive to mild hypoxia. *J Clin Invest* 1999; **103**:291–9.

67 Quinlan TR, Li D, Laubach VE *et al.* eNOS-deficient mice show reduced pulmonary vascular proliferation and remodelling to chronic hypoxia. *Am J Physiol Lung Cell Mol Physiol* 2000;**279**:L641–50.

68 Champion HC, Bivalacqua TJ, Greenberg SS *et al.* Adenoviral gene transfer of endothelial nitric-oxide synthase (eNOS) partially restores normal pulmonary arterial pressure in eNOS deficient mice. *Proc Natl Acad Sci USA* 2002; **99**:13248–53.

69 Tyler RC, Muramatsu M, Abman SH *et al.* Variable expression of endothelial NO synthase in three forms of rat pulmonary hypertension. *Am J Physiol Lung Cell Mol Physiol* 1999; **276**:L297–303.

70 Resta TC, Chicoine LG, Omdahl JL *et al.* Maintained upregulation of pulmonary eNOS gene and protein expression during recovery from chronic hypoxia. *Am J Physiol Heart Circ Physiol* 1999;**276**:H699–708.

71 Everett AD, Le Cras TD, Xue C *et al.* eNOS expression is not altered in pulmonary vascular remodelling due to increased pulmonary blood flow. *Am J Physiol Lung Cell Mol Physiol* 1998;**274**:L1058–65.

72 Busch T, Bartsch P, Papert D *et al.* Hypoxia decreases exhaled nitric oxide in mountaineers susceptible to high-altitude pulmonary edema. *Am J Respir Crit Care Med* 2001;**163**: 368–73.

73 Duplain H, Sartori C, Lepori M *et al.* Exhaled nitric oxide in high-altitude pulmonary edema: role in the regulation of pulmonary vascular tone and evidence for a role against inflammation. *Am J Respir Crit Care Med* 2000;**162**:221–4.

74 Scherrer U, Vollenwieder L, Delbays A *et al.* Inhaled nitric oxide for high-altitude pulmonary edema. *N Engl J Med* 1996;**334**:624–9.

75 Droma Y, Hanaoka M, Ota M *et al.* Positive association of the endothelial nitric oxide synthase gene polymorphisms with high-altitude pulmonary edema. *Circulation* 2002;**106**: 826–30.

76 Lacolley P, Gautier S, Poirier O. Nitric oxide synthase gene polymorphisms, blood pressure and aortic stiffness in normotensive and hypertensive subjects. *J Hypertens* 1998; **16**:31–5.

77 Bartsch P, Haefeli WE, Gasse C. Lack of association of high altitude pulmonary edema and polymorphisms on the NO pathway. *High Alt Med Biol* 2002;**3**:105 (Abstract).

The diagnosis of pulmonary hypertension

7

Clinical features

ANDREW J PEACOCK

INTRODUCTION

Pulmonary hypertension is not a disease, but a syndrome in which the pressure in the pulmonary circulation is raised. The clinical features of this syndrome are mostly related to the degree of pulmonary artery pressure elevation and its effect on the right ventricle. Although primary pulmonary hypertension (PPH) is a very rare disease, pulmonary arterial hypertension (PAH) is remarkably common and is estimated to be the third most common cardiovascular syndrome after coronary artery disease and systemic hypertension. Pulmonary hypertension is common because raised blood pressure in the pulmonary circulation can accompany nearly all cardiac and pulmonary disease. Previous classifications of the causes of pulmonary hypertension distinguished between PPH, where there appears to be a primary histological vasculopathy but the cause is unknown, and secondary pulmonary hypertension (SPH) where pulmonary hypertension occurs in response to a known stimulus. This classification outlived its usefulness when it became clear that several types of 'secondary pulmonary hypertension' had similar histology to primary unexplained pulmonary hypertension, suggesting common biological pathways. Furthermore, with the advent of successful treatment for pulmonary hypertension it became clear that PPH and SPH due to connective tissue disease, HIV and portopulmonary syndromes responded in a similar fashion to intravenous therapies such as epoprostenol. This prompted the Evian Symposium in 1998 where physicians and scientists gathered from all over the world and spent time developing a new classification for pulmonary arterial hypertension (PAH) (see Chapter 12). In this classification, pulmonary hypertension is divided into pulmonary hypertension due to disease of the pulmonary arteries (PAH), e.g. PPH, connective tissue disease (CTD)-associated PAH, HIV-PAH, portopulmonary PAH, pulmonary hypertension associated with disorders of the respiratory system, pulmonary hypertension due to thrombotic or embolic disease and pulmonary venous hypertension. Within the general category of PAH, pathology and response to treatment may be similar, suggesting a common final pathobiological pathway (see Chapter 13A). The cellular processes may be primary but may also be a response to the deranged hemodynamics,[1] suggesting that the histological change may be, in some way, coupled to the vasomotor response.[2] Interestingly, despite similarities in histology, there may be marked differences in the rate of onset of the disease, its progression and its response to treatment. For example, congenital heart disease with left-to-right shunt causes a gradual increase in pulmonary vascular remodeling and hence pulmonary artery pressure, which can reach systemic levels. PPH is more rapidly progressive but the most rapidly progressive form of PAH is pulmonary hypertension associated with CREST syndrome, which also tends to be resistant to vasodilator therapy. The differences in progression and in etiology, whether familial, related to infection, related to autoimmune disease or related to anorexigen use have suggested the 'single, dual or multiple hit' hypothesis: a genetic susceptibility may exist which only results in clinical signs of disease when an additional factor exists, such as anorexigen use, exposure to high altitude, or pregnancy.

The main problem for clinicians interested in the pulmonary circulation has been the long delays between the onset of disease and its diagnosis. This delay may be because:

- Pulmonary hypertension is difficult to diagnose because the symptoms and signs are vague and basic investigations are unhelpful.
- Until the new era of treatment for pulmonary hypertension there was little urgency to establish the diagnosis, since the prognosis was bleak and the physicians were unable to offer much in the way of disease-modifying therapy.
- Pulmonary hypertension was considered to be a very rare condition and therefore did not prompt a high index of suspicion for the diagnostician.
- There is no sphygmomanometer for the pulmonary circulation. Measurements of pressure and flow could only be made invasively by right heart catheterization.

These obvious hurdles in the diagnostic pathway have meant that the average delay between onset of symptoms of pulmonary hypertension and diagnosis approaches 2 years in most studies.[3]

This delay is now being overcome and the reasons for improved diagnosis are as follows:

- The discovery of the gene for pulmonary hypertension. This is present in a high percentage of cases of familial primary pulmonary hypertension and approximately 25% of cases of sporadic primary pulmonary hypertension. Its discovery will eventually lead to genetic screening and has also prompted new avenues of pathobiological research (see Chapters 5 and 6).
- Non-invasive screening in the form of echocardiography is now widely available (see Chapter 8).
- The availability of non-invasive testing and the new classification of pulmonary hypertension allow us to screen more effectively for the presence of pulmonary hypertension even in the asymptomatic stage.
- The availability of effective treatment. The last few years have seen an explosion of effective treatments for pulmonary hypertension. The first was continuous intravenous epoprostenol (prostacyclin), followed by the prostacyclin analogs iloprost, beroprost, teprostinil and the endothelin receptor antagonist bosentan. At the time of writing, further trials are under way using phosphodiesterase inhibitors and arginine supplementation.
- We now have better techniques for evaluating the effectiveness of treatment, in particular sophisticated

studies of hemodynamics by cardiac catheter, echocardiography, magnetic resonance imaging or cardiopulmonary exercise testing.

This chapter examines the features of the epidemiology of pulmonary hypertension which enhance our clinical understanding of the various conditions whose common feature is an increase in pulmonary artery pressure. The clinical symptoms and signs associated with pulmonary hypertension and right heart dysfunction are discussed. Symptoms and signs that might lead to the diagnosis of the diseases associated with pulmonary hypertension are addressed. Lastly, those investigations that have improved our understanding of the clinical features of the pulmonary hypertension, both in terms of understanding the effects of a raised pulmonary vascular resistance *per se* and also our understanding of the various conditions that lead to a change in pulmonary vascular resistance are discussed.

EPIDEMIOLOGICAL FEATURES ASSISTING THE CLINICAL DIAGNOSIS OF PULMONARY HYPERTENSION

The syndrome of pulmonary hypertension has many causes, risk factors and associations. A thorough knowledge of these factors may allow improvement in the clinical diagnosis of pulmonary hypertension and also allow a better understanding of its clinical and pathobiological course.

Pulmonary arterial hypertension

GENETIC ASPECTS

A germ-line mutation in the gene for the bone morphogenetic protein receptor 2 (*BMPR2*) has been found in a number of families with primary pulmonary hypertension.[4–6] This mutation occurs in most cases of familial primary pulmonary hypertension but also occurs in 26% of patients with 'sporadic' primary pulmonary hypertension.[7] Furthermore, it is apparent that patients with 'sporadic' primary pulmonary hypertension can transmit the disease. *BMPR2* may not, however, be the only important genetic polymorphism. Mutation of the *ALK-1* gene, another member of the TGF-β superfamily (like *BMPR2*) is found in the rare condition of PPH associated with hereditary hemorrhagic telangectasia.[8] The deletion homozygote of the *ACE* gene may be important in patients who have chronic hypoxic lung disease[9] and is also associated with an inability to ascend to extreme altitude, possibly because of the excessive hypoxic pulmonary vasoconstriction limiting exercise. Finally, abnormalities of the serotonin transport gene promoter seems to be more common in patients with PPH, possibly because the increased transcription of serotonin transporter results in an increased take-up of serotonin into the cell where it can act as a growth promoter.[10] At present there is no large-scale program of screening the population for these genetic defects or indeed other genetic defects which may be important (e.g. NO synthase, endothelin receptors, etc.) but the evidence is good enough at present that family members of those with pulmonary hypertension should be screened for the presence of pulmonary hypertension. Progress has been made in this area, e.g. it has been shown that asymptomatic carriers of the gene have abnormal pulmonary artery pressure responses to exercise and hypoxia.[11] This, of course, raises three issues:

- **first**, should patients with abnormal gene mutations and polymorphisms be subjected to tests to indicate the presence of early pulmonary vascular disease;
- **second**, if early disease is found, should they be treated before symptoms develop;
- **third**, should they receive genetic counseling to try and ensure that the gene is not transmitted?

These are important ethical questions that are outside the remit of this chapter but, nevertheless, will require answers in the near future.

DEMOGRAPHICS

Primary pulmonary hypertension is more common in women. This has been thought to be due to the fact that males with the condition died *in utero* but, interestingly, in children the female to male ratio is 1:1 and then it becomes 1.7:1 in adults.[12] There appears to be no relationship between pulmonary hypertension and race. The mean age for developing the condition is 40 but 8% of patients are aged over 60.[12] There is evidence that elderly people have diastolic dysfunction of the heart and decreased compliance of both systemic and pulmonary vessels. It may be these features that act as triggers when there is an underlying tendency to pulmonary hypertension. Certainly, in this author's experience, it is common for patients to have a history of systemic hypertension. The association between the two is not yet understood and arteriosclerosis is extremely rare in the pulmonary circulation.

ENVIRONMENTAL FACTORS

The best-known external trigger to pulmonary hypertension is the anorectic drugs. It is ironic that the second WHO symposium was held at the time of the second epidemic of pulmonary hypertension associated with appetite suppressant usage. The first WHO symposium was held after the 1960s epidemic when the appetite suppressant aminorex was responsible for a 1000-fold increased risk of pulmonary hypertension. This lesson was not learned, however, and new anorectic drugs subsequently appeared; more than five million prescriptions were written for the fenfluramine anorectics before they were withdrawn from the market.[13] Luckily, the association was discovered early and a case-controlled study showed an overall increase in risk using these drugs of 6.3-fold, or 23-fold if they were used for more than 3 months.[14] Subsequently, a study of 579 patients in the USA[15] showed that the risk of primary pulmonary hypertension was increased by 7.5 times if anorectics were used for more than 6 months. Not surprisingly, there is an increased female to male ratio of pulmonary hypertension secondary to anorectic drugs, and this is particularly true in Belgium and France where the greatest number of prescriptions per capita were written.[16] The exact mechanism by which the anorexigens cause pulmonary hypertension is not understood (see Chapter 13E). A front-runner is likely to be the change in 5-HT transport that occurs in response to their use.[17]

CONNECTIVE TISSUE DISEASE

The fact that up to 10% of patients with PPH have Raynaud's phenomenon has prompted exhaustive investigation into the association between autoimmune disease and pulmonary hypertension. Interestingly, the rates of pulmonary hypertension in these diseases seem to vary from one study to another. For example, in France approximately 10% of patients with PAH have connective tissue disease.[12] However, in the recent treatment trials for PAH, approximately 50% of the patients had connective tissue disease-associated pulmonary hypertension. In order to decide whether or not to screen patients with connective tissue disease for the presence of pulmonary hypertension, it is necessary to look at the figures the other way round. This subject has been reviewed by Hoeper,[18] who found that approximately 5–10% of patients with systemic lupus erythematosus (SLE) had pulmonary arterial disease. This is higher in patients with the CREST variant of systemic sclerosis, where figures range between 10 and 30%; postmortem studies suggest that up to 50% of patients with CREST have pulmonary arterial disease. Figures from Japan suggest that 6% of patients with SLE[19] have pulmonary vascular disease and that it improves with treatment of the SLE using cyclophosphamide. The discrepancies between the clinical and the postmortem studies underscore the deficiency of our current methods for the diagnosis and assessment of patients with pulmonary arterial disease. Clearly, pulmonary vascular disease is more common than we have previously thought but only becomes manifest in those in whom the pulmonary vascular disease progresses faster and further (for review see Chapter 13D).

HIV INFECTION

The association of pulmonary hypertension with HIV infection has been known for a number of years (see Chapter 13G) but the mechanism remains unknown. The histological characteristics are similar to primary pulmonary hypertension, i.e. a plexogenic arteriopathy. The syndrome appears to be particularly prevalent in intravenous drug abusers,[12] suggesting that intravenous injection is an additional risk factor. The incidence of pulmonary hypertension in HIV infection in France is 0.6%. Survival of HIV pulmonary hypertension is poor, averaging 6 months in one study,[20] although, as with SLE, case reports have suggested that antiretroviral treatment may improve the pulmonary hypertension.[21]

PORTAL HYPERTENSION

The incidence of pulmonary hypertension occurring in the setting of cirrhosis and portal hypertension varies from 0.7% to 3.1%.[12,22] In the National Institutes of Health (NIH) Registry,[3] 8% of the patients with pulmonary arterial hypertension also had portal hypertension. Patients with cirrhosis but without portal hypertension do not develop pulmonary hypertension, suggesting that the development of pulmonary hypertension must be related to changes in the portal circulation (for review see Chapter 13F).

OTHERS

There are a number of other seemingly unrelated diseases and syndromes associated with pulmonary arterial hypertension and it is to be hoped that these associations will lead us to a clearer understanding of the pathobiology of the disease. For example, pulmonary arterial hypertension is associated with thyroid disease (in one study 22% of patients with primary pulmonary hypertension were hypothyroid),[23] with amyloid,[24] with hemoglobinopathies,[12] with splenectomy[25] and with the ingestion of toxic oil as in the infamous outbreak in Spain. Importantly, some of these syndromes are reversible. For example, approximately 8% of those with toxic oil syndrome developed pulmonary arterial hypertension but this regressed in 74%, suggesting that once the cause was removed the process was reversed. Also of interest was the high male to female ratio in the toxic oil syndrome. The cause of pulmonary arterial hypertension in the hemoglobinopathies is unknown. In patients with splenectomy it is possible that the abnormal red cells that would normally be cleared by the spleen result in platelet activation in the pulmonary vascular bed causing *in situ* thrombosis that is often difficult to distinguish from plexogenic pulmonary arteriopathy.

Hypoxic lung disease

It has been known since 1946 that alveolar hypoxia produces pulmonary hypertension. Interestingly, hypoxemia without alveolar hypoxia (such as in cyanotic heart disease) does not cause pulmonary hypertension to the same extent, suggesting that the oxygen sensor is indeed on the alveolar side of the small pulmonary arteries. Because hypoxia is a potent pulmonary vasoconstrictor, hypoxia-induced pulmonary hypertension can be found at altitude. It occurs in 5% of those residing between 3000 and 5000 m and 27% of those living between 4500 and 5000 m.[12] The most common cause of secondary pulmonary hypertension is chronic obstructive pulmonary disease, where it appears that a minimum daily level of hypoxia is necessary for its establishment.[26] There are several mechanisms by which hypoxia could cause pulmonary hypertension:

- hypoxia causes contraction of the entire pulmonary vascular bed, of isolated pulmonary arteries and even isolated pulmonary artery smooth muscle cells;
- hypoxia stimulates both the production of hypoxia-inducible factor-α (HIF-α) and the signaling pathways associated with the stress kinase p38. This raises the possibility that hypoxia may be an additional element in the development of the pulmonary arterial hypertension even when it is not its primary cause. To this end, it has been noted that patients with primary pulmonary hypertension tend to desaturate particularly at night, possibly related to reduced ventilation. It is also known that up to one-quarter of patients with obstructive sleep apnea develop pulmonary hypertension[27] (for review see Chapter 15B).

Thromboembolic pulmonary hypertension

Obstruction of the pulmonary arteries by a clot produces pulmonary hypertension. Since removal of the clot at surgery does not always cure the pulmonary hypertension, intrinsic abnormalities in the pulmonary vessel, in addition to the mechanical obstruction from the clot, may also be responsible (for review, see Chapter 17). Furthermore, controversy exists about whether the clot really migrated from peripheral veins or develops *in situ*.[28] To add to this debate it has been found that although thrombotic risk factors are not usually present in primary pulmonary hypertension, antiphospholipid antibodies are present in both primary pulmonary hypertension (10%) and thromboembolic pulmonary hypertension (20%).[12] The pathological variant of pulmonary hypertension known as thrombotic pulmonary hypertension likely results from thrombosis *in situ* due to low flow in the pulmonary circulation, resulting from endothelial damage, abnormal circulating platelets, or other elements. Since anticoagulants alone improve survival in primary pulmonary hypertension, thromboembolic pulmonary hypertension and primary pulmonary hypertension might be have more in common than previously suggested.

Congenital heart disease

Approximately 5% of patients with congenital heart disease will develop pulmonary hypertension. It is thought that, in the setting of inter-atrial or interventricular septal defects, left-to-right shunting results in high flow and higher pressure in the low-pressure right circulation, causing sheer stress and endothelial damage, leading to pulmonary vascular remodeling and pulmonary hypertension. However, in some cases the pulmonary hypertension is out of proportion to the degree of shunt,[29] suggesting that these pulmonary vessels have a propensity to develop histological changes in the presence of shunt-induced higher flow.

SYMPTOMS

The classical, albeit non-specific, symptom of pulmonary arterial hypertension is exertional breathlessness. The fact that breathlessness may not be associated with any additional symptoms of cardiopulmonary disease has led in the past to delays in diagnosis of up to 2 years,[3] a problem that persists.[14] A typical case might be a young woman in her 20s and slightly overweight who presents to her general practitioner with breathlessness. Initially this is put down to lack of physical fitness. Later it may be put down to hyperventilation syndrome and the diagnosis only becomes apparent when additional factors develop such as chest pain, syncope or ankle swelling.[3] The exertional breathlessness is probably due to the inability of the right heart to raise output on exercise. It is now becoming clear that cardiac index is the most useful prognostic factor in patients with pulmonary arterial hypertension. It is said that symptoms do not develop until the pulmonary artery pressure has doubled, but breathlessness can vary depending on the etiology and severity of the pulmonary hypertension. For example, Delcroix[16] showed that anorexigen-induced pulmonary hypertension is commonly associated with shortness of breath, but the severity is generally less than that seen in patients from the NIH Registry for the same degree of pulmonary arterial pressure. An interesting observation is that the duration of breathlessness appears, at least in one study, to be inversely related to the survival.[30] This

might suggest that the breathlessness is not simply related to the pulmonary vascular changes but has other causes; it is possible that an increased sensation of breathlessness might protect the patient from high exertion which, in turn, induces worsening vascular changes. While breathlessness is the most common symptom, the other two symptoms that usually lead to the diagnosis are syncope and chest pain.

Chest pain is thought to be due to relative ischemia of the right ventricular myocardium. The expression 'relative ischemia' is used because coronary artery anatomy is usually normal but, because of the grossly thickened right ventricle, there is inadequate coronary supply. Furthermore, the reduced cardiac output and reduced intra-aortic pressure also reduce the coronary artery perfusion pressure.

Syncope, which usually occurs on exercise, is thought to be due to right ventricular encroachment on the left ventricle, decreasing left ventricular stroke volume particularly on exercise, and thus reducing forward systemic cardiac flow. Syncope is usually thought of as an ominous sign because it indicates severe pulmonary arterial changes and dilating right ventricle.

Shortness of breath, chest pain and syncope are the classic symptoms of pulmonary hypertension but other symptoms related to right ventricular dysfunction may also be present, such as ankle swelling, ascites (which appears to occur in patients on prostacyclin even where there is very little ankle swelling, suggesting a local hepatic dysfunction) and anorexia, presumably due to gastric mucosal edema. Finally, there may be other symptomatic clues that are helpful: for example, the syndrome may have been brought on by triggers such as pregnancy [especially in atrial septal defect (ASD)], high altitude (particularly in pulmonary artery vascular abnormalities such as pulmonary artery atresia) and the use of anorexigens. There may also be symptoms of other underlying diseases that are known to be associated with pulmonary hypertension such as HIV infection, thyroid disease, connective tissue disease, venous thrombotic disease or primary cardiac disease (see Tables 7.1–7.3).

Table 7.1 *Symptoms of pulmonary hypertension*

Shortness of breath
Syncope
Chest pain

Table 7.2 *Symptoms of right heart dysfunction*

Breathlessness
Ascites
Ankle swelling
Poor appetite

Table 7.3 *Symptoms of disease associated with pulmonary hypertension*

Hypoxic lung disease
Congenital heart disease
Left heart disease
Thromboembolic disease
Thyroid disease
HIV
Cirrhosis of the liver

Table 7.4 *Signs associated with pulmonary hypertension*

Loud split P2
Right ventricular hypertrophy
Increased 'a' waves
Increased 'v' waves
Diastolic murmur (pulmonary valvular reflux)
Pansystolic murmur (tricuspid reflux)

Table 7.5 *Signs of right heart failure*

Poor peripheral perfusion
Raised right atrial pressure
Right ventricular third and fourth heart sounds
Tricuspid regurgitation
Ejection systolic murmur across the pulmonary valve

Table 7.6 *Signs of associated conditions*

Connective tissue disease, especially scleroderma
Hypoxic lung disease especially
 – Chronic obstructive pulmonary disease
 – Interstitial lung disease
 – Kyphoscoliosis
Signs of left heart disease
Signs of congenital disease
Signs of thyroid disease
Signs of portal hypertension

SIGNS

The clinical signs in pulmonary vascular disease should be considered in the same way as the clinical symptoms, i.e. the signs associated with pulmonary hypertension, the signs associated with right ventricular dysfunction and signs associated with primary disorders that cause pulmonary hypertension (Tables 7.4–7.6). Typically, the signs of pulmonary hypertension are difficult to discern even when the examiner already knows that the pulmonary artery pressure is high. Cyanosis can have two causes:

- the decrease in mixed venous oxygen tension that is characteristic of the low cardiac output in pulmonary hypertension, and
- the right-to-left shunt that may occur, particularly on exercise, when a patent foramen ovale opens.[31]

The jugular venous pressure may reveal enlarged 'a' waves thought to be secondary to poor compliance of the right ventricle and 'v'-waves due to tricuspid regurgitation. The tricuspid valve is a naturally leaky valve and the presence of the murmur of tricuspid reflux and the presence of 'v'-waves does not necessarily indicate right ventricular failure. Right ventricular hypertrophy can be determined from left parasternal or sub-xiphisternal pulsation although this may be absent when there is a relatively hyperinflated chest. Pulmonary hypertension produces a loud pulmonary component of the second heart sound,[3] often associated with 'normal' splitting of the second sound, i.e. the split widens on inspiration as blood is sucked into the chest and right ventricular preload increases. A shunt such as an ASD should be considered when the splitting of the second sound is fixed and wide. The signs of right ventricular dysfunction include raised jugular venous pressure, ascites and swollen ankles. All these features are due to backpressure on the right atrium from the dilated and dysfuntioning right ventricle. Interestingly, sometimes the signs are dissociated, for example in patients on prostacyclin it is not uncommon to find ascites, raising the possibility of primary liver disease. It may simply be that hepatic hemodynamics are changed by the prostacyclin.

There are a number of important points that can be made about the clinical signs.

- Where there is evidence of an intracardiac shunt it is important to consider whether the shunt is the cause of the pulmonary hypertension or simply coincidental.
- Where there are signs of connective tissue disease, one should determine whether the breathlessness and poor exercise tolerance is a consequence of the pulmonary arterial hypertension or associated interstitial lung disease.
- Where there is evidence of peripheral edema, it is important to consider whether this is due to raised right atrial pressure, hypoalbuminemia or vasodilators such as calcium antagonists, which are used to treat pulmonary hypertension.
- There is great confusion about the term cor pulmonale. The WHO definition is right ventricular hypertrophy as a consequence of pulmonary disease, but it has come to mean the presence of fluid retention in hypoxic lung disease. In hypoxic lung disease fluid retention is likely to be due to renal causes[32] because cardiac output in these patients is usually normal. However, when peripheral edema is

seen in the context of primary pulmonary hypertension, it is likely that right ventricular failure is the cause and this will be associated with a low cardiac index.

INVESTIGATION OF PULMONARY HYPERTENSION

When faced with a breathless patient, the cardiologist or respiratory physician will normally undertake a number of investigations including electrocardiogram, chest x-ray, pulmonary function tests, $\dot{V}/\dot{Q}$ scan, CT scan and echocardiography as well as routine blood tests and arterial blood gases. Therefore, these investigations are taken here as the starting point. They are divided into:

- those investigations that suggest the **presence** of pulmonary hypertension;
- those investigations that suggest the **cause** of pulmonary hypertension; and
- those investigations that give us some idea of the **severity** of pulmonary hypertension.

Investigations suggesting the presence of pulmonary hypertension

CHEST X-RAY

Classically, the chest x-ray would show enlargement of the right side of the heart, enlargement of the main pulmonary artery and enlargement of both hila due to enlarged pulmonary arteries. There may also be loss of vascularity in the peripheral lung due to diminished blood flow as a consequence of the high peripheral resistance. The lateral chest x-ray may show loss of the retrosternal space due to enlargement of the right ventricle. The chest x-ray is not, however, wholly reliable; although these features are common when there is severe pulmonary hypertension, the chest x-ray may be entirely normal when it is less severe (Figures 7.1 and 7.2).

ELECTROCARDIOGRAM

The electrocardiogram classically shows features of right atrial and right ventricular hypertension, i.e. large p-wave, especially in II, right axis deviation, tall R waves and ST depression in the right-sided chest leads. Once again these features may be absent (Figures 7.3 and 7.4). Patients are usually in sinus rhythm, possibly because arrhythmias are fatal.

PULMONARY FUNCTION TESTS

These are most useful to exclude chronic obstructive pulmonary disease (COPD) and interstitial lung disease.

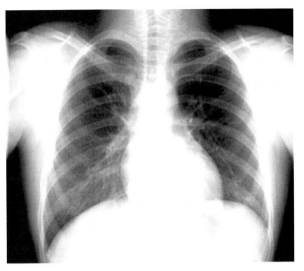

Figure 7.1 *Chest x-ray of a young man with severe thromboembolic pulmonary hypertension. There is little evidence of pulmonary hypertension on this x-ray.*

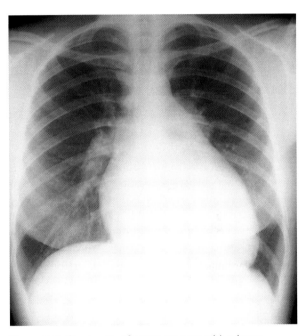

Figure 7.2 *Chest x-ray of a young woman with primary pulmonary hypertension who remains symptomatically well on continuous intravenous prostacyclin 7 years after the original diagnosis.*

In the NIH Registry study,[3] patients with primary pulmonary hypertension had mild restriction and diminished gas transfer. Similar results were seen in an Israeli study.[33] It has always been assumed that the loss of gas transfer is due to diminished pulmonary capillary blood volume, as a consequence of constriction of small peripheral pulmonary arteries, but studies where pulmonary capillary blood volume has been separated from gaseous diffusion have suggested that most of the loss of

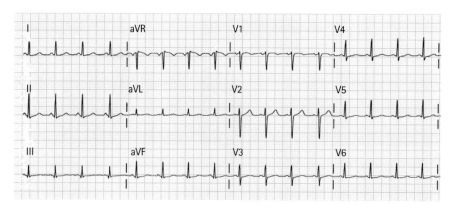

Figure 7.3 *Electrocardiogram of the young man from Figure 7.1 with thromboembolic pulmonary hypertension. There is little evidence of a right ventricular response to his high pulmonary artery pressures.*

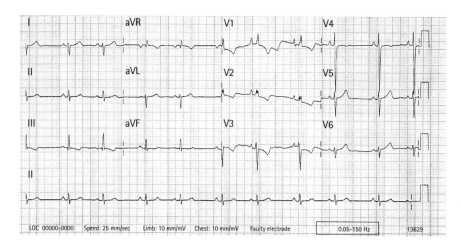

Figure 7.4 *Electrocardiogram of the young woman in Figure 7.2 showing right ventricular hypertrophy with right axis deviation.*

DLCO (diffuse capacity for carbon monoxide) in primary pulmonary hypertension and chronic thromboembolic pulmonary hypertension is due to a decrease in the diffusion at the membrane level.[34] The mild restriction to ventilation is not really understood but could be due to the thickening of peripheral vessels, which diminishes lung compliance. Other studies have also shown mild airflow obstruction in primary pulmonary hypertension, particularly at the level of peripheral airways, with changes in the flow independent section of the flow/volume loop.[35] The reason for this peripheral airflow obstruction is not understood.

VENTILATION/PERFUSION SCAN

The ventilation/perfusion scan is classically used as a means for distinguishing pulmonary thromboembolism from other causes of breathlessness. The situation in pulmonary arterial hypertension is, however, more complicated because there may be *in situ* thrombosis in primary pulmonary hypertension, which can closely mimic pulmonary embolism.[36–38] Generally, however, the loss of perfusion is segmental in fashion and asymmetric in quality in thromboembolic pulmonary hypertension (Figures 7.5 and 7.6).

CT SCAN

The main purpose of the CT scan is to distinguish pulmonary hypertension from other causes of progressive breathlessness, particularly emphysema and interstitial lung disease.[39,40] In 'pure' primary pulmonary hypertension, the CT scan will demonstrate enlarged pulmonary arteries with diminished peripheral vascularity.

BLOOD TESTS

Typically, arterial PO_2 is low and there is an accompanying decrease in arterial PCO_2 due to increased ventilation. The low PO_2 is a consequence of low mixed venous O_2, in turn a consequence of the poor cardiac index. There is probably no significant defect in gaseous diffusion despite abnormalities in DLCO as described above.

ECHOCARDIOGRAM

This is the definitive screening test for the presence of pulmonary hypertension and is dealt with elsewhere (Chapter 8). The echocardiogram will demonstrate right ventricular dilation; an estimate of pulmonary artery systolic pressure can be obtained from a measurement of tricuspid regurgitant jet wave velocity.

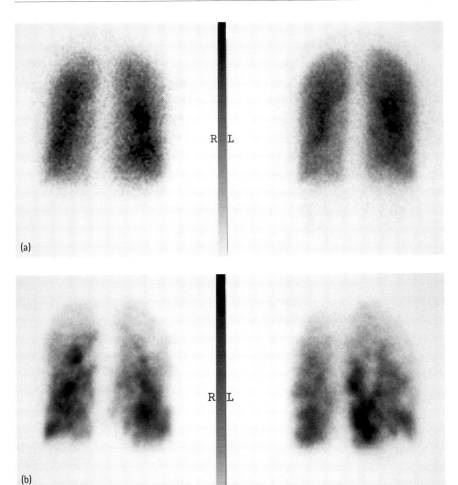

Figure 7.5 *Ventilation (a) and perfusion (b) scans from patient with primary pulmonary hypertension showing patchy ('motheaten') appearance of the perfusion images. These changes are thought to represent pulmonary artery thrombosis.*

Investigations suggesting the cause of pulmonary arterial hypertension

From the classification of pulmonary hypertension (see Chapter 12) it is clear that there are many causes, some of which can be determined by basic investigation. Since pulmonary hypertension is difficult to treat, it is very important to establish a diagnosis if there is a causative disease which can be independently treated with benefit to the pulmonary circulation (particularly in SLE, HIV, COPD and left heart dysfunction).

CHEST X-RAY

The chest x-ray may show evidence of COPD, interstitial lung disease or abnormalities of the chest wall causing hypoventilation.

ECHOCARDIOGRAM

The electrocardiogram may demonstrate ischemic heart disease or systemic hypertension.

PULMONARY FUNCTION TESTS

These may show the presence of COPD, restriction due to chest wall disease or restriction due to interstitial lung disease. The patients with 'pure' primary pulmonary hypertension will also have restriction and low gas transfer. Clearly, it can be difficult to determine whether or not there is significant interstitial lung disease from the pulmonary function tests and whether this is contributing to the restriction and loss of gas transfer. Careful evaluation of the pulmonary function tests in conjunction with the high resolution of the chest and clinical examination is necessary.

VENTILATION PERFUSION SCAN

The $\dot{V}/\dot{Q}$ scan will show patchy loss of ventilation in primary lung disease[36-38] and the presence of asymmetric perfusion defects in thromboembolic pulmonary hypertension, but there can be confusion because of a similar appearance that occurs in the thrombotic variant of primary pulmonary hypertension. The perfusion scan may

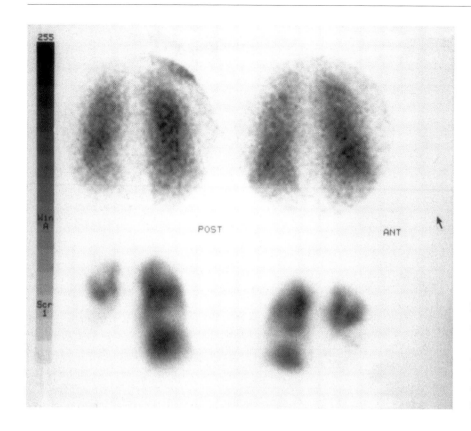

Figure 7.6 *Ventilation/perfusion scan from patient with thromboembolic pulmonary hypertension showing normal ventilation (upper panels) but abnormal perfusion (lower panels) due to vascular obstruction by clot.*

also give some clue about the presence of pulmonary veno-occlusive disease. This variant was thought to be rare but is now believed to be more common. It is very important to make the diagnosis because treatment with standard vasodilators may be fatal.[41]

ECHOCARDIOGRAPHY

The echocardiogram may show evidence of left ventricular disease (either hypertrophy or dysfunction), the presence of proximal thromboembolism or the presence of left-to-right cardiac shunt.

CT SCAN

It is our practice to perform a high resolution CT (HRCT) scan to look for evidence of interstitial lung disease or pulmonary veno-occlusive disease,[40,42–44] where the presence of lymphadenopathy, nodular opacities, septal lines and small pleural effusions typical of this disease may be apparent, since it is so difficult to diagnose otherwise, even on cardiac catheterization. We would also perform CT pulmonary angiography to look for proximal, surgically removable clots.[43,44]

BLOOD TESTS

Arterial blood gases do not help to find the cause of pulmonary hypertension but other blood tests can be helpful. In particular, there may be thrombocytopenia

and raised antineutrophil cytoplasmic antibody (ANCA) in CTD, and HIV serology will be positive in HIV-associated pulmonary hypertension.

ABDOMINAL ULTRASOUND

This should be performed in all patients with PAH and abnormal liver function to exclude cirrhosis of the liver with or without portal hypertension.

Investigations indicating the severity of pulmonary arterial hypertension

The principal complaint of patients with pulmonary hypertension is breathlessness on exertion; thus some form of functional test performed on exertion is going to give the most useful information about the severity of pulmonary hypertension. This should be compared with assessments of quality of life in order to determine the functional severity of disease and to determine the impact of therapy. After the 1998 Evian Symposium, a classification of breathlessness was formed based on the New York Heart Association Criteria and this is given in Chapter 12. All recent treatment trials in pulmonary hypertension used some measure of quality of life; while none is perfect, these have included: the medical outcomes trust shortform 12 (SF12) and 36 (SF36); the EQ-5D and, for most of the trials, a modification of the Minnesota Living with Heart Failure Questionnaire. None of these quality of life tests was developed specifically for pulmonary hypertension and in future when we consider the end points for trials with vasodilators in pulmonary hypertension we will need better quality of life studies in association with better estimation of the physiological responses to exercise. Basic static investigations that give some idea of severity are as follows.

CHEST X-RAY

An enlarging heart indicates that it is failing in response to the high-outflow impedance.

ELECTROCARDIOGRAM

There is some evidence that size of p-wave amplitude and the development of features of right ventricular hypertrophy relate to prognosis in primary pulmonary hypertension.[45]

PULMONARY FUNCTION TESTS

The only pulmonary function variable related to severity is the gas transfer, which has been found to be proportional to the VO_{2max}, the oxygen pulse and the V/VCO_2 slope at anaerobic threshold.[46]

V/Q SCAN

This is also essentially a description of the anatomic derangement of the pulmonary circulation but one study reported a perfusion index from the perfusion scans that was proportional to mean pulmonary artery pressure and right ventricular ejection fraction in patients with primary pulmonary hypertension.[47]

ECHOCARDIOGRAPHY

This investigation would appear to be the non-invasive investigation of choice for looking at the severity of pulmonary hypertension. It is possible using echocardiography to measure right ventricular size (rather inaccurate) and pulmonary artery systolic pressure (usually with considerable accuracy). Since severity of pulmonary hypertension is only partly related to these two variables, there have been attempts to get more information from echocardiography (see Chapter 8). Two studies are worth mentioning here. The Derived Right Ventricular index was the only independent predictor of mortality in 53 patients with pulmonary hypertension.[48] In addition, a poor outcome could be predicted by the presence of pericardial effusion and increased right atrial size.[49] In an attempt to improve the morphological description given by echocardiography, Menzel et al.[50] used three-dimensional echo to develop measurements of right ventricular size and systolic function that improved after surgery for thromboembolic disease.

MAGNETIC RESONANCE IMAGING (MRI)

MRI has much greater potential than echocardiography to measure right ventricular mass, right ventricular morphology, pulmonary artery morphology and pulmonary artery physiology in the form of velocity profiles. At present, these investigations are still in their infancy but it is known that right ventricular mass is proportional to mean pulmonary artery pressure.[51] In the future we may be able to measure the benefit of therapy by improvements in right ventricular mass. At present, physiological variables derived from MRI appear to have poor correlation with invasive hemodynamics,[52] but increasingly sophisticated measures of pulse wave profile, reflective waves and other variables may improve this non-invasive assessment.

EXERCISE TESTING

The 6-minute walk test has been widely used in all the trials of the effectiveness of vasodilators in pulmonary hypertension. This test has the advantages of being low tech, easy to administer, and relatively reproducible.[53–55] Despite its widespread use, there have been remarkably few publications of its value in the assessment of pulmonary hypertension. During the 6-minute walk, measurements are made of arterial oxygen saturation (SaO_2), heart rate and the distance walked. It is the distance walked that has been used to evaluate the effectiveness of therapy and the prognosis of patients with these diseases. There appears to be no linear correlation between distance walked and mortality from pulmonary hypertension,[54] but there does appear to be a threshold, i.e. if patients can walk more than a certain distance (332 m),[55] their survival is a great deal better. This fits very well with the data from invasive cardiac index studies, which have shown that the resting cardiac index is the best predictor of exercise tolerance and prognosis. Indeed, it has been suggested that the 6-minute walk distance is determined by the cardiac output response to exercise.[56]

CARDIOPULMONARY EXERCISE TESTING

It would seem obvious that cardiopulmonary exercise testing would be the most useful way of looking at exercise tolerance in pulmonary hypertension. Measurements are normally made of ventilation, CO_2 production, oxygen consumption, respiratory rate and tidal volume. From these variables oxygen pulse, ventilatory equivalents for O_2 and CO_2 and maximum oxygen uptake are calculated.

Not surprisingly, exercise tolerance is dictated by VO_{2max}, which is always diminished in these patients. VO_{2max} may also be a very good way of looking at the response to therapy: for example, it has been shown that by increasing the dose of intravenous prostacyclin it is possible to further increase the cardiac output without improving VO_{2max}. This suggests that the drug is opening up shunts in the skin and visceral organs without further improvement in oxygen delivery.

Since pulmonary hypertension is associated with loss of vascularity in the periphery, there is $\dot{V}/\dot{Q}$ mismatching with a high physiological dead space and hence wasted ventilation. This is reflected in changes in slope of the VE/VCO_2 and VE/VO_2 curves. It has recently been shown that the slope of these curves relates directly to the pulmonary artery pressure measured by high fidelity micromanometer tipped catheter during exercise.[57] Cardiopulmonary exercise testing will also show an increase in right-to-left shunt when a patent foramen ovale opens due to the high pressures in the pulmonary circulation developed on exercise. This is detected by changes in VO_2 and VCO_2.[46] At present, it seems we will get the most information from VO_{2max}, heart rate, VO_2 curves[46] and the slopes of the VE/VCO_2 and VE/VO_2 curves.[57]

All the investigations described above are, of course, invasive and ultimately we would hope that the investigation and management of these patients can be conducted in a non-invasive fashion. However, at present, right heart catheterization is mandatory for all these patients in order to make a diagnosis of the presence of pulmonary hypertension, a measure of the severity of pulmonary hypertension and to look for possible other causes of pulmonary hypertension.

RIGHT HEART CATHETERIZATION

This is normally performed using a triple lumen, fluid-filled Swan–Ganz thermodilution catheter. Measurements are made of right atrial and ventricular pressures, pulmonary artery pressure and cardiac output at baseline and after a vasodilator.[58,59] Fluid-filled catheters are notorious for the poor frequency-to-noise ratio and, because of the external transducer, poor reliability if there is any patient movement. These problems have been overcome by the development of the micromanometer-tipped high fidelity catheter where the transducer is on the tip of the catheter and hence movement of the patient makes no difference to the pressure obtained. Also, because there is no fluid in the catheter, the results are much more accurate. These catheters have been exploited to make measurements in the pulmonary circulation under conditions of changes in posture, changes in exercise, changes in inhaled gases[60] and have also been used to generate pressure/flow lines which are far more useful than single measurements of pressure or flow. For example, it has been shown that whereas the pressure and flow measured at rest on the catheter table may be identical for a patient before and after prolonged treatment with prostacyclin even though the patient has noted considerable clinical benefit, the slope of the pressure/flow curve is improved by the drug.[61]

It is likely that solid–state catheters will prove to be more useful in the assessment of patients with pulmonary hypertension, particularly since they can be inserted for up to 48 hours with recordings downloaded to a small computer carried on a waistband. Ultimately, however, these invasive tests must be used to correlate with non-invasive measurements that can be performed routinely to follow up patients with pulmonary vascular disease. One of the advantages of catheterization is being able to obtain accurate measurements of cardiac index. It has been shown that cardiac index in response to exercise correlates with the 6-minute walk and a study of our patients has shown that cardiac index is the most important predictor of survival in patients with pulmonary hypertension regardless of cause.[30]

PROGNOSIS AND SURVIVAL

There have been several studies of the prognosis in pulmonary arterial hypertension, some of which were performed in the 'pre-prostacyclin' era and some performed subsequently. The NIH Registry in the USA included 194 patients collected between 1981 and 1985. The median survival of these patients was 2.8 years and appeared to relate to cardiac index, right atrial pressure and pulmonary artery pressure.[62] A small study in the UK of 34 patients showed a mean survival of 7.3 years,[63] but these patients are unusual. In Mexico, the median survival in 61 patients diagnosed between 1977 and 1991 was 4 years.[64] In Japan, the median survival of 223 patients diagnosed between 1980 and 1990 was 32 months.[65] It appears that the expected median survival for primary pulmonary hypertension is between 2.5 and 4 years. However, when the pulmonary hypertension is due to other conditions, the prognosis may be quite different. For example, the prognosis is worse in anorexigen-induced pulmonary hypertension; in a USA study, the 3-year survival was only 17%, versus 60% for sporadic PPH.[66] Survival of HIV-associated pulmonary hypertension is also poor but in a study of 82 patients in France, a combination of antiretroviral therapy and prostacyclin was found to diminish that mortality.[67] In connective tissue disease, the prognosis also appears to be poor. Although disability from the disease and exercise tolerance can be improved by intravenous prostacyclin (see Chapter 13D), mortality is not improved by therapy and remains worse than primary pulmonary hypertension.

Prognosis in pulmonary arterial hypertension in the original NIH study was related to cardiac index, right atrial pressure and mean pulmonary artery pressure.[62] In the Swiss Registry study of 106 patients, survival was related to 6-minute walk distance, the New York Heart Association (NYHA) criteria and mixed venous oxygen tension. In a recent French study, prognosis of patients receiving prostacyclin related to a history of right heart failure, the presence of NYHA grade 4 breathlessness, a 6-minute walk distance of less than 250 meters and a right atrial pressure of more than 12 mmHg.[68] A study of our own group of approximately 90 patients suggested that cardiac index is the most important predictor of survival and, interestingly, this is true no matter what the cause of the pulmonary hypertension.[30] While the bulk of evidence suggests that factors related to hemodynamics and cardiac responses dictate survival, a study in 90 patients with pulmonary hypertension showed that serum uric acid levels are proportional to pulmonary vascular resistance and mortality and inversely proportional to cardiac output. Possibly the poor oxygen delivery from the diminished cardiac output causes a rise in uric acid level.[68] Furthermore, plasma brain natriuretic protein (BNP) is also an independent predictor of survival.[70] While we presently need an invasive measurement of cardiac output and pulmonary hemodynamics, preferably on exercise, to predict prognosis, in the future we may be able to obtain similar information from measurements of circulating levels of hormones or other markers of disease severity.

SCREENING FOR PULMONARY HYPERTENSION

From the above it is evident that we now understand the natural history of severe pulmonary arterial hypertension quite well. Since there is treatment available for these patients, we should try and diagnose them earlier. However, the symptoms and signs of pulmonary arterial hypertension are vague and the basic investigations are often unhelpful. If we had screening tests (particularly non-invasive screening tests) it would allow us to make an earlier diagnosis before hemodynamics are changed and therapy becomes difficult. The questions are: who should we screen and how should we screen them? At the Evian meeting 1999 it was agreed that we should screen the following:

- first-degree relatives of those with pulmonary hypertension
- patients with connective tissue disease
- patients with suspected portopulmonary hypertension if being considered for transplantation.

In other groups it was suggested that we should only screen those who developed symptoms suggesting pulmonary hypertension. At present, the gold standard for screening is echocardiography. It is non-invasive and can usually demonstrate the presence of right ventricular dilatation and/or an increase in pulmonary artery pressure. In future, blood tests, changes in cardiopulmonary exercise tests, and changes in MRI may prove more useful than echocardiography.

KEY POINTS

Causative factors

- Since the histology in pulmonary arterial hypertension from various causes such as PPH, HIV-associated PAH, CTD-associated PAH, portal hypertension PAH is similar, it is likely that these conditions share pathoetiology. This is consistent with the 'double-hit' hypothesis, i.e. an initial propensity and a subsequent secondary trigger.
- Since in some cases the pulmonary arterial hypertension will regress with treatment of the underlying disease as in SLE or HIV, it is possible that the histological lesions seen in pulmonary hypertension can regress provided that the causative stimulus is removed.
- There is clearly an interaction within the pulmonary circulation between vasospasm, histological changes and the presence of intravascular thrombosis. Understanding the link between these will be critical if we are to unravel the pathobiological pathways for pulmonary hypertension and develop treatments that will reverse these pathways.

Symptoms and signs

- Symptoms and signs of pulmonary arterial hypertension are vague and are often missed.
- The symptom of excessive exertional breathlessness in association with 'normal' physical examination should alert the physician to the possibility of pulmonary arterial disease.
- Resting pulmonary artery pressure has already risen considerably by the time symptoms due to pulmonary hypertension develop – methods for earlier screening are necessary.
- The clue to the presence of pulmonary hypertension is often given by the associated condition such as connective tissue disorder, congenital heart disease or hypoxic lung disease. Patients with any of these syndromes should be examined with a view to determining the functional status of the pulmonary circulation.

Investigations

- Basic investigations may be unhelpful.
- Pulmonary function tests showing normal lung volumes and spirometry but diminished gas transfer should arouse suspicion.

- Exercise tolerance and survival in pulmonary hypertension appears to relate to cardiac output.
- Echocardiography remains the screening investigation of choice for those at risk from pulmonary hypertension.

REFERENCES

1 Botney MD. Role of hemodynamics in pulmonary vascular remodeling, implications for primary pulmonary hypertension. *Am J Respir Crit Care Med* 1999;**159**:361–4.

◆2 Scott PH, Peacock AJ. Cell signalling in pulmonary vascular cells: do not shoot the messenger. *Thorax* 1996;**51**:864–6.

◆3 Rich S, Dantzker DR, Ayres SM *et al.* Primary pulmonary hypertension. *Ann Intern Med* 1987;**107**:216–23.

●4 Lane KB, Machado RD, Paucilo MW *et al.* Heterozygous germline mutations in *BMPR2*, encoding a TGF-beta receptor, cause familial primary pulmonary hypertension to chromosome 2q31–2. *Nat Genet* 2000;**26**:81–4.

●5 Deng Z, Morse JH, Slager SL. Familial primary pulmonary hypertension (gene *PPH*) is caused by mutations in the bone morphogenetic protein receptor-II gene. *Am J Hum Genet* 2000;**67**:737–44.

●6 Newman JH, Wheeler L, Lane K B *et al.* Mutation in the gene for bone morphogenetic protein receptor II as a cause of primary pulmonary hypertension in a large kindred. *N Engl J Med* 2001;**345**:319–24.

●7 Thomson JR, Machado RD, Paucilo MW. Sporadic primary pulmonary hypertension is associated with germline mutations of the gene encoding BMPR-II, a receptor member of the TGF-beta family. *J Med Genet* 2000;**37**:741–5.

8 Trembath RC, Thomson JR, Machado RD *et al.* Clinical and molecular genetic features of pulmonary hypertension in patients with hereditary hemorrhagic telangectasia. *N Engl J Med* 2001;**345**:325–34.

●9 Montgomery HE, Marshall R, Hemmingway H *et al.* Human gene for physical performance. *Nature* 1998;**393**:221–2.

●10 Eddahibi S, Humbert M, Fadel E *et al.* Serotonin transporter overexpression is responsible for pulmonary artery smooth muscle hyperplasia in primary pulmonary hypertension. *J Clin Invest* 2001;**108**:1141–50.

11 Grunig E, Janssen B, Mereles D *et al.* Abnormal pulmonary artery pressure response in asymptomatic carriers of primary pulmonary hypertension gene. *Circulation* 2000;**102**:1145–50.

◆12 Humbert M, Nunes H, Sitbon O *et al.* Risk factors for pulmonary arterial hypertension. *Clin Chest Med* 2001;**22**:459–75.

13 Voelkel NF, Clarke WR, Higenbotham T. Obesity, dexfenfluramine and pulmonary hypertension. *Am J Respir Crit Care Med* 1997;**155**:786–8.

●14 Abenheim L, Moride Y, Brenot F *et al.* Appetite suppressant drugs and the risk of pulmonary hypertension. *N Engl J Med* 1996;**335**:609–16.

15 Rich S, Rubin L, Walker AM *et al.* Anorexigens and pulmonary hypertension in the United States. *Chest* 2000;**117**:870–4.

16 Delcroix M, Kurz X, Walckiers D *et al.* High incidence of primary pulmonary hypertension associated with appetite suppresants in Belgium. *Eur Respir J* 1998;**12**:271–6.

17 Eddahibi S, Adnot S. Anorexigen-induced pulmonary hypertension and the serotonin (5-HT) hypothesis: lessons for the future in pathogenesis. *Respir Res* 2002;**3**:9.

◆18 Hoeper MM. Pulmonary hypertension in collagen vascular disease. *Eur Respir J* 2002;**19**:571–6.

19 Tanaka E, Harigai M, Tanaka M *et al.* Pulmonary hypertension in systemic lupus erythematosus: evaluation of clinical characteristics and response to immuno-suppressive treatment. *J Rheumatol* 2002;**29**:282–7.

20 Mehta NJ, Khan IA, Mehta RN *et al.* HIV-related pulmonary hypertension. *Chest* 2000;**118**:1133–41.

21 Speich R, Jenni R, Opravil M *et al.* Regression of HIV-associated pulmonary arterial hypertension and long-term survival during antiretroviral therapy. *Swiss Med Wkly* 2001;**131**:663–5.

22 Yang YY, Lin HC, Lee WC *et al.* Portopulmonary hypertension: distinctive hemodynamic and clinical manifestations. *J Gastroenterol* 2001;**36**:181–6.

23 Curncock AL, Dweik RA, Higgins BH *et al.* High prevalence of hypothyroidism in patients with primary pulmonary hypertension. *Am J Med Sci* 1999;**318**:289–92.

24 Dingli D, Utz JP, Gertz MA. Pulmonary hypertension in patients with amyloidosis. *Chest* 2001;**120**:1735–8.

25 Hoeper MM, Niedermeyer J, Hoffmeyer F *et al.* Pulmonary hypertension after splenectomy. *Ann Intern Med* 1999;**130**:506–9.

26 Weizenblum E, Chaouat A. Hypoxic pulmonary hypertension in man: what minimum daily duration of hypoxaemia is required? *Eur Respir J* 2001;**18**:251–3.

27 Yamakawa H, Shiomi T, Sasanabe R *et al.* Pulmonary hypertension in patients with severe sleep apnea. *Psychiatry Clin Neurosci* 2002;**56**:311–12.

28 Fedullo PF, Rubin LJ, Kerr KM *et al.* The natural history of acute and chronic thromboembolic disease: the search for the missing link. *Eur Respir J* 2000;**15**:435–6.

◆29 Rich S, Rubin LJ, Abenheim L. Executive summary. From the World Symposium on Primary pulmonary hypertension. World Health Organization publication via the internet (http://www.who.int/ncd/cvd/pph.html).

30 Impey V, Crozier A, Hamilton G *et al.* Cardiac index is the most important predictor of survival in patients with all types of pulmonary hypertension. *Am J Respir Crit Care Med* 2002;**165**:A97.

31 Sun XG, Hansen JG, Oudiz RJ *et al.* Gas exchange detection of exercise-induced right to left shunt in patients with pulmonary hypertension. *Circulation* 2002;**105**:54–60.

◆32 MacNee W. Pathophysiology of cor pulmonale in chronic obstructive pulmonary disease. *Am J Respir Crit Care Med* 1994;**150**:833–52.

33 Applebaum L, Yigla M, Bendayan D *et al.* Primary pulmonary hypertension in Israel. *Chest* 2001;**119**:1801–6.

34 Steenhuis LH, Groen HJM, Koeter GH *et al.* Diffusion capacity and haemodynamics in primary and chronic thromboembolic pulmonary hypertension. *Eur Respir J* 2000;**16**:276–81.

35 Meyer FJ, Ewert R, Hoeper MM *et al.* Peripheral airway obstruction in primary pulmonary hypertension. *Thorax* 2002;**57**:473–6.

●36 D'Alonzo GE, Bower JS, Dantzker DR. Differentiation of patients with primary and thromboembolic pulmonary hypertension. *Chest* 1984;**85**:457–61.

37 Azarian R, Brenot F, Sitbon O *et al.* [Pulmonary arterial hypertension of chronic thromboembolic origin; therapeutic indications]. *Arch Mal Coeur Vaiss* 1994; **87**:1709–13.

◆38 Moser KM, Auger WR, Fedullo PF *et al.* Chronic thromboembolic pulmonary hypertension: clinical picture and surgical treatment. *Eur Respir J* 1992; **5**:334–42.

39 Pauwels RA, Buist AS, Calverley P *et al.* Global strategy for the diagnosis, management and prevention of chronic obstructive pulmonary disease. *Am J Respir Crit Care Med* 2001;**163**:1256–76.

40 Kazerooni EA, Martinez FJ, Flint A *et al.* Thin-section CT obtained at 10-mm increments versus limited three-level thin-section CT for idiopathic pulmonary fibrosis: correlation with pathological scoring. *Am J Roentgenol* 1997;**169**:977–83.

41 Bailey CL, Channick RN, Auger WR *et al.* 'High probability' perfusion lung scans in pulmonary venoocclusive disease. *Am J Respir Crit Care Med* 2000;**162**:1974–8.

42 Reston A, Maitre S, Humbert M *et al.* Pulmonary arterial hypertension: thin-section CT predictors of epoprostenol therapy failure. *Radiology* 2002;**222**:782–8.

43 Swensen SJ, Tashjian JH, Myers JL *et al.* Pulmonary venocclusive disease: CT findings in eight patients. *Am J Roentgenol* 1996;**167**:937–40.

●44 Remy-Jardin M, Remy J, Deschildre F *et al.* Diagnosis of pulmonary embolism with spiral CT: comparison with pulmonary angiography and scintigraphy. *Radiology* 1996;**200**:699–706.

45 Bossone E, Paciocco G, Iarussi D *et al.* The prognostic role of the ECG in primary pulmonary hypertension. *Chest* 2002;**121**:513–18.

46 Sun X-G, Hansen JE, Oudiz R *et al.* Heart rate (HR) – oxygen uptake (VO₂) hysteresis during incremental exercise and recovery in primary pulmonary hypertension (PPH). *Am J Crit Care Med* 2002;**165**:A573.

47 Fukuchi K, Hayashida K, Inubushi M *et al.* Quantative analysis of lung perfusion in patients with primary pulmonary hypertension. *J Nucl Med* 2002;**43**:757–61.

●48 Yeo TC, Dujardin KS, Tei C *et al.* Value of a Doppler-derived index combining systolic and diastolic time intervals in predicting outcome in primary pulmonary hypertension. *Am J Cardiol* 1998;**81**:1157–61.

49 Raymond RJ, Hinderliter AL, Willis PW *et al.* Echocardiographic predictors of adverse outcomes in primary pulmonary hypertension. *J Am Coll Cardiol* 2002;**39**:1214–19.

50 Menzel T, Wagner S, Kramm T *et al.* Pathophysiology of impaired right and left ventricular function in chronic embolic pulmonary hypertension. *Chest* 2000; **118**:897–903.

51 Saba TS, Foster J, Cockburn M *et al.* Ventricular mass index using magnetic resonance imaging accurately estimates pulmonary artery pressure. *Eur Respir J* 2002; **20**:1519–24.

52 Tardivon AA, Mousseaux E, Brenot F *et al.* Quantification of hemodynamics in primary pulmonary hypertension with magnetic resonance imaging. *Am J Respir Crit Care Med* 1994;**150**:1075–80.

53 Kadikar A, Maurer J, Kesten S. The six-minute walk test: a guide to assessment for lung transplantation. *J Heart Lung Transplant* 1997;**16**:313–19.

54 Paciocco G, Martinez FJ, Bossone E *et al.* Oxygen desaturation on the six minute walk test and mortality in untreated primary pulmonary hypertension. *Eur Respir J* 2001;**17**:647–52.

●55 Miyamoto S, Nagaya N, Satoh T *et al.* Clinical correlates and prognostic significance of 6 minute walk test in patients with primary pulmonary hypertension. *Am J Crit Care Med* 2000;**161**:487–92.

56 Chabot F, Schrijen F, Borgna M *et al.* Six minutes walking test is related to pulmonary hemodynamic data on exercise in patients with primary pulmonary hypertension. *Am J Respir Crit Care Med* 2002;**165**:A37.

57 Raeside DA, Smith A, Brown A *et al.* Pulmonary artery pressure measurement during exercise testing in patients with suspected pulmonary hypertension. *Eur Respir J* 2000;**16**:282–7.

58 Galie N, Ussia G, Passarelli P *et al.* Role of pharmacologic tests in the treatment of primary pulmonary hypertension. *Am J Cardiol* 1995;**75**:55A–62A.

●59 Sitbon O, Humbert M, Jagot JL *et al.* Inhaled nitric oxide as a screening agent for safely identifying responders to oral calcium-channel blockers in primary pulmonary hypertension. *Eur Respir J* 1998;**12**: 265–70.

60 Raeside DA, Chalmers G, Clelland J *et al.* Pulmonary artery pressure variation in patients with connective tissue disease: 24 hour ambulatory pressure monitoring. *Thorax* 1998;**53**:857–62.

61 Chastelain V, Chemla D, Humbert M *et al.* Pulmonary artery pressure-flow relations after prostacyclin in primary pulmonary hypertension. *Am J Crit Care Med* 2002; **165**:338–40.

●62 D'Alonzo GE, Barst RJ, Ayres SM *et al.* Survival in patients with primary pulmonary hypertension. *Ann Intern Med* 1991;**115**:343–9.

63 Rozkovec A, Montanes P, Oakley CM. Factors that influence the outcome of primary pulmonary hypertension. *Br Heart J* 1986;**55**:449–58.

●64 Sandoval J, Bauerle O, Palomar A *et al.* Survival in primary pulmonary hypertension. *Circulation* 1994; **89**:1733–44.

65 Okada O, Tanabe N, Yasinda J *et al.* Prediction of life expectancy in patients with primary pulmonary hypertension. *Intern Med* 1999;**38**:12–16.

66 Rich S, Shillington A, McLaughlin VV. Prognosis of patients with primary pulmonary hypertension induced by fenfluramine diet pills. *Am J Respir Crit Care Med* 2002; **165**:A37.

67 Nunes H, Humbert M, Sitbon O *et al.* Declining mortality from HIV-associated pulmonary arterial hypertension with combined use of highly active antiretroviral therapy and long-term epoprostenol infusion. *Am J Respir Crit Care Med* 2002;**165**:B81.

●68 Sitbon O, Humbert M, Nunes H *et al.* Intravenous infusion of epoprostenol in severe primary pulmonary hypertension (PPH): long-term survival and prognostic factors. *Am J Respir Crit Care Med* 2002;**165**:C49.

69 Nagaya N, Uematsu M, Satoh T *et al.* Serum uric acid levels correlate with the severity and the mortality of pulmonary hypertension. *Am J Respir Crit Care Med* 1999;**160**:487–92.

70 Nagaya N, Nishikima T, Uematsu M *et al.* Plasma brain natriuretic peptide as a prognostic indicator in patients with pulmonary hypertension. *Circulation* 2000; **102**:865–70.

8

Echocardiography

ADAM TORBICKI AND MARCIN KURZYNA

Echocardiography proved highly reliable in the assessment of the dynamic morphology of cardiac and vascular structures. Moreover, it offers the possibility to record and measure flow velocities using pulsed and continuous-wave Doppler in preselected sites within the cardiovascular system. All this makes echocadiography useful for the non-invasive evaluation of right heart chambers and pulmonary hemodynamics.

This chapter focuses on the role of echocardiography in:

- the assessment of pulmonary arterial pressure
- the diagnosis of pulmonary hypertension.

The potential role of echocardiography in the differential diagnosis and evaluation of prognosis in patients with pulmonary hypertension is also discussed.

ASSESSMENT OF PULMONARY ARTERIAL PRESSURE (PAP)

Increased PAP results in several morphological and functional changes detectable with echocardiography. Unfortunately, only a few are specific for pulmonary hypertension (PH) or correlate with its severity. Echocardiographic signs of PH may be modified by the duration and character of underlying changes within the pulmonary vascular bed as well as by the right ventricular (RV) pre-load, contractility and dynamic coupling to the arterial system. Therefore, non-invasive assessment of PAP with echocardiography should always take into account the coexisting clinical and pathophysiological context.

Right ventricular morphology

The detailed two-dimensional echocardiographic analysis of the morphology of the RV, validated using casts of human ventricles as well as the range of normal values derived from healthy adults, was described almost three decades ago.[1–3] The most widely used measurement is the maximum short axis diameter assessed in the apical or subcostal four-chamber view (Figure 8.1). When increased, RV end-diastolic dimension, either alone or indexed for body surface area, was reported to correlate with mean PAP in patients with chronic PH.[4–6] However, RV dilation may be also caused by its primary failure and/or increased pre-load. Despite low specificity, a dilated RV at transthoracic echocardiography should always prompt a more specific diagnostic process, including non-invasive estimation of PAP.

Increased thickness of the RV free wall might support suspicion of its chronic pressure overload. Unfortunately, trabeculation of the RV endocardial surface affects reproducibility of the measurements.[7] Calculations of the RV mass is even less practical due to the complex RV shape.[3] Therefore, prior to introduction of Doppler echocardiography, differential diagnosis of RV dilatation was difficult and mostly based on the analysis of systolic and diastolic position of the interventricular septum. In pure RV pressure overload, interventricular septal (IVS) flattening was reported to be most marked in end-systole, while increased RV pre-load resulted in predominantly diastolic leftward IVS displacement.[8] Even among patients with primary RV volume overload due to ASD, those with significant PH could be identified on the basis of leftward displacement of the interventricular septum persisting until end-systole.[9] The degree of this displacement can be expressed by the left ventricular eccentricity index (LVEI). To assess eccentricity index (EI), the left ventricle (LV) should be imaged in short axis and measured perpendicularly (D2) and in parallel (D1) to the interventricular

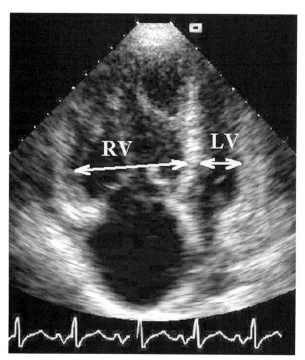

Figure 8.1 *Apical four-chamber view. Enlarged right ventricle (RV) and compressed left ventricle (LV) in a patient with severe primary pulmonary hypertension. Right ventricle is usually measured in end-diastole at the place of its maximum widths, with left ventricle measured along the same line.*

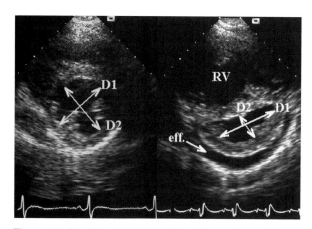

Figure 8.2 *Parasternal short axis view. Left panel: normal morphology of both ventricles. Right panel: Flattening of interventricular septum and compression of the left ventricle by severely enlarged right ventricle (RV). Diastolic dimensions of left ventricle measured perpendicularly (D2) and in parallel (D1) to the septum for assessment of its eccentricity index (LVEI = D1/D2); eff., pericardial effusion.*

septum (Figure 8.2). In healthy adults, systolic and diastolic LVEI calculated as D1/D2 was 1.00 ± 0.06 and 1.01 ± 0.04, respectively. Patients with RV volume overload had normal systolic but elevated diastolic LVEI (1.02 ± 0.04 and 1.26 ± 0.12, respectively) while patients with RV pressure overload presented with more markedly increased systolic than diastolic LVEI (1.44 ± 0.16 and 1.26 ± 0.11, respectively).[8]

Eccentricity index provides information on the severity of RV overload as well as on the degree of secondary LV compression and/or underfilling.[10,11] This explains its correlation with hemodynamic and functional compromise observed in patients with PH and expressed by the distance covered during the 6-minute walk test[12] or by adverse effects of nifedipine administration during vasoreactivity testing.[13]

Blood velocity across orifices

Doppler echocardiography, by allowing for measurement of instantaneous velocity of blood within the heart, provides excellent means for clinically useful non-invasive assessment of PAP. Best correlation was reported for calculations of pressure gradients derived from continuous-wave Doppler measurements of peak velocities of blood traversing orifices within the cardiovascular system. The pressure gradient (PG) driving blood through an orifice can be calculated according to a simplified Bernoulli equation as $PG = 4V^2$ (mmHg). While the jet of pulmonary insufficiency[14] as well as peak flow velocities across ventricular septal defect (VSD)[15,16] and patent ductus arteriosus (PDA)[17] allow for calculations of PAP, tricuspid valve regurgitant jets are by far most widely used for this purpose[18] (Figure 8.3).

Even a trivial tricuspid valve regurgitation permits calculation of the systolic pressure gradient between the contracting right ventricle and the right atrium (tricuspid insufficiency pressure gradient, TIPG). Even beat-to-beat changes in directly measured pressure are reflected in TIPG changes.[19] For calculation of pulmonary arterial systolic pressure (PASP), RV outflow stenosis must be excluded and an estimate of the right atrial pressure (RAP) should be added to the pressure gradient: PASP = TIPG + estimated RAP.

The reliability of such assessment of PASP has been extensively verified (Table 8.1). Reported correlation was invariably excellent ($r = 0.89$–0.97), which was partly due to the broad spectrum of PASPs ranging from normal to suprasystemic levels in the studied groups. Unfortunately, the standard error of estimation was relatively high (4.9–8.0 mmHg), making precise estimation of PAP in an individual patient with PH less reliable.[12] Such inaccuracies could only partially be attributed to non-simultaneous invasive and Doppler-derived measurements,[18,20,21] or to subjectivity of velocity measurements. In fact, inter-observer and intra-observer variability reported in a landmark trial were low, with mean ± SD discrepancy of −1.8 ± 4.9 mmHg and −0.2 ± 3.4 mmHg, respectively.[18] Different timing of peak RV and right atrial pressures might affect the precision

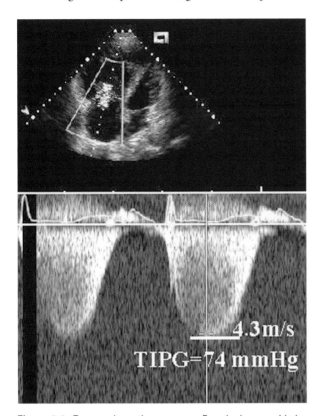

Figure 8.3 *Top panel: continuous-wave Doppler beam guided by 'color-coded' Doppler visualization of the jet of tricuspid insufficiency. Bottom panel: Doppler measurement of the peak velocity of the jet. According to the Bernoulli equation, a velocity of 4.3 m/s indicates a maximum systolic pressure gradient between the right ventricle and atrium of 74 mmHg.*

of Doppler-derived calculations.[22] Furthermore, orifice geometry and blood viscosity are not accounted for by the simplified version of Bernoulli equation.[22,23]

However, reliability of PASP estimation with the tricuspid jet method depends mostly on the quality of Doppler spectrum, which must allow measurement of peak velocity. Even before two-dimensional ('color-coded') Doppler echocardiography was introduced tricuspid jets were often recorded in healthy people, and almost always in patients with PH (Table 8.1). A learning curve and technical progress probably explain a reported linear increase in the percentage of patients with otherwise normal echograms in whom TIPG was measured in 1990 (9%) and in 1999 (59%) in a tertiary referral echocardiographic laboratory of Massachusetts General Hospital.[24] In a recent trial involving patients with COPD, who are particularly difficult to assess with echocardiography due to lung hyperinflation, tricuspid jet velocity was measurable in 77% of cases[25] compared to 25–65% reported in earlier landmark trials.[26–28] Moreover, the Doppler spectrum can be enhanced by intravenous injection of echocardiographic contrast, further increasing the number of technically adequate tracings.[29,30]

Assessment of right atrial pressure

Several approaches to account for right atrial pressure (RAP), required for estimation of PASP from TIPG, have been reported. They were mostly based on the presence and level of jugular vein congestion.[18,22] Currie *et al.*[19] compared this approach with two other methods: based on a regression equation and based on assumption of fixed right atrial pressure of 10 mmHg. All three methods performed equally well in their study population recruited from patients referred for cardiac catheterization (r = 0.89–0.90, SEE 8–9 mmHg). More recently, estimation of RAP based on echocardiographic inferior

Table 8.1 *Correlations of directly measured pressures with non-invasive pressure estimate based on measurement of peak velocity of tricuspid jet and Bernoulli equation*

Author (year)	n	% patients with measurable peak jet velocity	r	versus	SEE	Comments
Yock Popp (1984)[18]	62	87	0.93	RVSP	8 mmHg	
Berger (1985)[88]	69	59	0.97	PASP	4.9 mmHg	
Skjaerpe (1986)[22]	70	?	0.96	RVSP	7.1 mmHg	
Currie (1985)[19]	127	75	0.89	PASP	8 mmHg	
Laaban (1986)[26]	34	65	0.65	PASP	(-)	COPD
Torbicki (1989)[27]	70	25	0.92	PASP	7.7 mmHg	Lung diseases
Himelman (1989)[64]	36	56%		PASP	(-)	COPD
		92*	0.98*			Contrast*

COPD, chronic obstructive pulmonary disease; PASP, pulmonary artery systolic pressure; RVSP, right ventricular systolic pressure; SEE, standard error of estimate.
*After saline contrast enhancement of Doppler spectrum.

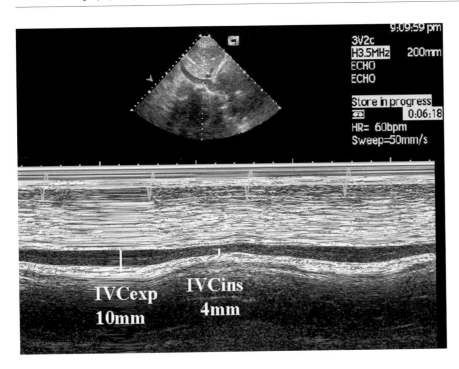

Figure 8.4 *Inferior vena cava measured at expiration (IVCexp) and inspiration (IVCins) to calculate its collapsibility index: IVCCI = (IVCexp − IVCins)/ IVCexp = 60%.*

vena cava collapsibility index (IVCCI) has been suggested (Figure 8.4). This index is calculated by subtracting inspiratory from expiratory and dividing the result by expiratory IVC diameter. In one study, IVCCI <50% was 89% specific for RAP ≥10 mmHg.[31] Pepi *et al.*[32] used an IVCCI index of >45%, 35–45% and <35% to assign to RAP the values of 6, 9 and 16 mmHg, respectively. In this study, PASP calculation based on IVCCI performed better than methods using a fixed RAP of 10 mmHg or a regression equation.[32] More complex methods based on echocardiographic monitoring of IVC diameter during controlled inspiratory effort (sonospirometry) did not gain popularity.[33] Whenever IVC is measured, the position of the patient during the examination should be considered and standardized, as it has an important influence on the shape of this vessel.[34]

Available evidence and personal experience indicate several specific issues that should be considered when using tricuspid jet velocity for estimation of PASP in clinical practice:

- Suboptimal spectral tracings should be discarded. Even a small inaccuracy in jet velocity measurement (e.g. 5.0 instead of 4.5 m/s) translates into a substantial error in calculated pressure gradient (100 mmHg instead of 80 mmHg, respectively).
- Angle correction based on the difference between the direction of Doppler beam and regurgitant jet should be discouraged. Angles below 10° do not affect the calculations.[18] Those exceeding 20° in most cases result in a suboptimal spectral envelope and should in any case be discarded.

- During inspiration, the Doppler spectrum may be more clearly recorded but the peak velocity of the jet might be slightly higher due to increased RV pre-load and enhanced RV contractility.[18] Therefore, RV jet recordings for velocity measurements should be made either during relaxed expiration or averaged over 5–10 consecutive cycles during quiet respiration. This helps to avoid false diagnosis of PH in patients with borderline TIPG.
- Whilst TIPG is a straightforward measurement, calculation of PASP requires assumption of RAP which may introduce additional error. Therefore, if an estimated PASP is quoted in the echocardiographic report, the method that was used to account for RAP should be clearly stated. This is essential for reproducibility of results.
- For reasons that are not clear, the Doppler TIPG method slightly underestimates PASP in patients with severe PH. During a simultaneous study, TIPG underestimated systolic pressure gradient assessed with high fidelity tip-transducers by up to 20–30 mmHg.[20]
- False diagnosis of mild PH was reported with the tricuspid jet method.[35] However, when the above rules are followed, clinically significant overestimation of PASP based on TIPG is unlikely.

Whilst peak velocity of the jet of tricuspid regurgitation is related to PASP, end-diastolic velocity of the pulmonary regurgitant jet is related to diastolic pulmonary arterial pressure (PADP).[14] In a study of 32 patients,

Table 8.2 *Comparison of Doppler methods used for assessment of pulmonary arterial pressure: patients with cardiovascular diseases (Currie et al., 1987; n = 50)[89]*

Method used	Success rate (%)	Correlation Coefficient (r)	With	SEE (mmHg)
TVR jet velocity	72	0.89	PASP	7.4
AcT	88	−0.66	PAMP	10
(AcT*)	(52)	(−0.85)		(7)
RVIRT	64	−		
(RVIRT**)	(22)		(PASP)	(11)

AcT, acceleration time of right ventricular ejection; PAMP, mean pulmonary arterial pressure; PASP, systolic pulmonary arterial pressure; RVIRT, right ventricular isovolumic relaxation time; SEE, standard error of estimate; TVR, tricuspid valve regurgitation.
*Patients with heart rate between 60 and 100/min.
**Patients in sinus rhythm.

Table 8.3 *Comparison of Doppler methods used for assessment of pulmonary arterial pressure: patients with respiratory diseases (Torbicki et al., 1989; n = 70)[27]*

Method used	Success rate (%)	Correlation Coefficient (r)	With	SEE (mmHg)
TVR jet velocity	25	0.91	PASP	7.9
AcT	97	−0.72	PAMP	8.3
RVIRT*	84	0.66	PASP	11.6

AcT, acceleration time of right ventricular ejection; PAMP, mean pulmonary arterial pressure; PASP, systolic pulmonary arterial pressure; RVIRT, right ventricular isovolumic relaxation time; SEE, standard error of estimate; TVR, tricuspid valve regurgitation.
*Patients in sinus rhythm.

the peak diastolic and end-diastolic pulmonary to RV pressure gradients derived from the Doppler flow profiles correlated well with the catheter measurements (r = 0.95 and r = 0.95, respectively).[36] As PAP increased, the peak velocity of the pulmonary regurgitant jet became higher, with a linear relationship between mean PAP and Doppler-derived peak diastolic pressure gradient (r = 0.94). Based on peak diastolic gradients of <15, 15–30 or >30 mmHg, patients could be separated into those with mild, moderate or severe PH, respectively (P < 0.05). A correlation was also observed between PADP and Doppler-derived end-diastolic pressure gradient (r = 0.91).[36] However, when directly compared in the same patients, Doppler-derived pressure calculations based on diastolic velocities across the pulmonary valve were less accurate than those based on tricuspid jet velocity measurements (r = 0.83 versus 0.98, respectively).[37] The reported prevalence of pulmonary regurgitation on Doppler echocardiography ranged from 22% in healthy women to 86% in patients with PH.[14,38]

If both tricuspid and pulmonary regurgitant jets are clearly recorded and superimposed, a complete PASP curve can be reconstructed, and mean PAP can be calculated. However, despite reported excellent correlations with catheterization data (r = 0.97), this approach was probably too cumbersome to gain popularity.[37]

Other jets have been used for the assessment of RVP and PASP, mostly in infants and newborns. Peak flow velocity through a VSD reflected a systolic pressure gradient between contracting ventricles whilst peak flow velocity across a PDA in newborns correlated with the pressure gradients between the aorta and pulmonary artery.[16,17] In both cases systemic arterial pressure had to be added to the gradient in order to calculate PAP. Clearly, right and left ventricular outflow must be checked for the presence of additional gradients. If present, these gradients should be appropriately considered in the calculations.

In general, echocardiographic methods estimating RVP and PAP based on peak velocity of jets within the heart and proximal arteries are firmly established in clinical practice. In studies directly comparing various echocardiographic methods, the tricuspid jet method was the most precise in predicting PAP in patients with both cardiovascular and respiratory pathology (Tables 8.2 and 8.3).[27,39]

Right ventricular systolic and diastolic time intervals

Estimation of PAP from echocardiographically measured classic right ventricular systolic and diastolic time intervals, such as pre-ejection or isovolumetric relaxation time,[27,40–42] has been reported but is of questionable clinical value. Pulsed-wave Doppler analysis of time intervals derived from the flow velocity curve in the RV outflow tract or proximal PA received more attention. With increasing PAP, the interval between the onset and peak velocity of RV ejection (acceleration time, AcT) was reported to decrease.[43] Furthermore, in severe pulmonary hypertension, mid-systolic deceleration of RV ejection to the pulmonary artery was often noted, and occurred earlier with higher PAPs[44] (Figure 8.5). Reports suggesting excellent correlations of AcT and PAP followed, offering regression equations that permitted non-invasive pressure calculations. However, significant differences in suggested equations precluded their

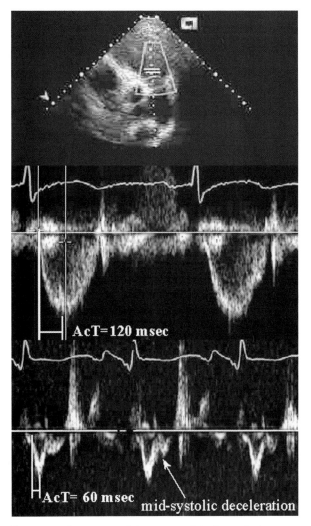

Figure 8.5 *Assessment of the pattern of the flow velocity curve in the right ventricular outflow tract just below the level of the pulmonary valve. Tracing from a healthy individual (upper panel) with normal acceleration time (AcT) compared with severely disturbed pattern characterized by short AcT and the presence of mid-systolic deceleration of flow recorded in a patient with PH.*

universal applications.[45] While heart rate[46] and the presence of tricuspid regurgitation apparently did not affect AcT,[47] several other factors did. For the same level of PAP, AcT tended to be longer in patients with low cardiac index[48] and with increased pulmonary flow due to pre-tricuspid shunts.[47] Conversely, AcT tended to be shorter with more distal Doppler sample volume positions,[49,50] in individuals with body surface area $>2.0 \, m^2$ and in adults >30 years old.[51] Also, proximal pulmonary emboli, especially when acute, profoundly disturbed the flow velocity curve, resulting in particularly short AcT and prominent mid-systolic deceleration, regardless of the level of pulmonary arterial pressure.[52]

Whilst correlation of simultaneous AcT and PAP measurements were reported,[53] acutely induced changes in PAP were not accurately reflected by AcT changes in a simultaneous Doppler-catheter study.[54]

Taken together, available data coming from clinical and experimental studies indicate that AcT is not directly related to PAP.[44,47,52,55–58] Differences in dynamic coupling between the ejecting right ventricle and pulmonary arterial bed with its characteristic impedance and reflected pressure waves probably account for much of the observed variability of the flow velocity pattern. Therefore, information contained in the dynamics of RV ejection into the pulmonary artery may be even more closely related to the true RV afterload than variables measured during standard right heart catheterization.[23]

DIAGNOSING AND SCREENING FOR PULMONARY HYPERTENSION

Echocardiographic definitions of PH

Standard definition of pulmonary hypertension (PH) is based on catheter-derived assessment of mean PAP exceeding 20–25 mmHg at rest or 30 mmHg during exercise. Unfortunately, mean PAP cannot be reliably estimated with echocardiography while definition of PH based on PASP was lacking.

Arbitrarily set criteria for non-invasive diagnosis of PH in the presence of TIPG ≥ 30 mmHg have been used by some authors.[59,60] In a recent summary from the PPH symposium held in Evian in 1998, mild pulmonary hypertension was defined, always arbitrarily, as tricuspid jet velocity between 2.8 and 3.4 m/s, which corresponds to TIPG 31–46 mmHg and to PASP 36–51 mmHg (assuming fixed RAP of 5 mmHg for its calculation).[61] Several studies attempted to define the upper limits of tricuspid jet velocity at rest. In 53 healthy non-smokers aged 14–55 years, TIPG ranged from 12.6 to 29.3 mmHg (mean 19.3 ± 4.0);[62] Dib *et al.*[63] selected 134 echocardiographic Doppler examinations considered as normal but allowing measurement of the PASP with the simplified Bernoulli equation. There was a highly significant correlation between PASP and the age of the patient ($r = 0.47$, $P = 0.0001$). Systolic PAP increased progressively with age from 13 ± 5 mmHg between 20 and 29 years old to 22 ± 6 mmHg when 80 years old or more.[63] The Massachusetts General Hospital echocardiographic database was recently analyzed for tricuspid jet velocities in patients with otherwise normal transthoracic examination and no clinically suspected diseases potentially leading to elevated PAP.[25] Among 3212 such patients, mean peak tricuspid jet velocity was 2.61 m/s and TIPG 18.0 ± 4.7 mmHg, with 95% confidence interval (CI) 8.8–27.2 mmHg. Multiple linear regression revealed that age, body mass index (BMI), gender, left ventricular ejection fraction (LVEF) and clinical referral category independently influenced tricuspid velocity. In patients aged over 60 years and/or presenting with BMI >30 kg/m², the 95% confidence interval (CI) for pressure gradient derived from tricuspid jet velocity measurement slightly exceeded 30 mmHg (Table 8.4).

Thus, based on existing evidence, it appears justified to consider tricuspid jet velocities exceeding at rest 2.8 m/s, and corresponding to TIPG ≥ 31 mmHg, as elevated, except for elderly and/or very obese patients. However, there are no data on the clinical outcome of patients with diagnosis of PH made according to these criteria.

Despite multiple factors influencing the relationship between PAP and AcT, several authors assessed the clinical value of this variable for diagnosing PH both in cardiovascular and lung diseases (Table 8.5). Reported results indicate that, if interpreted with caution, short AcT may be a reliable sign of PH, especially useful when tricuspid jet cannot be clearly recorded and measured. Conversely, a long AcT suggests normal PAP, provided that no intracardiac shunt is present.[47]

Echocardiographic tests for latent PH

Similarly to catheter evaluation, Doppler echocardiography may also be performed during exercise to estimate PAP. Though technically difficult, tricuspid jets were recorded and its velocity could be measured during supine exercise, especially after tilting the patient to the left during pedaling or enhancing the jet signal with peripheral saline contrast injection. The correlation with simultaneously performed catheter measurements of PASP seemed excellent ($r = 0.98$).[64] Exercise echo was used to assess systolic PAP in several specific groups of patients: with chronic lung diseases, after heart transplantation,[65] with atrial septal defect (ASD),[66] as well as in individuals susceptible to high altitude lung edema[67] and in asymptomatic carriers of a PPH gene mutation.[68] In all these groups studied, PASP significantly increased on exercise when compared to controls. Prolonged hypoxia (fraction of inspired oxygen, FiO_2 12.5%) was also used to induce PH which could be quantified with Doppler echocardiography.[67]

In healthy controls, PASP, as assessed with the Doppler tricuspid jet method, remained low despite exercise and averaged: 31 ± 7 mmHg, 20.5 ± 3.8 mmHg, 19 ± 8 mmHg, 36 ± 3 mmHg and 37 ± 3 mmHg, for the five studies listed above, respectively. One of the groups arbitrarily defined PASP ≤ 40 mmHg, calculated after assuming fixed RAP of 5 mmHg, as a normal hemodynamic reaction during stress echocardiography. Interestingly, athletes were reported to generate higher PAP when exercising under the same workload as non-athletes when assessed with tricuspid jet method[69] (Table 8.6).

Another approach to latent PH was attempted with the pulsed-wave Doppler method assessing the flow velocity curve in the RV outflow tract during various interventions. Acceleration time showed divergent trends during RV pre-load challenge induced by passive leg

Table 8.4 *Reference ranges for normal systolic pressure gradients assessed with Doppler between right ventricle and right atrium (TIPG) according to McQuillan et al. (2001)[24]*

| Age (years) | n | 95% CI for TIPG (mmHg) | |
		Women (n = 2065)	Men (n = 1147)
<20	856	8.6–24.2	8.2–26.2
20–29	669	9.2–24.4	9.9–26.3
30–39	650	9.3–25.7	8.7–27.5
40–49	494	9.9–27.5	9.1–28.3
50–59	344	10.2–29.4	11.0–30.6
>60	19	10.5–32.1	11.2–33.6

Table 8.5 *Sensitivity and specificity of diagnosis of pulmonary hypertension (PH) with acceleration time (AcT) and related time intervals*

Author (year)	Definition of PH; mean PAP =	Cut-off value	Sensitivity (%)	Specificity (%)	Comments
Matsuda (1986)[47]	>25; 'prominent PH'	AcT ≤ 90 ms	(-)	100	
Isobe (1986)[48]	≥20 mmHg	PEP/AcT > 1.1	93	97	
Torbicki (1989)[27]	≥20 mmHg	AcT < 90 ms	79	78	COPD
		PEP/AcT > 1.0	93	69	

COPD, chronic obstructive pulmonary disease; PAP pulmonary arterial pressure; PEP, right ventricular pre-ejection time.

Table 8.6 *Reference ranges for systolic pressure gradients assessed at rest and during exercise in athletes and healthy non-athletes with Doppler between right ventricle and right atrium (TIPG) according to Bossone et al.*[89]

Workload (watts)	95% CI for TIPG (mmHg)	
	Athletes (n = 26)	Non–athletes (n = 14)
Rest	17.5–23.2	9.0–12.1
40	21.7–29.4	9.9–26.3
120	26.6–36.0	17.8–29.4
240	38.4–55.4	12.3–26.6

raising in patients with normal and abnormal pulmonary circulation.[69–71]

DIFFERENTIAL DIAGNOSIS OF PULMONARY HYPERTENSION

Echocardiography may reveal the cause of PH, such as left ventricular dysfunction, mitral valve disease, or intracardiac shunt, if present. However, some congenital defects potentially leading to PH may be missed during transthoracic examination. These include atypically located ASD, especially of sinus venosus type, anomalous pulmonary venous drainage, PDA and atypical interventricular septal defects.[72] Additional data which significantly altered surgical therapy were found at transesophageal echocardiography (TEE) in 25% (12 out of 48) of patients awaiting lung transplantation for severe PH.[73] Therefore, complete echocardiographic work-up of unexplained PH should probably include transesophageal evaluation. In some patients, TEE may disclose centrally located PA thrombi. Such a finding usually suggests chronic thromboembolic PH, suitable for surgical treatment.[74] However, in cases of severe PH with RV dysfunction and stagnant flow in dilated proximal pulmonary arteries, secondary *in situ* thrombi have been described.[75] Whether intrapulmonary pressure gradients found at TEE can help in assessing the hemodynamic significance of thrombi, in this way assisting in surgical qualification, remains to be verified.

Short AcT (<60 ms) in the presence of TIPG <60 mmHg, a so-called '60/60 sign', as well as isolated hyperkinesis of the apical part of an otherwise hypokinetic RV ('McConnell sign'), strongly suggest transient PH caused by acute pulmonary embolism.[52,76]

FOLLOW–UP AND PROGNOSIS

Echocardiography, as a non-invasive method which permits assessment of several independent variables related

to right heart hemodynamics, seems to be perfectly suited for follow-up of patients with PH. In fact, spectacular echocardiographic improvement was observed after lung transplantation or pulmonary thrombendarteriectomy.[77–80] Pharmacological treatment of primary PH usually results in changes in PAPs, which are too small to be reliably followed in individual patients even by tricuspid jet method.[12] Limited clinical experience seems to indicate that echocardiographic indices related to RV systolic and left ventricular diastolic function might be more useful to follow the effects of treatment than echocardiographic estimates of PAP. RV size, left ventricular eccentricity index and diastolic filling pattern all seem related to functional improvement observed with current pharmacological treatment of pulmonary hypertension.[81] For prognostic significance, leftward shifting of the interventricular septum, right atrial area and pericardial effusion were all reported to independently increase the risk of death or transplantation among 81 PPH patients followed up for a mean of 36.9 ± 15.4 months.[82] The presence of pericardial effusion on echocardiography was consistently reported to indicate poor prognosis in patients with PPH, while prognostic significance of its resolution with effective treatment of PH remains speculative.[83,84]

The RV function might be expected to correlate with prognosis. Echocardiographic estimation of RV ejection fraction is difficult.[3,7] Assessment of RV dP/dt from the rate of rise of tricuspid jet velocity is feasible with Doppler but this index of contractility is influenced by PAP.[85] Doppler index of global RV dysfunction was suggested by Tei *et al.*[86] It is calculated by subtraction of RV ejection time (ET) from total RV systolic time (the latter measured as the interval between cessation and reappearance of tricuspid diastolic flow). In such a way combined duration of systolic and diastolic isovolumetric time intervals of RV (ICT and IRT, respectively) can be assessed. In a retrospective study involving 55 PPH patients, this index of myocardial dysfunction, calculated as (ICT + IRT)/ET was independent of heart rate, RV pressure, dilation, or tricuspid regurgitation but correlated with symptoms and survival.[86,87] In an even smaller group of 26 PPH patients, multivariate analysis identified two Doppler-derived indices related to left and right ventricular filling, suggesting diastolic dysfunction as independent predictors of survival.[81,84]

KEY POINTS

- Enlarged or dominating right ventricle on echocardiography may indicate PH, and requires differential diagnosis.

- Continuous-wave Doppler measurement of peak velocity of the jet of tricuspid regurgitation is the most reliable non-invasive method of assessing PASP.
- Normal ranges of tricuspid jet velocity at rest and on exercise are becoming better defined by recent trials. This should make formal and reliable non-invasive diagnosis of mild, moderate and hopefully also latent PH possible in the near future.
- Other Doppler and echocardiographic variables have a supporting role in the assessment of PAP, but usually contain relevant pathophysiological information regarding pulmonary circulation.
- Follow-up of patients with PH should probably focus on echocardiographic indices of right ventricular systolic and left ventricular diastolic function, rather than on attempts at estimation of changes in PAP.

REFERENCES

1 Bommer W, Weinert L, Neumann A et al. Determination of right atrial and right ventricular size by two-dimensional echocardiography. Circulation 1979;60:91–100.

2 Levine RA, Gibson TC, Aretz T et al. Echocardiographic measurement of right ventricular volume. Circulation 1984;69:497–505.

3 Foale R, Nihoyannopoulos P, McKenna W et al. Echocardiographic measurement of the normal adult right ventricle. Br Heart J 1986;56:33–44.

4 Zenker G, Forche G, Harnoncourt K. Two-dimensional echocardiography using a subcostal approach in patients with COPD. Chest 1985;88:722–25.

5 Danchin N, Cornette A, Henriquez A et al. Two-dimensional echocardiographic assessment of the right ventricle in patients with chronic obstructive lung disease. Chest 1987;92:229–33.

6 Oswald-Mammosser M, Oswald T, Nyankiye E et al. Non-invasive diagnosis of pulmonary hypertension in chronic obstructive pulmonary disease. Comparison of ECG, radiological measurements, echocardiography and myocardial scintigraphy. Eur J Respir Dis 1987;71:419–29.

7 Prakash R, Matsukubo H. Usefulness of echocardiographic right ventricular measurements in estimating right ventricular hypertrophy and right ventricular systolic pressure. Am J Cardiol 1983;51:1036–40.

●8 Ryan T, Petrovic O, Dillon JC et al. An echocardiographic index for separation of right ventricular volume and pressure overload. J Am Coll Cardiol 1985;5:918–27.

●9 Shimada R, Takeshita A, Nakamura M. Noninvasive assessment of right ventricular systolic pressure in atrial septal defect: analysis of the end-systolic configuration of the ventricular septum by two-dimensional echocardiography. Am J Cardiol 1984;53:1117–23.

10 Louie EK, Rich S, Brundage BH. Doppler echocardiographic assessment of impaired left ventricular filling in patients with right ventricular pressure overload due to primary pulmonary hypertension. J Am Coll Cardiol 1986;8: 1298–306.

11 Louie EK, Lin SS, Reynertson SI et al. Pressure and volume loading of the right ventricle have opposite effects on left ventricular ejection fraction. Circulation 1995;92:819–24.

●12 Hinderliter AL, Willis PW, Barst RJ et al. Effects of long-term infusion of prostacyclin (epoprostenol) on echocardiographic measures of right ventricular structure and function in primary pulmonary hypertension. Primary Pulmonary Hypertension Study Group. Circulation 1997;95:1479–86.

13 Ricciardi MJ, Bossone E, Bach DS et al. Echocardiographic predictors of an adverse response to a nifedipine trial in primary pulmonary hypertension: diminished left ventricular size and leftward ventricular septal bowing. Chest 1999; 116:1218–23.

●14 Masuyama T, Kodama K, Kitabatake A et al. Continuous-wave Doppler echocardiographic detection of pulmonary regurgitation and its application to noninvasive estimation of pulmonary artery pressure. Circulation 1986;74:484–92.

●15 Matsuoka Y, Hayakawa K. Noninvasive estimation of right ventricular systolic pressure in ventricular septal defect by a continuous wave Doppler technique. Jpn Circ J 1986; 50:1062–70.

●16 Marx GR, Allen HD, Goldberg SJ. Doppler echocardiographic estimation of systolic pulmonary artery pressure in pediatric patients with interventricular communications. J Am Coll Cardiol 1985;6:1132–7.

●17 Musewe NN, Poppe D, Smallhorn JF et al. Doppler echocardiographic measurement of pulmonary artery pressure from ductal Doppler velocities in the newborn. J Am Coll Cardiol 1990;15:446–56.

●18 Yock PG, Popp RL. Noninvasive estimation of right ventricular systolic pressure by Doppler ultrasound in patients with tricuspid regurgitation. Circulation 1984;70:657–62.

●19 Currie PJ, Seward JB, Chan KL et al. Continuous wave Doppler determination of right ventricular pressure: a simultaneous Doppler-catheterization study in 127 patients. J Am Coll Cardiol 1985;6:750–6.

●20 Brecker SJ, Gibbs JS, Fox KM et al. Comparison of Doppler derived haemodynamic variables and simultaneous high fidelity pressure measurements in severe pulmonary hypertension. Br Heart J 1994;72:384–9.

21 Richards AM, Ikram H, Crozier IG et al. Ambulatory pulmonary arterial pressure in primary pulmonary hypertension: variability, relation to systemic arterial pressure, and plasma catecholamines. Br Heart J 1990;63:103–8.

●22 Skjaerpe T, Hatle L. Noninvasive estimation of systolic pressure in the right ventricle in patients with tricuspid regurgitation. Eur Heart J 1986;7:704–10.

◆23 Naeije R, Torbicki A. More on the noninvasive diagnosis of pulmonary hypertension: Doppler echocardiography revisited [editorial]. Eur Respir J 1995;8:1445–9.

●24 McQuillan BM, Picard MH, Leavitt M et al. Clinical correlates and reference intervals for pulmonary artery systolic pressure among echocardiographically normal subjects. Circulation 2001;104:2797–802.

25 Higham MA, Dawson D, Joshi J *et al.* Utility of echocardiography in assessment of pulmonary hypertension secondary to COPD. *Eur Respir J* 2001;**17**:350–5.

26 Laaban JP, Diebold B, Zelinski R *et al.* Noninvasive estimation of systolic pulmonary artery pressure using Doppler echocardiography in patients with chronic obstructive pulmonary disease. *Chest* 1989;**96**:1258–62.

●27 Torbicki A, Skwarski K, Hawrylkiewicz I *et al.* Attempts at measuring pulmonary arterial pressure by means of Doppler echocardiography in patients with chronic lung disease. *Eur Respir J* 1989;**2**:856–60.

●28 Tramarin R, Torbicki A, Marchandise B *et al.* Doppler echocardiographic evaluation of pulmonary artery pressure in chronic obstructive pulmonary disease. A European multicentre study. Working Group on Noninvasive Evaluation of Pulmonary Artery Pressure. European Office of the World Health Organization, Copenhagen. *Eur Heart J* 1991;**12**:103–11.

●29 Beard JT, Byrd BF, III. Saline contrast enhancement of trivial Doppler tricuspid regurgitation signals for estimating pulmonary artery pressure. *Am J Cardiol* 1988;**62**:486–8.

30 Himelman RB, Struve SN, Brown JK *et al.* Improved recognition of cor pulmonale in patients with severe chronic obstructive pulmonary disease. *Am J Med* 1988;**84**:891–8.

●31 Kircher BJ, Himelman RB, Schiller NB. Noninvasive estimation of right atrial pressure from the inspiratory collapse of the inferior vena cava. *Am J Cardiol* 1990; **66**:493–6.

●32 Pepi M, Tamborini G, Galli C *et al.* A new formula for echo-Doppler estimation of right ventricular systolic pressure. *J Am Soc Echocardiogr* 1994;**7**:20–6.

33 Simonson JS, Schiller NB. Sonospirometry: a new method for noninvasive estimation of mean right atrial pressure based on two-dimensional echographic measurements of the inferior vena cava during measured inspiration. *J Am Coll Cardiol* 1988;**11**:557–64.

●34 Nakao S, Come PC, McKay RG *et al.* Effects of positional changes on inferior vena caval size and dynamics and correlations with right-sided cardiac pressure. *Am J Cardiol* 1987;**59**:125–32.

●35 Vachiery JL, Brimioulle S, Crasset V *et al.* False-positive diagnosis of pulmonary hypertension by Doppler echocardiography. *Eur Respir J* 1998;**12**:1476–8.

36 Lei MH, Chen JJ, Ko YL *et al.* Reappraisal of quantitative evaluation of pulmonary regurgitation and estimation of pulmonary artery pressure by continuous wave Doppler echocardiography. *Cardiology* 1995;**86**:249–56.

●37 Ensing G, Seward J, Darragh R *et al.* Feasibility of generating hemodynamic pressure curves from noninvasive Doppler echocardiographic signals. *J Am Coll Cardiol* 1994; **23**:434–42.

38 Michelsen S, Hurlen M, Otterstad JE. Prevalence of tricuspid and pulmonary regurgitation diagnosed by Doppler in apparently healthy women. Possible influence on their physical performance? *Eur Heart J* 1988;**9**:61–7.

●39 Chan KL, Currie PJ, Seward JB *et al.* Comparison of three Doppler ultrasound methods in the prediction of pulmonary artery pressure. *J Am Coll Cardiol* 1987;**9**:549–54.

40 Boyd MJ, Williams IP, Turton CW *et al.* Echocardiographic method for the estimation of pulmonary artery pressure in chronic lung disease. *Thorax* 1980;**35**:914–19.

41 Stevenson JG, Kawabori I, Guntheroth WG. Noninvasive detection of pulmonary hypertension in patent ductus arteriosus by pulsed Doppler echocardiography. *Circulation* 1979;**60**:355–9.

42 Torbicki A, Hawrylkiewicz I, Zielinski J. Value of M-mode echocardiography in assessing pulmonary arterial pressure in patients with chronic lung disease. *Bull Eur Physiopathol Respir* 1987;**23**:233–9.

●43 Kitabatake A, Inoue M, Asao M *et al.* Noninvasive evaluation of pulmonary hypertension by a pulsed Doppler technique. *Circulation* 1983;**68**:302–9.

●44 Turkevich D, Groves BM, Micco A *et al.* Early partial systolic closure of the pulmonic valve relates to severity of pulmonary hypertension. *Am Heart J* 1988;**115**:409–18.

◆45 Robinson PJ, Macartney FJ, Wyse RK. Non-invasive diagnosis of pulmonary hypertension. *Int J Cardiol* 1986;**11**:253–9.

46 Mallery JA, Gardin JM, King SW *et al.* Effects of heart rate and pulmonary artery pressure on Doppler pulmonary artery acceleration time in experimental acute pulmonary hypertension. *Chest* 1991;**100**:470–3.

●47 Matsuda M, Sekiguchi T, Sugishita Y *et al.* Reliability of non-invasive estimates of pulmonary hypertension by pulsed Doppler echocardiography. *Br Heart J* 1986;**56**:158–64.

48 Isobe M, Yazaki Y, Takaku F *et al.* Prediction of pulmonary arterial pressure in adults by pulsed Doppler echocardiography. *Am J Cardiol* 1986;**57**:316–21.

49 Okamoto M, Miyatake K, Kinoshita N *et al.* Analysis of blood flow in pulmonary hypertension with the pulsed Doppler flowmeter combined with cross sectional echocardiography. *Br Heart J* 1984;**51**:407–15.

●50 Panidis IP, Ross J, Mintz GS. Effect of sampling site on assessment of pulmonary artery blood flow by Doppler echocardiography. *Am J Cardiol* 1986;**58**:1145–7.

51 Gardin JM, Davidson DM, Rohan MK *et al.* Relationship between age, body size, gender, and blood pressure and Doppler flow measurements in the aorta and pulmonary artery. *Am Heart J* 1987;**113**:101–9.

●52 Torbicki A, Kurzyna M, Ciurzynski M *et al.* Proximal pulmonary emboli modify right ventricular ejection pattern. *Eur Respir J* 1999;**13**:616–21.

53 Marangoni S, Quadri A, Dotti A *et al.* Noninvasive assessment of pulmonary hypertension: a simultaneous echo-Doppler hemodynamic study. *Cardiology* 1988;**75**:401–8.

●54 Torbicki A, Tramarin R, Fracchia F *et al.* Reliability of pulsed wave Doppler monitoring of acute changes in pulmonary artery pressure in patients with chronic obstructive pulmonary disease. *Progr Respir Res* 1990;**26**:133–41.

55 Furuno Y, Nagamoto Y, Fujita M *et al.* Reflection as a cause of mid-systolic deceleration of pulmonary flow wave in dogs with acute pulmonary hypertension: comparison of pulmonary artery constriction with pulmonary embolisation. *Cardiovasc Res* 1991;**25**:118–24.

●56 Laskey WK, Ferrari VA, Palevsky HI *et al.* Pulmonary artery hemodynamics in primary pulmonary hypertension. *J Am Coll Cardiol* 1993;**21**:406–12.

57 Laskey WK, Ferrari VA, Palevsky HI *et al.* Ejection characteristics in primary pulmonary hypertension. *Am J Cardiol* 1993;**71**:1111–14.

58 Castelain V, Herve P, Lecarpentier Y *et al*. Pulmonary artery pulse pressure and wave reflection in chronic pulmonary thromboembolism and primary pulmonary hypertension. *J Am Coll Cardiol* 2001;**37**:1085–92.

59 Murata I, Takenaka K, Yoshinoya S *et al*. Clinical evaluation of pulmonary hypertension in systemic sclerosis and related disorders. A Doppler echocardiographic study of 135 Japanese patients. *Chest* 1997;**111**:36–43.

60 Elstein D, Klutstein MW, Lahad A *et al*. Echocardiographic assessment of pulmonary hypertension in Gaucher's disease. *Lancet* 1998;**351**:1544–6.

◆61 McGoon MD. The assessment of pulmonary hypertension. *Clin Chest Med* 2001;**22**:493–508, ix.

62 Aessopos A, Farmakis D, Taktikou H *et al*. Doppler-determined peak systolic tricuspid pressure gradient in persons with normal pulmonary function and tricuspid regurgitation. *J Am Soc Echocardiogr* 2000;**13**:645–9.

63 Dib JC, Abergel E, Rovani C *et al*. The age of the patient should be taken into account when interpreting Doppler assessed pulmonary artery pressures. *J Am Soc Echocardiogr* 1997;**10**:72–3.

64 Himelman RB, Stulbarg M, Kircher B *et al*. Noninvasive evaluation of pulmonary artery pressure during exercise by saline-enhanced Doppler echocardiography in chronic pulmonary disease. *Circulation* 1989;**79**:863–71.

65 Barbant SD, Redberg RF, Tucker KJ *et al*. Abnormal pulmonary artery pressure profile after cardiac transplantation: an exercise Doppler echocardiographic study. *Am Heart J* 1995;**129**:1185–92.

66 Oelberg DA, Marcotte F, Kreisman H *et al*. Evaluation of right ventricular systolic pressure during incremental exercise by Doppler echocardiography in adults with atrial septal defect. *Chest* 1998;**113**:1459–65.

●67 Grunig E, Mereles D, Hildebrandt W *et al*. Stress Doppler echocardiography for identification of susceptibility to high altitude pulmonary edema. *J Am Coll Cardiol* 2000;**35**:980–7.

●68 Grunig E, Janssen B, Mereles D *et al*. Abnormal pulmonary artery pressure response in asymptomatic carriers of primary pulmonary hypertension gene. *Circulation* 2000;**102**:1145–50.

●69 Bossone E, Avelar E, Bach DS *et al*. Diagnostic value of resting tricuspid regurgitation velocity and right ventricular ejection flow parameters for the detection of exercise induced pulmonary arterial hypertension. *Int J Card Imaging* 2000;**16**:429–36.

70 Torbicki A, Tramarin R, Fracchia F *et al*. Effect of increased right ventricular preload on pulmonary artery flow velocity in patients with normal or increased pulmonary artery pressure. *Am J Noninvas Cardiol* 1994;**8**:151–5.

71 Ohashi M, Sato K, Suzuki S *et al*. Doppler echocardiographic evaluation of latent pulmonary hypertension by passive leg raising. *Coron Artery Dis* 1997;**8**:651–5.

72 Chen WJ, Chen JJ, Lin SC *et al*. Detection of cardiovascular shunts by transesophageal echocardiography in patients with pulmonary hypertension of unexplained cause. *Chest* 1995;**107**:8–13.

73 Gorcsan J, III, Edwards TD, Ziady GM *et al*. Transesophageal echocardiography to evaluate patients with severe pulmonary hypertension for lung transplantation. *Ann Thorac Surg* 1995;**59**:717–22.

74 Pruszczyk P, Torbicki A, Pacho R *et al*. Noninvasive diagnosis of suspected severe pulmonary embolism: transesophageal echocardiography vs spiral CT. *Chest* 1997;**112**:722–8.

75 Moser KM, Fedullo PF, Finkbeiner WE *et al*. Do patients with primary pulmonary hypertension develop extensive central thrombi? *Circulation* 1995;**91**:741–5.

●76 McConnell MV, Solomon SD, Rayan ME *et al*. Regional right ventricular dysfunction detected by echocardiography in acute pulmonary embolism. *Am J Cardiol* 1996;**78**:469–73.

77 Ritchie M, Waggoner AD, Davila-Roman VG *et al*. Echocardiographic characterization of the improvement in right ventricular function in patients with severe pulmonary hypertension after single-lung transplantation. *J Am Coll Cardiol* 1993;**22**:1170–4.

78 Katz WE, Gasior TA, Quinlan JJ *et al*. Immediate effects of lung transplantation on right ventricular morphology and function in patients with variable degrees of pulmonary hypertension. *J Am Coll Cardiol* 1996;**27**:384–91.

79 Dittrich HC, Nicod PH, Chow LC *et al*. Early changes of right heart geometry after pulmonary thromboendarterectomy. *J Am Coll Cardiol* 1988;**11**:937–43.

80 Menzel T, Wagner S, Mohr-Kahaly S *et al*. Reversibility of changes in left and right ventricular geometry and hemodynamics in pulmonary hypertension. Echocardiographic characteristics before and after pulmonary thromboendarterectomy. *Z Kardiol* 1997;**86**:928–35.

●81 Hinderliter AL, Willis PW, Long W *et al*. Frequency and prognostic significance of pericardial effusion in primary pulmonary hypertension. PPH Study Group. Primary pulmonary hypertension. *Am J Cardiol* 1999;**84**:481–4, A10.

●82 Raymond RJ, Hinderliter AL, Willis PW *et al*. Echocardiographic predictors of adverse outcomes in primary pulmonary hypertension. *J Am Coll Cardiol* 2002;**39**:1214–19.

●83 Eysmann SB, Palevsky HI, Reichek N *et al*. Two-dimensional and Doppler-echocardiographic and cardiac catheterization correlates of survival in primary pulmonary hypertension. *Circulation* 1989;**80**:353–60.

84 Galie N, Hinderliter AL, Torbicki A *et al*. Effects of the oral endothelin-receptor antagonist bosentan on echocardiographic and doppler measures in patients with pulmonary arterial hypertension. *J Am Coll Cardiol* 2003;**41**:1380–6.

85 Pai RG, Bansal RC, Shah PM. Determinants of the rate of right ventricular pressure rise by Doppler echocardiography: potential value in the assessment of right ventricular function. *J Heart Valve Dis* 1994;**3**:179–84.

●86 Tei C, Dujardin KS, Hodge DO *et al*. Doppler echocardiographic index for assessment of global right ventricular function. *J Am Soc Echocardiogr* 1996;**9**:838–47.

●87 Yeo TC, Dujardin KS, Tei C *et al*. Value of a Doppler-derived index combining systolic and diastolic time intervals in predicting outcome in primary pulmonary hypertension. *Am J Cardiol* 1998;**81**:1157–61.

88 Berger M, Haimowitz A, Van Tosh A *et al*. Quantitative assessment of pulmonary hypertension in patients with tricuspid regurgitation using continuous wave Doppler ultrasound. *J Am Coll Cardiol* 1985;**6**:359–65.

●89 Bossone E, Rubenfire M, Bach DS *et al*. Range of tricuspid regurgitation velocity at rest and during exercise in normal adult men: implications for the diagnosis of pulmonary hypertension. *J Am Coll Cardiol* 1999;**33**:1662–6.

Imaging

RICHARD COULDEN

Options for imaging pulmonary hypertension are almost as diverse as the disease processes that cause it. As each new imaging modality is introduced, algorithms for investigation perversely become more complex rather than more straightforward. Many imaging tests involve exposure to ionizing radiation and its inherent risks. Some are associated with significant morbidity and mortality. Performing all tests on all patients with suspected pulmonary hypertension is not an option, even if our health care systems could afford it. This chapter examines:

- the imaging techniques available
- the radiological features of each major condition as seen in different imaging techniques
- possible algorithms for the investigation of suspected pulmonary hypertension.

The description of radiographic abnormalities for each condition (see Radiological Features) is divided into categories as per the WHO classification of pulmonary hypertension (see Chapter 12) (Table 9.1).[1] This is a descriptive classification rather than a pathological one and is ideally suited to a discussion of imaging and imaging algorithms as they might be used in suspected pulmonary hypertension.

IMAGING TECHNIQUES

Chest radiography

The chest radiograph is inexpensive, non-invasive and frequently overlooked. It provides invaluable information about heart size, the pulmonary vasculature and the presence or absence of lung disease. It often provides the first indication of pulmonary hypertension.

The initial examination should include a frontal and lateral view. The lateral is helpful for assessment of cardiac chamber size, calcification of valves, vessels and pericardium and localization of pathology. Having established a baseline, follow-up examinations often require only a frontal view.

Echocardiography

Like chest radiography, echocardiography is widely available, non-invasive and relatively inexpensive (see Chapter 8). It is the ideal 'next test' after the chest radiograph once pulmonary hypertension is suspected. By combining the assessment of anatomy with function, it can either confirm or refute the presence of right-sided chamber dilatation and through the use of Doppler, provide an estimate peak pulmonary artery pressure. When an intracardiac shunt or valve disease is responsible for pulmonary hypertension, it will also provide a definitive diagnosis.

A detailed description of echocardiography and its role in the diagnosis and assessment of pulmonary hypertension is given elsewhere.

Ventilation/perfusion scintigraphy

Diagnostic scintigraphy is primarily for the diagnosis of pulmonary emboli. Areas of the lung subtended by occluded vessels appear as perfusion defects on a perfusion study, while the pulmonary parenchyma usually remains intact and appears normal on a ventilation

Table 9.1 *Classification of pulmonary hypertension according to the WHO 1998*

Pulmonary arterial hypertension
Primary pulmonary hypertension
Sporadic, familial
Related to
Collagen vascular disease
Congenital systemic to pulmonary shunts
Portal hypertension
IV infection
Drugs/toxins, i.e. anorexigens (aminorex, fenfluramine, dexfenfluramine)
Persistent pulmonary hypertension of the newborn
Other

Pulmonary venous hypertension
Left-sided atrial or ventricular heart disease
Left-sided valvar heart disease
Extrinsic compression of the central pulmonary veins
Fibrosing mediastinitis, adenopathy/tumors
Pulmonary veno-occlusive disease
Other

Pulmonary hypertension associated with disorders of the respiratory system and/or hypoxemia
Chronic obstructive lung disease
Interstitial lung disease
Sleep-disordered breathing
Alveolar hypoventilation disorders
Chronic exposure to high altitude
Neonatal lung disease
Alveolar capillary dysplasia
Other

Pulmonary hypertension due to chronic thrombotic and/or embolic disease
Thromboembolic obstruction of proximal pulmonary arteries
Obstruction of distal pulmonary arteries
Pulmonary embolism (thrombus, tumor, ova/parasites, foreign material)
In situ thrombosis
Sickle cell disease

study. The discrepancy between the two, ventilation/perfusion ($\dot{V}/\dot{Q}$) mismatch, is the hallmark of embolic disease.

Perfusion scanning is performed after injection of radioactive particles (size 10–100 μm) that are trapped in the pulmonary vasculature following intravenous injection. Macroaggregates of human serum albumin (MAA) labelled with technetium-99 m (^{99m}Tc) are usually used. In patients with a right-to-left shunt there is a theoretical risk of systemic embolization, although the risk is very low. Similarly, in patients with pulmonary hypertension there is a theoretical risk of further occlusion of an already compromised pulmonary microcirculation. However, given that the number of vessels in the pulmonary capillary bed (300 million) far outstrips the number of particles injected (200 000–500 000), the risk is very low.

Ventilation scanning can be performed using inert radioactive gases (xenon-133 or krypton-108) or an aerosol of ^{99m}Tc bound to diethylenediaminepentaacetic acid (DTPA). ^{99m}Tc DTPA is generally preferred, as the radiation characteristics of ^{99m}Tc are ideally suited to gamma camera imaging, it is cheap and it is readily available. As with ^{99m}Tc perfusion imaging, imaging after administration of a radioactive aerosol represents ventilation at a moment in time. The aerosol is deposited in the peripheral airways. This contrasts with radioactive gases that wash in and out with each breath, providing a dynamic assessment of ventilation. For imaging pulmonary emboli, wash-in/wash-out is often a source of confusion rather than an advantage.

In patients with chronic airway obstruction, abnormal airflow leads to deposition and pooling of aerosol in the central airways. This accentuates regional variations in ventilation and produces ventilation defects on subsequent imaging. These defects are not matched by pulmonary parenchymal abnormalities on the chest radiograph and are a source of interpretative error. Once deposited, whether in the central or peripheral airways, ^{99m}Tc DTPA dissolves in respiratory mucus and crosses the alveolar-capillary membrane. In normal, non-smoking, subjects ^{99m}Tc DTPA is cleared from the lung with a half-life of approximately 80 minutes. In smokers or patients with an alveolitis, this can be two to four times faster.[2] When a ventilation study is performed before the perfusion study, any ^{99m}Tc DTPA that has been absorbed into the bloodstream will have been excreted by the kidneys and may be seen in the renal tract. Tracer deposited in the mouth or central airways of patients with chronic airways obstruction may be swallowed and appear in the upper gastrointestinal tract.

The absorbed radiation dose attributable to a $\dot{V}/\dot{Q}$ study (1–1.5 mSv) is largely due to the perfusion study and is equivalent to 50–75 chest radiographs.[3] If a $\dot{V}/\dot{Q}$ study is needed in pregnancy, this should be performed with little hesitation, as the dose to the fetus is small and the risk of unnecessary anticoagulation is high. A perfusion study alone may be adequate if the chest radiograph is normal. As ^{99m}Tc is excreted in breast milk, nursing mothers should avoid breast-feeding for 48 hours.[4]

Computed tomography

In the last 10 years, the role of computed tomography (CT) in pulmonary hypertension has been revolutionized by the introduction of spiral CT.[5] Faster scan times, more efficient use of intravascular contrast enhancement and reduced motion artifact have all added to image quality. In the last 3 years, these benefits have been further enhanced by the development of multislice spiral acquisition.

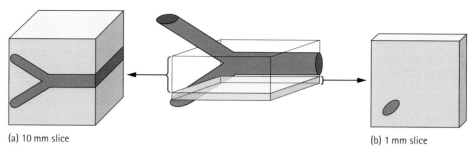

(a) 10 mm slice   (b) 1 mm slice

Figure 9.1 *Diagramatic representation of a thick slice (10 mm) imaging voxel – **vo**lume **el**ement – which contains a branching vessel. The thick voxel averages the attenuation of the branching structure across the whole 10 mm losing through-plane resolution when viewed end on (a). The thin-slice voxel (1 mm) only contains a small part of the branching structure (b). If multiple thin slices are obtained, the fine detail of the original through-plane branching structure is maintained.*

On CT, as in chest radiography, the attenuation of x-rays by blood and soft tissue is very similar. Intravenous contrast enhancement is needed to raise the attenuation value of blood and so provide the necessary blood pool to soft tissue contrast to see the vessel lumen. Conventional iodinated contrast media move quickly from the blood pool into the extracellular space and imaging must be completed during its first pass. Scanning speed is therefore critical. Using a standard single-slice spiral CT scanner and a slice thickness of 3 mm (table travel 5 mm/s), it is possible to image 12 cm of mediastinum (aortic arch to lower pulmonary veins) in 24 seconds. By comparison, using a multislice scanner with a fourfold increase in speed, the same distance can be covered in 6 seconds or the whole chest can be imaged in 1 mm thick slices in the same 24 seconds.

The in-plane resolution of a CT scanner is defined by the number picture elements (pixels) that make up the field of view, i.e. for a 25 cm field of view with 512 pixels in each direction; the size of each pixel is approximately 0.5 mm. Through-plane or long axis resolution, however, depends on slice thickness. As many pulmonary vessels lie in the transaxial plane, they are difficult to demonstrate by CT. To maximize through-plane resolution, the thinnest possible slice thickness is needed (Figure 9.1).[6] Using 1-mm thick CT slices and overlapping reconstruction, through-plane resolution can be reduced to 0.5 mm, i.e. the resolution in all three orthogonal planes is similar. For the first time in its history, CT may be considered to be truly multiplanar.

Multislice CT, by providing thinner slices and wider coverage, brings other benefits:

- the whole lung will be imaged;
- high-resolution images of the lung (HRCT) can be reconstructed specifically to look at lung detail in every patient without the need for additional radiation;
- the heart will be included in the area imaged.

In the past, conventional CT has not been considered to be useful for cardiac imaging but fast scan times have the added benefit of reducing blurring due to cardiac motion.[7] Cardiac chamber size, wall thickness and general anatomy are all easily assessed and careful review of the heart must not be ignored.

The absorbed radiation dose attributable to CT pulmonary angiography (CTPA) is 8 mSv. This is equivalent to 400 chest radiographs,[3] substantially more than a $\dot{V}/\dot{Q}$ scintigram. When choosing which of these tests to use, the benefit of higher diagnostic yield from CT must be balanced against the increased radiation burden. This is particularly true in young patients who are likely to live long enough to experience the full radiation risk.

Magnetic resonance imaging

Magnetic resonance imaging (MRI) of the chest has been available for many years but its inclusion into mainstream cardiothoracic imaging has been slow. Access to MRI has been limited and image acquisition and postprocessing has been slow and laborious. New developments with faster gradients, new sequences and more efficient surface coils have addressed many of these issues. MRI, however, unlike CT can assess structure and function without the need for ionizing radiation.

ANATOMY

Anatomic imaging in the chest can be performed using either a 'black blood' (spin echo, SE) or 'white blood' (gradient refocused echo, GRE) technique. Both require electrocardiogram (ECG) gating to allow data to be collected over multiple heartbeats. The number of radiofrequency excitations/data acquisitions needed to create an image depends on the spatial and contrast resolution required. For most cardiac purposes, this would be 256 or 512 and for conventional sequences would take 256 or

512 heartbeats. 'Fast' versions of both sequences are now widely available and can be performed in a breath-hold of 4–16 heartbeats.[8,9] Image quality is similar to CT although tissue contrast mechanisms are very different.

VENTRICULAR FUNCTION

The major advantage of MR over CT lies not in anatomic imaging, but in its capacity to assess ventricular function and flow. Multiphase cine images can be obtained in any plane providing both qualitative and quantitative assessment of ventricular function and wall motion. Echocardiography and contrast ventriculography, while most commonly used for this purpose, are at best qualitative. By defining both epicardial and endocardial borders, ventricular volumes, muscle volume and hence muscle mass, regional wall motion and systolic wall thickening can all be measured.[10,11] With respect to the right ventricle, its pyramidal shape and thin free wall make it almost impossible to assess quantitatively by any other method. MRI is now the 'gold standard' for measurement of ventricular function and muscle mass. Although radionuclide ventriculography can match the reproducibility of MRI in measuring ejection fraction, absolute volumes are rarely available and radiation exposure limits repeat investigation.

FLOW MEASUREMENT

Using a modified gradient echo sequence, MR estimates of blood velocity and flow can be made. As blood flows through a magnetic field gradient, its hydrogen protons acquire a phase shift relative to stationary tissue that is proportional to its velocity. By measuring blood velocity at multiple time points throughout the cardiac cycle (cine phase contrast imaging – cine PC),[12,13] the velocity profile for any vessel can be calculated (Figure 9.2). In many respects, cine PC is the MR equivalent of Doppler ultrasound. MRI, however, is independent of acoustic window and can examine any vessel in any plane. It also has the advantage of being able to combine measurements of vessel cross-sectional area with mean velocity and so calculate absolute flow (mL/min). Numerous applications have been described, including the measurement of right and left ventricular stroke volume (main pulmonary artery and aortic root flow),[14] calculation of intracardiac shunt fractions (comparison of aortic root and main pulmonary artery flow)[15] and the calculation of flow in individual pulmonary arteries.[16]

MAGNETIC RESONANCE ANGIOGRAPHY

Magnetic resonance angiography (MRA) has been available in different guises for many years. Early applications involved the use of two-dimensional time-of-flight sequences to maximize the conspicuity of flowing blood.

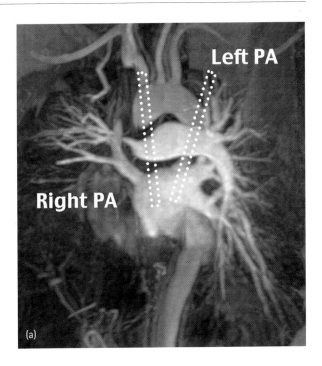

(a)

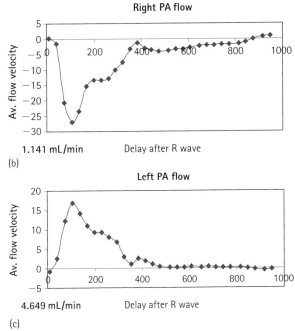

Figure 9.2 *(a) Contrast-enhanced magnetic resonance angiogram in a patient with severe chronic thromboembolic pulmonary hypertension (CTEPH). The right lung is particularly affected with only one segment to the upper lobe patent. Dotted blocks show planes for acquisition of cine PC data from which blood flow to the right lung (b) and the left lung (c) can be calculated. PA, pulmonary artery.*

Magnetic resonance systems were slow and pulmonary MRA required multiple long breath-holds. It was not until the introduction of faster scanners with stronger gradients that pulmonary MRA became a practical possibility.

Now that an entire chest can be imaged in a breath-hold, intravenous contrast medium may be used to enhance vascular signal during its first pass (contrast-enhanced MRA, CEMRA).[17,18] Multislice CT and CEMRA produce pulmonary angiograms of similar quality although MR is technically more demanding to perform. MRA, however, involves no ionizing radiation and is more suited to repeat investigation in patients requiring serial studies.

PULMONARY ANGIOGRAPHY

Like all angiographic procedures, pulmonary angiography carries a recognized morbidity and mortality. This, surprisingly, is much lower than most doctors believe. In the PIOPED study, there were only five deaths in 1111 patients (0.5%)[19] and in a large meta-analysis of 5320 patients there were only 15 deaths.[20] Death as a result of pulmonary angiography is rare and when it does occur it is almost always associated with pulmonary hypertension.[21] The most common non-fatal complication is arrhythmia, which is a consequence of pulmonary hypertension and right ventricular hypertrophy.[22]

Despite its risks, conventional pulmonary angiography continues to have advantages over competitive techniques:

- ability to perform direct pressure measurements and Swan–Ganz estimation of cardiac output as part of the same examination;[23]
- capacity to proceed immediately with a therapeutic procedure if the patient is found to have major pulmonary emboli, i.e. using a thrombolyser or intra-arterial clot lysis;
- temporal resolution. Each image is acquired in a few milliseconds compared with seconds for CT and MRI. This minimizes cardiac and respiratory motion artifact and avoids venous contamination of the arterial image, i.e. overlapping arteries and veins on the same image spatial resolution. Resolution of cut film is in the order of 0.1 mm compared with 0.5 mm for CT and MRI. Digital subtraction angiography (DSA) with a 1024 matrix and 30 cm field of view is 0.3 mm.

RADIOLOGICAL FEATURES

Pulmonary hypertension – general

Pulmonary hypertension is a function of blood flow and resistance across the pulmonary vascular bed. As the vascular bed has considerable inherent overcapacity, resistance only rises when a large proportion of the vascular bed is excluded (50–60%)[24] or increased flow exceeds maximal pulmonary vasodilatation.

For most causes of pulmonary hypertension, the same signs are seen on chest radiography, i.e. cardiac enlargement, dilatation of the right-sided cardiac chambers and enlargement of the proximal pulmonary arteries (to segmental level). Peripheral vessels are disproportionately tapered, giving rise to 'peripheral pruning'. Only in pulmonary hypertension associated with a large left-to-right shunt are the peripheral vessels also large. Dilated peripheral vessels (plethora) are usually only recognized when the pulmonary to systemic flow ratio is greater than 2:1.[25]

Heart size is best assessed by the cardiothoracic ratio (CTR),[25,26] the ratio between cardiac transverse diameter and maximum width of the thorax above the costophrenic angles (Figure 9.3). The upper limit of normal for a standard posteroanterior (PA) chest in inspiration is 0.50, rising to 0.57 for a supine anteroposterior (AP) film. On the AP film, the short film to x-ray source focus distance (usually 100 cm) increases magnification.[27] In children, CTR may be over 0.5 (0.6 in neonates). CTR varies inversely with age and must be taken into account when making serial measurements in children with congenital heart disease. When dilatation of the right atrium is associated with elevated pressure, the cavae and azygos vein also dilate. The degree of azygos dilatation broadly correlates with mean right atrial pressure.[28]

Proximal pulmonary arteries are measured at the hilar point and should be no more than 17 mm in diameter.[29] Although pulmonary artery dilatation is reasonably specific, it is neither sensitive nor well correlated with the severity of hypertension. Dilatation also occurs as a consequence of pulmonary valve disease. In pulmonary stenosis, dilatation involves only the pulmonary trunk and left pulmonary artery, the right pulmonary artery is usually spared (Figure 9.4).[30]

Pulmonary arterial hypertension

PRIMARY PULMONARY HYPERTENSION (PPH)

Radiographic features are those of pulmonary hypertension (right-sided cardiac chamber enlargement, dilated proximal pulmonary arteries and abrupt peripheral vascular pruning).[31] When pulmonary hypertension has been prolonged, the vessels also appear tortuous, probably as a result of remodeling and elongation. The absence of pulmonary artery dilatation does not exclude it. V̇/Q̇ scintigraphy may be normal or show heterogenous perfusion with mismatched perfusion defects (Figure 9.5).[32–34] This is in sharp contrast to chronic thromboembolic disease, which will invariably show multiple large areas of perfusion mismatch. The PPH pattern of heterogeneous lung perfusion is also recognized on HRCT; small areas of increased centrilobular attenuation clearly visible relative to areas of vasoconstriction.[35] There is no interlobular septal thickening. This finding, together with a normal

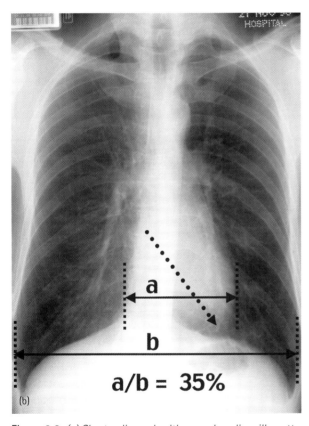

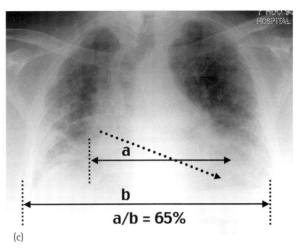

Figure 9.3 (continued).

Figure 9.3 *(a) Chest radiograph with normal cardiac silhouette showing calculation of cardiothoracic ratio (CTR) (black arrows) and pulmonary artery diameter (white arrows). Dotted black arrow shows normal cardiac axis in inspiration. In lung disease causing large lung volume (b) or small lung volume (c), cardiac axis will change and result in a low CTR (b) or high CTR (c) even when the heart is normal.*

pulmonary capillary wedge pressure (PCWP), helps to distinguish PPH from veno-occlusive disease, which in other respects is very similar. Pulmonary angiography is not needed except to exclude other diagnoses.

COLLAGEN VASCULAR DISEASE

Walcott *et al.* suggest that up to 30% of patients presenting with apparent PPH have evidence of collagen vascular disease.[36] Features are those of pulmonary hypertension with addition of features specific to the connective tissue disease (see Chapter 13D). While rheumatoid vasculitis may cause pulmonary hypertension, this complication is more frequently a late manifestation of rheumatoid interstitial lung disease.[37,38]

Pulmonary hypertension in systemic sclerosis is common but independent of the florid interstitial pulmonary fibrosis with which it is also associated.[39,40]

A large number of very rare vasculitides are known to produce pulmonary hypertension. The majority of these involve small vessels although pulmonary hypertension may also occur in large vessel vasculitis (Takayasu's disease).

Takayasu's arteritis is predominantly a disease of young women, involving the pulmonary arteries in approximately 50% of cases.[41,42] When present, pulmonary hypertension is mild and symptoms are overshadowed by involvement of systemic vessels (coronary, carotid, renal and aorto-iliac arteries). The same is true of the chest radiograph where features of aortitis predominate (irregularity of the aortic outline, focal ectasia and rib notching if descending thoracic aortic stenosis is present).[43] On pulmonary angiography, stenoses in the lobar and segmental pulmonary arteries can be mistaken for chronic thromboembolic pulmonary hypertension (CTEPH), although the clinical picture allows the correct diagnosis to be made. On CTPA, pulmonary stenoses are shown to be due to focal thickening of the vessel wall. As with aortitis, these areas show delayed contrast enhancement, confirming their inflammatory nature.[44] Pulmonary vascular obstruction gives rise to perfusion abnormalities on scintigraphy identical to those seen in thromboembolic disease.

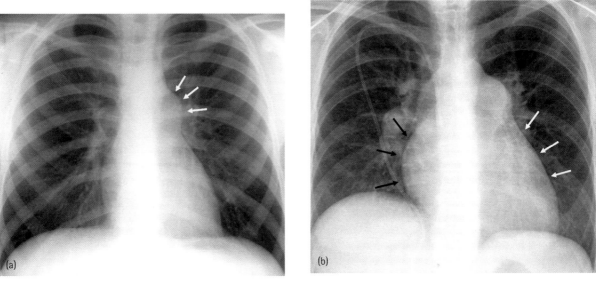

Figure 9.4 *(a) Chest radiograph showing dilated pulmonary outflow (arrows) with lower lobe pulmonary arteries of normal size in a patient with pulmonary stenosis. This contrasts with a dilated pulmonary outflow and dilated lower lobe arteries in a patient with PPH (b). Bulging upper left heart border (white arrows) and right heart border (black arrows) due to right ventricular and right atrial enlargement, respectively.*

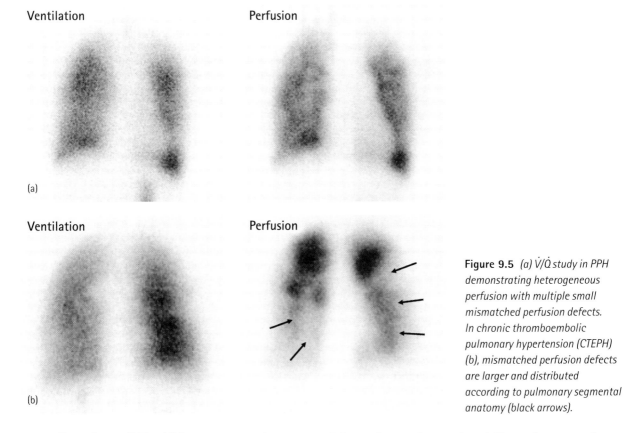

Figure 9.5 *(a) V̇/Q̇ study in PPH demonstrating heterogeneous perfusion with multiple small mismatched perfusion defects. In chronic thromboembolic pulmonary hypertension (CTEPH) (b), mismatched perfusion defects are larger and distributed according to pulmonary segmental anatomy (black arrows).*

Small vessel vasculitides fall into two categories:

- those associated with antineutrophil cytoplasmic antibody (ANCA) and
- those associated that are immune complex mediated.

Wegener's granulomatosis and Churg–Strauss syndrome are the best known of the ANCA-positive conditions. Both are multisystem disorders with different spectra of involvement. Both conditions typically involve the lung, although in neither is pulmonary hypertension an important feature.

The main pulmonary manifestations of Wegener's are of necrotizing granulomatous pulmonary masses,[45] pulmonary hemorrhage[46] and stenosis of the trachea and main bronchi.[47] Churg–Strauss syndrome, at the other end of the ANCA disease spectrum, is characterized by transient, multifocal, non-segmental consolidation.[48,49] As might be anticipated, appearances are indistinguishable from pulmonary eosinophilia. Unlike Wegener's, however, cavitation is rare. In both conditions, the imaging findings are dominated by the underlying condition and pulmonary hypertension often goes unnoticed.

Immune complex diseases (Henoch–Schönlein pupura, necrotizing sarcoidal angiitis and Behçet's disease) are not direct causes of pulmonary hypertension although Behçet's disease is associated with thrombophlebitis and venous thromboembolism.[50] Pulmonary artery aneurysms, which may be multiple, give rise to hemoptysis and/or pulmonary infarction. When thrombosed, they are a cause of $\dot{V}/\dot{Q}$ mismatch on scintigraphy.[51] The presence of pulmonary aneurysms carries a very poor prognosis and is more frequently associated with thrombophlebitis than is usual in Behçet's disease.[52]

CONGENITAL SYSTEMIC TO PULMONARY SHUNTS

When flow through the pulmonary vascular bed is increased, pulmonary hypertension can occur without a rise in pulmonary vascular resistance. For practical purposes, this only occurs in left-to-right shunts, the most common of which are atrial septal defect (ASD), ventricular septal defect (VSD) and patent ductus arteriosus (PDA) (see Chapter 13H). Pulmonary hypertension in these conditions is mild until pulmonary vascular resistance rises. The radiographic features, in the absence of significant pulmonary hypertension, are cardiomegaly due to volume overload and pulmonary plethora (Figure 9.6). If pulmonary hypertension intervenes, these changes will be superimposed on the features of pulmonary hypertension.

As pulmonary artery pressure rises, the left-to-right shunt diminishes, eventually reversing when pulmonary artery pressure exceeds systemic pressure (Eisenmenger reaction). Vessels that were initially plethoric become progressively 'pruned', giving the same end-stage appearance as pulmonary hypertension from other causes. Confusingly, during the transition from plethora to constriction, there is a period when vessel caliber may be normal and so mask the underlying process.

In Eisenmenger ASD, there is often massive dilatation of the proximal pulmonary arteries with rapid tapering beyond the hila. Right-sided chambers and the left atrium are enlarged but the left ventricle is normal. Left ventricular dilatation only occurs when there is a septum primum defect associated with significant mitral regurgitation. This contrasts with a VSD where all four cardiac chambers experience the volume overload and are dilated.

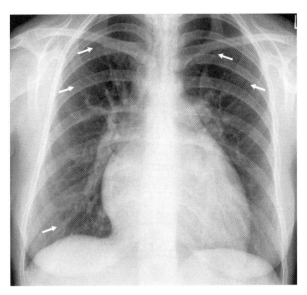

Figure 9.6 *Chest radiograph showing cardiomegaly and configuration of right-sided cardiac chamber enlargement (bulging right heart border and superior left heart border). Pulmonary arteries are large but do not taper. They are dilated to the periphery of the lung (arrows), indicating plethora in this patient with an atrial septal defect (ASD).*

Pulmonary artery dilatation in VSD and PDA is generally less marked than in an ASD. It is suggested that in an ASD, pulmonary vascular resistance is low, even in large shunts well into adult life. Despite high flow, the pulmonary vascular tree develops normally and the arterial walls that are thickened and muscular in the fetus are allowed to involute. In a VSD, pulmonary vascular resistance is high from birth. The presence of early pulmonary hypertension may prevent regression of the arterial wall and thereby reduce compliance. The end result is less pulmonary artery dilatation.[53]

In PDA, the ascending aorta and arch are large with dilatation of the main pulmonary artery. Dilatation of the right and left pulmonary artery is less marked. Main pulmonary artery dilation is largely a consequence of the aortopulmonary jet which is being directed anteriorly from the patent ductus. Both atria and ventricles are dilated.

Echocardiography is central to the investigation of congenital heart disease and in the majority of cases will provide a firm diagnosis. Certain areas, however, are difficult to visualize even by transesophageal echocardiography. These include entry of the pulmonary veins into the left atrium (anomalous pulmonary venous drainage and sinus venosus ASD) and the aortic arch (PDA). For these conditions, CTPA and MRA can be helpful (Figure 9.7), MRA having the additional advantage of being able to assess ventricular function and estimate shunt fraction as part of the same examination.

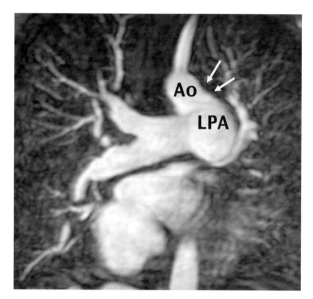

Figure 9.7 *Coronal section from a magnetic resonance angiogram showing a large patent ductus arteriosus (arrows), which was unsuspected in this patient with pulmonary hypertension. Ao, aorta; LPA, left pulmonary artery.*

HEPATOPULMONARY SYNDROME

Patients with severe cirrhotic liver disease develop pulmonary 'spider nevi' and right-to-left intrapulmonary shunting in up to 20% of cases (hepatopulmonary syndrome).[54,55] Nevi occur throughout the lung but are rarely seen on the plain chest radiograph.[56] Indeed, even on HRCT, they may be hard to identify. While pulmonary angiography has sufficient spatial resolution to show the nevi, it is rarely needed to make the diagnosis. The lungs are otherwise normal and interstitial pulmonary fibrosis is not associated (see Chapter 27).

Shunts are best detected and quantified by perfusion scintigraphy which shows tracer uptake in the renal parenchyma; radioactive macroaggregates shunting through the lung, reach the systemic circulation and are trapped by the kidneys.[57] By measuring relative uptake of tracer in the lungs and kidneys, shunt fraction can be estimated. Hepatopulmonary syndrome is one of the few causes of pulmonary hypertension which can be treated surgically. Successful liver transplantation leads to regression of nevi, reduction in shunt fraction and hypoxia and normalization of pulmonary artery pressure.

Pulmonary venous hypertension

When pulmonary venous pressure is consistently elevated above 25 mmHg, there is a disproportionate rise in pulmonary artery pressure. The mechanism for the increase in pulmonary vascular resistance is unclear but both structural and physiological vasoconstriction are involved (see Chapter 14A).

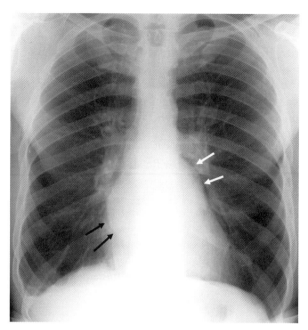

Figure 9.8 *Chest radiograph in mitral stenosis showing dilated left atrium (double right heart border, black arrows; left atrial appendage, white arrows). Proximal pulmonary arteries are large, indicating pulmonary hypertension.*

On plain radiography, mitral stenosis is characterized by left atrial (LA) enlargement without left ventricular (LV) dilatation. The presence of LV dilatation indicates significant mitral regurgitation in addition to stenosis. Pulmonary venous hypertension is associated with upper zone vascular redistribution,[58] septal lines (Kerly A and B lines) and pulmonary edema.[59] Frank pulmonary edema is not normally a feature of chronic venous hypertension unless there is an acute predisposing cause, i.e. acute myocardial infarction. Although the chest radiograph may suggest the diagnosis of mitral valve disease, echocardiography is essential to confirm the diagnosis and assess severity (Figure 9.8). The plain film cannot distinguish between mitral stenosis, atrial myxoma or cor triatriatum. These are also echocardiographic diagnoses.

Pulmonary veno-occlusive disease is a rare condition of unknown etiology, which is almost invariably fatal (see Chapter 14B). It results from thrombosis and intimal hyperplasia of the small pulmonary veins leading to venous hypertension, pulmonary edema and secondary pulmonary hypertension.[60] Interstitial fibrosis and interstitial pneumonitis are often associated, although honeycomb change does not occur. The radiographic appearances are of pulmonary hypertension associated with varying degrees of pulmonary edema.[61] Distinction from other causes of venous hypertension is based on the normal size of the left atrium and normal PCWP on right heart catheterization. The CT findings mirror those of the chest radiograph, i.e. pulmonary edema without left

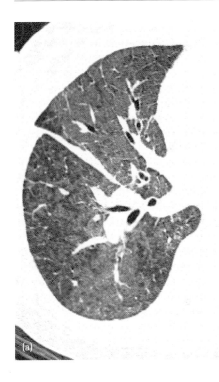

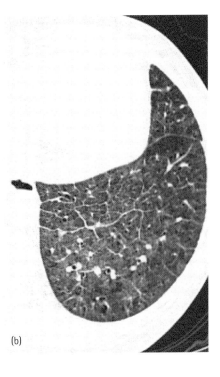

Figure 9.9 *High-resolution computed tomography in primary pulmonary hypertension (a) and veno-occlusive disease (b). In both conditions there may be heterogeneous ground-glass shadowing, but veno-occlusive disease also leads to smooth interlobular septal thickening (black arrows) and pleural effusions, thereby mimicking left ventricular failure.*

atrial hypertension. Smooth interlobular septal thickening, pleural effusions and peri-bronchovascular airspace shadowing are characteristic of end-stage disease (Figure 9.9).[62] Mediastinal adenopathy may also occur. The large pulmonary veins often appear normal on CT, as they do on late-phase pulmonary angiography. Conventional pulmonary angiography is of no diagnostic value.

Pulmonary hypertension associated with disorders of the respiratory system and/or hypoxemia

PULMONARY HYPERTENSION SECONDARY TO LUNG DISEASE

The features of pulmonary hypertension secondary to lung disease reflect both the underlying lung condition and pulmonary hypertension (see Chapter 15A). Plain film assessment of heart size may be particularly difficult. As lung disease leads to an increase (emphysema) or decrease (interstitial fibrosis) in lung volume, diaphragms may fall or rise, respectively. This alters cardiac axis and CTR measurements may be spuriously low or high. In this setting, any discrepancy between clinical and radiographic findings should lead to echocardiography or MRI to assess cardiac function. The latter may be necessary if echocardiography in the presence of lung disease is technically difficult, i.e. limited acoustic window. On HRCT, the absence of a recognizable lung abnormality in a patient with pulmonary hypertension effectively excludes lung disease as a cause.

SLEEP DISORDERS AND ALVEOLAR HYPOVENTILATION

Hypoventilation results in small volume lungs without underlying lung disease, i.e. the appearances are of expiration. The hemidiaphragms are elevated and there is plate atelectasis in the lower zones. Plate atelectasis is more easily recognized on HRCT, which also shows a generalized increase in lung attenuation. This reflects the reduced ratio of air to soft tissue that results from reduced lung volume. Obstructive sleep apnea (see Chapter 15B) results from loss of pharyngeal or palatal tone and leads to upper airway obstruction during sleep. Although more common in obesity, it may also occur in those of normal weight. In the absence of neuromuscular disease or chest wall deformity, wakeful hypoventilation is almost always associated with obesity. Increased intra-abdominal fat leads to splinting of the chest and diaphragm and reduced effective lung volume.

Pulmonary hypertension due to chronic thrombotic and/or embolic disease

ACUTE PULMONARY EMBOLISM

The features of acute pulmonary embolism (PE) on the chest radiograph are well described.[63,64] They are, however, subtle and even in the presence of massive PE, the plain film may be normal.[65] The chest radiograph is performed to exclude conditions that might mimic PE rather than make the diagnosis. The most important of these are pneumonia, pneumothorax and rib fracture, all of which may present with dyspnea and chest pain.

Pulmonary infarction complicating acute PE is relatively uncommon. The signs of PE without infarction therefore relate to the embolus itself, i.e. oligemia beyond an occluded vessel and increase in size of the main and/or descending pulmonary arteries proximal to the occlusion. The diaphragm may be elevated and there is often linear atelectasis even in the absence of infarction.[66] This is presumed to be a consequence of impaired ventilation or reduced surfactant.[67] Pulmonary infarcts give rise to areas of subpleural consolidation which are often multifocal and basal. Although large emboli may occlude lobar arteries, lobar consolidation is rare. Opacities usually develop within 12–24 hours but may take months to resolve, often leaving a subpleural scar. This contrasts with pulmonary hemorrhage (without infarction) that clears in days and pneumonia that clears patchily over weeks. Cavitation is rare and suggests a septic origin or secondary infection.

After the chest radiograph, V̇/Q̇ scanning has been the first line investigation for PE for many years. A normal V̇/Q̇ scan in a patient with a low clinical suspicion of PE reliably excludes the diagnosis (prevalence of PE in this patient group is 4%),[18] whereas a high probability scan in someone with a high clinical suspicion can confirm the diagnosis (prevalence of PE 96%). A V̇/Q̇ study giving a normal or high probability result is very useful. Unfortunately, between 40% and 60% of patients with suspected acute PE have a low or intermediate probability V̇/Q̇ result (prevalence of PE of 10–40% depending on whether an outpatient or inpatient population is being considered). Add to this an inter-observer variability of 25–30% for reporting intermediate and low probability scans and nearly two-thirds of patients will have an indeterminate result. These patients need a further test, which, until recently, was pulmonary angiography as the only practical alternative (for review see Chapter 16A).

Pulmonary angiography is the 'gold standard' for the investigation of PE. Sensitivity and specificity are high (98% and 97%, respectively)[68] and many diagnostic algorithms advocate its use when V̇/Q̇ scanning gives an indeterminate result. Availability, however, is limited (<30% of UK hospitals are able to perform a pulmonary angiogram). It is expensive and many clinicians perceive it as dangerous. The actual risk is small, even in pulmonary hypertension, but the misconception may explain why fewer pulmonary angiograms are performed than are clinically indicated. Fewer than 15% of patients with an inconclusive V̇/Q̇ scan go on to angiography. This means that many patients without PE are being anticoagulated inappropriately and many who have pulmonary emboli are not.

Ultrasound of the pelvic and leg veins is inexpensive, non-invasive and widely available. Sensitivity and specificity to thrombus above the knee is high (94% and 99%, respectively)[69] and in many centers ultrasound has replaced conventional venography. Sensitivity to below-knee deep venous thrombosis (DVT), however, is poor

(60%) and a negative ultrasound does not exclude a thrombus. Furthermore, as an indirect test looking for a source of emboli, ultrasound can neither confirm nor refute the presence of pulmonary emboli. This fact is reflected in the lack of impact that ultrasound has had in reducing the need for additional tests.

The initial reports of CTPA were so promising that many believed the 'holy grail' of diagnostic tests for PE had been reached.[70] As a non-invasive examination which is widely available and relatively inexpensive, it fulfilled the criteria for the ideal test. Unfortunately, time has shown that sensitivity and specificity are not as high as originally hoped and a significant proportion of examinations continue to be unsatisfactory.[71] Intense contrast enhancement is required to detect peripheral emboli and most investigators advocate using 150 ml of contrast medium with a high flow rate and thin slice collimation (≤3 mm slice thickness).[72] Using this approach, a large European multicenter trial has shown a sensitivity and specificity of 88% and 94%, respectively (Figure 9.10).[73] The most common sources of diagnostic error are listed in Table 9.2. The diagnostic problem of emboli limited to subsegmental vessels, however, remains.

When compared with pulmonary angiography, the accuracy of single slice CTPA for subsegmental emboli is only 17–25%,[74] and yet subsegmental emboli are common. It is suggested that emboli may be purely subsegmental in as many as 30% of patients.[75] Is this important? At subsegmental level, not even pulmonary angiography is perfect; wide inter-observer variability in reporting subsegmental disease is a well reported.[76] Untreated patients from the PIOPED study with a negative pulmonary angiogram had a PE rate of 0.6% in the following year. Some of these patients must have had subsegmental emboli at the time of their initial investigation, indicating that small emboli have little impact on subsequent health. Similarly, a negative CTPA is associated with an excellent outcome in patients who do not receive anticoagulation (<1% risk of subsequent PE during a 6-month follow-up).[77]

Not all patients presenting with dyspnea, chest pain and hemoptysis will prove to have pulmonary emboli. A negative scintigram or pulmonary angiogram merely excludes PE; they do not provide alternative diagnoses. This is not true for CTPA, which frequently identifies causes for chest pain other than PE.[78] CT is not organ specific; therefore it is far more versatile. The same CTPA examination that is used to look for a PE can be tailored to examine the systemic venous system looking for DVT. There is no benefit in looking for the source of emboli once the diagnosis of PE has been made, but identifying venous thrombus following a negative CTPA will still alter management. CT venography (CTV) of the IVC and iliofemoral veins (umbilicus to knees) is easily achieved using the same bolus of contrast medium that

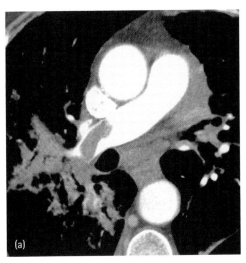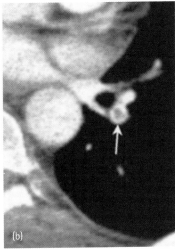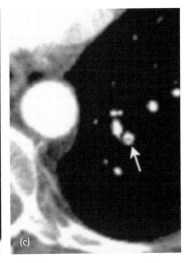

Figure 9.10 *Computed tomography pulmonary angiography in acute pulmonary embolism showing a large central thrombus (a), smaller segmental thrombus (b) and small subsegmental thrombus (c). In all cases the thrombus (arrows) is largely surrounded by bright blood-pool contrast, indicating an acute embolus rather than chronic mural thrombus.*

Table 9.2 *Causes of false-positive and false-negative diagnoses of pulmonary embolism on spiral computed tomography*

- Inadequate opacification of pulmonary arteries
- Respiratory and cardiac motion
- Partial volume effect with vessels running in-plane
- Low signal-to-noise ratio when imaging large patients
- Small hilar and bronchopulmonary nodes simulating occluded arteries
- Fluid-filled bronchi simulating occluded arteries
- Reduced vascularity in regions of hypoventilation (severe air trapping or consolidation)
- Emboli limited to subsegmental arteries

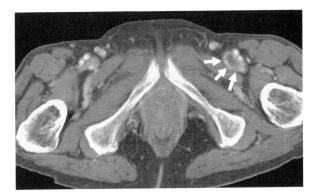

Figure 9.11 *Computed tomography of the iliofemoral veins 3 minutes after contrast injection for computed tomography pulmonary angiography (CTPA). This shows thrombus within the left common femoral vein (arrows) in a patient with no evidence of pulmonary embolism on CTPA.*

was injected for the CTPA. Imaging after a delay of 3 minutes from the start of the injection provides good systemic venous enhancement and will either confirm or refute the presence of DVT (Figure 9.11).[79] Early reports indicate a sensitivity and specificity of nearly 100% compared with Doppler ultrasound for above-knee DVT.[80] Katz et al.[81] recently showed that 6% of patients undergoing CTPA for suspected PE had no evidence of PE but did have a DVT. The routine inclusion of CTV in a department's CTPA protocol would therefore obviate the need for Doppler ultrasound of the legs in patients in whom there is a clinical suspicion of venous thromboembolism.

It is only with the introduction of CEMRA that the magnetic resonance has become sufficiently robust to compete with CTPA.[82] Reported sensitivity and specificity are similar to CTPA, although the number of patients in published series is small. Difficulties related to cardiac motion artifact in the lower lobe vessels have yet to be addressed[83] and monitoring of critically ill patients in the magnetic environment remains a problem. Time will tell

whether the early promise of initial studies is sustained in the long term. In the meantime, limited availability and high cost make it unlikely that MRI will play a significant role in the diagnosis of acute PE in the short term.

CHRONIC PULMONARY EMBOLI (SEE CHAPTER 17)

The chest radiograph shows cardiomegaly and right-sided chamber dilatation. The central pulmonary arteries are large and abrupt 'cut-off' is common.[84,85] Peripheral pulmonary vessels are disorganized rather than simply tapered. Although pulmonary vascular changes are more common than in acute PE, they may be subtle and can be masked or mimicked by underlying chronic airways obstruction. As in acute PE, areas of peripheral oligemia can be seen and correlate well with areas of reduced vascularity on angiography and hypoperfusion on scintigraphy.

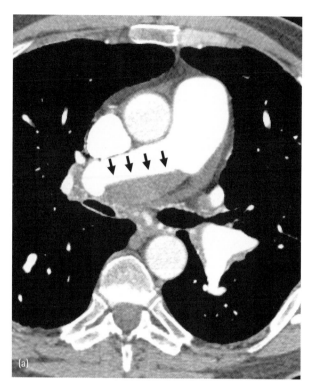

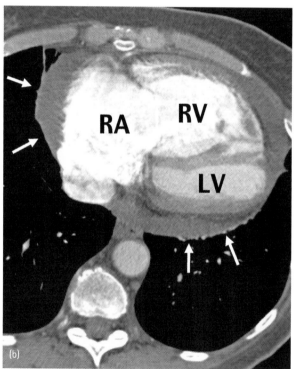

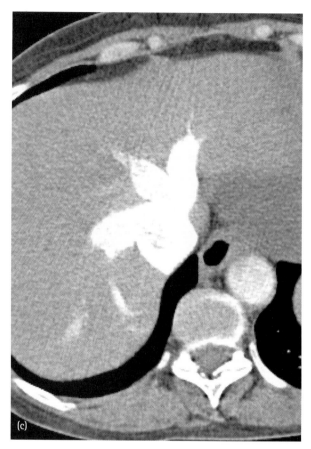

Figure 9.12 *Three images from a computed tomography pulmonary angiography examination in chronic thromboembolic pulmonary hypertension. There is laminated thrombus (black arrows) in the right main pulmonary artery (a). The right ventricle and atrium are dilated and hypertrophied displacing the left ventricle posteriorly (b). Small pericardial effusions are common in pulmonary hypertension (white arrows). Tricuspid regurgitation is indicated by contrast refluxing into the inferior vena cava and hepatic veins during its first pass (c).*

Normal or near-normal vascularity does not exclude the diagnosis. Pleural thickening, pleural effusions, plate atelectasis and small peripheral foci of consolidation are common, albeit non-specific, associations of CTEPH.

$\dot{V}/\dot{Q}$ scintigraphy in chronic pulmonary embolism will show multiple mismatched perfusion defects which are indistinguishable from those seen in acute PE.[86] Unlike acute PE, however, the perfusion defects will not resolve on sequential imaging. The combination of a plain film suggesting pulmonary hypertension and a $\dot{V}/\dot{Q}$ scan with multiple mismatched perfusion defects is diagnostic of CTEPH.

In recent years CTPA has become the mainstay of diagnosis. Pulmonary artery size, patency and the presence of mural thrombus are well shown. Right-sided cardiac chambers can be easily assessed, using the degree of dilation as broad guide to function. Reflux of contrast into the IVC during its first pass indicates tricuspid regurgitation; the extent of reflux correlates well with the severity of TR on echocardiography (Figure 9.12).[87]

Recanalization of acute occlusive thrombus often leads to the creation of short stenoses or webs. Webs in the lower lobe vessels lie in the transaxial plane and as such are difficult to demonstrate by CT. They are only seen when the best technique is used, i.e. thin-slice multislice

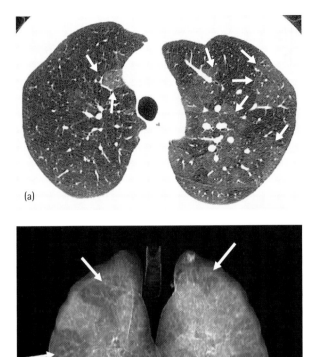

(a)

(b)

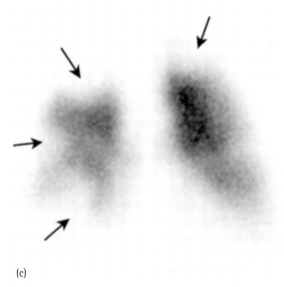

(c)

Figure 9.13 (continued).

Figure 9.13 *High-resolution computed tomography in a patient with chronic thromboembolic pulmonary hypertension showing mosaic perfusion (a). Areas of pulmonary hyperperfusion are of increased attenuation (white arrows) and are associated with large vessels, whereas areas of hypoperfusion are of low attenuation and contain small vessels. On a three-dimensional reconstruction of the lung parenchyma from a thin-slice computed tomography pulmonary angiography examination (b), hypoperfused areas correlate well with perfusion defects seen on perfusion scintigraphy (c).*

CT, with the data being examined by multiplanar reformat. As thrombus becomes organized, it is incorporated into the vessel wall and has a smooth luminal surface.[88] Late calcification is common and must be distinguished from calcification occurring in atheroma. Atheroma in the pulmonary arteries is identical to that seen in the systemic circulation but only occurs in the presence of pulmonary hypertension. In some patients with very slow pulmonary flow and giant pulmonary arteries, laminated thrombus may develop *in situ* in the proximal pulmonary arteries. This is not usually associated with peripheral emboli and can be distinguished from CTEPH by the absence of webs or peripheral occlusions. The underlying

cause for the giant pulmonary arteries is also often apparent, e.g. an ASD.

On HRCT, areas of low attenuation are frequently seen in the pulmonary parenchyma. These are associated with small pulmonary vessels and correspond to areas of hypoperfusion seen on perfusion scintigraphy (Figure 9.13). The intervening 'normal' lung is of high attenuation due to focal hyperperfusion. Vessels in the 'normal' areas are large. This pattern of mosaic perfusion is virtually pathognomonic of chronic thromboembolic disease,[89] although its absence does not exclude it. The variation in attenuation between regions of hypo- and hyper-perfusion is broadly related to the degree of pulmonary hypertension. Following successful surgical thromboendarterectomy, treated areas of hypoperfusion rise to normal attenuation values with a concomitant reduction in attenuation values in areas of hyperperfusion. Untreated areas of hypoperfusion also show an improvement. This suggests that the intensity of the mosaic pattern is dependent on the degree of pulmonary hypertension, hyperperfusion of 'normal' areas being as abnormal as hypoperfusion in regions subtended by occluded vessels.[90]

Focal hypoventilation, hypoxia and pulmonary vasoconstriction can also give rise to mosaic attenuation in small airways disease.[91] The distinction between chronic thromboembolic mosaic attenuation and air trapping is made on expiratory imaging. On expiratory HRCT, mosaic attenuation due to air trapping is exaggerated, whereas mosaic perfusion due to chronic thromboembolic disease is not (Figure 9.14). Bronchial dilatation, possibly related to ischemia, may also occur in CTEPH.[92] It arises in areas of hypoperfusion but is not associated with the small airways disease, thereby allowing distinction from true bronchiectasis, which frequently is.[93]

Whilst the role of pulmonary angiography in other conditions causing pulmonary hypertension has declined, pulmonary angiography remains the technique of choice for demonstrating the webs and occlusions of chronic thromboembolism (Figure 9.15). Non-invasive techniques can be valuable in making the diagnosis, but surgical planning in patients being considered for thromboendarterectomy still requires conventional angiography. Its advantages in terms of temporal and spatial resolution continue to outweigh the small risk of an invasive procedure. As with any cause of chronic pulmonary hypoperfusion, bronchial artery dilatation is common and frequently recognized on CTPA or MRA. While a large bronchial blood supply may complicate surgical endarterectomy, it implies that the peripheral pulmonary vasculature is patent and is therefore a good predictor of outcome.[94]

Pulmonary artery sarcoma is a rare tumor of the pulmonary arterial wall (see Chapter 18). In many respects

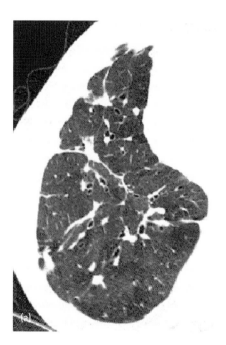
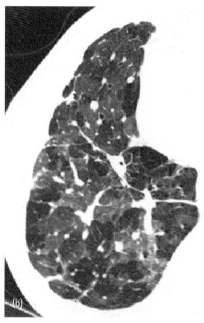

Figure 9.14 *Inspiratory (a) and expiratory (b) high-resolution computed tomography images in obliterative bronchiolitis showing mosaic attenuation, which is exaggerated on expiration due to air trapping.*

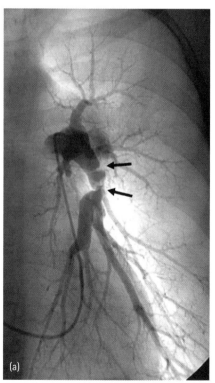
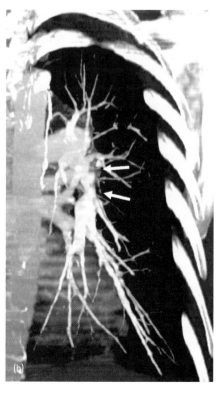

Figure 9.15 *Selective left pulmonary angiogram (a) and matching three-dimensional reconstruction of the left pulmonary vasculature from a multislice CT data set (b) in a patient with chronic thromboembolic pulmonary hypertension (CTEPH). Tight webs, typical of CTEPH, are shown well on conventional angiography (arrows) and correlate with the computed tomography pulmonary angiography reconstruction.*

it is indistinguishable from mural thrombus in CTEPH. Patients present with progressive symptoms of pulmonary hypertension. On CTPA there is a soft tissue mass lying within dilated pulmonary arteries. Pulmonary arterial occlusions and right-sided chamber dilatation with hypertrophy are common. These tumors are not metabolically active and there is little evidence of delayed enhancement following intravenous contrast. Extension beyond the arterial wall at the time of presentation is also uncommon. The only features that may help to distinguish CTEPH from pulmonary artery sarcoma are:

- sarcomas usually arise in the main pulmonary artery and may extend proximally through the pulmonary valve into the RV outflow tract, and
- the intraluminal surface of a sarcoma is often irregular.

Despite these pointers, the diagnosis is often not made until surgical thromboendarterectomy is performed or the patient dies.

SICKLE CELL DISEASE

Sickle cell anemia is frequently associated with episodes of pneumonia or pulmonary infarction.[95] The two conditions can be difficult to separate clinically and the more general term of acute chest syndrome (ACS) is applied.[96] ACS is characterized by fever, cough, chest pain and hypoxia. It is one of the most frequent causes of hospitalization in sickle cell disease.

Just as the clinical distinction between pneumonia and pulmonary infarction is difficult, so it is on chest radiography. There may be areas of confluent lobar or segmental consolidation and pleural effusions are common.[97] As a result of the radiographic abnormality, $\dot{V}/\dot{Q}$ scintigraphy is unhelpful, with many examinations falling into the indeterminate category. When pulmonary shadowing develops late after the onset of symptoms, this favors infarction rather than pneumonia. Interstitial shadowing in a patient with fever is more in keeping with a viral pneumonia or mycoplasma. Heart failure, as a direct result of sickle cell infarction, iron overload or opiate analgesia, may be difficult to distinguish from other causes of pulmonary shadowing. Repeated episodes of ACS eventually result in pulmonary fibrosis and infarction, which is best shown by HRCT.[98] Mosaic perfusion (mimicking CTEPH) has also been described.[99]

ALGORITHMS FOR INVESTIGATION

As with all areas of medicine, greater sophistication in imaging does not necessarily mean easier decision-making. The wider the choice, the greater is the duplication. The more tests available, the more a rational approach to their use becomes important. Pulmonary hypertension is a relatively common problem and the pool of patients requiring investigation is large. If the investigation of pulmonary hypertension is not to consume the resources of the entire radiology department, a diagnostic strategy must be in place and must be adhered to. Diagnostic algorithms abound; there is no consensus view and, correspondingly, no right answer. The following description details our local approach in two areas:

- the investigation of suspected pulmonary hypertension (Figure 9.16) and
- the investigation of suspected acute PE (Figure 9.17).

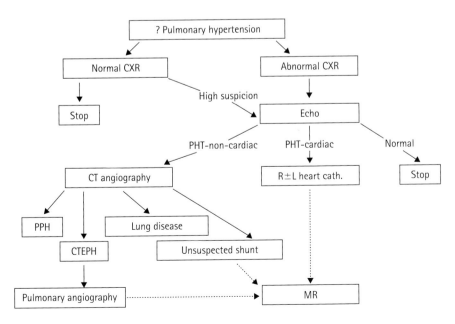

Figure 9.16 *Algorithm for the investigation of suspected pulmonary hypertension. CT, computed tomography; CTEPH, chronic thromboembolic pulmonary hypertension; CXR, chest x-ray; MR, magnetic resonance; PHT, pulmonary hypertension, PPH, primary pulmonary hypertension.*

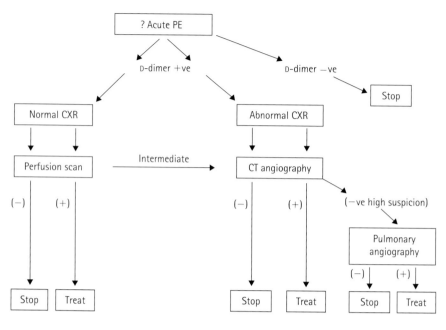

Figure 9.17 *Algorithm for the investigation of suspected acute pulmonary embolism (PE). CT, computed tomography; CXR, chest x-ray.*

They are based on published literature and local experience, but most importantly they have the approval of our referring physicians.

Suspected pulmonary hypertension

Patients presenting with dyspnea, chest pain, cough or lethargy will invariably have a chest radiograph at their first clinic visit. The presence of cardiomegaly, with or without pulmonary artery enlargement, will require further investigation by echocardiography. If the radiograph is normal but the history or physical examination suggests cardiopulmonary disease, an echocardiogram is still indicated. No other imaging should be requested until the result of the echocardiogram is available (see Chapter 8). This result determines the direction of subsequent imaging.

A normal echocardiogram excludes significant pulmonary hypertension and no further investigation is indicated. The only exception to this rule is when the echocardiogram is technically poor, e.g. lung disease and poor acoustic window, and the result is in doubt. In this case, cardiac MRI is a good alternative.

In a small number of patients with a cardiac cause for pulmonary hypertension, MRI is required. This is either in addition to, or instead of, cardiac catheterization. Patients in this group would include those with mild pulmonary hypertension in whom surgery is unlikely to be necessary, e.g. small left-to-right shunt through an ASD. For some patients in whom surgery is planned, further anatomic information is needed before operation, e.g. atrial myxoma for assessment of site of tumor attachment, or complex congenital heart disease

to establish pulmonary venous drainage or pulmonary arterial anatomy.

In patients with right-sided chamber dilatation for which no cause can be found on echocardiography, the next step is CTPA. A multislice CT scanner should be used where possible. This allows coverage of the whole lung and includes an HRCT examination without additional radiation exposure. For institutions with a single-slice spiral CT, CTPA of 12–15 cm of the mediastinum should be combined with a separate HRCT examination of the lungs. The combination of HRCT and CTPA will allow a diagnosis to be made in the majority of patients. Any further investigation will depend on the outcome of CTPA. Patients with obstructive lung disease or HRCT evidence of a collagen vascular disease or vasculitis will need lung function tests, auto-antibody screen, etc. A diagnosis of CTEPH will warrant assessment for possible surgical thromboendarterectomy, i.e. right ± left heart catheterization and pulmonary angiography. Pulmonary CEMRA may be indicated in these patients if it is to be used repeatedly for reassessment during post-surgical follow-up. Portopulmonary hypertension is usually suspected before investigation because of a history of liver disease. Even if unsuspected, however, CT of much of the liver is included on the CTPA examination and should suggest cirrhosis and portal hypertension.

Occasionally, an unsuspected left-to-right shunt is discovered as a cause for pulmonary hypertension on CTPA, e.g. sinus venosus ASD or anomalous pulmonary venous drainage. These cases will need to be investigated further by right heart catheterization and/or MRI. PPH is a diagnosis of exclusion, although in some patients subtle heterogenous lung attenuation on HRCT and abruptly tapered and tortuous pulmonary vessels may suggest it. In its early stages, CT appearances of veno-occlusive disease may be indistinguishable from PPH. As both conditions require right heart catheterization to assess severity, to determine prognosis and to plan treatment, this is unimportant. Right heart catheterization will usually provide the diagnosis.

The V̇/Q̇ scintigram is reserved for problem-solving. It is no longer part of the routine investigation of pulmonary hypertension. It can be a useful non-invasive method for assessing right-to-left shunts in hepatopulmonary syndrome or Eisenmenger reactions but even here, MRI has usurped its role. Routine use of V̇/Q̇ scintigraphy is limited to the investigation of a selected group of patients with suspected acute PE.

Suspected acute pulmonary embolism

For a discussion of suspected acute pulmonary embolism, see Chapter 16A.

SUMMARY

Pulmonary hypertension is a relatively common manifestation of a broad range of disease processes. Many of the conditions respond well to treatment and some can be cured. Accurate diagnosis is essential and requires judicious use of the many investigations now available.

In patients with suspected PE, a low clinical suspicion and a normal chest radiograph, i.e. outpatients, perfusion scintigraphy is often sufficient. When suspicion is high and the chest radiograph is abnormal, i.e. inpatients, CTPA should be the first imaging test. Pulmonary angiography should be used as a problem solver when other tests are inconclusive. Magnetic resonance angiography is now a practical alternative to the other investigations but high cost and limited access continue to be a problem.

The chest radiograph is usually the first indication of disease in patients presenting with symptoms of pulmonary hypertension. Echocardiography will either confirm or refute the diagnosis, and in those patients with a cardiac cause will provide a firm diagnosis. In patients with echocardiographic features of pulmonary hypertension but no apparent cause, CTPA combined with HRCT should be used. This will provide a definitive diagnosis in the majority of cases and direct subsequent investigation. V̇/Q̇ scintigraphy, MRI and cardiac catheterization are reserved for solving diagnostic problems, planning treatment and establishing prognosis. Their use depends on local access and expertise but as with acute PE, the rapid development and expansion of MRI is likely to change diagnostic algorithms in coming years.

KEY POINTS

- Risk of further pulmonary occlusion in patients with pulmonary hypertension by V̇/Q̇ scanning is very low.
- Fast (multislice) CT scanning is now an accepted technique for cardiac imaging.
- MR has the potential to assess structure and function of the right heart and major pulmonary vessels without the need for ionizing radiation.
- A chest radiograph often provides the first clues in patients with symptoms caused by pulmonary hypertension.
- A normal echocardiogram refutes the diagnosis of pulmonary hypertension.
- In patients with echocardiographic evidence of pulmonary hypertension but no obvious cause, CTPA and HRCT should be the next steps. They will provide diagnosis in the majority of cases and direct further investigations such as V̇/Q̇, MRI and cardiac catheterization.

REFERENCES

●1 Rich S (ed.) Executive summary. *Primary pulmonary hypertension.* Geneva: World Health Organization, 2001.
2 O'Doherty MJ, Peters AM. Pulmonary Tc-99m DTPA aerosol clearance as an index of lung injury. *Eur J Nucl Med* 1997;**24**:81–7.
●3 *Making the best use of a radiology department: guidelines for doctors,* 4th edn. London: Royal College of Radiologists, 1998.
4 Mountford PJ, Oakley AJ. A review of the secretion of radioactivity in human breast milk: data, quantitative analysis and recommendations. *Nucl Med Commun* 1989;**10**:15–27.
●5 Kalender WA, Seissler W, Klotz E et al. Spiral volumetric CT with single breath-hold technique, continuous transport and continuous scanner rotation. *Radiology* 1990;**176**:1881–3.
6 Remy-Jardin M, Remy J, Artaud D et al. Spiral CT of pulmonary embolism: technical considerations and interpretative pitfalls. *J Thorac Imaging* 1997;**12**:103–17.
7 Brown SJ, Hayball MP, Coulden RA. Impact of motion artefact on the measurement of coronary calcium score. *Br J Radiol* 2000;**73**:956–62.
8 Simonetti OP, Finn JP, White RD et al. 'Black blood' T2-weighted inversion-recovery MR imaging of the heart. *Radiology* 1996;**199**:49–57.
9 Atkinson DJ, Edelman RR. Cineangiography of the heart in a single breath hold with a segmented TurboFLASH sequence. *Radiology* 1991;**178**:357–60.
10 Katz J, Milken MC, Stray-Gunderson J et al. Estimation of human myocardial mass with MR imaging. *Radiology* 1988;**169**:495–8.

11 Longmore DB, Klipstein RH, Underwood SR *et al.* Dimensional accuracy of magnetic resonance in studies of the heart. *Lancet* 1985;**1**:1360–2.

●12 Firmin DN, Naylor GL, Kilner PJ *et al.* The applications of phase shifts in NMR for flow measurements. *Magn Reson Med* 1990;**14**:230–41.

13 Spritzer CE, Pelc NJ, Lee JN *et al.* Rapid MR imaging of blood flow with a phase sensitive, limited-flip-angle, radiant recalled pulse sequence: preliminary experience. *Radiology* 1990;**176**:255–62.

14 Kondo C, Caputo GR, Semelka R *et al.* Right and left ventricular stroke volume velocity measurements with velocity encoded cine NMR imaging: *in vivo* and *in vitro* evaluation. *AJR Am J Roentgenol* 1991;**157**:9–16.

15 Arheden H, Holmquist C, Thilen U *et al.* Left-to-right cardiac shunts: comparison of measurements obtained with MR velocity mapping and with radionuclide angiography. *Radiology* 1999;**211**:453–8.

16 Coulden RA, Butt YA, Hayball M *et al.* Patterns of pulmonary artery blood flow in thrombo-embolic pulmonary hypertension: a study using cine phase contrast MRI. *Eur Respir J* 1995;**8**(Suppl 19):176.

●17 Prince MR. Gadolinium enhanced MR aortography. *Radiology* 1994;**191**:155–64.

18 Leung JA, Debatin JF. Three-dimensional contrast-enhanced magnetic resonance angiography of the thoracic vasculature. *Eur Radiol* 1997;**7**:981–9.

●19 PIOPED investigators. Value of the ventilation perfusion scan in acute pulmonary embolism. *JAMA* 1990;**263**:2753–9.

20 Stein PD, Athanasoulis C, Alavi A *et al.* Complications and validity of pulmonary angiography in acute pulmonary embolism. *Circulation* 1992;**85**:462–8.

◆21 Goodman PC. Pulmonary angiography. *Clin Chest Med* 1984;**5**:465–77.

22 Zuckerman DA, Sterling KM, Oser RF. Safety of pulmonary angiography in the 1990s. *J Vasc Intervent Radiol* 1996;**7**:199–205.

23 Ganz W, Donoso R, Marcus HS *et al.* A new technique for measurement of cardiac output by thermodilution in man. *Am J Cardiol* 1971;**27**:392–5.

24 Harrison RW, Adams WE, Beuhler W *et al.* Effects of acute and chronic reduction of lung volumes on cardiopulmonary reserve. *Arch Surg* 1957;**75**:546–62.

25 Jefferson K, Rees S. *Clinical cardiac radiology*, 2nd edn. London: Butterworths, 1980.

26 Ungerleider HE, Gubner R. Evaluation of heart size measurements. *Am Heart J* 1942;**24**:494–8.

27 Milne ENC, Burnett K, Aufrichtig D *et al.* Assessment of cardiac size on portable chest films. *J Thoracic Imaging* 1988;**3**:64–9.

28 Pistolesi M, Milne ENC, Miniati M *et al.* The vascular pedicle of the heart and the azygos vein. Part II: In acquired heart disease. *Radiology* 1984;**152**:9–17.

29 Chang CH. The roentgenographic measurement of the right pulmonary artery in 1085 cases. *AJR Am J Roentgenol* 1993;**87**:926–35.

◆30 Coulden RA, Lipton MJ. Radiological examination in valvular heart disease. In: Al Zaibag M, Duran CMG (eds), *Valvular heart disease*. New York: Marcel Dekker, 1994.

31 Boxt LM, Rich S, Fried R *et al.* Automated morphologic evaluation of pulmonary arteries in primary pulmonary hypertension. *Invest Radiol* 1986;**21**:906–9.

32 Fishman AJ, Moser KM, Fedullo PF. Perfusion lung scans vs. pulmonary angiography in evaluation of suspected pulmonary hypertension. *Chest* 1983;**84**:679–83.

33 Powe JE, Palevski HI, McCarthy KE *et al.* Pulmonary arterial hypertension: value of perfusion scintigraphy. *Radiology* 1987;**164**:727–30.

34 Rich S, Pietra GG, Kieras K *et al.* Primary pulmonary hypertension: angiographic and scintigraphic patterns of histologic subtypes. *Ann Intern Med* 1986;**105**:449–502.

35 Engeler CE, Kuni CC, Tashjian JH *et al.* Regional alterations in lung ventilation in primary pulmonary hypertension: correlation between CT and scintigraphy. *AJR Am J Roentgenol* 1995;**164**:831–5.

◆36 Walcott B, Burchell HB, Brown AL. Primary pulmonary hypertension. *Am J Med* 1970;**70**:49–58.

37 Balagopal VP, da Costa P, Greenstone MA. Fatal pulmonary hypertension and rheumatoid vasculitis. *Eur Respir J* 1995;**8**:331–3.

38 Turner-Warwick M, Evans RC. Pulmonary manifestations of rheumatoid disease. *Clin Rheum Dis* 1977;**3**:549–64.

39 Battle RW, Davitt MA, Cooper SM *et al.* Presence of pulmonary hypertension in limited and diffuse scleroderma. *Chest* 1996;**110**:1515–19.

40 Trell E, Lindstrom C. Pulmonary hypertension in systemic sclerosis. *Ann Rheum Dis* 1971;**30**:390–400.

41 Lupi-Herrera E, Sanchez-Torres G, Marcushamer J *et al.* Takayasu's arteritis: clinical study of 107 cases. *Am Heart J* 1997;**93**:94–103.

42 Kawai C, Ishikaw K, Kato M *et al.* 'Pulmonary pulseless disease': pulmonary involvement in so called Takayasu's disease. *Chest* 1978;**73**:651–7.

43 Yamoto M, Lecky JW, Hiramatsu K *et al.* Takayasu's arteritis: radiographic and angiographic findings in 59 patients. *Radiology* 1986;**161**:329–34.

44 Park JH, Chung JW, Im JG *et al.* Takayasu's arteritis: evaluation of mural changes in the aorta and pulmonary artery with CT angiography. *Radiology* 1993;**196**:89–93.

◆45 Farelli CA. Wegener's granulomatosis: a radiological review of the pulmonary manifestations at initial presentation and during relapse. *Clin Radiol* 1982;**33**:545–51.

46 Frazier AA, Rosado-de-Christenson ML, Gavin JR *et al.* Pulmonary angiitis and granulomatosis: radiologic-pathologic correlation. *Radiographics* 1998;**18**:687–710.

47 Langford CA, Sneller MC, Hallahan CW *et al.* Clinical features and therapeutic management of subglottic stenosis in patients with Wegener's granulomatosis. *Arthritis Rheum* 1996;**39**:1754–60.

48 Lanham JG, Elkon KB, Pusey CD *et al.* Systemic vasculitis with asthma and eosinophilia: a clinical approach to the Churg-Strauss syndrome. *Medicine* 1984;**63**:65–81.

49 Masi AT, Hunder GG, Lie JT *et al.* The American College of Rheumatology 1990 criteria for the classifiaction of Churg-Strauss allergic granulomatosis and angiitis. *Arthritis Rheum* 1990;**33**:1094–100.

50 Erkan F, Cavdar T. Pulmonary vasculitis in Behcet's disease. *Am Rev Respir Dis* 1992;**146**:232–9.

51 Gibson RN, Morgan SH, Krausz T *et al*. Pulmonary artery aneurysms in Behcet's disease. *Br J Radiol* 1985;**58**:79–82.

52 Raz I, Okon E, Chajek-Shaul T. Pulmonary manifestations in Behcet's syndrome. *Chest* 1989;**95**:585–9.

53 Harris P, Heath D. *The human pulmonary circulation*, 2nd edn. London: Churchill Livingstone, 1986.

54 Berthalot P, Walker JG, Sherlock S *et al*. Arterial changes in the lungs in cirrhosis of the liver – lung spider nevi. *N Engl J Med* 1966;**274**:291–8.

55 Robin ED, Horn B, Goris ML *et al*. Detection, quantification and physiology of lung spiders. *Trans Assoc Am Physicians* 1975;**88**:202–16.

56 Stanley NN, Woodgate DG. Mottled chest radiograph and gas transfer defect in chronic liver disease. *Thorax* 1972; **27**:315–23.

57 Bank ER, Thrall JH, Dantzker DR. Radionuclide demonstration of intrapulmonary shunting in cirrhosis. *AJR Am J Roentgenol* 1983;**140**:967–9.

58 Friedman WF, Braunwald E. Alterations in regional pulmonary blood flow in mitral valve disease studied by radioisotope scanning: a simple non-traumatic technique for estimation of left atrial pressure. *Circulation* 1966;**34**: 363–40.

●59 Kerley P. Radiology in heart disease. *Br Med J* 1933;**2**:594–8.

60 Wagenvoort CA, Wagenvoort N. The pathology of pulmonary veno-occlusive disease. *Virchows Arch [Pathol Anat]* 1974;**364**:69–79.

61 Rambihar VS, Fallen EL, Cairns JA. Pulmonary veno-occlusive disease: antemortem diagnosis from roentgenographic and hemodynamic findings. *Can Med Assoc J* 1979;**120**:1519–22.

62 Swensen SJ, Tashjian JH, Myers JL *et al*. Pulmonary venoocclusive disease: CT findings in eight patients. *AJR Am J Roentgenol* 1996;**167**:937–40.

63 Talbot S, Worthington BS, Roebuck EJ. Radiographic signs of pulmonary embolism and infarction. *Thorax* 1973;**28**: 198–203.

64 Greenspan RH, Ravin CE, Polanski SM *et al*. Accuracy of the chest radiograph in diagnosis of pulmonary embolism. *Invest Radiol* 1982;**17**:539–43.

65 Wenger NK, Stein PD, Willis PW. Massive acute pulmonary embolism: the deceivingly non-specific manifestations. *JAMA* 1972;**220**:843–4.

66 Wescott JL, Cole S. Plate atelectasis. *Radiology* 1985;**155**:1–9.

◆67 Moser KM. Venous thromboembolism: state of the art. *Am Rev Respir Dis* 1990;**141**:235–49.

68 van Erkel AR, van Rossum AB, Bloem JB *et al*. Spiral CT angiography for suspected pulmonary embolism: a cost-effectiveness analysis. *Radiology* 1996;**201**:29–36.

69 Cronan JJ, Doriman GS, Scola FH *et al*. Deep venous thrombosis: ultrasound assessment using vein compression. *Radiology* 1987;**152**:191–4.

●70 Remy-Jardin M, Remy J, Wattine L *et al*. Central pulmonary thromboembolism: diagnosis with spiral volumetric CT with single breathold technique – comparison with pulmonary angiography. *Radiology* 1992;**185**:381–7.

71 Remy-Jardin M, Remy-Jardin-J. Spiral CT angiography of the pulmonary circulation. *Radiology* 1999;**212**:615–36.

72 Remy-Jardin M, Remy J, Artaud D *et al*. Peripheral pulmonary arteries: optimisation of the spiral CT acquisition protocol. *Radiology* 1997;**204**:157–63.

73 Herold CJ, Remy-Jardin M, Grenier PA *et al*. Prospective evaluation of pulmonary embolism: initial results of the European multicentre trial (ESTIPEP). *Radiology* 1998;**209**(P):299.

∗74 van Rossum AB, Treurniet FEE, Keift GJ *et al*. Role of spiral volumetric computed tomographic scanning in the assessment of patients with suspected pulmonary embolism and in abnormal ventilation-perfusion lung scan. *Thorax* 1996;**51**:23–8.

75 Oser RF, Zuckerman DA, Gutierrez RF *et al*. Anatomic distribution of pulmonary emboli at pulmonary angiography: implications for cross-sectional imaging. *Radiology* 1996; **199**:31–5.

76 Stein PD. Henry JW. Gottschalk A. Reassessment of pulmonary angiography for the diagnosis of pulmonary embolism: relation of interpreter agreement to the order of the involved pulmonary arterial branch. *Radiology* 1999; **210**:689–91.

∗77 Goodman LR, Lipchik RJ, Kuzo RS *et al*. Subsequent pulmonary embolism: risk after a negative helical CT pulmonary angiogram – prospective comparison with scintigraphy. *Radiology* 2000;**215**:535–42.

●78 Coche EE, Müller NL, Kim K-I *et al*. Acute pulmonary embolism: ancillary findings at spiral CT. *Radiology* 1998;**207**:753–60.

79 Yankelevitz DF, Gamsu G, Shah A *et al*. Optimization of combined CT pulmonary angiography with lower extremity CT venography. *AJR Am J Roentgenol* 2000;**174**:67–9.

●80 Loud PA, Katz DS, Klippenstein RA *et al*. Combined CT venography and pulmonary angiography in suspected thromboembolic disease: diagnostic accuracy for deep venous evaluation. *AJR Am J Roentgenol* 2000;**174**:61–5.

81 Katz DS, Loud PA, Klippenstein RA *et al*. Extrathoracic findings on the venous phase of combined computed tomography venography and pulmonary angiography. *Clin Radiol* 2000;**55**:177–88.

●82 Meaney JFM, Weg JG, Chenevert TL *et al*. Diagnosis of pulmonary embolism with magnetic resonance angiography. *N Engl J Med* 1997;**336**:1422–7.

83 Coulden RA, Graves MJ, Tasker AD *et al*. Contrast enhanced pulmonary MRA in pulmonary hypertension: comparison with CT angiography, pulmonary angiography and $\dot{V}/\dot{Q}$ scanning in the diagnosis of chronic pulmonary thromboembolism. *Radiology* 1998;**209**(P):451.

84 Anderson G, Reid L, Simon G. The radiographic appearances in primary and in thromboembolic pulmonary hypertension. *Clin Radiol* 1973;**24**:113–20.

85 Schmidt HC, Kauczor HU, Schild HH *et al*. Pulmonary hypertension in patients with chronic thromboembolism: chest radiograph and CT evaluation before and after surgery. *Eur Radiol* 1996;**6**:818–25.

86 Lisbona R, Kreisman H, Novales-Diaz J *et al*. Diffusion lung scanning: differentiation of primary from thromboembolic pulmonary hypertension. *AJR Am J Roentgenol* 1985;**144**:27–30.

87 Collins MA, Pidgeon JW, Fitzgerald R. Computed tomography manifestations of tricuspid regurgitation. *Br J Radiol* 1995;**68**:1058–60.

88 Schwickert HC, Schweden F, Schild HH *et al*. Pulmonary arteries and lung parenchyma in chronic pulmonary

embolism: preoperative and postoperative CT findings. *Radiology* 1994;**191**:351–7.

●89 Bergin CJ, Rios G, King MA *et al*. Accuracy of high resolution CT in identifying chronic pulmonary thromboembolic disease. *AJR Am J Roentgenol* 1996;**166**:1371–7.

90 Martin KW, Sagel SS, Siegel BA. Mosaic oligaemia simulating pulmonary infiltrates on CT. *AJR Am J Roentgenol* 1986;**147**:670–3.

91 Chen D, Webb WR, Storto ML *et al*. Assessment of air trapping using postexpiratory high-resolution computed tomography. *J Thorac Imaging* 1998;**13**:135–43.

92 Remy-Jardin, M, Remy J, Louvegny S *et al*. Airway changes in chronic pulmonary embolism: CT findings in 33 patients. *Radiology* 1997;**203**:355–60.

93 Kang EY, Miller RR, Muller NL. Bronchiectasis: comparison of pre-operative thin-section CT and pathologic findings in resected specimens. *Radiology* 1995;**195**:649–54.

94 Kauczor H-U, Schwickert HC, Mayer E *et al*. Spiral CT of bronchial arteries in chronic thromboembolism. *J Comput Assis Tomogr* 1994;**6**:855–60.

◆95 Haupt HM, Moore W, Bauer TW *et al*. The lung in sickle cell disease. *Chest* 1982;**81**:332–7.

96 Barrett-Connor E. Pneumonia and pulmonary infarction in sickle cell anemia. *JAMA* 1973;**224**:997–1000.

97 Smith JA. Cardiopulmonary manifestations of sickle cell disease in childhood. *Semin Roentgenol* 1987;**22**:160–7.

98 Powars D, Weidman JA, Odom-Maryon T *et al*. Sickle cell chronic lung disease: prior morbidity and the risk of pulmonary failure. *Medicine (Baltimore)*1988;**67**:66–76.

99 Powars DR. Sickle cell anemia and major organ failure. *Hemoglobin* 1990;**14**:573–98.

10

Cardiac catheterization of patients with pulmonary hypertension

BERTRON M GROVES AND DAVID B BADESCH

INTRODUCTION

Patients referred for cardiac catheterization to evaluate pulmonary hypertension are clinically categorized as having primary ('unexplained') pulmonary hypertension or pulmonary arterial hypertension associated with a condition known to cause pulmonary hypertension. In addition to characterizing the patient's pulmonary hemodynamics, the catheterization procedure should be designed to safely answer the following questions:

- Is the pulmonary hypertension predominantly due to elevation of the pulmonary arterial wedge pressure secondary to left-sided cardiac disease, or is the pulmonary hypertension 'precapillary' due to pulmonary arterial/arteriolar obstructive disease?
- Does the patient have a left-to-right shunt which might explain the presence of pulmonary hypertension as a result of increased pulmonary flow secondary to an atrial septal defect (ASD), ventricular septal defect (VSD), or patent ductus arteriosus (PDA) which may or may not have progressed to the 'end stage' with reversed right-to-left shunting as a manifestation of Eisenmenger's syndrome? Is isolated surgical or percutaneous transcatheter correction of the congenital heart defect possible or will the patient require simultaneous lung or heart/lung transplantation?

- Does the patient have an intracardiac right-to-left shunt via a patent foramen ovale which markedly increases the challenge of accurately measuring pulmonary/systemic blood flow ($\dot{Q}P/\dot{Q}S$)?
- Does the patient have sufficient acute pulmonary vasoreactivity to warrant a long-term trial of vasodilator treatment, or does such a trial subject the patient to significant risk with minimal benefit?
- In patients with pulmonary hypertension secondary to left ventricular cardiomyopathy who are undergoing evaluation as potential candidates for heart transplantation, is there enough reversibility of the elevated pulmonary vascular resistance for the patient to be accepted as a heart transplant recipient?

PRECATHETERIZATION EVALUATION

To address all issues of importance for a pulmonary hypertensive patient's hemodynamic assessment, a thorough precatheterization evaluation is performed in all patients (see Chapters 7–9). Since we do not perform selective pulmonary arteriography in our cardiac catheterization laboratories, patients who are suspected of having pulmonary thromboembolic disease as the etiology of their pulmonary hypertension undergo this procedure in interventional radiology before or after their cardiac catheterization to determine if they are candidates for surgical thrombo-endarterectomy (see Chapter 9).

INITIAL CARDIAC CATHETERIZATION PROCEDURE

We perform each patient's first catheterization in our laboratory using a 'standardized' procedure as detailed below to confirm the diagnosis of PPH[1] or PAH associated with another condition,[2] before proceeding with assessment of pulmonary vasoreactivity using vasodilators.

Sedation

We do not routinely use sedation prior to or during the cardiac catheterization procedure since pulmonary hypertensive patients can react adversely to any sedative. When local anesthesia is insufficient for an anxious patient, we currently use reduced dosages of intravenous midazolam, which works well and has an intravenous antidote if needed.

Percutaneous placement of venous sheath for right heart catheterization

Most of the right heart catheterization procedures we performed in pulmonary hypertensive patients in the past used the percutaneous right femoral vein approach. Influenced by our increased experience in recent years using outpatient percutaneous right internal jugular (RIJ) vein cannulation for follow-up right heart catheterization and right ventricular endomyocardial biopsy procedures in cardiac transplant patients, we now perform over 95% of our pulmonary hypertension catheterizations as an outpatient procedure using the 'anterior' RIJ vein approach. To assist in cannulating the internal jugular vein, we find it useful to use a two-dimensional, near-range, ultrasonic probe to locate and cannulate the internal jugular vein (Site-Rite II Ultrasound System, Dymax, Pittsburg, PA, USA). This device can provide excellent visualization of the internal jugular vein and adjacent carotid artery **while needle puncture is being performed**. We frequently use this probe to locate and confirm patency of the RIJ vein before the neck is prepped and draped, and then perform the venous cannulation without simultaneous ultrasonic visualization. However, we routinely use the device with a sterile transducer cover during internal jugular venous cannulation when technical difficulties are expected or encountered. We prefer to avoid the subclavian vein approach, which is associated with a small incidence of pneumothorax, which can be life-threatening in pulmonary hypertensive patients.

Since catheter manipulation into the pulmonary artery is much easier from the neck, an 8.0 Fr sheath with a self-sealing hemostatic valve and side-arm port is satisfactory for the internal jugular vein approach in most pulmonary hypertensive patients when a 7.5 Fr standard or 'guidewire' Swan–Ganz thermodilution catheter is used. If an 8.0 Fr oximetric balloon-tipped pulmonary artery catheter (Opticath, P7110-EP8-H, Abbott Laboratories, Chicago, IL, USA) is used, a 9.0 Fr sheath is needed to accommodate the larger catheter size. Owing to the increased technical difficulty that is frequently encountered secondary to marked enlargement of the right atrium (RA) and right ventricle (RV) in association with severe tricuspid and/or pulmonary valvular regurgitation when the femoral venous approach is used, we prefer to use a straight 8.0 Fr sheath with no side-arm port or hemostatic valve in these technically difficult patients. To provide hemostasis and optimal freedom of catheter manipulation through this femoral venous sheath, an adjustable Luer lock adapter (PMLLA-UCC-L, Cook Cardiology, Bloomington, IN, USA) is used.

Following RIJ venous catheterization, patients who are hemodynamically stable are discharged directly from the cardiac catheterization laboratory without the need for further observation. When femoral venous catheterization is performed, patients are observed in the supine position in a recovery unit for 1 hour following removal of the sheath to ensure adequate venous hemostasis prior to ambulation and discharge.

'GUIDEWIRE' SWAN–GANZ THERMODILUTION CATHETER

Hemodynamic evaluation of patients with severe pulmonary hypertension is frequently difficult due to marked enlargement of the right atrium and right ventricle associated with severe tricuspid regurgitation which has a tendency to prolapse a standard balloon-tipped Swan–Ganz catheter from the right ventricle back into the right atrium. To overcome these difficulties, we developed a 'guidewire' Swan–Ganz balloon-tipped thermodilution catheter (93A-821H, Baxter Healthcare, Irvine, CA, USA) in collaboration with the American Edwards Co. in 1983.[3] The idea for this catheter was derived from our experience, which taught us that 'loading' the 'distal lumen' of a standard Swan–Ganz balloon-tipped catheter with a 0.025 inch Teflon-coated guidewire would frequently stiffen the catheter shaft sufficiently to allow advancement into the pulmonary artery.

We reasoned that a 'blind-end' lumen which would allow an indwelling guidewire to be advanced to or retracted from the distal end of the catheter would be more helpful in advancing the catheter into the pulmonary artery and in maintaining its position within the pulmonary artery for prolonged periods of monitoring. The 'guidewire' lumen of this catheter ends proximal to

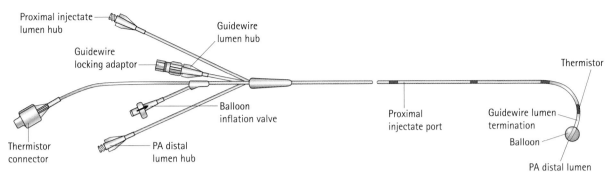

Figure 10.1 *'Guidewire' Swan–Ganz catheter design. The anatomy of this catheter is identical to the Venous Infusion Port (VIP) Swan–Ganz balloon-tipped thermodilution catheter with the exception that the VIP port is used as the guidewire lumen, which is a blind-end lumen that terminates near the thermistor. The guidewire lumen is preloaded with an 0.028 inch guidewire before the catheter is inserted into the venous access sheath to stiffen the shaft of the catheter for navigation through an enlarged, hypertensive right ventricle that is usually associated with moderate to severe tricuspid valvular regurgitation. Once the tip of the catheter is positioned appropriately in the right or left pulmonary artery, the guidewire is retracted approximately 10 cm from the tip of the catheter so that it still traverses the pulmonary valve but softens the catheter tip enough to prevent inadvertent wedging that could cause a life-threatening pulmonary infarction in patients with severe pulmonary hypertension. The guidewire locking adaptor is then tightened to secure the desired guidewire position within the catheter.*

the location of the thermistor near the end of the thermodilution balloon-tipped catheter (Figure 10.1). The blind lumen accommodates a 0.025–0.028 inch guidewire that does not come into contact with blood and does not allow exit of the guidewire outside the catheter, which could initiate arrhythmias or cause perforation of the heart. Once the catheter is properly positioned within the right or left pulmonary artery, it can readily be inflated to allow recording of a wedge pressure, which we also had noted was very difficult or impossible using a standard balloon-tipped catheter in many patients with severe pulmonary hypertension. After optimal positioning of this catheter is accomplished, we recommend that the guidewire be retracted approximately 10 cm from the tip of the catheter to soften its distal segment and minimize the likelihood of prolonged entrapment in the wedge position that could produce life-threatening pulmonary infarction or rupture of the pulmonary artery with excessive balloon inflation in patients with severe pulmonary hypertension.

Once the baseline wedge pressure has been proven to be normal, it is not essential to rewedge the catheter during each recording of the pulmonary arterial pressures, since we have observed that patients with 'precapillary' pulmonary hypertension do not develop elevated mean wedge pressures during vasodilator trials. Therefore, if repeated wedge pressure measurements are technically difficult (requiring manipulation under fluoroscopic guidance), serial measurements of total pulmonary resistance (mean PA pressure/cardiac output) can be substituted for measurements of pulmonary vascular resistance (mean PA pressure − mean wedge pressure/cardiac output).

In the rare patient in whom the pulmonary arterial wedge pressure cannot be successfully obtained from the 'guidewire' Swan–Ganz balloon-tipped catheter, the left ventricular end-diastolic pressure (LVEDP) is measured directly by using percutaneous femoral arterial cannulation to advance a 5 Fr pigtail catheter retrogradely across the aortic valve into the left ventricle. A normal LVEDP associated with echocardiographic evidence of a normal left atrium and mitral valve excludes 'left-sided' etiologies of pulmonary hypertension.

Percutaneous systemic arterial catheterization

We perform most of our hemodynamic studies without using percutaneous insertion of an intra-arterial catheter in pulmonary hypertensive patients who are hemodynamically stable. The systemic arterial pressure and oxygen saturation are monitored non-invasively using a combined automated brachial arterial blood pressure cuff and finger pulse oximeter (Propaq 104, Protocol Systems, Beaverton, OR, USA). However, in hemodynamically unstable patients with decreased systemic arterial pressure, we recommend placement of a 20 gauge percutaneous radial or brachial arterial cannula which has a flexible guidewire stylet (RA-04120, Arrow International, Reading, PA, USA) for continuous systemic arterial pressure monitoring. In such patients, the systemic arterial oxygen saturation is continuously monitored using a finger pulse oximeter to ensure adequate oxygenation. This combination also optimizes patient comfort and mobility and provides painless monitoring of arterial blood gases if subsequent hemo-dynamic monitoring in the intensive care unit (ICU) is required.

Echo/Doppler detection of intracardiac shunting

Prior to cardiac catheterization, transthoracic echo-cardiography with Doppler color flow and intravenous injection of agitated saline (shunt 'bubble study') to detect intracardiac shunting is performed routinely in all patients with pulmonary hypertension (see Chapter 8).

Methods used to detect and quantify left-to-right intracardiac shunts during cardiac catheterization

OXIMETRY 'SERIES'

If the precatheterization echo/Doppler study suggests the presence of an ASD, it is our preference to perform the right heart catheterization using the femoral vein approach in order to facilitate inter-atrial trans-septal catheterization using an endhole multipurpose catheter loaded with a 0.035 inch J guidewire. Small samples of 0.5–1.0 ml whole blood are withdrawn for measurement of O_2 saturation and O_2 content (Hemoximeter OSM 3, Radiometer, Copenhagen, Denmark) from multiple sites including: high superior vena cava (SVC), low SVC, high RA, mid-RA, low RA, high inferior vena cava (IVC), low IVC, left atrium (LA) (if trans-septal catheter passage is possible through a patent foramen ovale or ASD), pulmonary vein (usually technically accessible from the LA via retro-grade catheterization when a patent foramen ovale or ASD is present), RV, main pulmonary artery (PA) and right or left PA, and aorta (AO) (by finger pulse oxime-try). If there is a physiologically significant left-to-right shunt, there will be a $\geq$5–7% 'step-up' in O_2 saturation in the chamber into which the shunt flows compared to the 'mixed venous' or average O_2 saturation proximal to that chamber. Because of the relative imprecision of this technique secondary to streaming and inadequate mix-ing in the RA and RV, especially in the presence of severe tricuspid regurgitation, a small left-to-right shunt may be undetected or falsely identified as being present by analysis of oximetry data. To detect and quantify left-to-right shunting from an atrial septal defect, we recommend compensating for the known higher oxygen saturation of 'high' IVC blood (due to the contribution of renal vein blood, which normally contains a higher oxygen satura-tion than systemic venous blood sampled from the SVC or 'low' IVC) when computing the 'mixed venous' O_2 sat-uration by using the Flamm equation:[4]

$$\text{Mixed venous} \atop O_2 \text{ saturation} = \frac{(\text{SCV } O_2 \text{ sat} \times 3) + (\text{IVC } O_2 \text{ sat} \times 1)}{4}$$

The standard Fick equation is used to calculate $\dot{Q}P$ and $\dot{Q}S$ from the measured (or estimated) oxygen con-sumption and oxygen contents obtained from the oxi-metry series.[4] A physiologically significant left-to-right shunt will have a $\dot{Q}P/\dot{Q}S$ ratio of $\geq$1.5/1.0. Patients with the Eisenmenger reaction from an ASD or VSD second-ary to severe pulmonary hypertension usually have a $\dot{Q}P/\dot{Q}S$ <1.0 secondary to right-to-left intracardiac shunting.

ANGIOGRAPHY

Contrast injection with angiographic imaging of antegrade flow can also be used to localize and semiquantify left-to-right shunts. An injection into the aortic arch will opacify a PDA, a left ventricular injection in the left anterior oblique (LAO) projection with cranial angulation (parallel to the interventricular septum) will localize a VSD with contrast streaming through the defect into the RV and/or PA, and injection of contrast into the left atrium or pulmonary artery with levophase angiography will demonstrate con-trast flowing from the left atrium into the right atrium through an ASD. (Note: for historic reference, we previ-ously described the use of hydrogen curves and indocya-nine green dye dilution curves to detect intracardiac shunts in the first edition of this book.[5] However, hydrogen gas is no longer allowed for use in our hospital because of its potential explosive hazard and the commercial availability of indocyanine green dye has been limited. Therefore, both these methods have been abandoned in our laboratory.)

Catheterization methods used to detect and quantify right-to-left shunts

OXIMETRY SERIES

Using oximetry data from the sites sampled above for detection of a left-to-right shunt, one can also detect and quantify the size of a right-to-left shunt which is reflected by a 'step-down' in oxygen saturation between the pul-monary vein and the left-sided chamber which receives the right-to-left shunt:

- left atrium (LA) if an ASD or patent foramen ovale is present;
- left ventricle if there is a VSD; or
- descending thoracic aorta when a PDA is present.

Most commonly, right-to-left shunts in pulmonary hypertensive adults occur at the atrial level via an ASD or patent foramen ovale that has been stretched open, resulting in a drop in O_2 saturation from $\geq$95% in the pulmonary veins to a lower level in the LA depending upon the size of the right-to-left shunt. If a pulmonary vein cannot be sampled through the ASD, the room air pul-monary vein saturation can be estimated as 95–98% for the purpose of shunt calculation. The LV and AO will have approximately the same saturation as the LA; however,

LA sampling is susceptible to 'streaming' or incomplete mixing artifacts. In the presence of significant intracardiac shunting, the thermodilution cardiac output method is unreliable. Therefore, we recommend that the Fick method be used to measure pulmonary and systemic flow and vascular resistances in these patients.

HYPEROXIA

If the oximetry series is suggestive of a right-to-left shunt, we have found it useful to administer 100% oxygen for 10 minutes and repeat the arterial blood gases and hemodynamics. If the arterial partial pressure of oxygen (PaO_2) exceeds 300 mmHg in our laboratory, which is 1609 meters above sea level, there is no physiologically significant right-to-left shunt. Conversely, if the PaO_2 is <300 mmHg, a right-to-left shunt is likely present and warrants fur-ther investigation. At sea level, the PaO_2 should exceed 400 mmHg in the absence of a right-to-left shunt.

ANGIOGRAPHY

Injection of contrast into the right-sided chamber which produces right-to-left shunting into the left-sided chambers will visualize the right-to-left shunt in patients with Eisenmenger's syndrome. An ASD or patent foramen ovale with right-to-left shunting causes contrast injected into the RA to opacify the LA directly, a VSD opacifies the LV directly if the RV is injected, and a PDA causes the descending thoracic AO to be visualized early if contrast injection into the main pulmonary artery is performed.

Hemodynamic evaluation

MEASURED VARIABLES

Baseline invasive pressures [RA, RV, PA and pulmonary arterial 'wedge' (PAWP)] and the brachial arterial cuff pressure are recorded in a computerized physiological recorder (Prucka Mac-Lab 7000 Cath Lab Physiological Monitoring System; General Electric Medical Systems, Milwaukee, WI, USA). Cardiac output is measured by the thermodilution technique using a small portable computer (Edwards COM-2, Baxter, Irvine, CA, USA). In a study of pulmonary hypertensive patients, we found the thermodilution cardiac output to be an overestimate when compared to simultaneously measured Fick cardiac output if the thermodilution value was <3.5 L/min.[6] On the other hand, we observed that the thermodilution cardiac outputs which were >3.5 L/min compared favorably to measured Fick cardiac outputs even in the presence of significant tricuspid regurgitation. Therefore, for multiple repeat cardiac output measurements during the titration of vasodilator drugs, we use serial thermodilution cardiac output measurements to avoid excessive blood loss and logistical difficulties which are inherent in the measured Fick technique. For comparison with the thermodilution cardiac output, we calculate a baseline Fick cardiac output by estimating the oxygen consumption and measuring the $A - V O_2$ difference using the classic Fick equation:

$$\text{Fick cardiac output} = \text{oxygen consumption (estimated or measured)}/(\text{arterial } O_2 \text{ content} - \text{mixed venous } O_2 \text{ content})$$

where cardiac output is in L/min; oxygen consumption is in mL/min; O_2 content is in vol%; mixed venous is pulmonary artery in the absence of a left-to-right shunt.

In the presence of a left-to-right shunt, the thermodilution cardiac output reflects $\dot{Q}P$ and not $\dot{Q}S$. A right-to-left shunt invalidates the thermodilution method for measurement of pulmonary flow since some of the indicator (that is, 'cold') is shunted from the RA to LA if an ASD or patent foramen ovale is present, or RV to LV if a VSD is present. Therefore, the area beneath the curve is reduced and the calculated thermodilution pulmonary flow is erroneously increased.

DERIVED VARIABLES

In addition to quantifying the severity of any patient's pulmonary hypertension by directly measuring the pulmonary artery pressure, **pulmonary vascular resistance** (PVR) should be calculated according to the following equation:

$$PVR = \frac{(PAM - PAWM)}{CO}$$

where PVR is pulmonary vascular resistance in Wood units; PAM is pulmonary artery mean pressure (mmHg); PAWM is pulmonary artery wedge mean pressure (mmHg); and CO is cardiac output (L/min). PVR can be expressed as dyn s/cm^5 by multiplying Wood units by 80.

The normal resting pulmonary vascular resistance ranges between 0.3 and 1.6 Wood units or approximately 24–128 dyn s/cm^5.

SYSTEMIC OXYGEN TRANSPORT

Systemic oxygen transport (SO_2T) is an important measurement for monitoring oxygen delivery to the tissues and organs of the body which is calculated by the following equation:

$$SO_2T = aO_2 \text{ content} \times CO$$

where SO_2T is systemic oxygen transport (oxygen delivery in mL/min); aO_2 content is arterial oxygen content (mL/L); and CO is cardiac output (L/min).

When measurement of the cardiac output is not readily available, the dynamic physiological status of the pulmonary hypertensive patient can be inferred from following the $A - V O_2$ **content difference** (arterial − mixed venous oxygen contents in vol%). If an oximetric balloon-tipped catheter (Opticath P7110-EP8-H, Abbott Laboratories, Chicago, IL, USA) and optical module (Oximetric 3 SO_2/CO computer, Abbott Laboratories) are used to monitor the pulmonary arterial pressure, oxygen saturation and thermodilution cardiac output, and a pulse oximeter is used for monitoring systemic arterial oxygen saturation, the $A - V O_2$ content difference can be calculated and monitored as a meaningful parameter to assess a pulmonary hypertensive patient's hemodynamic response to vasodilator treatment in the acute setting. This approach also eliminates the necessity for repetitive withdrawal of blood.

$$\text{Oxygen content (vol\%)} = \text{Hb (g\%)} \times 1.36 \times O_2 \text{ sat} \times 100$$

where $1.36 = O_2$ carrying capacity/g Hb and $A - V O_2$ content difference (vol%) is systemic arterial − mixed venous O_2 content.

As the cardiac output decreases, the pulmonary arterial (that is, mixed venous) O_2 content falls and the $A - V O_2$ content difference widens. Conversely, when a pulmonary hypertensive patient responds favorably to a pulmonary vasodilator, the pulmonary arterial pressure decreases, cardiac output increases, $A - V O_2$ content difference narrows as systemic oxygen transport is increased.

ASSESSING PULMONARY VASOREACTIVITY

Varying the fraction of inspired oxygen (FiO₂)

If the pulmonary hypertensive patient being evaluated for the first time in our cardiac catheterization laboratory does not have significant resting hypoxemia, we prefer to perform all resting hemodynamic measurements with the patient breathing **room air**. If the patient is being treated with chronic **supplemental oxygen therapy** at home, the initial hemodynamics are measured while the patient continues receiving his prescribed supplemental oxygen dosage – usually 2–4 L/min via nasal cannulae. If the history indicates chronic residency at high altitude (above 1829 meters) or suggests the possibility of hypoxic pulmonary vasoconstriction, we may repeat all hemodynamics including measurement of the cardiac output with the patient breathing a **hypoxic gas mixture containing 16% oxygen** for 10 minutes using a noseclip and mouthpiece with a one-way valve. At our altitude of 1609 meters, this simulates an altitude exposure of approximately 3353 meters. At sea level, to achieve a similar level of hypoxic challenge, 14% oxygen has been used. Once a full set of hypoxic hemodynamic and blood gas measurements have been collected, we replace the hypoxic mixture with **100% oxygen** for 10 minutes and repeat the hemodynamic and blood gas measurements.

Some patients with PPH also have superimposed hypoxic pulmonary vasoconstriction which can be treated effectively with a calcium blocker.[7] The PPH patients in whom we observed hypoxic pulmonary vasoconstriction did not demonstrate pulmonary vasodilation when hyperoxia hemodynamics were compared to baseline measurements made while breathing ambient air. We have also had several PPH patients referred to us after their initial cardiac catheterization in a referral hospital had been interpreted as showing pulmonary vasodilatory benefit from 100% oxygen based upon observed lowering of the mean pulmonary artery pressure with no cardiac output measurement having been repeated during hyperoxia. When we subsequently readministered 100% oxygen to those patients, we confirmed a lowering of mean pulmonary artery pressure that was associated with a decrease in heart rate and cardiac output that resulted in no significant decrease in PVR.

Therefore, if one is attempting to assess the effect of any pharmacological intervention on the pulmonary circulation, we consider it **mandatory that pressure *and* flow be measured** to allow calculation of the PVR for comparison with baseline hemodynamics. Dr Naeije and others have appropriately emphasized the value of measuring the pulmonary artery pressure over a range of flows (see Chapter 1).

Patients with pulmonary arterial hypertension secondary to pulmonary thromboembolic disease, alveolar hypoventilation or chronic obstructive lung disease, may demonstrate marked improvement in pulmonary hemodynamics (including a reduction in the mean PAP without a concomitant fall in cardiac output) in response to acute hyperoxia. Cardiac output in these patients may increase in response to 100% oxygen. It is also important to reassess such patients after prolonged home oxygen therapy, since the improvement in pulmonary hemodynamics may require weeks or months to achieve the maximal benefit, which is not always predicted by the response to acute hyperoxia.

Exercise

Some patients with mild resting pulmonary hypertension and preserved cardiac output complain of severe symptoms during exercise. In such patients, we try to simulate the level of exercise that was described as provoking the symptoms. The most strenuous exercise workload that can be achieved during supine clinical cardiac catheterization is **leg exercise** using a cycle ergometer with a variable workload. However, most clinical cardiac catheterization laboratories, including our own, have abandoned the costly and time-consuming usage of supine cycle ergometers and oxygen consumption computers to perform exercise studies. We have found **supine straight-arm-raising exercise** using small weighted bar-bells in each hand is a satisfactory alternative form of exercise.

In pulmonary hypertensive patients, we have been able to achieve satisfactory exercise workloads by having the supine patient hold a small 1, 2 or 3 pound bar-bell (secured with Velcro straps around the back of the hand) in each hand while rapidly raising the extended arms to a position of apposition directly above the chest and lowering the extended arms to a position level with the mid-axillary line. We apply an appropriate sized blood pressure cuff to the thigh for recording the popliteal arterial pressure while monitoring arterial saturation with a pulse oximeter attached to a toenail on the opposite foot. During exercise the patient is instructed to signal approximately 2 minutes before he/she anticipates having to stop from exhaustion so that we can rapidly record the RA, PA, wedge and popliteal arterial (cuff) pressures, thermodilution cardiac output, and sample PA (mixed venous) and arterial oxygen saturation (using the toe pulse oximeter) during peak exercise. We currently use this form of exercise to simplify and shorten the duration of these procedures. Many laboratories also use supine **straight-leg-raising exercise** as a satisfactory alternative that requires no special equipment and achieves an adequate workload.

During **strenuous exercise in normal athletic men**, the PAP can increase in response to marked elevation of the cardiac output without a concomitant increase in pulmonary vascular resistance. In a sea level study of eight normal, conditioned, male athletes who had a resting mean pulmonary artery pressure of 15.0 ± 0.9 mmHg, mean cardiac output of 6.7 L/min, and pulmonary vascular resistance of 1.2 Wood units, we observed an increase in cardiac output during extreme upright cycle ergometric exercise to a mean value of 27.2 ± 2.0 L/min (range 19.1–35.9), which was associated with an increase in the mean pulmonary artery pressure to 33 ± 1 mmHg (range 25–45).[8] The mean pulmonary arterial wedge pressure in these subjects also increased to 21 mmHg during extreme exercise and contributed to the elevation of the pulmonary artery pressure. Therefore, despite having a significant increase in pulmonary arterial pressure during extreme exercise, the pulmonary vascular resistance was decreased to 0.4 Wood units in these conditioned athletes. In pulmonary hypertensive patients, we have observed that symptom-limited exercise is usually not associated with more than a twofold increase in cardiac output and we have never observed an increase in the mean wedge pressure above the normal range unless there was associated left ventricular disease.

ACUTE VASODILATOR ASSESSMENT OF PULMONARY VASOREACTIVITY

Intravenous vasodilators with short duration of action
Background Daoud reported in 1978 that acutely administered intravenous isoproterenol could be used to assess pulmonary vasoreactivity in patients with PPH.[9] We also found that intravenous isoproterenol produced pulmonary vasodilation in some PPH patients; however, its potent inotropic and chronotropic effects frequently produced marked sinus tachycardia, increased cardiac output, and higher PAP. Thus, patients were prone to experience ischemic-like chest pain (presumed to be secondary to right ventricular ischemia reflecting an imbalance in myocardial oxygen supply and demand), despite having a significant decrease in pulmonary vascular resistance. Rubin reported a beneficial acute vasodilatory effect of intravenous hydralazine in PPH patients in 1980.[10]

Prostaglandins
Prostacyclin In 1982, Rubin reported that intravenous prostacyclin (PGI_2) produced acute pulmonary vasodilation in patients with PPH.[11] The hemodynamic effects of prostacyclin were subsequently reported to be similar to, but more potent than, intravenous hydralazine.[12] Between 1981 and 1988, we studied 44 PPH patients in whom we were able to compare the acute intravenous response to PGI_2 with oral diltiazem or nifedipine.[13] Prostacyclin was titrated from 1.0 to a maximum of 12.0 ng/kg·min with the mean tolerated dosage being 8.0 ng/kg·min. The mean hemodynamic effects of PGI_2 included a 14% increase in heart rate, a 5% decrease in mean PA pressure, a 47% increase in cardiac output, and a 32% decrease in pulmonary resistance. We defined a favorable individual patient response to PGI_2 to be a >30% decrease in pulmonary resistance **and** a >10% decrease in mean pulmonary artery pressure that was observed in 30% of the untreated PPH patients. Side effects including cutaneous flushing, headache, nausea, systemic hypotension and vomiting were observed, but cleared within 10–15 minutes after stopping prostacyclin. The response to intravenous PGI_2 was predictive of the subsequent response to oral calcium blocker treatment.

Iloprost Between 1988 and 1994 we used intravenous iloprost, a more stable analogue of prostacyclin, in a similar protocol for assessing acute pulmonary vasoreactivity in 26 untreated patients with PPH.[14] Intravenous iloprost was titrated from 1.0 to a maximum of 8.0 ng/kg·min with the mean tolerated dosage being 4.0 ng/kg·min. The mean hemodynamic responses to intravenous iloprost included an 11% increase in heart rate, a 9% decrease in mean PA pressure, a 40% increase in cardiac output, and a 31% decrease in pulmonary resistance. A favorable vasodilatory response to intravenous iloprost (using the same arbitrary definition of >30% decrease in pulmonary resistance **and** a >10% decrease in mean pulmonary artery pressure) was observed in 42% of the PPH patients. Side effects were similar to those noted above for intravenous prostacyclin and cleared within 15–30 minutes after stopping iloprost. Thus, we consider intravenous PGI_2 and iloprost to be effective and safe vasodilators in acutely assessing pulmonary vasoreactivity in PPH patients. Similar hemo-dynamic results have been obtained when we have administered either intravenous PGI_2 or intravenous iloprost to patients with pulmonary arterial hypertension associated with diverse conditions known to cause pulmonary hypertension.

In the USA, neither intravenous nor inhaled iloprost has been approved for clinical use in the assessment or treatment of pulmonary hypertension. Therefore, since 1994, we have routinely used intravenous prostacyclin for the acute assessment of pulmonary vasoreactivity in our laboratory for all pulmonary hypertensive patients without left-sided disease. We have had no fatal compli-cations from the acute intravenous administration of prostacyclin or iloprost in pulmonary hypertensive patients during our 21-year experience.

Adenosine Other reports have indicated that adenosine injected into the pulmonary artery[15,16] or intra-venously[17] is another pulmonary vasodilator which is attractive because of its potency on the pulmonary circu-lation and short duration of action. Since adenosine is rapidly destroyed by adenosine deaminase in endothelial cells and erythrocytes, it has a limited effect on the systemic circulation. Thus, intravenous adenosine titrated from 50 to 500 $\mu g/kg \cdot min$ is a desirable alternative agent for acutely assessing pulmonary vasoreactivity that is predictive of subsequent responsiveness to oral calcium blocker treatment in pulmonary hypertensive patients.[17]

Nitrates

Nitroglycerin Intravenous nitroglycerin has also been used in assessing pulmonary vasoreactivity in pulmonary hypertensive patients,[18] but is generally considered to be a less potent pulmonary vasodilator in comparison with intravenous prostacyclin, iloprost, or adenosine in pul-monary hypertensive patients.

Nitroprusside Intravenous nitroprusside has been established as being useful in evaluating the reversibility of pulmonary arterial hypertension in patients with left ventricular decompensation from ischemic or idiopathic cardiomyopathy who are undergoing pre-cardiac trans-plantation evaluation.[19] In our laboratory, we administer intravenous nitroprusside to all patients being considered for cardiac transplantation who have pulmonary hyper-tension with a pulmonary vascular resistance above 2.5 Wood units. We begin the intravenous nitroprusside infusion at 0.1 $\mu g/kg \cdot min$ and increase the dosage by 0.2 $\mu g/kg \cdot min$ every 3 minutes until either the PVR falls below 2.5 Wood units, based upon serial thermodilution cardiac output measurements, or the mean systemic arterial pressure falls below 65 mmHg. Arterial saturation is monitored continuously by finger pulse oximetry and the $A - V O_2$ content difference is measured at the peak nitroprusside dosage. An occassional patient with refractory congestive heart failure and systemic arterial

hypotension requires the administration of concurrent intravenous dobutamine to maintain an adequate systemic arterial pressure to allow intravenous nitroprusside to be used for assessing pulmonary vasoreactivity in potential cardiac transplantation candidates. Patients whose PVR can be decreased to ≤ 2.5 Wood units are listed for cardiac transplantation.

Inhaled vasodilators

Nitric oxide Inhaled nitric oxide (NO) is another agent with proven efficacy for acutely assessing pulmonary vasoreactivity in pulmonary hypertensive patients during cardiac catheterization.[20–22] The dosage of inhaled NO for these studies ranged from 10 to 80 p.p.m. In our laboratory, we have adopted a modified Stanford University protocol for testing acute pulmonary vasore-activity using low-dose inhaled NO. The delivery of NO is regulated using an INOvent delivery system (Daytex-Ohmeda, Inc., Madison, WI, USA) that can deliver 1–80 p.p.m NO via an airtight mask with the patient breathing room air or supplemental oxygen from 21% to 100%. After baseline hemodynamics are recorded with the patient breathing room air, inhaled NO is administered at 5 p.p.m for 15 minutes and 20 p.p.m for 15 minutes. The 20 p.p.m inhaled NO is continued for another 15 minutes during 100% oxygen breathing. Complete pulmonary hemodynamics and methemo-globin are measured at the end of each condition to assess the patient's acute pulmonary vasoreactivity. Since inhaled NO is rapidly inactivated by hemoglobin conversion to methemo-globin, it has minimal effects on the systemic vascular resistance. The acute response to inhaled NO in patients with pulmonary hypertension has been reported to be predictive of their responsiveness to oral calcium blocker treatment.[21] Persistent pulmonary hypertension of the newborn formerly requiring extracorporeal membrane oxygenation (ECMO) may also be responsive to NO inhalation therapy.[23]

Iloprost In Europe, inhaled iloprost has been reported to be a safe and effective agent for acutely assessing pulmonary vasoreactivity in pulmonary hypertensive patients[24] and is becoming widely utilized for both acutely testing pulmonary vasoreactivity and chronic treatment of pulmonary hypertension.[25,26]

COMPLICATIONS OF CARDIAC CATHETERIZATION

Complications which are particularly important in patients with severe pulmonary hypertension and rela-tively 'fixed' low cardiac outputs include the following:

- Vasovagal reactions with bradycardia and systemic hypotension are life threatening and must be treated immediately with intravenous atropine and volume expansion.

- Supraventricular tachycardias (SVTs) including paroxysmal atrial tachycardia and atrial fibrillation can be induced by guidewire and/or catheter manipulation through the right heart. The rapid rate during SVT with inadequate ventricular filling or loss of atrial contraction during atrial fibrillation with a rapid ventricular response can quickly cause right ventricular decompensation, which requires immediate electrical cardioversion to sustain an adequate systemic blood pressure.
- A large hematoma at an arterial catheter entry site with significant blood loss can produce systemic hypotension requiring immediate intravenous fluid administration.
- With the exception of inhaled nitric oxide and inhaled iloprost, pulmonary vasodilators are also systemic vasodilators. Therefore, if the pulmonary vascular resistance is relatively 'fixed' and the systemic vascular resistance is responsive to the acute administration of a vasodilator, systemic hypotension is a potential side effect of any intravenous or oral vasodilator treatment trial. For this reason, vasodilators with a short duration of action are favored for acutely assessing pulmonary vasoreactivity.

FOLLOW-UP OUTPATIENT CARDIAC CATHETERIZATION PROCEDURES

These procedures are designed to assess efficacy of chronic treatment. Prior to the follow-up repeat cardiac catheterization procedure, we obtain a repeat chest x-ray, electrocardiogram (ECG), and a cardiac echo/Doppler study to evaluate regression of pulmonary hypertension and enlargement of the right atrium and right ventricle. The patient is instructed to continue his/her usual dosage of vasodilator therapy prior to reporting to the catheterization laboratory to ensure the hemodynamic data obtained reflect the steady-state efficacy of the current therapeutic regimen. The hemodynamic measurements are the same as the initial catheterization procedure. After the resting hemodynamics are measured, we consider the possibility of acutely adding intravenous prostacyclin to determine whether or not there might be additional pulmonary vasoreactivity which is not being achieved with the current vasodilator at the current dosage. Our experience has taught us that such data are clinically useful in adjusting the dosage of the vasodilator the patient is already taking, or in considering the possibility of adding an additional agent to achieve multidrug therapy analogous to the common management of patients with systemic hypertension who require multiple simultaneous antihypertensive medications. During the repeat hemodynamic evaluation, we also consider including an assessment of the added physiological effect of hypoxia, hyperoxia and/or exercise if the initial catheterization demonstrated significant abnormalities which may have been improved by vasodilator treatment.

Unfortunately, 70–75% of patients with pulmonary arterial hypertension do not demonstrate significant pulmonary vasoreactivity acutely and are refractory to the chronic administratioin of oral calcium channel antagonists. However, chronic treatment of these acutely nonresponsive patients has advanced dramatically in the past decade, and is covered in detail in other chapters. Briefly, these refractory patients often respond hemodynamically and clinically to chronic therapy with continuous intravenous prostacyclin,[27,28] oral bosentan (a dual endothelin receptor antagonist),[29,30] subcutaneously infused treprostinil (a prostacyclin analogue),[31] or inhaled iloprost (which is not currently approved for use in the USA).[25,26] Clinical trials are also anticipated soon to evaluate the treatment safety and efficacy for combinations of agents such as inhaled iloprost and oral sildenafil, a phosphodiesterase inhibitor,[32–34] or the addition of oral bosentan to chronic intravenous prostacyclin. Repeat right heart catheterization with direct measurement of the pulmonary arterial pressure and cardiac output is helpful for the objective assessment of the efficacy of all treatment modalities of pulmonary hypertension.

SUMMARY

In summary, cardiac catheterization contributes to the clinical evaluation of the patient with pulmonary hypertension in two important ways, both of which are useful in guiding therapy: it helps to establish the severity and etiology, and it can determine whether or not there is a significant component of pulmonary vasoreactivity to aid in the selection of appropriate therapy. Right heart catheterization should only be performed in the context of a complete evaluation of the pulmonary hypertensive patient. Patients with severe pulmonary hypertension present unique technical challenges due to the elevation of right-sided pressures, marked dilation of the right ventricle and atrium, and coexistent severe tricuspid and/or pulmonary valvular regurgitation. Catheterization of such patients requires the use of techniques to detect and quantify intracardiac shunts. Invasive procedures in pulmonary hypertensive patients are associated with increased morbidity because of hemodynamic intolerance to significant bradycardia and/or hypovolemia. Proper patient preparation for the catheterization procedure minimizes the risk taken and maximizes the information obtained.

KEY POINTS

- We now perform more than 95% of our pulmonary hypertension catheterizations as an outpatient procedure using the 'anterior' right internal jugular vein approach.
- Hemodynamic evaluation of patients with severe pulmonary hypertension is frequently difficult due to marked enlargement of the right atrium and right ventricle associated with severe tricuspid regurgitation, which has a tendency to prolapse a standard balloon-tipped Swan–Ganz catheter from the right ventricle back into the right atrium.
- Patients with 'precapillary' pulmonary hypertension do not develop elevated wedge pressures during vasodilator trials.
- The systemic arterial pressure and oxygen saturation can be monitored non-invasively using a combined automated brachial arterial blood pressure cuff and finger pulse oximeter.
- After intervention, it is **mandatory that pressure and flow be measured** to allow calculation of the PVR for comparison with baseline hemodynamics and ideally the pulmonary artery pressure should be measured over a range of flows.
- If resting PAP is normal, then exercise (straight-leg raising, supine ergometry or straight-arm raising loaded with bar-bells) can be used to reveal exercise-induced pulmonary hypertension.
- In pulmonary hypertensive patients, we have observed that symptom-limited exercise is usually not associated with more than a twofold increase in cardiac output and we have never observed an increase in the mean wedge pressure above the normal range unless there was associated left ventricular disease.
- For acute vasodilator trials, inhaled nitric oxide is the safest and most widely used agent but, unfortunately, 70–75% of patients with pulmonary arterial hypertension do not demonstrate significant pulmonary vasoreactivity acutely and are refractory to the chronic administration of oral calcium channel antagonists.

REFERENCES

1 Rich S, Dantzker DR, Ayres SM et al. Primary pulmonary hypertension – a national prospective study. Ann Intern Med 1987;107:216–23.

2 Rich S (ed.) Primary pulmonary hypertension: Executive summary from the World Symposium – PPH, 1998. Available from the World Health Organization via the Internet (www.who.int/ncd/cvd/pph.html).

3 Groves BM, Ditchey RV, Reeves JT et al. Multicenter trial of a new guidewire thermodilution catheter. J Am Coll Cardiol 1984;3:599.

4 Grossman W. Shunt detection and quantification. In: Baim DS, Grossman W (eds), Grossman's cardiac catheterization, angiography and intervention, 6th edn. Philadelphia: Lippincott Williams & Wilkins, 2000;179–91.

5 Groves BM, Badesch DB. Cardiac catheterization of patients with pulmonary hypertension. In: Peacock A J (ed.), Pulmonary circulation, a handbook for clinicians. London: Chapman and Hall Medical, 1996;5–67.

6 van Grondelle A, Ditchey RV, Groves BM et al. Thermodilution method overestimates low cardiac output in humans. Am J Physiol 1993;14:H690–2.

7 Groves BM, Donnellan K, Robertson AD et al. Diltiazem inhibits hypoxic pulmonary vasoconstriction in primary pulmonary hypertension. In: Sutton JR, Coates G, Remmers JE (eds), Hypoxia: the adaptations. Toronto: BC Decker Inc., 1990;163–9.

8 Groves BM, Reeves JT, Sutton JR et al. Operation Everest II: elevated high altitude pulmonary resistance unresponsive to oxygen. J Appl Physiol 1986;63:521–30.

9 Daoud FS, Kelly DB, Reeves JT. Isoproterenol as a potential pulmonary vasodilator in primary pulmonary hypertension. Am J Cardiol 1978;42:817–23.

10 Rubin LJ, Peter RH. Oral hydralazine therapy for primary pulmonary hypertension. N Engl J Med 1980;302:69–73.

11 Rubin LJ, Groves BM, Reeves JT et al. Prostacyclin induced acute pulmonary vasodilation in pulmonary hypertension. Circulation 1982;66:334–8.

12 Groves BM, Rubin LJ, Frosolono MF et al. A comparison of the hemodynamic effects of prostacyclin and hydralazine in primary pulmonary hypertension. Am Heart J 1985;110:1200–4.

13 Groves BM, Badesch DB, Turkevich D et al. Correlation of acute prostacyclin response in primary (unexplained) pulmonary hypertension with efficacy of treatment with calcium channel blockers and survival. In: Weir EK, Hume JR, Reeves JT (eds), Ion flux in pulmonary vascular control. New York: Plenum Publishing Corporation, 1993;317–30.

14 Groves BM, Badesch DB, Donnellan K et al. Acute hemodynamic effects of iloprost in primary (unexplained) pulmonary hypertension. Semin Respir Crit Care Med 1994;15:230–7.

15 Morgan JM, McCormack DG, Griffiths MB et al. Adenosine as a vasodilator in primary pulmonary hypertension. Circulation 1991;84:1145–9.

16 Reeves JT, Groves BM, Weir EK. Adenosine and selective reduction of pulmonary vascular resistance in primary pulmonary hypertension. Circulation 1991;84:1437–9.

17 Schrader BJ, Inbar S, Kaufmann L et al. Comparison of the effects of adenosine and nifedipine in pulmonary hypertension. J Am Coll Cardiol 1992;19:1060–4.

18 Pearl RG, Rosenthal MH, Schroeder JS et al. Acute hemodynamic effects of nitroglycerin in pulmonary hypertension. Ann Intern Med 1983;99:9–13.

19 Costard-Jackle A, Fowler MB. Influence of preoperative pulmonary artery pressure on mortality after heart transplantation: testing of potential reversibility of

pulmonary hypertension with nitroprusside is useful in defining a high-risk group. *J Am Coll Cardiol* 1992;**19**:48–54.

20 Pepke-Zaba J, Higenbottam TW, Dinh-Xuan AT *et al.* Inhaled nitric oxide as a cause of selective pulmonary vasodilation in pulmonary hypertension. *Lancet* 1991;**338**:1173–4.

21 Ricciardi MJ, Knight BP, Martinez FJ *et al.* Inhaled nitric oxide in primary pulmonary hypertension. A safe and effective agent for predicting response to nifedipine. *J Am Coll Cardiol* 1998;**32**:1068–73.

22 Hoeper MM, Olschewski H, Ghofrani HA *et al.* A comparison of the acute hemodynamic effects of inhaled nitric oxide and aerosolized iloprost in primary pulmonary hypertension. *J Am Coll Cardiol* 2000;**35**:176–82.

23 Kinsella JP, Neish SR, Shaffer E *et al.* The effect of low-dose inhalational NO in pulmonary hypertension of the newborn. *Lancet* 1992;**340**:819–20.

24 Olschewski H, Walmrath D, Schermuly R *et al.* Aerosolized prostacyclin and iloprost in severe pulmonary hypertension. *Ann Intern Med* 1996;**124**:820–4.

25 Hoeper MM, Schwarze M, Ehlerding S *et al.* Long-term treatment of primary pulmonary hypertension with aerosolized iloprost, a prostacyclin analogue. *N Engl J Med* 2000;**342**:1866–70.

26 Olschewski H, Ghofrani HA, Schmehl T *et al.* Inhaled iloprost to treat severe pulmonary hypertension. An uncontrolled trial. German PPH Study Group. *Ann Intern Med* 2000;**132**:435–43.

27 Barst RJ, Rubin LJ, Long WA *et al.* for the Primary Pulmonary Hypertension Study Group. A comparison of continuous intravenous epoprostenol (prostacyclin) with conventional therapy for primary pulmonary hypertension. *N Engl J Med* 1996;**334**:296–301.

28 Badesch DB, Tapson VF, McGoon MD *et al.* Continuous intravenous epoprostenol for pulmonary hypertension due to the scleroderma spectrum of disease. A randomized controlled trial. *Ann Intern Med* 2000;**132**:425–34.

29 Channick RN, Simonneau G, Sitbon O *et al.* Effects of the dual endothelin receptor antagonist bosentan in patients with pulmonary hypertension: a randomized placebo-controlled study. *Lancet* 2001;**358**:1119–23.

30 Rubin LJ, Badesch DB, Barst RJ *et al.* on behalf of the BREATHE-1 Study Group. Bosentan in patients with pulmonary arterial hypertension. *N Engl J Med* 2002;**346**:896–903.

31 Simonneau G, Barst RJ, Galie N *et al.* Continuous subcutaneous infusion of treprostinil, a prostacyclin analogue, in patients with pulmonary arterial hypertension: a double-blind, randomized, placebo-controlled trial. *Am J Respir Crit Care Med* 2002;**165**:800–4.

32 Schermuly RT, Krupnik E, Tenor H *et al.* Coaerosolization of phosphodiesterase inhibitors markedly enhances the pulmonary vasodilatory response to inhaled iloprost in experimental pulmonary hypertension. Maintenance of lung selectivity. *Am J Respir Crit Care Med* 2001;**164**:1694–700.

33 Wilkens H, Guth A, Konig J *et al.* Effect of inhaled iloprost plus oral sildenafil in patients with primary pulmonary hypertension. *Circulation* 2001;**104**:1218–22.

34 Ghofrani HA, Wiedemann R, Rose F *et al.* Combination therapy with oral sildenafil and inhaled iloprost for severe pulmonary hypertension. *Ann Intern Med* 2002;**136**:515–22.

11

An integrated approach to the diagnosis of pulmonary hypertension*

MICHAEL D McGOON

INTRODUCTION

The diagnosis of pulmonary hypertension (PH) entails two stages: detection and characterization (Figure 11.1). **Detection** refers to the process of establishing the presence of PH. The purpose of this phase is to determine a cause of symptoms or to detect the presence of PH in a high-risk patient. PH may also be discovered incidentally during the course of general evaluation. **Characterization** refers to the process of determining the specific clinical context of the PH, including causal factors, associated diseases or substrates, hemodynamic perturbations and their localization, and sequelae. The purpose of this stage of diagnosis is to identify optimal treatment strategies and to estimate prognosis. **Detection** requires awareness of the clinical presentation and maintenance of a high level of suspicion when circumstances warrant. **Characterization** demands understanding the appropriate utilization and capabilities of a broad range of investigational modalities.

The tools for the assessment of PH range from the physical examination and basic laboratory studies to various imaging procedures and hemodynamic analyses.

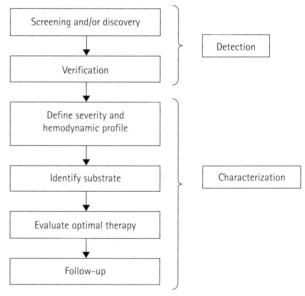

Figure 11.1 *General approach to evaluation of pulmonary arterial hypertension.*

Figure 11.2 is a diagnostic flow chart showing a strategy for integrating these tools into the evaluation of PH or possible PH. Although specific circumstances may justify modifying this schema, the general approach may be broadly applied. This chapter discusses the range of diagnostic tools that are pertinent for applying these guidelines. Further details about each procedure can be found in the respective chapter describing it.

---

*Portions of this text were originally published in McGoon MD. The assessment of pulmonary hypertension. *Clin Chest Med* 2001;**22**:493–508. By permission of WB Saunders Company. © Copyright 2002 Mayo Foundation.

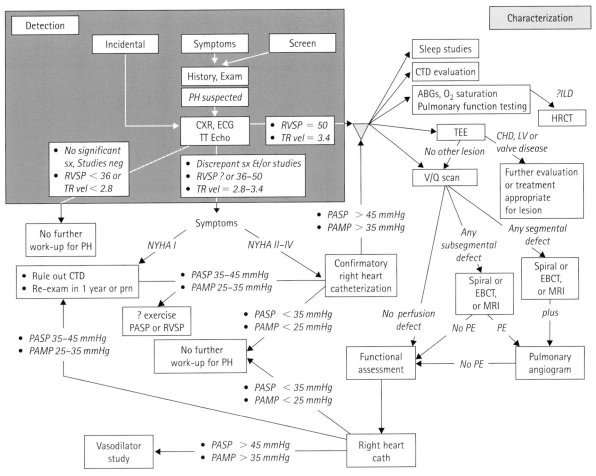

Figure 11.2 *Guideline for general strategy of evaluating pulmonary hypertension. Abbreviations: ABGs, arterial blood gases; CHD, congenital heart disease; CTD, connective tissue disease; CXR, chest x-ray; EBCT, electron-beam computed tomography; ECG, electrocardiogram; HRCT, high-resolution computed tomography of the chest; ILD, interstitial lung disease; LV, left ventricular; MRI, magnetic resonance imaging; NYHA, New York Heart Association; PASP, pulmonary arterial systolic pressure; PAMP, pulmonary arterial mean pressure; PE, pulmonary embolism; PH, pulmonary hypertension; RVSP, right ventricular systolic pressure; sx, symptoms; TEE, transesophageal echocardiography; TR vel, tricuspid regurgitant jet velocity; TT echo, transthoracic two-dimensional Doppler echocardiogram; V̇/Q̇ scan, lung ventilation and perfusion scintigraphy. (From McGoon MD. The assessment of pulmonary hypertension. Clin Chest Med 2001;22:493–508. By permission of W B Saunders Company.)*

DETECTION

The initial consideration of PH as a potential diagnosis in an individual patient may arise from one of three general scenarios:

- evaluation of symptoms for which PH is in the differential diagnosis;
- screening for the presence of PH in a high-risk individual without suggestive symptoms; or
- the incidental discovery of PH as a consequence of a general evaluation for unrelated issues.

The context of the discovery of PH may have an impact on the further strategy of diagnosis and treatment.

Symptom evaluation

Since PH is less prevalent than many other types of cardiovascular diseases that are associated with the same non-specific symptoms, a high level of suspicion directs further evaluation. Among the symptoms that should raise the possibility of PH, exertional dyspnea is most common, occurring in almost 100% of symptomatic patients. Quantification of subjective activity tolerance should be documented to provide a baseline for serial follow-up of disease progression, response to treatment, and prognostication. Fatigue, weakness, angina, syncope, peripheral edema, and abdominal distension, particularly in patients without typical signs of underlying ischemic or other cardiopulmonary diseases, should raise the possibility of PH.

Screening

Risk factors for PH include a history of appetite suppressant use, liver disease with portal hypertension, past pulmonary thromboembolism, residence at high altitude, connective tissue disease, congenital heart disease or human immunodeficiency virus (HIV) infection, chronic hypoxic restrictive or obstructive lung disease, sleep apnea, and a family history of primary PH. Periodic assessment of patients with an underlying predisposition may be warranted so that therapy can be introduced at an early stage or so that more aggressive surveillance can be initiated to detect progression.

Incidental discovery

Discovery of unsuspected PH, especially of milder degrees, has become more frequent with the widespread use of Doppler echocardiographic techniques. The clinical significance and natural history of asymptomatic or mild PH is unclear, and so the implications for further assessment and treatment remain uncertain. The observation of PH should prompt an attempt to define or exclude possible causes, since it may be the first evidence of a modifiable substrate. However, the severity of the PH and the reliability of the measurement should temper the aggressiveness of the evaluation. Possible explanations for mildly increased pulmonary artery systolic pressure detected by echocardiography or right heart catheterization include:

- overestimation of the pulmonary artery pressure in a patient with normal pressure;
- serendipitous observation of a rare transient pressure increase in an otherwise healthy individual;
- discovery of stable, mild PH, possibly of long duration; and
- discovery of early progressive PH in a patient with intrinsic pulmonary vascular disease.

Physical examination

The findings on physical examination, though they can be subtle and are never independently diagnostic, may be the first step in narrowing the extensive differential diagnosis raised by presenting symptoms.

Chest x-ray

A chest x-ray showing central pulmonary and right ventricular enlargement supports the possibility of PH. Since a chest x-ray is an integral part of general screening examinations and the assessment of dyspnea, it is seldom omitted, though significant clues may be overlooked.

Careful attention to radiographic findings on plain x-ray, as described in Chapter 9, may provide an early pointer toward the cause of symptoms or the substrate for PH.

Electrocardiography

Electrocardiography may support the diagnosis of PH by revealing evidence of right ventricular hypertrophy and right atrial enlargement.

Transthoracic echocardiography

If screening or preliminary evaluation of symptoms supports the possibility of PH, validation and initial exploration of severity and the underlying cause are pursued by Doppler echocardiographic techniques. Echo cardiography is useful for the evaluation of the right heart and pulmonary hemodynamics because of its ability to assess the morphology of cardiac and vascular structures and to record flow velocities at selected sites. Doppler echocardiography contributes clinical data for both detection and characterization in a single examination. These include semiquantitative right ventricular size and function and right atrial size, tricuspid regurgitant velocity for estimation of right ventricular systolic pressure (RVSP), left ventricular systolic and diastolic function, morphology and function of all cardiac valves, and intracardiac or intrapulmonary shunt.

Doppler echocardiography is the most sensitive noninvasive method for detection of PH or right ventricular pressure overload. As described in detail in Chapter 8, continuous-wave Doppler determination of tricuspid regurgitant jet velocity and application of the modified Bernoulli equation permit estimation of right ventricular systolic pressure. Tricuspid regurgitant Doppler signals are present in 95% of unselected cardiovascular patients.[1] Doppler RVSP correlates well with invasively measured pulmonary systolic pressure.[2–11] If appropriately performed, the likelihood of a clinically important error in the estimation of RVSP is low. Incorrect estimation of right atrial pressure will yield an incorrect RVSP. Echocardiographic assessment of inferior vena cava diameter and hepatic vein velocity curves to approximate right atrial pressure may minimize this source of inaccuracy.[12]

RVSP in normal patients has been well characterized. Among a broad population of male and female subjects ranging from 1 to 89 years of age, it was reported as 28.3 ± 4.9 mmHg (range 15–57 mmHg). Average RVSP increases with age and body mass index.[13] Athletically conditioned men also have higher resting RVSP than normal men.[14]

Defining the normal distribution of RVSP does not *ipso facto* define the point at which an elevated RVSP is clinically important or is predictive of future consequences.

Although there is high correlation with invasively measured pulmonary artery pressure, Doppler RVSP estimates pulmonary artery pressure at a single time. Because of a possible discrepancy in individual cases, the results should be interpreted in the light of additional data, including physical examination and echocardiographic right ventricular function. The global clinical scenario, and **not** the RVSP, is the object of analysis and treatment.

CHARACTERIZATION

Once PH is suspected or has been confirmed, evaluation to define the nature and severity of the disease is warranted.

Transthoracic echocardiography

Doppler echocardiographic examination conceptually consists of the detection aspect (see above), which discovers or confirms the probability of PH, and the aspect of characterizing the severity and possible causes of the hemodynamic abnormality.

ASSESSMENT OF SEVERITY OF PH

Estimation of RVSP is the most commonly used method to quantitate the severity of PH. Doppler echocardiography can also estimate both diastolic and mean pulmonary artery pressures (Chapter 8), which may provide useful additional information in some patients or may provide the only non-invasive pressure quantification for patients in whom tricuspid regurgitant velocity cannot be measured accurately.

DIFFERENTIAL DIAGNOSIS OF PH

Two-dimensional transthoracic echocardiography may elucidate causes underlying PH, such as left ventricular dysfunction, mitral valve disease, and intracardiac shunt. The amplitude of pulmonary artery 'pulse pressure', as assessed with Doppler in patients with significant PH, helps distinguish between patients with primary PH and those with proximal chronic pulmonary thromboembolism.[15]

ASSESSMENT OF RIGHT VENTRICULAR FUNCTION AND RIGHT VENTRICULAR-TO-PULMONARY ARTERIAL COUPLING

It is important to assess the right ventricle, as the 'end organ' most directly affected, during the evaluation of PH. Complex right ventricular geometry precludes reliable echocardiographic assessment of ejection fraction and related indices. Consequently, quantitative assessment of right ventricular function using other Doppler echo-cardiographic techniques has been explored. One index of right ventricular dysfunction is the right ventricular index of myocardial performance.[16] This index (Chapter 8) reflects global right ventricular dysfunction and is not significantly affected by heart rate, right ventricular pressure, right ventricular dilatation, or tricuspid regurgitation. It correlates with symptoms and survival in patients with primary PH.[17]

Although the right ventricular index of myocardial performance describes the global function of the ventricle, pulsed-wave Doppler assessment of the systolic flow velocity curve in the right ventricular outflow tract may provide insight into the coupling of the right ventricular to the pulmonary arterial system.

RIGHT VENTRICULAR MORPHOLOGY AND FUNCTION

Techniques for measuring right ventricular volume and function have been described but are limited because of the complexity of the formulas derived and the difficult imaging imposed by the crescentic shape of the right ventricle. Even qualitative descriptions of right ventricular size and function impart useful impressions about the severity and consequences of the hemodynamic abnormality.

EVALUATION OF PROGNOSIS AND RESPONSE TO TREATMENTS

Echocardiographic data have prognostic relevance. Parameters including elevated pulmonary artery pressure, increased right atrial pressure, and decreased cardiac output were found to identify patients with PH and poor survival.[18] In addition, pericardial effusions (which occur frequently in primary PH[19]) and short acceleration time correlate with poor prognosis.[20] Pulmonary artery systolic pressure correlates poorly with survival. Echocardiographic and Doppler indices of right ventricular pressure overload and dysfunction improve after successful treatment of chronic severe PH either by thromboendarterectomy[21] or by continuous intravenous infusion of prostacyclin.[22]

FOLLOW-UP

Patients with high-quality echocardiographic studies and good correlation of non-invasively measured pulmonary hemodynamics with catheterization data can be followed with serial echocardiograms to assess progression of disease or response to treatment. Despite high correlation with catheter-measured pulmonary artery pressures in populations with PH, however, operator technique and interpretation may introduce errors in measurement. Consequently, comparison of measurements over time in a single person should be considered in the light of corroborative data and the experience of the echocardiographic laboratory. Data regarding pulmonary resistance and cardiac output cannot be reliably evaluated by echocardiography, and, if necessary for clinical decision-making, right heart catheterization is needed.

Transesophageal echocardiography (TEE)

TEE is useful in the detection of otherwise occult intracardiac shunts, especially atrial septal defects. Some congenital defects may be missed if TEE techniques are not used. These disorders include atypically situated atrial septal defects, especially of the sinus venosus type with abnormal pulmonary venous drainage.

TEE can detect central pulmonary emboli, including chronic thromboemboli causing PH.[23,24] It can be performed safely in patients with severe PH, and it provides data that may alter treatment in up to 25% of patients.[25]

Specific blood tests for evaluation of PH

Antinuclear antibody (ANA) titer to screen for connective tissue disease and HIV serology should be obtained in all cases of undifferentiated PH. Screening for HIV status is predicated on the recognition that a substantial portion of patients with primary PH may be HIV positive,[26] and the development of primary PH after HIV infection has been reported.[27–31]

For patients with known or suspected thromboembolic PH, evaluation of a potential clotting diathesis is warranted. Assessment may include antiphospholipid antibodies (lupus anticoagulant, anticardiolipin antibody). The presence of a lupus anticoagulant has been identified in about 10% of patients with chronic pulmonary embolism.[32] Specific evaluation of other disorders of the coagulation system includes bleeding time, coagulation factors (VIII, VII, II and V), von Willebrand factors, and proteins C and S. Factor V Leiden mutation (the most common cause of activated protein C resistance) has been implicated as a risk factor for idiopathic venous thromboembolism,[33] though not specifically for pulmonary embolism[34] or chronic thromboembolic PH.[35] Serum viscosity, serum protein electrophoresis, hemoglobin electrophoresis, quantitative immunoglobulins, or fractionated plasma catecholamines may be required under certain circumstances.

Markers of endothelial dysfunction, such as endothelin levels in the plasma, have been shown to correlate with the degree of pulmonary hemodynamic abnormality.[36–39] Whether such markers will serve a clinically useful role in establishing and following disease severity and response to treatment is not yet clear.

Hyperthyroid[40–42] and hypothyroid[43,44] disorders have been implicated as being associated with, and possibly causal in, some forms of PH, perhaps because of an autoimmune mechanism, high cardiac output, endothelial dysfunction, or altered metabolism of endogenous pulmonary vasodilators. Conversely, the possibility has been raised that treatment of PH may induce hyperthyroidism in some patients.[42] Assessment and follow-up of thyroid function in patients with PH is advised.

Hyperuricemia occurs with high frequency in patients with PH[45] and correlates with hemodynamic abnormalities (especially right atrial pressure)[46] and mortality in primary PH.[47] Although the significance of this association is uncertain, obtaining a serum uric acid level may lead to the discovery of a hyperuricemic condition that requires treatment.

Ventilation/perfusion scintigraphy

Ventilation/perfusion scanning is a widely available screening modality to detect chronic pulmonary thromboemboli. Lung scans in chronic pulmonary embolism usually show at least one segmental-sized or larger perfusion defect. Most patients have several segmental or lobar defects bilaterally, which are typically mismatched and larger than ventilation abnormalities.[32] Large perfusion defects that are not segmental or lobar in distribution are not indicative of pulmonary embolism, especially when in the lower lung distribution, but may be due to diversion of flow to upper lung zones in patients with high left-sided filling pressures and secondary lower-zone vasoconstriction.[48]

Non-homogeneous flow patterns are very unlikely to represent chronic pulmonary embolism, and such patients are more likely to have primary PH.[49–53] Patchy, non-segmental, diffuse defects are less specific but may be associated with thromboembolic disease.[54] Perfusion scans consistently tend to underestimate the degree of severity of large-vessel obstruction in PH.[55]

Computed tomography (CT)

The CT scanning measurements that correlate with severity of pulmonary hypertension are the cross-sectional area of the pulmonary artery,[56] the diameter of the main pulmonary artery, the ratio of the diameter of the artery to the bronchus,[57] the ratio of the diameter of the pulmonary artery to that of the pulmonary vein,[58] the ratio of the main pulmonary artery to the aortic diameter,[59] and the presence of pericardial thickening or effusion.[60] A mosaic pattern of lung attenuation in a non-contrast CT scan raises the possibility of chronic thromboembolism.[61] Although such observations may be useful in non-invasively adding strength to a diagnosis of PH and assessment of severity, they do not take the place of more precise and validated Doppler echocardiographic measurements. Rather, the role of CT is to explore possible etiological factors.

The main utility of contrast-enhanced CT scans is evaluation for possible chronic thromboembolism, and it is considered by many as more useful than ventilation/perfusion scans, especially for detecting disease that is amenable to surgical treatment. Spiral (or helical) CT,[62] or electron-beam CT (EBCT)[63] can visualize central chronic pulmonary thromboemboli, in some cases more accurately than angiography or magnetic resonance imaging (MRI).[64] CT features of chronic thromboembolic disease are complete occlusion of pulmonary arteries, eccentric filling defects consistent with thrombi, recanalization, and stenoses or webs.[65]

EBCT can provide clues to the presence of pulmonary venous obstruction, such as stricture or hypoplasia in children with congenital heart disease.[66] Other signs of possible pulmonary vein obstruction, including pulmonary veno-occlusive disease, are smooth thickening of interlobular septa, peribronchovascular cuffing, and alveolar ground-glass opacification.[66,67]

High-resolution CT

High-resolution CT scanning is most commonly used to determine whether interstitial lung disease is a contributor to both symptoms and PH, especially when pulmonary function tests suggest restrictive disease. A mosaic pattern of the lung parenchyma and variation of segmental vessel size are suggestive of chronic thromboembolic disease.[68] Features of high-resolution CT scans may be helpful in suggesting diagnoses that might otherwise not be suspected. Diffuse bilateral thickening of the interlobular septa and the presence of small, centrilobular, poorly circumscribed nodular opacities suggest pulmonary capillary hemangiomatosis. Patients with pulmonary veno-occlusive disease may demonstrate diffuse, predominantly central ground-glass opacification and thickening of interlobular septa.[69]

Magnetic resonance imaging (MRI)

MRI can provide non-invasive clues to the presence of PH by the evaluation of right ventricular chamber size, shape, and volume; myocardial thickness and mass; and the presence of fat or edema.[70] MRI-measured right ventricular systolic and diastolic volumes are significantly increased and left ventricular end-diastolic volume is decreased in patients with primary PH. In addition, right and left ventricular ejection fractions are depressed in primary PH, and right ventricular stroke volume index is higher than left stroke volume index as a result of tricuspid regurgitation.[71]

Mean pulmonary artery pressure correlates linearly with MRI-measured right ventricular wall thickness, inferior vena cava diameter and main pulmonary artery diameter,[72] and right ventricular mass index,[73] although correlation coefficients are not sufficient for any of these parameters for accurate estimation of pressure. MRI-measured parameters can yield an estimate of mean pulmonary artery pressure based on regression analysis of the measured dimensions of the main pulmonary artery and mid-descending thoracic aorta.[74] Velocity-encoded MRI, which provides two-dimensional velocity maps of a vessel cross-section, has a higher ratio of maximal change in pulmonary flow rate during ejection to acceleration volume in PH compared with normal; it is proportional to pulmonary resistance, suggesting that this technique may be useful as a means of non-invasively estimating pulmonary resistance.[75] Complex assessment of the pulmonary arterial-reflected pressure wave velocity using velocity-encoded MR techniques has been used with a fair degree of accuracy to estimate mean pulmonary artery pressure in patients with PH,[76] but it needs to be validated and its clinical utility has yet to be determined. MRI techniques can also be used to delineate anatomic abnormalities of the pulmonary arteries,[77] including the presence of chronic thromboemboli.[78] The use of contrast refines the image distinction between blood and thrombi, though accurate visualization is technique dependent.[79]

Pulmonary angiography

Pulmonary angiography is important in confirming or excluding a diagnosis of chronic pulmonary embolism and in defining the extent and location of thrombus. It can be performed safely in patients with severe PH and right ventricular failure when appropriate safeguards are used.[80,81] These include using a brachial or jugular approach (to reduce risk of femoral thrombus), continuous monitoring of the electrocardiogram and arterial saturation, single injections into the right (using posterior-anterior projection) and the left (using slight left anterior-oblique projection) main pulmonary arteries, non-ionic contrast, and pretreatment with atropine, 1 mg intravenously.

Chronic thrombi appear different from acute thrombi and occur in highly variable locations, often incorporated into and retracting the vessel wall. Obstruction can take the form of bands or webs, sometimes with post-stenotic dilatation. Irregular intimal surface, rounded or pouch-like termination of segmental branches, luminal narrowing of the central vessel, and odd-shaped pulmonary arteries all may indicate the presence of chronic pulmonary embolism.[82]

Pulmonary function testing

Pulmonary function testing is required to exclude or characterize the contribution of underlying airway or parenchymal lung disease. Although obstructive pulmonary disease with hypoxemia may be confirmed by testing, abnormalities may occur in other types of PH. Approximately 20% of patients with chronic pulmonary embolism have a restrictive defect (a reduction in lung volumes to <80% of normal),[32] and they may have near-normal diffusing capacity for carbon monoxide (DLCO).[83] More often, however, low DLCO may be an early and important clue to the presence of pulmonary hypertensive arterial disease. Twenty per cent of patients with systemic sclerosis have an isolated reduction in DLCO,[84] which, when severe (<55% of predicted), may be associated with future development of PH in the limited cutaneous form (CREST).[85]

Arterial blood gas measurement

Arterial oxygen desaturation is both a promoter and a consequence of PH but is in itself non-specific regarding underlying cause. It may signal abnormal gas exchange, right-to-left shunting and ventilation/perfusion mismatching, interstitial fibrosis or other parenchymal lung disease, or hypoventilation. Failure to normalize with high FIO_2 oxygen inhalation supports a component of right-to-left shunting.

A search for abnormal oxygenation is warranted even when resting oxygen saturation is unremarkable. Arterial blood gas measurement or oximetry during exercise may disclose desaturation, requiring supplemental oxygen treatment to improve exercise capacity and promote pulmonary vasodilation. Overnight oximetry may disclose disordered sleep with frequent desaturations and may be the first clue to sleep apnea sufficient to contribute to PH. Nocturnal hypoxemia occurs in more than 75% of patients with primary PH, independently of the occurence of apnea or hypopnea, and many also have hypoxemia with walking.[86] Since hypoxia is a potent pulmonary vasoconstrictor, all patients with unexplained PH require assessment of both sleep and exercise oxygen saturation.

Exercise assessment

Assessment of exercise capacity is an integral part of the evaluation of PH. The goals of exercise testing include: searching for alternative or contributory reasons for symptoms, such as myocardial ischemia; determining maximal exercise tolerance; characterizing the comfortable activity level (functional capacity) of the patient; obtaining predictive data; establishing a baseline measure of exercise capacity and following the response to therapy; assessing the interaction of the circulatory and ventilatory systems; and attempting to discover abnormal pulmonary hemodynamic responses to exercise before clinically evident PH at rest.

The most commonly used exercise tests for the evaluation of PH are: the 6-minute walk test; standard treadmill exercise test utilizing a low-intensity, graduated exercise protocol; cardiopulmonary exercise testing; exercise testing in conjunction with non-invasive Doppler echocardiographic assessment of pulmonary artery pressure; and exercise testing with right heart catheterization.

The 6-minute walk test is reproducible, correlates with other measures of functional status, and is predictive of survival.[87,88] It has been used as a primary end point in a number of clinical drug treatment trials. At the Mayo Clinic, unencouraged 6-minute walk tests are performed on a 20-meter back-and-forth course during monitoring by a trained pulmonary hypertension nurse specialist. Measured parameters are distance walked, baseline and peak oxygen saturation by finger or earlobe oximetry, supplemental oxygen flow rate if used, baseline and peak blood pressure and pulse, number of breaks, and self-reported Borg dyspnea scale rating.

Cardiopulmonary exercise testing using cycle ergometry can be performed safely in adults[89,90] and children[91] with PH. The mechanisms of exercise limitation in primary PH are ventilation/perfusion mismatching, lactic acidosis at a low work rate, arterial hypoxemia, and inability to adequately increase stroke volume and cardiac output.[89,90]

Exercise and ambulatory invasive pulmonary hemodynamic measurements show marked increases in pulmonary arterial pressure during exertion in patients with dyspnea or suspected PH.[92–94] However, the value of exercise hemodynamic studies in predicting future outcomes or worsening of PH remains uncertain. The observation of a substantial increase of PH in dyspneic patients with minimal hemodynamic abnormalities at rest and no alternative explanation for symptoms justifies treatment for PH, as discussed elsewhere.

Exercise non-invasive hemodynamic assessment using Doppler echocardiography has been utilized to evaluate pulmonary artery pressure responses in different patient populations with varying degrees of baseline PH.[95–97] In healthy men, tricuspid regurgitant velocity increases from an average of 1.72 m/s at baseline to a peak of 2.46 m/s at mid-level exercise and to 2.27 m/s at peak exercise (240 watts); in trained athletes, the baseline value is 2.25 m/s, which increases to 3.41 m/s at peak exercise.[14] As with invasive exercise studies, the degree of abnormal pressure response to exercise which may reliably be considered a cause of symptoms or have prognostic significance has not been well established.

Right heart hemodynamic catheterization

Catheter measurement of mean pulmonary artery pressure (PAP, mmHg), pulmonary arterial blood flow ($\dot{Q}\dot{P}$,

L/min), pulmonary capillary wedge pressure (PCWP, mmHg), right atrial pressure, and mixed venous oxygen saturation provides the most definitive characterization of pulmonary hemodynamics. Right heart catheterization is required before a diagnosis of any type of PH can be regarded as secure.

ASSESSMENT OF SHUNT

Although significant right-to-left shunting can most often be excluded by bubble-contrast echocardiography, right heart catheterization may be required to exclude left-to-right shunting and thus the presence of a potentially treatable intracardiac or extracardiac shunt.

MEASUREMENT OF PULMONARY ARTERY WEDGE (OCCLUSION) PRESSURE

Assessment of pulmonary vein pressure and transpulmonary gradient is needed for calculation of pulmonary arteriolar resistance. This requires knowing pulmonary artery occlusion pressure. If necessary, left atrial pressure or left ventricular end-diastolic pressure should be measured. An increased pulmonary arterial occlusion pressure supports the presence of left heart disease or pulmonary vein obstruction but is very insensitive for pulmonary veno-occlusive disease.[67]

MEASUREMENT OF PULMONARY RESISTANCE

PAP and $\dot{Q}P$ provide the basis for calculating total pulmonary vascular resistance (TPR [U] = PAP/$\dot{Q}P$) and pulmonary arterial resistance {PAR [U] = (PAP − PCWP)/$\dot{Q}P$}. Blood flow and resistance can be indexed to body surface area (m^2). Calculation of $\dot{Q}P$ by the Fick method and thermodilution correlate reasonably well, including in patients with low cardiac output or tricuspid regurgitation, so that either technique may be used in most cases,[98] though the Fick technique is preferable in cases with significant tricuspid regurgitation. This calculation, however, reflects an artificial situation applicable to steady flow in a system of smooth-walled, regular, non-distensible conduits with laminar flow. In such a system, pressure increases proportionately with flow and the slope of the increase defines the resistance (which is constant).[99] More accurate interpretations of physiological pulmonary vascular resistance have been advocated since the pulmonary vasculature is compliant and recruitable, and flow is pulsatile, but these have not found wide use in clinical assessment.

MEASUREMENT OF PULMONARY VASODILATOR RESPONSE

A vasodilator study should be performed whenever PH is discovered or confirmed during right heart catheterization

of patients in whom symptoms or severity of hypertension would warrant treatment (Chapter 10). All patients in whom vasodilator treatment is to be initiated require hemodynamic monitoring for detection of either beneficial or detrimental effects of acute treatment. A decrease in PAP and PAR of 20–26% is required before the effect can confidently be attributed to an intervention.[100, 101]

PROGNOSTICATION

Baseline hemodynamic measurements provide information that can be used to estimate the natural history of the disease in an individual patient. The probability of survival P(t) 1, 2 or 3 years after diagnosis can be estimated as $P(t) = [H(t)]^{A(x,y,z)}$, where $H(t) = [0.88 − 0.14t + 0.01t^2]$, $A(x,y,z) = e^{(0.007325x + 0.0526y − 0.3275z)}$, t is in years, x is mean pulmonary artery pressure (mmHg), y is mean right atrial pressure (mmHg), and z is cardiac index (L/min·m^2).[18] Other logistic regression equations have been reported to predict survival or death within 1 year.[102]

SELECTION OF TREATMENT

The acute pulmonary hemodynamic effect of intravenously administered short-acting vasodilators predicts the hemodynamic response to oral long-acting vasodilators. Thus, the efficacy of the short-acting drug can be used to determine optimal treatment.[103–109] Short-acting vasodilators reportedly used in this capacity are prostacyclin,[105,110–114] nitric oxide,[115] adenosine,[105,108,116] acetylcholine,[105] and L-arginine.[117] For patients who respond with a reduction in mean pulmonary artery pressure of 10 mmHg with no change or an increase in cardiac output, a trial of oral medications is warranted. For nonresponders, a trial of bosentan may be warranted, but long-term intravenous prostacyclin should be considered early in view of observations that hemodynamic, symptomatic, and survival benefit may occur in spite of the absence of a significant acute beneficial effect.[87,118]

Abrupt development of pulmonary edema during acute vasodilator testing suggests the presence of pulmonary veno-occlusive disease.[119]

Lung biopsy

Open or thoracoscopic lung biopsy entails substantial risk of morbidity and mortality.[120] Because of the low likelihood of its altering the clinical diagnosis, routine biopsy is discouraged. Histopathological findings in small pulmonary arteries obtained at biopsy may not even reliably distinguish between chronic thrombo-embolic disease and primary PH.[121] Under certain circumstances, histopathological diagnosis may provide useful information by excluding or establishing a diagnosis of active vasculitis, granulomatous pulmonary disease, pulmonary veno-occlusive disease, interstitial lung disease, or bronchiolitis.

CONCLUSION

A variety of functional, imaging, and laboratory testing procedures are available to detect, characterize, and follow the course of PH, its consequences, and its response to treatment. Optimal management requires that the evaluation of the patient proceed in an orderly fashion with assimilation of data into a coherent picture of the patient's clinical status. No single test or result fully defines a diagnosis; rather, the entire body of information must be considered and discrepant results accounted for in the light of all the information available. A clear conceptual 'game plan,' based on the strategy outlined in Figure 11.1 and the guidelines in Figure 11.2, and in understanding of the implications of the tests, as discussed more fully in other chapters, provide the infrastructure for appropriate and optimal treatment.

KEY POINTS

- Pulmonary hypertension of a clinically significant degree can be suspected by careful attention to history and examination, coupled with appropriate interpretation of chest x-ray and electrocardiogram. Failure to appropriately diagnose pulmonary hypertension or to attribute symptoms to it accounts for the largest delay in initiating treatment in these patients.
- Detection of pulmonary hypertension of mild degree generally warrants further evaluation for confirmation, identification of potentially treatable causes, initiation of the monitoring of progression, and treatment of related symptoms.
- Detection and confirmation of pulmonary hypertension of moderate or severe degree requires full evaluation of underlying causes and identification of an optimal treatment regimen.
- Full Doppler echocardiographic examination is pivotal in characterizing pulmonary hypertension and screening for a broad range of potential causes.
- Left-sided cardiac disease and chronic thromboembolism are the most frequently treatable causes of pulmonary hypertension and must be fully evaluated as potential causes.
- The diagnostic process should ideally occur at referral centers where complex treatment regimens can most effectively be initiated and followed.

REFERENCES

*1 Borgeson DD, Seward JB, Miller FA Jr et al. Frequency of Doppler measurable pulmonary artery pressures. J Am Soc Echocardiogr 1996;9:832–7.

*2 Currie PJ, Seward JB, Chan KL et al. Continuous wave Doppler determination of right ventricular pressure: a simultaneous Doppler-catheterization study in 127 patients. J Am Coll Cardiol 1985;6:750–6.

3 Laaban JP, Diebold B, Zelinski R et al. Noninvasive estimation of systolic pulmonary artery pressure using Doppler echocardiography in patients with chronic obstructive pulmonary disease. Chest 1989;96:1258–62.

4 Chan KL, Currie PJ, Seward JB et al. Comparison of three Doppler ultrasound methods in the prediction of pulmonary artery pressure. J Am Coll Cardiol 1987;9:549–54.

5 Chapoutout L, Metz D, Jolly D et al. Diagnostic, prognostic and therapeutic value of Doppler echocardiography in pulmonary embolism. Apropos of 41 cases [French]. Ann Cardiol Angiol (Paris) 1989;38:523–9.

6 Kosturakis D, Goldberg SJ, Allen HD et al. Doppler echocardiographic prediction of pulmonary arterial hypertension in congenital heart disease. Am J Cardiol 1984;53:1110–15.

7 Isobe M, Yazaki Y, Takaku F et al. Prediction of pulmonary arterial pressure in adults by pulsed Doppler echocardiography. Am J Cardiol 1986;57:316–21.

8 Marchandise B, De Bruyne B, Delaunois L et al. Noninvasive prediction of pulmonary hypertension in chronic obstructive pulmonary disease by Doppler echocardiography. Chest 1987;91:361–5.

9 Marangoni S, Quadri A, Dotti A et al. Noninvasive assessment of pulmonary hypertension: a simultaneous echo-Doppler hemodynamic study. Cardiology 1988;75:401–8.

10 Torbicki A, Skwarski K, Hawrylkiewicz I et al. Attempts at measuring pulmonary arterial pressure by means of Doppler echocardiography in patients with chronic lung disease. Eur Respir J 1989;2:856–60.

11 Brecker SJ, Gibbs JS, Fox KM et al. Comparison of Doppler derived haemodynamic variables and simultaneous high fidelity pressure measurements in severe pulmonary hypertension. Br Heart J 1994;72:384–9.

12 Ommen SR, Nishimura RA, Hurrell DG et al. Assessment of right atrial pressure with 2-dimensional and Doppler echocardiography: a simultaneous catheterization and echocardiographic study. Mayo Clin Proc 2000;75:24–9.

*13 McQuillan BM, Picard MH, Leavitt M et al. Clinical correlates and reference intervals for pulmonary artery systolic pressure among echocardiographically normal subjects. Circulation 2001;104:2797–802.

14 Bossone E, Rubenfire M, Bach DS et al. Range of tricuspid regurgitation velocity at rest and during exercise in normal adult men: implications for the diagnosis of pulmonary hypertension. J Am Coll Cardiol 1999;33:1662–6.

15 Nakayama Y, Sugimachi M, Nakanishi N et al. Noninvasive differential diagnosis between chronic pulmonary thromboembolism and primary pulmonary hypertension by means of Doppler ultrasound measurement. J Am Coll Cardiol 1998;31:1367–71.

*16 Tei C, Dujardin KS, Hodge DO et al. Doppler echocardiographic index for assessment of global right ventricular function. J Am Soc Echocardiogr 1996;9:838–47.

17 Yeo TC, Dujardin KS, Tei C et al. Value of a Doppler-derived index combining systolic and diastolic time intervals in predicting outcome in primary pulmonary hypertension. Am J Cardiol 1998;81:1157–61.

18 D'Alonzo GE, Barst RJ, Ayres SM et al. Survival in patients with primary pulmonary hypertension. Results from a national prospective registry. Ann Intern Med 1991;115:343–9.

19 Hinderliter AL, Willis PW, IV, Long W et al. Frequency and prognostic significance of pericardial effusion in primary pulmonary hypertension. PPH Study Group. Primary pulmonary hypertension. Am J Cardiol 1999;84:481–4, A10.

20 Eysmann SB, Palevsky HI, Reichek N et al. Two-dimensional and Doppler-echocardiographic and cardiac catheterization correlates of survival in primary pulmonary hypertension. Circulation 1989;80:353–60.

21 Menzel T, Wagner S, Mohr-Kahaly S et al. Reversibility of changes in left and right ventricular geometry and hemodynamics in pulmonary hypertension. Echocardiographic characteristics before and after pulmonary thrombo-endarterectomy [German]. Z Kardiol 1997;86:928–35.

22 Hinderliter AL, Willis PW, IV, Barst RJ et al. Effects of long-term infusion of prostacyclin (epoprostenol) on echocardio-graphic measures of right ventricular structure and function in primary pulmonary hypertension. Primary Pulmonary Hypertension Study Group. Circulation 1997;95:1479–86.

23 Pruszczyk P, Torbicki A, Pacho R et al. Noninvasive diagnosis of suspected severe pulmonary embolism: transesophageal echocardiography vs spiral CT. Chest 1997;112:722–8.

24 Wittlich N, Erbel R, Eichler A et al. Detection of central pulmonary artery thromboemboli by transesophageal echocardiography in patients with severe pulmonary embolism. J Am Soc Echocardiogr 1992;5:515–24.

25 Gorcsan J, III, Edwards TD, Ziady GM et al. Transesophageal echocardiography to evaluate patients with severe pulmonary hypertension for lung transplantation. Ann Thorac Surg 1995;59:717–22.

26 Petitpretz P, Brenot F, Azarian R et al. Pulmonary hypertension in patients with human immunodeficiency virus infection. Comparison with primary pulmonary hypertension. Circulation 1994;89:2722–7.

27 Speich R, Jenni R, Opravil M et al. Primary pulmonary hypertension in HIV infection. Chest 1991;100:1268–71.

28 Mette SA, Palevsky HI, Pietra GG et al. Primary pulmonary hypertension in association with human immunodeficiency virus infection. A possible viral etiology for some forms of hypertensive pulmonary arteriopathy. Am Rev Respir Dis 1992; 145:1196–200.

29 Polos PG, Wolfe D, Harley RA et al. Pulmonary hypertension and human immunodeficiency virus infection. Two reports and a review of the literature. Chest 1992;101:474–8.

30 de Chadarevian JP, Lischner HW, Karmazin N et al. Pulmonary hypertension and HIV infection: new observations and review of the syndrome. Mod Pathol 1994;7:685–9.

31 Mani S, Smith GJ. HIV and pulmonary hypertension: a review. South Med J 1994;87:357–62.

32 Viner SM, Bagg BR, Auger WR et al. The management of pulmonary hypertension secondary to chronic thromboembolic disease. Prog Cardiovasc Dis 1994;37:79–92.

33 Ridker PM, Miletich JP, Stampfer MJ et al. Factor V Leiden and risks of recurrent idiopathic venous thromboembolism. Circulation 1995;92:2800–2.

34 Manten B, Westendorp RG, Koster T et al. Risk factor profiles in patients with different clinical manifestations of venous thromboembolism: a focus on the factor V Leiden mutation. Thromb Haemost 1996;76:510–13.

35 Lang IM, Klepetko W, Pabinger I. No increased prevalence of the factor V Leiden mutation in chronic major vessel thromboembolic pulmonary hypertension (CTEPH). Thromb Haemost 1996;76:476–7.

36 Stewart DJ, Levy RD, Cernacek P et al. Increased plasma endothelin-1 in pulmonary hypertension: marker or mediator of disease? Ann Intern Med 1991;114:464–9.

37 Nootens M, Kaufmann E, Rector T et al. Neurohormonal activation in patients with right ventricular failure from pulmonary hypertension: relation to hemodynamic variables and endothelin levels. J Am Coll Cardiol 1995;26:1581–5.

38 Cody RJ, Haas GJ, Binkley PF et al. Plasma endothelin correlates with the extent of pulmonary hypertension in patients with chronic congestive heart failure. Circulation 1992;85:504–9.

*39 Rubens C, Ewert R, Halank M et al. Big endothelin-1 and endothelin-1 plasma levels are correlated with the severity of primary pulmonary hypertension. Chest 2001;120:1562–9.

40 Arroliga AC, Dweik RA, Rafanan AL. Primary pulmonary hypertension and thyroid disease. Chest 2000;118:1224–5.

41 Nakchbandi IA, Wirth JA, Inzucchi SE. Pulmonary hypertension caused by Graves' thyrotoxicosis: normal pulmonary hemodynamics restored by ^{131}I treatment. Chest 1999;116:1483–5.

42 Ferris A, Jacobs T, Widlitz A et al. Pulmonary arterial hypertension and thyroid disease. Chest 2001;119:1980–1.

43 Curnock AL, Dweik RA, Higgins BH et al. High prevalence of hypothyroidism in patients with primary pulmonary hypertension. Am J Med Sci 1999;318:289–92.

44 Badesch DB, Wynne KM, Bonvallet S et al. Hypothyroidism and primary pulmonary hypertension: an autoimmune pathogenetic link? Ann Intern Med 1993;119:44–6.

45 Leyva F, Lambiase P, Rakhit R et al. Hyperuricemia in pulmonary hypertension and thromboembolic disease (abstract). Circulation 1998;98(Suppl 1): 1-272.

46 Voelkel MA, Wynne KM, Badesch DB et al. Hyperuricemia in severe pulmonary hypertension. Chest 2000;117:19–24.

47 Nagaya N, Uematsu M, Satoh T et al. Serum uric acid levels correlate with the severity and the mortality of primary pulmonary hypertension. Am J Respir Crit Care Med 1999;160:487–92.

48 Au VW, Jones DN, Slavotinek JP. Pulmonary hypertension secondary to left-sided heart disease: a cause for ventilation-perfusion mismatch mimicking pulmonary embolism. Br J Radiol 2001;74:86–8.

49 D'Alonzo GE, Bower JS, Dantzker DR. Differentiation of patients with primary and thromboembolic pulmonary hypertension. Chest 1984;85:457–61.

50 Fishman AJ, Moser KM, Fedullo PF. Perfusion lung scans vs pulmonary angiography in evaluation of suspected primary pulmonary hypertension. *Chest* 1983;**84**:679–83.

51 Hull RD, Hirsh J, Carter CJ *et al.* Pulmonary angiography, ventilation lung scanning, and venography for clinically suspected pulmonary embolism with abnormal perfusion lung scan. *Ann Intern Med* 1983;**98**:891–9.

52 Chapman PJ, Bateman ED, Benatar SR. Primary pulmonary hypertension and thromboembolic pulmonary hypertension – similarities and differences. *Respir Med* 1990;**84**:485–8.

53 Worsley DF, Palevsky HI, Alavi A. Ventilation-perfusion lung scanning in the evaluation of pulmonary hypertension. *J Nucl Med* 1994;**35**:793–6.

54 Rich S, Pietra GG, Kieras K *et al.* Primary pulmonary hypertension: radiographic and scintigraphic patterns of histologic subtypes. *Ann Intern Med* 1986;**105**:499–502.

55 Ryan KL, Fedullo PF, Davis GB *et al.* Perfusion scan findings understate the severity of angiographic and hemodynamic compromise in chronic thromboembolic pulmonary hypertension. *Chest* 1988;**93**:1180–5.

56 Kuriyama K, Gamsu G, Stern RG *et al.* CT-determined pulmonary artery diameters in predicting pulmonary hypertension. *Invest Radiol* 1984;**19**:16–22.

57 Tan RT, Kuzo R, Goodman LR *et al.* Utility of CT scan evaluation for predicting pulmonary hypertension in patients with parenchymal lung disease. Medical College of Wisconsin Lung Transplant Group. *Chest* 1998;**113**:1250–6.

58 Choe KO, Hong YK, Kim HJ *et al.* The use of high-resolution computed tomography in the evaluation of pulmonary hemodynamics in patients with congenital heart disease: in pulmonary vessels larger than 1 mm in diameter. *Pediatr Cardiol* 2000;**21**:202–10.

59 Ng CS, Wells AU, Padley SP. A CT sign of chronic pulmonary arterial hypertension: the ratio of main pulmonary artery to aortic diameter. *J Thorac Imaging* 1999;**14**:270–8.

60 Baque-Juston MC, Wells AU, Hansell DM. Pericardial thickening or effusion in patients with pulmonary artery hypertension: a CT study. *AJR Am J Roentgenol* 1999;**172**:361–4.

61 King MA, Bergin CJ, Yeung DW *et al.* Chronic pulmonary thromboembolism: detection of regional hypoperfusion with CT. *Radiology* 1994;**191**:359–63.

62 Remy-Jardin M, Remy J, Wattinne L *et al.* Central pulmonary thromboembolism: diagnosis with spiral volumetric CT with the single-breath-hold technique – comparison with pulmonary angiography. *Radiology* 1992;**185**:381–7.

63 Teigen CL, Maus TP, Sheedy PF, II *et al.* Pulmonary embolism: diagnosis with electron-beam CT. *Radiology* 1993;**188**:839–45.

64 Bergin CJ, Sirlin CB, Hauschildt JP *et al.* Chronic thromboembolism: diagnosis with helical CT and MR imaging with angiographic and surgical correlation. *Radiology* 1997;**204**:695–702.

∗65 Remy-Jardin M, Remy J. Spiral CT angiography of the pulmonary circulation. *Radiology* 1999;**212**:615–36.

66 Chen SJ, Wang JK, Li YW *et al.* Validation of pulmonary venous obstruction by electron beam computed tomography in children with congenital heart disease. *Am J Cardiol* 2001;**87**:589–93.

67 Holcomb BW, Jr, Loyd JE, Ely EW *et al.* Pulmonary veno-occlusive disease: a case series and new observations. *Chest* 2000;**118**:1671–9.

68 Bergin CJ, Rios G, King MA *et al.* Accuracy of high-resolution CT in identifying chronic pulmonary thromboembolic disease. *AJR Am J Roentgenol* 1996;**166**:1371–7.

69 Dufour B, Maitre S, Humbert M *et al.* High-resolution CT of the chest in four patients with pulmonary capillary hemangiomatosis or pulmonary venoocclusive disease. *AJR Am J Roentgenol* 1998;**171**:1321–4.

∗70 Boxt LM. MR imaging of pulmonary hypertension and right ventricular dysfunction. *Magn Reson Imaging Clin North Am* 1996;**4**:307–25.

71 Boxt LM, Katz J, Kolb T *et al.* Direct quantitation of right and left ventricular volumes with nuclear magnetic resonance imaging in patients with primary pulmonary hypertension. *J Am Coll Cardiol* 1992;**19**:1508–15.

72 Frank H, Globits S, Glogar D *et al.* Detection and quantification of pulmonary artery hypertension with MR imaging: results in 23 patients. *AJR Am J Roentgenol* 1993;**161**:27–31.

73 Katz J, Whang J, Boxt LM *et al.* Estimation of right ventricular mass in normal subjects and in patients with primary pulmonary hypertension by nuclear magnetic resonance imaging. *J Am Coll Cardiol* 1993; **21**:1475–81.

74 Murray TI, Boxt LM, Katz J *et al.* Estimation of pulmonary artery pressure in patients with primary pulmonary hypertension by quantitative analysis of magnetic resonance images. *J Thorac Imaging* 1994;**9**:198–204.

75 Mousseaux E, Tasu JP, Jolivet O *et al.* Pulmonary arterial resistance: noninvasive measurement with indexes of pulmonary flow estimated at velocity-encoded MR imaging – preliminary experience. *Radiology* 1999;**212**:896–902.

76 Laffon E, Laurent F, Bernard V *et al.* Noninvasive assessment of pulmonary arterial hypertension by MR phase-mapping method. *J Appl Physiol* 2001; **90**:2197–202.

77 Tardivon A, Mousseaux E, Tasu JP *et al.* Morphological and functional study of pulmonary arteries by MRI [French]. *Ann Radiol* 1995;**38**:98–110.

78 Hatabu H, Gefter WB, Axel L *et al.* MR imaging with spatial modulation of magnetization in the evaluation of chronic central pulmonary thromboemboli. *Radiology* 1994;**190**:791–6.

∗79 Wielopolski PA. Magnetic resonance pulmonary angiography. *Coron Artery Dis* 1999;**10**:157–75.

∗80 Rich S, Dantzker DR, Ayres SM *et al.* Primary pulmonary hypertension. A national prospective study. *Ann Intern Med* 1987;**107**:216–23.

81 Nicod P, Peterson K, Levine M *et al.* Pulmonary angiography in severe chronic pulmonary hypertension. *Ann Intern Med* 1987;**107**:565–8.

∗82 Auger WR, Fedullo PF, Moser KM *et al.* Chronic major-vessel thromboembolic pulmonary artery obstruction: appearance at angiography. *Radiology* 1992;**182**:393–8.

83 Moser KM, Auger WR, Fedullo PF *et al.* Chronic thromboembolic pulmonary hypertension: clinical picture and surgical treatment. *Eur Respir J* 1992;**5**:334–42.

84 Owens GR, Fino GJ, Herbert DL *et al.* Pulmonary function in progressive systemic sclerosis. Comparison of CREST syndrome variant with diffuse scleroderma. *Chest* 1983;**84**:546–50.

85 Steen VD, Graham G, Conte C et al. Isolated diffusing capacity reduction in systemic sclerosis. Arthritis Rheum 1992;35:765–70.

86 Rafanan AL, Golish JA, Dinner DS et al. Nocturnal hypoxemia is common in primary pulmonary hypertension. Chest 2001;120:894–9.

*87 Barst RJ, Rubin LJ, Long WA et al. A comparison of continuous intravenous epoprostenol (prostacyclin) with conventional therapy for primary pulmonary hypertension. The Primary Pulmonary Hypertension Study Group. N Engl J Med 1996;334:296–302.

88 Miyamoto S, Nagaya N, Satoh T et al. Clinical correlates and prognostic significance of six-minute walk test in patients with primary pulmonary hypertension. Comparison with cardiopulmonary exercise testing. Am J Respir Crit Care Med 2000;161:487–92.

*89 Sun XG, Hansen JE, Oudiz RJ et al. Exercise pathophysiology in patients with primary pulmonary hypertension. Circulation 2001;104:429–35.

90 Riley MS, Porszasz J, Engelen MP et al. Responses to constant work rate bicycle ergometry exercise in primary pulmonary hypertension: the effect of inhaled nitric oxide. J Am Coll Cardiol 2000;36:547–56.

91 Garofano RP, Barst RJ. Exercise testing in children with primary pulmonary hypertension. Pediatr Cardiol 1999;20:61–4.

92 James KB, Maurer J, Wolski K et al. Exercise hemodynamic findings in patients with exertional dyspnea. Tex Heart Inst J 2000;27:100–5.

93 Raeside DA, Chalmers G, Clelland J et al. Pulmonary artery pressure variation in patients with connective tissue disease: 24 hour ambulatory pulmonary artery pressure monitoring. Thorax 1998;53:857–62.

94 Raeside DA, Smith A, Brown A et al. Pulmonary artery pressure measurement during exercise testing in patients with suspected pulmonary hypertension. Eur Respir J 2000;16:282–7.

*95 Bach DS. Stress echocardiography for evaluation of hemodynamics: valvular heart disease, prosthetic valve function, and pulmonary hypertension. Prog Cardiovasc Dis 1997;39:543–54.

96 Himelman RB, Stulbarg MS, Lee E et al. Noninvasive evaluation of pulmonary artery systolic pressures during dynamic exercise by saline-enhanced Doppler echocardiography. Am Heart J 1990;119:685–8.

97 Kuecherer HF, Will M, da Silva KG et al. Contrast-enhanced Doppler ultrasound for noninvasive assessment of pulmonary artery pressure during exercise in patients with chronic congestive heart failure. Am J Cardiol 1996;78:229–32.

98 Hoeper MM, Maier R, Tongers J et al. Determination of cardiac output by the Fick method, thermodilution, and acetylene rebreathing in pulmonary hypertension. Am J Respir Crit Care Med 1999;160:535–41.

99 McGregor M, Sniderman A. On pulmonary vascular resistance: the need for more precise definition. Am J Cardiol 1985;55:217–21.

100 Rich S, D'Alonzo GE, Dantzker DR et al. Magnitude and implications of spontaneous hemodynamic variability in primary pulmonary hypertension. Am J Cardiol 1985;55:159–63.

101 Simonneau G, Hervé P, Petitpretz P et al. Detection of a reversible component in primary pulmonary hypertension: value of prostacyclin acute infusion (abstract). Am Rev Respir Dis 1986;133(Suppl):A223.

102 Okada O, Tanabe N, Yasuda J et al. Prediction of life expectancy in patients with primary pulmonary hypertension. A retrospective nationwide survey from 1980–1990. Intern Med 1999;38:12–16.

103 Nootens M, Schrader B, Kaufmann E et al. Comparative acute effects of adenosine and prostacyclin in primary pulmonary hypertension. Chest 1995;107:54–7.

104 Groves BM, Rubin LJ, Frosolono MF et al. A comparison of the acute hemodynamic effects of prostacyclin and hydralazine in primary pulmonary hypertension. Am Heart J 1985;110:1200–4.

105 Palevsky HI, Long W, Crow J et al. Prostacyclin and acetylcholine as screening agents for acute pulmonary vasodilator responsiveness in primary pulmonary hypertension. Circulation 1990;82:2018–26.

106 Galie N, Ussia G, Passarelli P et al. Role of pharmacologic tests in the treatment of primary pulmonary hypertension. Am J Cardiol 1995;75:55A–62A.

107 Shapiro SM, Oudiz RJ, Cao T et al. Primary pulmonary hypertension: improved long-term effects and survival with continuous intravenous epoprostenol infusion. J Am Coll Cardiol 1997;30:343–9.

108 Morgan JM, McCormack DG, Griffiths MJ et al. Adenosine as a vasodilator in primary pulmonary hypertension. Circulation 1991;84:1145–9.

109 Sitbon O, Brenot F, Denjean A et al. Inhaled nitric oxide as a screening vasodilator agent in primary pulmonary hypertension. A dose-response study and comparison with prostacyclin. Am J Respir Crit Care Med 1995;151:384–9.

110 Weir EK, Rubin LJ, Ayres SM et al. The acute administration of vasodilators in primary pulmonary hypertension. Experience from the National Institutes of Health Registry on Primary Pulmonary Hypertension. Am Rev Respir Dis 1989;140:1623–30.

111 Barst RJ. Pharmacologically induced pulmonary vasodilatation in children and young adults with primary pulmonary hypertension. Chest 1986;89:497–503.

112 Jones DK, Higenbottam TW, Wallwork J. Treatment of primary pulmonary hypertension intravenous epoprostenol (prostacyclin). Br Heart J 1987;57:270–8.

113 Rubin LJ, Groves BM, Reeves JT et al. Prostacyclin-induced acute pulmonary vasodilation in primary pulmonary hypertension. Circulation 1982;66:334–8.

*114 Rubin LJ, Mendoza J, Hood M et al. Treatment of primary pulmonary hypertension with continuous intravenous prostacyclin (epoprostenol). Results of a randomized trial. Ann Intern Med 1990;112:485–91.

115 Pepke-Zaba J, Higenbottam TW, Dinh-Xuan AT et al. Inhaled nitric oxide as a cause of selective pulmonary vasodilatation in pulmonary hypertension. Lancet 1991;338:1173–4.

116 Inbar S, Schrader BJ, Kaufmann E et al. Effects of adenosine in combination with calcium channel blockers in patients with primary pulmonary hypertension. J Am Coll Cardiol 1993;21:413–18.

117 Mehta S, Stewart DJ, Langleben D *et al.* Short-term pulmonary vasodilation with L-arginine in pulmonary hypertension. *Circulation* 1995;**92**:1539–45.

*118 McLaughlin W, Genthner DE, Panella MM *et al.* Reduction in pulmonary vascular resistance with long-term epoprostenol (prostacyclin) therapy in primary pulmonary hypertension. *N Engl J Med* 1998;**338**:273–7.

119 Palmer SM, Robinson LJ, Wang A *et al.* Massive pulmonary edema and death after prostacyclin infusion in a patient with pulmonary veno-occlusive disease. *Chest* 1998;**113**:237–40.

120 Nicod P, Moser KM. Primary pulmonary hypertension. The risk and benefit of lung biopsy. *Circulation* 1989;**80**:1486–8.

121 Moser KM, Bloor CM. Pulmonary vascular lesions occurring in patients with chronic major vessel thromboembolic pulmonary hypertension. *Chest* 1993;**103**:685–92.

PART 4

Disorders associated with pulmonary hypertension: pathobiology, diagnosis and treatment

12

Classification and clinical features of PHT

STUART RICH

INTRODUCTION

Pulmonary hypertension, in its simplest sense, refers to any elevation in the pulmonary arterial pressure above normal. The presence of pulmonary hypertension may reflect a serious underlying pulmonary vascular disease, which can be progressive and fatal, or simply an obligatory passive elevation in the pulmonary artery pressure in response to elevated pressures in the left heart. Consequently, an accurate diagnosis of the cause of pulmonary hypertension in a patient is essential in order to establish an effective treatment plan.

Because pulmonary hypertension can occur from diverse etiologies, a classification of the disease has been very helpful. The original classification, established at a World Health Organization Symposium in 1973,[1] classified pulmonary hypertension into groups based on the known cause and defined primary pulmonary hypertension (PPH) as a separate entity of unknown cause. PPH was then classified into three histopathological patterns:

- plexogenic arteriopathy
- recurrent thromboembolism
- veno-occlusive disease.

In 1998, a new classification for pulmonary hypertension was developed which focused on the biological expression of the disease and etiologic factors in an attempt to group these illnesses based on clinical similarities.[2]

This classification (Table 12.1) serves as a useful guide to the clinician in organizing the evaluation of a patient with pulmonary hypertension and developing a treatment plan. In addition, a functional classification (Table 12.2) patterned after the New York Heart Association (NYHA) Functional Classification for heart disease, was developed to allow comparisons of patients with respect to the clinical severity of the disease process.

The diagnosis of pulmonary hypertension relies on establishing an elevation in pulmonary artery pressure above normal. Published norms have come from cardiac catheterizations performed in young subjects at rest without any evidence of cardiopulmonary disease.[3] The upper limit of normal for pulmonary artery mean pressure is 19 mmHg. However, this assumes that there are no abnormalities in downstream pressures of the left atrium or left ventricle, or an increased cardiac output. That is why a patient can have pulmonary hypertension from the standpoint of an elevated pulmonary artery pressure, but normal pulmonary vascular resistance (Figure 12.1). Recently, parameters for normal pulmonary arterial systolic pressure derived by echo Doppler studies have been published which suggest that the upper limit of normal of pulmonary arterial systolic pressure in the general population may be higher than previously appreciated.[4] Importantly, however, the study characterized changes based on age and found a modest increase in pulmonary arterial pressure with age similar to that which exists in the systemic circulation.

Table 12.1 *WHO classification of pulmonary arterial hypertension*

1 Pulmonary arterial hypertension
  1.1 Primary pulmonary hypertension
    (a) Sporadic
    (b) Familial
  1.2 Related to:
    (a) Collagen vascular disease
    (b) Congenital systemic-to-pulmonary shunts
    (c) Portal hypertension
    (d) HIV infection
    (e) Drugs/toxins
      (i) Anorexigens
      (ii) Other
    (f) Persistent pulmonary hypertension of the newborn
    (g) Other

2 Pulmonary venous hypertension
  2.1 Left-sided atrial or ventricular heart disease
  2.2 Left-sided valvular heart disease
  2.3 Extrinsic compression of central pulmonary veins
    (a) Fibrosing mediastinitis
    (b) Adenopathy/tumors
  2.4 Pulmonary veno-occlusive disease
  2.5 Other

3 Pulmonary hypertension associated with disorders of the respiratory system and/or hypoxemia
  3.1 Chronic obstructive pulmonary disease
  3.2 Interstitial lung disease
  3.3 Sleep-disordered breathing
  3.4 Alveolar hypoventilation disorders
  3.5 Chronic exposure to high altitude
  3.6 Neonatal lung disease
  3.7 Alveolar-capillary dysplasia
  3.8 Other

4 Pulmonary hypertension due to chronic thrombotic and/or embolic disease
  4.1 Thromboembolic obstruction of proximal pulmonary arteries
  4.2 Obstruction of distal pulmonary arteries
    (a) Pulmonary embolism (thrombus, tumor, ova and/or parasites, foreign material)
    (b) *In situ* thrombosis
    (c) Sickle cell disease

5 Pulmonary hypertension due to disorders directly affecting the pulmonary vasculature
  5.1 Inflammatory
    (a) Schistosomiasis
    (b) Sarcoidosis
    (c) Other
  5.2 Pulmonary capillary hemangiomatosis

Table 12.2 *WHO functional classification of pulmonary hypertension*

- Class I – Patients with pulmonary hypertension but without resulting limitation of physical activity. Ordinary physical activity does not cause undue dyspnea or fatigue, chest pain or near syncope
- Class II – Patients with pulmonary hypertension resulting in slight limitation of physical activity. They are comfortable at rest. Ordinary physical activity causes undue dyspnea or fatigue, chest pain or near syncope
- Class III – Patients with pulmonary hypertension resulting in marked limitation of physical activity. They are comfortable at rest. Less than ordinary activity causes undue dyspnea or fatigue, chest pain or near syncope
- Class IV – Patients with pulmonary hypertension with inability to carry out any physical activity without symptoms. These patients manifest signs of right heart failure. Dyspnea and/or fatigue may even be present at rest. Discomfort is increased by any physical activity

A.	Pulmonary hypertension in a patient with PPH	
	Pulmonary artery pressure (mmHg)	60/20 (35)
	Pulmonary wedge pressure (mmHg)	10
	Cardiac output (L/min)	5.0
	Pulmonary vascular resistance (units)	5
B.	Pulmonary hypertension in a patient with LV diastolic failure	
	Pulmonary artery pressure (mmHg)	60/20 (35)
	Pulmonary wedge pressure (mmHg)	20
	Cardiac output (L/min)	5.0
	Pulmonary vascular resistance (units)	3
C.	Pulmonary hypertension in a patient with high output heart failure	
	Pulmonary artery pressure	60/20 (35)
	Pulmonary wedge pressure	15
	Cardiac output	10.0
	Pulmonary vascular resistance	2

Figure 12.1 *The hemodynamic profiles of three hypothetical patients with similar levels of pulmonary artery pressure elevation are illustrated. (A) This patient has hemodynamics consistent with primary pulmonary hypertension with a pulmonary vascular resistance of 5 units. (B) This is a patient with left ventricular diastolic failure. The pulmonary artery diastolic and left ventricular end diastolic pressures are the same. The pulmonary vascular resistance is much less than in (A), despite the same level of pulmonary hypertension. Although the etiology is clearly related to high filling pressure of the left ventricle, morphological changes in the pulmonary venous and arteriolar beds may raise pulmonary artery pressure even further over time. (C) A high cardiac output state, with modest elevations in ventricular filling pressures, can easily cause pulmonary hypertension in the face of a near-normal pulmonary vascular resistance. These profiles illustrate why obtaining a right heart catheterization with measurements of ventricular diastolic pressures and cardiac output is absolutely essential in making the correct diagnosis of pulmonary hypertension.*

There are patients whose resting hemodynamics are normal, but in whom marked elevations in pulmonary pressure occur with exercise. It has been presumed that this represents an early stage of pulmonary vascular disease.[5] However, as patients may have a hypertensive response to exercise with respect to the systemic vasculature, a similar type of response can occur in the pulmonary vasculature. Thus, whether exercise-induced pulmonary hypertension represents true pulmonary vascular disease or reduced compliance of an otherwise normal pulmonary circulation can be difficult to ascertain.

PULMONARY ARTERIAL HYPERTENSION

Patients with pulmonary arterial hypertension characteristically present with effort dyspnea which can have a slowly progressive course.[6] The onset of right ventricular failure, manifest by a reduction in cardiac output and/or elevation in right atrial pressure, is usually associated with a marked clinical deterioration and poor prognosis.[7] The rapidity in which this occurs in highly variable, and is often related to the age of onset and associated conditions. Thus, patients with pulmonary arterial hypertension associated with congenital heart defects will more commonly have a slow, insidious onset of symptoms and develop right heart failure after decades, whereas patients with the calcinosis, Raynaud's, sclerodactyly and telangectasia (CREST) syndrome present later in life with a progressive downhill course.

Primary pulmonary hypertension

Patients with PPH are subcategorized into sporadic and familial. The diagnosis of familial PPH is made through a patient's family history, as there are no clinical or pathological features that separate these two entities.[8] Although the prevalence of familial PPH had been published as being 12% at the time of the NIH Registry, this underestimates the true familial prevalence.[7] Because of incomplete penetrance of the gene, it may skip several generations and would not be uncovered unless the physician were to take an in-depth look at the patient's family medical histories. The *PPH1* gene, which has been recently described, has been reported to be present in approximately half the patients with familial PPH.[9] Those without the *PPH1* gene may have other genetic mutations that have not yet been discovered or may have a gene that cannot be determined by current techniques. Patients with sporadic PPH have also been noted to test positive for the *PPH1* gene in about 25%.[10] These patients actually may be familial but mischaracterized as sporadic because of the lack of a supporting family history, or may indeed represent point mutations.

Collagen vascular disease

Patients with pulmonary arterial hypertension related to the collagen vascular diseases will have clinical features representing both entities. It is most common for the collagen vascular disease to manifest itself years before the onset of pulmonary hypertension, but on occasion the opposite has occurred. Many patients with PPH will have elevated titers of antinuclear antibodies.[11] Whether this represents a *forme fruste* of a collagen vascular disease, or is just a clinical feature of PPH, has been debated. The high incidence of pulmonary hypertension in patients with CREST and scleroderma has supported the recommendation that these patients be screened periodically with echocardiography.[2]

Congenital heart disease

Congenital systemic-to-pulmonary shunts can cause pulmonary hypertension believed to be related to the increased blood flow and pressure transmitted to the pulmonary circulation. In most instances this entity is reversible if detected early and the shunt is corrected. In some instances, however, pulmonary hypertension develops very rapidly at the early stages of the disease and precludes any surgical correction. Some patients present with a remote history of a patent ductus arteriosis that was ligated, or an atrial septal defect that was relatively small with coexisting pulmonary vascular disease. Whether the shunt and the pulmonary hypertension are related or coincidental has been a matter of debate.[12] Right-to-left shunting through a patent foramen ovale needs to be distinguished from congenital heart disease. It is uncommon for a patent foramen ovale to be associated with significant right-to-left shunting at rest but it can contribute to exercise-induced hypoxemia. When uncertainty exists, transesophageal echocardiography should distinguish a foramen ovale from an atrial septal defect. If necessary, the distinction can be made during catheterization by sizing the defect with the balloon from a pulmonary artery catheter.

Portal hypertension

The association between liver disease and pulmonary hypertension appears to be related to portal hypertension, and not liver disease itself.[13] Why portal hypertension leads to pulmonary hypertension has never been fully understood. Making the diagnosis of portal hypertension in a patient with pulmonary hypertension can be problematic. The diagnosis of portal hypertension, an elevation in portal pressure, can be made by direct wedge pressure determination of the portal vein at the time of cardiac catheterization. An elevation of portal pressure above 10 mmHg from a normal right atrial pressure defines portal hypertension.[14] It is has never been determined, however, what gradient is necessary to make this diagnosis in a patient with an elevated right atrial pressure, which is commonly found in patients with pulmonary hypertension. Thus, the clinical diagnosis of portal hypertension may need to be made by other indirect determinations such as the presence of esophageal varices or an abnormal flow pattern in the hepatic veins determined by Doppler.[15]

HIV infection

It is well established that the presence of the HIV virus can induce pulmonary hypertension, probably through activation of cytokine or growth factor pathways.[16] There has been no association made between the viral load or the type of antiviral therapy, and the severity of the pulmonary hypertension.[17] As antiviral therapy against HIV improves over time, it will be of interest to note whether or not the coexisting pulmonary hypertension resolves with treatment.

Drugs/toxins

Although several drugs and toxins have been associated with the development of pulmonary hypertension, a causal relationship with many of these remain uncertain. The strongest association between drug ingestion and the development of pulmonary hypertension has been made with the fenfluramines.[18] Although the syndrome is indistinguishable from primary pulmonary hypertension, our experience suggests these patients tend to have a more aggressive disease with a poorer prognosis than similar patients with PPH. This may be a result of the fenfluramines triggering a unique molecular pathway that produces pulmonary vasculopathy.

Pulmonary hypertension of the newborn

Persistent pulmonary hypertension of the newborn should be distinguished from congenital abnormalities of the heart and pulmonary vasculature.[19] It represents an entity similar to PPH and is typically somewhat more responsive to acute and chronic vasodilator therapies.[20] Untreated it can be rapidly fatal.

PULMONARY VENOUS HYPERTENSION

Pulmonary venous hypertension represents a clinical entity that has a pathophysiology and clinical course that is markedly different from pulmonary arterial hypertension. Orthopnea and paroxysmal nocturnal dyspnea are characteristic features, which may precede effort dyspnea. These patients often have a chronic history of congestive heart failure and/or recurring pulmonary edema, which then becomes obscured when right ventricular failure ensues.

Pulmonary venous hypertension is the most common cause of pulmonary hypertension in clinical practice. Because blood by necessity flows through the pulmonary vascular bed into the left heart, any elevation of the filling pressure of the left side of the heart will result in an increase in pulmonary artery pressure. Although often this is quite apparent, there are some circumstances

where the situation is confusing. For example, chronic pulmonary venous hypertension can lead to morphological changes in the pulmonary arterial and venous bed, resulting in further elevation of the pulmonary artery pressure beyond that which was initially a result of the elevated left-sided pressure implying pulmonary vasoconstriction or a vasculopathy triggered by the elevation in pulmonary venous pressure.[21] Often, the physician must try to ascertain whether or not two processes are ongoing, or the chronic result of a single process.

Another scenario are patients who have a longstanding history of left heart disease and develop pulmonary hypertension and severe right heart failure. At the time of cardiac catheterization these patients may have a normal pulmonary capillary wedge or left ventricular end-diastolic pressure in the presence of a low cardiac output. Thus, they may have the hemodynamic profile of a patient with PPH because one is unable to determine what the left ventricular end-diastolic pressure would be in the face of a normal cardiac output.

Although the pulmonary capillary wedge pressure measurement is used by most clinicians as a measure of left ventricular filling pressure, our experience suggests this is frequently unreliable. Despite the methods available to determine whether or not the pulmonary capillary wedge pressure is a true reflection of left ventricular filling pressure, we often encounter patients in whom a pulmonary capillary wedge tracing fulfils all these criteria and yet is inconsistent with the left ventricular end-diastolic pressure. For that reason, it is the standard in our practice to always measure directly a left ventricular end-diastolic pressure in every patient undergoing an initial assessment of the etiology of their pulmonary hypertension.

Pulmonary venous obstruction at several levels may present with pulmonary hypertension. The diagnosis of extrinsic compression of the pulmonary veins presents a challenge because selective pulmonary venous involvement may create pulmonary hypertension, which will not be apparent from the capillary wedge tracing in a non-involved pulmonary vein. Similarly, the hemodynamic diagnosis of pulmonary veno-occlusive disease can be difficult since, like extrinsic compression of an isolated pulmonary vein, the pulmonary wedge pressure may be normal or elevated depending on the segment of the lung that is measured.[22] For the patient in whom extrinsic compression of the pulmonary veins is felt to be the etiology, the diagnosis can be confirmed with either computed tomography or magnetic resonance imaging. For the patient with pulmonary veno-occlusive disease, however, it may difficult to make the diagnosis with certainty on clinical grounds. In our experience, these patients often have a very abnormal perfusion lung scan without any evidence of pulmonary thromboembolic disease.[23] Another common, but inconsistent feature, is an elevation in pulmonary capillary wedge pressure following the challenge of an infusion of adenosine or prostacyclin at the time of catheterization.[24]

PULMONARY HYPERTENSION ASSOCIATED WITH DISORDERS OF THE RESPIRATORY SYSTEM AND/OR HYPOXEMIA

Although hypoxemia may coexist in all forms of pulmonary hypertension, it is the hallmark of these conditions. These patients are often dyspneic at rest as well as with minimal activity, with only subtle clinical features of pulmonary hypertension. Supplemental oxygen will usually provide substantial clinical improvement.[25]

Although a wide constellation of lung diseases can produce pulmonary hypertension, for the most part it arises as a consequence of the effect of chronic hypoxemia from the disease process itself. Chronic hypoxemia produces pulmonary capillary vasoconstriction and pulmonary hypertension, but as a rule, it is of a much lesser degree than seen in pulmonary arterial hypertension.[26] The most common finding in these disorders is a reduced systemic arterial oxygen saturation, often at rest but typically dramatically worsened with exercise. A marked reduction in diffusing capacity is also characteristic. Pulmonary function tests may reveal restrictive physiology, but they tend to be both non-specific and insensitive. High-resolution chest CT is also helpful, but significant interstitial lung disease may exist in a relatively normal appearing chest CT scan.[27] On occasion, lung biopsy is required to make a diagnosis.

There exists a subset of patients who present with severe elevations in pulmonary artery pressure beyond which is typically seen in these disease entities.[28] Whether this represents an extreme manifestation of the underlying disease, or a different disease process characteristic of pulmonary arterial hypertension that has been triggered by a common pathway, is currently unknown. Clinically, it can be difficult to sort out the basis of a patient's complaint of dyspnea. In addition, even successful treatment of the pulmonary hypertensive component of the problem may not render the patient clinically improved if the hypoxemia persists. Of great concern is that some therapies directed towards the pulmonary hypertension can worsen gas exchange and make the hypoxemia even worse.[29,30]

PULMONARY HYPERTENSION DUE TO CHRONIC THROMBOTIC OR EMBOLIC DISEASE

These patients will often present with clinical signs and symptoms that are indistinguishable from pulmonary arterial hypertension. Unless a thorough work-up is conducted to exclude these diseases, patients may be misdiagnosed and inappropriately treated. Chronic proximal thromboembolic obstruction of the pulmonary arteries is a well characterized clinical entity that has been extensively studied.[31] Because it is potentially reversible, it needs to be excluded in every patient who presents with pulmonary hypertension irrespective of the lack of an antecedent history of deep vein thrombosis or pulmonary thromboembolism.

Obstruction of the distal pulmonary arteries can be either embolic or thrombotic. Recurrent microthromboembolism does not appear to be a clinical entity since current evidence points to thrombosis *in situ* as being responsible for the thrombotic changes noted in the arteriolar bed in patients with pulmonary arterial hypertension.[32] Thrombotic obstruction, however, can occur anywhere from the pulmonary capillary bed to the main pulmonary arteries and may reflect a continuum of a disease process. This makes it difficult to ascertain the cause of pulmonary hypertension in a patient with clear evidence of pulmonary thromboembolism involving a relatively small number of vessels. It appears that in some of these patients thrombotic obstruction of the pulmonary arteries leads to chronic pathological changes in the uninvolved vasculature.[33] Diffuse pulmonary embolism can occur on rare occasion from metastatic tumors, parasitic disease, or from foreign material through intravenous injection.[34]

PULMONARY HYPERTENSION DUE TO DISORDERS DIRECTLY AFFECTING THE PULMONARY VASCULATURE

These very rare entities require a high of index suspicion in order for a diagnosis to be made. Schistosomiasis, for example, is probably the most common cause of pulmonary hypertension worldwide, although it is virtually never seen in westernized countries.[34] It should be kept in mind, when patients are referred from developing countries, as a potential underlying etiology.

Sarcoidosis can cause extensive destruction of the pulmonary parenchyma and pulmonary vascular bed and cause pulmonary hypertension merely by lung destruction and resulting hypoxemia.[35] In addition, these patients may develop pulmonary hypertension presumed to be on the basis of involvement of the pulmonary circulation from the sarcoid process. It is unlikely that this is due to local gramuloma formation within the pulmonary vasculature, and more likely the result of growth factors triggering the same process that is seen in pulmonary arterial hypertension. Some of these patients may respond very favorably to chronic intravenous epoprostenol.[36]

Pulmonary capillary hemangiomatosis is an extremely rare disorder involving the pulmonary capillary bed and can present in different stages.[37] It is often associated with frequent hemoptysis, severe pulmonary hypertension, and a progressive fatal course in a short period of time. The diagnosis can be made with pulmonary angiography in the hands of an experienced radiologist.

KEY POINTS

- Pulmonary hypertension can be classified based on clinical etiologies.
- Categories of pulmonary hypertension share distinctive features.
- A careful evaluation, including cardiac catheterization, is essential to make the correct diagnosis.
- Some patients will present with confusing clinical features making a correct diagnosis difficult.

REFERENCES

1 Hatano S, Strasser T. *Primary pulmonary hypertension.* Report on a WHO Meeting. Geneva: World Health Organization, 1975.

●2 Rich S. Primary pulmonary hypertension. The World Symposium – Primary Pulmonary Hypertension 1998. Available from the World Health Organization via the Internet (www.who.int/ncd/cvd/pph.html).

3 Braunwald E, Zipes DP, Libby P (eds). *Heart disease*, 6th edn. Philadelphia: WB Saunders, 2001;359–86.

4 McQuillan B, Picard M, Leavitt M *et al.* Clinical correlates and reference intervals for pulmonary artery systolic pressure among echocardiographical normal subjects. *Circulation* 2001;**104**:2797–802.

5 Raeside D, Smith A, Brown A *et al.* Pulmonary artery pressure measurement during exercise testing in patients with suspected pulmonary hypertension. *Eur Respir J* 2000; **16**:282–7.

◆6 Rich S. Primary pulmonary hypertension. *Prog Cardiovasc Dis* 1988;**31**:205–38.

●7 Rich S, Dantzker DR, Ayres SM *et al.* Primary pulmonary hypertension: a national prospective study. *Ann Intern Med* 1987;**107**:216–23.

◆8 Barst R, Loyd J. Genetics and immunogenetic aspects of primary pulmonary hypertension. *Chest* 1998;**114**:231S–6S.

9 Deng Z, Haghighi F, Helleby L *et al.* Fine mapping of PPH1, a gene for familial primary pulmonary hypertension, to a 3-cM region on chromosome 2q33. *Am J Respir Crit Care Med* 2000;**161**:1055–9.

10 Newman J, Wheeler L, Lane K *et al.* Mutation in the gene for bone morphogenetic protein receptor II as a cause of primary pulmonary hypertension in a large kindred. *N Engl J Med* 2001;**345**:319–24.

11 Rich S, Kieras K, Hart K *et al.* Antinuclear antibodies in primary pulmonary hypertension. *J Am Coll Cardiol* 1986;**8**:1307–11.

12 Brickner M, Hillis L, Lange R. Congenital heart disease in adults. First of two parts. *N Engl J Med* 2000;**342**:256–63.

13 Herve P, Lebrec D, Brenot F *et al.* Pulmonary vascular disorders in portal hypertension. *Eur Respir J* 1998;**11**:1153–66.

14 Bosch J, Navasa M, Garcia-Pagan J *et al.* Portal hypertension. *Med Clin North Am* 1989;**73**:931–49.

15 Kuo P, Plotkin J, Johnson L *et al.* Distinctive clinical features of portopulmonary hypertension. *Chest* 1997;**112**:980–6.

16 Opravil M, Pechere M, Speich R *et al.* HIV-associated primary pulmonary hypertension: a case control study. *Am J Respir Crit Care Med* 1997;**155**:990–5.

17 Pellicelli A, Palmieri F, Cicalini S *et al.* Pathogenesis of HIV-related pulmonary hypertension. *Ann NY Acad Sci* 2001;**946**:82–94.

18 Abenhaim L, Moride Y, Brenot F *et al.* Appetite-suppressant drugs and the risk of primary pulmonary hypertension. *N Engl J Med* 1996;**335**:609–16.

19 Steinhorn R. Persistent pulmonary hypertension of the newborn. *Acta Anaesthesiol Scand Suppl* 1997;**111**:135–40.

20 Clark R, Kueser T, Walker M *et al.* Low-dose nitric oxide therapy for persistent pulmonary hypertension of the newborn. *N Engl J Med* 2000;**34**:469–74.

21 Edwards EN. The pathology of secondary pulmonary hypertension. In: Fishman AP (ed.), *The pulmonary circulation: normal and abnormal.* Philadelphia: University of Pennsylvania Press, 1990;329–42.

22 Holcomb B, Loyd J, Ely E *et al.* Pulmonary veno-occlusive disease. A case series and new observations. *Chest* 2000;**118**:1671–9.

23 Bailey C, Channick R, Auger W *et al.* 'High probability' perfusion lung scans in pulmonary veno-occlusive disease. *Am J Respir Crit Care Med* 2000;**162**:1974–8.

24 Palmer S, Robinson L, Wang A *et al.* Massive pulmonary edema and death after prostacyclin infusion in a patient with pulmonary veno-occlusive disease. *Chest* 1998;**113**:237–40.

25 Nocturnal Oxygen Therapy Trial Group. Continuous or nocturnal oxygen therapy in hypoxemic chronic obstructive lung disease. *Ann Intern Med* 1980;**93**:391–8.

26 Oswald-Mammosser M, Apprill M, Bachez P *et al.* Pulmonary hemodynamics in chronic obstructive pulmonary disease of the emphysematous type. *Respiration* 1991;**58**:304–10.

27 Orens J, Kazerooni E, Martinez F *et al.* The sensitivity of high-resolution CT in detecting idiopathic pulmonary fibrosis proved by open lung biopsy: a prospective study. *Chest* 1995;**108**:109–15.

28 Stevens D, Sharma K, Szidon P *et al.* Severe pulmonary hypertension associated with COPD. *Ann Transplant* 2000;**5**:8–12.

29 Domenighetti G, Saglini V. Short- and long-term hemodynamic effects of oral nifedipine in patients with pulmonary hypertension secondary to COPD and lung fibrosis. *Chest* 1992;**102**:708–14.

30 Keller C, Shepard J, Chun D *et al.* Effects of hydralazine on hemodynamics, ventilation, and gas exchange in patients with chronic obstructive pulmonary disease and pulmonary hypertension. *Am Rev Respir Dis* 1984;**130**:606–11.

◆31 Fedullo P, Auger W, Kerr K *et al.* Chronic thromboembolic pulmonary hypertension. *N Engl J Med* 2001;**345**:1465–72.

◆32 Pietra GG, Edward WD, Kay JM *et al.* Histopathology of primary pulmonary hypertension: a qualitative and quantitative study of pulmonary blood vessels from 58 patients in the National Heart, Lung, and Blood Institute Primary Pulmonary Hypertension Registry. *Circulation* 1989;**80**:1198–206.

33 Moser KM, Bloor CM. Pulmonary vascular lesions occurring in patients with chronic major vessel thromboembolic pulmonary hypertension. *Chest* 1993;**103**:684–92.

34 Morris W, Knauer C. Cardiopulmonary manifestations of schistosomiasis. *Semin Respir Infect* 1997;**12**:159–70.

35 Lynch J, Kazerooni E, Gay S. Pulmonary sarcoidosis. *Clin Chest Med* 1997;**18**:755–85.

36 McLaughlin VV, Genthner DE, Panella MM *et al.* Compassionate use of continuous prostacyclin in the management of secondary pulmonary hypertension: a case series. *Ann Intern Med* 1999;**130**:740–3.

37 Magee F, Wright JL, Kay MJ *et al.* Pulmonary capillary hemangiomatosis. *Am Rev Respir Dis* 1985;**132**:922–5.

13

Pulmonary arterial hypertension

Pathobiology of pulmonary arterial hypertension

NORBERT F VOELKEL AND CARLYNE D COOL

TRADITIONAL PATHOPHYSIOLOGICAL CONCEPTS

Concepts and hypotheses are children of their times, and it was Albert Einstein who told us that 'only a hypothesis permits us to see what can be seen'. When Ernst Romberg wrote his paper, 'On Sclerosis of the Pulmonary Artery', in 1891,[1] describing a patient with what would later be called 'primary' pulmonary hypertension, he described a patient who was cyanotic, had a small pulse, and when he examined postmortem the patient's heart, he stated: 'Of the left ventricle, almost nothing is visible.' Microscopically he found that the right ventricle had in several places foci of cellular infiltrations and connective tissue scars. He noted that the small pulmonary arteries were sclerotic and that the intima at all of the **branch points** showed more or less developed sclerotic changes and 'several irregularities of the most different forms and sizes covering the surface of the vascular lumen'.

The pioneers of the middle of the twentieth century, Heath, Edwards and the Wagenvoorts,[2–6] had better microscopes, they described many cases of severe pulmonary hypertension and they also performed animal experiments from which they concluded that vasoconstriction, intense and lasting, must be the initiating event. Early on, Paul Wood, motivated by the need to identify patients with mitral stenosis and pulmonary hypertension, which were operable, found that certain patients responded to acute infusion of acetylcholine with a decrease in their pulmonary vascular resistance.[7] Then, vasoconstriction, pressure and flow provided the conceptual framework for our understanding of severe pulmonary hypertension.

Until recently, many investigators insisted on a categorical distinction between primary, or unexplained pulmonary hypertension, and secondary forms of pulmonary hypertension. Today, it is clear that the complex vascular abnormalities, which include the so-called plexiform lesions, occur in many forms of severe pulmonary hypertension and a consensus is developing of identical treatment – whether medical or surgical – of many of these forms of severe pulmonary hypertension.[8] Once the dogma that severe vasoconstriction or elevated blood flow were the principal initiating events causing some ill-defined vascular damage had been challenged, the door was open for new ideas such as 'altered vascular cell phenotypes', 'cell growth' and 'angiogenesis'.[9–14] Figure 13A.1 attempts to contrast the traditional and present concepts.

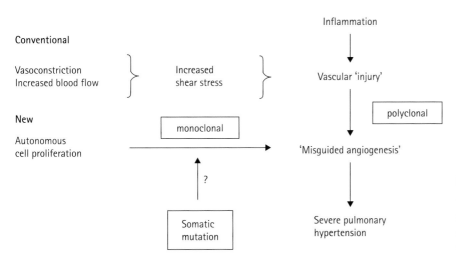

Figure 13A.1 *Comparison between the conventional pathogenetic concept of severe pulmonary hypertension and the concept of endothelial cell growth.*

SEVERE PULMONARY HYPERTENSION ASSOCIATED WITH PLEXIFORM LESIONS: THE CANCER PARADIGM AND THE ALTERED VASCULAR CELL PHENOTYPE

Tuder and colleagues described the exuberant endothelial cell growth in the plexiform lesions observed in the lungs from patients with primary pulmonary hypertension and he compared these lesions morphologically to the lesions of the brain tumor glioblastoma multiforme.[9] Because some of these early endovascular endothelial cell accumulations are reminiscent of tumorlets,[9] it became of interest whether indeed these lesions – or at least some of these lesions – developed from one single cell, i.e. were monoclonal. This was shown in 1998 by Lee and colleagues, only for the plexiform lesions found in the lungs from patients with primary but not secondary pulmonary hypertension.[15] Monoclonality of endothelial cell growth implies mutational alterations of endothelial cell genes.

If one applies the criteria of the cancer cell phenotype as published by Hanahan and Weinberg,[16] then the cell growth in the complex vascular lesions in severe pulmonary hypertension fulfils four of the six criteria stated in Table 13A.1. Because vascular endothelial growth factor (VEGF) and its VEGF receptor II (KDR), are expressed in the highly vascularized glioblastoma multiforme lesions and because tumor growth and angiogenesis are intimately related, evidence for an angiogenesis-related process involved in the formation of plexiform lesions was sought. In addition to VEGF and VEGF RII (KDR) the hypoxia-inducible factor HIF-1α and its binding partner ARNT were identified in many of the plexiform lesions.[10] These features are compatible with an angiogenic process, and if indeed nitric oxide is the ultimate angiogenesis factor, then overexpression of the endothelial nitric oxide synthase (eNOS) in PPH plexiform lesions have been documented[17] The endoluminal clustering of endothelial cells of different phenotypes[18–20] that eventually leads to lumen

Table 13A.1 *Hallmark features of the cancer cell phenotype*

Feature	Plexiform lesions
Disregard of signals to stop proliferating	Yes
Disregard of signals to differentiate	Yes
Capacity for sustained proliferation	No
Evasion of apoptosis	Yes
Invasion	No
Angiogenesis	Yes

Modified after Hanahan and Weinberg.[16]

obliteration indicates that the 'law of the monolayer' has been broken.[21] Which critical control mechanisms have to break down for endothelial cells to disregard the law of the monolayer is unknown, but they likely include factors which control cell anchorage and appropriate neighborly contacts.[22] It is known that VEGF, which is over-expressed in the vascular lesions, can stimulate the expression of endothelial cell derived proteases, including matrix metalloproteases, and proteolytic degradation of the vascular basement membrane is clearly a feature of angiogenesis and sprout formation. We see the complex endovascular lesions as a product of misguided angiogenesis.[10,23] Tumor suppressor genes may function, in part, as suppressors of angiogenesis[13] and VEGF and its downstream intracellular events may be essential in triggering a recapitulation of a vascular development program.[24,25]

Using TUNEL staining, a striking absence of TUNEL-positive apoptotic cells is found in all of the plexiform lesions from patients with severe pulmonary hypertension and in general the number of TUNEL-positive apoptotic cells in lung tissue of these patients is lower than found in normal lung tissues.[26]

Recently, Michael Yeager, after close reading of the cancer literature, decided to examine plexiform lesions in the lungs from patients with PPH for mutations in the TGF-β receptor II gene. He reported that 50% of the microdissected plexiform lesions in PPH, but not in normal lung tissue and not in lung tissue from patients with congenital heart disease, are microsatellite unstable as assessed by the presence of microsatellite instability within the BAT-26 region in the DNA repair enzyme Mut/S homolog 2 gene. The TGF-β RII gene point mutation is predicted to cause a truncated protein that cannot signal. Although the single nucleotide loss within exon 3 of the TGF-β RII gene, which had been described for several human cancers, was observed in only 32% of the PPH lesions sampled, approximately 80% of the PPH plexiform lesions did not express the TGF-β RII protein by immunohistochemistry, whereas the plexiform lesions from patients with secondary PH did express this protein.[21,27] We postulate that additional epigenetic gene silencing plays a role in the loss of TGF-β RII protein expression in PPH.

Cool and associates examined three-dimensionally reconstructed plexiform lesions (Plate 13A.1) and by using multiple immune histochemical probes found loss of staining for the cell cycle control protein p27 in endothelial cells within the core of the lesions;[18] more recently we found that plexiform lesions are lacking the expression of

Table 13A.2 *Evolution of the cancer paradigm*

Exuberant endothelial cell growth in PPH (1994)[9]

Monoclonal endothelial cell growth in PPH (1998)[15]

Multiple endothelial cell phenotypes in plexiform lesions (1999)[18]

Expression of angiogenesis-related molecules in plexiform lesions (2001)[10]

Microsatellite instability of endothelial cell growth and apoptosis genes in PPH (2001)[27]

Loss of tumor suppressor gene expression in plexiform lesions (1999, 2002)[18–21,27,28]

Evolution of an apoptosis-resistant proliferating endothelial cell phenotype in a rat model of severe PH (2001)[64]

Table 13A.3 *Markers of altered phenotypes of the cells in plexiform lesions*

	Direction of change	Reference
VEGF	↑	10
KDR	↑	18
5-LO	↑	56
FLAP	↑	56
ET	↑	75
HOX	↑	76
RANTES	↑	57
PGI$_2$-S	↓	63
PGI$_2$-R	↓	29
PPARγ	↓/absent	20
Caveolin-1 and -2	↓/absent	19
p27	↓/absent	18

VEGF, vascular endothelial growth factor; KDR, VEGF receptor II; 5-LO, 5-lipoxygenase; FLAP, 5-lipoxygenase-activating protein; ET, endothelin; HOX, homeobox; PGI$_2$-S, prostacyclin synthase; PGI$_2$-R, prostacyclin receptor; PPARγ, nuclear peroxisome proliferator activator receptor γ.

other tumor suppressor genes, namely the expression of caveolin-1 and of PPARγ (Table 13A.2).[18–20,27,28] Loss of caveolin-1 expression has been documented in several cancers and also loss of PPARγ expression. Moreover, expression of PPARγ in human umbilical vein endothelial cells caused apoptosis.

Clearly, although the cancer paradigm has emerged mainly by comparison of plexiform lesions from patients with sporadic, unexplained or primary pulmonary hypertension with the plexiform lesions from patients with severe secondary forms of pulmonary hypertension, PPARγ protein staining is also absent in the plexiform lesions from patients with secondary pulmonary hypertension, and we propose that most, if not all, of the phenotypic alterations which have been described for the cells that constitute the plexiform lesions are shared between primary and secondary PH forms (Table 13A.3), and are therefore not restricted to the monoclonal endothelial cell phenotype.

One possible explanation for the decreased expression of tumor suppressor genes in plexiform lesions may be epigenetic silencing via hypermethylation of target suppressor gene promoter regions this could also be the consequence of viral infection. However, it remains surprising that the typical, complex vascular lesions which can be observed in severe pulmonary hypertension associated with as diverse conditions as anorexigen use, collagen vascular diseases (such as the CREST variant of scleroderma) and severe pulmonary hypertension associated with AIDS share some of the same phenotypic markers – even if the complex vascular endothelial cells are not monoclonal.

Less is known, at the present time, about the molecular alterations that characterize the phenotypically abnormal smooth muscle cells in the vascular lesions. A recent study investigated small pulmonary arteries from patients with sporadic severe pulmonary hypertension and pulmonary hypertension associated with congenital heart disease and found that there was no difference in the relative proportions of ET$_A$ and ET$_B$ receptors in distal pulmonary arteries and parenchyma in sections of lungs from hypertensive patients compared with controls.[14] In contrast, VSMC prostacyclin receptor protein expression is drastically decreased in lung precapillary arterioles in severe PH (Plate 13A.2).[29]

THE ROLE OF MEMBERS OF THE TGF-β SUPERFAMILY IN SEVERE PH

Although the complex vascular lesions in severe PH – primary or secondary – share phenotypic alterations of their endothelial and smooth muscle cells, we do not understand the common underlying molecular events. One postulate is that members of the TGF-β superfamily are involved. Both the bone morphogenic protein receptor (BMPR2),[30–33] as well as endoglin and ALk-1 – which are involved in hereditary hemorrhagic telangiectasia[34] – are members of the large TGF-β superfamily, which includes many multifunctional cytokines and growth factors.[35] The highly similar isoforms TGF-β1, TGF-β2 and TGF-β3 inhibit the proliferation of many cell types (including endothelial cell growth) but stimulate the growth of most mesenchymal cells and the synthesis of extracellular matrix proteins (Table 13A.4; for review see references 35 and 36). Whereas BMP[37] signaling is likely important in the maintenance of vascular homeostasis, it is unclear how **germline** mutations of the *BMPR2* gene[30] contribute to the development of plexiform lesions. Most likely a 'second hit' is required.[21,27]

In general terms, TGF-β factors signal by assembling receptor type I and type II complexes that activate Smad transcription factors.[38,39] Two branches of the Smad pathway mediate signaling by the two main groups of TGF-β ligands. The TGF-βs, activins and nodals engage receptors which phosphorylate Smad 2 and Smad 3, whereas the BMPs and related growth and differentiation factors (GDFs) engage receptors which signal via Smad 1, 5 and 8. The complexity of the system is greatly enhanced because some ligands share their type II receptors, and because soluble binding proteins tightly control access of the ligand to the receptors; for example, latency-associated protein, LAP, binds TGF-β and noggin, chordin, caronte and others bind BMPs.[35] In contrast, betaglycan (the TGF-β RIII) enhances TGF-β binding to its receptors, as does endoglin. Other levels of complexity and control are due to links to the Erk MAP kinase which (via phosphorylation) attenuates nuclear accumulation of the Smads.[35]

This brief and cursory overview of the multilayered and interconnected TGF-β system may just give the first impression of the great number of factors involved and an idea about the consequences of mutational alterations of one or several genes of the TGF-β family – specifically if one considers that TGF-β stimulation of certain cells affects approximately 1% of their transcripts.[35] Inactivating mutations in the TGF-β RII occur in ovarian cancers,[35] and the inactivating point mutation in TGF-β RII, as described by us,[27] occurs in most colorectal cancers. Smad 4 mutations have been found in association with TGF-β

RII mutations in colon cancer. Missense mutations in noggin, the gene product of which antagonizes BMP/GDF receptor binding (see above) are associated with proximal symphalangism of the proximal anterophalangeal and carpal joints of the hands. Mutations of the human GDF5 ortholog CDMP1 (cartilage-derived morphogenetic protein-1) are associated with several chondrodysplastic disorders including brachydactyly.[35] In this context, the

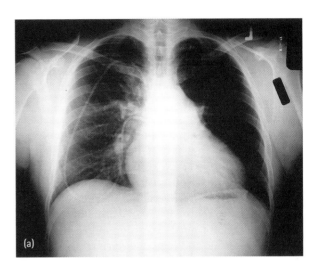

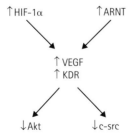

Figure 13A.2 *Hypoxia-inducible factor 1α (HIF-1α), vascular endothelial growth factor (VEGF) and the VEGF receptor VEGF-RII (KDR) are up-regulated, but intracellular signaling proteins Akt and c-src are decreased in their expression in PPH. ARNT, aryl hydrocarbon receptor nuclear translocator.*

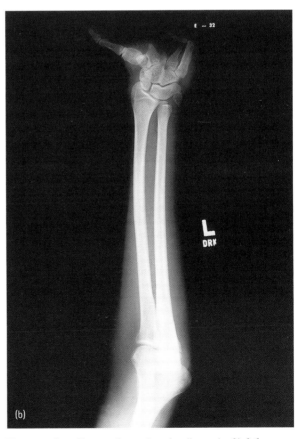

Figure 13A.3 *Chest radiograph and radiograph of left forearm and hand of a patient with primary pulmonary hypertension and brachydactyly.*

Table 13A.4 *Actions of transforming growth factor- β (TGF-β)*

Inhibition of epithelial cell growth[35]
Expression of a ryanodine receptor Ca^{2+} channel[77]
Tumor suppressor[13,35]
Via Smad-4, decreased VEGF expression[13]
Endothelial cell apoptosis[78,79]
Inhibition of VSMC migration and proliferation
Promotion of myofibroblast differentiation[80]
Inhibition of NO synthase induction[81]

VEGF, vascular endothelial growth factor; VSMC, vascular smooth muscle cell.

association in one of our patients of severe unexplained PH and brachydactyly and left-sided pectoralis major muscle agenesis (Figure 13A.2) is remarkable. When examined, this patient did not have any of the known *BMPR2* mutations (unpublished own observation).

It is also of interest that TGF-β plays a fundamental role in several connective tissue disorders,[40,41] which overlap and associate with severe PH.

In conclusion, *BMPR2* germline mutations,[30] somatic cell mutations of one or several members of the TGF-β superfamily[27] and altered expression of genes encoding TGF-β networking and binding proteins[28] may all – or in combination – be involved in tipping the cell growth/ apoptosis balance and tripping the phenotypic switch of the vascular cells in severe PH.

ANOREXIGENS, SEROTONIN AND SEVERE PULMONARY HYPERTENSION

Anorexigen intake has been clearly associated with the development of severe pulmonary hypertension[42–45] and there have been reports of elevated plasma serotonin levels in patients with primary pulmonary hypertension;[46] yet, whether the molecular mechanisms involve serotonin is not understood. Both aminorex fumarate (Menocil) and more recently fenfluramine and dexfenfluramine[43] have caused severe pulmonary hypertension that is histologically indistinguishable from the so-called 'primary' pulmonary hypertension. Recent cell and animal experiments have focused on issues of serotonin uptake, release and transport[47–49] and although serotonin can (in cell culture) stimulate proliferation of vascular smooth muscle cells[50] and potentiate the development of pulmonary hypertension in chronically hypoxic rats,[47] at time of writing, in spite of many attempts by many laboratories, no animal model of severe chronic pulmonary hypertension has been generated after treatment of animals with either aminorex or fenfluramine.

We interpret this failure of investigators to cause severe pulmonary hypertension in animals after anorexigen drug treatment as evidence supporting a unique human susceptibility (constellation of uniquely **human** genetic factors)

that is the 'conditio sine qua non' for the development of severe pulmonary hypertension in humans. This condition or these conditions must, in principle, reside in the patient's lung since the disease does not recur in transplanted lungs. Elevated plasma serotonin levels in patients with PPH could possibly be explained by impaired first-pass uptake of circulating serotonin by damaged pulmonary vascular endothelial cells. However, plasma serotonin levels apparently are not elevated in patients with HIV-associated severe pulmonary hypertension (Philip Herve, personal communication).

Whether plasma serotonin levels are high in patients with portal hypertension-related pulmonary hypertension or severe pulmonary hypertension associated with the CREST syndrome is unclear. Whether serotonin is critically involved in the development of all forms of severe pulmonary hypertension is doubtful, but elevated plasma levels could worsen the disease. No information is available regarding the crosstalk between serotonin, serotonin receptors or transporters and members of the TGF-β superfamily. One report finds that BMP-6 induces the production of serotonergic neuronal cells, which includes the up-regulation of the plasma membrane 5-hydroxytryptamine transporter.[51]

INFLAMMATION AND ROLE OF INFLAMMATORY MEDIATORS

There is clear evidence that elements of inflammation, i.e. inflammatory cells, are present in the remodeled vasculature in pulmonary hypertension.[52,53] For example, mast cell infiltration of plexiform lesions has been known for more than 25 years. In addition, clusters of macrophages accumulate in the perivascular space and growth factors, cytokines and key enzymes involved in production of lipid mediators have been identified in the vascular lesions. Humbert and coworkers documented increased serum concentrations of interleukin (IL)-1 and IL-6 in patients with severe pulmonary hypertension, and possibly these elevated serum levels reflect increased cytokine production by the pulmonary hypertensive lung tissue.[54] Since hypoxia causes increased cytokine release from macrophages, one possibility is that decreased tissue oxygenation in microareas of the hypertensive lung contributes to the increased cytokine release. Both hypoxia and IL-1 can induce the expression of the VEGF gene[10,55] and thus hypoxia and inflammation can both contribute to angiogenesis. Usually, endothelial cells do not express 5-lipoxygenase, but Wright and colleagues found that pulmonary hypertensive arteries and plexiform lesion endothelial cells express both 5-lipoxygenase and the 5-lipoxygenase-activating protein (FLAP),[56] and recently Dorfmuller and colleagues[57] detected high expression of RANTES in plexiform lesions.

Recently, our group demonstrated, using mass spectroscopy, that indeed lung tissue from patients with primary pulmonary hypertension contains increased amounts of 5-hydroxyeicosotetraenoic acid (5-HETE), but not in the tissues obtained from patients chronically treated with prostacyclin infusion. Prostacyclin may reduce inflammation but, without having data, we doubt that inflammation provides the inciting event in the pathobiology of severe PH. Rather, based on animal experiments (see below) we postulate that endothelial cell apoptosis, as has been shown in scleroderma,[58] is the initiating event. The engulfment and phagocytosis of apoptosed cells and the subsequent release of TGF-β and VEGF into the environment may generate inflammation[59] and further stimulate angiogenesis. It remains to be seen whether drugs designed to decrease the activity of inflammatory cells or the release of inflammatory mediators have any value in the treatment of severe pulmonary hypertension.

THE PULMONARY HYPERTENSION RESPONSE MODIFIERS PROSTACYCLIN, NO AND ENDOTHELIN: IMPORTANCE FOR TREATMENT OF SEVERE PH

It is now clear from experiments with genetically altered mice that the major vasodilatory arachidonic acid metabolite prostacyclin is an important modifier of pulmonary hypertension and pulmonary hypertensive vascular remodeling.[60–62] Unfortunately, in severe pulmonary hypertension the endogenous lung tissue prostacyclin synthesis is likely reduced because of severe decrease in the expression of the critical enzyme protein prostacyclin synthase[63] and importantly, also the therapy of patients with severe pulmonary hypertension with chronic intravenous infusion of prostacyclin finds an impaired target since there is a decreased or lacking expression of the prostacyclin receptor protein in many of the plexiform lesions and precapillary arterioles.[29]

In our opinion, these changes, i.e. decrease in the expression of both the prostacyclin synthase and prostacyclin receptor proteins, as well as the overexpression of nitric oxide synthase and of endothelin in the plexiform lesions in PPH, are not the cause, but the consequence of the angioproliferative process, which produces cells of an altered, quasi-malignant phenotype.[9,15,18,64] Although decrease of lung tissue prostacyclin and nitric oxide and increase in endothelin may all facilitate cell growth and make the vascular disease worse, these factors may remain at the sidelines of the playing field as disease modifiers. Theoretically, prostacyclin treatment will prevent platelet aggregation, *in situ* thrombosis and may possess an anti-inflammatory action. Yet, it is now clear that many patients fail long-term prostacyclin treatment and go on to lung or heart/lung transplantation. In those patients who failed chronic prostacyclin treatment, the pulmonary vasculature and the plexiform lesions are indistinguishable from those who did not receive chronic prostacyclin treatment.[65] In this context, it may be important that prostacyclin increases VEGF gene expression.[61] VEGF ligand binding to its VEGF-RII triggers endothelial cell prostacyclin and NO production.

Nitric oxide, via cGMP, is a potent vasodilator, and exhaled NO is clearly decreased in patients with primary pulmonary hypertension, yet NO synthase is overexpressed in the plexiform lesions.[17] Whereas the mechanism whereby exhaled NO in patients with PPH is reduced is unclear, NO is considered by some as the ultimate angiogenesis factor, and lung tissue from patients with severe pulmonary hypertension shows immunohistochemically a great abundance of nitrotyrosine (Plate 13A.3). Thus, the NO generated in the pulmonary hypertensive lung may undergo a number of chemical reactions, some of which result in nitrotyrosine formation; this could be one mechanism whereby the exhaled air NO concentration becomes decreased and nitrosation and nitrosylation could render critical signaling proteins and effector proteins inactive. One example is the NO-related inactivation of the critical enzyme prostacyclin synthase.

ANIMAL MODELS OF SEVERE PULMONARY HYPERTENSION ARE NEEDED FOR THE DESIGN OF PRECLINICAL STUDIES

The time-proven models of chronic hypoxia or single subcutaneous injection of monocrotaline reliably produce moderate pulmonary hypertension in rats, but they do not produce lumen obliterating endothelial cell proliferation. Botney and colleagues developed a rat model of pulmonary hypertension based on the combination of pneumonectomy plus monocrotaline;[66] however, whether, in these animals, endothelial cell proliferation developed still remains unclear. We have developed in our laboratory a rodent model based on the blockade of the VEGF receptor II (KDR) combined with chronic hypoxia. A single dose of a lipophilic VEGF receptor antagonist, SU5416, is deposited subcutaneously and subsequently animals are exposed to chronic hypoxia for 3 weeks. The injection of SU5416 alone causes emphysema and a small increment in the pulmonary artery pressure.[67] However, when combined with chronic hypoxia, severe pulmonary hypertension, right ventricular hypertrophy and lumen obliterating vascular lesions develop. The lumen is obliterated by factor VIII-positive and KDR-positive endothelial cells resulting in a mean pulmonary arterial pressure of 50 mmHg or greater.[64] Glenny recently showed that similar lesions occur when SU5416 is injected into rats following right-sided pneumonectomy (unpublished observations). This indicates to us that it is not the combination of hypoxia and

SU5416 that causes the lesions to develop, but rather the combination of the VEGF receptor blocker plus increased shear stress. Because in the model of combined VEGF receptor blockade and chronic hypoxia there is the establishment of severe pulmonary hypertension and pulmonary precapillary arterial lumen obliteration, which persist after the cessation of the hypoxic exposure, we believe that this model more closely resembles the human disease of severe and progressive pulmonary hypertension. Preclinical prevention and intervention trials have been conducted with this model. If the SU5416-treated and hypoxia-exposed animals also receive daily doses of a broad-spectrum caspase antagonist, both severe pulmonary hypertension and lumen obliteration by proliferating endothelial cells can be prevented.[64] However, the real challenge posed by this model is whether any single agent or combination therapy can remove existing endovascular lesions and reduce established severe pulmonary hypertension. Plate 13A.4 shows the lung histology of an animal with established severe pulmonary hypertension and for comparison the histology of the lung from an animal that had received daily injections of simvastatin for 3 weeks. This intervention also reduces the pulmonary hypertension (unpublished data).

Knowledge gaps and loose ends

Challenges and questions to be answered are many. Perhaps the most perplexing aspect of severe pulmonary hypertensive disorders remains the manifestation of identical vascular lesions as a consequence of pulmonary hypertension associated with as varied disorders as HIV and HHV-8() infection, collagen vascular disorders and portal hypertension. The question then arises whether there are distinct pathways – and how many – which can be 'used' to achieve the identical vascular lesion outcome (angiogenic response). In an elegant and thought-provoking series of experiments Sundberg et al.[23] generated glomeruloid vascular lesions which were generated and maintained by VEGF. Both VEGF and nitric oxide.[68–70] may be fundamentally involved in the growth and maintenance of the complex vascular lesions in severe human PH. In human disease, it is almost certain that we will never be privy to observing the initiating event and to know for certain what kind of vascular endothelial cell damage occurs and whether apoptosis of endothelial cells is indeed the initiating event. It is now clear, but still astonishing, that in the complex pulmonary vascular lesions in **established** disease, there is a complete absence of apoptotic events.[67] One can postulate that shear stress is a very important apoptosis inhibiting participating factor in the pathogenesis of severe pulmonary hypertension; but there must be other factors. Another question is whether severe pulmonary hypertensive disorders, if one considers the cancer paradigm, also display a metastatic aspect, since there are increased numbers of abnormal circulating endothelial cells found in the peripheral blood of patients with severe pulmonary hypertension.[71–73] Lastly, we need to ask which are the appropriate cell models that can be investigated in order to understand the molecular details of the phenotypic switch of pulmonary vascular cells that apparently can occur rapidly in some forms of severe pulmonary hypertension.[44]

KEY POINTS

- Severe pulmonary hypertension constitutes a group of diseases. One of the challenging aspects of our understanding of the complexities of the pathobiology of these diseases is the fact that histologically indistinguishable vascular lesions – or histopathology end points – can be triggered by factors and conditions germane to collagen vascular disorders, high fluid shear stress or viral infections.
- The group of severe pulmonary hypertensive diseases can no longer be understood by simply implying only hemodynamic factors, such as vasoconstriction.
- The angiogenic or angioproliferative disease component is in many aspects distinct from atherosclerosis; for example, atherosclerotic plaques show many cell apoptotic events, whereas the complex vascular lesions in severe PH show complete absence of apoptotic cells.
- In idiopathic forms of severe PH vascular lesions can show monoclonal cell expansion and evidence for infection of the lung tissue with human herpes virus (HHV-8) also known as Kaposi's sarcoma virus KSV.[74] Viral infections can epigenetically silence gene expression, possibly decreasing the expression of the TGF-βRII gene, which is also mutated in many plexiform lesions endothelial cells.
- The inflammatory and immune competency component of the group of severe pulmonary hypertensive disorders is poorly understood.
- Animal models relevant to severe pulmonary hypertensive human diseases should display pulmonary vascular endothelial cell proliferation, not just vascular smooth muscle cell hypertrophy.
- New treatment strategies for severe human pulmonary hypertensive disorders likely will include anti-angioproliferative measures.

REFERENCES

1 Romberg E. Ueber Sklerose de Lungenarterie: aus der medicinischen klinik zu Leipzig. *Dtsch Arch Klin Med* 1891;**48**:197–206.

●2 Wagenvoort CA, Wagenvoort N. Primary pulmonary hypertension. A pathologic study of the lung vessels in 156 clinically diagnosed cases. *Circulation* 1970;**42**:1163–84.

3 Heath D, Wagenvoort CA. Classification and nomenclature. In: Hatano S, Strasser T (eds), *Primary pulmonary hypertension: report on a WHO meeting, October 15–17, 1973*. Geneva: World Health Organization, 1975;15–17.

4 Wagenvoort CA, Wagenvoort N. Normal pulmonary and bronchial vasculature. In: Wagenvoort CA, Wagenvoort N (eds), *Pathology of pulmonary hypertension*. New York: John Wiley and Sons, 1977;17–55.

●5 Wagenvoort CA, Wagenvoort N. Unexplained plexogenic pulmonary arteriopathy: primary pulmonary hypertension. In: Wagenvoort CA, Wagenvoort N (eds), *Pathology of pulmonary hypertension*. New York: John Wiley and Sons, 1977;119–42.

6 Heath D, Edwards JE. Pathology of hypertensive pulmonary vascular disease: a description of six grades of structural changes in the pulmonary arteries with special references to congenital cardiac septal defects. *Circulation* 1958;**18**:533.

7 Wood P. Pulmonary hypertension with special reference to the vasoconstrictive factor. *Br Heart J* 1959;**21**:557.

◆8 Voelkel NF, Tuder RM. Severe pulmonary hypertensive diseases: a perspective. *Eur Respir J* 1999;**14**:1246–50.

●9 Tuder RM, Groves BM, Badesch DB *et al.* Exuberant endothelial cell growth and elements of inflammation are present in plexiform lesions of pulmonary hypertension. *Am J Pathol* 1994;**144**:275–85.

●10 Tuder RM, Chacon M, Alger L *et al.* Expression of angiogenesis-related molecules in plexiform lesions in severe pulmonary hypertension: evidence for a process of disordered angiogenesis. *J Pathol* 2001;**195**:367–74.

11 Liekens S, De Clercq E, Neyts J. Angiogenesis: regulators and clinical applications. *Biochem Pharm* 2001;**61**:253–70.

12 Pettersson A, Nagy JA, Brown LF *et al.* Heterogeneity of the antigenic response induced in different normal adult tissues by vascular permeability factor/vascular endothelial growth factor. *Lab Invest* 2000;**80**:99–115.

13 Schwarte-Waldhoff I, Volpert OV, Bouck NP *et al.* Smad4/DPC4-mediated tumor suppression through suppression of angiogenesis. *Proc Natl Acad Sci USA* 2000;**97**:9624–9.

14 Davie N, Haleen SJ, Upton PD *et al.* ETA and ETB receptors modulate the proliferation of human pulmonary artery smooth muscle cells. *Am J Respir Crit Care Med* 2002;**165**:398–405.

●15 Lee SD, Shroyer KR, Markham NE *et al.* Monoclonal endothelial cell proliferation is present in primary but not secondary pulmonary hypertension. *J Clin Invest* 1998;**101**:927–34.

16 Hanahan D, Weinberg RA. The hallmarks of cancer. *Cell* 2000;**100**:57–70.

17 Mason NA, Springall DR, Burke M *et al.* High expression of endothelial nitric oxide synthase in plexiform lesions of pulmonary hypertension. *J Pathol* 1998;**185**:313–18.

●18 Cool CD, Stewart JS, Werahera P *et al.* Three-dimensional reconstruction of pulmonary hypertension using cell specific markers: evidence for a dynamic and heterogeneous process of pulmonary endothelial cell growth. *Am J Pathol* 1999; **155**:411–19.

19 Achcar ROD, Voelkel NF, Kasper M *et al.* Loss of caveolin-1 expression in phenotypically altered endothelial cells and smooth muscle cells in severe pulmonary hypertension. *Am J Pathol* (in press).

20 Ameshima S, Golpon H, Cool C *et al.* Peroxisome proliferator-activated receptor gamma (PPARγ) expression is decreased in pulmonary hypertension and affects endothelial cell growth. *Circ Res* 2003;**92**:1162–9.

◆21 Tuder RM, Yeager ME, Geraci M *et al.* Severe pulmonary hypertension after the discovery of the familial primary pulmonary hypertension gene. *Eur Respir J* 2001;**17**:1065–9.

●22 Watanabe Y, Dvorak HF. Vascular permeability factor/vascular endothelial growth factor inhibits anchorage-disruption-induced apoptosis in microvessesl endothelial cells by inducing scaffold formation. *Exp Cell Res* 1997;**233**:340–9.

23 Sundberg C, Nagy JA, Brown LF *et al.* Glomeruloid microvascular proliferation follows adenoviral vascular permeability factor/vascular endothelial growth factor-164 gene delivery. *Am J Pathol* 2001;**158**:1145–60.

24 Lassus P, Turanlahti M, Heikkila P *et al.* Pulmonary vascular endothelial growth factor and Flt-1 in fetuses, in acute and chronic lung disease, and in persistent pulmonary hypertension of the newborn. *Am J Respir Crit Care Med* 2001;**164**:1981–7.

25 Bhatt AJ, Pryhuber GS, Huyck H *et al.* Disrupted pulmonary vasculature and decreased vascular endothelial growth factor, Flt-1, and TIE-2 in human infants dying with bronchopulmonary dysphasia. *Am J Respir Crit Care Med* 2001;**164**:1971–80.

26 Kasahara Y, Tuder RM, Cool CD *et al.* Endothelial cell death and decreased expression of vascular endothelial growth factor and vascular endothelial growth factor receptor 2 in emphysema. *Am J Respir Crit Care Med* 2001;**163**:737–44.

27 Yeager ME, Halley GR, Golpon HA *et al.* Microsatellite instability of endothelial cell growth and apoptosis genes within plexiform lesions in primary growth and apoptosis genes within plexiform lesions in primary pulmonary hypertension. *Circ Res* 2001;**88**:E8–11.

●28 Geraci MW, Moore M, Gesell T *et al.* Gene expression patterns in the lungs of patients with primary pulmonary hypertension: a gene micro array analysis. *Circ Res* 2001;**88**:555–62.

29 Bishop AE, Geraci MW, Mason NA *et al.* Reduced expression of membrane prostacyclin receptor in pulmonary hypertension. *J Pathol* (in press).

●30 Lane KB, Machado RD, Pauciulo MW *et al.* Heterozygous germline mutations in *BMPR2*, encoding a TGF-β receptor, cause familial primary pulmonary hypertension. *Nature Genet* 2000;**26**:81–4.

●31 Deng Z, Morse JH, Slager SL *et al.* Familial primary pulmonary hypertension (gene *PPH1*) is caused by mutations in the bone morphogenetic protein receptor II gene. *Am J Hum Genet* 2000;**67**:737–44.

32 Thomson JR, Machado RD, Pauciulo MW *et al.* Sporadic primary pulmonary hypertension is associated with germline

mutations of the gene encoding BMPR-II, a receptor member of the TGF-β family. *J Med Genet* 2000;**37**:741–5.

33 Scott J. Pulling apart pulmonary hypertension. *Nature Genet* 2000;**26**:3–4.

34 McAllister KA, Grogg KM, Johnson DW *et al*. Endoglin, a TGF-β binding protein of endothelial cells, is the gene for hereditary hemorrhagic telangiectasia type 1. *Nature Genet* 1994;**8**:345–51.

35 Massague J, Blain SW, Lo RS. TGF-beta signaling in growth control, cancer and heritable disorders. *Cell* 2000;**103**: 295–309.

36 Massague J, Wotton D. Transcriptional control of the TGF-beta/SMAD signaling system. *EMBO J* 2000;**19**:1745–54.

37 Nakaoka T, Gonda K, Ogita T *et al*. Inhibition of rat vascular smooth muscle proliferation *in vitro* and *in vivo* by bone morphogenetic protein-2. *J Clin Invest* 1997;**100**:2824–32.

38 Zhang Y, Feng XH, Wu RY *et al*. Receptor-associated Mad homologues synergize as effectors of the TGF-β response. *Nature* 1996;**282**:168–72.

39 Piek E, Heldin CH, Ten Dijke P. Specificity, diversity and regulation in TGF-β superfamily signaling. *FASEB J* 1999;**13**:2105–24.

40 Trojanowska M. Molecular aspects of scleroderma. *Bront Biosci* 2002;**7**:D608–18.

41 Ihn H, Yamane K, Kubo M *et al*. Blockade of endogenous transforming growth factor beta signaling prevents up-regulated collagen synthesis in scleroderma fibroblasts: association with increased expression of transforming growth factor beta receptors. *Arthritis Rheum* 2001;**44**:474–80.

42 Gahl K, Fabel H, Greiser E *et al*. Primary vascular pulmonary hypertension. Report on 21 patients. *Z Kreislaufforsch* 1970;**59**:868–83.

43 Abenhaim L, Moride Y, Brenot F *et al*. Appetite-suppressant drugs and the risk of primary pulmonary hypertension. *N Engl J Med* 1996;**335**:609–16.

44 Mark EJ, Patalas ED, Chang HT *et al*. Fatal pulmonary hypertension associated with short-term use of fenfluramine and phentermine. *N Engl J Med* 1997;**337**:602–6.

45 Voelkel NF. Appetite suppressants and pulmonary hypertension. *Thorax* 1997;**52**:563–7.

46 Herve P, Launay JM, Scrobohaci ML *et al*. Increased plasma serotonin in primary pulmonary hypertension. *Am J Med* 1995;**99**:249–54.

47 Eddahibi S, Raffestin B, Pham I *et al*. Treatment with 5-HT potentiates development of pulmonary hypertension in chronically hypoxic rats. *Am J Physiol* 1997;**272**:H1173–81.

◆48 Egermayer P, Town I, Peacock AJ. Role of serotonin in the pathogenesis of acute and chronic pulmonary hypertension. *Thorax* 1999;**54**:161–8.

49 Eddahibi S, Hanoun N, Lanfumey L *et al*. Attenuated hypoxic pulmonary hypertension in mice lacking the 5-hydroxytryptamine transporter gene. *J Clin Invest* 2000;**105**:1555–62.

50 Fanburg BL, Lee SL. A new role for an old molecule: serotonin as a mitogen. *Am J Physiol* 1997;**272**:L795–806.

51 Galter D, Bottner M, Grieglstein K *et al*. Differential regulation of distinct phenotypic features of serotonergic neurons by bone morphogenetic proteins. *Eur J Neurosci* 1999;**11**:2444–52.

●52 Tuder RM. Voelkel NF. Pulmonary hypertension and inflammation. *J Lab Clin Med* 1998;**132**:16–24.

53 Tuder RM, Zaiman AL. Pathology of pulmonary vascular disease. In: Peacock AJ, Rubin LJ (eds), *Pulmonary circulation*, 2nd edn. London: Arnold, 2004.

54 Humbert M, Monti G, Brenot F *et al*. Increased interleukin-1 and interleukin-6 serum concentrations in severe primary pulmonary hypertension. *Am J Respir Crit Care Med* 1995;**151**:1629–31.

55 Forsythe JA, Jiang BH, Iyer NV *et al*. Activation of vascular endothelial growth factor gene transcription by hypoxia-inducible factor 1. *Mol Cell Biol* 1996;**16**:4604–13.

●56 Wright L, Tuder RM, Wang UJ *et al*. 5-Lipoxygenase and 5-lipoxygenase activating protein (FLAP) immunoreactivity in lungs from patients with primary pulmonary hypertension. *Am J Respir Crit Care Med* 1998;**157**:219–29.

57 Dorfmuller P, Zarka V, Durand-Gasselin I *et al*. Chemokine RANTES in severe pulmonary arterial hypertension. *Am J Respir Crit Care Med* 2002;**165**:449–56.

●58 Sgonc R, Gruschwitz MS, Dietrich H *et al*. Endothelial cell apoptosis is a primary pathogenetic event underlying skin lesions in avian and human scleroderma. *J Clin Invest* 1996;**98**:785–92.

●59 McDonald PP, Fadok VA, Bratton D *et al*. Transcriptional and translational regulation of inflammatory mediator production by endogenous TGF-beta in macrophages that have ingested apoptotic cells. *J Immunol* 1999;**163**:6164–72.

●60 Owen NE. Prostacyclin can inhibit DNA synthesis in vascular smooth muscle cells. In: Bailey JM (ed), *Prostaglandins, leukotrienes and lipoxins.* New York: Plenum Press, 1985;193–204.

61 Voelkel NF, Badesch DB, Zapp LM *et al*. Impaired prostacyclin synthesis of endothelial cells derived from hypertensive calf pulmonary arteries. In: Widimsky J, Herget J (eds), *Pulmonary blood vessels in lung disease.* Progress in Respiration Research. Basel: Karger, 1990;**26**:63–9.

●62 Hoshikawa Y, Voelkel NF, Gesell TL *et al*. Prostacyclin receptor-dependent modulation of pulmonary vascular remodeling. *Am J Respir Crit Care Med* 2001;**164**:314–18.

●63 Tuder RM, Cool CD, Geraci MW *et al*. Prostacyclin synthase expression is decreased in lungs from patients with severe pulmonary hypertension. *Am J Respir Crit Care Med* 1999;**159**:1925–32.

●64 Taraseviciene-Stewart L, Kasahara Y, Alger L *et al*. Inhibition of the VEGF receptor 2 combined with chronic hypoxia causes cell death-dependent pulmonary endothelial cell proliferation and severe pulmonary hypertension. *FASEB J* 2001;**15**:427–38.

65 Achcar R, Cool CD, Saffer HL *et al*. Chronic prostacyclin infusion does not affect the vascular alterations in severe pulmonary hypertension. *Am J Respir Crit Care Med* 2002. Abstract.

66 Botney M. Vascular remodeling in primary pulmonary hypertension: what role for transforming growth factor-beta. *Semin Respir Crit Care Med* 1994;**15**:215–25.

67 Kasahara Y, Tuder RM, Taraseviciene-Stewart L *et al*. Inhibition of VEGF receptors causes lung cell apoptosis and emphysema. *J Clin Invest* 2000;**106**:1311–19.

68 Celletti FL, Waugh JM, Amabile PG *et al*. Vascular endothelial growth factor enhances atherosclerotic plaque progression. *Nat Med* 2001;**7**:425–43.

●69 He H, Venema VJ, Gu X *et al.* Vascular endothelial growth factor signals endothelial cell production of nitric oxide and prostacyclin through flk-1/KDR activation of c-SRC. *J Biol Chem* 1999;**274**:25130–5.

●70 Dimmeler S, Zeiher AM. Nitric oxide – an endothelial cell survival factor. *Cell Death Differ* 1999;**6**:964–8.

71 Bull TM, Golpon H, Hebbel RP *et al.* Circulating endothelial cells in pulmonary hypertension. *Thromb Haemost* 2003;**90**: 698–703.

●72 Lin Y, Weisdorf DJ, Solovey A *et al.* Origins of circulating endothelial cells and endothelial outgrowth from blood. *J Clin Invest* 2000;**105**:71–7.

◆73 Rafii S. Circulating endothelial precursors: mystery, reality and promise. *J Clin Invest* 2000;**105**:17–19.

74 Cool CD, Rai PR, Yeager ME *et al.* Human herpes virus 8 (HHV-8) expression in primary pulmonary hypertension. *N Engl J Med* 2003; **349**:1113–22.

●75 Giaid A, Yanagisawa M, Langleben D *et al.* Expression of endothelin-1 in the lungs of patients with pulmonary hypertension. *N Engl J Med* 1993; **328**:1732–9.

76 Golpon HA, Geraci MW, Moore MD *et al.* HOX genes in human lung: altered expression in primary pulmonary

hypertension and emphysema. *Am J Pathol* 2001; **158**:955–66.

77 Giannini G, Clementi E, Ceci R *et al.* Expression of a ryanodine receptor-Ca^{2+} channel that is regulated by TGF-β. *Science* 1992;**257**:91–4.

78 Schuster N, Krieglstein K. Mechanisms of TGF-β-mediated apoptosis. *Cell Tissue Res* 2002;**307**:1–14.

79 Levkau B, Koyama H, Raines EW *et al.* Cleavage of p21Cip1/ Waf1 and p27 Kip1 mediates apoptosis in endothelial cells through activation of Cdk2: role of a caspase cascade. *Mol Cell* 1998;**1**:553–63.

80 Vaughan MB, Howard EW, Tomasek JJ. Transforming growth factor-beta1 promotes the morphological and functional differentiation of the myofibroblast. *Exp Cell Res* 2000;**257**:180–9.

81 Schini VB, Durante W, Elizondo E *et al.* The induction of nitric oxide synthase activity is inhibited by TGF-β_1, $PDGF_{AB}$ and $PDGF_{BB}$ in vascular smooth muscle cells. *Eur J Pharm* 1992;**216**:379–83.

82 Badesch DB, Tapson VF, McGoon MD *et al.* Continuous intravenous epoprostenol for pulmonary hypertension due to the scleroderma spectrum of disease. A randomized, controlled trial. *Ann Intern Med* 2000;**132**:425–34.

Primary pulmonary hypertension: pathophysiological and clinical aspects

LEWIS J RUBIN

Primary pulmonary hypertension (PPH) is a disease of unclear etiology that is characterized by a mean pulmonary arterial pressure >25 mmHg at rest or >30 mmHg with exercise, in the absence of other potential causes. PPH can be clinically diagnosed only when pulmonary arterial hypertension is present in patients without other defined risk factors. These include significant parenchymal lung disease, chronic thromboembolic disease, left-sided valvular or myocardial disease, congenital heart disease, or systemic connective tissue disease.[1–4]

A World Health Organization symposium proposed that pulmonary hypertension might be considered to be present when echocardiographic estimates of systolic pulmonary artery pressure exceed 40 mmHg, which corresponds to a tricuspid regurgitant velocity on Doppler echocardiography of 3.0–3.5 m/s.[5]

The pathophysiology and clinical characteristics of primary pulmonary hypertension are briefly reviewed here. The treatment and prognosis of this disorder are discussed separately (see Chapter 13K).

ETIOLOGY AND PATHOGENESIS

It is likely that PPH and related disorders represent a final common response to a number of potential inciting factors, likely in conjunction with a genetically determined susceptibility (see Chapter 6).

Familial PPH

While most cases of PPH are sporadic, a familial predisposition has been noted in approximately 10% of cases. In this setting, the disease appears to be genetically transmitted as an autosomal dominant trait with incomplete penetrance.[4,6] A gene responsible (*PPH1*) has been localized to chromosome 2 at locus 2q33,[7,8] resulting in defective function of the bone morphogenetic protein receptor type II (BMPR2).[9,10] One study of 19 patients with familial PPH found mutations likely to disrupt function of the BMPR2 in nine.[9] Abnormal pulmonary vascular responses to exercise characterized by increases in pulmonary artery systolic pressure estimated by Doppler echocardiography have been documented in asymptomatic carriers of *PPH1*[11] and may signify the presence of early, subclinical disease (see Chapter 13C).

The bone morphogenetic protein family of proteins is related to TGF-β family and consists of at least 10 peptides that are produced by many different cells with multiple actions on growth and development.[12] The BMPR2 pathway induces apoptosis in some types of cells, and it has been hypothesized that diminution of signaling via this pathway may result in abnormal endothelial cell growth and proliferation in response to a variety of injuries[9,13] (see Chapters 5 and 13A).

A registry of 67 of the 98 known families with familial PPH suggests that familial PPH may be underdiagnosed.[14] Almost 400 subjects from five apparently unrelated families were linked by pedigree analysis to a pair of common ancestors in the 1850s. Familial PPH was diagnosed based upon identical *BMPR2* mutations in 18 patients. Twelve of these subjects had been initially classified as having sporadic PPH. In addition to underdiagnosis because of the unrecognized family history, initial misdiagnosis of PPH as another cardiopulmonary disease was noted in 7 of the 18 subjects.

Risk factors for sporadic PPH

BMPR2 abnormalities are present in up to 25% of patients with sporadic (non-familial) PPH.[15] Other individuals with sporadic PPH or secondary pulmonary hypertension appear to have specific abnormalities that interfere with BMPR2 function. A recent study found that angiopoietin-1, a protein involved in smooth muscle recruitment and vascular development, is over-expressed in patients with sporadic or secondary pulmonary hypertension and profoundly down-regulates the expression of BMPR2 mRNA.[16] In addition, angiopoietin-1 protein levels in lung tissue were closely correlated with pulmonary vascular resistance and the degree of vascular smooth muscle hyperplasia in histological samples. These findings suggest a unifying mechanism by which both primary and secondary pulmonary hypertension are perpetuated, and may have implications for future drug development.

The inability to normally terminate the proliferative response to injury may explain the observation that endothelial cell proliferation within plexiform lesions of patients with PPH tends to be monoclonal. Lee *et al.* have demonstrated monoclonal endothelial cell proliferation within 17 of 22 plexiform lesions from four patients with PPH, in contrast to none of 19 plexiform lesions from four patients with other forms of pulmonary hypertension.[17]

It is likely that many of the observed risk factors for PPH have in common their ability to damage the pulmonary artery endothelium. Such damage could provoke an endothelial proliferative response which, if dysregulated, could progress to clinical PPH or similar conditions. Initiating conditions are discussed below, and include the use of anorectic drugs, cocaine, amphetamines, portal hypertension and HIV infection.[1]

ANORECTIC DRUG USE

There is an increased risk of developing pulmonary arterial hypertension when the fenfluramine appetite-suppressant medications have been taken for the treatment of obesity,[18–21] and monoclonal endothelial proliferation has been observed in this setting[22] (see Chapter 13E). In one retrospective study, 15 of 73 patients (20%) with PPH had used fenfluramine; in 10, there was a close temporal relationship between drug use and the onset of dyspnea.[20] The International Primary Pulmonary Hypertension Study (IPPHS), a case control study of 95 patients, found that 32% used an appetite suppressant (primarily dexfenfluramine and fenfluramine) compared to 7% of controls.[18] The adjusted odds ratio for pulmonary hypertension in users of appetite suppressants for more than 3 months was 23. The absolute risk was estimated at 28 cases per million person-years of exposure. It is also possible that fenfluramine use may accelerate the development of secondary pulmonary hypertension when they are used by patients with underlying predisposing conditions, such as chronic obstructive pulmonary disease, sleep apnea, or connective tissue disease.[23]

Pulmonary arterial hypertension can occur even after short-term use of these drugs. For example, death occurred due to primary pulmonary hypertension in a 29-year-old woman 8 months after taking fenfluramine plus phentermine for only 23 days.[24] Some of the increase in mortality from PPH observed in the USA between 1979 and 1996 may relate to the introduction of anorexigens during this period.[25]

COCAINE OR AMPHETAMINES

Chronic use of cocaine or amphetamines, either inhaled or intravenous, has also been associated with pulmonary hypertension,[26,27] with an adjusted odds ratio of 2.8 in the IPPHS report of 95 patients.[18] More recently, pulmonary hypertension has also been linked to the recreational use of the designer amphetamine analog 4-methyl-aminorex ('ice', 'euphoria', or 'U-4-E-uh'), which has a chemical structure similar to that of the anorectic drug aminorex.[28]

PORTAL HYPERTENSION

Some patients with portal hypertension, due either to intrinsic liver disease or abnormalities of the portal circulation, develop pulmonary hypertension that is pathologically identical to PPH.[29] Portopulmonary hypertension may be due to failure of the liver to remove vasoactive substances such as serotonin or other amines from the portal circulation, resulting in toxic concentrations that reach the pulmonary arterial endothelium[30–32] (see Chapter 13F).

HIV INFECTION

Plexogenic arteriopathy can be seen in patients who test positive for antibodies to the human immunodeficiency virus (HIV), even in the absence of AIDS.[33,34] The frequency of this complication is not known but has been estimated at 1 in 200 patients based upon several small case series.[35–37] In a case–control study, the presence of HIV-associated pulmonary arterial hypertension contributed to overall mortality.[38] Over a median follow-up of 1.3 years, treatment with antiretroviral agents in a small number of patients with HIV-associated pulmonary hypertension appeared to have a beneficial effect on hemodynamics, whereas hemodynamics worsened in patients who were untreated. More recently, additional therapy with continuous intravenous epoprostenol has been shown to produce clinical improvement[39] (see Chapter 13G).

Studies in HIV-infected patients and simian immuno-deficiency virus (SIV)-infected monkeys suggest that HIV may damage the pulmonary endothelium by a mechanism unrelated to vasoactive amines.[35] Viral nucleic acids have not been recovered from involved pulmonary endothelial cells to suggest direct infection by HIV or other infectious agents; rather, it has been hypothesized that HIV-infected macrophages may release cytokines that lead sequentially to leukocyte adherence, growth factor secretion, and endothelial proliferation. Alternatively, leukocyte adherence and activation may damage endothelial cells and trigger dysregulated proliferation in susceptible individuals.

Observed abnormalities in endothelial function

Several studies suggest that abnormalities in endothelial function may be present in PPH, including impaired production of prostacyclin and nitric oxide, and excessive synthesis of endothelin.[40–45] These abnormalities could lead to vasoconstriction and vascular growth and remodeling. However, it is unknown whether these abnormalities cause the disease or are the result of progressive vascular damage as the disease advances (see Chapters 5 and 13A).

Some data suggest that PPH may result from functional impairment of the voltage-gated potassium channel (Kv) in pulmonary artery smooth muscle cells[46,47] that could lead sequentially to a change in resting membrane potential, elevation of the intracytoplasmic free calcium concentration, and an increase in pulmonary vascular tone. The Kv activity is lower among patients with PPH than among those with secondary pulmonary hypertension or non-hypertensive pulmonary diseases (e.g. lung cancer), and in comparison with lung transplant donor tissue, apparently because of decreased transcription and/or decreased mRNA stability of the Kv 1.5 α-subunit gene.[48]

Kv dysfunction may also play an important role in the genesis of pulmonary hypertension secondary to chronic hypoxia or following the use of the anorectic agents fenfluramine, dexfenfluramine, and the older drug aminorex.[49–51] Thus, it is possible that some individuals with PPH possess defects in the sensing of hypoxia or in the normal transcription and mRNA processing of the Kv gene.

CLINICAL PRESENTATION

Most patients with PPH present with exertional dyspnea, which is indicative of an inability to increase cardiac output with exercise.[52] Exertional chest pain, syncope and edema are indications of more severe pulmonary hypertension and impaired right heart function. The mean age at diagnosis of PPH is 36, although the syndrome can occur at any age.[4] Unfortunately, establishing the diagnosis of PPH is frequently delayed, due to the subtle findings on physical examination and the non-specific symptoms experienced by most patients (see Chapters 7 and 11).

DIAGNOSTIC EVALUATION

The diagnosis of PPH rarely requires histopathological confirmation because:

- There are no pathological features that are diagnostic of PPH.
- Invasive procedures carry an increased risk in this population.

The diagnosis of PPH can be made on clinical grounds, based on a comprehensive evaluation that includes pulmonary function testing, connective tissue serology, echocardiography, complete cardiac catheterization, ventilation/perfusion lung scanning, and/or pulmonary angiography (see Chapter 11).

Echocardiography (see Chapter 8) is usually the first diagnostic test suggesting the presence of pulmonary vascular disease, typically showing evidence of right heart chamber enlargement, paradoxic motion of the interventricular septum, and tricuspid insufficiency. Trace-to-moderate pericardial effusions may be visualized and correlate with elevations in right atrial pressure.[53]

The pulmonary artery systolic pressure can be estimated non-invasively using Doppler techniques, although these measurements are not uniformly accurate compared with invasive measurements, particularly when performed by less experienced individuals.

Chest radiographs typically demonstrate enlarged central pulmonary arteries and right heart dilation.

The electrocardiogram shows right axis deviation and right ventricular hypertrophy with a strain pattern. Electrocardiographic changes are generally not helpful in assessing disease severity or prognosis.[54,55]

Pulmonary function testing is often slightly abnormal, with over half of all patients demonstrating a mild-to-moderate decrease in FEV_1 and FVC compared to age- and sex-matched control subjects.[56] The diffusing capacity for carbon monoxide (DLCO) is typically reduced; lung volume measurements may reveal an increase in residual volume, consistent with airway obstruction.[56,57]

References 169

Complete cardiac catheterization (see Chapter 10) is ultimately necessary to establish the diagnosis by excluding other cardiovascular conditions that can cause pulmonary hypertension. Pulmonary arteriography should be performed when the perfusion lung scan does not exclude unresolved chronic thromboembolic disease, since patients with proximal chronic thromboembolic disease may be candidates for pulmonary thromboendarterectomy (see Chapter 17).

Pulmonary veno-occlusive disease, an unusual form of pulmonary hypertension, may be suggested on clinical grounds when severe pulmonary artery hypertension, accompanied by normal pulmonary capillary wedge and left ventricular diastolic pressures, is associated with evidence of venous congestion on chest radiograph and a patchy appearance of tracer activity on a perfusion scan.[1,58] Occasionally, a lung biopsy or findings at postmortem examination are often required to confirm the diagnosis (see Chapter 14B).

KEY POINTS

- Primary pulmonary hypertension is a rare disease that can be diagnosed on clinical grounds only when pulmonary artery hypertension is documented in the absence of other demonstrable cause.
- A mutation in the *BMPR2* gene appears to be responsible for some cases of familial PPH.
- Other conditions, such as portopulmonary hypertension, HIV-associated pulmonary hypertension, and pulmonary artery hypertension associated with anorexigen use may result in pulmonary vascular disease through common pathways of vascular injury.

REFERENCES

1 Rubin LJ, Barst RJ, Kaiser LR et al. Primary pulmonary hypertension. ACCP Consensus Report. Chest 1993; 104:236–50.
◆2 Rubin LJ. Primary pulmonary hypertension. N Engl J Med 1997;336:111–17.
◆3 Gaine SP, Rubin LJ. Primary pulmonary hypertension. Lancet 1998;352:719–25.
●4 Rich S, Dantzker DR, Ayres SM et al. Primary pulmonary hypertension: a national prospective study. Ann Intern Med 1987;107:216–23.
5 Rich S (ed.) Executive summary from the World Symposium on Primary Pulmonary Hypertension, Evian, France, September 6–10, 1998, co-sponsored by The World Health Organization. (http://www.who.int/ncd/cvd/pph.html).
6 Loyd JE, Primm RK, Newman JH. Transmission of familial primary pulmonary hypertension. Am Rev Respir Dis 1984;129:194–7.
7 Nichols WC, Koller DL, Slovis B et al. Localization of the gene for familial primary pulmonary hypertension to chromosome 2q31–32. Nat Genet 1997;15:277–80.
8 Deng Z, Haghighi F, Helleby L et al. Fine mapping of PPH1, a gene for familial primary pulmonary hypertension, to a 3-cM region on chromosome 2q33. Am J Respir Crit Care Med 2000;161:1055–9.
9 Deng Z, Morse JH, Slager SL et al. Familial primary pulmonary hypertension (gene PPH1) is caused by mutations in the bone morphogenetic protein receptor-II gene. Am J Hum Genet 2000;67:737–44.
●10 Lane KB, Machado RD, Pauciulo MW et al. Heterozygous germline mutations in BMPR2, encoding a TGF-beta receptor, cause familial primary pulmonary hypertension. Nat Genet 2000;26:81–4.
11 Grunig E, Janssen B, Mereles D et al. Abnormal pulmonary artery pressure response in asymptomatic carriers of primary pulmonary hypertension gene. Circulation 2000;102:1145–50.
12 Centrella M, Horowitz MC, Wozney et al. Transforming growth factor-β gene family members and bone. Endocr Rev 1994;15:27–39.
13 Kimura N, Matsuo R, Shibuya H et al. BMP2-induced apoptosis is mediated by activation of the TAK1-p38 kinase pathway that is negatively regulated by Smad6. J Biol Chem 2000;275:17 647–52.
14 Newman JH, Wheeler L, Lane KB et al. Mutation in the gene for bone morphogenetic protein receptor II as a cause of primary pulmonary hypertension in a large kindred. N Engl J Med 2001;345:319–24.
15 Thomson JR, Machado RD, Pauciulo MW et al. Sporadic primary pulmonary hypertension is associated with germline mutations of the gene encoding BMPR-II, a receptor member of the TGF-beta family. J Med Genet 2000;37:741–5.
16 Du L, Sullivan CC, Chu D et al. Signaling molecules in nonfamilial pulmonary hypertension. N Engl J Med 2003;348:500–9.
17 Lee SD, Shroyer KR, Markham NE et al. Monoclonal endothelial cell proliferation is present in primary but not secondary pulmonary hypertension. J Clin Invest 1998;101:927–34.
●18 Abenhaim L, Moride Y, Brenot F et al. for the Primary Pulmonary Hypertension Study Group. Appetite-suppressant drugs and risk of primary pulmonary hypertension. N Engl J Med 1996;335:609–16.
19 Voelkel NF, Clarke WR, Higenbottam T. Obesity, dexfenfluramine, and pulmonary hypertension. A lesson not learned? Am J Respir Crit Care Med 1997;155:786–8.
20 Brenot F, Herve P, Petitpretz P et al. Primary pulmonary hypertension and fenfluramine use. Br Heart J 1993;70:537–54.
21 Delcroix M, Kurz X, Walckiers D et al. High incidence of primary pulmonary hypertension associated with appetite suppressants in Belgium. Eur Respir J 1998;12:271–6.
22 Tuder RM, Radisavljevic Z, Shroyer KR et al. Monoclonal endothelial cells in appetite suppressant-associated pulmonary hypertension. Am J Respir Crit Care Med 1998;158:1999–2001.
23 Rich S, Rubin L, Walker AM et al. Anorexigens and pulmonary hypertension in the United States: results from the

surveillance of North American pulmonary hypertension. *Chest* 2000;**117**:870–4.

24 Mark EJ, Patalas ED, Chang HT *et al.* Fatal pulmonary hypertension associated with short-term use of fenfluramine and phentermine. *N Engl J Med* 1997;**337**:602–6.

25 Lilienfeld DE, Rubin LJ. Mortality from primary pulmonary hypertension in the United States, 1979–1996. *Chest* 2000;**117**:796–800.

26 Schaiberger PH. Pulmonary hypertension associated with long-term inhalation of 'crack' methamphetamine. *Chest* 1993;**104**:614–16.

27 Albertson TE, Walby WF, Derlet RW. Stimulant-induced pulmonary toxicity. *Chest* 1995;**108**:1140–9.

28 Gaine SP, Rubin LJ, Kmetzo JJ *et al.* Recreational use of aminorex and pulmonary hypertension. *Chest* 2000;**118**:1496–7.

29 Edwards BS, Weir EK, Edwards WD *et al.* Coexistent pulmonary and portal hypertension: Morphologic and clinical features. *J Am Coll Cardiol* 1987;**10**:1233–8.

30 Egermayer P, Town GI, Peacock AJ. Role of serotonin in the pathogenesis of acute and chronic pulmonary hypertension. *Thorax* 1999;**54**:161–8.

31 Mandell MS, Groves BM. Pulmonary hypertension in chronic liver disease. *Clin Chest Med* 1996;**17**:17–33.

32 Salvi SS. Alpha1-adrenergic hypothesis for pulmonary hypertension. *Chest* 1999;**115**:1708–19.

33 Petitpretz P, Brenot F, Azartam R *et al.* Pulmonary hypertension in patients with human immunodeficiency virus infection: comparison with primary pulmonary hypertension. *Circulation* 1994;**89**:2722–7.

34 Mehta NJ, Khan IA, Mehta RN *et al.* HIV-related pulmonary hypertension: analytic review of 131 cases. *Chest* 2000;**118**:1133–41.

35 Mesa RA, Edell ES, Dunn WF *et al.* Human immunodeficiency virus infection and pulmonary hypertension: two new cases and a review of 86 reported cases. *Mayo Clin Proc* 1998;**73**:37–45.

36 Himelman RB, Dohrmann M, Goodman P *et al.* Severe pulmonary hypertension and cor pulmonale in the acquired immunodeficiency syndrome. *Am J Cardiol* 1989;**64**:1396–9.

37 Speich R, Jenni R, Opravil M *et al.* Primary pulmonary hypertension and HIV infection. *Chest* 1991;**100**:1268–71.

38 Opravil M, Pechere M, Speich R *et al.* HIV-associated primary pulmonary hypertension. A case control study. *Am J Respir Crit Care Med* 1997;**155**:990–5.

39 Aguilar RV, Farber HW. Epoprostenol (prostacyclin) therapy in HIV-associated pulmonary hypertension. *Am J Respir Crit Care Med* 2000;**162**:1846–50.

●40 Christman BW, McPherson CD, Newman JH *et al.* An imbalance between the excretion of thromboxane and prostacyclin metabolites in pulmonary hypertension. *N Engl J Med* 1992;**327**:70–5.

●41 Giaid A, Yanagisawa M, Langleben D *et al.* Expression of endothelin-1 in the lungs of patients with pulmonary hypertension. *N Engl J Med* 1993;**328**:1732–9.

42 Giaid A, Saleh D. Reduced expression of endothelial nitric oxide synthase in the lungs of patients with pulmonary hypertension. *N Engl J Med* 1995;**333**:214–21.

43 Archer SL, Djaballah K, Humbert M *et al.* Nitric oxide deficiency in fenfluramine- and dexfenfluramine-induced pulmonary hypertension. *Am J Respir Crit Care Med* 1998;**158**:1061–7.

44 Tuder RM, Cool CD, Geraci MW *et al.* Prostacyclin synthase expression is decreased in lungs from patients with severe pulmonary hypertension. *Am J Respir Crit Care Med* 1999;**159**:1925–32.

45 Bauer M, Wilkens H, Langer F *et al.* Selective upregulation of endothelin B receptor gene expression in severe pulmonary hypertension. *Circulation* 2002;**105**:1034–6.

46 Yuan XJ, Wang J, Juhaszova M *et al.* Attenuated K^+ channel gene transcription in primary pulmonary hypertension. *Lancet* 1998;**351**:726–7.

47 Archer S, Rich S. Primary pulmonary hypertension: a vascular biology and translational research 'work in progress'. *Circulation* 2000;**102**:2781–91.

48 Yuan JXJ, Aldinger AM, Juhaszova M *et al.* Dysfunctional voltage-gated K^+ channels in pulmonary artery smooth muscle cells of patients with primary pulmonary hypertension. *Circulation* 1998;**98**:1400–6.

49 Wang J, Juhaszova M, Rubin LJ *et al.* Hypoxia inhibits gene expression of voltage-gated K^+ channel alpha subunits in pulmonary artery smooth muscle cells. *J Clin Invest* 1997;**100**:2347–53.

50 Gelband CH, Gelband H. Ca^{++} release from intracellular stores is an initial step in hypoxic pulmonary vasoconstriction of rat pulmonary artery resistance vessels. *Circulation* 1997;**96**:3647–54.

51 Weir EK, Reeve HL, Huang JMC *et al.* Anorexic agents aminorex, fenfluramine and dexfenfluramine inhibit potassium current in rat pulmonary vascular smooth muscle and cause pulmonary vasoconstriction. *Circulation* 1996;**94**:2216–20.

52 Peacock AJ. Primary pulmonary hypertension. *Thorax* 1999;**54**:1107–18.

53 Hinderliter AL, Willis PW 4th, Long W *et al.* Frequency and prognostic significance of pericardial effusion in primary pulmonary hypertension. PPH Study Group. Primary pulmonary hypertension. *Am J Cardiol* 1999; **84**:481–4.

54 Bossone E, Paciocco G, Iarussi D *et al.* The prognostic role of the ECG in primary pulmonary hypertension. *Chest* 2002;**121**:513–8.

55 Ahearn GS, Tapson VF, Rebeiz A *et al.* Electrocardiography to define clinical status in primary pulmonary hypertension and pulmonary arterial hypertension secondary to collagen vascular disease. *Chest* 2002;**122**:524–7.

56 Sun XG, Hansen JE, Oudiz RJ *et al.* Pulmonary function in primary pulmonary hypertension. *J Am Coll Cardiol* 2003;**41**:1028–35.

57 Meyer FJ, Ewert R, Hoeper MM *et al.* Peripheral airway obstruction in primary pulmonary hypertension. *Thorax* 2002;**57**:473–6.

58 Mandel J, Mark EJ, Hales CA. Pulmonary veno-occlusive disease. *Am J Respir Crit Care Med* 2000;**162**:1964–73.

Familial primary pulmonary hypertension

JAMES R RUNO, JOHN H NEWMAN AND JAMES E LOYD

INTRODUCTION

Primary pulmonary hypertension (PPH) is a progressive disorder characterized by elevated pulmonary artery pressures in the absence of a secondary cause. PPH was defined in the National Institutes of Health (NIH) registry by a mean pulmonary artery pressure of more than 25 mmHg at rest, or 30 mmHg with exertion.[1] Pathologically, PPH is defined by the obstruction of small pulmonary arteries in association with plexiform lesions, medial hypertrophy, concentric laminar intimal fibrosis, fibrinoid degeneration, and thrombotic lesions.[2–4] PPH can be subdivided into a sporadic form and a familial form. For many years, physicians thought sporadic PPH was the rule and familial disease was the exception. It has only been in the last 15 years that familial PPH has taken on a greater interest culminating in the recent discovery of a gene responsible for PPH. This chapter discusses investigations of familial primary pulmonary hypertension (FPPH) and how they have helped further knowledge of PPH including pathology, clinical symptoms and etiology. Recent studies that advance our understanding of the pathogenesis of PPH and the ability to detect patients with familial disease are emphasized.

HISTORICAL PERSPECTIVE

Dresdale first used the term primary pulmonary hypertension in 1951.[5] In 1954, he reported the first documented case of FPPH in a mother and son with elevated pulmonary artery (PA) pressures at right heart catheterization.[6] The mother's sister was clinically diagnosed by meeting electrocardiographic and radiographic criteria for right ventricular hypertrophy. Another family member, the mother's brother, died early of an unknown heart ailment, bringing the total number of possibly involved family members to four.

A review of multiple families with PPH was published in 1984.[7] We successfully contacted nine of the 13 previously reported families in the literature, finding eight new cases in five of the families, and a newly discovered family with six deaths over two generations. From the accumulated data, we hypothesized that many cases of apparently sporadic PPH are in fact familial cases with a lack of sufficient family histories. Based on this study, an NIH-funded registry of FPPH was founded to identify PPH families by patient referrals, family histories and comparisons of family pedigrees. At present, this registry contains 103 US families.

INCIDENCE

In 1981, the NIH started a national prospective study to collect data on PPH and reported the clinical and survival data of 187 patients from 32 medical centers.[1] The prevalence of FPPH was 6%, but recent data suggests that the actual proportion of FPPH is likely to be much

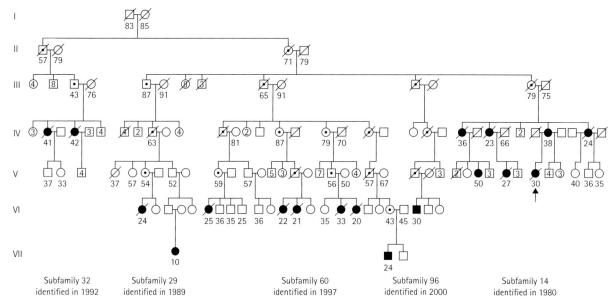

Figure 13C.1 *Abbreviated pedigree of a large kindred comprising five subfamilies over seven generations and 394 known descendants of generation I. The propositus (arrow), a woman in generation V of subfamily 14 who died at the age of 30, received her diagnosis from one of us in 1980. Details of the discovery and linkage of these subfamilies are given in the Methods and Results sections of reference 8. There are at least 200 descendants at varying degrees of risk for primary pulmonary hypertension. Familial primary pulmonary hypertension has been diagnosed in 18 members (16 women and 2 men), and at least 23 (12 women and 11 men, 20 of whom are shown in the figure) are known to carry the gene for the disease. Open symbols indicate unaffected members, solid symbols members with primary pulmonary hypertension, symbols with dots carriers, squares male family members, circles female family members, and slashes deceased members. Numbers inside the symbols indicate the number of members of that gender; numbers under the symbols indicate the age at death or at the time of this writing. (From Newman JH, Wheeler L, Lane KB et al. Mutations in the gene for bone morphogenetic protein receptor II as a cause of primary pulmonary hypertension in a large kindred. N Engl J Med 2001;345:319–24, with permission. Copyright © 2001 Massachusetts Medical Society. All rights reserved.)*

higher. We recently detailed a large family of 394 members spanning seven generations and, by careful pedigree analysis, discovered that five PPH subfamilies were actually related by common ancestors (Figure 13C.1).[8] Within this large kindred, 18 members have been diagnosed with PPH, with 12 who were thought initially to have sporadic PPH and seven first misdiagnosed as another cardiopulmonary disorder. Patients were initially thought to have sporadic PPH because the disease skipped generations and because of misclassification due to inadequate family history.

Further evidence for a higher percentage of familial cases comes from work by Elliot *et al.*[9] Family pedigrees of 13 patients with sporadic PPH were examined with the grandparents' ancestral records being available for seven of these individuals. It was discovered that two of these seven people had shared ancestors. To rule out that the finding was by chance alone, the authors calculated a coefficient of kinship (C_K) for the 13 individuals that was highly significant when compared with the average C_K from 500 random controls in the Utah Population Database. The

authors concluded that familial cases are more common than generally accepted.

EPIDEMIOLOGY AND GENETIC INHERITANCE

Since the first reports of FPPH, several works have helped elucidate the genetic characteristics. Kingdon and associates published an account of a father and son with PPH diagnosed by autopsy and a daughter with PPH diagnosed by right heart catheterization.[10] Symptoms began in the father at around 55 years compared with 20 and 25 years in the son and daughter, respectively. The writers hypothesized that FPPH may show genetic anticipation, or the onset of a more severe form of the disease at an earlier age in successive generations. This article in the mid-1960s was prior to the knowledge that genetic anticipation could have a molecular basis.

In the previously mentioned FPPH study,[7] 14 kindreds were analyzed with 52 cases of PPH found. The mode of inheritance was autosomal dominant with incomplete

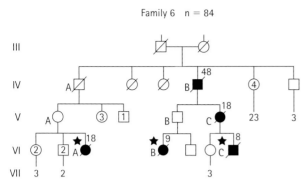

Figure 13C.2 *Pedigree of family 6. Circles are females, squares males, lines through symbols indicate deceased family members, numbers inside symbols the number of persons of that sex in subsequent generations, numbers below symbols the number of persons of either gender in subsequent generations, numbers above deceased individuals indicate age at death, darkened symbols indicate proven primary pulmonary hypertension cases, and shaded symbols indicate probable primary pulmonary hypertension cases. The propositus was individual (IV-B). Asterisks indicate new cases. (From Loyd JE, Primm RK, Newman JH. Familial primary pulmonary hypertension: clinical patterns. Am Rev Respir Dis 1984;129:194–7. Official Journal of the American Thoracic Society. © American Lung Association.)*

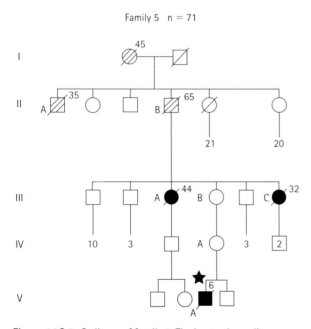

Figure 13C.3 *Pedigree of family 5. The key to the pedigree is the same as in Figure 13C.2. The propositus was individual (III-C). Asterisk indicates new case. (From Loyd JE, Primm RK, Newman JH. Familial primary pulmonary hypertension: clinical patterns. Am Rev Respir Dis 1984;129:194–7. Official Journal of the American Thoracic Society. © American Lung Association.)*

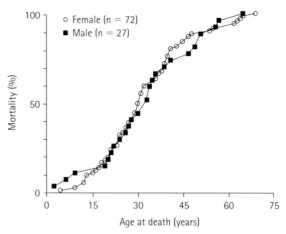

Figure 13C.4 *Cumulative mortality curves of 72 female and 27 male patients with familial primary pulmonary hypertension. There is no difference between the curves. (From Loyd JE, Butler MG, Foroud TM et al. Genetic anticipation and abnormal gender ratio at birth in familial primary pulmonary hypertension. Am J Respir Crit Care Med 1995;152:93–7. Official Journal of the American Thoracic Society. © American Lung Association.)*

penetrance. X-linkage was excluded by father-to-son transmission and by a granddaughter receiving the gene from a grandfather through her father (Figure 13C.2). Also found in the pedigree analysis was the common occurrence of the disease skipping generations (Figure 13C.3). Clinical expression differed widely from one family to another with significant variabilities in the reduced penetrance. The female-to-male ratio was elevated at 2:1 and, as in Kingdon's study,[10] genetic anticipation was observed.

A subsequent study with a larger cohort of 24 families included a total of 429 individuals, 124 known to carry the gene, and 99 with actual disease.[11] Among 282 progeny from individuals known to carry the gene for FPPH, 160 (57%) were female and 122 (43%) were male. This gender ratio was aberrant, as 167 males would be predicted to be born for every 160 females, thus leading the investigators to postulate increase in male fetal wastage. Effects of the PPH gene on development or selective ability between X and Y sperm to reach and fertilize the egg may explain the abnormal gender ratio. Penetrance calculations based on number with disease versus number at risk of disease was 62% for females and 28% for males. However, the absolute numbers of asymptomatic obligate heterozygotes for the PPH gene was similar at 12 females and 13 males. The female-to-male ratio was again elevated at 2.7:1 but there were no differences in age at PPH death between the 72 females and 27 males (Figure 13C.4). As noted in the earlier studies,[7,10] genetic anticipation was seen with earlier age of onset in successive generations, with the mean age at death decreasing from 45.6 years in the earliest generation to 36.3 years in the next and 24.2 years in the most recent generation (Figure 13C.5).

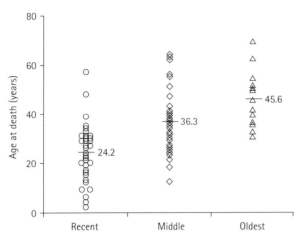

Figure 13C.5 *Age at death versus generation in familial primary pulmonary hypertension. The mean age at death was significantly different for each generation, POP < 0.05. (From Loyd JE, Butler MG, Foroud TM et al. Genetic anticipation and abnormal gender ratio at birth in familial primary pulmonary hypertension. Am J Respir Crit Care Med 1995;152:93–7. Official Journal of the American Thoracic Society. © American Lung Association.)*

ETIOLOGY

Bone morphogenetic protein receptor II (*BMPR2*) gene has recently been established as a PPH gene (*PPH1*), (see Chapter 13A).[12,13] Before discovery of a gene, several theories were presented for the etiology of PPH. Inglesby *et al.* found abnormalities in the fibrinolytic system in a family of 10, five of whom had evidence for PPH.[14] They suggested that a propensity to form microthrombi in the pulmonary arteries may lead to the development of PPH. Tests from seven of the family members revealed increased antiplasmin activity. Rich *et al.* described a family with PPH in association with a variant β-chain hemoglobinopathy (Hb Warsaw) with elevated fibrinopeptide A levels.[15] Wille and associates described another family with a different low-oxygen affinity β-chain hemoglobinopathy (Hb Washtenaw).[16] Both groups hypothesized that a gene for FPPH may lie in close proximity to the β-globin gene on chromosome 11 and serve in linkage analyses.

Linkage of PPH with the major histocompatibility complex has also been discussed. One study compared four children with PPH, two of whom had FPPH, with 13 children with secondary pulmonary hypertension from congenital defects and found an increased incidence of HLA class II alleles DR3, DRw52 and DQw2 and a decreased incidence of DR5 in the PPH children.[17] Another investigation found an increased prevalence of DR3, DRw52, and DQw2 in seven of eight individuals with FPPH from three families.[18]

A relationship between estrogen and the risk of developing PPH for carriers of the gene has been postulated given the higher penetrance of the gene in females. One report described a 64-year-old woman known to be an obligate carrier of the FPPH gene prescribed hormone replacement therapy (HRT) with an estrogen/progesterone mixture 8 months after having a normal echocardiogram. Three months after starting HRT, the patient had evidence of pulmonary hypertension by echocardiogram and cardiac catheterization.[19] Whether estrogen activates modifying genes or stimulates promoter regions of *PPH1* is unknown. However, until these questions are determined, the utilization of oral contraceptives and HRT in women at risk for FPPH can only be assessed on an individual basis.

PATHOLOGY

Early pathology studies attempted to classify PPH cases into either plexogenic arteriopathy or thromboembolic arteriopathy. Wagenvoort described lung biopsy specimens from 40 patients with unexplained pulmonary hypertension diagnosed with PPH clinically.[4] Two major subdivisions were found: plexogenic arteriopathy with concentric laminar intimal fibrosis, fibrinoid necrosis, pulmonary arterial medial hypertrophy, and plexiform lesions; and thromboembolic arteriopathy with eccentric intimal fibrosis, organized thrombi, and medial hypertrophy. Bjornsson and Edwards pathologically categorized 80 cases of unexplained pulmonary hypertension placing 56% in thromboembolic changes and 28% in plexogenic arteriopathy.[3] They hypothesized that *in situ* thrombosis may occur as they could not distinguish between emboli and thrombi in their specimens. Furthermore, they often found thrombotic and plexiform changes in the same samples. Fifty-eight patients from the NIH registry had lung tissue examined and also were classified into plexiform lesions (43%) and thrombotic changes (33%).[2] Nine specimens with plexogenic arteriopathy also had thrombi present. All the above studies attempted to differentiate clinical characteristics and mortality based on pathology with the assumption that the disease processes or pathogenesis of plexogenic and thrombotic arteriopathy were distinct.

We, along with Pietra, analyzed postmortem lung specimens of 23 patients with known FPPH from 13 families and categorized all pulmonary artery lesions according to predefined criteria.[20] Organized thrombi and plexiform lesions were present in 14 patients and within samples from the same family. Heterogeneity of vascular lesions was also noted among members in each family. These observations suggest that these patterns of vascular pathology do not represent distinct clinical or pathogenic

Table 13C.1 *Presenting symptoms at the time of diagnosis of patients with familial primary pulmonary hypertension (FPPH) versus patients with sporadic primary pulmonary hypertension. Functional studies*

Study outcome	% of patients	
	FPPH	NIH PPH (n = 187)
Echocardiogram		
RV enlargement	84	75
RA/RV enlargement	36	n/a
CXR		
Normal	10	6
Enlarged PA	90	94
V̇/Q̇		
Normal	74	42
Diffuse mottling	13	44
Segmental defects	6	11

From Gaddipati R, Wheeler L, Lane KB *et al.* Clinical characteristics of 160 patients in 89 families with primary pulmonary hypertension. *Am J Respir Crit Care Med* 2000;**161**:A140. Official Journal of the American Thoracic Society. © American Lung Association; and Rich S, Dantzker DR, Ayres SM *et al.* Primary pulmonary hypertension: a national prospective study. *Ann Intern Med* 1987;**107**:216–23, with permission.

entities but rather that they are pleiotropic manifestations of one disorder. In the future, detailed pathological analyses will be of great interest to ascertain if the specific molecular mutation influences its histological findings.

CLINICAL PRESENTATION

Patients with familial disease appear identical to those with sporadic disease in both clinical symptoms and objective findings. In the NIH prospective study involving 187 PPH patients, the 12 individuals with FPPH had no differences in their ages or hemodynamic data.[1] However, the FPPH patients were diagnosed sooner after symptom onset than the sporadic patients (0.68 years versus 2.56 years, respectively). To more precisely determine whether clinical differences exist between sporadic and familial cases, Gaddipati *et al.* analyzed data from the sporadic cases in the NIH study above[1] and compared them with 160 patients from a FPPH registry.[21] Clinical symptoms at onset (Table 13C.1), chest radiographs, ventilation/perfusions lung scans, echocardiograms and hemodynamic findings were not significantly different between the sporadic and familial groups. The mean survival after diagnosis was comparable at 2.8 years in sporadic cases and 2.96 years in familial cases. As supported in an earlier study,[11] age at death was not different for females and males with FPPH in the present study.[21] The female-to-male ratio ranges from 2:1 to 2.7:1 in familial disease[7,11,21] compared with 1.7:1 in sporadic disease.[1]

GENETICS

The culmination of working with families affected by PPH was the discovery of *PPH1*, the gene for FPPH. *PPH1* has an autosomal dominant mode of transmission, reduced penetrance, and genetic anticipation.[7,11] By employing short tandem repeat markers to search the genome, linkage analysis on 19 individuals with FPPH from six families yielded localization of *PPH1* to the long arm of chromosome 2.[22] More specific markers then isolated a 25 centiMorgan (cM) region encompassing chromosome 2q31–32. Separate investigation concurrently isolated the location of *PPH1* to a 27 cM interval on chromosome 2q31–32 by employing linkage analysis of two families with PPH and later to a 3 cM region on chromosome 2q33.[23,24]

The International PPH Consortium detected heterogeneous germline mutations in the gene encoding bone morphogenetic protein receptor II (BMPR2) including two frameshift, two nonsense and three missense mutations in seven of eight PPH kindreds.[13] Deng *et al.* identified five premature termination and two missense mutations in the gene for BMPR2 in nine of 19 families with PPH.[12] These genetic studies confirmed that the BMPR2 gene is responsible for FPPH and is *PPH1*.

BMPR2 is one of several receptors in the transforming growth factor-β (TGF-β) receptor superfamily which bind cytokines, including TGF-β, bone morphogenetic protein (BMP), activins and inhibins.[25] BMPR2 binds along with BMPR1a or BMPR1b in a heterodimer complex to BMP on the cell surface, resulting in the phosphorylation of BMPRIa/b through a serine/threonine kinase. This type I receptor then phosphorylates Smad 1, 5, or 8, which act as pathway-restricted Smads for BMP signaling. The pathway-restricted Smads bind to the common-mediator Smad 4 to form hetero-oligomers that translocate into the nucleus to initiate/inhibit transcription of target genes (Figure 13C.6).[25–27] BMPs are important in embryogenesis, development, cell differentiation and proliferation, apoptosis and bone growth.[28,29] One possible mechanism for pathogenesis of the phenotypic expression of FPPH by *BMPR2* mutations is haploinsufficiency, in which expression of less than 50% of a gene product will result in disease.[30] A dominant-negative mechanism could also be a contributor in that if one of the *BMPR2* receptors is dysfunctional, it could disable the whole receptor complex's ability to transmit a signal.[31] Precisely how mutations in *BMPR2* affect cell signaling and lead to the manifestations of PPH should be forthcoming from future investigations.

As previously discussed, *PPH1* displays genetic anticipation as onset and death occur at an earlier age in subsequent generations. It is possible that genetic anticipation in FPPH is simply due to one of several ascertainment biases, but features suggest it has a biological basis that

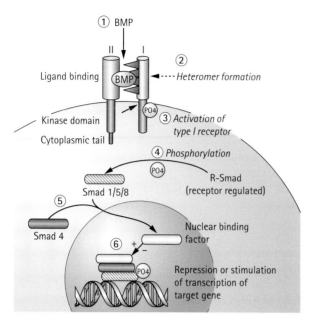

Figure 13C.6 *Signaling pathway for the bone morphogenetic proteins. Bone morphogenetic protein binds to the extracellular domain of BMPR-II, resulting in the formation of a heteromeric complex with BMPR-I. BMPR-II then phosphorylates the transmembrane region of BMPR-I, activating its kinase domain. The activated BMPR-I phosphorylates a receptor Smad (R-Smad), one or more receptor-dependent cytoplasmic Smad proteins (Smad1, Smad5 and Smad8), which bind with Smad4 and migrate to the nucleus. This Smad complex interacts with a nuclear binding factor in the nucleus and either stimulates or represses gene transcription by interacting with DNA.*

has not yet been elucidated. Trinucleotide repeat expansion disorders such as Huntington's disease also share this characteristic of genetic anticipation.[32] Recently, a pentanucleotide repeat expansion causing spinocerebellar ataxia type 10 has been uncovered in five Mexican families.[33] Possible explanations for the pathogenesis in expansions of repeat sequences involve errors in DNA replication or repair systems.[32,34] To date, no evidence of nucleotide repeat expansion has been found in the *BMPR2* gene. However, repeat expansions could be present in modifier genes that may contribute to disease pathogenesis.

INVESTIGATIONS

Mutations in the gene for BMPR2 are found not only in familial PPH, but also in sporadic cases. Thomson *et al.* sequenced the *BMPR2* gene in 50 patients with sporadic PPH and discovered 11 heterozygous mutations in 13 (26%) individuals.[35] Sequencing for *BMPR2* was performed on five parents revealing parental transmission in three cases and *de novo* mutations in the other two cases.

The authors concluded that at least 26% of sporadic cases are due to *BMPR2* mutations and that familial disease is more common than reported. *BMPR2* mutations also may be more prevalent as the sequencing methods utilized would not find promoter mutations, large deletions, or rearrangements.

Plexiform lesions are pathological hallmarks of pulmonary hypertension with exuberant endothelial cell growth.[2,3,36] Lee and associates examined plexiform lesions from four female PPH and four female secondary pulmonary hypertension (three congenital heart disease and one CREST) patients.[37] Methylation of the human androgen receptor gene on the X chromosome was determined for endothelial cells in the plexiform lesions to assess for monoclonal versus polyclonal cell populations. For the PPH samples, 17 of 22 (77%) lesions were monoclonal populations compared with none of 19 secondary pulmonary hypertension samples which exhibited polyclonality. Vascular smooth muscle cells from pulmonary arteries were also analyzed for methylation patterns and found not to demonstrate clonality.

Yeager *et al.* further investigated endothelial cell proliferation.[38] Plexiform lesions were microdissected from 13 PPH and seven secondary pulmonary hypertension (three congenital heart disease, two cirrhosis, one CREST and one scleroderma) patients and assessed for microsatellite instability (MSI) in endothelial cells. MSI was discovered in 50% of PPH plexiform lesions compared with none in secondary pulmonary hypertension lesions for human MutS Homolog 2 gene (*hMSH2*), a DNA repair enzyme. MSI in *BAX*, a proapoptotic gene, was present in 21% of PPH samples versus none found in the secondary pulmonary hypertension group. Finally, 32% of PPH lesions but none of the secondary pulmonary hypertension lesions displayed at least one allelic mutation in exon 3 microsatellite of the TGF-β receptor II gene. This would theoretically reduce TGF-β signaling which has been shown to inhibit endothelial cell proliferation.[26] The genetic alterations found in endothelial cells from PPH plexiform lesions may provide a growth advantage which was lacking in samples from secondary pulmonary hypertension patients.

Difficulties in producing nitric oxide at baseline or during times of stress may also predispose to the development of clinical PPH. Pearson *et al.* found that levels of plasma arginine and nitric oxide metabolites were lower in neonates with respiratory distress and pulmonary hypertension compared with control neonates with respiratory distress but without pulmonary hypertension.[39] Arginine is a precursor for nitric oxide production and is produced by the urea cycle, with the enzyme carbamoyl-phosphate synthetase (CPS) being the rate-limiting step of the urea cycle. The authors concluded that infants with pulmonary hypertension were predisposed due to inability to adequately produce nitric oxide in a stressed situation as evidenced by low levels of the precursor, arginine, and metabolites of nitric oxide. Interestingly, no infant with pulmonary hypertension had a homozygous polymorphism in CPS, which substitutes asparagine for threonine at position 1405 in the critical N-acetylglutamate-binding domain. This polymorphism has been shown to have higher enzymatic activity and thus may protect against pulmonary hypertension due to its ability to produce precursors for nitric oxide at a faster rate.[39]

We also speculated that CPS genotype may modify the penetrance of BMPR2 in FPPH. We determined CPS genotype in 75 individuals from 37 FPPH kindreds with BMPR2 mutations.[40] This pilot study showed a significantly skewed distribution of CPS genotypes.

FAMILIAL PULMONARY VENO–OCCLUSIVE DISEASE AND FAMILIAL PULMONARY CAPILLARY HEMANGIOMATOSIS

Pulmonary veno-occlusive disease (PVOD) is a rare disorder of unknown etiology that presents similar to PPH with progressive dyspnea and elevated pulmonary artery pressures.[41] The primary pathological lesion is obliteration of the small pulmonary vein and venules from intimal fibrosis and thrombosis.[42] Pulmonary arteries show changes of medial hypertrophy and absence of plexiform lesions.[42] The incidence of PVOD is much lower than PPH and the sex ratio is equal.[41] Wagenvoort reported two brothers with PVOD[42] and Voordes discussed these two siblings in detail in a later publication.[43] The proband developed cyanosis and failure to grow at 2 weeks of age with a PA pressure of 78/40 mmHg. Lung biopsy revealed PVOD and the child died days later. A brother died 2 years earlier at the age of 2 months from PVOD. Earlier, Rosenthal and coworkers reported on a 13 year-old-girl who presented with dyspnea, fatigue and cyanosis for 18 months and was found to have a PA pressure of 80/36 mmHg.[44] The patient died of right heart failure soon thereafter with autopsy revealing histological changes consistent with PVOD. Interestingly, the patient's brother had died earlier at the age of 2 years old from 'Eisenmenger's syndrome'. Davies and Reid also described a brother and sister who both died from PVOD that was confirmed histologically at autopsy.[45] Given its similar clinical characteristics to PPH and pathological involvement of part of the pulmonary vascular bed, it seems likely that the pathogenesis of PVOD may be similar to PPH, with an abnormality in the TGF-β pathway or related mechanism. Furthermore, the incidence of familial PVOD may be higher than expected due to its low prevalence and lack of sufficient family history, as observed in FPPH. In addition, the absence of documented vertical transmission in familial PVOD could indicate a common environmental exposure as a trigger.

Pulmonary capillary hemangiomatosis (PCH) is a rare disease with unknown pathogenesis leading to pulmonary hypertension and eventual death.[46] Pathologically it is identified by proliferation of capillaries infiltrating the walls of pulmonary blood vessels, especially the veins and venules, as well as the interlobular septae.[47,46] Langleben and associates described three siblings of 11 who died from pulmonary hypertension with two siblings displaying PCH on lung biopsy.[48] To our knowledge this is the only reported finding of familial PCH. The authors hypothesized that PCH may be an autosomal recessive disorder as the parents and forebears did not manifest any disorders resembling pulmonary hypertension. PCH represents another pulmonary vascular disorder which may have its origin from a mutation in the TGF-β superfamily.

HEREDITARY HEMORRHAGIC TELANGIECTASIA

Hereditary hemorrhagic telangiectasia (HHT) or Osler–Weber–Rendu disease is an autosomal dominant disorder presenting with recurrent bleeding from telangiectasias and arteriovenous malformations.[49] In 1994, the first reported case of a mutation in a TGF-β receptor family member was reported for the gene encoding endoglin on chromosome 9, which leads to HHT type 1.[49] Endoglin facilitates binding of TGF-β to type 1 and type 2 receptors on the cell membrane.[26] The investigators hypothesized that a mutated endoglin receptor would decrease the TGF-β signal and permit endothelial cell proliferation and formation of arteriovenous channels. Later, Johnson et al. discovered three mutations in four families with HHT type 2 in the gene for activin receptor-like kinase 1 (ALK1), a type 1 receptor in the TGF-β superfamily,[27] on chromosome 12.[50] The authors suggested that a mutated ALK1 would exert a dominant-negative effect on TGF-β signaling.[50]

A recent investigation examined five families and one individual with HHT from which a total of 10 individuals had pulmonary hypertension.[51] Novel ALK1 mutations were found in the probands with pulmonary hypertension from four of the five families and one individual with HHT but BMPR2 mutations were not discovered. The proband without an ALK1 mutation did not have HHT but only pulmonary hypertension. Analysis of her BMPR2 gene revealed a partial deletion inherited from her mother, who was not descended from the HHT bloodline, and thus likely represented a chance occurrence. Lung pathology from four patients with ALK1 mutations showed plexogenic lesions characteristic for PPH. Analysis of 11 FPPH and 24 sporadic PPH patients known to be negative for mutations in BMPR2 did not reveal any ALK1 mutations. Because mutations in members of the TGF-β superfamily (BMPR2 and

ALK1) have been demonstrated in PPH, it seems reasonable to speculate that other members may also participate.

SCREENING FOR DISEASE

Stress echocardiography may be useful to screen for asymptomatic gene carriers. Grunig *et al.* examined 48 members of two large families with FPPH with exercise echocardiography and defined normal as a PA systolic pressure <25 mmHg at rest and <40 mmHg with exercise.[52] Normal responses were seen in 27 patients, while abnormal responses were noted in 14 patients. Right heart catheterizations of two normal and seven abnormal responders correlated well with echocardiographic results. Both groups had similar exercise capacity, cardiac output, heart rate, blood pressure, and right and left ventricular function responses at rest and with exercise. Linkage analysis to chromosome 2q31–32 found disease haplotypes in 14 abnormal, two normal, and two undetermined responders, giving stress echocardiography a sensitivity of 87.5% and specificity of 100% in identifying asymptomatic carriers of the gene.

As *BMPR2* mutations have not been found in all FPPH cases, Janssen and coworkers looked at five families with FPPH and performed microsatellite analysis for linkage to *BMPR2* on chromosome 2q33 on 87 members.[53] They discovered only two of five families had linkage to *BMPR2* and the other three linked to a more centromeric region of chromosome 2q31–32. *BMPR2* mutations were excluded in these three families by DHPLC (WAVE) and SSCP analysis. The authors concluded that at least one more PPH gene exists and designated the locus as *PPH2*. This study raises the possibility of one or more genes contributing to the pathogenesis of PPH. In addition, environmental factors such as estrogen and other gene modifiers may also play a critical role in the development of PPH. Resolution of the question of whether other genes cause PPH should be possible in the near future.

TREATMENT AND COMPLICATIONS

Treatment of familial PPH is the same as for sporadic PPH. It is improving rapidly and is discussed extensively in other chapters. One caveat that may be encountered in the future treatment of FPPH could be families' requests for genetic testing of asymptomatic individuals. Currently, there is no clinically approved genetic method for screening of asymptomatic people who may be obligate gene carriers, but appropriate methods are being developed. As mentioned earlier, there is also no method to determine whether obligate carriers will later develop symptomatic disease. The penetrance of the *BMPR2* mutation is low and the role of possible environmental factors, such as estrogen, and existence of modifier genes are yet to be determined.

FUTURE DIRECTIONS

The mechanisms by which mutations in *BMPR2* lead to the phenotypic expression of elevated PA pressures and PPH are not yet known. Haploinsufficiency and dominant-negative mechanisms have been proposed as models for *BMPR2* mutations.[30,31] Reduction in BMP signaling may lead to loss of antiproliferative or apoptotic mechanisms in the pulmonary circulation. Evidence for this explanation exists as mutations in TGF-β receptors have been identified in clonal populations in atherosclerotic lesions and in hereditary polyposis colon cancer.[54–56] Identification of modifier gene(s) and elucidation of the promoter region of *BMPR2* are also essential to understanding the pathogenesis of disease. The primary pathological cell responsible also has yet to be determined. Endothelial cells are a principal component of plexiform lesions and often display monoclonality in plexiform lesions.[36,37] Whether the endothelial cell, or another such as the vascular smooth muscle, is responsible for the changes observed in PPH is still unanswered. Clearly the TGF-β receptor family has a role in pulmonary vascular disease, with mutations in endoglin and *ALK1* causing HHT.[49,50] In addition, familial disease has been reported in PVOD and PCH,[42–45,48] raising the possibility of a TGF-β receptor mutation in these PPH-related disorders. Hopefully, future research will enlighten our understanding of PPH and pulmonary vascular disease and eventually lead to more direct therapeutic interventions.

KEY POINTS

- The proportion of primary pulmonary hypertension that has a familial basis is higher than expected.
- FPPH is inherited in an autosomal dominant fashion with reduced penetrance and genetic anticipation.
- Familial PPH patients present with the same clinical symptoms and have similar outcomes as sporadic patients.
- Mutations in the gene for bone morphogenetic protein receptor II (*PPH1*) are responsible for 50% of familial and 25% of sporadic cases.

ACKNOWLEDGEMENT

This work was supported by the grants HL 48164 and HL 07123 from the National Institutes of Health, National Heart, Lung and Blood Institute.

REFERENCES

●1 Rich S, Dantzker DR, Ayres SM *et al*. Primary pulmonary hypertension: a national prospective study. *Ann Intern Med* 1987;**107**:216–23.

2 Pietra GG, Edwards WD, Kay JM *et al*. Histopathology of primary pulmonary hypertension. A qualitative and quantitative study of pulmonary blood vessels from 58 patients in the National Heart, Lung, and Blood Institute, primary pulmonary hypertension registry. *Circulation* 1989;**80**:1198–206.

3 Bjornsson J, Edwards WD. Primary pulmonary hypertension. A histopathologic study of 80 cases. *Mayo Clin Proc* 1985;**60**:16–25.

4 Wagenvoort CA. Lung biopsy specimens in the evaluation of pulmonary vascular disease. *Chest* 1980;**77**:614–25.

●5 Dresdale DT, Schultz M, Michtom RJ. Primary pulmonary hypertension. I. Clinical and hemodynamic study. *Am J Med* 1951;**11**:686–701.

6 Dresdale DT, Michtom RJ, Schultz M. Recent studies in primary pulmonary hypertension, including pharmacodynamic observations on pulmonary vascular resistance. *Bull NY Acad Med* 1954;**30**:195–207.

7 Loyd JE, Primm RK, Newman JH. Familial primary pulmonary hypertension: clinical patterns. *Am Rev Respir Dis* 1984;**129**:194–7.

8 Newman JH, Wheeler L, Lane KB *et al*. Mutation in the gene for bone morphogenetic protein receptor II as a cause of primary pulmonary hypertension in a large kindred. *N Engl J Med* 2001;**345**:319–24.

9 Elliott G, Alexander G, Leppert M *et al*. Coancestry in apparently sporadic primary pulmonary hypertension. *Chest* 1995;**108**:973–7.

10 Kingdon HS, Cohen LS, Roberts WC *et al*. Familial occurrence of primary pulmonary hypertension. *Arch Intern Med* 1966;**118**:422–426.

11 Loyd JE, Butler MG, Foroud TM *et al*. Genetic anticipation and abnormal gender ratio at birth in familial primary pulmonary hypertension. *Am J Respir Crit Care Med* 1995;**152**:93–7.

●12 Deng Z, Morse JH, Slager SL *et al*. Familial primary pulmonary hypertension (gene *PPH1*) is caused by mutations in the bone morphogenetic protein receptor-II gene. *Am J Hum Genet* 2000;**67**:737–44.

●13 Lane KB, Machado RD, Pauciulo MW *et al*. for the International PPH Consortium. Heterozygous germline mutations in *BMPR2*, encoding a TGF-β receptor, cause familial primary pulmonary hypertension. *Nat Genet* 2000;**26**:81–4.

14 Inglesby TV, Singer JW, Gordon DS. Abnormal fibrinolysis in familial pulmonary hypertension. *Am J Med* 1973;**55**:5–13.

15 Rich S, Hart K. Familial pulmonary hypertension in association with an abnormal hemoglobin. Insights into the pathogenesis of primary pulmonary hypertension. *Chest* 1991;**99**:1208–10.

16 Wille RT, Krishan K, Cooney KA *et al*. Familial association of primary pulmonary hypertension and a new low-oxygen affinity B-chain hemoglobinopathy, Hb Washtenaw. *Chest* 1996;**109**:848–50.

17 Barst RJ, Flaster ER, Menon A *et al*. Evidence for the association of unexplained pulmonary hypertension in children with the major histocompatibility complex. *Circulation* 1992;**85**:249–58.

18 Morse JH, Barst RJ, Fotino M. Familial pulmonary hypertension. Immunogenetic findings in four caucasian kindreds. *Am Rev Respir Dis* 1992;**145**:787–92.

19 Morse JH, Horn EM, Barst RJ. Hormone replacement therapy. A possible risk factor in carriers of familial primary pulmonary hypertension. *Chest* 1999;**116**:847.

20 Loyd JE, Atkinson JB, Pietra GG *et al*. Heterogeneity of pathologic lesions in familial primary pulmonary hypertension. *Am Rev Respir Dis* 1988;**138**:952–7.

21 Gaddipati R, Wheeler L, Lane KB *et al*. Clinical characteristics of 160 patients in 89 families with primary pulmonary hypertension. *Am J Respir Crit Care Med* 2000;**161**:A140.

22 Nichols WC, Koller DL, Slovis B *et al*. Localization of the gene for familial primary pulmonary hypertension to chromosome 2q31–32. *Nat Genet* 1997;**15**:277–80.

23 Morse JH, Jones AC, Barst RJ *et al*. Mapping of familial primary pulmonary hypertension locus (*PPH1*) to chromosome 2q31-q32. *Circulation* 1997;**95**:2603–6.

24 Deng Z, Haghighi F, Helleby L *et al*. Fine mapping of *PPH1*, a gene for familial primary pulmonary hypertension, to a 3-cM region on chromosome 2q33. *Am J Respir Crit Care Med* 2000;**161**:1055–9.

25 Heldin C, Miyazono K, Dijke P. TGF-beta signalling from cell membrane to nucleus through SMAD proteins. *Nature* 1997;**390**:465–71.

26 Blobe GC, Schiemann WP, Lodish HF. Role of transforming growth factor B in human disease. *N Engl J Med* 2000;**342**:1350–8.

27 Massague J, Blain SW, Lo RS. TGFB signaling in growth control, cancer, and heritable disorders. *Cell* 2000;**103**:295–309.

28 Dale L, Jones CM. BMP signalling in early *Xenopus* development. *BioEssays* 1999;**21**:751–60.

29 Hogan BLM. Bone morphogenetic proteins. Multifunctional regulators of vertebrate development. *Genes Dev* 1996;**10**:1580–94.

30 Machado RD, Pauciulo MW, Thomson JR *et al*. BMPR2 haploinsufficiency as the inherited molecular mechanism for primary pulmonary hypertension. *Am J Hum Genet* 2001;**68**:92–102.

◆31 Thomas AQ, Gaddipati R, Newman JH *et al*. Genetics of primary pulmonary hypertension. *Clin Chest Med* 2001;**22**:477–91.

32 Cummings CJ, Zoghbi HY. Fourteen and counting. Unraveling trinucleotide repeat diseases. *Hum Mol Genet* 2000;**9**:909–16.

33 Matsuura T, Yamagata T, Burgess DL *et al*. Large expansion of the ATTCT pentanucleotide repeat in spinocerebellar ataxia type 10. *Nat Genet* 2000;**26**:191–4.

34 Sinden RR. Neurodegenerative diseases. Origins of instability. *Nature* 2001;**411**:757–8.

35 Thomson JR, Machado RD, Pauciulo MW *et al.* Sporadic primary pulmonary hypertension is associated with germline mutations of the gene encoding BMPR-II, a receptor member of the TGF-β family. *J Med Genet* 2000;**37**:741–5.

36 Tuder RM, Groves B, Badesch DB *et al.* Exuberant endothelial cell growth and elements of inflammation are present in plexiform lesions of pulmonary hypertension. *Am J Pathol* 1994;**144**:275–85.

37 Lee S, Shroyer KR, Markham NE *et al.* Monoclonal endothelial cell proliferation is present in primary but not secondary pulmonary hypertension. *J Clin Invest* 1998;**101**:927–34.

38 Yeager ME, Halley GR, Golpon HA *et al.* Microsatellite instability of endothelial cell growth and apoptosis genes within plexiform lesions in primary pulmonary hypertension. *Circ Res* 2001;**88**:e2–l1.

39 Pearson DL, Dawling S, Walsh WF *et al.* Neonatal pulmonary hypertension. Urea-cycle intermediates, nitric oxide production, and carbamoyl-phosphate synthetase function. *N Engl J Med* 2001;**344**:1832–8.

40 Thomas AQ, Summar M, Scott N *et al.* Penetrance of familial primary pulmonary hypertension may be modified by carbamoyl phosphate synthetase I (CPSI) genotype. *Am J Respir Crit Care Med* 2001;**163**:A113.

◆41 Mandel J, Mark EJ, Hales CA. Pulmonary veno-occlusive disease. *Am J Respir Crit Care Med* 2000;**162**:1964–73.

42 Wagenvoort CA, Wagenvoort N. The pathology of pulmonary veno-occlusive disease. *Virchows Arch A Pathol Anat Histol* 1974;**364**:69–79.

43 Voordes CG, Kuipers JRG, Elema JD. Familial pulmonary veno-occlusive disease. A case report. *Thorax* 1977;**32**:763–6.

44 Rosenthal A, Vawter G, Wagenvoort CA. Intrapulmonary veno-occlusive disease. *Am J Cardiol* 1973;**31**:78–85.

45 Davies P, Reid L. Pulmonary veno-occlusive disease in siblings. Case reports and morphometric study. *Hum Pathol* 1982;**13**:911–15.

46 Magee F, Wright JL, Kay JM *et al.* Pulmonary capillary hemangiomatosis. *Am Rev Respir Dis* 1985;**132**:922–5.

47 Wagenvoort CA, Beetstra A, Spijker J. Capillary haemangiomatosis of the lungs. *Histopathology* 1978;**2**:401–6.

48 Langleben D, Heneghan JM, Batten AP *et al.* Familial pulmonary capillary hemangiomatosis resulting in primary pulmonary hypertension. *Ann Intern Med* 1988;**109**:106–9.

●49 McAllister KA, Grogg KM, Johnson DW *et al.* Endoglin, a TGF-β binding protein of endothelial cells, is the gene for hereditary haemorrhagic telangiectasia type 1. *Nat Genet* 1994;**8**:345–51.

●50 Johnson DW, Berg JN, Baldwin MA *et al.* Mutations in the activin receptor-like kinase I gene in hereditary haemorrhagic telangiectasia type 2. *Nat Genet* 1996;**13**:189–95.

51 Trembath RC, Thomson JR, Machado RD *et al.* Clinical and molecular genetic features of pulmonary hypertension in patients with hereditary hemorrhagic telangiectasia. *N Engl J Med* 2001;**345**:325–34.

52 Grunig E, Janssen B, Mereles D *et al.* Abnormal pulmonary artery pressure response in asymptomatic carriers of primary pulmonary hypertension gene. *Circulation* 2000;**102**:1145–50.

53 Janssen B, Rindermann M, Barth U *et al.* Linkage analysis in a large family with primary pulmonary hypertension: genetic heterogeneity and a second primary pulmonary hypertension locus on 2q31–32. *Chest* 2002;**121**:54–6.

54 McCaffrey TA, Du B, Consigli S *et al.* Genomic instability in the type II TGF-β1 receptor gene in atherosclerotic and restenotic vascular cells. *J Clin Invest* 1997;**100**:2182–8.

55 Lu SL, Zhang WC, Akiyama Y *et al.* Genomic structure of the transforming growth factor beta type II receptor gene and its mutations in hereditary nonpolyposis colorectal cancers. *Cancer Res* 1996;**56**:4595–8.

56 Akiyama Y, Iwanaga R, Saitoh K *et al.* Transforming growth factor beta type II receptor gene mutations in adenomas from hereditary nonpolyposis colorectal cancer. *Gastroenterology* 1997;**112**:33–9.

Pulmonary hypertension associated with connective tissue disease

KAREN A FAGAN AND DAVID B BADESCH

INTRODUCTION

Pulmonary arterial hypertension is a complication of several connective tissue diseases leading to significant morbidity and mortality. Scleroderma (both diffuse and limited scleroderma – the CREST syndrome), systemic lupus erythematosus (SLE), mixed connective tissue disease (MCTD) and less commonly rheumatoid arthritis (RA) and dermatomyositis/polymyositis have been associated with the development of pulmonary hypertension. This chapter reviews the incidence of pulmonary hypertension in association with connective tissue disease, potential etiologies, clinical presentation and treatment options.

INCIDENCE

Pulmonary hypertension can occur in association with several connective tissue diseases (Table 13D.1). Scleroderma is a progressive, multisystem disease manifest by connective tissue and vascular lesions in many organs including lung, kidney, and skin. Vascular lesions are prominent in affected tissues.[1,2] Pulmonary manifestations include pulmonary arterial hypertension, interstitial fibrosis, and, less commonly, restriction of the chest wall due to skin changes, chronic aspiration due to esophageal dysfunction, and possibly increased susceptibility to lung neoplasms.[3] Pulmonary complications are the most frequent cause of death in patients with scleroderma,[3,4] particularly with the presence of pulmonary vascular disease.[5]

Table 13D.1 *Connective tissue diseases associated with pulmonary arterial hypertension*

- Scleroderma
  - Diffuse
  - Limited – CREST
- Systemic lupus erythematosis
- Mixed connective tissue disease
- Rheumatoid arthritis
- Polymyositis
- Dermatomyositis

The incidence of pulmonary hypertension in scleroderma varies between 6 and 60% depending on the report and the method used to identify pulmonary hypertension.[6–8] Two-thirds of patients with scleroderma may have pathological evidence of pulmonary vascular involvement, manifest by intimal proliferation and smooth muscle hyperplasia with medial hypertrophy, although not all have clinically significant pulmonary arterial hypertension.[2,6–9] Pulmonary hypertension, both isolated and in association with interstitial lung disease, occurs in up to 33% of patients with diffuse scleroderma.[6,8,10–12] In patients with limited scleroderma or the CREST (calcinosis cutis, Raynaud's phenomenon, esophageal dysfunction, sclerodactyly, and telangectasias) syndrome, pulmonary hypertension is found in up to 60% of patients.[7,8,10,12,13] In both cases, the presence of pulmonary arterial hypertension significantly worsens prognosis. Stupi reported 2-year survival in patients with CREST without pulmonary

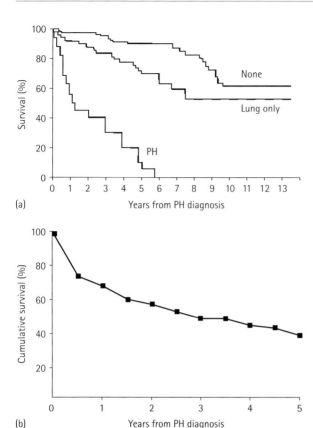

Figure 13D.1 *(a) Survival in patients with scleroderma without organ involvement (none), with lung involvement only, and with pulmonary hypertension (PH). Adapted from Koh et al.[5] by permission of Oxford University Press. (b) Survival in patients with primary pulmonary hypertension. Adapted from D'Alonzo et al.[14] by permission of the American College of Physicians.*

hypertension to be greater than 80%, while patients with CREST and pulmonary hypertension had a 2-year survival of 40%.[7] Sacks reported an overall survival of approximately 50% in patients with pulmonary hypertension and either diffuse or limited scleroderma.[11] Koh reported 40% survival in patients with scleroderma and pulmonary hypertension, contrasting with higher survival in scleroderma patients without organ failure or with interstitial lung disease without pulmonary hypertension.[5] This compares similarly to the registry data demonstrating slightly greater than 50% 2-year survival of patients diagnosed with primary pulmonary hypertension[14] (Figure 13D.1).

Systemic lupus erythematosus (SLE) is also associated with pulmonary hypertension, although the incidence may be less than in patients with scleroderma. Pulmonary hypertension has been reported in 4–14% of patients with SLE, with an overall mortality rate of 25–50% at 2 years from the time of diagnosis of pulmonary hypertension.[15–21] In one study, 14% of patients with SLE had pulmonary hypertension; at follow-up 5 years later the incidence had increased to 43%.[20] In SLE, the pulmonary vasculature may be directly involved or

pulmonary hypertension may be related to interstitial lung disease, diffuse alveolar hemorrhage, airways disease, or thromboembolic disease.[15,18,22]

Mixed connective tissue disease (MCTD) represents a clinical entity where patients may have features of several different rheumatological diseases including SLE, scleroderma, rheumatoid arthritis, and polymyositis.[23,24] During the course of their illness, patients may develop a definable connective tissue disease[25,26] or remain diagnosed with MCTD as a distinct entity.[27] The incidence of pulmonary hypertension in patients with MCTD is not certain: one report suggested that more than 50% of MCTD patients had evidence of pulmonary hypertension.[28] As with SLE, MCTD-associated pulmonary hypertension may be due to direct involvement of the pulmonary circulation or as a consequence of interstitial fibrosis or thromboembolic disease.[23] The prognosis of MCTD-associated pulmonary hypertension is also uncertain, but pulmonary hypertension is frequently cited as a cause of death.[28–31]

Rheumatoid arthritis (RA) affects up to 5% of the population over age 65. Pulmonary complications include interstitial fibrosis, rheumatoid nodules, pleural effusions and pulmonary hypertension. In a recent report, 21% of patients with RA had echocardiographic evidence of mild pulmonary hypertension in the absence of other pulmonary or cardiac disease.[32] The prognosis for RA-associated pulmonary hypertension is not known. Other connective tissue diseases including dermatomyositis/polymyositis are also associated with pulmonary arterial hypertension, often in association with interstitial lung disease. The incidence and prognosis are also not known.[33]

ETIOLOGY

Similar to primary pulmonary hypertension, the etiology of pulmonary hypertension in the connective tissue diseases remains obscure. Some cases are related to severe pulmonary parenchymal disease, such as interstitial fibrosis with hypoxemia. In addition, diastolic dysfunction of the left ventricle, possibly due to fibrosis, has been associated with scleroderma and may lead to pulmonary hypertension[34–36] Pulmonary hypertension may also arise from thromboembolic disease and the hypercoagulable state associated with some connective tissue diseases (see Chapter 17). Pathologically, pulmonary hypertension associated with connective tissue disease is manifest by intimal hyperplasia, smooth muscle hypertrophy, and medial thickening, similar to that seen in primary pulmonary hypertension[2] (see Chapter 3).

Several etiologies have been proposed for the development of connective tissue disease associated pulmonary hypertension (Table 13D.2). Given the frequent occurrence of positive antinuclear antibodies (ANA) in patients with

Table 13D.2 *Potential etiologies of connective tissue disease-associated pulmonary arterial hypertension*

- Idiopathic
- Underlying parenchymal lung disease
  - Interstitial lung disease
- Cardiac involvement
  - Myositis
  - Fibrosis
- Autoimmunity
  - Anti-fibrillarin antibodies
  - Anti-endothelial cell antibodies
  - Anti-tPA antibodies
  - Anti-centromere antibodies
  - Anti-histone antibodies
  - Anti-topoisomerase antibodies
  - HLA-DQ7
  - HLA-B35
- Enhanced vasoreactivity
  - 'Pulmonary Raynaud's'
  - Endothelial dysfunction
- Increased ET-1
- Vascular injury
- Platelet activation
- Oxidant stress
- Genetic – *BMPR2*

primary pulmonary hypertension, autoimmune processes have been proposed in the etiology of primary pulmonary hypertension.[37] Indeed, pulmonary hypertension can occur years before the onset of an identifiable connective tissue disease diagnosis.[38] Several specific antibody patterns have been reported more commonly in patients with connective tissue diseases and pulmonary hypertension: anti-fibrillarin antibodies (also known as anti-U3-RNP) are frequently found in patients with scleroderma and are more common in patients with diffuse disease also accompanied by pulmonary hypertension.[39,40] Anti-fibrillarin antibodies are also found in patients with pulmonary hypertension and SLE.[41] Anti-endothelial antibodies (aECA) are present in 28% of patients with scleroderma (40% in diffuse disease and 13% in limited disease) and are associated with higher incidence of pulmonary hypertension and digital infarcts.[42] aECAs are also associated with pulmonary hypertension in SLE patients.[31] In CREST patients, antibodies to fibrin-bound tissue type plasminogen activator (tPA) are more common in patients with pulmonary hypertension[43] and may also be more common in patients with primary pulmonary hypertension and HLA-DQ7 antigen.[44] Anti-centromere and anti-histone antibodies have also been associated with vascular disease in patients with scleroderma.[45] Recently, anti-topoisomerase II-alpha antibodies have been found more commonly in patients with scleroderma and pulmonary hypertension, particularly when

accompanied by HLA-B35 antigen.[46] Anti-phospholipid antibodies are found commonly in patients with lupus and pulmonary hypertension in the absence of evidence of thromboembolic disease.[41,47]

Raynaud's phenomenon (RP) is commonly observed in patients with scleroderma and SLE. One report found that all CREST patients with pulmonary hypertension had RP, compared with an incidence of RP of 68% in CREST patients without pulmonary hypertension.[7] Another report found that up to 75% of patients with SLE and pulmonary hypertension had RP.[17,41] RP is also common in patients with MCTD and pulmonary hypertension.[48] By contrast, only 10–14% of patients with primary pulmonary hypertension have RP.[49] While RP is seen in patients with RA, there is no clear association with pulmonary hypertension.[32] The high prevalence of RP in patients with connective tissue disease-associated pulmonary hypertension has led to the hypothesis that regulation of pulmonary vascular tone is abnormal – the 'pulmonary Raynaud's' hypothesis.[50,51] Wise reported that patients with RP and scleroderma failed to increase pulmonary diffusing capacity (DLCO) when exposed to cold air compared to patients with RP without scleroderma.[47] By contrast, Shuck found no evidence of pulmonary vasospasm in patients with RP and scleroderma.[52] It has also been suggested that hypoxic pulmonary vasoconstriction may be more pronounced in patients with scleroderma-associated pulmonary hypertension than primary pulmonary hypertension.[53] Thus, while not certain, several reports suggest that dysregulation of pulmonary vascular tone may contribute to connective tissue disease-related pulmonary hypertension.

In support of this concept, endothelial dysfunction in connective tissue disease patients may lead to altered regulation of pulmonary vascular tone and the development of pulmonary hypertension.[54,55] Defective endothelial-dependent, but not endothelial-independent, vasodilation was reported in patients with scleroderma without pulmonary hypertension,[56] a finding consistent with reports of decreased NO production in the lungs of patients with scleroderma and pulmonary hypertension.[57,58] Decreased expression of endothelial nitric oxide synthase (eNOS) in lungs of patients with severe pulmonary hypertension has been reported, although the expression in the lung of patients with connective tissue disease-associated pulmonary hypertension is not known.[59,60] In patients with scleroderma, decreased expression of eNOS in dermal microvascular endothelial cells may play a role in the systemic vascular disease.[61] In addition, pulmonary endothelial expression of prostacyclin synthase is decreased in patients with severe pulmonary hypertension, possibly including those with connective tissue disease-associated pulmonary hypertension.[62]

Endothelin-1 (ET-1) levels are increased in serum of patients with scleroderma, both diffuse and limited[63,64] and correlate with survival,[65] although the levels in scleroderma are not higher in those with pulmonary hypertension compared to those without.[63] By contrast, patients with SLE and pulmonary hypertension have higher serum endothelin levels than non-pulmonary hypertensive SLE patients.[19] Endothelin may also play a role in enhanced vascular reactivity since plasma ET-1 levels increase significantly during cold pressor testing in patients with scleroderma compared to controls.[66] The potential role of ET-1 in the pathogenesis of pulmonary hypertension has led to the therapeutic use of endothelin receptor antagonists in patients with connective tissue disease-associated pulmonary hypertension[67,68] (see Chapters 13P and 13T).

Activation of pulmonary endothelial cells *in vitro* in response to autoantibodies found in patients with connective tissue diseases has been reported.[69] However, evidence of endothelial activation in patients with connective tissue diseases is less clear.[70] Inflammatory cytokines from blood monocytes may activate endothelial cells in patients with MCTD.[71] Thrombomodulin, a marker of vascular injury, is increased in both primary pulmonary hypertension[72,73] and scleroderma-associated pulmonary hypertension.[74] Similarly, circulating levels of von Willibrand's factor, a marker for vascular injury and severity of disease, is increased in patients with pulmonary hypertension and may also be increased in patients with scleroderma, particularly those with pulmonary vascular disease.[77] This marker of endothelial injury improved in patients with primary pulmonary hypertension following treatment with intravenous epoprostenol.[78,79]

Serotonin is released by platelet activation and may also play a role in the pathogenesis of pulmonary hypertension, both primary and in association with connective tissue disease. In patients with systemic sclerosis and RP, platelet serotonin concentrations are decreased[80] and serum levels are increased,[81] respectively. Impaired pulmonary endothelial metabolic activity, with decreased pulmonary capillary angiotensin converting enzyme activity, has also been reported in diffuse and limited scleroderma.[82] Increased oxidant stress has also been found in patients with scleroderma.[83]

The recent demonstration that mutations in the *BMPR2* (bone morphogenetic receptor 2) gene are present in >60% of cases of familial primary pulmonary hypertension and up to 50% of sporadic cases of pulmonary hypertension may provide insights into the pathogenesis not only of PPH but also of other forms of pulmonary hypertension.[84–86]

CLINICAL PRESENTATION AND EVALUATION

As in other forms of pulmonary hypertension, dyspnea is the most common presenting symptom of connective tissue disease-associated pulmonary hypertension (see Chapter 7). Unfortunately, many patients do not seek medical care until symptoms have become advanced. History and physical examination also often reveal findings consistent with the underlying connective tissue disease (i.e. Raynaud's phenomenon, telangectasias, rash, synovitis, interstitial lung disease).

Autoimmune evaluations should be considered when an underlying connective tissue disease is suspected as the cause of pulmonary hypertension. In patients with a suspected diagnosis of connective tissue disease, positive ANA and other, more specific, positive antibody titers in the disease-specific pattern are found, as described previously in this chapter.

The evaluation of suspected pulmonary arterial hypertension in patients with connective tissue disease is similar to that in patients with primary pulmonary hypertension. The most common pulmonary function abnormality in pulmonary hypertension in association with connective disease is a decrease in diffusing capacity of the lung and may prompt an evaluation for both pulmonary vascular disease and interstitial disease.[87] Since patients with scleroderma should be considered at risk for developing pulmonary hypertension, echocardiography, perhaps exercise echocardiography, may reveal right ventricular hypertrophy and dilatation prior to the development of symptoms.[88,89] As with primary pulmonary hypertension, right heart catheterization with a hemodynamically monitored assessment of vasoreactivity is needed to confirm the diagnosis, assess hemodynamic severity, and exclude other possible contributing factors such as an occult congenital heart defect or increased pulmonary venous pressure.

TREATMENT

Treatment options for patients with connective tissue disease-associated pulmonary hypertension are similar

Table 13D.3 *Current and future potential therapeutic options for treatment of connective tissue disease-associated pulmonary arterial hypertension*

- Vasodilators
  - Calcium channel antagonists
  - Intravenous epoprostenol
  - Subcutaneous epoprostenol
  - Inhaled iloprost
- Endothelin-1 antagonists
- Serotonin antagonists
- Immunomodulators
  - Corticosteroids
  - Cyclophosphamide
  - Bone marrow transplantation
- Lung transplantation

to those for primary pulmonary hypertension and are outlined in Table 13D.3 and in Chapters 13K–13P, and 13T.

Oral vasodilators (calcium channel antagonists, angiotensin converting enzyme inhibitors, and α-adrenergic antagonists) have been reported to improve pulmonary hypertension in patients with scleroderma and MCTD.[90–93] These agents may have the greatest utility in patients with favorable acute vasodilator responses. Although calcium channel blockers may improve survival in some patients with scleroderma-associated pulmonary hypertension, only a small percentage of these patients respond favorably to these agents.[90,93–95] Angiotensin converting enzyme inhibitors have also been used with some success both acutely and long term, although controlled trials are lacking.[19,96]

Since a decrease in the production of endogenous vasodilators such as NO and prostacyclin is present in pulmonary hypertension, replacement therapy with these agents is an attractive approach. To date, there have not been any reports of long-term use of NO in the treatment of connective tissue disease-associated pulmonary hypertension, although NO is useful in acute pulmonary vasodilator testing.[97]

Chronic intravenously infused epoprostenol (Flolan) improves functional status and survival in patients with primary pulmonary hypertension.[98] In a randomized, multicenter study, we reported short-term improvement in patients with pulmonary hypertension due to scleroderma treated with intravenous epoprostenol.[99] 111 patients with scleroderma (70% limited disease, 13% diffuse disease, 11–14% overlap syndrome, and 5% with features of scleroderma) were randomized to receive continuous intravenous infusion of epoprostenol versus conventional treatment and followed for 12 weeks. Exercise capacity, cardiopulmonary hemodynamics, NYHA functional class, and Borg dyspnea score improved in the epoprostenol treated group. This study was not powered to detect a mortality benefit as had been seen in the same treatment duration with primary pulmonary hypertension. Long-term follow-up of the patients in the study has suggested that epoprostenol may improve survival compared to historical controls (Figure 13D.2);[5] however, patients with scleroderma treated with epoprostenol have poorer survival compared to patients with primary pulmonary hypertension (Figure 13D.3). Others have also reported both short- and long-term success with intravenous epoprostenol.[100–102]

Intravenous epoprostenol has also been used in SLE-associated pulmonary hypertension. Robbins reported short- and long-term hemodynamic and functional class improvement in six patients with SLE-associated pulmonary hypertension[103] and Horn reported successful treatment of six patients with SLE-associated pulmonary hypertension, although this was complicated by severe, refractory thrombocytopenia in four.[104]

Iloprost has also been used in the treatment of connective tissue disease associated pulmonary hypertension. Five patients with CREST and severe pulmonary hypertension were treated with aerosolized iloprost. At one year, quality of life, functional class and hemodynamics were improved and this was maintained at 2 years in three patients.[105] Recently, treprostinil, a stable prostacyclin analog, was approved for use in patients with pulmonary arterial hypertension.[106] Beraprost sodium, an orally active prostacyclin analog, was recently reported to improve the 6-minute walk distance in patients with primary pulmonary hypertension but not in the subgroup of patients with connective tissue disease.[107]

Complicating the use of vasodilators, especially intravenous epoprostenol, is pulmonary edema following both

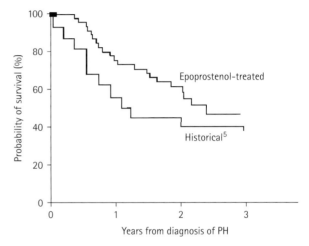

Figure 13D.2 *Survival in patients with scleroderma treated with continuous infusion of epoprostenol compared to historical controls. Data from scleroderma epoprostenol extension trial (GlaxoSmithKline) and adapted from Koh et al.[5] with permission of Oxford University Press and GlaxoSmithKline.*

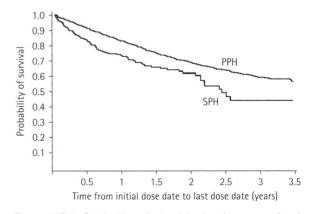

Figure 13D.3 *Survival in patients with scleroderma-associated pulmonary hypertension (SPH) compared to patients with primary pulmonary hypertension (PPH) treated with epoprostenol. Data from manufacturer (GlaxoSmithKline) from 1996 to 1999, reproduced with permission.*

acute and chronic administration therapy, possibly due to the presence of pulmonary capillary hemangiomatosis or pulmonary veno-occlusive disease.[108–110] While very rare, pulmonary veno-occlusive disease may be more common in patients with connective tissue disease[111] (see Chapters 14B and 14C).

Given the increased levels of endothelin in patients with primary pulmonary hypertension and scleroerma, the therapeutic use of endothelin receptor antagonists in the treatment of pulmonary arterial hypertension was recently studied. Rubin *et al.* report the results of a multicenter, randomized, double-blinded placebo-controlled trial of bosentan (Tracleer™) for the treatment of pulmonary arterial hypertension.[68] 213 patients with pulmonary hypertension, either primary or due to connective tissue disease (scleroderma and lupus) were randomized to receive placebo or bosentan at 125 or 250 mg orally twice daily. After 16 weeks, exercise capacity (as measured by the 6-minute walk test) improved in patients receiving bosentan, although there was no significant difference between the two doses tested. Functional class, Borg dyspnea index, and time to clinical worsening also improved. Approximately 30% of patients enrolled had a diagnosis of connective tissue disease. In the patients with scleroderma, bosentan prevented the deterioration in walking distance compared to placebo-treated patients, who had significant worsening of exercise capacity. By contrast, patients with primary pulmonary hypertension had significant improvement in exercise capacity, suggesting that, overall, patients with scleroderma did less well. This study was not designed to test survival. Most patients tolerated the drug, with headache being the most common complaint. Dose-dependent hepatotoxicity occurred in 14% of patients receiving high-dose bosentan. Following review of this trial, bosentan was licensed for the treatment of moderate to severe pulmonary arterial hypertension.

Serotonergic blockade with the selective receptor 2-antagonist ketanserin acutely improved pulmonary artery pressure and cardiac output in patients with pulmonary hypertension and systemic sclerosis.[112] Sarpogrelate, another receptor 2 antagonist, was administered orally for 12 months to patients with systemic sclerosis, leading to increased diffusing capacity of carbon monoxide, decreased mean pulmonary arterial pressure, and increased right ventricular ejection fraction.[113] Although a randomized, controlled trial of these agents has not been done, these reports suggest a potential role for serotonin in the pathogenesis of scleroderma-associated pulmonary arterial hypertension.

Immunomodulatory treatments for patients with connective tissue disease associated pulmonary hypertension have also been investigated. Long-term plasma exchange,[114] corticosteroids with and without cyclophosphamide[21] and autologous stem cell transplantation[115] have been reported to improve or stabilize pulmonary hypertension in patients with scleroderma. However, these represent case reports or retrospective case studies, and no prospective study of immunosuppressive therapy has been completed.

Finally, surgical or interventional options including atrial septostomy[116] and lung or heart/lung transplantation may be considered in patients with severe pulmonary arterial hypertension in association with connective tissue disease (see Chapters 13R and 13S). Careful consideration must be given to the presence of other organ involvement, particularly renal disease, in patients being considered for transplant. In one series, survival in patients undergoing lung or heart/lung transplantation with connective tissue disease was no different than survival in patients with primary pulmonary hypertension.[117]

KEY POINTS

- Pulmonary arterial hypertension is associated with several connective tissue diseases and is associated with significant morbidity and mortality.
- Multiple etiologies for the development of connective tissue disease related pulmonary hypertension have been proposed but, similarly, patients with primary pulmonary hypertension do not know the exact etiology.
- Evaluation of patients with connective tissue disease related pulmonary arterial hypertension is similar to patients with primary pulmonary hypertension.
- Therapy for patients with connective tissue disease-related pulmonary hypertension is similar to patients with primary pulmonary hypertension. However, while patients with connective tissue disease may not respond as well to therapy as patients with primary pulmonary hypertension, aggressive therapy may improve functional status and quality of life.

REFERENCES

●1 al-Sabbagh MR, Steen VD, Zee BC *et al.* Pulmonary arterial histology and morphometry in systemic sclerosis: a case-control autopsy study. *J Rheumatol* 1989;**16**:1038–42.
2 Young RH, Mark GJ. Pulmonary vascular changes in scleroderma. *Am J Med* 1978;**64**:998–1004.
◆3 Minai OA, Dweik RA, Arroliga AC. Manifestations of scleroderma pulmonary disease. *Clin Chest Med* 1998;**19**:713–31, viii–ix.
4 Arroliga AC, Podell DN, Matthay RA. Pulmonary manifestations of scleroderma. *J Thorac Imaging* 1992;**7**:30–45.
●5 Koh ET, Lee P, Gladman DD *et al.* Pulmonary hypertension in systemic sclerosis: an analysis of 17 patients. *Br J Rheumatol* 1996;**35**:989–93.

6 Battle RW, Davitt MA, Cooper SM *et al.* Prevalence of pulmonary hypertension in limited and diffuse scleroderma. *Chest* 1996;**110**:1515–19.

7 Stupi AM, Steen VD, Owens GR *et al.* Pulmonary hypertension in the CREST syndrome variant of systemic sclerosis. *Arthritis Rheum* 1986;**29**:515–24.

8 Ungerer RG, Tashkin DP, Furst D *et al.* Prevalence and clinical correlates of pulmonary arterial hypertension in progressive systemic sclerosis. *Am J Med* 1983;**75**:65–74.

9 Yousem SA. The pulmonary pathologic manifestations of the CREST syndrome. *Hum Pathol* 1990;**21**:467–74.

10 MacGregor AJ, Canavan R, Knight C *et al.* Pulmonary hypertension in systemic sclerosis: risk factors for progression and consequences for survival. *Rheumatology (Oxford)* 2001;**40**:453–9.

11 Sacks DG, Okano Y, Steen VD *et al.* Isolated pulmonary hypertension in systemic sclerosis with diffuse cutaneous involvement: association with serum anti-U3RNP antibody. *J Rheumatol* 1996;**23**:639–42.

12 Thurm CA, Wigley FM, Dole WP *et al.* Failure of vasodilator infusion to alter pulmonary diffusing capacity in systemic sclerosis. *Am J Med* 1991;**90**:547–52.

13 Salerni R, Rodnan GP, Leon DF *et al.* Pulmonary hypertension in the CREST syndrome variant of progressive systemic sclerosis (scleroderma). *Ann Intern Med* 1977;**86**:394–9.

●14 D'Alonzo GE, Barst RJ, Ayres SM *et al.* Survival in patients with primary pulmonary hypertension. Results from a national prospective registry. *Ann Intern Med* 1991;**115**:343–9.

15 Asherson RA, Higenbottam TW, Dinh Xuan AT *et al.* Pulmonary hypertension in a lupus clinic: experience with twenty-four patients. *J Rheumatol* 1990;**17**:1292–8.

16 Badui E, Garcia-Rubi D, Robles E *et al.* Cardiovascular manifestations in systemic lupus erythematosus. Prospective study of 100 patients. *Angiology* 1985;**36**:431–41.

17 Li EK, Tam LS. Pulmonary hypertension in systemic lupus erythematosus: clinical association and survival in 18 patients. *J Rheumatol* 1999;**26**:1923–9.

18 Orens JB, Martinez FJ, Lynch JP, 3rd. Pleuropulmonary manifestations of systemic lupus erythematosus. *Rheum Dis Clin North Am* 1994;**20**:159–93.

19 Shen JY, Chen SL, Wu YX *et al.* Pulmonary hypertension in systemic lupus erythematosus. *Rheumatol Int* 1999;**18**:147–51.

20 Simonson JS, Schiller NB, Petri M *et al.* Pulmonary hypertension in systemic lupus erythematosus. *J Rheumatol* 1989;**16**:918–25.

◆21 Tanaka E, Harigai M, Tanaka M *et al.* Pulmonary hypertension in systemic lupus erythematosus: evaluation of clinical characteristics and response to immunosuppressive treatment. *J Rheumatol* 2002;**29**:282–7.

22 Love PE, Santoro SA. Antiphospholipid antibodies: anticardiolipin and the lupus anticoagulant in systemic lupus erythematosus (SLE) and in non-SLE disorders. Prevalence and clinical significance. *Ann Intern Med* 1990;**112**:682–98.

◆23 Prakash UB. Respiratory complications in mixed connective tissue disease. *Clin Chest Med* 1998;**19**:733–46, ix.

24 Sharp GC, Irvin WS, Tan EM *et al.* Mixed connective tissue disease – an apparently distinct rheumatic disease syndrome associated with a specific antibody to an extractable nuclear antigen (ENA). *Am J Med* 1972;**52**:148–59.

25 Kallenberg CG. Overlapping syndromes, undifferentiated connective tissue disease, and other fibrosing conditions. *Curr Opin Rheumatol* 1995;**7**:568–73.

26 van den Hoogen FH, Spronk PE, Boerbooms AM *et al.* Long-term follow-up of 46 patients with anti-(U1)snRNP antibodies. *Br J Rheumatol* 1994;**33**:1117–20.

27 Lundberg I, Nyman U, Pettersson I *et al.* Clinical manifestations and anti-(U1)snRNP antibodies: a prospective study of 29 anti-RNP antibody positive patients. *Br J Rheumatol* 1992;**31**:811–17.

28 Sullivan WD, Hurst DJ, Harmon CE *et al.* A prospective evaluation emphasizing pulmonary involvement in patients with mixed connective tissue disease. *Medicine (Baltimore)* 1984;**63**:92–107.

29 Burdt MA, Hoffman RW, Deutscher SL *et al.* Long-term outcome in mixed connective tissue disease: longitudinal clinical and serologic findings. *Arthritis Rheum* 1999;**42**:899–909.

30 Prakash UB, Luthra HS, Divertie MB. Intrathoracic manifestations in mixed connective tissue disease. *Mayo Clin Proc* 1985;**60**:813–21.

31 Yoshio T, Masuyama J, Sumiya M *et al.* Antiendothelial cell antibodies and their relation to pulmonary hypertension in systemic lupus erythematosus. *J Rheumatol* 1994;**21**:2058–63.

32 Dawson JK, Goodson NG, Graham DR *et al.* Raised pulmonary artery pressures measured with Doppler echocardiography in rheumatoid arthritis patients. *Rheumatology (Oxford)* 2000;**39**:1320–5.

33 Denbow CE, Lie JT, Tancredi RG *et al.* Cardiac involvement in polymyositis: a clinicopathologic study of 20 autopsied patients. *Arthritis Rheum* 1979;**22**:1088–92.

34 Aguglia G, Sgreccia A, Bernardo ML *et al.* Left ventricular diastolic function in systemic sclerosis. *J Rheumatol* 2001;**28**:1563–7.

35 Coghlan JG, Mukerjee D. The heart and pulmonary vasculature in scleroderma: clinical features and pathobiology. *Curr Opin Rheumatol* 2001;**13**:495–9.

36 Giunta A, Tirri E, Maione S *et al.* Right ventricular diastolic abnormalities in systemic sclerosis. Relation to left ventricular involvement and pulmonary hypertension. *Ann Rheum Dis* 2000;**59**:94–8.

37 Rich S, Kieras K, Hart K *et al.* Antinuclear antibodies in primary pulmonary hypertension. *J Am Coll Cardiol* 1986;**8**:1307–11.

38 Gurubhagavatula I, Palevsky HI. Pulmonary hypertension in systemic autoimmune disease. *Rheum Dis Clin North Am* 1997;**23**:365–94.

39 Okano Y, Steen VD, Medsger TA, Jr. Autoantibody to U3 nucleolar ribonucleoprotein (fibrillarin) in patients with systemic sclerosis. *Arthritis Rheum* 1992;**35**:95–100.

40 Tormey VJ, Bunn CC, Denton CP *et al.* Anti-fibrillarin antibodies in systemic sclerosis. *Rheumatology (Oxford)* 2001;**40**:1157–62.

41 Asherson RA, Oakley CM. Pulmonary hypertension and systemic lupus erythematosus. *J Rheumatol* 1986;**13**:1–5.

42 Negi VS, Tripathy NK, Misra R *et al.* Antiendothelial cell antibodies in scleroderma correlate with severe digital ischemia and pulmonary arterial hypertension. *J Rheumatol* 1998;**25**:462–6.

43 Fritzler MJ, Hart DA, Wilson D et al. Antibodies to fibrin bound tissue type plasminogen activator in systemic sclerosis. *J Rheumatol* 1995;**22**:1688–93.

44 Morse JH, Barst RJ, Fotino M et al. Primary pulmonary hypertension, tissue plasminogen activator antibodies, and HLA-DQ7. *Am J Respir Crit Care Med* 1997;**155**:274–8.

45 Martin L, Pauls JD, Ryan JP et al. Identification of a subset of patients with scleroderma with severe pulmonary and vascular disease by the presence of autoantibodies to centromere and histone. *Ann Rheum Dis* 1993;**52**:780–4.

46 Grigolo B, Mazzetti I, Meliconi R et al. Anti-topoisomerase II alpha autoantibodies in systemic sclerosis - association with pulmonary hypertension and HLA-B35. *Clin Exp Immunol* 2000;**121**:539–43.

47 Wise RA, Wigley F, Newball HH et al. The effect of cold exposure on diffusing capacity in patients with Raynaud's phenomenon. *Chest* 1982;**81**:695–8.

48 Ueda N, Mimura K, Maeda H et al. Mixed connective tissue disease with fatal pulmonary hypertension and a review of literature. *Virchows Arch A Pathol Anat Histopathol* 1984;**404**:335–40.

◆49 Rich S, Dantzker DR, Ayres SM et al. Primary pulmonary hypertension. A national prospective study. *Ann Intern Med* 1987;**107**:216–23.

50 Fahey PJ, Utell MJ, Condemi JJ et al. Raynaud's phenomenon of the lung. *Am J Med* 1984;**76**:263–9.

51 Rozkovec A, Bernstein R, Asherson RA et al. Vascular reactivity and pulmonary hypertension in systemic sclerosis. *Arthritis Rheum* 1983;**26**:1037–40.

52 Shuck JW, Oetgen WJ, Tesar JT. Pulmonary vascular response during Raynaud's phenomenon in progressive systemic sclerosis. *Am J Med* 1985;**78**:221–7.

53 Morgan JM, Griffiths M, du Bois RM et al. Hypoxic pulmonary vasoconstriction in systemic sclerosis and primary pulmonary hypertension. *Chest* 1991;**99**:551–6.

54 Kahaleh B, Matucci-Cerinic M. Raynaud's phenomenon and scleroderma. Dysregulated neuroendothelial control of vascular tone. *Arthritis Rheum* 1995;**38**:1–4.

55 Wigley FM. Raynaud's phenomenon and other features of scleroderma, including pulmonary hypertension. *Curr Opin Rheumatol* 1996;**8**:561–8.

56 Cailes J, Winter S, du Bois RM et al. Defective endothelially mediated pulmonary vasodilation in systemic sclerosis. *Chest* 1998;**114**:178–84.

57 Kharitonov SA, Cailes JB, Black CM et al. Decreased nitric oxide in the exhaled air of patients with systemic sclerosis with pulmonary hypertension. *Thorax* 1997;**52**:1051–5.

58 Rolla G, Colagrande P, Scappaticci E et al. Exhaled nitric oxide in systemic sclerosis: relationships with lung involvement and pulmonary hypertension. *J Rheumatol* 2000;**27**:1693–8.

59 Giaid A, Saleh D. Reduced expression of endothelial nitric oxide synthase in the lungs of patients with pulmonary hypertension. *N Engl J Med* 1995;**333**:214–21.

60 Mason NA, Springall DR, Burke M et al. High expression of endothelial nitric oxide synthase in plexiform lesions of pulmonary hypertension. *J Pathol* 1998;**185**:313–18.

61 Romero LI, Zhang DN, Cooke JP et al. Differential expression of nitric oxide by dermal microvascular endothelial cells from patients with scleroderma. *Vasc Med* 2000;**5**:147–58.

62 Tuder RM, Cool CD, Geraci MW et al. Prostacyclin synthase expression is decreased in lungs from patients with severe pulmonary hypertension. *Am J Respir Crit Care Med* 1999;**159**:1925–32.

63 Morelli S, Ferri C, Polettini E et al. Plasma endothelin-1 levels, pulmonary hypertension, and lung fibrosis in patients with systemic sclerosis. *Am J Med* 1995;**99**:255–60.

64 Yamane K. Endothelin and collagen vascular disease: a review with special reference to Raynaud's phenomenon and systemic sclerosis. *Intern Med* 1994;**33**:579–82.

65 Galie N, Grigoni F, Bacchi-Reggiani L et al. Relation of endothelin-1 to survival in patients with primary pulmonary hypertension. *Eur J Clin Invest* 1996;**26**(Suppl 1):48.

66 Danese C, Parlapiano C, Zavattaro E et al. ET-1 plasma levels during cold stress test in sclerodermic patients. *Angiology* 1997;**48**:965–8.

67 Channick RN, Simonneau G, Sitbon O et al. Effects of the dual endothelin-receptor antagonist bosentan in patients with pulmonary hypertension: a randomised placebo-controlled study. *Lancet* 2001;**358**:1119–23.

●68 Rubin LJ, Badesch DB, Barst RJ et al. Bosentan therapy for pulmonary arterial hypertension. *N Engl J Med* 2002; **346**:896–903.

69 Okawa-Takatsuji M, Aotsuka S, Fujinami M et al. Up-regulation of intercellular adhesion molecule-1 (ICAM-1), endothelial leucocyte adhesion molecule-1 (ELAM-1) and class II MHC molecules on pulmonary artery endothelial cells by antibodies against U1-ribonucleoprotein. *Clin Exp Immunol* 1999;**116**:174–80.

70 Stratton RJ, Coghlan JG, Pearson JD et al. Different patterns of endothelial cell activation in renal and pulmonary vascular disease in scleroderma. *Q J Med* 1998;**91**:561–6.

71 Okawa-Takatsuji M, Aotsuka S, Uwatoko S et al. Enhanced synthesis of cytokines by peripheral blood monocytes cultured in the presence of autoantibodies against U1-ribonucleoprotein and/or negatively charged molecules: implication in the pathogenesis of pulmonary hypertension in mixed connective tissue disease (MCTD). *Clin Exp Immunol* 1994;**98**:427–33.

72 Hoeper MM, Sosada M, Fabel H. Plasma coagulation profiles in patients with severe primary pulmonary hypertension. *Eur Respir J* 1998;**12**:1446–9.

73 Welsh CH, Hassell KL, Badesch DB et al. Coagulation and fibrinolytic profiles in patients with severe pulmonary hypertension. *Chest* 1996;**110**:710–17.

74 Stratton RJ, Pompon L, Coghlan JG et al. Soluble thrombomodulin concentration is raised in scleroderma associated pulmonary hypertension. *Ann Rheum Dis* 2000;**59**:132–4.

75 Lopes AA, Maeda NY. Circulating von Willebrand factor antigen as a predictor of short-term prognosis in pulmonary hypertension. *Chest* 1998;**114**:1276–82.

76 Lopes AA, Maeda NY, Goncalves RC et al. Endothelial cell dysfunction correlates differentially with survival in primary and secondary pulmonary hypertension. *Am Heart J* 2000; **139**:618–23.

77 Scheja A, Eskilsson J, Akesson A et al. Inverse relation between plasma concentration of von Willebrand factor and CrEDTA clearance in systemic sclerosis. *J Rheumatol* 1994;**21**:639–42.

78 Friedman R, Mears JG, Barst RJ. Continuous infusion of prostacyclin normalizes plasma markers of endothelial cell injury and platelet aggregation in primary pulmonary hypertension. *Circulation* 1997;**96**:2782-4.

79 Veyradier A, Nishikubo T, Humbert M *et al.* Improvement of von Willebrand factor proteolysis after prostacyclin infusion in severe pulmonary arterial hypertension. *Circulation* 2000;**102**:2460-2.

80 Klimiuk PS, Grennan A, Weinkove C *et al.* Platelet serotonin in systemic sclerosis. *Ann Rheum Dis* 1989;**48**:586-9.

81 Biondi ML, Marasini B, Bianchi E *et al.* Plasma free and intraplatelet serotonin in patients with Raynaud's phenomenon. *Int J Cardiol* 1988;**19**:335-9.

82 Orfanos SE, Psevdi E, Stratigis N *et al.* Pulmonary capillary endothelial dysfunction in early systemic sclerosis. *Arthritis Rheum* 2001;**44**:902-11.

83 Stein CM, Tanner SB, Awad JA *et al.* Evidence of free radical-mediated injury (isoprostane overproduction) in scleroderma. *Arthritis Rheum* 1996;**39**:1146-50.

●84 Deng Z, Morse JH, Slager SL *et al.* Familial primary pulmonary hypertension (gene *PPH1*) is caused by mutations in the bone morphogenetic protein receptor-II gene. *Am J Hum Genet* 2000;**67**:737-44.

●85 Lane KB, Machado RD, Pauciulo MW *et al.* Heterozygous germline mutations in *BMPR2*, encoding a TGF-beta receptor, cause familial primary pulmonary hypertension. The International PPH Consortium. *Nat Genet* 2000;**26**:81-4.

●86 Thomson JR, Machado RD, Pauciulo MW *et al.* Sporadic primary pulmonary hypertension is associated with germline mutations of the gene encoding BMPR-II, a receptor member of the TGF- beta family. *J Med Genet* 2000;**37**:741-5.

87 Scheja A, Akesson A, Wollmer P *et al.* Early pulmonary disease in systemic sclerosis: a comparison between carbon monoxide transfer factor and static lung compliance. *Ann Rheum Dis* 1993;**52**:725-9.

88 Denton CP, Cailes JB, Phillips GD *et al.* Comparison of Doppler echocardiography and right heart catheterization to assess pulmonary hypertension in systemic sclerosis. *Br J Rheumatol* 1997;**36**:239-43.

89 Grunig E, Janssen B, Mereles D *et al.* Abnormal pulmonary artery pressure response in asymptomatic carriers of primary pulmonary hypertension gene. *Circulation* 2000;**102**:1145-50.

90 Alpert MA, Pressly TA, Mukerji V *et al.* Acute and long-term effects of nifedipine on pulmonary and systemic hemodynamics in patients with pulmonary hypertension associated with diffuse systemic sclerosis, the CREST syndrome and mixed connective tissue disease. *Am J Cardiol* 1991;**68**:1687-91.

91 Glikson M, Pollack A, Dresner-Feigin R *et al.* Nifedipine and prazosin in the management of pulmonary hypertension in CREST syndrome. *Chest* 1990;**98**:759-61.

92 Sfikakis PP, Kyriakidis MK, Vergos CG *et al.* Cardiopulmonary hemodynamics in systemic sclerosis and response to nifedipine and captopril. *Am J Med* 1991;**90**:541-6.

93 Shinohara S, Murata I, Yamada H *et al.* Combined effects of diltiazem and oxygen in pulmonary hypertension of mixed connective tissue disease. *J Rheumatol* 1994;**21**:1763-5.

94 O'Brien JT, Hill JA, Pepine CJ. Sustained benefit of verapamil in pulmonary hypertension with progressive systemic sclerosis. *Am Heart J* 1985;**109**:380-2.

●95 Rich S, Kaufmann E, Levy PS. The effect of high doses of calcium-channel blockers on survival in primary pulmonary hypertension. *N Engl J Med* 1992;**327**:76-81.

96 Alpert MA, Pressly TA, Mukerji V *et al.* Short- and long-term hemodynamic effects of captopril in patients with pulmonary hypertension and selected connective tissue disease. *Chest* 1992;**102**:1407-12.

97 Williamson DJ, Hayward C, Rogers P *et al.* Acute hemodynamic responses to inhaled nitric oxide in patients with limited scleroderma and isolated pulmonary hypertension. *Circulation* 1996;**94**:477-82.

●98 Barst RJ, Rubin LJ, Long WA *et al.* A comparison of continuous intravenous epoprostenol (prostacyclin) with conventional therapy for primary pulmonary hypertension. The Primary Pulmonary Hypertension Study Group. *N Engl J Med* 1996;**334**:296-302.

●99 Badesch DB, Tapson VF, McGoon MD *et al.* Continuous intravenous epoprostenol for pulmonary hypertension due to the scleroderma spectrum of disease. A randomized, controlled trial. *Ann Intern Med* 2000;**132**:425-34.

100 Humbert M, Sanchez O, Fartoukh M *et al.* Treatment of severe pulmonary hypertension secondary to connective tissue diseases with continuous IV epoprostenol (prostacyclin). *Chest* 1998;**114**(1 Suppl):80S-2S.

101 Klings ES, Hill NS, Ieong MH *et al.* Systemic sclerosis-associated pulmonary hypertension: short- and long-term effects of epoprostenol (prostacyclin). *Arthritis Rheum* 1999;**42**:2638-45.

102 Menon N, McAlpine L, Peacock AJ *et al.* The acute effects of prostacyclin on pulmonary hemodynamics in patients with pulmonary hypertension secondary to systemic sclerosis. *Arthritis Rheum* 1998;**41**:466-9.

●103 Robbins IM, Gaine SP, Schilz R *et al.* Epoprostenol for treatment of pulmonary hypertension in patients with systemic lupus erythematosus. *Chest* 2000;**117**:14-18.

104 Horn EM, Barst RJ, Poon M. Epoprostenol for treatment of pulmonary hypertension in patients with systemic lupus erythematosus. *Chest* 2000;**118**:1229-30.

105 Launay D, Hachulla E, Hatron PY *et al.* Aerosolized iloprost in CREST syndrome related pulmonary hypertension. *J Rheumatol* 2001;**28**:2252-6.

●106 Simonneau G, Barst RJ, Galie N *et al.* Continuous subcutaneous infusion of treprostinil, a prostacyclin analogue, in patients with pulmonary arterial hypertension: a double-blind, randomized, placebo-controlled trial. *Am J Respir Crit Care Med* 2002;**165**:800-4.

●107 Galie N, Humbert M, Vachiery JL *et al.* Effects of beraprost sodium, an oral prostacyclin analogue, in patients with pulmonary arterial hypertension: a randomized, double-blind, placebo-controlled trial. *J Am Coll Cardiol* 2002;**39**:1496-502.

108 Farber HW, Graven KK, Kokolski G *et al.* Pulmonary edema during acute infusion of epoprostenol in a patient with pulmonary hypertension and limited scleroderma. *J Rheumatol* 1999;**26**:1195-6.

109 Palmer SM, Robinson LJ, Wang A *et al.* Massive pulmonary edema and death after prostacyclin infusion in a patient with pulmonary veno-occlusive disease. *Chest* 1998; **113**:237-40.

110 Preston IR, Klinger JR, Houtchens J *et al.* Pulmonary edema caused by inhaled nitric oxide therapy in two patients with

pulmonary hypertension associated with the CREST syndrome. *Chest* 2002;**121**:656–9.

111 Mandel J, Mark EJ, Hales CA. Pulmonary veno-occlusive disease. *Am J Respir Crit Care Med* 2000;**162**:1964–73.

112 Seibold JR, Molony RR, Turkevich D *et al.* Acute hemodynamic effects of ketanserin in pulmonary hypertension secondary to systemic sclerosis. *J Rheumatol* 1987;**14**:519–24.

113 Kato S, Kishiro I, Machida M *et al.* Suppressive effect of sarpogrelate hydrochloride on respiratory failure and right ventricular failure with pulmonary hypertension in patients with systemic sclerosis. *J Int Med Res* 2000;**28**:258–68.

114 Ferri C, Emdin M, Storino FA *et al.* Isolated pulmonary hypertension in diffuse cutaneous systemic sclerosis

115 Binks M, Passweg JR, Furst D *et al.* Phase I/II trial of autologous stem cell transplantation in systemic sclerosis: procedure related mortality and impact on skin disease. *Ann Rheum Dis* 2001;**60**:577–84.

116 Allcock RJ, O'Sullivan JJ, Corris PA. Palliation of systemic sclerosis-associated pulmonary hypertension by atrial septostomy. *Arthritis Rheum* 2001;**44**:1660–2.

117 Rosas V, Conte JV, Yang SC *et al.* Lung transplantation and systemic sclerosis. *Ann Transplant* 2000;**5**:38–43.

successfully treated with long-term plasma exchange. *Scand J Rheumatol* 2000;**29**:198–200.

Pulmonary hypertension related to appetite suppressants

OLIVIER SITBON, MARC HUMBERT AND GÉRALD SIMONNEAU

INTRODUCTION

A new diagnostic classification of pulmonary hypertension was proposed at the 1998 WHO Pulmonary Hypertension Meeting held in Evian, France.[1] This classification reflects recent advances in the understanding of pulmonary hypertensive diseases, and recognizes the similarity between 'unexplained' pulmonary hypertension ['primary' pulmonary hypertension (PPH)] and pulmonary arterial hypertension (PAH) associated with several conditions and diseases, such as connective tissue diseases, portal hypertension, congenital left-to-right cardiac shunts, HIV infection, and exposure to toxins and drugs, including appetite suppressants. Among anorectic drugs, aminorex fumarate and fenfluramine derivatives (Figure 13E.1) have been reported to be associated with the development of PAH and are considered as definite risk factors for PAH, playing a causal role.

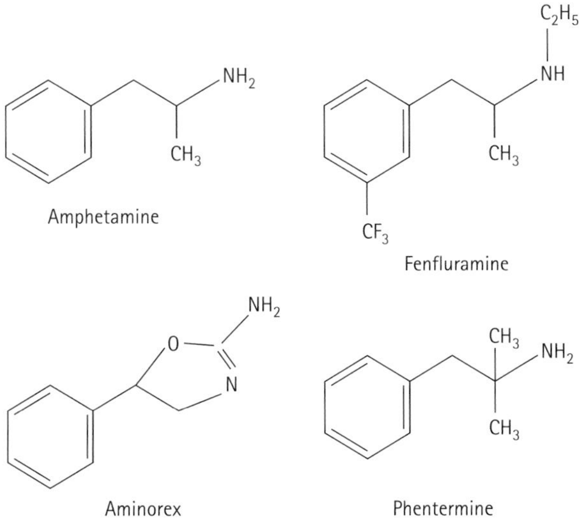

Figure 13E.1 *Chemical structure of amphetamine and related anorectic drugs (aminorex, fenfluramine and phentermine).*

DEFINITION OF A RISK FACTOR FOR PULMONARY ARTERIAL HYPERTENSION

A risk factor for PAH is any factor or condition that is suspected to play a causal or facilitating role in the development of the disease.[1] Because risk factors relate to the probability of occurrence of the disease, they must be present prior to the onset of the disease. Risk factors may include drugs, chemical products, diseases or a clinical state (age, gender). When it is not possible to determine whether a factor was present before the onset of pulmonary hypertension, and thus it is unclear whether it played a causal role the term 'associated condition' is used.[1] Given the fact that the absolute risk is generally

Table 13E.1 *Consensus on drugs and toxins as risk factors for pulmonary arterial hypertension*

- Definite
  - Aminorex
  - Fenfluramine
  - Dexfenfluramine
  - Toxic rapeseed oil
- Very likely
  - Amphetamines
  - L-Tryptophan
- Possible
  - Meta-amphetamines
  - Cocaine
  - Chemotherapeutic agents
- Unlikely
  - Antidepressants
  - Oral contraceptives
  - Estrogen therapy
  - Cigarette smoking

Risk factors are categorized based on the strength of the association with PAH and their probable causal role. 'Definite' indicates an association based on several concordant observations, including a major controlled study or a clear epidemic. Definite risk factors are considered to play a causal role in the development of the disease. 'Very likely' indicates several concordant observations (including large case series and studies) that are not attributable to considered biases, or a general consensus among experts. 'Possible' indicates an association based on case series, registries, or expert opinions. 'Unlikely' indicates risk factors that have been proposed but have not been found to have any association from controlled studies.[1]

low with the known risk factors of PAH, factors of individual susceptibility are likely to play an important role. These elements have been classified according to the strength of the association with pulmonary hypertension and their probable facilitating role.[1] 'Definite' indicates an association based on several concordant observations, including a major controlled study or a clear epidemic. Definite risk factors are considered to play a causal role in the development of the disease. 'Very likely' indicates several concordant observations (including large case series and studies) that are not attributable to considered biases, or a general consensus among experts. 'Possible' indicates an association based on case series, registries, or expert opinions. 'Unlikely' indicates risk factors that have been proposed but have not been found to have any association from controlled studies. The 1998 Evian meeting reviewed this topic and a consensus statement was established.[1] Table 13E.1 summarizes this consensus.

AMINOREX FUMARATE

The question of a relation between some drug ingestion and pulmonary hypertension was first raised in the late 1960s, when a 20-fold increase of unexplained pulmonary

hypertension was reported in Switzerland, Austria and West Germany.[2–4] A dramatic increase in the number of diagnoses of 'primary' pulmonary hypertension was first noted in a Swiss medical clinic in 1967; diagnoses rose from 0.87% to 13.5% of adults who underwent cardiac catherization. There were no apparent changes in either size or composition of the population, or of diagnostic procedures. About half the patients were more or less overweight, with a female preponderance. Afterwards, 582 cases were identified in a study conducted in Germany, Switzerland and Austria.[3,4] This epidemic just followed the introduction in these countries of the appetite depressant aminorex fumarate (2-amino-5-phenyl-2-oxazoline), and subsided shortly after the drug had been banned from the market (Figure 13E.2). Approximately 2% of the population who had taken aminorex developed pulmonary arterial hypertension,[2,4,5] but 61% of the 582 patients who were identified as new cases of PPH gave a history of aminorex intake, either alone or in combination with other anorectic agents.[3,4] In a cohort of 731 patients known to have taken aminorex and who were covered by a single health insurance company, 3% developed PPH.[6] The number of cases varied geographically, consistent with the marketing, and temporally with the intake of aminorex. The relative risk of developing pulmonary hypertension in aminorex users was estimated to be 52:1 compared with patients without any exposure to the drug.[3,4] The clinical manifestations, hemodynamic measures, and pathological changes were reported to be indistinguishable from those of PPH. At that time, controversial conclusions were raised regarding the relationship between the total individual dose and the risk of developing the disease, whereas there was no correlation between the disease severity and the number of tablets each individual patient had taken.[3,4] Despite the fact that a dose–response effect between aminorex intake and severity of pulmonary hypertension has not been established, and that the evidence has not been substantiated by an animal model, it is widely accepted that the epidemic of pulmonary hypertension was due to aminorex. During follow-up, some authors felt that after discontinuation of the drug, patients with a history of aminorex intake had a better long-term survival than 'unexposed' patients with primary pulmonary hypertension, whereas other authors did not report differences in the survival rates.[3,4,6]

Aminorex resembles epinephrine and amphetamine (Figure 13E.1), and a release of catecholamines from endogenous stores by this drug has been suggested, as well as a mechanism involving lung serotonin release. However, all attempts from experimental work to produce chronic pulmonary hypertension and to demonstrate the effect of the chronic administration of aminorex in any species have failed. This has been explained, first, by the low incidence of pulmonary hypertension in test animals as well as in humans, and second, by the fact that a prerequisite

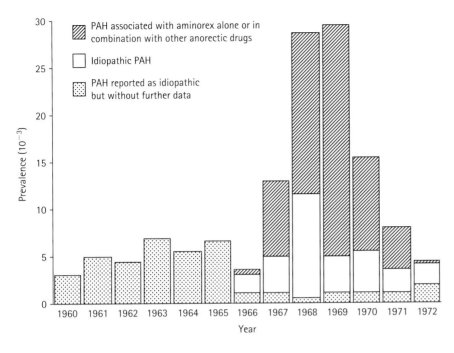

Figure 13E.2 *Prevalence of aminorex-associated pulmonary arterial hypertension (PAH) in Switzerland, Austria and West Germany. (Adapted from reference 3.)*

for the pulmonary circulation to constrict or proliferate when exposed to an offending agent is probably a genetic susceptibility.

FENFLURAMINE DERIVATIVES

Fenfluramine derivatives (D,L-fenfluramine and dexfenfluramine) are phenylethylanine derivatives that have been widely prescribed as anorectic drugs since the early 1960s.[7]

Several cases of fenfluramine-associated pulmonary arterial hypertension have been reported since 1981.[8–20] For some patients, the condition resolved completely after withdrawal of the drug, although reversibility is debatable.[8,9,15] In 1981, Douglas and coworkers published two case of fenfluramine-associated PAH in women who had taken fenfluramine over 8 months for weight reduction.[8] In these patients, symptoms occurred, respectively, 35 weeks and 18 months after fenfluramine commencement. After drug discontinuation, both symptoms and electrocardiographic signs of pulmonary hypertension disappeared within 6 and 3 weeks, respectively. In one patient, pulmonary hypertension recurred 6 weeks later after rechallenge with fenfluramine. In 1990, Pouwels reported the case of a 58-year-old woman who developed severe pulmonary hypertension after 11 months of fenfluramine intake; in this patient, symptoms disappeared within 3 weeks after fenfluramine withdrawal and pulmonary artery pressure returned to normal value within 3 months.[10]

In 1993, Brenot and coworkers studied a group of 73 'PPH' patients and found that about 25% of them had been exposed to fenfluramine.[13] This marked increase

followed the large increase in the sales of fenfluramines in France after the introduction of dexfenfluramine in the market (1985–92). All of the 15 patients reported were women who had been exposed to fenfluramine derivatives for at least 3 months with a close temporal relation between fenfluramine derivative use and development of symptoms related to pulmonary hypertension. Eight patients developed dyspnea approximately 12 months after the beginning of fenfluramine therapy. There were nine current users in whom symptoms suggestive of PPH had appeared or worsened during fenfluramine use, and six previous users whose symptoms developed after fenfluramine discontinuation. The time between onset of symptoms and diagnosis of pulmonary hypertension was about 20 months. The outcome of pulmonary hypertension was not favorable in most of patients, even after drug withdrawal. In fatal cases the lungs showed pulmonary arteriopathy with plexiforms lesions.[9,11,13]

Finally, the International Primary Pulmonary Hypertension Study (IPPHS) found a clear association between appetite suppressants and pulmonary hypertension, with an odds ratio (relative risk estimates) of 6.3 (95% CI: 3.0–13.2).[14] Ninety per cent of cases for whom a defined product could be traced had used a fenfluramine derivatives.[14] The risk increased markedly with duration of use (relative risk estimate of 23.1, for more than 3 months, 95% CI: 6.9–77.7; Figure 13E.3) and decreased after cessation of the drug.[14] Belgian investigators showed that in the absence of any restriction to the prescription of appetite suppressants, more than half the patients with PPH presented with a history of previous intake of these drugs.[18] In this study, patients with previous intake of appetite suppressants appeared to be more severely ill,

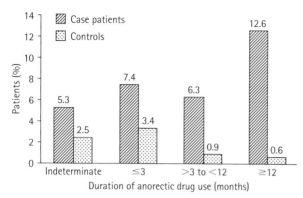

Figure 13E.3 *Duration of exposure to anorectic drugs in patients before the onset of symptoms of pulmonary hypertension. The risk increased markedly with duration of anorectic drug use (relative risk estimate of 23.1, for more than 3 months, 95% confidence interval: 6.9–77.7). (Adapted from reference 14© 2004 Massachusetts Medical Society. All rights reserved.)*

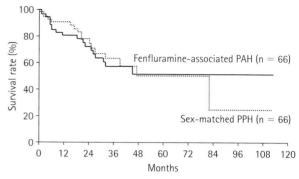

Figure 13E.4 *Overall survival of a group of 66 patients with fenfluramine-associated pulmonary arterial hypertension (PAH; solid line) compared with that of a sex-matched group of 66 primary pulmonary hypertension patients (PPH; dashed line). Survival rates in the two patient populations are similar of about 65% at 2 years and 50% at 5 years. In each group, one half of patients have been treated with long-term epoprostenol infusion. (Adapted from references 17 and 21.)*

with a more rapid progression of the disease and a reduced survival.[18] Between 1986 and 1998, 66 patients with fenfluramine-associated PAH were referred to our institution.[17,21] This group of fenfluramine-exposed patients did not differ from a sex-matched PPH control group in terms of clinical presentation, severity, hemodynamics at diagnosis and overall survival (Figure 13E.4). Only the rate of responders to acute vasodilator challenge was lower in the fenfluramine-associated PAH.[17,21] In France, the regulations regarding the prescription of appetite suppressants have been changed as recently as June 1995, leading to a major restriction of their use. In September 1997, fenfluramine and dexfenfluramine were recalled from the global world market. In our institution, the annual incidence of fenfluramine-associated PAH increased from 1986 to reach a maximum in 1994. Since the beginning of 1997, the incidence has dropped sharply with less than 3 cases per year (Figure 13E.5).

Similar cases of fenfluramine- or dexfenfluramine-induced pulmonary arterial hypertension were reported in the USA after the introduction of these agents in the market and/or after the large increase in the use of the combination of fenfluramine and phentermine ('phen-fen').[15,22,23] The Surveillance of North American Pulmonary Hypertension (SNAP) Study recently confirmed a clear association between the use of fenfluramine derivatives and the diagnosis of pulmonary hypertension.[23] The withdrawal of these agents in September 1997 may well have aborted an incipient epidemic in North America, all the more since the risk of developing the condition increases with the duration of use of fenfluramines. Moreover, these anorexigens also may have precipitated the occurrence of pulmonary arterial hypertension in patients with other underlying conditions such as collagen vascular diseases.[23]

The pathogenetic mechanisms of pulmonary hypertension associated to fenfluramine derivatives remain unknown.[17] However, it appears that alteration of the serotonin (5-hydroxytryptamine, 5-HT) pathway might be a common denominator.[7,24,25] Serotonin is known to be a powerful pulmonary vasoconstrictor and can induce platelet aggregation.[25] Moreover, serotonin is also a potent factor stimulating pulmonary smooth muscle proliferation.[26] Recent studies support the hypothesis that fenfluramine derivatives may contribute to pulmonary arterial hypertension by increasing serotonin availability and/or by interacting with serotonin receptors, thus promoting pulmonary vascular smooth muscle proliferation, pulmonary arterial vasoconstriction and local microthrombosis.[25] Under normal conditions, the lung vascular bed is not exposed to excessive serotonin levels, because virtually all blood serotonin is stored in the platelets and free serotonin is rapidly metabolized by the endothelial monoamine oxidase in the liver and the lung endothelium. By interacting with the serotonin transporter, fenfluramine derivatives release serotonin from platelets and inhibit its reuptake into platelet and pulmonary endothelial cells.[7] As a consequence, blood free serotonin concentration increases with fenfluramine treatment.[24] There is some evidence to indicate that such abnormality in platelet serotonin storage is a trigger factor in the development of pulmonary arterial hypertension in susceptible patients:

• A decrease in platelet serotonin storage with enhanced blood concentration of free serotonin has been reported in sporadic case of PPH, and in numerous disorders occasionally associated with PAH, including portal hypertension, Raynaud's phenomenon, collagen vascular disease, and platelet storage pool disease.[25,27,28]

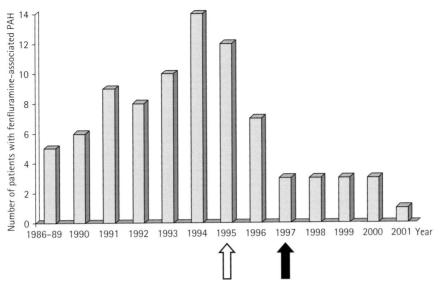

Figure 13E.5 *Annual incidence of fenfluramine-associated pulmonary arterial hypertension (PAH) cases in Paris-Sud University (1986–2001). In France, the regulations regarding the prescription of appetite suppressants have been changed as recently as June 1995 (white arrow) leading to a major restriction of their use. In September 1997 (black arrow), fenfluramine and dexfenfluramine were recalled from the global world market. (Adapted from references 17 and 21.)*

- Platelet serotonin storage remains impaired in PPH patients after heart/lung transplantation, whereas it is normal in patients with secondary pulmonary hypertension, indicating that this platelet dysfunction is not secondary to the pulmonary vascular disease.[28]
- The fawn-hooded rat, which has a genetic defect in serotonin platelet storage, develops severe pulmonary hypertension upon exposure to modest hypoxia.[25]
- Fenfluramine in association, or not, with phentermine has been shown to induce a valvular heart disease very similar to those observed after exposure to serotonin-like drugs such as ergotamine and methysergide, and with increased serotonin levels associated with carcinoid disease.[29] Interestingly, one-third of these patients with valvular heart disease had coexisting pulmonary hypertension.[29] All these observations suggest that fenfluramine may trigger pulmonary hypertension by aggravating or inducing impairment in platelet serotonin storage.

Additional mechanisms seem to be involved in triggering the occurrence of fenfluramine derivative-associated pulmonary hypertension:

- Aminorex and fenfluramine derivatives inhibit potassium current flux in rat pulmonary vascular smooth muscle and may therefore stimulate pulmonary vasoconstriction.[30] This inhibition is implicated in the pulmonary artery vasoconstriction observed in rat and dog lungs after fenfluramine or serotonin exposure.[30,31]
- Because inhibition of nitric oxide synthase markedly potentiated the vasoconstrictor effect of

fenfluramine in isolated rat lung, it has been speculated that patients who develop pulmonary hypertension while taking an anorectic agent could have a pre-existing diminished nitric oxide activity.[30] Such a defect has been demonstrated in a small series of patients suffering with severe fenfluramine-associated pulmonary hypertension.[32]
- Lastly, poor metabolizers of fenfluramine derivatives may have a more pronounced exposure to the drug and therefore may be more prone to develop the condition, as recently suggested.[33] Fenfluramine and dexfenfluramine are metabolized by cytochrome P450-2D6, an enzyme that shows a marked genetic polymorphism. Lack of the functional enzyme (poor metabolizers), occurs in 8% of the general Caucasian population. Higenbottam and colleagues have shown that the frequency of the poor metabolizer genotype of cytochrome P450-2D6 was greater in patients with PAH who had taken fenfluramine or dexfenfluramine (6/26; 23%), compared to PPH patients (1/39; 3%), pulmonary hypertension associated with other disease (2/26; 8%) and healthy control (15/201; 7%).[33]

Only a minority of individuals exposed to fenfluramine derivatives will develop pulmonary hypertension, suggesting that this subset of patients could have a genetic susceptibility.[14,17] Recent genetic studies have identified mutations in the bone morphogenetic protein receptor 2 gene (*BMPR2*) – a receptor member of the transforming growth factor-β (TGF-β) family – in a majority of familial cases of PPH.[34,35] Interestingly, more than 25% of patients displaying sporadic PPH have mutations in the *BMPR2*

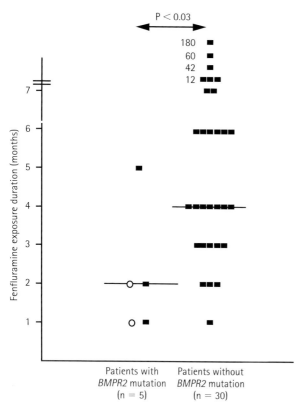

Figure 13E.6 *Duration of fenfluramine derivatives exposure in* BMPR2 *mutants (n = 5) versus patients without* BMPR2 *mutations (n = 30). The duration of exposure to fenfluramine derivatives (fenfluramine or dexfenfluramine) was significantly shorter in* BMPR2 *mutants compared to patients without* BMPR2 *mutations (P < 0.03). Circles indicate familial cases (two sisters), and squares indicate sporadic cases.[38]*

gene, emphasizing the relevance of genetic susceptibility for this severe condition.[36] Other molecular processes behind the complex vascular changes associated with pulmonary arterial hypertension are currently being investigated, including vasoconstrictor/vasodilator imbalance, thrombosis, misguided angiogenesis, and inflammation.[1,37] In PPH, the distinctive vascular changes are found in the precapillary arteries. The same pathology is found in pulmonary arterial hypertension of various origins such as collagen vascular diseases, HIV infection, portal hypertension, congenital systemic-to-pulmonary shunts, and anorexigen exposure.[1] A recent study sought to determine if patients developing pulmonary arterial hypertension after exposure to appetite suppressants fenfluramine and dexfenfluramine have mutations in the *BMPR2* gene, as reported in PPH.[38] *BMPR2* mutations were determined in 33 unrelated patients with sporadic pulmonary arterial hypertension plus two sisters with familial pulmonary arterial hypertension, all of whom had taken fenfluramine derivatives, as well as in 130 normal controls. Three new *BMPR2* mutations predicting changes in the primary

structure of the *BMPR2* protein were found in three of the 33 unrelated patients (9%), and a fourth new mutation was found in the two sisters. No *BMPR2* mutations were identified in the 130 normal controls. This difference in frequency was statistically significant (P = 0.015). Moreover, the mutation-positive patients had a somewhat shorter duration of fenfluramine exposure before illness than the mutation-negative patients, a difference that was statistically significant when the two sisters were included in the analysis. *BMPR2* mutations appear to be rare in the general population but may combine with exposure to fenfluramine derivatives to greatly increase the risk of developing severe PAH. The difference in exposure time suggested that these drugs could provide a risk factor for pulmonary hypertension in those patients with mutations even after a short exposure (Figure 13E.6).[38] Nevertheless, most patients had no *BMPR2* mutations, suggesting that other genetic or environmental factors could be involved in this condition. The authors further concluded that the onset of disease may require 'two events', namely the presence of a heterozygous germline mutation followed by the use of a fenfluramine derivative. Also, other genes and mechanisms associated with appetite suppressant pulmonary hypertension remain to be characterized.

AMPHETAMINES

Phentermine has been used as an appetite suppressant since the 1960s. During the aminorex epidemic, a survey found that cases of pulmonary hypertension had used phentermine.[39] In the mid-1990s, a large increase in the use of phentermine occurred in the USA due to the popular 'phen-fen' combination.[22] A few cases of PPH with phentermine use alone have been reported (LJ Rubin, personal communication).

Chlorphentermine and phenmetrazine were suggested to contribute to the development of pulmonary hypertension, but no report has been issued in humans since 1972.[40]

In our institution, several patients with an isolated exposure to amphetamine derivatives such as amfepramone and clobenzorex have been clearly identified.[21] In contrast to fenfluramine-associated PAH, no close temporal relationship between the onset of amphetamine intake and that of symptoms related to pulmonary hypertension was clearly demonstrated. Furthermore, it is not yet clear whether amphetamines alone can cause the disease.[19]

OTHER SEROTONIN REUPTAKE INHIBITORS

The effects of the selective serotonin reuptake inhibitor antidepressant drugs such as fluoxetine on platelet serotonin uptake are very similar to those of fenflu-ramine.[17] However, despite large worldwide use, no case of pulmonary hypertension or valvular heart disease has been yet reported with these drugs. In contrast to fenflu-ramine derivatives, which are serotonin receptors ago-nists in the brain, these antidepressants do not stimulate serotonin receptors. This suggests that the increase in serotonin availability is not the unique mechanism of fenfluramine-associated pulmonary hypertension, and that fenfluramine derivatives might induce pulmonary arterial hypertension by interacting also with serotonin receptors located in the pulmonary arterial wall.[17]

OBESITY

Many detractors of the fact that appetite suppressants could play a role in pulmonary hypertension assumed that obesity by itself was a confounding risk factor for this condition. The international primary pulmonary hyper-tension study (IPPHS) investigators indeed considered whether the association between the use of appetite suppressants and pulmonary hypertension could be explained by the confounding effect of obesity or that of any hidden factor associated with obesity. However, the odds ratio for anorexic agents was similar whether or not the logistic-regression models were adjusted for high body mass index.[14,19,20] The effect of appetite suppres-sants was the same whether patients had a high body mass index or not.[14,19,20] Neither weight-loss behavior of another type nor the use of thyroid extracts was positively associated with the risk of pulmonary hypertension, as would have been expected if obesity accounted for the odds ratio observed for anorexic agents.[14,19,20]

CONCLUSION

The use of fenfluramine derivatives is an established risk factor for pulmonary arterial hypertension. The relative risk is low but does increase markedly in some situations such as long-term use. Therefore, wide-spread uncontrolled use of these drugs could lead to an epidemic of PAH. The pathophysiological link between fenfluramine derivative intake and the develop-ment of PAH remains unclear. However, accumulating evidence suggests a possible role for serotonin. Most patients with fenfluramine-associated PAH had no *BMPR2* mutations, suggesting that other genetic or envi-ronmental factors could be involved in this condition. Unfortunately, the absence of experimental animal models is an important limitation for a better understanding of this condition.

KEY POINTS

- Among anorectic drugs, aminorex fumarate and fenfluramine derivatives are considered as definite risk factors for pulmonary arterial hypertension (PAH), playing a causal role.
- Aminorex was responsible of a epidemic of PAH in the late 1960s.
- Clinical presentation, severity, hemodynamics and overall survival in patients with fenfluramine-associated PAH are very similar to those in patients with primary pulmonary hypertension.
- Reversibility of pulmonary hypertension after appetite suppressant withdrawal is uncommon.
- The pathogenetic mechanisms of pulmonary hypertension associated with fenfluramine derivatives remain unknown. However, it appears that alteration of the serotonin pathway might be a common denominator. By interacting with the serotonin transporter, fenfluramine derivatives release serotonin from platelets and inhibit its reuptake into platelet and pulmonary endothelial cells.
- Only a minority of individuals exposed to fenfluramine derivatives will develop pulmonary hypertension, suggesting that this subset of patients could have a genetic susceptibility. Bone morphogenetic protein receptor 2 mutations were found in only 9% of PAH patients with a history of fenfluramine intake. Nevertheless, most patients had no *BMPR2* mutations, suggesting that other genetic or environmental factors could be involved in this condition.
- Several cases of amphetamine-associated PAH have been reported. However, it is not yet clear whether amphetamines alone can cause the disease.

REFERENCES

●1 Rich S (ed.) *Primary pulmonary hypertension: executive summary from the World Symposium – Primary Pulmonary Hypertension 1998.* Available from the World Health Organization via the Internet (http://www.who.int/ncd/cvd/pph.html).

2 Kay JM, Smith P, Heath D. Aminorex and the pulmonary circulation. *Thorax* 1971;**26**:262–70.

●3 Gurtner HP. Pulmonary hypertension, plexogenic pulmonary arteriopathy and the appetite depressant drug aminorex: post or propter? *Bull Physiopathol Respir (Nancy)* 1979;**15**:897–923.

◆4 Gurtner HP. Aminorex and pulmonary hypertension. A review. *Cor Vasa* 1985;**27**:160–71.

5 Follath F, Burrart F, Schweizer W. Drug-induced pulmonary hypertension? *Br Med J* 1971;**1**:265–6.

6 Loogen F, Worth H, Schwan G *et al.* Long-term follow-up of pulmonary hypertension in patients with and without anorectic drug intake. *Cor Vasa* 1985;**27**:111–24.

◆7 McTavish D, Heel RC. Dexfenfluramine. A review of its pharmacological properties and therapeutic potential in obesity. *Drugs* 1992;**43**:713–33.

8 Douglas JG, Munro JF, Kitchin AH *et al.* Pulmonary hypertension and fenfluramine. *Br Med J (Clin Res Ed)* 1981;**283**:881–3.

9 McMurray J, Bloomfield P, Miller HC. Irreversible pulmonary hypertension after treatment with fenfluramine [letter]. *Br Med J* 1986;**293**:51–2.

10 Pouwels HM, Smeets JL, Cheriex EC *et al.* Pulmonary hypertension and fenfluramine. *Eur Respir J* 1990;**3**:606–7.

11 Atanassoff PG, Weiss BM, Schmid ER *et al.* Pulmonary hypertension and dexfenfluramine. *Lancet* 1992;**339**:436–7.

12 Roche N, Labrune S, Braun JM *et al.* Pulmonary hypertension and dexfenfluramine. *Lancet* 1992;**339**:436.

13 Brenot F, Hervé P, Petitpretz P *et al.* Primary pulmonary hypertension and fenfluramine use. *Br Heart J* 1993;**70**:537–41.

●14 Abenhaim L, Moride Y, Brenot F *et al.* Appetite-suppressant drugs and the risk of primary pulmonary hypertension. International Primary Pulmonary Hypertension Study Group. *N Engl J Med* 1996;**335**:609–16.

15 Mark EJ, Patalas ED, Chang HT *et al.* Fatal pulmonary hypertension associated with short-term use of fenfluramine and phentermine. *N Engl J Med* 1997;**337**:602–6.

16 Voelkel NF, Clarke WR, Higenbottam T. Obesity, dexfenfluramine, and pulmonary hypertension. A lesson not learned? *Am J Respir Crit Care Med* 1997;**155**:786–8.

17 Simonneau G, Fartoukh M, Sitbon O *et al.* Primary pulmonary hypertension associated with the use of fenfluramine derivatives. *Chest* 1998;**114**:195S–9S.

18 Delcroix M, Kurz X, Walckiers D *et al.* High incidence of primary pulmonary hypertension associated with appetite suppressants in Belgium. *Eur Respir J* 1998;**12**:271–6.

19 Abenhaim L, Rich S, Benichou J *et al.* Primary pulmonary hypertension and anorectic drugs. *N Engl J Med* 1999;**340**:481.

◆20 Abenhaim L, Humbert M. Pulmonary hypertension related to drugs and toxins. *Curr Opin Cardiol* 1999;**14**:437–41.

21 Fartoukh M, Sitbon O, Humbert M *et al.* Primary pulmonary hypertension associated with the use of anorectic drugs. *Eur Respir J* 1998;**12**:141s (abstract).

◆22 Fishman AP. Aminorex to fen/phen: an epidemic foretold. *Circulation* 1999;**99**:156–61.

23 Rich S, Rubin L, Walker AM *et al.* Anorexigens and pulmonary hypertension in the United States: results from the surveillance of North American pulmonary hypertension. *Chest* 2000;**117**:870–4.

24 Martin F, Artigas F. Simultaneous effects of *p*-chloramphetamine, D-fenfluramine, and reserpine on free blood and stored 5-HT in brain and blood. *J Neurochem* 1992;**59**:1138–44.

◆25 Egermayer P, Town GI, Peacock AJ. Role of serotonin in the pathogenesis of acute and chronic pulmonary hypertension. *Thorax* 1999;**54**:161–8.

26 Fanburg BL, Lee SL. A new role for an old molecule: serotonin as a mitogen. *Am J Physiol* 1997;**16**:795–806.

27 Herve P, Drouet L, Dosquet C *et al.* Primary pulmonary hypertension in a patient with a familial platelet storage pool disease: role of serotonin. *Am J Med* 1990;**89**:117–20.

28 Herve P, Launay JM, Scrobohaci ML *et al.* Increased plasma serotonin in primary pulmonary hypertension. *Am J Med* 1995;**99**:249–54.

●29 Connolly HM, Crary JL, McGoon MD *et al.* Valvular heart disease associated with fenfluramine-phentermine. *N Engl J Med* 1997;**337**:581–8.

30 Weir EK, Reeve HL, Huang JM *et al.* Anorexic agents aminorex, fenfluramine, and dexfenfluramine inhibit potassium current in rat pulmonary vascular smooth muscle and cause pulmonary vasoconstriction. *Circulation* 1996;**94**:2216–20.

31 Naeije R, Wauthy P, Maggiorini M *et al.* Effects of dexfenfluramine on hypoxic pulmonary vasoconstriction and embolic pulmonary hypertension in dogs. *Am J Respir Crit Care Med* 1995;**151**:692–7.

32 Archer SL, Djaballah K, Humbert M *et al.* Nitric oxide deficiency in fenfluramine- and dexfenfluramine-induced pulmonary hypertension. *Am J Respir Crit Care Med* 1998;**158**:1061–7.

33 Higenbottam T, Humbert M, Simonneau G *et al.* Subjects deficient for CYP2D6 expression (poor metabolizers) are over-represented among patients with anorectic associated pulmonary hypertension. *Am J Respir Crit Care Med* 1999;**159**:A165 (abstract).

34 Deng Z, Morse JH, Slager SL *et al.* Familial primary pulmonary hypertension (gene *PPH1*) is caused by mutations in the bone morphogenetic protein receptor-II gene. *Am J Hum Genet* 2000;**67**:737–44.

●35 The International PPH Consortium. Heterozygous germline mutations in *BMPR2*, encoding a TGF-β receptor, cause familial primary pulmonary hypertension. *Nat Genet* 2000;**26**:81–4.

36 Thomson JR, Machado RD, Pauciulo MW *et al.* Sporadic primary pulmonary hypertension is associated with germline mutations of the gene encoding BMPR-II, a receptor member of the TGF-β family. *J Med Genet* 2000;**37**:741–5.

◆37 Voelkel NF, Tuder RM. Cellular and molecular mechanisms in the pathogenesis of severe pulmonary hypertension. *Eur Respir J* 1995;**8**:2129–38.

38 Humbert M, Deng Z, Simonneau G *et al.* BMPR2 germline mutations in pulmonary hypertension associated with fenfluramine derivatives. *Eur Respir J* 2002;**20**:518–23.

39 Backman R. Primäre pulmonale hypertonie. In: Steinkopff D (ed.), *Verhandlungen der deutschen Gesellschaft für Kreislaufforschungh.* Darmstadt: Verlag, 1972;134–41.

40 Fuller RW. Serotonin uptake inhibitors: use in clinical therapy and in laboratory research. *Prog Drug Res* 1995;**45**:167–204.

Pulmonary hypertension associated with portal hypertension

PHILIPPE HERVÉ, GÉRALD SIMONNEAU, MARC HUMBERT AND OLIVIER SITBON

DEFINITION

The diagnosis of portopulmonary hypertension (POPH) is based on pulmonary hemodynamic criteria obtained via right heart catheterization. POPH can be defined as a pulmonary arterial hypertension (PAH) associated with portal hypertension with or without hepatic disease. Diagnostic criteria include a mean pulmonary artery pressure (PAP) > 25 mmHg at rest or 30 mmHg during exercise, with pulmonary artery occlusion pressure (PAOP) under 15 mmHg. A moderate increase in mean PAP (25–35 mmHg) is frequent in up to 20% of patients with cirrhosis and portal hypertension.[1–3] This increase in PAP is mainly passive (with minimum pulmonary vascular remodeling) in relation to the increases in cardiac output and/or blood volume, and is associated with near-normal pulmonary vascular resistance (PVR) and normal or increased PAOP. By contrast, a severe PAH with extensive pulmonary vascular remodeling and elevated PVR is more rarely observed in patients with portal hypertension. This latter condition represents the entity of POPH and is associated with poor outcome. To distinguish between these two forms of PH the following criteria have been proposed[4,5] for the diagnosis of POPH:

- increase in mean mean PAP at rest > 25 mmHg;
- increase in PVR > 120 dyn s/cm^5 [PVR being calculated as (mean PAP − mean PAOP)/(cardiac output) × 80]; and
- normal PAOP < 15 mmHg.

PH associated with cirrhosis and/or portal hypertension was initially subclassified in the 1981 NIH Registry for Characterization of Primary PH (PPH)[6] as a clinical subset of PPH. POPH was classified in 1993 as a form of secondary PH in the PH Consensus Statement of the American College of Chest Physicians.[7] In 1998, at the second World Symposium on PPH,[8] POPH was classified as one of the forms of PAH associated with various causes including: collagen vascular disease, congenital systemic-to-pulmonary shunts, portal hypertension, HIV infection, drugs/toxins and anorexigens. This new classification is based on the observations that the pathological features of PAH associated with these causes are indistinguishable from those observed in PPH.

Incidence and epidemiology

The first retrospective autopsy study showed that in 17 901 autopsied patients the prevalence of PAH was 0.73% in patients with portal hypertension or cirrhosis,[9] as compared with only 0.13% in the general population. In a clinical study in 2459 patients with biopsy-proven cirrhosis, the prevalence of clinical PH was 0.61%.[9] Two prospective hemodynamic studies conducted by Naeije et al.[10] and Hadengue et al.[11] in patients with portal hypertension found a prevalence of 2%. Recent studies[12–15] indicated a 3.1–4.7% incidence of moderate POPH in patients with severe liver disease. Taken together, these studies suggest an incidence of less than 1% of **severe** PAH in portal hypertension.

Portal hypertension is a causative factor in a about 10% of the cases of PAH. Among the 735 patients with suspected PAH referred from 1981 to 1999 to our pneumology department, 11.1% had portal hypertension. In 1995, a case–control study[16] found that cirrhosis was present in 7.3% of the patients with PAH versus none in the controls.

HISTOLOGY

Pulmonary pathology in patients with POPH consists of the same patterns of pulmonary arteriopathy as in patients with PPH or PAH associated with various causes.[18] Two rare histological patterns of PH, namely pulmonary veno-occlusive disease and pulmonary capillary hemangiomatosis, have not been reported in POPH.

ETIOLOGY

Portal hypertension induces systemic inflammatory changes and increased vascular wall shear stress, which may trigger a cascade of intracellular signals and/or cause activation or repression of various genes in the endothelial and/or smooth muscle cells that could lead to pulmonary vascular remodeling in susceptible patients.

Mutations in BMPR2[18] and ALK-1,[19] genes that encode members of the transforming growth factor-β (TGF-β) receptor superfamily, recently reported in familial and sporadic PPH, have not been found in patients with POPH (M Humbert personal communication, 2002).

Compared with controls, patients with PPH more frequently carry the LL variant of serotonin transporter.[20] This was not found in POPH (S Adnot, personal communication).

Increased levels of several inflammatory mediators, cytokines, or growth factors have been demonstrated in patients with portal hypertension.[21] The incidence of bacterial translocation, i.e. dissemination of gut lumen bacteria within the body, is increased in cirrhosis.[22] Normally, the lung vascular bed is not exposed to large amounts of bacterial products: these are filtered out by the liver, whose Kupffer cells clear nearly all gut bacteria and bacterial endotoxins from the bloodstream.[23] In cirrhosis, the development of portosystemic shunts and the dramatic decrease in the phagocytic capacity of the liver allow circulating bacteria or bacterial endotoxins to enter the pulmonary circulation. In rats with biliary cirrhosis, the lungs clear the blood of gut bacteria and endotoxins,[23] thereby compensating for the decrease in liver phagocytic function. This increase in pulmonary phagocytic activity is ascribable to extensive accumulation of pulmonary intravascular macrophages that adhere to the pulmonary endothelium of the pulmonary arteries and capillaries.[24] During phagocytosis, activated macrophages release numerous secretory products into the extracellular environment, including cytokines, growth factors and nitric oxide (NO).[25] This pulmonary phagocytosis has been demonstrated in cirrhotic patients,[26] suggesting that induction of pulmonary intravascular macrophages might contribute to development of pulmonary vascular disease seen in these patients, such as hepatopulmonary syndrome (HPS) and POPH. Interestingly, several studies lend support also to the presence of activated macrophages in patients with other form of PAH.[27–29]

Alternatively, it has been hypothesized that a substance which exits the liver via the hepatic veins may control angiogenesis. Patients with congenital heart disease develop diffuse pulmonary arteriovenous malformations after anastomosis of the superior vena cava to the right pulmonary artery.[30] No such abnormalities have been reported after total cavopulmonary anastomosis, which directs the entire systemic venous return, including hepatic venous blood to the pulmonary arterial bed. Moreover, redirection of hepatic venous flow to the pulmonary bed either by surgical inclusion of hepatic vein,[31] or by heart transplantation can reverse these vascular abnormalities.[32,33] These findings suggest that the absence of a hepatic agent in the pulmonary vasculature, by virtue of either poor hepatic synthetic function or decreased hepatic venous blood flow, results in exaggerated angiogenesis. This factor could be the angiogenesis inhibitor endostatin because the liver is the major source of collagen XVIII, the precursor of the endostatin.[34]

CLINICAL PRESENTATION

Our patients with POPH were older than those reported in the literature[1] in relation to the higher prevalence of alcoholic cirrhosis. The sex ratio was 1.1:1, whereas there was a 2:1 female bias in our patients with PPH, in agreement with other studies of patients with POPH.[1,35] Given the male preponderance of alcoholic cirrhosis, this suggests that female hormones may be an independent risk factor for POPH.

In our series, antinuclear antibodies were present in 19% of patients with POPH and 14% of those with PPH. Other serological markers for autoimmune disorders were also positive in a significant number of patients with POPH.[1]

A non-hepatic cause of portal hypertension was present in 10% of our patients, including three with Budd–Chiari syndrome. This is consistent with other series and case reports,[1] indicating that portal hypertension rather than liver disease is the key factor for the development of POPH. The severity of liver failure, as estimated by the

Child Pugh's score, was not correlated with PVR in our experience as well as in the study by Hadengue *et al.*[11] In most series, the diagnosis of portal hypertension antedated that of POPH in the majority of the patients.

In the study of Hadengue *et al.*,[11] 60% of patients with POPH were asymptomatic, and PVR values were lower in asymptomatic patients. In our series, NYHA grades of dyspnea were lower in the patients with portal hypertension than in those with PPH. There were no significant differences in the frequency of chest pain, syncope, or hemoptysis.

Mean PAP was lower in our patients with POPH (n = 100) than with PPH (n = 300), (55 ± 11 versus 63 ± 12 mmHg, respectively, P = 0.02), whereas cardiac index and mixed venous oxygen saturation were higher (2.9 ± 0.7 versus 2.2 ± 0.6 L/min·m^2, and 66 ± 10 versus 58 ± 8 %, P = 0.0004), yielding lower calculated total PVR values (30 ± 9 versus 21 ± 7 mmHg/L/min·m^2). The other hemodynamic values were similar in the two groups. These findings are comparable to those previously reported.[35]

The results of pharmacological vasodilation testing using inhaled NO were different in our two groups, with decreases from baseline in mean total PVR of 26 ± 9% versus 3 ± 7%, and of mean PAP of 9 ± 9% versus 3 ± 3% in POPH and PPH (P < 0.001 for both), respectively. According to Kneussl *et al.*,[36] 16% of patients were classified as responders (reduction of total PVR ≥ 20% and reduction of mean mean PAP ≥ 20%) in the PPH group and none in the POPH group. This could be related to persistent lung NO overproduction in POPH.

Patients with POPH are generally believed to have substantially shorter survival rate than PPH patients.[1] By contrast, actual survivals at 1, 2 and 5 years in our POPH and PPH groups were 76% versus 64%, 72% versus 54% and 50% versus 25%, respectively (P < 0.05). Similar findings were reported in a recent study.[14]

The diagnosis of POPH based on clinical presentation is challenging because many of the symptoms of POPH are present in patients with advanced liver disease without POPH. Moreover, many POPH patients are asymptomatic at the time of diagnosis. Two-dimensional and Doppler echocardiography should be routinely performed as a primary screening procedure, especially in patients undergoing a preoperative liver transplant evaluation. When suspected of POPH, these patients should undergo right heart catheterization.

MANAGEMENT AND TREATMENT

Medical treatment

Anticoagulation is not recommended in POPH patients with high risk of bleeding from the gastrointestinal tract.

Beta-blocking agent therapy is not advisable because it can further decrease cardiac output.

Long-term prostacyclin or epoprostenol therapy given by continuous intravenous infusion improves exercise tolerance, quality of life and survival in patients with PPH independently of the presence of a positive response to NO.[37] Although randomized controlled trials have not been performed, several case series have shown substantial improvement of exercise tolerance with compassionate use of prostacyclin in NYHA class III or IV POPH patients.[38–40] In our patients with severe POPH (NYHA class III and IV), 2-year prostacyclin treatment (mean dosage 28 ± 8 ng/kg·min) improved pulmonary hemodynamic and exercise tolerance to a greater magnitude than in our patients with PPH of similar severity. The 6-minute walking distance improved by 157 ± 55 meters, pulmonary arterial pressure decreased by 25 ± 10%, cardiac index increased by 43 ± 10% and the total PVR decreased by 45 ± 8%. The 5-year actuarial survival rate was similar in these POPH patients treated with prostacyclin as compared with POPH patients under conventional treatment. It has been recently reported that continuous prostacyclin was followed by the development of progressive splenomegaly, with worsening thrombocytopenia and leukopenia in four POPH patients. This complication may limit the usefulness of prostacyclin in POPH patients.[41] Inhaled iloprost and oral beraprost may be used in class I and II POPH patients.[42,43] Because of hepatic safety concerns, the endothelin receptor antagonist bosentan should not be administered to patients with POPH.[37]

Liver transplantation

There have been reports of improvement, persistence, or development of POPH following liver transplantation.[1] In the retrospective studies from Taura *et al.*,[13] Castro *et al.*[12] and Starkel *et al.*,[44] postoperative complications and mortality were similar in the patients with and without moderate POPH. Krowka *et al.*[45] have recently established recommendations on the advisability of liver transplantation at different levels of POPH. The risk of mortality was 100% for the patients with a mean PAP > 50 mmHg, 50% with mean PAP between 35 and 50 mmHg and PVR > 250 dyn s/cm^5, and 0% with mean pulmonary arterial pressure < 35 mmHg. The management of patients with POPH requires early diagnosis and chronic therapy with intravenous prostacyclin to decrease PVR. A reduction of PVR under 250 dyn s/cm^5 and an increase to normal value of cardiac index with intravenous prostacyclin may facilitate successful liver transplantation. Further studies of outcomes are needed to determine the role of liver transplantation in patients with POPH. In the patients with refractory POPH, combined liver and (heart/)lung transplantation remains the only therapeutic option.[46]

HPS AND POPH

Vachiery et al.[47] recently showed that patients with hypoxemia did not have POPH, and vice versa. In a recent prospective study, Swanson and Krowka[48] reported that hypoxemia was usually mild even in the setting of moderate-to-severe POPH.

Severe hypoxemia and POPH has been reported however, in patients with right-to-left intracardiac shunt through a patent foramen ovale,[49] or with intrapulmonary shunt,[50–58] indicating that HPS and POPH are not mutually exclusive complications of portal hypertension. POPH usually occurs in patients with a pre-existing HPS and is associated with a marked improvement in dyspnea and gas exchange with normalization of the intrapulmonary shunt.[49]

SUMMARY

The pathophysiology of portopulmonary hypertension (POPH) may involve an imbalance between factors inhibiting and stimulating pulmonary vascular cells proliferation. POPH is not an uncommon complication of portal hypertension. Intravenous prostacyclin improves hemodynamics, exercise tolerance and survival and may facilitate liver transplantation that has an uncertain effect in POPH.

KEY POINTS

- The incidence of severe pulmonary arterial hypertension in patients with cirrhosis and/or portal hypertension is about 1%.
- Since portopulmonary hypertension have been reported in patients with non-hepatic portal hypertension, the common factor that determines its development must be portal hypertension.
- Patients with portopulmonary hypertension do not usually respond to acute vasodilator testing with NO, whereas they benefit from long-term intravenous prostacyclin treatment.
- Orthotopic liver transplantation does not resolve portopulmonary hypertension in the vast majority of cases.

REFERENCES

◆1 Mandell SM, Groves BM. PH in liver disease. Clin Chest Med 1996;**17**:17–33.
●2 Castro M, Krowka MJ, Schroeder DR et al. Frequency and clinical implications of increased mean PAPs in liver transplantation. Mayo Clin Proc 1996;**71**:543–51.
●3 Auletta M, Oliviero U, Iasiuolo L et al. PH associated with liver cirrhosis: an echocardiographic study. Angiology 2000;**51**:1013–20.
◆4 Krowka MJ. HPS and portoPH: distinctions and dilemmas. Hepatology 1997;**25**:1282–4.
●5 Kuo PC, Plotkin JS, Johnson LB et al. Distinctive clinical features of portoPH. Chest 1997;**112**:980–6.
●6 Rich S, Dantzker DR, Ayres SM. Primary PH: a national prospective study. Ann Intern Med 1987;**107**:216–23.
◆7 Rubin LJ. Primary PH. ACCP consensus statement. Chest 1993;**104**:236–50.
◆8 Fishman AP. Clinical classification of PH. Clin Chest Med 2001;**22**:385–91.
●9 McDonnel PJ, Toye PA, Hutchins GM. Primary PH and cirrhosis: are they related? Am Rev Respir Dis 1983;**127**:437–41.
●10 Naeije R, Melot C, Hallemans R et al. Pulmonary hemodynamics in liver cirrhosis. Semin Respir Med 1985;**7**:164–70.
●11 Hadengue A, Benhayoun MK, Lebrec D et al. PH complicating portal hypertension: prevalence and relation to splanchnic hemodynamics. Gastroenterology 1991;**100**:520–8.
●12 Castro M, Krowka MJ, Schroeder DR et al. Frequency and clinical implications of increased mean PAPs in liver transplantation. Mayo Clin Proc 1996;**71**:543–51.
●13 Taura P, Garcia-Valdecasas JC, Beltran J et al. Moderate primary PH in patients undergoing liver transplantation. Anesth Analg 1996;**83**:675–80.
●14 Yang YY, Lin HC, Hou MC et al. PortoPH: distinctive hemodynamic and clinical manifestations. J Gastroenterol 2001;**36**:181–6.
●15 Toregrossa M, Genesca J, Gonzalez A et al. Role of Doppler echocardiography in the assessment of portoPH liver transplantation candidates. Transplantation 2001;**71**:572–4.
●16 Abenhaim L, Moride Y, Brenot F et al. Appetite-suppressant drugs and the risk of primary PH. N Engl J Med 1996;**335**:609–16.
◆17 Mandell SM, Groves BM. PH in liver disease. Clin Chest Med 1996;**17**:17–33.
●18 Lane KB, Machado RD, Pauciulo MW et al. Heterozygous germline mutations in BMPR2, encoding a TGF-beta receptor, cause familial primary PH. The International PPH Consortium. Nat Genet 2000;**26**:81–4.
●19 Trembath RC, Thomson JR, Machado RD et al. Clinical and molecular genetic features of PH in patients with hereditary hemorrhagic telangiectasia. N Engl J Med 2001;**345**:325–34.
●20 Eddahibi S, Humbert M, Fadel E et al. Serotonin transporter overexpression is responsible for pulmonary artery smooth muscle hyperplasia in primary PH. J Clin Invest 2001;**108**:1141–50.
◆21 Panos RJ, Backer SK. Mediators, cytokines, and growth factors in liver-lung interactions. Clin Chest Med 1996;**17**:151–69.
◆22 Herve P, Lebrec D, Brenot F et al. Pulmonary vascular disorders in portal hypertension. Eur Respir J 1998;**11**:1153–66.
●23 Miot-Noirault E, Faure L, Guichard Y et al. Scintigraphic in vivo assessment of the development of pulmonary

intravascular macrophages in liver disease: experimental study in rats with biliary cirrhosis. *Chest* 2001;**120**:941–7.

●24 Nunes H, Lebrec D, Mazmanian M *et al.* Role of nitric oxide in HPS in cirrhotic rats. *Am J Respir Crit Care Med* 2001;**164**:879–85.

●25 Laffy G, Foschi M, Simoni A *et al.* Increased production of nitric oxide by neutrophils and monocytes from patients with ascites and hyperdynamic circulation. *Hepatology* 1995;**22**:1666–73.

●26 Keyes JW, Wilson GA, Quinonest JD. An evaluation of lung uptake of colloid during liver imaging. *J Nucl Med* 1973;**14**:687–91.

●27 Galiè NF, Grigioni L, Uguccioni V. Increased levels of TNF-in patients with primary PH. *Eur Heart J* 1997;**18**:A528.

●28 Humbert M, Monti G, Brenot F *et al.* Increased interleukin-1 and interleukin-6 serum concentrations in severe primary PH. *Am J Respir Crit Care Med* 1995;**151**:1628–31.

●29 Raychaudhuri B, Dweik R, Connors MJ *et al.* Nitric oxide blocks nuclear factor-β activation in alveolar macrophages. *Am J Respir Cell Mol Biol* 1999;**21**:311–16.

●30 Srivastava D, Preminger T, Lock JE *et al.* Hepatic venous blood and the development of pulmonary arteriovenous malformations in congenital heart disease. *Circulation* 1995;**92**:1217–22.

●31 Shah MJ, Rychick J, Fogel MA *et al.* Pulmonary arteriovenous malformations after superior cavopulmonary connection: resolution after inclusion of hepatic veins in the pulmonary circulation. *Ann Thorac Surg* 1997;**63**:960–3.

32 Graham K, Sonheimer H, Schaffer M. Resolution of cavopulmonary shunt-associated pulmonary arteriovenous malformation after heart transplantation. *J Heart Transplant* 1997;**16**:1271–4.

33 Lamour JM, Hsu DT, Kichuk MR *et al.* Regression of pulmonary arteriovenous malformations following heart transplantation. *Pediatr Transplant* 2000;**4**:280–4.

●34 Clement B, Musso O, Lietard J *et al.* Homeostatic control of angiogenesis: a newly identified function of the liver? *Hepatology* 1999;**29**:621–3.

◆35 Groves BM, Brundage BH, Elliot CG *et al.* PH associated with hepatic cirrhosis. In: Fishman AP (ed.), *The pulmonary circulation: normal and abnormal.* Philadelphia: University of Pennsylvania Press, 1990;359–69.

◆36 Kneussl MP, Lang IM, Brenot FP. Medical management of primary PH. *Eur Respir J* 1996;**9**:2401–9.

37 Hoeper MM, Galie N, Simonneau G *et al.* New treatments for PAH. *Am J Respir Crit Care Med* 2002;**165**:1209–16.

∗38 McLaughlin VV, Genthner DE, Panella MM *et al.* Compassionate use of continuous prostacyclin in the management of secondary PH: a case series. *Ann Intern Med* 1999;**130**:740–3.

∗39 Krowka MJ, Frantz RP, McGoon MD *et al.* Improvement in pulmonary hemodynamics during intravenous epoprostenol (prostacyclin): a study of 15 patients with moderate to severe portoPH. *Hepatology* 1999; **30**:641–8.

∗40 Kuo PC, Johnson LB, Plotkin JS *et al.* Continuous intravenous infusion of epoprostenol for the treatment of portoPH. *Transplantation* 1997;**63**:604–6.

●41 Findlay JY, Plevak DJ, Krowka MJ *et al.* Progressive splenomegaly after epoprostenol therapy in portoPH. *Liver Transpl Surg* 1999;**5**:362–5.

∗42 Schroeder RA, Rafii AA, Plotkin JS *et al.* Use of aerosolized inhaled epoprostenol in the treatment of portoPH. *Transplantation* 2000;**70**:548–50.

∗43 Galie N, Humbert M, Vachiery JL *et al.* Arterial PH and Beraprost European (ALPHABET) Study Group. Effects of beraprost sodium, an oral prostacyclin analogue, in patients with PAH: a randomized, double-blind, placebo-controlled trial. *J Am Coll Cardiol* 2002;**39**:1496–502.

∗44 Starkel P, Vera A, Gunson B *et al.* Outcome of liver transplantation for patients with PH. *Liver Transpl* 2002;**8**:382–8.

45 Krowka MJ, Plevak DJ, Findlay JY *et al.* Pulmonary hemodynamics and perioperative cardiopulmonary-related mortality in patients with portoPH undergoing liver transplantation. *Liver Transpl* 2000;**6**:443–50.

∗46 Pirenne J, Verleden G, Nevens F *et al.* Combined liver and heart-lung transplantation in liver transplant candidates with refractory portoPH. *Transplantation* 2002;**73**:140–2.

●47 Vachiery F, Moreau R, Hadengue A *et al.* Hypoxemia in patients with cirrhosis: relationship with liver failure and hemodynamic alterations. *J Hepatol* 1997;**27**:492–5.

●48 Swanson KL, Krowka MJ. Arterial oxygenation associated with portoPH. *Chest* 2002;**121**:1869–75.

●49 Raffy O, Sleiman C, Vachiery F *et al.* Refractory hypoxemia during liver cirrhosis: HPS or 'primary PH'. *Am J Respir Crit Care Med* 1996;**153**:1169–71.

●50 Mal H, Burgiere O, Durand F *et al.* PH following HPS in a patient with cirrhosis. *J Hepatol* 1999;**31**:360–4.

●51 Chongsrisawat V, Vivatvakin B, Suwangool P *et al.* Non-cirrhotic portal fibrosis associated with pulmonary arteriovenous communication and PAH. *Southeast Asian J Trop Med Public Health* 1998;**29**:76–9.

●52 Kolan C, Ghuysen A, Lambermont B *et al.* Clinical case of the month. Porto-PH syndrome associated with severe hypoxemia. *Rev Med Liege* 2001;**56**:543–7.

●53 Kaspar MD, Ramsay MA, Shuey CB Jr *et al.* Severe PH and amelioration of HPS after liver transplantation. *Liver Transpl Surg* 1998;**4**:177–9.

●54 Sasaki T, Hasegawa T, Kimura T *et al.* Development of intrapulmonary arteriovenous shunting in postoperative biliary atresia: evaluation by contrast-enhanced echocardiography. *J Pediatr Surg* 2000;**35**:1647–50.

●55 Jones FD, Kuo PC, Johnson LB *et al.* The coexistence of portoPH and HPS. *Anesthesiology* 1999;**90**:626–9.

●56 Krowka MJ, Cortese DA. Pulmonary aspect of liver disease and liver transplantation. *Clin Chest Med* 1989; **10**:593–616.

●57 Dawson A, Elias DJ, Rubenson D *et al.* PH developing after aglucerase therapy in two patients with type I Gaucher disease complicated by the HPS. *Ann Intern Med* 1996;**125**:901–4.

●58 Tasaka S, Kanazawa M, Nakamura H *et al.* An autopsied case of primary PH complicated by HPS. *Nippon Kyobu Shikkan Gakkai Zasshi* 1995;**33**:90–4.

Pulmonary hypertension related to HIV infection

RUDOLF SPEICH

INTRODUCTION

Human immunodeficiency virus (HIV) infection is associated with numerous infectious and non-infectious complications. During the first years of the HIV epidemic, non-infectious conditions such as cardiovascular diseases remained mostly undetected because they were overshadowed by HIV-related opportunistic infections and malignancies. The advent of highly active antiretroviral therapy (HAART) and the increase in survival time of HIV-infected patients saw the emergence of non-infectious complications, such as cardiovascular diseases, including dilated cardiomyopathy, pericardial effusion, non-bacterial thrombotic endocarditis and accelerated atherosclerosis.

In 1987, pulmonary hypertension was reported for the first time, by Kim and Factor,[1] in a 40-year-old homosexual white man with AIDS and membranoproliferative glomerulonephritis. Autopsy of the lungs revealed plexiform lesions. An immune-mediated pathogenesis was postulated, but in contrast to the findings of the glomerular immunohistochemistry, no IgG deposits were found in the pulmonary vessels. One year later, Goldsmith and coworkers described 'primary' pulmonary hypertension in five HIV-infected hemophiliacs and suggested a possible pathogenetic role of treatment with low-purity factor VIII.[2]

Subsequently, two groups reported six cases, each with pulmonary hypertension clinically and pathologically resembling primary pulmonary hypertension (PPH) out of a cohort of 1200 HIV-infected patients, thus both estimating a cumulative incidence of 0.5%.[3,4] Considering the

annual incidence of PPH of 1–2 per million in the general population, these findings strongly suggested an association between HIV infection and pulmonary hypertension. Moreover, the occurrence of the disorder in patients who did not have other possible confounding factors such as use of intravenous drugs, cocaine or amphetamine corroborated the relationship of the two disorders. Therefore, in accordance with these two and further case series,[5–8] the executive summary of the Second World Symposium on Primary Pulmonary Hypertension concluded that HIV infection is a definite risk factor for the development of pulmonary hypertension.[9] Despite the similarity in the clinical and pathological presentation of HIV-related pulmonary hypertension and sporadic PPH, the experts decided from a semantic point of view to use the term pulmonary arterial hypertension related to HIV infection (PAHRH) for the former disorder.

DEFINITIONS

The diagnostic criteria of PAHRH are based on the presence of a sustained elevation of the pulmonary artery pressure without any demonstrable cause. In accordance with the National Institutes of Health (NIH) registry, the diagnosis is based on a mean pulmonary artery pressure of more than 25 mmHg at rest, or more than 30 mmHg on exercise.[10] Furthermore, other known causes for pulmonary hypertension, including congenital or left-sided valvular heart disease, myocardial disease, any significant respiratory, connective-tissue, or chronic thromboembolic disease, and the use of appetite-suppressant agents should be ruled out.

The diagnosis of HIV infection is based on standard serological testing. For classification, the 1993 Revised Centers for Disease Control and Prevention (CDC) Classification System for HIV Infection is still used most widely.[11]

EPIDEMIOLOGY

The risk for the development of pulmonary hypertension is definitely increased in HIV-infected subjects. A large case–control study involving 3349 HIV-infected patients over a period of 5.5 years demonstrated a cumulative incidence of pulmonary hypertension of 0.57%, resulting in an annual incidence of about 0.1%. Compared with the annual incidence of PPH in the general population of 1.7 per million,[12] HIV infection carries a relative risk of pulmonary hypertension of more than 500.

Based on date from the Swiss HIV cohort (Figure 13G.1), the annual incidence of PAHRH remained constant through the past decade with a median value of 0.1% (range 0.04–0.20%). Despite the increase in the proportion of patients treated with HAART, there was no clear trend towards a lower incidence of PAHRH. An Italian study even found an increase in its cumulative incidence from 0.7% in patients treated with nucleoside reverse transcriptase inhibitors to 2.0% in those receiving HAART, in contrast to a significant decrease in the other HIV-related cardiovascular complications.[13] However, the authors do not mention the total number of observed HIV-infected patients and the higher cumulative incidence of PAHRH under HAART may simply reflect the recommendation

known at that time that all patients with PAHRH should be treated with HAART.

ETIOLOGY

PAHRH is characterized clinically and pathologically by the typical features of PPH. Histopathological findings were available from 43 literature cases. Of these, 36 patients (83%) demonstrated plexiform lesions (Plate 13G.1), 5 (12%) medial hypertrophy and intimal fibrosis, and 2 (5%) *in situ* thrombotic changes in addition to the features of PPH. In addition, there are two literature reports of pulmonary veno-occlusive disease in HIV-infected patients.[14,15]

Because of the similarities between PAHRH and PPH, other concomitant risk factors associated with PPH have to be considered. Even though intravenous drug use is frequently associated with PAHRH, according to the second WHO conference only the use of amphetamines is a very likely secondary cause of PAH.[9] In contrast, cocaine is just regarded as a possible risk factor for PAH by these experts. The occurrence of pulmonary hypertension in HIV-negative cocaine users is highly unusual. There are only nine case reports in literature, in which the hemodynamic changes usually were mild[16] and transient.[17] Injection of small particles containing talc may cause granulomas within small pulmonary arteries and lead to increased pulmonary vascular resistance, as shown in autopsy studies.[18] However, several studies conducted in the pre-AIDS era have extensively demonstrated that ordinary heroin does not contain enough crystalline debris to induce pulmonary angiothrombosis.[19] This observation was also confirmed by autoptic studies on intravenous drug users.[20] Moreover, histological specimens of patients with PAHRH showed only occasional birefringent talc particles that usually were located adjacent to and not within the plexiform lesions (Plate 13G.2). In addition, their amount was incongruous with the severity of the vascular changes.[21]

Liver cirrhosis was present in at least 11 of the literature cases of PAHRH. Since there is a very likely association of PAH and portal hypertension secondary to liver cirrhosis with a reported coincidence of up to 2%,[22] liver disease might have contributed at least in part to the development of PAH in some patients.

In more than one-third of the cases described in literature, HIV infection was the sole potential risk factor for PAH. Therefore, it was hypothesized that HIV itself could play a direct role in the pathogenesis of PAHRH. The development of pulmonary hypertension not attributable to chronic hypoxia has been demonstrated in a murine model of AIDS.[23] Recently, human pulmonary artery smooth muscle cells were successfully transfected by a

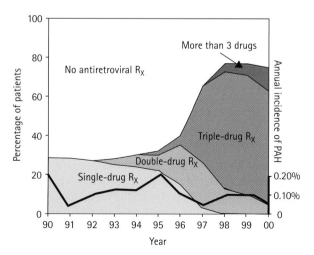

Figure 13G.1 *Annual incidence of PAHRH in the Swiss HIV cohort compared with the percentage of the various antiretroviral treatments (M Opravil, personal communication).*

vesicular stomatitis virus G protein pseudotyped HIV vector *in vitro*.[24] However, neither HIV-1 p24 antigen, Tat protein nor *gag* RNA were found in the affected pulmonary vessels of six cases documented in literature.[25–27] In a study of open lung biopsy specimens from three HIV-infected homosexuals, Mette *et al.* found tuboloreticular structures on electron microscopy and speculated that PAHRH might be caused by a mediator release associated with HIV infection rather than direct endothelial infection.[27] This may be underscored by the increased frequency of HLA-DR52 and HLA-DR6 in patients with PAHRH,[28] since the latter HLA allele is associated with the diffuse infiltrative CD8 lymphocytosis syndrome, which resembles autoimmune Sjögren's disease. A case–control study of two groups of 19 HIV-infected patients each with and without PAH, however, found no difference with respect to various autoantibodies, except for a higher prevalence of anti-SS B in the PAHRH group.[6] In contrast to the absence of HIV in the pulmonary vasculature, there is a single case report of a patient with AIDS and pulmonary hypertension who showed extensive microvascular endothelialitis caused by cytomegalovirus at autopsy.[29]

Another possibility is that PAHRH results from the production of growth factors, either directly related to HIV or mediated through infected T cells, which may cause pulmonary arteriolar endothelial cell proliferation. A regulatory gene from the HIV-1 triggering the growth of dermal lesions resembling Kaposi's sarcoma in transgenic mice[30] and a growth factor elaborated by HIV-infected T cells that stimulates Kaposi's sarcoma cells in culture[31] have been described. However, the risk of developing Kaposi's sarcoma seems not to be increased in patents with PAHRH since this complication was described in only two of the literature cases.[3,32] Recently, Humbert *et al.* found an increased expression of platelet-derived growth factor (PDGF) in perivascular cells of two patients with PAHRH.[26] PDGF has the ability to induce the proliferation and migration of smooth muscle cells and fibroblasts, and it has been proposed to be a key mediator in several fibroproliferative disorders including hypoxic pulmonary vasoconstriction.

Mutations of the bone morphogenetic protein receptor type II gene (*BMPR2*), a component of the transforming growth factor-β (TGF-β) family have recently been identified to cause familial PPH. It is well known that BMPs regulate growth, differentiation and apoptosis in a diverse number of cell lines, including mesenchymal and epithelial cells. It was hypothesized that the *BMPR2* mutation may lead to an abnormal response of the pulmonary vasculature to various endogenous or exogenous stimuli predisposing to the development of PPH.[33] Interestingly, the *BMPR2* mutation of familial PPH could also be detected in 13 out of 50 cases of sporadic PPH.[34] Thus, in at least one-quarter of the sporadic PPH cases a genetic predisposition plays an important pathogenetic role. However, it is

unlikely that this is the case for PAHRH since in none of the 30 patients tested so far the *BMPR2* mutation could be detected (G Simonneau and R Trembath, personal communication).

In analogy to PPH, endothelin-1 may play a role in the pathogenesis of PAHRH. Ehrenreich *et al.* could demonstrate that the HIV-1 envelope glycoprotein gp120 stimulates the secretion of endothelin-1 from macrophages in a concentration-dependent manner.[35] Furthermore, they found that in HIV-infected individuals circulating monocytes show a distinct expression of the endothelin-1 gene which is not detectable in healthy controls, indicating chronic activation of this gene in HIV-infection. So far, however, elevated endothelin-1 immunoreactivity has been demonstrated only for the HIV-associated retinal microangiopathic syndrome.[36] Further evidence for a pathogenetic role of endogenous vasoactive substances stems from a recent study, which showed a marked reduction in the expression of prostacyclin synthase in two patients with PAHRH, comparable to the findings in PPH.[37] The hypothesis of an endothelial dysfunction in patients with PAHRH is further substantiated by the observation of an own patient (Plate 13G.3) and three literature cases[38,39] with concurrent thrombotic thrombocytopenic purpura and PAHRH. Other vascular abnormalities associated with PAHRH include cryoglobulinemia[40,41] and membranoproliferative glomerluonephritis[1,42,43] in three patients each, and one own case with purpura fulminans (Plate 13G.4).

CLINICAL PRESENTATION

A total of 202 cases of PAHRH were reported up to the end of 2001. In addition to previous reviews,[5,44,45] the present analysis includes some single case reports and three larger recent series.[46–48] The mean age at the time of diagnosis was 33 years (Table 13G.1). This is comparable to the 36 years of the NIH patients with PPH but significantly lower than the mean age of 41 years of the 112 PPH patients from the large French series.[7,47] Unlike PPH, there was a slight male preponderance, probably reflecting the gender distribution of the HIV population. In contrast, the frequency of HIV risk factors in the PAHRH patients was different from the general experience, with intravenous drug use being the most common in more than half the cases, followed by homosexual contacts and heterosexual transmission. With respect to the CD4 cell count at the time of diagnosis, all three CDC categories were involved, and the mean value was 265/μL. Two-fifths of the patients had CD4 cell count below 200/μL and in about one-third, AIDS-indicator conditions were present.

Progressive shortness of breath was the presenting symptom in more than 90% of the patients. Less common symptoms were peripheral edema or syncope in about 30%, and non-productive cough, chest pain or Raynaud's

Table 13G.1 *Clinical characteristics of 165 literature cases of HIV-related pulmonary arterial hypertension*

• Age, years	33 ± 8 (2–57)
• Sex (male-to-female ratio)	54:46
• HIV risk factors (%)	
– Intravenous drug use	56
– Homosexual contacts	20
– Heterosexual transmission	12
– Hemophilia	6
– Transfusion-related	4
– Congenital	2
• Right ventricular systolic pressure (mmHg)	62 ± 17 (35–120)
• CD4 cell counts (/μL)	265 ± 243 (0–937)
– Counts below 200/μL (%)	41
– Counts between 200 and 500/μL (%)	38
– Counts over 500/μL (%)	21
– AIDS-indicator conditions (%)	31

phenomenon in about 15%.[7,44,47] The interval between onset of symptoms and diagnosis was only 6–10 months for the PAHRH group compared with 20–30 months in sporadic PPH.[7,10,44,47] This might be due to a higher awareness with respect to PAHRH and/or a more aggressive course of the disease in this patient group.

The findings on physical examination were described only sporadically in the case reports and included a loud P2, a right-sided S3 gallop, murmurs of tricuspid and pulmonic regurgitation, increased jugular venous pressure, ascites and peripheral edema.[44] Electrocardiogram and chest radiograph findings were reported in about half the patients, and they demonstrated the typical features of pulmonary hypertension such as right ventricular hypertrophy, right-axis deviation or right atrial abnormality and cardiomegaly or enlargement of the pulmonary artery, respectively, in more than 90% of the cases. However, this might be an overestimate due to a reporting bias, since in one of the largest single-center series, 20% of the patients had either a normal ECG or a normal chest radiograph.[6]

Diagnosis of HIV-related disease was made by Doppler echocardiography in most cases. Right ventricular systolic pressure (RVSP) given either as an invasively measured value or the pressure gradient between right ventricle and atrium determined by echocardiography was 62 ± 17 (range 35–120) mmHg. Right heart catheterization was performed in less than one-quarter of the patients reported in the literature. It uniformly confirmed the presence of an elevated pulmonary vascular resistance of 983 ± 429 (range 490–1943) dyn s/cm[5].[44] There was no correlation between the CD4 cell count and RSVP (Spearman R = 0.024; P = NS). RSVP was comparable in AIDS patients (71 ± 19 mmHg) versus non-AIDS patients (74 ± 19 mmHg; P = NS), in female (72 ± 20 mmHg) versus male patients (75 ± 17 mmHg; P = NS), as well as in intravenous drug users (70 ± 17 mmHg) versus other HIV risk categories (73 ± 17 mmHg; P = NS).

Ventilation/perfusion scans, if reported, were negative for pulmonary embolism. A mildly restrictive pattern with variably reduced diffusing capacity was present in cases where pulmonary function tests were performed.

INVESTIGATIONS

Diagnosis of PAHRH is usually made by Doppler echocardiography. Assuming a right atrial pressure of at least 5 mmHg, a RSVP gradient higher than 30 mmHg is generally considered to represent pulmonary hypertension.[4] In addition to the diagnosis of PAHRH, echocardiography is helpful in ruling out congenital, valvular, myocardial and pericardial diseases. Pulmonary function tests serve to exclude a significant restrictive or obstructive ventilatory impairment. Chest radiographs may indicate secondary causes that lead to pulmonary hypertension such as parenchymatous or veno-occlusive lung disease. Ventilation/perfusion scans are necessary to exclude pulmonary embolism, which may be a cause of chronic pulmonary hypertension in HIV-infected patients.[49] Liver function tests, viral hepatitis serology and abdominal ultrasound should be performed if liver cirrhosis is suspected. In patients with hepatitis C virus infection, the presence of cryoglobulinemia should be considered. If there is otherwise unexplained thrombocytopenia, the peripheral blood may show microangiopathic changes associated with thrombotic thrombocytopenic purpura in addition to the clinical findings of purpura, renal failure and neurological disturbances.

With respect to modern vasodilator therapy, right heart catheterization and acute vasodilator testing should be performed in all patients suitable for this therapeutic option.

MANAGEMENT

The medical therapy of PAHRH is comparable to that of PPH.[9] Oral anticoagulation is recommended in compliant patients without contraindications. Lung transplantation is generally not considered in HIV-infected patients.

The response to calcium antagonists in PAHRH is even poorer than in PPH. Only 2 of 20 cases documented in the literature showed a favorable acute response.[44,50] Serious adverse events including a case of cardiogenic shock have been reported.[51]

In contrast, the effect of intravenous prostacyclin seems more promising. Petitpretz *et al.* demonstrated a favorable acute response in 11 (58%) of their patients with PAHRH, which was comparable to their PPH patients.[7] Overall, two-thirds of the 39 literature cases tested with intravenous prostacyclin showed a positive acute response without significant adverse effects. In seven patients long-term follow-up was available.[46,52] Their median survival was 35 months, with a maximum of 6 years. All improved in their NYHA class, and in four cases repeat right heart catheterization documented a further improvement or maintenance of the hemodynamics. Three patients died, but none because of PAHRH.

There are only limited data on the effect of inhaled prostaglandins. Stricker *et al.* have reported two cases of PAHRH which showed a favorable short- and long-term response with improvement in hemodynamics and 6-minute walk distance with inhaled prostacyclin and iloprost, respectively.[53] Recently, a favorable acute response to the oral administration of sildenafil, a specific inhibitor of the phosphodiesterase isoform 5, has been demonstrated in two patients with PAHRH.[54] One of them was treated for more than 3 months with a persisting clinical improvement and decrease in pulmonary artery pressures.

The role of antiretroviral treatment in the management of PAHRH remains to be established. In the study by Opravil *et al.*[6] seven of the 13 patients who had a follow-up echocardiography received either zidovudine or didanosine. Their RVSP dropped by 3.2 mmHg, while it rose an average of 19 mmHg among those not receiving antiretroviral therapy. The median survival, however, was 2 years in both groups. Pellicelli *et al.* treated four patients with PAHRH with HAART and reported a worsening of the pulmonary artery pressure in two of them, but both patients survived for more than 1 year.[55] The only patient who died in their series did not respond to HAART. Further evidence for a potential beneficial effect of HAART stems from two case reports. One showed a decrease in RVSP from 75 to 40 mmHg and a survival of more than 2 years,[8] the other an improvement from 96 to 49 mmHg and a survival of more than 6 years[56] with HAART and without the use of any vasodilating agents.

PROGNOSIS

PAHRH contributes significantly to the mortality of HIV-infected patients. A case–control study comparing 19 cases of PAHRH with a well-matched HIV-infected group of patients without PAHRH demonstrated a median survival of 1.3 years in the PAHRH cases versus 2.6 years in the control subjects (P < 0.05 in the log rank test).[6] The survival data of this study are exactly the same as the present Kaplan–Meier analysis of the literature cases (Figure 13G.2). Thus, the overall survival of PAHRH is significantly shorter than the median survival of patients with PPH in the NIH series.[57] This is confirmed by the largest series comparing 56 patients with PAHRH and 112 with PPH. Although the authors initially reported a similar

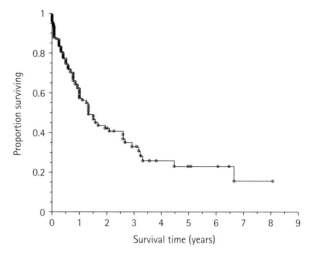

Figure 13G.2 *Kaplan–Meier survival analysis of 143 of the 202 literature cases in whom specific data were available. Median survival was 485 days (1.3 years).*

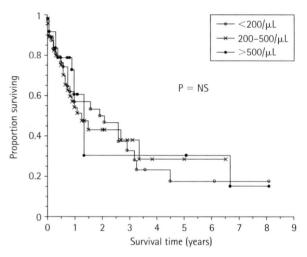

Figure 13G.3 *Kaplan–Meier estimates of 117 of the 202 literature cases comparing three patient groups with respect to their CD4 cell counts: values below 200/µL (open circles; median survival 1.6 years), values between 200 and 500/µL (crosses; median survival 1.2 years), and values greater 500/µL (filled circles; median survival 1.3 years; P = NS).*

2-year survival rate of 46% and 53%, respectively,[7] a recent update showed a 4-year survival of 13% and 48%, respectively.[47]

Interestingly, the survival of patients with PAHRH was affected neither by the CD4 cell count (Figure 13G.3), nor the level of the RSVP (Figure 13G.4). The latter was 75 ± 19 in the patients who died compared with 71 ± 18 in the survivors (P = NS). The reason for the lack of correlation between hemodynamics and survival as shown for sporadic PPH is unclear, but may be due to a bias in the literature reports or the more aggressive course of PAHRH. In contrast to the literature data, a

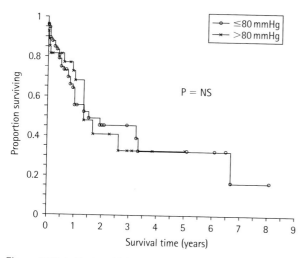

Figure 13G.4 *Kaplan–Meier estimates of 100 of the 202 literature cases comparing two patient groups with respect to their RSVP: values of 80 mmHg or lower (open circles; median survival 1.5 years), and values greater than 80 mmHg (crosses; median survival 1.3 years; P = NS).*

recent multivariate analysis on 82 patients with PAHRH assessing patient age, gender, intravenous drug use, CD4 cell count, viral load, 6-minute walk test, hemodynamic parameters, treatment with warfarin (80%), calcium channel blockers (13%), intravenous prostacyclin (24%) and HAART (48%), demonstrated that only a CD4 cell count $>212/\mu L$ remained independently associated with a better survival (G Simonneau, personal communication).

FUTURE DIRECTIONS

Additional studies are needed to better define the effect of HAART on PAHRH. Screening of HIV-infected patients by echocardiography would be interesting to determine the exact incidence of PAHRH and to note whether a measurable change occurs with the increased use of HAART. Investigations of the effects of novel vasodilating agents such as inhaled prostaglandins, oral beraprost, subcutaneous uniprost and bosentan are mandatory.

KEY POINTS

- PAH is definitely associated with HIV infection with an annual incidence of at least 0.1% and a relative risk of more than 500 compared with the general population.
- PAHRH occurs at any HIV stage independently of the CD4 cell count.

- PAHRH has a worse prognosis than sporadic PPH and significantly affects outcome of HIV-infected patients.
- The pathogenesis of PAHRH remains unknown.
- The optimal treatment strategy is not established yet. Whereas intravenous prostacyclin seems effective in these patients, the importance of HAART is less clear.
- Screening with echocardiography of all HIV-infected persons with unexplained shortness of breath or syncope is mandatory.

REFERENCES

●1 Kim KK, Factor SM. Membranoproliferative glomerulonephritis and plexogenic pulmonary arteriopathy in a homosexual man with acquired immunodeficiency syndrome. *Hum Pathol* 1987;**18**:1293–6.

●2 Goldsmith GH, Jr, Baily RG, Brettler DB *et al.* Primary pulmonary hypertension in patients with classic hemophilia. *Ann Intern Med* 1988;**108**:797–9.

●3 Himelman RB, Dohrmann M, Goodman P *et al.* Severe pulmonary hypertension and cor pulmonale in the acquired immunodeficiency syndrome. *Am J Cardiol* 1989;**64**:1396–9.

●4 Speich R, Jenni R, Opravil M *et al.* Primary pulmonary hypertension in HIV infection. *Chest* 1991;**100**:1268–71.

◆5 Mesa RA, Edell ES, Dunn WF *et al.* Human immunodeficiency virus infection and pulmonary hypertension: two new cases and a review of 86 reported cases. *Mayo Clin Proc* 1998;**73**:37–45.

●6 Opravil M, Pechere M, Speich R *et al.* HIV-associated primary pulmonary hypertension. A case control study. Swiss HIV Cohort Study. *Am J Respir Crit Care Med* 1997; **155**:990–5.

●7 Petitpretz P, Brenot F, Azarian R *et al.* Pulmonary hypertension in patients with human immunodeficiency virus infection. Comparison with primary pulmonary hypertension. *Circulation* 1994;**89**:2722–7.

8 Petureau F, Escamilla R, Hermant C *et al.* Hypertension artérielle pulmonaire ches le toxicomane VIH+. A propos de 10 cas. *Rev Mal Respir* 1998;**15**:97–102.

*9 Rich S (ed.) Executive summary from the World Symposium on Primary Pulmonary Hypertension, Evian, France, September 6–10, 1998, co-sponsored by The World Health Organization. http://www.who.int/ncd/cvd/pph.html.

10 Rich S, Dantzker DR, Ayres SM *et al.* Primary pulmonary hypertension. A national prospective study. *Ann Intern Med* 1987;**107**:216–23.

11 Centers for Disease Control and Prevention. 1993 revised classification system for HIV infection and expanded surveillance case definition for AIDS among adolescents and adults. *MMWR* 1992;**41**:1–17.

12 Abenhaim L, Moride Y, Brenot F *et al.* Appetite-suppressant drugs and the risk of primary pulmonary hypertension. *N Engl J Med* 1996;**335**:609–16.

13 Pugliese A, Isnardi D, Saini A et al. Impact of highly active antiretroviral therapy in HIV-positive patients with cardiac involvement. J Infect 2000;40:282–4.

14 Escamilla R, Hermant C, Berjaud J et al. Pulmonary veno-occlusive disease in a HIV-infected intravenous drug abuser. Eur Respir J 1995;8:1982–4.

15 Ruchelli ED, Nojadera G, Rutstein RM et al. Pulmonary veno-occlusive disease. Another vascular disorder associated with human immunodeficiency virus infection? Arch Pathol Lab Med 1994;118:664–6.

16 Yakel DL, Jr, Eisenberg MJ. Pulmonary artery hypertension in chronic intravenous cocaine users. Am Heart J 1995; 130:398–9.

17 Collazos J, Martinez E, Fernandez A et al. Acute, reversible pulmonary hypertension associated with cocaine use. Respir Med 1996;90:171–4.

18 Kringsholm B, Christoffersen P. Lung and heart pathology in fatal drug addiction: a consecutive autopsy study. Forensic Sci Int 1987;34:39–51.

19 Overland ES, Nolan AJ, Hopewell PC. Alteration of pulmonary function in intravenous drug abusers. Prevalence, severity, and characterization of gas exchange abnormalities. Am J Med 1980;68:231–7.

20 Tomashefski JE, Hirsch CS. The pulmonary vascular lesions of intravenous drug abuse. Hum Pathol 1980;11:133–45.

21 Polos PG, Wolfe D, Harley RA et al. Pulmonary hypertension and human immunodeficiency virus infection. Two reports and a review of the literature. Chest 1992;101:474–8.

22 Hadengue A, Benhayoun MK, Lebrec D et al. Pulmonary hypertension complicating portal hypertension: prevalence and relation to splanchnic hemodynamics. Gastroenterology 1991;100:520–8.

23 Gillespie MN, Hartsfield CL, O'Connor WN et al. Pulmonary hypertension in a murine model of the acquired immunodeficiency syndrome. Am J Respir Crit Care Med 1994;150:194–9.

24 Li SL, Zhang XY, Ling H et al. A VSV-G pseudotyped HIV vector mediates efficient transduction of human pulmonary artery smooth muscle cells. Microbiol Immunol 2000;44:1019–25.

25 Conraads VM, Colebunders RL, Boshoff C et al. Primary pulmonary hypertension in a patient with HIV infection. Acta Cardiol 1998;53:367–9.

26 Humbert M, Monti G, Fartoukh M et al. Platelet-derived growth factor expression in primary pulmonary hypertension: comparison of HIV seropositive and HIV seronegative patients. Eur Respir J 1998;11:554–9.

27 Mette SA, Palevsky HI, Pietra GG et al. Primary pulmonary hypertension in association with human immunodeficiency virus infection. A possible viral etiology for some forms of hypertensive pulmonary arteriopathy. Am Rev Respir Dis 1992;145:1196–200.

28 Morse JH, Barst RJ, Itescu S et al. Primary pulmonary hypertension in HIV infection: an outcome determined by particular HLA class II alleles. Am J Respir Crit Care Med 1996;153:1299–301.

29 Smith FB, Arias JH, Elmquist TH et al. Microvascular cytomegalovirus endothelialitis of the lung: a possible cause of secondary pulmonary hypertension in a patient with AIDS. Chest 1998;114:337–40.

30 Vogel J, Hinrichs SH, Reynolds RK et al. The HIV tat gene induces dermal lesions resembling Kaposi's sarcoma in transgenic mice. Nature 1988;335:606–11.

31 Nakamura S, Salahuddin SZ, Biberfeld P et al. Kaposi's sarcoma cells: long-term culture with growth factor from retrovirus-infected CD4+ T cells. Science 1988;242:426–30.

32 Coplan NL, Shimony RY, Ioachim HL et al. Primary pulmonary hypertension associated with human immunodeficiency viral infection. Am J Med 1990;89:96–9.

33 Rudarakanchana N, Trembath RC, Morrell NW. New insights into the pathogenesis and treatment of primary pulmonary hypertension. Thorax 2001;56:888–90.

34 Thomson JR, Machado RD, Pauciulo MW et al. Sporadic primary pulmonary hypertension is associated with germline mutations of the gene encoding BMPR-II, a receptor member of the TGF-beta family. J Med Genet 2000;37:741–5.

35 Ehrenreich H, Rieckmann P, Sinowatz F et al. Potent stimulation of monocytic endothelin-1 production by HIV-1 glycoprotein 120. J Immunol 1993;150:4601–9.

36 Rolinski B, Geier SA, Sadri I et al. Endothelin-1 immuno-reactivity in plasma is elevated in HIV-1 infected patients with retinal microangiopathic syndrome. Clin Invest 1994;72:288–93.

37 Tuder RM, Cool CD, Geraci MW et al. Prostacyclin synthase expression is decreased in lungs from patients with severe pulmonary hypertension. Am J Respir Crit Care Med 1999; 159:1925–32.

38 Fiorencis R, Zonzin P, Carraro M et al. Pulmonary hypertension associated with human immunodeficiency virus infection. Report of two cases and review of the literature. G Ital Cardiol 1998;28:1404–8.

39 Monsuez JJ, Auperin I, Vittecoq D et al. Pulmonary hypertension associated with thrombotic thrombocytopaenic purpura in AIDS patients. Eur Heart J 1997;18:1036–7.

40 Leautez S, Boutoille D, Renard B et al. Hypertension artérielle pulmonaire et infection à VIH. Rev Mal Respir 2001;18:432–5.

41 Mani S, Smith GJ. HIV and pulmonary hypertension: a review. South Med J 1994;87:357–62.

42 de Chadarevian JP, Lischner HW, Karmazin N et al. Pulmonary hypertension and HIV infection: new observations and review of the syndrome. Mod Pathol 1994;7:685–9.

43 Reiser P, Opravil M, Pfaltz M et al. Primäre pulmonale Hypertonie und mesangioproliferative Glomerulonephritis bei HIV-Infektion. Dtsch Med Wochenschr 1992; 117:815–18.

◆44 Mehta NJ, Khan IA, Mehta RN et al. HIV-Related pulmonary hypertension: analytic review of 131 cases. Chest 2000;118: 1133–41.

◆45 Pellicelli AM, Barbaro G, Palmieri F et al. Primary pulmonary hypertension in HIV patients: a systematic review. Angiology 2001;52:31–41.

●46 Aguilar RV, Farber HW. Epoprostenol (prostacyclin) therapy in HIV-associated pulmonary hypertension. Am J Respir Crit Care Med 2000;162:1846–50.

●47 Nunez H, Humbert M, Jagot JL et al. Hypertension artérielle pulmonaire primitive et infection par le VIH. Sang Thrombose Vaisseaux 1998;10:555–62.

●48 Valencia Ortega ME, Ortega Millan G, Guinea Esquerdo J et al. Hipertension pulmonar en los patientes con la infeccion por el virus de la inmunodeficiencia humana. Estudio de 14 casos. *Med Clin (Barc)* 2000;**115**:181–4.

49 Maliakkal R, Friedman SA, Sridhar S. Progressive pulmonary thromboembolism in association with HIV disease. *N Y State J Med* 1992;**92**:403–4.

50 Bragulat E, Garcia F, Fernandez F *et al*. Effecto de los antagonistas de los canales de calcio en la hipertension pulmonar primaria asociada al virus de la inmunodeficiencia humana. *An Med Interna* 1998;**15**:114.

51 Louis M, Thorens JB, Chevrolet JC. Calcium-channel blockers testing for primary pulmonary hypertension associated with HIV infection. [abstract] *Am Rev Respir Dis* 1993;**147**:A536.

52 Farber HW. HIV-associated pulmonary hypertension. *AIDS Clin Care* 2001;**13**:53–5, 9.

53 Stricker H, Domenighetti G, Mombelli G. Prostacyclin for HIV-associated pulmonary hypertension. *Ann Intern Med* 1997;**127**:1043.

54 Schumacher YO, Zdebik A, Huonker M *et al*. Sildenafil in HIV-related pulmonary hypertension. *AIDS* 2001;**15**:1747–8.

55 Pellicelli AM, Palmieri F, D'Ambrosio C *et al*. Role of human immunodeficiency virus in primary pulmonary hypertension – case reports. *Angiology* 1998;**49**: 1005–11.

56 Speich R, Jenni R, Opravil M *et al*. Regression of HIV-associated pulmonary arterial hypertension and long-term survival during antiretroviral therapy. *Swiss Med Wkly* 2001;**131**:663–5.

57 D'Alonzo GE, Barst RJ, Ayres SM *et al*. Survival in patients with primary pulmonary hypertension. *Ann Intern Med* 1991;**115**:343–55.

Pulmonary hypertension in association with congenital systemic-to-pulmonary shunts

SHEILA G HAWORTH

INTRODUCTION

Pulmonary hypertension is a major complicating factor in the management of many types of congenital heart disease associated with a left-to-right shunt, preventing intracardiac repair in those with established pulmonary vascular disease. The rate at which pulmonary vascular disease develops varies according to the type of intracardiac abnormality, and an appreciation of the natural history usually makes it possible to prevent the development of significant disease by timely operative intervention. With the increasing sophistication of surgery and cardiopulmonary bypass it has now become accepted practice to carry out a primary intracardiac repair in early infancy and so prevent the development of pulmonary vascular obstructive disease. In patients who present later in life, predicting the outcome of intracardiac repair in the presence of an elevated pulmonary vascular resistance calls for fine clinical judgment. Is an early improvement in quality of life worth the risk of reducing long-term survival? For those with irreversible pulmonary vascular disease, medical treatment remains largely empirical. Ultimately, the only 'cure' for advanced pulmonary vascular obstructive disease is lung transplantation. For the minority of patients offered lung transplantation, the long-term outlook can also be uncertain. Transplantation should only be offered when the probability of survival with a satisfactory quality of life is better than that without transplantation.

Fifteen to twenty years ago research activities focused on understanding the evolution of pulmonary vascular disease in the different intracardiac abnormalities and on improving the accuracy with which long-term outcome could be predicted, with and without intracardiac repair. It soon became apparent that children with potentially reversible pulmonary vascular disease were at risk of dying in the postoperative period with pulmonary hypertensive crises and the emphasis shifted to studying the functional manifestations of pulmonary vascular disease, particularly the developmental pharmacology of the immature pulmonary circulation. The advent of nitric oxide revolutionized postoperative care. Our priorities today include:

- improved non-invasive assessment of the pulmonary vasculature;
- reducing the lability of the pulmonary circulation in potentially operable patients by preoperative therapy;
- structural remodeling of the pulmonary vasculature in the 'borderline' operable case in order to operate safely;
- arresting inoperable pulmonary vascular disease therapeutically and at least improving quality of life and survival.

To achieve these goals requires greater understanding of the pathobiology of pulmonary vascular disease in the presence of a systemic–pulmonary shunt, particularly the early postnatal origins of disease and the molecular basis of the response to a high pulmonary blood flow. Advances in the genetics and treatment of primary pulmonary hypertension open up new lines of enquiry into the pathogenesis and treatment of this and other forms of pulmonary hypertension.

Definitions

Pulmonary hypertension is defined as a pulmonary arterial pressure >25 mmHg at rest or 30 mmHg on exercise, although pulmonary hypertension in childhood is usually associated with considerably higher pressures. Pulmonary hypertension can be described as either primary, being of unknown etiology, or secondary resulting from cardiac or parenchymal lung disease. However, this description is unsatisfactory since it takes no account of the similarities in pathobiology and response to treatment between primary and certain other types of pulmonary hypertension. It narrows our perspective. A new classification was proposed at a WHO Symposium in 1998, based on anatomy, clinical features and an appreciation of the commonality of at least some of the underlying mechanisms.[1] Primary pulmonary hypertension (PPH) and pulmonary hypertension related to congenital heart disease, persistent pulmonary hypertension of the newborn (PPHN), connective tissue disease, HIV infection, drugs and toxins were grouped together as 'pulmonary arterial hypertension'. This new classification encourages the extension of therapeutic modalities known to be effective in primary pulmonary hypertension to other forms of hypertension, in both adults and children.

Further clarification is necessary in children with congenital heart disease. In the majority of children, pulmonary arterial hypertension is usually caused and driven by a cardiac abnormality, which leads to the development of the Eisenmenger syndrome, but in some children the abnormality is, and always has been, hemodynamically insignificant. Clinically, these children behave as though they have primary pulmonary hypertension, and can be treated as such.

PATHOBIOLOGY

Pathology of pulmonary hypertension

EVOLUTION OF PULMONARY VASCULAR DISEASE: GENERAL FEATURES

Children are occasionally born with pulmonary vascular disease, but this is rare. Pulmonary vascular disease usually begins at birth when the vasculature fails to adapt normally to extrauterine life (Plate 13H.1).[2] An increase in pulmonary blood flow with little increase in pressure causes peripheral extension of muscle from differentiating pericytes and intermediate cells in precapillary vessels (Figure 13H.1).[3] Simultaneously, the media of larger arteries increases in thickness as smooth muscle cells hypertrophy and excessive connective tissue is deposited in both the media and adventitia. The normal postnatal increase in contractile myofilaments is accelerated and the myofilament concentration normally present by 6 months is achieved during the first weeks of life.[2] In the endothelial cells, microfilament disarray is seen in early infancy. Some of the cells become partially detached from the basement membrane, and scanning electron microscopy reveals a ridged, irregular surface to which activated leukocytes and platelets adhere. There is abundant evidence of early endothelial dysfunction.

If the pulmonary arterial pressure is allowed to remain elevated, marked differences in smooth muscle cell phenotype become apparent between the inner and outer part of the media in infancy. The innermost smooth muscle cells have a more synthetic phenotype than the outermost cells, cease to express many smooth-muscle-specific contractile and cytoskeletal proteins, and appear

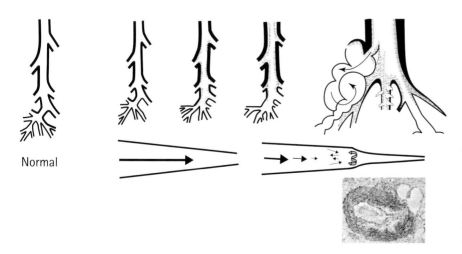

Normal

Figure 13H.1 *Diagram illustrating the evolution of pulmonary vascular disease showing the early reduction in number of arteries, increase in muscularity, and development of intimal proliferation accompanied by a reduction in peripheral muscularity. Flow becomes progressively more turbulent. Inset: Photomicrograph of artery showing dilation lesion, stained for γ-actin (magnification × 200).*

to migrate through gaps in the internal elastic lamina to produce intimal proliferation. Heightened activity of a proteolytic enzyme, endogenous vascular elastase, is thought to help induce structural remodeling and cause disruption of the internal elastic lamina to facilitate smooth muscle cell migration.[4] The rate at which these changes occur depends upon the type of intracardiac abnormality, and intimal proliferation can develop rapidly in certain abnormalities. In transposition of the great arteries with ventricular septal defect, for example, severe obstructive intimal proliferation increases resistance to flow during the first months of life. In such babies, intimal proliferation is cellular and exuberant, obstructing and even occluding the lumen before there has been sufficient time to achieve neat, circumferential intimal fibrosis, known as the onion skin picture, seen in older patients.[5] The veins show a slight increase in wall thickness, commensurate with the increase in pulmonary arterial wall thickness.

The intimal obstruction to flow is strategically placed at the entrance to each respiratory unit (Figure 13H.1).[6] As intimal proliferation increases in severity in the small muscular arteries, it narrows the lumen and the medial thickness of the more peripheral respiratory unit arteries decreases. The transitory near-normal appearance of the peripheral intra-acinar arteries can be misleading, but it reflects the severity of more proximal obstruction in patients with a high pressure and resistance (Figure 13H.1). Therefore, in order to interpret a lung biopsy with confidence, it is important that the biopsy be sufficiently deep to include some of the pre-acinar and terminal bronchiolar arteries in which intimal proliferation first develops.[6,7] This predilation stage in the evolution of pulmonary vascular disease is associated with an increase in mortality and morbidity at, and after, intracardiac repair.[7] The number of intra-acinar arteries is reduced in severe pulmonary hypertension. Ultrastructural examination reveals many occluded vessels.[8] This is an early change and can be seen in young infants with a low resistance. Whether or not there is also a primary failure of postnatal angiogenesis is unknown, but seems possible given that the vasculature is exposed to a high pressure before it is fully developed. In the normal child, approximately 50% of the arteries accompanying the alveoli form after birth.

In children with a sustained, high pulmonary arterial pressure, the obstruction to flow increases with age and dilatation lesions develop from the walls of small muscular arteries. The smooth muscle cells of the thick-walled arteries continue to synthesize TGF-β, a potent mitogen. The walls of both the original vessels and the dilatation lesions contain smooth-muscle-specific contractile proteins and regulatory proteins, but how these vessels function in relation to each other is unknown (Figure 13H.1). The structurally abnormal, dysfunctioning endothelium expresses vascular endothelial growth factor (VEGF), even when covering a thick layer of intimal proliferation. The dilatation lesions contain abundant VEGF (see Chapter 3). *In vitro*, VEGF induces endothelium-dependent relaxation[9] and its presence in unobstructed pulmonary arteries and in dilatation lesions may help ensure continued perfusion of the capillary bed. VEGF co-localizes with TGF-β_1 in the endothelium of both the pulmonary arteries and dilatation lesions. VEGF is a potent angiogenic factor, and TGF-β up-regulates its angiogenic activity *in vitro*.[10] Plexiform lesions accompany or follow the appearance of dilatation lesions and they also contain abundant VEGF. The role of VEGF in the pathogenesis of pulmonary vascular disease is unclear, but it may have an angiogenic effect after peripheral pulmonary arterial occlusion. Obstructive intimal proliferative tissue shows intense tenascin expression and tenascin co-localizes with epidermal growth factor and indices of cell replication.[11] Expression of fibronectin is widespread. These findings are consistent with *in vitro* studies showing that tenascin modulates epidermal growth factor-dependent neointimal smooth muscle cell proliferation.

When the pulmonary arterial pressure remains elevated after birth, whatever the reason, the structure of the pulmonary trunk retains its fetal appearance and contains long, thick elastin fibers. If pulmonary hypertension develops later in life, the pulmonary trunk becomes thicker due to the deposition of connective tissue and smooth muscle cell hypertrophy in a normally adapted vessel.

PULMONARY VASCULAR DISEASE IN COMMON TYPES OF INTRACARDIAC ABNORMALITY

In most children with severe pulmonary hypertension, the rate at which pulmonary vascular disease progresses depends upon the type of intracardiac abnormality. Disease progression is accelerated in a minority of patients who are thought to have a genetic predisposition to develop pulmonary vascular disease, rather as in primary pulmonary hypertension, the high pulmonary blood flow acting as the trigger.

In children with an isolated hypertensive **ventricular septal defect** the pulmonary vasculature fails to develop normally after birth.[7,12] Intimal proliferation tends to develop towards the end of the first year and fibrosis during the third year of life. Patients with severe pulmonary hypertension and a large defect should therefore be operated upon before their first birthday and certainly before the age of 2 years if the pulmonary resistance is to become normal after repair. Progression is relatively slow in most patients and grade IV pulmonary vascular disease seldom occurs in young children. Intimal obstruction does not usually reduce peripheral muscularity until the teenage years (Figure 13H.2).

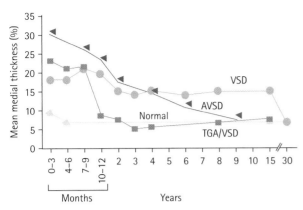

Figure 13H.2 *Mean percentage medial thickness of intra-acinar arteries 50–100 μm in diameter in the normal, in 90 children with a ventricular septal defect (VSD), 38 with an atrioventricular septal defect (AVSD) and 28 with transposition of the great arteries (TGA) and VSD at different ages. Peripheral arterial muscularity decreases at a younger age in TGA/VSD > AVSD > VSD.*

In transposition of the great arteries patient outcome correlates with the pulmonary arterial pressure.[13] With a large **ventricular septal defect**, the pulmonary vasculature does not remodel normally after birth, and this failure to remodel marks the onset of rapidly progressive pulmonary vascular obstructive disease (Figure 13H.2). Intimal proliferation is seen from 2 months of age and is abundant by 5 months.[5] As the intimal obstruction increases in severity, the muscularity decreases in more distal vessels. After 7–9 months of age the medial thickness is normal or even less than normal in the distal vessels. These patients have a high resistance and are usually inoperable. A **patent ductus arteriosus** also leads to the early development of pulmonary vascular disease in children with transposition, and should have been closed therapeutically, if not spontaneously, by 3 months of age. With an **intact ventricular septum**, the pulmonary circulation usually adapts normally to extrauterine life. The bronchial circulation is enlarged, making a substantial but unknown contribution to total pulmonary blood flow, probably from birth. An enlarged bronchial circulation can sometimes persist after successful intracardiac repair. Patients are now operated on soon after birth and nearly all patients with transposition and an intact ventricular septum undergo intracardiac repair with a relatively normal pulmonary vasculature. Exceptionally, babies who have had an apparently successful arterial switch operation later develop severe progressive pulmonary vascular disease, and can be treated as though they have primary pulmonary hypertension. In the days before an intracardiac repair could be carried out in early infancy, children developed severe polycythemia and pulmonary thrombo-embolism, and some became pulmonary hypertensive.

In infants with an **atrioventricular septal defect**, cellular intimal proliferation develops earlier and is more severe than in those with an isolated ventricular septal defect, but develops more slowly than in those with transposition and ventricular septal defect (Figure 13H.2). Severe medial hypertrophy and intimal proliferation can be present by 6 or 7 months of age, and intracardiac repair should be carried out in early infancy.[14] Pulmonary vascular structure can be particularly difficult to evaluate in complete atrioventricular defect because of the varying degrees of incompetence of the left atrioventricular valve. When this is severe, the vein walls are abnormally thick and perivascular connective tissue deposition is excessive, particularly around the capillary bed and small veins.

Pulmonary hypertension rarely develops in children with a **secundum atrial septal defect**. Most children are asymptomatic but in the exceptional patient who develops cardiac failure the pulmonary arterial pressure is usually considerably higher than in an older patient in failure. The pulmonary vascular abnormalities resemble those of children with a hypertensive ventricular septal defect and such children are generally inoperable when they present.[15] An atrial septal defect may also precipitate the presentation of a child or young person with primary pulmonary hypertension, it usually being a protective feature in this condition. Such children fail to thrive but there is no suggestion of the pulmonary blood flow ever having been elevated. In adults, the pathological features of a pulmonary hypertensive atrial septal defect are unlike those seen in children. The preacinar arteries are dilated and usually undergo a modest increase in pulmonary arterial muscularity. The dominant change at the periphery is fibrotic occlusion of small alveolar duct and the alveolar wall arteries, leading to a reduction in the capacity of the peripheral pulmonary vascular bed.

THE EFFECT OF PALLIATIVE SURGERY ON THE LUNG

In patients with congenital heart disease causing pulmonary hypoperfusion, insertion of a systemic–pulmonary shunt may lead to pulmonary hypertension. In patients with complex congenital heart disease associated with systemic–pulmonary shunting and hypertension, banding the pulmonary trunk may be carried out as an initial procedure to protect the pulmonary vasculature, but this fails to reduce the pulmonary arterial pressure and flow adequately. Following either procedure, a moderate increase in pulmonary arterial medial thickness may have little or no effect on the outcome of a repair in which there will be a subpulmonary ventricle. However, the risk of a Fontan procedure is significantly increased, since outcome is largely determined by the ease with which blood can flow through the lung at systemic venous pressure.

Correlations between structural and hemodynamic findings

In 1958, Heath and Edwards published their classical papers on the evolution of pulmonary vascular disease.[16,17] They classified pulmonary vascular disease into six grades, in order of increasing severity. Grades I–III were said to indicate a 'low-resistance, high-reserve', still labile pulmonary vascular bed. The pulmonary arterial pressure is high, the pulmonary blood flow is high and the direction of the shunt is left to right. Grades V–VI indicate a 'high-resistance, low-reserve' pulmonary vascular bed which is no longer labile because the lumen of many arteries is occluded. Pulmonary arterial pressure is higher than in patients with grades I–III pulmonary vascular disease, flow is low and the direction of the shunt is predominantly right to left. Grade IV represents a transitional stage. However, although grades I–III reflect a succession of structural changes, grades IV–VI probably do not. Necrotizing arteritis can precede the development of plexiform lesions, but is rare in pulmonary hypertensive congenital heart disease. None of these advanced lesions is thought to carry a more severe prognosis than others, save for the plexiform lesion.

All the patients with congenital heart disease in the Heath and Edwards study were at least 10 months of age, and most had either an atrial or ventricular septal defect or a patent ductus arteriosus. They were the self-selected survivors. Our problems are now with patients with more complex types of congenital heart disease, many of whom develop pulmonary vascular obstructive disease during the first months of life. In certain anomalies, exuberant cellular intimal proliferation obstructs and even occludes the lumen of small muscular and terminal bronchiolar arteries. The Heath and Edwards classification of grade II disease would suggest a less dangerous situation. The Heath and Edwards classification is not helpful in young children but has been, and still is, useful in the management of older children and adults with pulmonary hypertension. A more recent classification system concentrated on the early structural changes before intimal damage appears. It emphasized the importance of assessing the muscularity, size and number of vessels in a pulmonary vascular bed that is still developing.[3] Both classifications are helpful when describing a group of patients, but when evaluating an individual lung biopsy it is wiser to describe all the abnormalities present rather than to try to classify them, and then relate the structural findings to the clinical and hemodynamic data. We still know too little about the cells that compose the vessel walls and about how the pulmonary circulation functions to make definitive correlations between structure and function, much less growth potential.

It is more difficult to relate the structural findings in the pulmonary vasculature to hemodynamic observations and to outcome in young children than it is in older patients. Medial hypertrophy is usually associated with a low pulmonary vascular resistance and is potentially reversible. However, in young children the resistance may be elevated, and the children can die in the postoperative period after a technically successful intracardiac repair owing to pulmonary hypertensive crises. Medial hypertrophy, although a potentially reversible lesion, is therefore not necessarily a safe lesion.[5] At the other extreme, extensive dilatation plus the other features of classical grade IV pulmonary vascular disease is invariably associated with a high resistance and a poor prognosis. In practice, most patients fall between the two extremes.

Early in the course of the disease, pulmonary arterial medial thickness correlates with pulmonary arterial pressure, but as intimal proliferation increases in small muscular arteries, the medial thickness of more peripheral arteries decreases. Resistance becomes inversely proportional to peripheral arterial muscularity (Figures 13H.1 and 13H.2). In practice, it is usually possible to predict the structural changes present in the pulmonary vascular bed from the hemodynamic findings, when these findings are considered in conjunction with the age of the patient and the type of intracardiac abnormality. The effect of associated lesions, such as coarctation of the aorta, must also be taken into account, even when they have been repaired earlier. If there is doubt about the likely outcome of surgical repair, then an open lung biopsy should clarify the position.

Derangements in vascular function

In the presence of a high pulmonary blood flow, endothelial dysfunction is present early, in young children who are potentially operable. The relaxation response to acetylcholine is impaired even with little increase in pulmonary pressure, and becomes more abnormal as pulmonary resistance rises.[18] The blood nitrate and nitrate concentrations, however, increased in a group of infants with pulmonary hypertension who were in heart failure, suggesting enhanced basal release of nitric oxide (NO) early in the course of the disease.[19] Such children have high circulating levels of thrombomodulin, an endothelial glycoprotein released by injured cells. The thromboxane: prostacyclin ratio is increased, tipping the balance between these two physiological mediators of vascular tone in favor of vasoconstriction and platelet aggregation.[20] Expression of angiotension converting enzyme is increased on the endothelium of intra-acinar arteries. Plasma epinephrine increases as resistance rises. Impaired endothelium-independent relaxation in response to the NO donor sodium nitroprusside occurs later in association with a higher resistance and more advanced structural disease.[18]

The diseased pulmonary vasculature is extremely vulnerable to the traumatic effects of cardiopulmonary bypass.[21] Circulating levels of vasoconstrictor substances such as endothelin-1, catecholamines and thromboxane increase. Nitrate anion levels reflecting NO release are not increased, and cGMP levels can be reduced, while prostacyclin levels rise. The changes are complex. Cardiopulmonary bypass evokes a generation of cascades of contractile agonists and the response to any vasodilator agonist is dependent upon the nature of the predominant contractile stimulus. A delay in meeting this challenge with intrinsic vasodilators seems very likely, and pulmonary hypertensive crises would seem to support this hypothesis.

The biology of flow – experimental studies

The endothelium is instrumental in regulating vascular tone and structural remodeling, and the signals it transmits are determined by the physical stresses imposed upon it. The high-flow, high-pressure circulation associated with a left-to-right shunt exposes the endothelium to an increase in shear stress, pressure and stretch. The healthy endothelium has a protective barrier function, an anticoagulant surface which inhibits adherence of leukocytes and platelets, it exerts a restraining influence on smooth muscle proliferation and extracellular matrix synthesis, and influences vascular tone. The endothelial cell membrane can sense an acute change in shear stress and transduces the signal(s) throughout the cell, to neighboring cells and to the underlying matrix.[22] The signal(s) is transduced into a well-ordered cascade of events.[22] Nitric oxide and prostacyclin are released in the first minute, and this would increase lumen diameter rapidly and help restore shear stress to its original level. Phosphorylation of eNOS can increase by 210% within one minute.[23] Almost simultaneously, biochemical cascades are instigated. These include mobilization of phosphoinositol derivatives, release of intracellular free calcium, and G-protein activation. These changes overlap with the next phase in the response taking place within the next hour, the rapid activation of mitogen-activated protein kinases, particularly ERK-1/2.[22,24,25] ERK-1/2 is thought to regulate both dynamic responses and gene transcription. Shear stress activates shear stress response elements (SSREs) in the endothelial cell, principally related nuclear kappa B (NFκB) and nuclear factor activator protein-1 (AP1).[26,27] The NFκB p50–p65 complex binds to a SSRE, a consensus sequence GAGACC present in the promoters of PDGF-B, eNOS, ET-1, MCP-1 and others.

Soon after exposure to an increase in shear stress, the endothelial cells become realigned along the direction of flow, a process involving reorganization of actin and vimentin filaments. But the endothelial cytoskeleton has also been implicated in mechanotransduction, transmitting changes in extracellular forces to signaling molecules within and beyond the cell. The intermediate filament vimentin network is displaced within the first 3 minutes after the introduction of flow and the findings suggest mechanical continuity between adjacent cells.[28] Neighboring cells can, however, behave differently. In an endothelial cell monolayer exposed to an increase in shear stress, some cells showed an increase in expression of adhesion proteins, elevation of intracellular calcium and other changes, while neighboring cells did not.[22,24] This is thought to be related to variation in the sensing and transmission of environmental change caused by marked differences in cell surface topography, and hence in the distribution of shear stress gradients at the cell surface.[22] Extremes of shear stress were less in aligned than in non-aligned cells. Changes in endothelial cell surface topography occur early in the course of pulmonary vascular disease.

Within each cell, stress is transmitted via the cytoskeleton to the focal adhesions at the abluminal cell surface. Focal adhesions contain transmembrane proteins, integrins, which physically link the cytoskeleton of the endothelial cell to the underlying matrix. Using tandem-scanning confocal microscopy, real-time studies on living cells have shown that adhesion sites remodel and realign in the direction of luminal shear stress.[22] The rate and degree of alignment was related to the magnitude of the shear stress and the composition of the underlying matrix. The imposition of a shear stress for between 20 and 120 minutes was associated with the phosphorylation of focal adhesion kinase and other focal adhesion proteins such as paxillin (Plate 13H.1).[25,29] This leads to integrin clustering, focal adhesion formation and cytoskeletal reorganization. β_1-Integrins can act as mechanotransducers and enhance flow-induced increases in MAP kinase activity, whilst β_3-integrins are involved in the immediate NO-mediated vasodilator response.[30]

Changes in shear stress provoke marked changes in the interplay between the endothelial cell cytoskeleton, biochemical cascades, extracellular matrix and gene regulation. Gene expression profiling shows that the expression of flow-responsive genes is also regulated by the type of hemodynamic stress.[31,32] Whereas laminar flow up-regulates desirable genes such as eNOS, disturbed flow up-regulates proinflammatory, proapoptotic and procoagulant molecules.[33] In systemic arteries, turbulence at atheroma-prone arterial bifurcations is associated with the local up-regulation of vascular cell adhesion molecule 1 (VCAM-1) and intracellular adhesion molecule 1 (ICAM-1), encouraging leukocyte recruitment and activation.[34] Disturbed flow is not simply the absence of laminar flow but has a distinct, and usually detrimental, positive effect on gene expression.

Flow is thought to be predominantly laminar in the early stages of pulmonary vascular disease but as disease advances, obstructive intimal lesions increase resistance to flow, amplify wave reflection, and increase input impedance and right ventricular work (Figure 13H.1). Turbulence develops and experimental studies indicate that the biology of flow changes dramatically.

CLINICAL PRESENTATION

In children with a left-to-right shunt, the nature of the anatomic abnormality determines the clinical picture, but if pulmonary vascular disease is allowed to pursue its natural course, then most of the findings become common to all types of congenital heart disease. At the onset in childhood, a high pulmonary blood flow is frequently associated with feeding difficulties, failure to thrive and recurrent respiratory tract infections. Dilated, hypertensive pulmonary arteries compress the main and lobar bronchi in young children, leading to the familiar problem of recurrent collapse of different lobes or segments of lung. The respiratory complications of congenital heart disease may constitute an indication for corrective surgery in infancy. (After operation, the deformity of the bronchi may persist for some time and in some patients prolonged compression appears to be associated with bronchomalacia.) Cardiac failure may appear to improve as pulmonary vascular resistance increases. Without surgical intervention, the resistance continues to increase until the shunt becomes bidirectional or reversed. This physiological situation is known as the Eisenmenger complex, defined as pulmonary hypertension at systemic level due to a high pulmonary vascular resistance (over 10 Wood units or 800 dyn s/cm^5) with a reversed shunt at any level.[35,36] Patients have exercise intolerance, central cyanosis, clubbing, polycythemia, and can develop hemoptysis in early adult life. Dr Paul Wood described a series of 727 patients with congenital heart disease with a systemic–pulmonary connection of whom 17.5% developed the Eisenmenger reaction.[36] (This early study could not have taken into account a substantial, early attrition.) The physical signs include a small or normal volume pulse, a right (or sub-pulmonary) ventricular lift extending to the pulmonary artery, a loud pulmonary ejection click, followed by a short pulmonary systolic murmur, and a palpable, accentuated pulmonary component of the second heart sound. Eventually, a pulmonary regurgitant murmur and signs of tricuspid incompetence develop.

Patients who have undergone intracardiac repair in the presence of an elevated pulmonary vascular resistance require careful long-term follow-up, with recatheterization. If the resistance does not fall, and certainly if it starts to increase, they should be evaluated and treated as though they have primary pulmonary hypertension, without waiting for clinical deterioration. The aim is to improve quality of life and survival, deferring the need for transplantation, if possible indefinitely.

In patients who have been deemed inoperable or have severe postoperative pulmonary hypertension, and who have failed medical treatment and become so ill that they are likely to be offered a transplant in the foreseeable future, reassessment should include repeat cardiac catheterization. Conventionally, the clinical status determines the necessity for transplantation. In patients with advanced disease, however, survival can be predicted from the product of mean right atrial pressure and pulmonary vascular resistance.[37] The optimal time to offer transplantation is when the expected survival time is less than the expected time of survival after transplantation, bearing in mind the quality of life achieved.

INVESTIGATIONS

The chest radiograph

The chest radiograph is reassuringly plethoric when the resistance is sufficiently low to permit a high blood flow and it is depressingly attenuated when pulmonary vascular disease is advanced. Severe obstructive disease in the muscular pulmonary arteries leads to peripheral pruning and a hypertranslucent appearance in association with dilatation of the hilar and proximal vessels.

Electrocardiogram, with Holter monitoring, if clinically indicated

The features are determined by the nature of the underlying cardiac abnormality, with signs of pulmonary hypertension and hypertrophy of the sub-pulmonary ventricle (see Chapter 8).

Cross-sectional echocardiography with Doppler studies

These are the principal non-invasive investigations. Intracardiac anatomy is clarified. Estimations of right atrial and ventricular (sub-pulmonary) cavity size, right ventricular hypertrophy and function have to be considered in relation to the cardiac abnormalities present. The pulmonary arterial pressure can usually be reliably determined non-invasively by Doppler interrogation, but resistance cannot. Transesophageal echocardiography may be indicated to optimize assessment of the left atrioventricular valve if it is thought that incompetence of this valve may be contributing to the elevation in pulmonary arterial pressure.

Magnetic resonance spectroscopy

Atrial and ventricular morphology and function, and the direction and volume of shunting can be determined. Velocity-encoded magnetic resonance imaging and other approaches can distinguish a high from a low resistance but further discrimination for reliable, routine use has proved difficult.

Cardiac catheterization

A conventional study to determine intracardiac anatomy, and the site, direction and magnitude of the shunt(s) is carried out, and if the resistance is elevated then acute vasodilator testing follows. Patients are best studied under light general anaesthesia, with respiratory gas analysis. Using measured oxygen consumption together with arteriovenous oxygen difference (bound and dissolved) cardiac output is calculated and pulmonary vascular resistance determined. The lowest determination of pulmonary arterial pressure and vascular resistance is conventionally accepted as a guide to surgical outcome. This is based on the premise that if the predominant structural abnormality in the pulmonary circulation is an increase in muscularity, then the circulation will respond to vasodilator substances. To this end, the patient is usually given 100% oxygen to breathe, with or without prostacyclin.[38] Giving both vasodilator agents together may produce a greater fall in resistance than if either is given alone. Inhaled NO, a specific pulmonary vasodilator, is frequently the most potent vasodilator. In one study, inhalation of NO at 40 p.p.m. reduced the resistance from a mean of 8.6 to 5.7 units/m^2.[39] Used together, NO and a high oxygen concentration can produce a greater fall in resistance than either used alone.[40] Endothelial-dependent and independent vasodilatation can be studied by the sequential infusion of acetylcholine and sodium nitroprusside.[18] Endothelial-dependent vasodilatation is impaired early in children with pulmonary hypertensive congenital heart disease and a high pulmonary blood flow, but the response to sodium nitroprusside is preserved. Endothelial-independent dilatation is diminished in patients with an elevated pulmonary vascular resistance.[18] With any vasodilator, the release of vasoconstrictor tone will lower pulmonary vascular resistance, increase the magnitude of the left-to-right shunt and may lower the pulmonary arterial pressure, although not necessarily. Failure to achieve a vasodilator response implies fixed, organic obstruction of the pulmonary circulation. Children with Down's syndrome are particularly difficult to assess because they often suffer from upper airway obstruction, which may contribute to the increased pulmonary vascular resistance determined at cardiac catheterization. The pathologist will then find less pulmonary vascular damage in a lung biopsy than expected for the increase in pulmonary arterial pressure and resistance.

In patients who have previously had an intracardiac repair and are pulmonary hypertensive, the approach is similar to that in patients with primary pulmonary hypertension. When extremely ill, cardiac catheterization should not be unduly prolonged but testing with at least 100% oxygen and inhaled nitric oxide is mandatory in all cases because long-term treatment (either a calcium antagonist or prostacyclin/prostacyclin analog/endothelin receptor antagonist) is based on the response. A positive response to acute vasodilator testing is defined as a 20% or greater fall in pulmonary arterial pressure in the presence of an unchanged or increased cardiac output. Atrial septostomy/septectomy should be considered at the time of diagnostic catheterization in severely ill children (particularly if there is a history of drop attacks) whose anatomy is such that there is no opportunity for right-to-left shunting to acutely decompress the right heart and improve systemic output.

Wedge angiography

Wedge angiography can be helpful in demonstrating advanced pulmonary vascular obstructive disease, but cannot help in discriminating between less severe degrees of disease when the patient may still be potentially operable. The abnormal pulmonary wedge angiogram is characterized by decreased arborization, reduced background opacification, and delayed venous filling. The arteries may appear tortuous, have segments of dilatation or constriction or marginal defects suggestive of obliterative disease. Quantitative wedge angiography represents an attempt to improve the correlation between structure and function.[41] In the normal lung, the pulmonary arteries taper towards the periphery, but the vessels narrow over a shorter distance when pulmonary vascular resistance is elevated. The rate of tapering can be related to the pulmonary arterial pressure and vascular resistance and to the structural changes found at lung biopsy. Abrupt tapering is associated with a resistance >3.5 units/m^2, but further discrimination is difficult.

Open lung biopsy

An open lung biopsy may be indicated in complex congenital heart disease, suspected veno-occlusive disease and vasculitis. Assessment includes quantitative morphometry to determine vascular development and a description of the pathological abnormalities. When evaluating an individual lung biopsy, it is wiser to describe all the abnormalities present rather than to try to classify them, and relate the structural findings to the clinical and hemodynamic data.

Exercise test

A 6-minute walk test or surrogate according to age and capacity, is used to measure the degree of functional impairment. These tests may have additional benefit in patients with postoperative pulmonary hypertension without a shunt. In PPH, exercise capacity correlates with right atrial pressure, pulmonary arterial pressure and cardiac index. Marked limitation (<10% predicted) is associated with increased risk at cardiac catheterization.

Oxygen saturation measurements

Oxygen saturation measurements, including a sleep assessment, are performed in those with inoperable and clinically advanced disease.

High-resolution computed tomography of the chest

This may be indicated to evaluate the lung parenchyma.

Pulmonary function tests

These may be indicated in patients with postoperative pulmonary hypertension, without a shunt. In PPH a reduction in the forced expiratory flow between 25% and 75% of vital capacity (FEV_{25-75}) reflects the clinical and hemodynamic status.

Other tests

Suspicion of acute or chronic **thromboembolism** is an indication for ventilation/perfusion scintigraphy, magnetic resonance imaging and possibly pulmonary angiography.

MANAGEMENT

Patients subjected to intracardiac repair: factors influencing early and late results

The outcome of a satisfactory intracardiac repair is largely determined by the state of the pulmonary vascular bed at the time of repair. In the perioperative period, the problems are associated with endothelial smooth muscle cell dysfunction. Late outcome is determined by the extent to which the structural abnormalities are reversible.

Pulmonary hypertensive crises are now a well-recognized complication of intracardiac repair. Hypoxia is probably only the commonest identifiable precipitating factor. Crises tend to cluster and can be fatal. Cardiopulmonary bypass is thought to cause further damage to the already traumatized pulmonary endothelium and excess reactivity is evidence of disturbed control of smooth muscle cell contractility. The ventilatory management of pulmonary hypertension involves manipulating factors which control pulmonary vascular resistance. These include alveolar oxygenation, blood pH and lung volume. Lung overdistension or low lung volume results in increased pulmonary vascular resistance. Normocapnia or mild hypocapnia, in addition to systemic alkalosis, should be used to achieve an alkalotic pH (pH 7.45–7.5). In patients with acute lung injury after cardiopulmonary bypass, high-frequency ventilation may be beneficial. Adequate analgesia and sedation are necessary to avoid severe pulmonary vasoconstriction in response to noxious stimuli such as endotracheal suctioning. Marked hyperventilation and hyperoxia should be avoided as these result in secondary lung injury from barotrauma and oxygen toxicity. The management of pulmonary hypertensive crises has been transformed by the introduction of NO therapy. The dose of NO is titrated against the pulmonary arterial pressure and the patient is then maintained on the lowest possible dose. A reduction in pulmonary arterial pressure and vascular resistance accompanies an increase in the plasma level of cGMP.[42] It can be difficult to wean some patients off NO, possibly because exogenous NO may depress the release of endogenous cGMP. This situation may be alleviated by adding a phosphodiesterase inhibitor, a combination that can be more effective in reducing pulmonary arterial pressure than NO alone. Rebound pulmonary hypertension can occur after discontinuing NO, but this usually settles after an hour or so unless there are other compromising factors present. Intravenous prostacyclin was used extensively to control pulmonary vascular resistance postoperatively before the advent of NO, despite its being a non-selective vasodilator and possibly prejudicing the systemic circulation. Recent studies, however, show that prostacyclin can be extremely helpful when given by inhalation and can reduce pulmonary vascular resistance postoperatively in a dose-dependent manner.[43]

After repair, extensive clinical and experimental evidence has shown that pulmonary arterial medial hypertrophy, even with a modest amount of cellular intimal proliferation and fibrosis, is potentially reversible. Complete obliteration of the arterial lumen by intimal proliferation, even when highly cellular, is not usually reversible. Plexiform lesions are regarded as irreversible. It is not entirely certain whether these lesions are irreversible when present in early childhood, but given the severity of obstructive pathology with which they are associated, reversibility seems unlikely. The reduction in small intra-acinar arteries seen particularly in young children with severe pulmonary hypertension is probably not reversible.

The age at which intracardiac repair is carried out is the most crucial factor. Several studies have shown that the pulmonary vascular resistance usually falls to normal in those children operated upon before the age of 1 year. Surgery soon after the age of 2 years is associated with a fall in resistance, but not usually to a normal level. In 1978, 67 children with different types of intracardiac abnormalities underwent lung biopsy at the time of intracardiac repair and on the day after operation, patients whose biopsies showed only a modest increase in pulmonary arterial smooth muscle generally had a normal or near-normal pulmonary arterial pressure.[3,44] Those whose biopsies showed severe arterial medial hypertrophy or a reduction in peripheral arterial number had an increase in pressure, which was greater in those who also had intimal proliferation. Those whose lung biopsy showed intimal fibrosis had a higher mean pulmonary arterial pressure of approximately 40 mmHg or more, irrespective of the morphometric findings. One year after repair, however, all those operated on before 9 months of age had a normal pressure and/or resistance, regardless of the severity of the pulmonary vascular lesions at the time of repair. These observations indicate vessel wall remodeling towards normality, continued growth and a demonstrable improvement in endothelial function.[20,45] Of the children repaired after 9 months of age, those who had extension of muscle and an increase in pulmonary arterial smooth muscle had normal hemodynamic findings one year later, whereas those with more advanced changes generally did not.

In patients considered 'borderline', high risk for intracardiac repair, therapeutic manipulation of the pulmonary vasculature to reduce resistance and risk may be considered. This approach has not been evaluated, although intravenous epoprostenol has been used to reduce resistance in patients with heart failure in whom it is preferable to do a heart rather than a heart/lung transplantation.

Repairing an intracardiac abnormality in the presence of established pulmonary vascular disease accelerates the progression of disease and the onset of right ventricular failure and death. An early study described a group of children with a ventricular septal defect who underwent intracardiac repair at a mean age of 4.8 years, with a pulmonary vascular resistance more than 25% of the systemic vascular resistance and in excess of 400 dynes s/cm^5 per m.[46] The operative mortality was high and 18% of those surviving the operation died at between 1 and 7 years after operation with the Eisenmenger syndrome, when they were 7–16 years old.

Emphasis in clinical management must be on the prevention of pulmonary vascular disease. When the natural history of the cardiac abnormality is that of rapidly progressive pulmonary vascular disease, the child should undergo corrective or palliative surgery soon after birth and other abnormalities should be corrected before 1 year of age if the pulmonary arterial pressure remains high.

Patients with postoperative pulmonary hypertension

The patient with repaired congenital heart disease has effectively been turned into a patient with PPH, with the added problem of a compromised myocardium. Survival is significantly worse in the untreated patient with PPH than in most patients with the Eisenmenger syndrome. Assuming that these patients cannot be helped by further surgery, they should generally be treated as though they had PPH, and without delay.

Patients with inoperable pulmonary vascular disease

For patients with the Eisenmenger syndrome, treatment is still largely empirical. Long-term domiciliary oxygen treatment gives subjective improvement and can increase survival. Dipyridamole is given to reduce platelet aggregation but it may also have a beneficial vasodilatory effect as a phosphodiesterase inhibitor. Since thrombi become superimposed on the obstructive lesions of pulmonary vascular disease, there is an argument for anticoagulating these patients. Venesection with plasma dilution in those with a high hematocrit is not used routinely but may afford symptomatic relief to some patients. Frequent venesections causing iron deficiency can increase the risk of cerebrovascular accidents.

Treatment with prostacyclin is tempting, but its efficacy is not yet proven in patients with the classical Eisenmenger syndrome. Given intravenously, this nonselective vasodilator can cause systemic hypotension in the presence of a pulmonary–systemic communication. Inhalation of a stable analog would be more appropriate. Patients with advanced pulmonary vascular obstructive disease may, like those with primary pulmonary hypertension, be unable to increase their NO production on exercise.[47] Chronic administration of L-arginine might be helpful if it could be shown conclusively that these patients have a relative substrate deficiency of NO production. Calcium channel blockers are not used.

Finally, the only effective treatment for the very sick patient is transplantation, either a combined heart/lung transplantation, or lung transplantation with intracardiac repair. Conventionally, transplantation is recommended when the patient's condition begins to deteriorate rapidly. But a more active approach is to be recommended, which includes recatheterization as part of the routine reassessment.[37] Survival has been found to correlate with the product of pulmonary vascular resistance and mean right atrial pressure, a relatively crude evaluation of right ventricular function. Since the results of lung transplantation are unsatisfactory, transplantation should only be considered when the expected survival time is less than the expected survival after transplantation. We would do well to remember how long many of these patients can live with a relatively good quality of life. The average age at death for untreated patients, reported in the 1950s, was 33 years for aortopulmonary and ventricular septal defects and 36 years for atrial defects.[36] The maximum age reached was 65 years for ventricular and atrial septal defects and 55 years for patent ductus arteriosus.

FUTURE DIRECTIONS OF THERAPY

A patient with a left-to-right shunt should be managed using an integrated medical and surgical therapeutic strategy, tailored to meet the individual needs of the patient. To achieve this end, the immediate aims are to:

- improve non-invasive evaluation of disease severity, progression and response to treatment, both medical and surgical and so ensure appropriate therapy;
- reduce pulmonary vascular lability preoperatively in order to reduce operative risk, to remodel the vasculature of patients considered 'borderline' for intracardiac repair and arrest inoperable pulmonary vascular disease therapeutically, and at least improve quality of life and survival;
- explore the extent to which new and evolving therapies designed to treat primary pulmonary hypertension can be applied to patients with pulmonary hypertensive congenital heart disease;
- develop therapeutic strategies to stimulate growth of new, normal vessels, particularly in the young who have developed pulmonary hypertension before the lung has fulfilled its growth potential and in whom growth potential is greater.

The long-term strategy must be to:

- understand how pulmonary hypertension alters the endothelial sensing of oxygen tension, stress and strain, how it alters the contractile and cytoskeletal apparatus of pulmonary vascular smooth muscle cells and how these and other abnormalities of structural remodeling integrate and translate into functional disturbances;
- Since pulmonary vascular obstructive disease usually begins at birth with abnormal structural remodeling, it is crucial to identify the early factors which are altered by pulmonary hypertension and which instigate the cascade of abnormal structural and functional changes that become increasingly difficult

to reverse with the passage of time. Clinical and experimental studies in newborns indicate that abnormal pulmonary vascular remodeling fails to resolve completely and that the response to a subsequent hypertensive insult will result in a disproportionately aggressive response. These observations suggest persistent abnormalities in gene expression and signal transduction, which we must understand if we are to modulate them and ensure the resumption of normal development.

KEY POINTS

- In the presence of a left-to-right shunt, pulmonary vascular disease starts soon after birth with failure of the pulmonary vasculature to adapt normally to extrauterine life.
- The rate at which pulmonary vascular disease develops is related to the type of intracardiac abnormality.
- Endothelial dysfunction is present early and can be demonstrated clinically.
- Early operative intervention is indicated to prevent established disease, timed according to functional status and the type of intracardiac abnormality.
- Prediction of outcome with and without intracardiac repair is based on: clinicopathological studies relating the preoperative clinical and hemodynamic findings to the preoperative structural abnormalities in the lung in groups of patients with different types of congenital heart disease; and long-term follow-up studies.
- Perioperative pulmonary hypertensive crises commonly occur in patients with potentially operable pulmonary vascular disease.
- Therapeutic manipulation of the vasculature is now feasible in patients thought 'borderline' for repair, in an attempt to reduce operative risk.
- For inoperable patients and those with postoperative pulmonary hypertension, the new medical treatments used to treat PPH successfully are now being trialled.
- New therapeutic approaches will depend on advances in understanding the biology of flow.

REFERENCES

●1 Rich S (ed.) Primary pulmonary hypertension: Executive summary from the World Symposium on Primary Pulmonary Hypertension 1998, Evian, France, 6–10 September 1998. 2002.

2 Hall SM, Haworth SG. Onset and evolution of pulmonary vascular disease in young children: abnormal postnatal remodelling studied in lung biopsies. *J Pathol* 1992;**166**:183–94.

●3 Rabinovitch M, Haworth SG, Castaneda AR *et al*. Lung biopsy in congenital heart disease: a morphometric approach to pulmonary vascular disease. *Circulation* 1978;**58**:1107–22.

4 Cowan KN, Heilbut A, Humpl T *et al*. Complete reversal of fatal pulmonary hypertension in rats by a serine elastase inhibitor. *Nat Med* 2000;**6**:698–702.

●5 Haworth SG, Radley-Smith R, Yacoub M. Lung biopsy findings in transposition of the great arteries with ventricular septal defect: potentially reversible pulmonary vascular disease is not always synonymous with operability. *J Am Coll Cardiol* 1987;**9**:327–33.

∗6 Haworth SG. Pulmonary vascular disease in different types of congenital heart disease. Implications for interpretation of lung biopsy findings in early childhood. *Br Heart J* 1984;**52**:557–71.

7 Haworth SG. Pulmonary vascular disease in ventricular septal defect: structural and functional correlations in lung biopsies from 85 patients, with outcome of intra-cardiac repair. *J Pathol* 1987;**152**:157–68.

8 Haworth SG, Hall SM. Occlusion of intra-acinar pulmonary arteries in pulmonary hypertensive congenital heart disease. *Int J Cardiol* 1986;**13**:207–17.

9 Ku DD, Zaleski JK, Liu S *et al*. Vascular endothelial growth factor induces EDRF-dependent relaxation in coronary arteries. *Am J Physiol* 1993;**265**:H586–92.

10 Leung DW, Cachianes G, Kuang WJ *et al*. Vascular endothelial growth factor is a secreted angiogenic mitogen. *Science* 1989;**246**:1306–9.

11 Jones PL, Cowan KN, Rabinovitch M. Tenascin-C, proliferation and subendothelial fibronectin in progressive pulmonary vascular disease. *Am J Pathol* 1997;**150**:1349–60.

12 Haworth SG, Sauer U, Buhlmeyer K *et al*. Development of the pulmonary circulation in ventricular septal defect: a quantitative structural study. *Am J Cardiol* 1977;**40**:781–8.

13 Leanage R, Agnetti A, Graham G *et al*. Factors influencing survival after balloon atrial septostomy for complete transposition of the great arteries. *Br Heart J* 1981;**45**:559–72.

14 Haworth S. Pulmonary vascular bed in children with complete atrioventricular septal defect: relation between structural and hemodynamic abnormalities. *Am J Cardiol* 1986;**57**:833–9.

15 Haworth SG. Pulmonary vascular disease in secundum atrial septal defect in childhood. *Am J Cardiol* 1983;**51**:265–72.

16 Heath D, Edwards JE. The pathology of hypertensive pulmonary vascular disease. A description of six grades of structural changes in the pulmonary artery with special reference to congenital cardiac septal defect. *Circulation* 1958;**18**:533–47.

●17 Heath D, Helmholz F, Burchell HB *et al*. Graded pulmonary vascular changes in cases of atrial and ventricular septal defect and patent ductus arteriosus. *Circulation* 1958;**18**:1155–66.

18 Celermajer DS, Cullen S, Deanfield JE. Impairment of endothelium-dependent pulmonary artery relaxation in children with congenital heart disease and abnormal pulmonary hemodynamics. *Circulation* 1993;**87**:440–6.

19 Seghaye MC, Serraf A, Planche C. Endogenous nitric oxide production and atrial natriuretic peptide biological activity in infants undergoing cardiac operations. *Crit Care Med* 1997;**25**:1063–70.

20 Adatia I, Barrow SE, Stratton PD *et al*. Thromboxane A2 and prostacyclin biosynthesis in children and adolescents with pulmonary vascular disease. *Circulation* 1993;**88**:2117–22.

21 Komai H, Haworth SG. The effect of cardiopulmonary bypass on the lung. In: Jonas R, Elliott M (eds), *Cardiopulmonary bypass for congenital heart disease*. London: Butterworths, 1994;242–263.

◆22 Davies PF, Barbee KA, Volin MV *et al*. Spatial relationships in early signaling events of flow-mediated endothelial mechanotransduction. *Annu Rev Physiol* 1997;**59**:527–49.

23 Corson MA, James NL, Latta SE *et al*. Phosphorylation of endothelial nitric oxide synthase in response to fluid shear stress. *Circ Res* 1996;**79**:984–91.

24 Takahashi M, Ishida T, Traub O *et al*. Mechanotransduction in endothelial cells: temporal signaling events in response to shear stress. *J Vasc Res* 1997;**34**:212–19.

25 Ishida T, Peterson TE, Kovach N *et al*. MAP kinase activation by flow in endothelial cells: role of β1 integrins and tyrosine kinases. *Circ Res* 1996;**79**:310–16.

26 Resnick N, Yahav H, Khachigian LM *et al*. Endothelial gene regulation by laminar shear stress. *Adv Exp Med Biol* 1997; **430**:155–64.

27 Khachigian LM, Resnick N, Gimbrone MA Jr *et al*. Nuclear factor-kappa B interacts functionally within the platelet-derived growth factor B-chain shear-stress response element in vascular endothelial cells exposed to fluid shear stress. *J Clin Invest* 1995;**96**:1169–75.

28 Helmke BP, Thakker DB, Goldman RD *et al*. Spatiotemporal analysis of flow-induced intermediate filament displacement in living endothelial cells. *Biophys J* 2001;**80**:184–94.

29 Wehrle-Haller B, Imhof BA. The inner lives of focal adhesions [Review]. *Trends Cell Biol* 2002;**12**:383–9.

30 Muller JM, Chilian WM, Davis MJ. Integrin signaling transduces shear stress-dependent vasodilation of coronary arterioles. *Circ Res* 1997;**80**:320–6.

◆31 Resnick N, Gimbrone MA Jr. Hemodynamic forces are complex regulators of endothelial gene expression. *FASEB J* 1995;**9**:874–82.

32 Garcia-Cardena G, Comander JI, Blackman BR *et al*. Mechanosensitive endothelial gene expression profiles: scripts for the role of hemodynamics in atherogenesis? *Ann N Y Acad Sci* 2001;**947**:1–6.

33 Brooks AR, Lelkes PI, Rubanyi GM. Gene expression profiling of human aortic endothelial cells exposed to disturbed flow and steady laminar flow. *Physiol Genomics* 2002;**9**:27–41.

34 Walpola PL, Gotlieb AI, Cybulsky MI *et al*. Expression of ICAM-1 and VCAM-1 and monocyte adherence in arteries exposed to altered shear stress. *Arterioscler Thromb Vasc Biol* 1995;**15**:3–20.

●35 Wood P. The Eisenmenger syndrome or pulmonary hypertension with reversed central shunt. *Br Med J* 1958;**2**: 701–9 and **9**:755–62.

36 Wood P. *Diseases of the heart and circulation*, 3rd edn. London: Eyre & Spottiswoode, 1968;976–7.

37 Clabby ML, Canter CE, Moller JH *et al.* Hemodynamic data and survival in children with pulmonary hypertension. *J Am Coll Cardiol* 1997;**30**:554–60.

38 Bush A, Busst C, Booth K *et al.* Does prostacyclin enhance the selective pulmonary vasodilator effect of oxygen in children with congenital heart disease? *Circulation* 1986;**74**:135–44.

39 Winberg P, Lundell BP, Gustafsson LE. Effect of inhaled nitric oxide on raised pulmonary vascular resistance in children with congenital heart disease. *Br Heart J* 1994;**73**:282–6.

*40 Roberts JD, Polaner DM, Todres ID *et al.* Inhaled nitric oxide (NO): a selective pulmonary vasodilator for the treatment of persistent pulmonary hypertension of the newborn (PPHN). *Circulation* 1991;**84**:321.

41 Rabinovitch M, Keane JF, Fellows KE *et al.* Quantitative analysis of the pulmonary wedge angiogram in congenital heart defects. Correlation with hemodynamic data and morphometric findings in lung biopsy tissue. *Circulation* 1981;**63**:152–64.

42 Goldman AP, Haworth SG, Macrae DJ. Does inhaled nitric oxide suppress endogenous nitric oxide production? *Cardiovasc Thorac Surg* 1996;**112**:541–2.

43 Haraldsson A, Kieler-Jensen N, Ricksten SE. Inhaled prostacyclin for treatment of pulmonary hypertension after cardiac surgery or heart transplantation: a pharmacodynamic study. *J Cardiothorac Vasc Anesth* 1997;**10**:864–8.

44 Rabinovitch M, Keane JF, Norwood WI *et al.* Vascular structure in lung tissue obtained at biopsy correlated with pulmonary hemodynamic findings after repair of congenital heart defects. *Circulation* 1984;**69**:655–67.

45 Adatia I, Barrow SE, Stratton PD *et al.* Effect of intracardiac repair on thromboxane A2 and prostacyclin biosynthesis in children with a left to right shunt. *Br Heart J* 1994;**72**:452–6.

46 Friedli B, Kidd BSL, Mustard WT *et al.* Ventricular septal defect with increased pulmonary vascular resistance. Late results of surgical closure. *Am J Cardiol* 1974;**33**:403–9.

47 Riley MS, Porszasz J, Miranda J *et al.* Exhaled nitric oxide during exercise in primary pulmonary hypertension and pulmonary fibrosis. *Chest* 1997;**111**:44–50.

48 Kitley RM, Hislop AA, Hall SM *et al.* Birth associated changes in pulmonary arterial connective tissue gene expression in the normal and hypertensive lung. *Cardiovasc Res* 2000;**46**:332–45.

49 Stenmark KR, Mecham RP. Cellular and molecular mechanisms of pulmonary vascular remodeling. *Annu Rev Physiol* 1997;**59**:89–144.

Pulmonary vasculitis

KARINA KEOGH AND SEAN P GAINE

INTRODUCTION

Vasculitis is inflammation involving the walls of blood vessels that may be localized to a single organ or can affect multiple different organs.[1-3] The primary vasculitic disorders may be categorized based on size of the vessel involved, into small, medium and large vessel vasculitides, as proposed at the Chapel Hill Consensus Conference in 1994 (Table 13I.1 and Figure 13I.1).[4] The large vessel diseases affect the aorta and its major branches. The medium vessel diseases affect predominantly, if not exclusively, the main visceral arteries including renal,

Table 13I.1 *Classification of the primary systemic vasculitides based on the size of the blood vessel involvement[1]*

- **Large vessel**
  - Takayasu's arteritis
  - Giant cell (temporal) arteritis
- **Medium-sized vessel**
  - Kawasaki's
  - Polyarteritis nodosa (PAN)
- **Small vessel**
  - Churg–Strauss syndrome (CSS)
  - Cutaneous leukocytoclastic vasculitis
  - Essential cryoglobulinemic vasculitis
  - Henoch–Schönlein purpura (HSP)
  - Microscopic polyangiitis (MPA)
  - Wegener's granulomatosis (WG)

Table 13I.2 *Vasculitis involving the lung*

Large vessel
Takayasu's arteritis
Giant cell (temporal) arteritis

Small vessel
ANCA related
   Wegener's granulomatosis (WG)
   Microscopic polyangiitis (MPA)
   Churg–Strauss syndrome (CSS)
   Isolated pauci-immune
Collagen vascular disorders
   Systemic lupus erythematosus
   Rheumatoid arthritis
   Polymyositis
   Scleroderma
   Mixed connective tissue disease
Pulmonary allograft rejection
Goodpasture's disease
Henoch–Schönlein purpura (HSP)
IgA nephropathy
Idiopathic pauci-immune glomerulonephritis
Behçet's disease
Antiphospholipid syndrome
Essential cryoglobulinemia
Drug-related hypersensitivity vasculitis
Infection related vasculitis
Paraneoplastic vasculitis
Sarcoid vasculitis
Myasthenia gravis
Ulcerative colitis
Autologous bone marrow transplantation

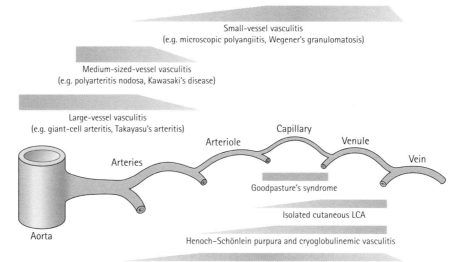

Figure 13I.1 *Preferred sites of vascular involvement by selected vasculitides. The widths of the trapezoids indicate the frequencies of involvement of various portions of the vasculature. LCA denotes leukocytoclastic angiitis. (From Jennette JC, Falk RJ. Small-vessel vasculitis. N Engl J Med 1997;337:1512–23, Figure 1, with permission.)*

hepatic, mesenteric and coronary arteries and their major branches. The small vessel vasculitides are distinguished by their involvement of arterioles, venules, and capillaries; however, they may also affect larger vessels.[1] Other forms of vasculitis not covered by this classification include vasculitis due to infection (e.g. *Rickettsia rickettsi*), medications (e.g. hydralazine), serum sickness and paraneoplastic syndromes.[1] Pulmonary involvement is most commonly associated with the small vessel vasculitides: Wegener's granulomatosis, microscopic polyangiitis, and Churg–Strauss syndrome (Table 13I.2).[5,6] Pulmonary involvement may rarely occur in the large vessel vasculitides, and thoracic aneurysms have been found in up to 17% of patients with temporal arteritis.[7,8] Pulmonary vasculitis may also be prominent in connective tissue diseases, such as systemic lupus erythematosus and rheumatoid arthritis.[6,9,10]

EPIDEMIOLOGY

Primary vasculitides are typically first diagnosed in middle life, although all ages may be affected. The average annual incidence has been estimated at 42–115 cases per million.[11–13] The incidence of individual vasculitic disorders may also vary with ethnicity. For example, Takayasu's arteritis is more common in Asians, whereas giant cell arteritis has a higher prevalence among northern Europeans.[14,15] Over the last decade, a trend towards an increased incidence of vasculitis has been reported,[16] though whether this is due to more accurate diagnosis

rather than a true increase in the incidence rate is unclear. Many of the vasculitides were once uniformly fatal, but with the advent of corticosteroid therapy and other immunosuppressive agents, significant improvements have been made.[17–24] However, particularly in the case of Wegener's and microscopic polyangiitis, there is still significant morbidity, and many patients experience one or more relapses.

PATHOLOGY

The hallmark of vasculitis is inflammation and necrosis involving the blood vessel wall. This can lead to two typical anatomical patterns; either there is sufficient inflammation to cause luminal narrowing and occlusion or alternatively, the extent of inflammation may cause sufficient weakening of the wall to cause aneurysm formation or vessel rupture. Vasculitic lesions are often both focal and segmental, meaning that the pathology will not be seen in all vessels of a similar size and even in those vessels that are affected, the lesions are generally not present in a uniform manner throughout. Parts of the vessel may be spared entirely. Inflammation may or may not extend through all vessel layers. Moreover, histologically there are only a limited number of patterns seen despite the many different etiologies and diffuse manifestations. Therefore, pathological findings are not generally diagnostic for a specific syndrome, although they may be suggestive, such as IgA and C3 deposition in Henoch–Schönlein purpura.[25]

In the lung, small vessel vasculitis affects the arterioles, venules and capillaries within the interstitial compartment The interstitial inflammation, as denoted by a neutrophilic infiltrate, edema and fibrin deposition, with fibrinoid necrosis of the capillary walls, is termed necrotizing pulmonary capillaritis. Damage to capillaries in the interstitium may cause leakage of blood into the alveolar spaces and diffuse alveolar hemorrhage. Arteriolar and capillary thrombosis can also be seen. In chronic cases there may be evidence of pulmonary fibrosis and/or changes consistent with emphysema.[6,26]

ETIOLOGY

A variety of pathophysiological processes have been implicated in the development of vasculitis, including immune-complex deposition, clonal lymphocyte expansion, cytokine production, autoantibody formation against neutrophilic granules and antigens presented by endothelial cells to circulating lymphocytes, thereby generating a localized immune response.[25,27–30] Within individual syndromes, it is felt that various different processes may lead to a final common pathway and therefore, similar histological pictures. The small vessel vasculitides that affect the lung are generally associated with antineutrophil cytoplasmic antibodies (ANCA).[29,31–33]

Antineutrophil cytoplasmic antibodies (ANCA)

Antineutrophil cytoplasmic antibodies (ANCA) were first described by Davies in 1982.[34] These antibodies react with antigens in neutrophil granules, and monocyte lysosomes resulting in two staining patterns on indirect immunofluorescence. Cytoplasmic ANCA (cANCA) cause a granular staining in the cytoplasm of ethanol-fixed neutrophils, while perinuclear ANCA (pANCA) give rise to perinuclear staining (Figure 13I.2). The target antigen for cANCA is almost always the serine protease PR-3, and is found in 80–95% of patients with Wegener's granulomatosis.[35] pANCA most commonly target MPO (myeloperoxidase) although there are a large number of other antigens with which it reacts, including many different neutrophil granule and cytoplasmic components as well as infection-related antigens (e.g. bactericidal permeability-increasing protein, BPI).[29] pANCA are reported to be positive in 50–80% of patients with Churg–Strauss syndrome[33,36] and in 40–80% with microscopic polyangiitis.[32,37,38] Furthermore, pANCA may also be present in a variety of connective tissue diseases such as rheumatoid arthritis, systemic lupus

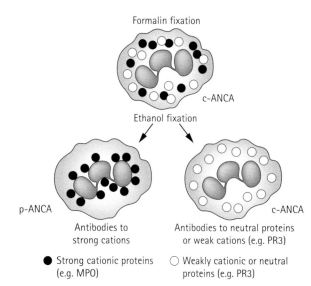

Figure 13I.2 *Antinuclear cytoplasmic antibodies (ANCA). The use of cross-linking fixatives (e.g. formalin) during the preparation of the neutrophil substrate results in ANCA-relevant antigens remaining in the cytoplasm. The pANCA fluorescent pattern represents an artifact of ethanol fixation. Ethanol fixation leads to alterations in granule membranes, allowing positively charged constituents to migrate to the negatively charged nuclear membrane. Because this does not occur with formalin fixation, use of both types of fixation allows the distinction of a true pANCA from an antinuclear antibody (ANA). With formalin-fixed neutrophils, antibodies that would cause pANCA patterns (on ethanol-fixed cells) will display diffuse granular cytoplasmic staining, whereas nuclear staining would indicate the presence of an ANA. MPO, myeloperoxidase; PR3, proteinase 3. (From Hoffman GS, Specks U. Antineutrophil cytoplasmic antibodies. Arthritis Rheum 1998;41(9):1521–37. Reprinted with permission from Wiley-Liss Inc., a subsidiary of John Wiley & Sons, Inc.)*

erythematosus and inflammatory bowel disease.[29,39–41] However, the presence of pANCA in patients with connective tissue disease does not necessarily indicate the presence of vasculitis. pANCA also appears to be induced by certain drugs (e.g. hydralazine)[42] and certain infections (e.g. pulmonary infections in patients with cystic fibrosis).[43]

There is evidence to suggest ANCA may play a direct pathogenic role in vasculitis. ANCA has been shown *in vitro* to have a proinflammatory effect on neutrophils, monocytes and endothelial cells (Figure 13I.3).[44] There are also animal studies where the majority of ANCA-positive mice develop vasculitis,[45] and where rats immunized with myeloperoxidase develop vasculitis.[46–48] Clinically, the correlation between ANCA positivity and disease activity would also support the theory that ANCA may play a pathogenic role.[29,49]

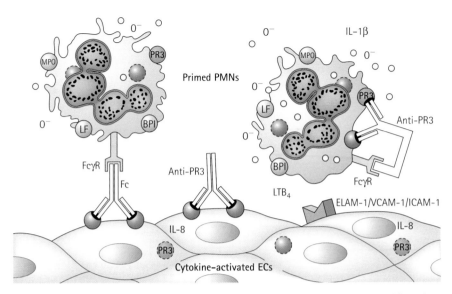

Figure 13I.3 *Hypothetical scheme for ANCA enhancement of vascular injury. In vitro activation of neutrophils and apoptosis is associated with translocation of numerous cytoplasmic proteins to the cell surface. Antibodies (e.g. anti-PR3) bound to appropriately displayed target antigens enhance neutrophil oxidative burst and degranulation. The magnitude of effect may be influenced by antibody specificity for different PR3 epitopes, IgG subclass, and the Fc(gamma) receptor [Fc(gamma)R] phenotype engaged. PR3 [and other proteins, e.g. elastase, lactoferrin (LF)] from degranulated neutrophils become bound to endothelial cells (ECs) and may cause enhanced expression of adhesion molecules and increased endothelial production of interleukin (IL)-8. ANCA have also been shown to enhance monocyte production of monocyte chemoattractant protein 1 and IL-8. Augmented chemotaxis and endothelial cell adhesion of leukocytes may follow, setting the stage for vascular injury. BPI, bactericidal/permeability-increasing protein; ELAM-1, endothelial leukocyte adhesion molecule 1; ICAM-1, intercellular adhesion molecule 1; LTB$_4$, leukotriene B$_4$; MPO, myeloperoxidase; PMN, polymorphonuclear cells; PR3, proteinase 3; VCAM-1, vascular cell adhesion molecule 1. (From Hoffman GS, Specks U. Antineutrophil cytoplasmic antibodies.* Arthritis Rheum *1998;41(9):1521–37. Reprinted with permission from Wiley-Liss, Inc., a subsidiary of John Wiley & Sons, Inc.)*

CLINICAL PRESENTATION

Common clinical manifestations of pulmonary vasculitis include dyspnea and cough with infiltrates (both localized and diffuse), or inflammatory nodules (often cavitatory) demonstrated radiologically. Hemoptysis secondary to alveolar hemorrhage occurs frequently in most types of pulmonary vasculitis and may be fatal.[6,50] However, significant alveolar hemorrhage may also occur in the absence of overt hemoptysis. In these patients, a diagnosis of diffuse alveolar hemorrhage may be made on the basis of bilateral alveolar infiltrates, a falling hematocrit, an elevated diffusion capacity on pulmonary function testing and a bronchoalveolar lavage showing aliquots that are sequentially more bloody and/or have hemosiderin-laden macrophages.[50] Pulmonary hypertension is rarely a feature in patients with pulmonary vasculitis but may be a feature in patients with more severe disease. Pulmonary vasculitis is also frequently associated with inflammatory involvement of the upper airways. Upper airway symptoms can include sinus pain, nasal discharge and epistaxis. Nasal erosions and crusting are frequently seen in patients with Wegener's or lymphomatoid granulomatosis. Oral ulcerations are characteristic of Behçet's

disease. In patients with tracheal involvement, tracheal stenosis may occur, and the presenting symptom may simply be stridor.

Although vasculitis can be localized to the respiratory tract, it more frequently occurs in the setting of systemic manifestations. These may include non-specific symptoms of fever, malaise, arthralgias or specific organ involvement.[1] The **skin** typically may reveal purpura, bullae or ulceration, livido reticularis and Raynaud's phenomenon.[51,52] **Renal** involvement is frequently found in the systemic vasculitic disorders. Wegener's granulomatosis commonly manifests with significant glomerulonephritis and may present with acute renal failure.[23,53] Renal disease less commonly occurs with Churg–Strauss syndrome and is rarely associated with significant loss of renal function.[32,54,55] **Central nervous system** involvement commonly occurs in giant cell arteritis and Takayasu's and to a lesser extent in Churg–Strauss syndrome and Wegener's granulomatosis.[56] **Peripheral nerve** lesions, such as mononeuritis multiplex, are common in polyarteritis nodosa and Churg–Strauss syndrome.[57,58] **Gastrointestinal disease** occurs frequently in patients with polyarteritis nodosa and to a lesser extent in Wegener's and Churg–Strauss.[53,55,59] Clinical manifestations range from abdominal pain (likely related to ischemia), bowel perforation, pancreatitis and bleeding. **Eye disease** is also frequently seen in Wegener's (sclero-uviitis) and Behçet's (iritis).

DIAGNOSTIC EVALUATION

Pulmonary function testing

The results of functional testing in patients with pulmonary vasculitis reflect the spectrum of clinical manifestations that can occur. In the absence of other pulmonary disease, pulmonary function testing may be normal or may show mildly reduced flow or lung volumes. Diffusing capacity is often reduced, though it may also be elevated in the setting of alveolar hemorrhage. Patients with Churg–Strauss will display typical reversible airflow obstruction of their associated asthma. Fixed obstructive flow patterns will be seen on the flow/volume loop of those patients with tracheal stenosis. Hypoxemia with or without hypocapnia is often seen in patients who develop an associated bronchiolitis obliterans.[23,60]

Radiological evaluation

The radiographic changes on chest x-ray and computed tomography are diverse. They include localized or diffuse infiltrates, solitary or multiple nodules (often cavitatory), or pseudotumor effects of lobar collapse. Pleural thickening or effusions secondary to inflammatory pleural disease may occur.[5] In those patients with chronic disease, a picture of interstial fibrosis may be seen. Even in those patients with no pulmonary symptoms, abnormalities on chest imaging are not uncommon.[23] Arterial narrowing and occlusion can be seen on pulmonary angiography in patients with large vessel vasculitides, e.g. Takayasu's arteritis (Figure 13I.4).[61] CT and MRI can also be used to image these lesions and may show thickened vessel walls and double ring attenuation. Perfusion lung scintigraphy, in these patients, often shows perfusion defects.[62–64]

Laboratory testing and biopsy

The vasculitides can rarely be diagnosed solely on clinical grounds, hence the importance of laboratory testing and biopsy. It is important to establish both the presence of vasculitis, and the exact type. In 1990, the American College of Rheumatology proposed criteria to define vasculitides for the purpose of clinical trials[65] and in 1994 the Chapel Hill Consensus Conference agreed upon definitions for the major vasculitides.[4] Although both these schemes are often

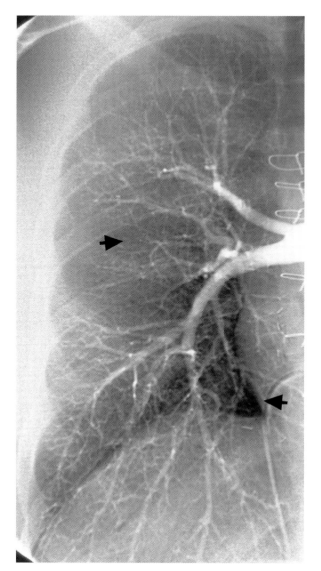

Figure 13I.4 *Radiology of Takayasu's arteritis. Pulmonary angiogram demonstrating diffusely narrowed vessels with areas of occlusion. (Image provided courtesy of the Mayo Foundation.)*

used in the diagnosis of individual patients, they were not originally intended to be used for this purpose and there are limited data on their suitability for this use.[66,67]

Investigation of patients with possible vasculitis include serological testing for ANCA, ANA, rheumatoid factor, complement, cryoglobulins, and viral serologies for hepatitis B and C as well as routine tests including full blood count, serum creatinine and electrolytes. If initial immunofluorescence testing for ANCA is positive, enzyme-linked immunoadsorbent assay (ELISA) testing for PR3 and MPO should be performed.[68] Urinalysis should be performed to assess for hematuria, red blood cell casts and proteinuria. Stool samples may be checked for occult blood. In the setting of neurological symptoms, an electromyogram may suggest a vasculitic etiology.

Ideally, the diagnosis would be confirmed with a biopsy, though in cases with classical symptomatology, particularly when supported by appropriate serology, it is not always necessary. A tissue diagnosis is not required to fulfill either the American College of Rheumatology criteria or the definitions of the Chapel Hill consensus conference. When a biopsy is necessary, it should be taken from the most accessible involved organ, such as the skin. In Wegener's granulomatosis, an upper airway biopsy is often diagnostic. The role of transbronchial biopsy in the diagnosis of pulmonary vasculitis is limited whereas open lung biopsy has a much higher yield.[23,69]

TREATMENT

The basis of pulmonary vasculitis treatment is immunosuppression with corticosteroids, generally at initial doses of 1 mg/kg·day of prednisone orally. Patients with alveolar hemorrhage or rapidly progressive glomerulonephritis should receive intravenous Solu-Medrol (methylprednisolone hemisuccinate) for the first 3 days. Cytotoxic therapy with cyclophosphamide is necessary in individuals with Wegener's granulomatosis who have significant pulmonary or renal disease.[70] Cyclophosphamide is generally started at 2 mg/kg·day orally, and is the preferred treatment; however, 'pulses' of intravenous cyclophosphamide every few weeks may also be given.[71] The intravenous route is used primarily where there is a particular need to limit side effects such as gonadal damage. Patients generally receive 750–1000 mg/m^2·month with pulse dosing, which is a smaller cumulative dose than they would receive in a month of oral cyclophosphamide.[72–74] In patients without life- or organ-threatening disease, a combination of prednisone and methotrexate can be used to induce remission. In other vasculitic diseases such as Churg–Strauss syndrome, cytotoxic agents are used in severe disease, especially if there is cardiac, CNS, renal or gastrointestinal involvement.[32] Cytotoxic therapies are also introduced if the patient fails to respond to initial therapy with corticosteroids. Immunosuppressive therapy places patients at risk for serious infections – in one study, 54% of patients with Wegener's granulomatosis developed opportunistic infection.[73] In addition, cyclophosphamide carries the risk of hematological malignancies, bladder cancer, hemorrhagic cystitis (the risk of this may be reduced by sufficient fluid intake and the co-administration of mesna) and infertility.[23]

Furthermore, the optimal duration of treatment is subject to ongoing investigation. In general, once the patient is in disease remission, has been stable for about 6 months, and has tolerated a steroid taper, they can be changed to less toxic agents such as azathioprine or methotrexate.[71] Patients should then remain on these immunosuppressants for at least 2 years, while their corticosteroid dose is slowly tapered. Some clinicians would continue immunosuppressant therapy indefinitely.[2] Relapse of Wegener's granulomatosis has been associated with infection of the upper respiratory tract[75] and there is some evidence that trimethoprim-sulfamethoxazole reduces the rate of relapse.[76–78] When patients do relapse, there is currently no consensus on the best treatment. Major relapses may necessitate a return to initial induction therapy. Other treatments that have been tried include cyclosporin, plasma exchanges[79] and the use of intravenous immunoglobulin.[80,81] Patients receiving long-term steroids should also receive prophylaxis against osteoporosis including: calcium, vitamin D and, where indicated, bisphosphonates. Prophylaxis against *Pneumocystis carinii* should be considered in any patient on chronic immunosuppressive therapy or corticosteroids in excess of 20 mg/day.[82,83]

SPECIFIC DISORDERS

Wegener's granulomatosis

Wegener's granulomatosis is the most common of the vasculitides that typically affect the lung, with an estimated prevalence of 3 per 100 000.[24] Moreover, the lung is the most frequently involved organ in Wegener's, with up to 90% of patients having pulmonary symptoms.[23,84]

The blood vessels involved in Wegener's granulomatosis are predominantly the small arteries and veins. Classically, the pathology shows a triad of necrotizing vasculitis, necrotizing granulomatous upper and lower respiratory tract inflammation, and necrotizing glomerulonephritis (Plate 13I.1).[85] However, limited forms may also occur.[86] The American College of Rheumatology criteria for the diagnosis of Wegener's granulomatosis are highlighted in Table 13I.3. Two out of four criteria must be met.[87]

More than 90% of patients with Wegener's are cANCA positive while a minority are pANCA positive. Wegener's granulomatosis presents most commonly in middle-aged men. Patients often present with non-specific symptoms such as fever and weight loss. They may have worsening sinusitis. Pulmonary involvement may cause chest pain, dyspnea, purulent sputum or hemoptysis. Airway stenosis occurs in 15% of adults and 50% of children secondary

Table 13I.3 *The American College of Rheumatology criteria for the diagnosis of Wegener's granulomatosis (two of four criteria are necessary)*[87]

1 Nasal or oral inflammation
2 Abnormal chest x-ray (nodules, fixed infiltrates or cavities)
3 Abnormal urinary sediment
4 Granulomatous inflammation on biopsy

to tracheal inflammation, most commonly in the sub-glottic region,[23] and presents with shortness of breath or stridor. Chest x-ray findings may be unilateral or bilateral and they include infiltrates (63%), nodules (31%) and cavitary lesions (20%). Endobronchial lesions have been identified in up to 59% of patients with pulmonary Wegener's undergoing bronchoscopy.[88] Hemoptysis (in 12–40%), increased DLCO or a fall in serum hemoglobin may indicate pulmonary hemorrhage. These patients have a high mortality due to either respiratory failure directly caused by the hemorrhage, or pulmonary fibrosis in the longer term. Upper respiratory tract involvement includes pain, purulent or bloody nasal discharge, perfo-ration and necrosis of the nasal septum leading to saddle nose deformity, and otitis media (involvement of the seventh cranial nerve leads to facial paralysis). Renal involvement is very common. In one large series 77% of patients developed glomerulonephritis.[23] Other organs that may be involved include the heart, skin, joints and both the peripheral and central nervous system.

Patient survival has improved dramatically from the original case series by Wegener, where all patients died within 7 months, to a 5-year mortality of less than 20%.[23,53] A significant proportion of the morbidity and mortality is now related to treatment. Treatment of Wegener's granulomatosis consists of both corticosteroids and cyclophosphamide from the time of presentation, as pre-viously outlined. Other agents which have been tried include: intravenous immunoglobulin, plasmapheresis, cyclosporin, antitumor necrosis factor, leflunomide, mycophenolate mofetil, tacrolimus and anti-CD20.[74,89–92] Subglottic stenosis may require mechanical dilatations and corticosteroid injections. Tracheostomy is now less commonly necessary. Direct involvement of the main pulmonary artery with stenosis and right heart failure has also been described (Figure 13I.5).[93]

Microscopic polyangiitis

Microscopic polyangiitis (MPA) is a non-granulomatous necrotizing vasculitis involving small and medium vessels that shares many features with Wegener's granulomatosis. The kidneys are invariably affected and, as in Wegener's, the renal disease may deteriorate rapidly. Pulmonary hem-orrhage may occur in 10–30% and may be fatal. Rashes and mononeuritis multiplex are less common, as is gastrointestinal involvement. Ocular and ENT symptoms are much less common than in Wegener's.[22,26,32,37,94,95] MPA was not widely accepted as an entity distinct from polyarteritis nodosa in the USA until the early 1990s, and is not included in the American College of Rheumatology classification scheme. It is defined as 'necrotizing vasculitis with few or no immune deposits affecting small vessels'.[4] It is generally diagnosed on the basis of renal biopsy

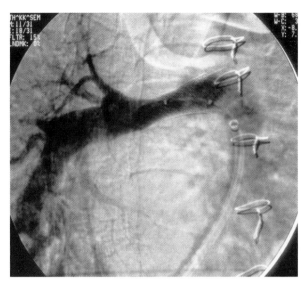

Figure 13I.5 *Radiology of pulmonary artery stenosis and stent. Stenosis of the right pulmonary artery in a patient with Wegener's granulomatosis corrected by the placement of an endovascular stent.*

showing focal pauci immune segmental glomerulonephri-tis, with extracapillary proliferation forming crescents. ANCA is present in 40–80% of patients with MPA and while in most studies the majority of patients are pANCA positive, cANCA positivity is reported at 10–50%. Skin biopsy generally shows leukocytoclastic vasculitis. There may be infiltrates on chest x-ray. Visceral angiogram is gen-erally unhelpful even in the setting of abdominal symp-toms as the involved vessels are too small to be visualized.[96]

Churg–Strauss syndrome

Churg–Strauss syndrome (CSS) is a necrotizing vasculi-tis of small and medium-sized vessels also commonly affecting the lung, but, unlike Wegener's granulomatosis and microscopic polyangiitis, it is typically associated with asthma and peripheral eosinophilia.[97,98] There may be three distinct phases of Churg–Strauss, the first being a prodromal asthmatic/allergic phase which tends to pre-cede the other features, often by many years. It may be associated with allergic rhinitis and nasal polyposis. The second is an eosinophilic phase with peripheral eosinophilia measured in excess of 1.5×10^9/L. This phase maybe associated with eosinophilic infiltrations of the lung (Loeffler's syndrome or eosinophilic pneumonia) or gastrointestinal tract (eosinophilic gastroenteritis). Finally there is a vasculitic phase of Churg–Strauss. It has been recognized, however, that all three phases are often not seen simultaneously in the same patient. Disease expression may also be modified by drug therapy and, increasingly, 'formes frustes' of CSS have been recog-nized.[99] The American College of Rheumatology criteria

Table 13I.4 *The American College of Rheumatology criteria for the diagnosis of Churg–Strauss syndrome (four of six criteria are necessary)*[100]

1 Asthma
2 Peripheral eosinophilia > 10% of the total white cell count
3 Peripheral neuropathy attributable to a systemic vasculitis
4 Transient pulmonary infiltrates on chest x-ray
5 Paranasal sinus disease
6 Biopsy containing a blood vessel with extravascular eosinophils

suggest the diagnosis of Churg–Strauss if four of six criteria are present (Table 13I.4).[100] Renal involvement in CSS is less prominent than in Wegener's and microscopic polyangiitis, and rarely leads to renal failure.[32,54,55] However, peripheral nerve involvement with mononeuritis multiplex is more common. Organs that may be involved include the skin, heart, peripheral and central nervous system and abdominal viscera. Churg–Strauss is typically pANCA positive, and ANCA status appears to correlate with disease activity, though not with organ manifestation.[33,36]

Recently, it has been suggested that the use of leukotriene receptor antagonists in the treatment of asthma may play a causative role in the development of CSS.[101–106] However, generally these agents allow for corticosteroid dose reduction and therefore may unmask pre-existing Churg–Strauss rather than play a primary 'vasculitogenic' role.[107,108] The mainstay of treatment is corticosteroids while the cytotoxic agent most commonly used is cyclophosphamide. Other drugs that have been used include azathioprine, methotrexate and interferon-alpha.[109]

Giant cell arteritis

Giant cell or temporal arteritis is a large vessel vasculitic disorder. It generally effects patients over the age of 50 and is more common in women and in those of Northern European origin.[13,110] A subacute onset may include early symptoms of malaise, fatigue, weight loss and fever associated with a very high erythrocyte sedimentation rate. Alternatively, an abrupt, painless visual loss may occur (in 15% of patients) due to vasculitic involvement of the ophthalmic or posterior ciliary artery.[110] Permanent blindness may be preceded by amaurosis fugax. Other common symptoms include headaches, tenderness over the temporal arteries and jaw claudication. Giant cell arteritis is frequently seen in association with polymyalgia rheumatica. Biopsy of the temporal arteries is diagnostic with pathology showing giant cells and lymphocytes, with intimal proliferation and destruction of the elastic membranes. Bilateral biopsies of the temporal arteries are generally obtained, as

there may be skip lesions.[111] The aortic arch and its branches are clinically involved in 10–15% of patients[112] and may lead to cough and aortic arch syndrome. There are several reports of pulmonary involvement.[113]

Isolated pauci–immune pulmonary capillaritis

There have been several reports of an isolated pauci-immune pulmonary capillaritis causing diffuse alveolar hemorrhage.[94,114,115] These patients have had variable pANCA positivity. In a series of 29 patients with mean follow-up of 43 months, there was no evidence for a systemic disease.[115]

Takayasu's arteritis

Takayasu's arteritis affects vessels with abundant elastic tissue such as the aorta and its major branches. The pulmonary vasculature has an elastic component to the peripheral lobular branches and these may be affected in up to 50% of patients with the disease, with almost 70% having moderate pulmonary hypertension.[61,64,116] Takayasu's arteritis is most common in Asian women and it almost universally occurs in those less than 50 years of age. Early symptoms include malaise and arthralgia. Later, symptoms of vascular obstruction become apparent, such as headaches, dizziness and visual disturbances. If the coronary ostia are involved, the patient may develop angina. There may be claudication in the arms or the legs due to involvement to the subclavian, or the distal aorta and the iliac vessels. Cerebral and intra-abdominal ischemia may also develop. On examination, almost all patients have an asymmetrical reduction in peripheral pulses, with blood pressure differences of >10 mmHg. They may also have bruits over the large vessels or a murmur of aortic insufficiency due to aortic root dilatation. Tests show normocytic anemia, a raised erythrocyte sedimentation rate and thrombocytosis. The electrocardiogram may show ischemia and the chest x-ray may show a dilated aortic arch. The diagnosis is generally confirmed on angiography that shows aneurysms with smooth tapered narrowings and occlusions of involved vessels (Figure 13I.4). CT and MRA are most commonly used in follow-up, rather than to make the initial diagnosis. Biopsy is rarely pursued because of the size of the vessels involved. These patients generally follow a chronic course, with a 15-year survival of greater than 80% with immunosuppressant therapy.[117]

Polyarteritis nodosa

Polyarteritis nodosa was the first form of vasculitis described in 1866 by Kussmaul and Maier.[118,119] It affects small and medium-sized muscular arteries, but not arterioles, venules or capillaries. Classically, polyarteritis nodosa affects the joints, gastrointestinal tract, including liver, and the peripheral and central nervous systems. While in the past pulmonary involvement has been reported, most, if not all, of these patients would now be classified as having Churg–Strauss syndrome or microscopic polyangiitis.

Miscellaneous causes of pulmonary vasculitis

Pulmonary vasculitis may also occur in a number of other diseases, including Goodpasture's disease, Henoch–Schönlein purpura, Behçet's disease and connective tissue diseases including rheumatoid arthritis and systemic lupus erythematosus.[120–124] It may also be seen in sarcoidosis and infectious processes such as with HIV and cytomegalovirus (CMV).[125–128]

KEY POINTS

- Vasculitis is inflammation and necrosis of blood vessel walls.
- Primary vasculitic disorders may be categorized based on size of vessel (small, medium, large).
- Pulmonary involvement in vasculitis is most commonly associated with small vessel vasculitides.
- The most common conditions are Wegener's granulomatosis, microscopic polyangiitis and Churg–Strauss syndrome.
- Pulmonary vasculitides are commonly associated with antineutrophilic cytoplasmic antibodies.
- Treatment involves steroids ± other immunosuppressants.

REFERENCES

♦1 Jennette JC, Falk RJ. Small-vessel vasculitis. *N Engl J Med* 1997;**337**:1512–23.

2 Savage CO, Harper L, Adu D. Primary systemic vasculitis. *Lancet* 1997;**349**:553–8.

3 Savage CO, Harper L, Cockwell P *et al*. ABC of arterial and vascular disease: vasculitis. *Br Med J* 2000;**320**:1325–8.

●4 Jennette JC, Falk RJ. Nomenclature of systemic vasculitides. *Arthritis Rheum* 1994;**37**:187–92.

5 Burns A. Pulmonary vasculitis. *Thorax* 1998;**53**:220–7.

♦6 Schwarz MI, Brown KK. Small vessel vasculitis of the lung. *Thorax* 2000;**55**:502–10.

7 Larson TS, Hall S, Hepper NG *et al*. Respiratory tract symptoms as a clue to giant cell arteritis. *Ann Intern Med* 1984;**101**:594–7.

8 Evans J, Hunder GG. The implications of recognizing large-vessel involvement in elderly patients with giant cell arteritis. *Curr Opin Rheumatol* 1997;**9**:37–40.

9 Zamora MR, Warner ML, Tuder R *et al*. Diffuse alveolar hemorrhage and systemic lupus erythematosus. Clinical presentation, histology, survival, and outcome. *Medicine (Baltimore)* 1997;**76**:192–202.

10 Schwarz MI, Zamora MR, Hodges TN *et al*. Isolated pulmonary capillaritis and diffuse alveolar hemorrhage in rheumatoid arthritis and mixed connective tissue disease. *Chest* 1998;**113**:1609–15.

11 Scott DG, Watts RA. Classification and epidemiology of systemic vasculitis. *Br J Rheumatol* 1994;**33**:897–9.

12 Haugeberg G, Bie R, Bendvold A *et al*. Primary vasculitis in a Norwegian community hospital: a retrospective study. *Clin Rheumatol* 1998;**17**:364–8.

♦13 Gonzalez-Gay MA, Garcia-Porrua C. Epidemiology of the vasculitides. *Rheum Dis Clin North Am* 2001;**27**:729–49.

14 Kerr GS, Hallahan CW, Giordano J *et al*. Takayasu arteritis. *Ann Intern Med* 1994;**120**:919–29.

15 Sala Felix J, Pereiro Alonso ME, Salas Anton C. Treatment of asthma with antileukotrienes and Churg-Strauss syndrome. *Arch Bronconeumol* 2001;**37**:48–50.

16 Watts RA, Gonzalez-Gay MA, Lane SE *et al*. Geoepidemiology of systemic vasculitis: comparison of the incidence in two regions of Europe. *Ann Rheum Dis* 2001;**60**:170–2.

17 Walton EW. Giant cell granuloma of the respiratory tract (Wegener's granulomatosis). *Br Med J* 1958;**2**:265–70.

18 Hollander D, Manning RT. The use of alkylating agents in the treatment of Wegener's granulomatosis. *Ann Intern Med* 1967;**67**:393–8.

●19 Fauci AS, Wolff SM. Wegener's granulomatosis: studies in eighteen patients and a review of the literature. *Medicine (Baltimore)* 1973;**52**:535–61.

20 Reza MJ, Dornfeld L, Goldberg LS *et al*. Wegener's granulomatosis. Long-term follow-up of patients treated with cyclophosphamide. *Arthritis Rheum* 1975;**18**:501–6.

●21 Fauci AS, Haynes BF, Katz P *et al*. Wegener's granulomatosis: prospective clinical and therapeutic experience with 85 patients for 21 years. *Ann Intern Med* 1983;**98**:76–85.

22 Savage CO, Winearls CG, Evans DJ *et al*. Microscopic polyarteritis: presentation, pathology and prognosis. *Q J Med* 1985;**56**:467–83.

●23 Hoffman GS, Kerr GS, Leavitt RY *et al*. Wegener granulomatosis: an analysis of 158 patients. *Ann Intern Med* 1992;**116**:488–98.

24 Cotch M, Hoffman G, Yerg D *et al*. The epidemiology of Wegener's granulomatosis: estimates of the five-year period prevalence, annual mortality, and geographic disease distribution from population-based data sources. *Arthritis Rheum* 1996;**39**:87–92.

25 Faille-Kuyber EH, Kater L, Kooiker CJ *et al*. IgA-deposits in cutaneous blood-vessel walls and mesangium in Henoch-Schonlein syndrome. *Lancet* 1973;**1**:892–3.

26 Mark EJ, Ramirez JF. Pulmonary capillaritis and hemorrhage in patients with systemic vasculitis. *Arch Pathol Lab Med* 1985;**109**:413–18.

27 Weyand CM, Schonberger J, Oppitz U *et al.* Distinct vascular lesions in giant cell arteritis share identical T cell clonotypes. *J Exp Med* 1994;**179**:951–60.

28 Weyand CM, Hicok KC, Hunder GG *et al.* Tissue cytokine patterns in patients with polymyalgia rheumatica and giant cell arteritis. *Ann Intern Med* 1994;**121**:484–91.

♦29 Hoffman GS, Specks U. Antineutrophil cytoplasmic antibodies. *Arthritis Rheum* 1998;**41**:1521–37.

30 Hughes CC, Savage CO, Pober JS. The endothelial cell as a regulator of T-cell function. *Immunol Rev* 1990;**117**:85–102.

31 Cohen Tervaert JW, Limburg PC, Elema JD *et al.* Detection of autoantibodies against myeloid lysosomal enzymes: a useful adjunct to classification of patients with biopsy-proven necrotizing arteritis. *Am J Med* 1991;**91**:59–66.

●32 Gayraud M, Guillevin L, le Toumelin P *et al.* Long-term followup of polyarteritis nodosa, microscopic polyangiitis, and Churg–Strauss syndrome: analysis of four prospective trials including 278 patients. *Arthritis Rheum* 2001;**44**:666–75.

33 Solans R, Bosch JA, Perez-Bocznegra C *et al.* Churg-Strauss syndrome: outcome and long-term follow-up of 32 patients. *Rheumatology (Oxford)* 2001;**40**:763–71.

34 Davies D, Moran J, Niall J. Segmental necrotizing glomerulonephritis with antineutrophil antibody: possible arbovirus aetiology. *Br Med J* 1982;**285**:606.

35 Specks U, Wiegert EM, Homburger HA. Human mast cells expressing recombinent proteinase 3 (PR3) as substrate for clincal testing for antineutophil cytoplasmic antibodies (ANCA). *Clin Exp Immunol* 1997;**109**:286–95.

36 Cohen Tervaert JW, Goldschmeding R, Elema JD *et al.* Antimyeloperoxidase antibodies in the Churg-Strauss syndrome. *Thorax* 1991;**46**:70–1.

37 Lauque D, Cadranel J, Lazor R *et al.* Microscopic polyangiitis with alveolar hemorrhage. A study of 29 cases and review of the literature. Groupe d'Etudes et de Recherche sur les Maladies 'Orphelines' Pulmonaires (GERM'O'P). *Medicine (Baltimore)* 2000;**79**:222–33.

●38 Guillevin L, Durand-Gasselin B, Cevallos R *et al.* Microscopic polyangiitis: clinical and laboratory findings in eighty-five patients. *Arthritis Rheum* 1999;**42**:421–30.

39 Savige JA, Gallicchio MC, Stockman A *et al.* Anti-neutrophil cytoplasm antibodies in rheumatoid arthritis. *Clin Exp Immunol* 1991;**86**:92–8.

40 Saxon A, Shanahan F, Landers C *et al.* A distinct subset of antineutrophil cytoplasmic antibodies is associated with inflammatory bowel disease. *J Allergy Clin Immunol* 1990;**86**:202–10.

41 Merkel PA, Polisson RP, Chang Y *et al.* Prevalence of antineutrophil cytoplasmic antibodies in a large inception cohort of patients with connective tissue disease. *Ann Intern Med* 1997;**126**:866–73.

42 Short AK, Lockwood CM. Antigen specificity in hydralazine associated ANCA positive systemic vasculitis. *Q J Med* 1995;**88**:775–83.

43 Aebi C, Theiler F, Aebischer CC *et al.* Autoantibodies directed against bactericidal/permeability-increasing protein in patients with cystic fibrosis: association with microbial respiratory tract colonization. *Pediatr Infect Dis J* 2000;**19**:207–12.

44 Russell KA, Specks U. Are antineutrophil cytoplasmic antibodies pathogenic? Experimental approaches to understand the antineutrophil cytoplasmic antibody phenomenon. *Rheum Dis Clin North Am* 2001;**27**:815–32, vii.

45 Harper JM, Thiru S, Lockwood CM *et al.* Myeloperoxidase autoantibodies distinguish vasculitis mediated by anti-neutrophil cytoplasm antibodies from immune complex disease in MRL/Mp- lpr/lpr mice: a spontaneous model for human microscopic angiitis. *Eur J Immunol* 1998;**28**:2217–26.

46 Harbeck RJ, Launder T, Staszak C. Mononuclear cell pulmonary vasculitis in NZB/W mice. II. Immunohistochemical characterization of the infiltrating cells. *Am J Pathol* 1986;**123**:204–11.

47 Foucher P, Heeringa P, Petersen AH *et al.* Antimyeloperoxidase-associated lung disease. An experimental model. *Am J Respir Crit Care Med* 1999;**160**:987–94.

48 Brouwer E, Huitema MG, Klok PA *et al.* Antimyeloperoxidase-associated proliferative glomerulonephritis: an animal model. *J Exp Med* 1993;**177**:905–14.

49 Pall AA, Savage CO. Mechanisms of endothelial cell injury in vasculitis. *Springer Semin Immunopathol* 1994;**16**:23–37.

50 Green RJ, Ruoss SJ, Kraft SA *et al.* Pulmonary capillaritis and alveolar hemorrhage. Update on diagnosis and management. *Chest* 1996;**110**:1305–16.

51 Blanco R, Martinez-Taboada VM, Rodriguez-Valverde V *et al.* Cutaneous vasculitis in children and adults. Associated diseases and etiologic factors in 303 patients. *Medicine (Baltimore)* 1998;**77**:403–18.

52 Gibson LE. Cutaneous vasculitis update. *Dermatol Clin* 2001;**19**:603–15, vii.

●53 Reinhold-Keller E, Beuge N, Latza U *et al.* An interdisciplinary approach to the care of patients with Wegener's granulomatosis: long-term outcome in 155 patients. *Arthritis Rheum* 2000;**43**:1021–32.

●54 Chumbley LC, Harrison RG, DeRemee RA. Allergic granulomatosis and angiitis (Churg-Strauss syndrome). *Mayo Clin Proc* 1977;**52**:477–84.

●55 Guillevin L, Cohen P, Gayraud M *et al.* Churg-Strauss syndrome. Clinical study and long-term follow-up of 96 patients. *Medicine (Baltimore)* 1999;**78**:26–37.

56 Ferro JM. Vasculitis of the central nervous system. *J Neurol* 1998;**245**:766–76.

57 Lhote F, Guillevin L. Polyarteritis nodosa, microscopic polyangiitis, and Churg-Strauss syndrome. Clinical aspects and treatment. *Rheum Dis Clin North Am* 1995;**21**:911–47.

58 Sehgal M, Swanson JW, DeRemee RA, Colby TV. Neurologic manifestations of Churg-Strauss syndrome. *Mayo Clin Proc* 1995;**70**:337–41.

59 Levine SM, Hellmann DB, Stone JH. Gastrointestinal involvement in polyarteritis nodosa (1986–2000): presentation and outcomes in 24 patients. *Am J Med* 2002;**112**:386–91.

60 Rosenberg DM, Weinberger SE, Fulmer JD *et al.* Functional correlates of lung involvement in Wegener's granulomatosis. Use of pulmonary function tests in staging and follow-up. *Am J Med* 1980;**69**:387–94.

61 Lie JT. Isolated pulmonary Takayasu arteritis: clinico-pathologic characteristics. *Mod Pathol* 1996;**9**:469–74.

62 Tanigawa K, Eguchi K, Kitamura Y *et al.* Magnetic resonance imaging detection of aortic and pulmonary artery wall thickening in the acute stage of Takayasu arteritis. Improvement of clinical and radiologic findings after steroid therapy. *Arthritis Rheum* 1992;**35**:476–80.

63 Takahashi K, Honda M, Furuse M *et al.* CT findings of pulmonary parenchyma in Takayasu arteritis. *J Comput Assist Tomogr* 1996;**20**:742–8.

64 Hara M, Sobue R, Ohba S *et al.* Diffuse pulmonary lesions in early phase Takayasu arteritis predominantly involving pulmonary artery. *J Comput Assist Tomogr* 1998;**22**:801–3.

65 Hunder GG, Arend WP, Bloch DA *et al.* The American College of Rheumatology 1990 criteria for the classification of vasculitis. Introduction. *Arthritis Rheum* 1990;**33**:1065–7.

66 Rao JK, Allen NB, Pincus T. Limitations of the 1990 American College of Rheumatology classification criteria in the diagnosis of vasculitis. *Ann Intern Med* 1998;**129**:345–52.

67 Hunder GG. The use and misuse of classification and diagnostic criteria for complex diseases. *Ann Intern Med* 1998;**129**:417–18.

68 Savige J, Gillis D, Benson E *et al.* International Consensus Statement on Testing and Reporting of Antineutrophil Cytoplasmic Antibodies (ANCA). *Am J Clin Pathol* 1999;**111**:507–13.

69 Schnabel A, Holl-Ulrich K, Dalhoff K *et al.* Efficacy of transbronchial biopsy in pulmonary vasculitides. *Eur Respir J* 1997;**10**:2738–43.

●70 Fauci AS, Wolff SM, Johnson JS. Effect of cyclophosphamide upon the immune response in Wegener's granulomatosis. *N Engl J Med* 1971;**285**:1493–6.

71 Hoffman GS. Treatment of Wegener's granulomatosis: time to change the standard of care? *Arthritis Rheum* 1997;**40**:2099–104.

72 Hoffman GS, Leavitt RY, Fleisher TA *et al.* Treatment of Wegener's granulomatosis with intermittent high-dose intravenous cyclophosphamide. *Am J Med* 1990;**89**:403–10.

73 Guillevin L, Cordier JF, Lhote F *et al.* A prospective, multicenter, randomized trial comparing steroids and pulse cyclophosphamide versus steroids and oral cyclophosphamide in the treatment of generalized Wegener's granulomatosis. *Arthritis Rheum* 1997;**40**:2187–98.

74 Regan MJ, Hellmann DB, Stone JH. Treatment of Wegener's granulomatosis. *Rheum Dis Clin North Am* 2001;**27**:863–86, viii.

75 Stegeman CA, Cohen Tervaert JW *et al.* Association of chronic nasal carriage of *Staphyloccus aureus* and higher relapse rates in Wegener's granulomatosis. *Ann Intern Med* 1994;**120**:12–17.

76 Ulmer M, Reinhold-Keller E, Gross WL. Alternative treatment strategies in Wegener's granulomatosis: first results of a prospective study. *APMIS Suppl* 1990;**19**:51.

●77 Stegeman CA, Tervaert JW, de Jong PE *et al.* Trimethoprim-sulfamethoxazole (co-trimoxazole) for the prevention of relapses of Wegener's granulomatosis. *N Engl J Med* 1996;**335**:16–20.

78 Reinhold-Keller E, De Groot K, Rudert H *et al.* Response to trimethoprim/sulfamethoxazole in Wegener's granulomatosis depends on the phase of disease. *Q J Med* 1996;**89**:15–23.

79 Reinhold-Keller E, Kekow J, Schnabel A *et al.* Influence of disease manifestation and antineutrophil cytoplasmic antibody titer on the response to pulse cyclophosphamide therapy in patients with Wegener's granulomatosis. *Arthritis Rheum* 1994;**37**:919–24.

80 Richter C, Schnabel A, Csernok E *et al.* Treatment of Wegener's granulomatosis with intravenous immunoglobulin. *Adv Exp Med Biol* 1993;**336**:487–9.

81 Jayne DR, Esnault VL, Lockwood CM. ANCA anti-idiotype antibodies and the treatment of systemic vasculitis with intravenous immunoglobulin. *J Autoimmun* 1993;**6**:207–19.

82 Godeau B, Mainardi JL, Roudot-Thoraval F *et al.* Factors associated with *Pneumocystis carinii* pneumonia in Wegener's granulomatosis. *Ann Rheum Dis* 1995;**54**:991–4.

83 Ognibene FP, Shelhamer JH, Hoffman GS *et al.* *Pneumocystis carinii* pneumonia: a major complication of immunosuppressive therapy in patients with Wegener's granulomatosis. *Am J Respir Crit Care Med* 1995;**151**(3 Pt 1):795–9.

84 Cordier JF, Valeyre D, Guillevin L *et al.* Pulmonary Wegener's granulomatosis. A clinical and imaging study of 77 cases. *Chest* 1990;**97**:906–12.

85 Godman GC, Churg J. Wegener's granulomatosis: pathology and review of the literature. *Arch Pathol* 1954;**58**:533–53.

86 Carrington CB, Liebow A. Limited forms of angiitis and granulomatosis of Wegener's type. *Am J Med* 1966;**41**:497–527.

●87 Leavitt RY, Fauci AS, Bloch DA *et al.* The American College of Rheumatology 1990 criteria for the classification of Wegener's granulomatosis. *Arthritis Rheum* 1990;**33**:1101–7.

88 Daum TE, Specks U, Colby TV *et al.* Tracheobronchial involvement in Wegener's granulomatosis. *Am J Respir Crit Care Med* 1995;**151**(2 Pt 1):522–6.

89 Jayne DR, Lockwood CM. Intravenous immunoglobulin as sole therapy for systemic vasculitis. *Br J Rheumatol* 1996;**35**:1150–3.

90 Gremmel F, Druml W, Schmidt P *et al.* Cyclosporin in Wegener granulomatosis. *Ann Intern Med* 1988;**108**:491.

91 Stone JH, Uhlfelder ML, Hellmann DB *et al.* Etanercept combined with conventional treatment in Wegener's granulomatosis: a six-month open-label trial to evaluate safety. *Arthritis Rheum* 2001;**44**:1149–54.

92 Specks U, Fervenza FC, McDonald TJ *et al.* Response of Wegener's granulomatosis to anti-CD20 chimeric monoclonal antibody therapy. *Arthritis Rheum* 2001;**44**:2836–40.

93 Case records of the Massachusetts General Hospital. Weekly clinicopathological exercises. Case 31-1986. A 39-year-old woman with stenosis of the subglottic area and pulmonary artery. *N Engl J Med* 1986;**315**:378–87.

94 Bosch X, Font J, Mirapeix E *et al.* Antimyeloperoxidase autoantibody-associated necrotizing alveolar capillaritis. *Am Rev Respir Dis* 1992;**146**(5 Pt 1):1326–9.

95 Niles JL, Bottinger EP, Saurina GR *et al.* The syndrome of lung hemorrhage and nephritis is usually an ANCA- associated condition. *Arch Intern Med* 1996;**156**:440–5.

96 Guillevin L, Lhote F. Distinguishing polyarteritis nodosa from microscopic polyangiitis and implications for treatment. *Curr Opin Rheumatol* 1995;**7**:20–4.

●97 Churg J, Strauss L. Allergic granulomatosis, allergic angiitis and periarteritis nodosa. *Am J Pathol* 1951; **27**:277–94.

●98 Lanham JG, Elkon KB, Pusey CD *et al.* Systemic vasculitis with asthma and eosinophilia: a clinical approach to the Churg-Strauss syndrome. *Medicine* 1984;**63**:65–81.

99 Churg A, Brallas M, Cronin SR *et al.* Formes frustes of Churg-Strauss syndrome. *Chest* 1995;**108**:320–3.

●100 Masi AT, Hunder GG, Lie JT *et al.* The American College of Rheumatology 1990 criteria for the classification of Churg-Strauss syndrome (allergic granulomatosis and angiitis). *Arthritis Rheum* 1990;**33**:1094–100.

101 Knoell DL, Lucas J, Allen JN. Churg-Strauss syndrome associated with zafirlukast. *Chest* 1998;**114**:332–4.

102 Churg J, Churg A. Zafirlukast and Churg-Strauss syndrome. *JAMA* 1998;**279**:1949–50.

103 Franco J, Artes MJ. Pulmonary eosinophilia associated with montelukast. *Thorax* 1999;**54**:558–60.

104 Wechsler ME, Pauwels R, Drazen JM. Leukotriene modifiers and Churg-Strauss syndrome: adverse effect or response to corticosteroid withdrawal? *Drug Saf* 1999;**21**:241–51.

105 Wechsler ME, Finn D, Gunawardena D *et al.* Churg-Strauss syndrome in patients receiving montelukast as treatment for asthma. *Chest* 2000;**117**:708–13.

106 Hashimoto M, Fujishima T, Tanaka H *et al.* Churg-Strauss syndrome after reduction of inhaled corticosteroid in a patient treated with pranlukast for asthma. *Intern Med* 2001;**40**:432–4.

♦107 Weller PF, Plaut M, Taggart V *et al.* The relationship of asthma therapy and Churg-Strauss syndrome: NIH workshop summary report. *J Allergy Clin Immunol* 2001;**108**:175–83.

108 Masi AT, Hamilos DL. Leukotriene antagonists: bystanders or causes of Churg-Strauss syndrome? *Semin Arthritis Rheum* 2002;**31**:211–17.

109 Tatsis E, Schnabel A, Gross WL. Interferon-alpha treatment of four patients with the Churg-Strauss syndrome. *Ann Intern Med* 1998;**129**:370–4.

110 Machado EB, Michet CJ, Ballard DJ *et al.* Trends in incidence and clinical presentation of temporal arteritis in Olmsted County, Minnesota, 1950–1985. *Arthritis Rheum* 1988;**31**:745–9.

111 Klein RG, Campbell RJ, Hunder GG *et al.* Skip lesions in temporal arteritis. *Mayo Clin Proc* 1976;**51**:504–10.

112 Lie JT. Aortic and extracranial large vessel giant cell arteritis: a review of 72 cases with histopathological documentation. *Semin Arthritis Rheum* 1995;**24**:422–31.

113 Glover MU, Muniz J, Bessone L *et al.* Pulmonary artery obstruction due to giant cell arteritis. *Chest* 1987;**91**:924–5.

114 Nierman DM, Kalb TH, Ornstein MH *et al.* A patient with antineutrophil cytoplasmic antibody-negative pulmonary capillaritis and circulating primed neutrophils. *Arthritis Rheum* 1995;**38**:1855–8.

115 Jennings CA, King TE, Jr, Tuder R *et al.* Diffuse alveolar hemorrhage with underlying isolated, pauciimmune pulmonary capillaritis. *Am J Respir Crit Care Med* 1997;**155**:1101–9.

116 Lupi E, Sanchez G, Horwitz S *et al.* Pulmonary artery involvement in Takayasu's arteritis. *Chest* 1975;**67**:69–74.

117 Ishikawa K, Maetani S. Long-term outcome for 120 Japanese patients with Takayasu's disease. Clinical and statistical analyses of related prognostic factors. *Circulation* 1994;**90**:1855–60.

●118 Kussmaul A, Maier R. On a previously undescribed peculiar arterial disease (periarteritis nodosa), accompanied by Bright's disease and rapidly progressive general muscle weakness. *Dtsch Arch Klin Med* 1866;**1**:484–518.

119 Matteson EL. *Commemorative translation of the 130-year anniversary of the original article by Adolf Kussmaul and Rudolf Maier.* Rochester, MN: Mayo Foundation, 1996.

120 Salama AD, Levy JB, Lightstone L *et al.* Goodpasture's disease. *Lancet* 2001;**358**:917–20.

121 Wright WK, Krous HF, Griswold WR *et al.* Pulmonary vasculitis with hemorrhage in anaphylactoid purpura. *Pediatr Pulmonol* 1994;**17**:269–71.

122 Erkan F, Cavdar T. Pulmonary vasculitis in Behçet's disease. *Am Rev Respir Dis* 1992;**146**:232–9.

123 Anaya JM, Diethelm L, Ortiz LA *et al.* Pulmonary involvement in rheumatoid arthritis. *Semin Arthritis Rheum* 1995;**24**:242–54.

124 Matthay RA, Schwarz MI, Petty TL *et al.* Pulmonary manifestations of systemic lupus erythematosus: review of twelve cases of acute lupus pneumonitis. *Medicine (Baltimore)* 1975;**54**:397–409.

125 Fernandes SR, Singsen BH, Hoffman GS. Sarcoidosis and systemic vasculitis. *Semin Arthritis Rheum* 2000;**30**:33–46.

126 Chetty R. Vasculitides associated with HIV infection. *J Clin Pathol* 2001;**54**:275–8.

127 Liu YC, Tomashefski JF, Jr, Tomford JW *et al.* Necrotizing *Pneumocystis carinii* vasculitis associated with lung necrosis and cavitation in a patient with acquired immunodeficiency syndrome. *Arch Pathol Lab Med* 1989;**113**:494–7.

128 Golden MP, Hammer SM, Wanke CA *et al.* Cytomegalovirus vasculitis. Case reports and review of the literature. *Medicine (Baltimore)* 1994;**73**:246–55.

Pulmonary hypertension in sickle cell disease and thalassemia

OSWALDO CASTRO

INTRODUCTION AND DEFINITIONS

Sickle cell disease and β-thalassemia are the most common genetic disorders of hemoglobin. Both are autosomal recessive and have worldwide distribution. Sickle cell disease affects primarily, but not exclusively, people of African descent.[1] The β-thalassemias occur in people of Mediterranean descent, from the Middle East, from the Indian Subcontinent, and from South East Asia.[2] In sickle cell disease, the genetic lesion is a point mutation that results in the synthesis of hemoglobin S, a structural variant that differs from normal hemoglobin (HbA) by the substitution of valine for glutamic acid in position 6 of the β-globin chain. Hemoglobin S polymerizes and aggregates upon deoxygenation. This leads to red cell rigidity and sickling which in turn cause chronic hemolysis, intermittent vascular occlusive episodes, and long-term damage to vital organs.[3,4] The main types of sickle cell disease are sickle cell anemia, or homozygous sickle cell disease (HbSS), sickle cell hemoglobin-C disease (HbSC) and the two common forms of sickle cell-β-thalassemia (Hb Sβ$^+$-thal and Hb Sβ^0-thal).[5]

Over 125 different genetic lesions, including point mutations, frameshift mutations, and deletions, can cause β-thalassemia, which is characterized by decreased (β$^+$-thalassemia) or absent (β^0-thalassemia) synthesis of the β-globin chain.[6] Hemoglobin tetramers are synthesized at a lower rate so that thalassemic erythrocytes are microcytic and hypochromic. More importantly, the lower rate of β-globin production also results in an imbalanced globin chain synthesis: there is an 'excess' of the normally synthesized α-globin chains. These chains are unstable when not joined to their non-α molecular partners (the β- or γ-globin chains) and they aggregate and precipitate causing membrane damage and death of the erythroid precursors in the bone marrow.[7] This pathological process is called ineffective erythropoiesis and is the principal cause of the severe, transfusion-dependent anemia that characterizes homozygous β-thalassemia. Those thalassemic erythrocytes that survive their bone marrow stage and enter the blood circulation also have a short intravascular life span, thus contributing to the anemia.[7]

Pulmonary arterial hypertension has been reported in patients with sickle cell disease and in those with β-thalassemia. The frequency of this association is much higher than expected if hemoglobinopathy patients merely had the coincidental occurrence of primary pulmonary hypertension. Therefore, hemoglobinopathy-related increases in pulmonary pressures should be considered as forms of secondary pulmonary hypertension. The mechanism by which hemoglobin disorders result in pulmonary hypertension is not known and, as discussed below, a variety of abnormalities common to sickle cell disease and thalassemia could play a role in increasing pulmonary artery pressures.

SICKLE CELL-RELATED PULMONARY HYPERTENSION

Incidence and risk factors

The prevalence of pulmonary hypertension in sickle cell disease appears to be increasing, particularly among adult patients. At the author's institution, the diagnosis of pulmonary hypertension was made in only about 5% of 57 adult sickle cell patients who died before 1990.[8] Pulmonary hypertension was not listed as an underlying condition in 209 patients who died during follow-up in the US Cooperative Study of Sickle Cell Disease (1978–88).[9] By contrast, over 30% of 58 adult sickle cell patients who died between 1990 and 1995 at our Center had this diagnosis.[8] Retrospective echocardiography (ECHO) studies in adult patients report pulmonary hypertension prevalence rates of 20–35%.[10,11] Four of 10 patients (40%) with cardiorespiratory symptoms had elevated pulmonary artery resistance at cardiac catheterization.[12] On the other hand, a prospective series reported no echocardiographic evidence of increased pulmonary pressure in 191 sickle cell patients, 71% of them children or young adults.[13] A more recent study of 25 sickle cell anemia patients ages 14–45 years showed normal pulmonary artery pressures, estimated by ECHO.[14] These widely varying prevalence figures probably reflect factors such as different ECHO diagnostic criteria, age differences, and selection bias. Results are now available from a prospective ECHO study of 195 unselected adult patients with sickle cell disease. Sixty-two of these patients (32%) had a tricuspid valve regurgitant jet velocity of 2.5 m/s or higher, corresponding to an estimated pulmonary artery systolic pressure of at least 35 mmHg. Nine per cent of these unselected patients had severe pulmonary hypertension. They had a tricuspid regurgitant jet velocity of ≥3.0 m/s, which corresponds to a pulmonary artery systolic pressure of 46 mmHg or higher.[15]

The risk factors for pulmonary hypertension in sickle cell disease have not yet been established and the limited information currently available derives largely from preliminary reports. In addition to older age, risk factors for pulmonary hypertension in sickle cell patients probably include the SS genotype and the degree of anemia. Gender does not appear to affect the prevalence of pulmonary hypertension.[16] Over 90% of the 50 pulmonary hypertension patients in the report by Al-Sukhun et al.[16] had the HbSS type. By comparison, the prevalence of the SS genotype among 696 patients followed at our institution is only 66%,[17] which is identical to that in the 3751 sickle cell patients who enrolled in the US Cooperative Study of Sickle Cell Disease.[18] The higher risk in SS patients is supported also by findings from an ongoing prospective study which suggest that the severity of the pulmonary pressure correlates with the degree of anemia.[15] Another risk factor could be the frequency of past episodes of acute chest syndrome (ACS). Some series found a relationship between frequent ACS episodes and chronic restrictive pulmonary disease, which can lead to cor pulmonale.[19] On the other hand, at least in children, past ACS episodes did not affect the pulmonary artery pressure estimated by ECHO.[20]

Etiology

The pathogenesis of pulmonary hypertension in sickle cell disease is not known but it is probably related in some way to HbS polymerization and red cell sickling. One or more of these factors could be operative:

- a sickle cell-related vasculopathy,[21]
- chronic oxygen desaturation and/or sleep hypoventilation,[22]
- pulmonary fibrosis from repeated episodes of chest syndrome,[19]
- recurrent episodes of thromboembolism,[23] or
- a high pulmonary blood flow secondary to the anemia.

The sickle cell-related vasculopathy may result not only from endothelial cell injury and proliferation secondary to adhesion and vascular obstruction by rigid sickle erythrocytes. Other factors, such as thrombocytosis, from the combination of functional or anatomic asplenia and marrow stimulation by hemolysis, are probably operative. Minter and Gladwin[24] postulate that hemolysis (some of which is intravascular in the hemoglobinopathies) also contributes to vasoconstriction and vascular injury through the liberation of free hemoglobin, heme and iron, which can scavenge nitric oxide and catalyze the production of reactive oxygen and nitrogen species. In fact, Reiter et al.[25] recently demonstrated that the small quantities of free hemoglobin present in the plasma of sickle cell patients substantially reduced their blood flow response to nitric oxide donor infusions. Table 13J.1 lists those features of sickle cell disease and thalassemia that probably play a role in the development of pulmonary hypertension in these disorders.

Table 13J.1 *Clinical features and complications of sickle cell disease and β-thalassemia that may play a role in the pathogenesis of pulmonary hypertension*

Abnormality	Sickle cell disease	β-Thalassemia*
Chronic hemolysis	+++	+++
Increased cardiac output	+++	+++
Splenectomy or autosplenectomy	+++	++
Thrombocytosis	+++	+++
Sickling-related vaso occlusion	+++	−
Restrictive lung disease/fibrosis	++	++
Chronic hypoxemia and hypoventilation	++	−
Thromboembolism	++	+++

*Non-regularly transfused patients with thalassemia intermedia.

Clinical presentation and diagnosis

The early stages of sickle cell-related pulmonary hypertension are not associated with specific symptoms. There may be fatigue but this is difficult to interpret in the setting of chronic anemia. The diagnosis should be suspected if the patient presents any of these findings:

- increased intensity of the second heart sound at the pulmonary auscultation point;
- right ventricular enlargement on chest x-ray, electrocardiogram or, more specifically, on two-dimensional echocardiography; and
- unexplained oxygen desaturation.

In many patients the pulmonary hypertension appears as the end-stage (stage 4) of sickle cell-related chronic lung disease.[19] Other abnormalities that may be observed in earlier stages include substernal pain and pulmonary fibrosis.

As pulmonary hypertension worsens, the patients have more frequent chest pain episodes, dyspnea and hypoxemia at rest. Oxygen desaturation is expected to increase the risk for more frequent vaso-occlusive events.[19] Other features of advanced pulmonary hypertension include right-sided heart failure (cor pulmonale), episodes of syncope and the risk of sudden death from pulmonary thromboembolism, systemic hypotension or cardiac arrhythmia.[26,27]

Echocardiography can establish pulmonary hypertension in patients who have tricuspid regurgitation and in whom the regurgitant jet velocity allows an estimate of the pulmonary artery systolic pressure. Other ECHO findings that suggest the diagnosis are:

- dilated right heart chambers with abnormal ventricular septal wall motion;
- notching of right ventricular outflow tract Doppler pattern with acceleration time of <100 ms; and
- dilated inferior vena cava with lack of inspiratory collapse.

However, the most reliable procedure for diagnosing or excluding pulmonary hypertension is right-sided heart catheterization with measurement of the pulmonary pressure.[28] The procedure is essential to measure the mean pulmonary arterial pressure, an elevation of which (above 25 mmHg) defines pulmonary hypertension,[29] and it can exclude or establish other forms of secondary pulmonary hypertension such as left ventricular failure or left-to-right shunt.

Few published data are available on cardiac catheterization findings in sickle cell patients with pulmonary hypertension. Their hemodynamic findings differ from those in primary pulmonary hypertension and in other forms of secondary hypertension. The pulmonary pressures are typically lower and the cardiac output is typically higher in sickle cell-related pulmonary hypertension than those in the primary form of the disease and in most types of secondary pulmonary hypertension.[8] Table 13J.2 compares the pulmonary pressures and cardiac outputs in pulmonary hypertension patients with hemoglobinopathy with those of patients with primary pulmonary hypertension. As a group, patients with sickle cell disease have lower pulmonary pressures than patients with β-thalassemia[30,31] and those with the primary form of pulmonary hypertension.[32,33]

Management and prognosis

Only recently has pulmonary hypertension been recognized as a frequent complication of the hemoglobinopathies and there are no evidence-based guidelines for its treatment. Those therapeutic measures that are effective in the primary form of pulmonary hypertension should be considered also in patients with sickle cell disease. At the time of cardiac catheterization, for example, administration of vasodilators or oxygen may reduce pulmonary pressure and this may predict the benefit of their long-term administration in sickle cell patients. In primary pulmonary hypertension, long-term, continuous

Table 13J.2 *Hemodynamic data from hemoglobinopathy patients with pulmonary hypertension and from patients with primary pulmonary hypertension*

	Sickle cell disease[40]	β-Thalassemia intermedia[30,31]	Primary pulmonary hypertension[32,33]
N	20	13	187
Age (years)	37.2 (21–59)	39.5 (26–65)	36.4
PASP (mmHg)	54.3 (36–80)	84.9 (55–120)	90.4 (males); 91.7 (females)
PADP (mmHg)	25.2 (13–40)	39.1 (25–54)	42.5 (males); 43.3 (females)
PAMP (mmHg)	36.0 (27–50)	52.0 (35–69)	60.7 (males); 60.3 (females)
Cardiac output (L/min)	8.6 (4.9–11.1)	7.5 (3.6–10.5)	3.0 (±0.3 SEM)*

Values in the columns are averages computed from individual cases in referenced publications. Unless otherwise specified, values in parentheses represent ranges.
PASP, pulmonary artery systolic pressure; PADP, pulmonary artery diastolic pressure; PAMP, pulmonary artery mean pressure.
*From reference 33.

intravenous infusion of prostacyclin was proven to lower pulmonary artery pressure and to improve survival.[34] Prostacyclin infusions may improve also various forms of secondary pulmonary hypertension.[35] At least acutely, this drug also lowered the pulmonary pressure in sickle cell patients at cardiac catheterization.[36] Intravenous prostacyclin administration requires the use of long-term vascular access devices which have a high frequency of infection and bacteremia.[34,37] For these reasons the long-term benefit of this treatment to sickle cell patients is unknown and needs to be examined in a controlled clinical trial.

Anticoagulation with warfarin [international normalized ratio (INR) 2.0–3.0] is used in primary pulmonary hypertension because of the known risk of thromboembolism,[34] a risk that may apply also to the sickle cell-related form of the disease.[23] Continuous oxygen administration decreases pulmonary artery pressure in most hypoxemic patients and should be used in sickle cell-related pulmonary hypertension, particularly if cardiac catheterization shows that it lowers the pulmonary pressure. Oxygen should be used also in all chronically hypoxemic patients (in the USA, medical insurance covers costs for continuous oxygen in patients with a PaO_2 of <60 mmHg, or with O_2 saturation lower than 90%). Preliminary reports suggest that sickle cell-related pulmonary hypertension improves with red cell transfusions[38] or with arginine administration.[39] Lung or heart/lung transplantation is probably too risky in patients with sickle cell disease.

There are no prospective studies of the survival of sickle cell patients with pulmonary hypertension. A retrospective analysis of a group of 20 sickle patients with pulmonary hypertension showed that their median survival was 25.6 months from the date of their cardiac catheterization diagnosis.[40] The preliminary report by Al-Sukhun et al. also showed a poor survival: 22 of 50 patients (44%) died 1–46 months after their ECHO diagnosis of pulmonary hypertension.[16] These retrospective data are likely to include more severely ill patients and those diagnosed at later stages of the disease. Furthermore, it is not clear that all of these patients died of pulmonary hypertension. It is possible that their pulmonary condition was a marker for severe vaso-occlusive disease, which is known to decrease survival, so that some patients may have died of another sickle cell disease complication. Nevertheless, pulmonary hypertension remains a serious threat to the life of sickle cell patients. Hemodynamically it is less severe than primary pulmonary hypertension, but sickle cell patients seem to have a low tolerance of even moderate elevations of pulmonary pressures.

Future therapeutic directions

A prostacyclin formulation suitable for subcutaneous infusion[41] is now available and its administration would be less invasive and less risky for all patients, including those with the hemoglobinopathies. The results with aerosolized prostacyclin treatment are conflicting,[42,43] but this non-invasive route of administration should be examined also in sickle cell patients with pulmonary hypertension. A recent and exciting development is the successful treatment of primary pulmonary hypertension with an oral preparation: the dual endothelin receptor antagonist bosentan.[44] The relatively low toxicity profile of this drug places it among the first candidates for prospective clinical trials in hemoglobinopathy patients with pulmonary hypertension. In sickle cell patients, bosentan could also decrease the frequency or severity of acute vaso-occlusive events since they may be mediated in part by endothelin.[45,46]

THALASSEMIA–RELATED PULMONARY HYPERTENSION

Incidence and risk factors

Patients with homozygous β-thalassemia usually have a severe, transfusion-dependent anemia from infancy and their clinical phenotype is designated as thalassemia major. Unless these patients' transfusional iron overload is managed effectively by iron chelation, they succumb to left ventricular cardiac failure and/or arrhythmias as a result of myocardial hemosiderosis.[7] Relatively few thalassemia major patients have pulmonary hypertension.[47,48] The thalassemia intermedia phenotype, which includes milder forms of homozygous β-thalassemia and Hb E-β-thalassemia, results in less severe anemia and such patients generally receive fewer transfusions. Pulmonary arterial obstructive lesions were found at autopsy in 19 of 44 South East Asian patients with Hb E-β-thalassemia[49] and most patients with this hemoglobinopathy who had cardiac catheterization were also diagnosed as having pulmonary hypertension.[50] A high prevalence of pulmonary hypertension in Greek adults with thalassemia intermedia was reported recently. Sixty-five of 110 such patients (59%) had this abnormality by ECHO criteria.[31] Most of them were not on regular transfusions. Older patients and those with previous splenectomy had a higher risk for pulmonary hypertension. However, degree of anemia, number of transfusions and serum ferritin levels did not appear to correlate with the pulmonary hypertension risk.[31]

Etiology, clinical presentation and diagnosis

Potential mechanisms for pulmonary hypertension in β-thalassemia are shown in Table 13J.1. In thalassemia intermedia, the most frequently reported abnormality is recurrent pulmonary thromboembolism[49] with platelet aggregates, particularly in patients with post-splenectomy thrombocytosis. Restrictive lung disease, secondary to pulmonary fibrosis or to tissue injury by free hydroxyl radicals from iron deposition, in combination with the anemia-related high cardiac output, also increases the pulmonary hypertension risk.[30]

Thalassemia patients with pulmonary hypertension tend to be diagnosed relatively late in the course of their disease. Hence, right-sided heart failure is a common presenting finding.[30,31] Hypoxemia,[51] which could also be the result of chronic restrictive pulmonary disease, is likely to be an early sign of pulmonary hypertension in thalassemia. Unfortunately, there are no prospective studies of the natural history of this complication in thalassemic patients. As in sickle cell disease, the diagnosis of pulmonary hypertension in thalassemia can be made through echocardiography but its definitive documentation or exclusion requires right-sided cardiac catheterization.

Management, prognosis, future directions

Pulmonary hypertension is not frequent in homozygous β-thalassemia patients who are transfused and chelated regularly. In fact, most thalassemic complications are prevented in these patients.[52] Therefore, early transfusion and iron chelation therapy should be offered to all thalassemic patients, including those with thalassemia intermedia. Children with hemoglobinopathies who have an HLA-compatible sibling can be cured by allogeneic bone marrow transplantation[53,54] before they have had a chance to develop abnormalities leading to pulmonary hypertension. No evidence-based treatment for thalassemia-related pulmonary hypertension has been described and management should be along the same lines discussed above for sickle cell disease. Starting a regular transfusion and iron chelation program to keep the Hb level close to normal ($>10 \, g/dL$) is recommended for managing pulmonary hypertension in thalassemia intermedia patients.[30] Since thromboembolism appears to have a prominent role in thalassemia intermedia patients with pulmonary hypertension,[50] long-term anticoagulation and/or antiplatelet therapy could be particularly useful. Lung or heart/lung transplantation as treatment of pulmonary hypertension has not been described in the hemoglobinopathies. They are likely to be followed by thalassemia-related injury to the transplanted organs unless a rigorous transfusion and iron chelation program is maintained. The future therapeutic developments discussed above for sickle cell disease should be applicable also to thalassemic patients with pulmonary hypertension.

KEY POINTS

- Pulmonary arterial hypertension occurs in one-third of adults with sickle cell disease and in about 60% of patients with thalassemia intermedia.
- The limited hemodynamic data available indicate that pulmonary hypertension patients with sickle cell disease have lower pressures (average PAm, 36.0 mmHg) and higher cardiac outputs (average, 8.6 L/min) than those reported in primary pulmonary hypertension.
- In thalassemia-related pulmonary hypertension, the pulmonary pressures (average PAm, 52.0 mmHg) are closer to those in the primary form of the disease but their cardiac outputs are also high (average 7.5 L/min).
- Despite their more favorable hemodynamic parameters, sickle cell patients with pulmonary hypertension have a short survival.
- Regular transfusions and iron chelation, if started in early childhood, prevent pulmonary hypertension in thalassemic patients.
- There are no published studies on treatment of pulmonary hypertension in the hemoglobinopathies. Management with vasodilators, anticoagulation and oxygen, as in other forms of pulmonary hypertension, seems the best approach at present.

REFERENCES

1 Nagel RL, Steinberg MH. Genetics of the β[S] gene: origins, genetic epidemiology, and epistasis in sickle cell anemia. In: Steinberg MH, Forget BG, Higgs DR et al. (eds), *Disorders of hemoglobin. Genetics, pathophysiology, and clinical management*. Cambridge, UK: Cambridge University Press, 2001;711–55.

2 Loukopolous D, Kollia P. Worldwide distribution of β-thalassemia. In: Steinberg MH, Forget BG, Higgs DR et al. (eds), *Disorders of hemoglobin. Genetics, pathophysiology, and clinical management*. Cambridge, UK: Cambridge University Press, 2001;861–984.

◆3 Bunn HF. Pathogenesis and treatment of sickle cell disease. *N Engl J Med* 1997;**337**:762–9.

◆4 Steinberg MH. Management of sickle cell disease. *N Engl J Med* 1999;**340**:1021–30.

5 Kinney TR, Ware RE. Compound heterozygous states. In: Embury SH, Hebbel RP, Mohandas N et al. (eds), *Sickle cell disease. Basic principles and clinical practice*. New York: Raven Press, 1994;437–51.

6 Forget BG. Molecular mechanisms of β-thalassemia. In: Steinberg MH, Forget BG, Higgs DR et al. (eds), *Disorders of hemoglobin. Genetics, pathophysiology, and clinical*

management. Cambridge, UK: Cambridge University Press, 2001;252–76.

◆7 Olivieri NF. The β-thalassemias. *N Engl J Med* 1999; **341**:99–109.

◆8 Castro O. Systemic fat embolism and pulmonary hypertension in sickle cell disease. *Hematol Oncol Clin North Am* 1996; **10**:1289–303.

●9 Platt OS, Brambilla DJ, Rosse WF *et al*. Mortality in sickle cell disease. Life expectancy and risk factors for early death. *N Engl J Med* 1994;**330**:1639–44.

10 Sutton LL, Castro O, Cross DJ *et al*. Pulmonary hypertension in sickle cell disease. *Am J Cardiol* 1994;**74**:626–8.

11 Simmons BE, Santhanam V, Castaner A *et al*. Sickle cell disease. Two-dimensional echo and doppler ultrasonographic findings in the hearts of adult patients with sickle cell anemia. *Arch Intern Med* 1988;**148**:1526–8.

12 Norris SL, Johnson C, Haywood LJ. Left ventricular filling pressure in sickle cell anemia. *J Assoc Acad Minor Phys* 1992;**3**:20–3.

13 Covitz W, Espeland M, Gallagher D *et al*. The heart in sickle cell anemia. The Cooperative Study of Sickle Cell Disease (CSSCD) *Chest* 1995;**108**:1214–19.

14 de Andrade-Martins W, Tinoco-Mesqita E, da Cunha DM *et al*. Doppler echocardiographic study of adolescents and young adults with sickle cell anemia. *Arq Bras Cardiol* 1999;**73**:469–74.

●15 Gladwin MT, Sachdev V, Jison ML *et al*. Pulmonary hypertension as a risk factor for death in patients with sickle cell disease. *N Engl J Med* 2004;**350**:886–95.

16 Al-Sukhun S, Aboubakr SE, Girgis RE *et al*. Pulmonary hypertension is present in 10–30% of adult patients with sickle cell disease. [Abstract] *Blood* 2000;**96**(Suppl 1):9a.

17 Dawkins FW, Kim KS, Squires RS *et al*. Cancer incidence and mortality rate in sickle cell disease patients at Howard Univer-sity Hospital: 1986–1995. *Am J Hematol* 1997;**55**:188–92.

18 Gaston M, Smith J, Gallagher D *et al*. Recruitment in the Cooperative Study of Sickle Cell Disease (CSSCD). *Control Clin Trials* 1987;**8**(4 Suppl):131S–40S.

19 Powars D, Weidman JA, Odom-Maryon T *et al*. Sickle cell chronic lung disease: prior morbidity and the risk of pulmonary failure. *Medicine* 1988;**67**:66–76.

20 Denbow CD, Chung EE, Serjeant GR. Pulmonary artery pressure and the acute chest syndrome in homozygous sickle cell disease. *Br Heart J* 1993;**69**:536–8.

21 Faller DV. Vascular modulation. In: Embury SH, Hebbel RP, Mohandas N *et al*. (eds), *Sickle cell disease. Basic principles and clinical practice*. New York: Raven Press, 1994;235–46.

22 Samuels MP, Stebbens VA, Davies SC *et al*. Sleep related upper airway obstruction and hypoxaemia in sickle cell disease. *Arch Dis Child* 1992;**67**:925–9.

23 Yung GL, Channick RN, Fedullo PF *et al*. Successful pulmonary thromboendarterectomy in two patients with sickle cell disease. *Am J Respir Crit Care Med* 1998;**157**:1690–3.

◆24 Minter KR, Gladwin MT. Pulmonary complications of sickle cell anemia: a need for increased recognition, treatment, and research. *Am J Respir Crit Care Med* 2001;**164**:2016–19.

●25 Reiter CD, Wang X, Tanus-Santos JE *et al*. Cell-free hemoglobin limits nitric oxide bioavailability in sickle-cell disease. *Nat Med* 2002;**8**:1383–9.

26 Case records of the Massachusetts General Hospital (Case 52–1983). *N Engl J Med* 1983;**309**:1627–33.

27 Clinicopathologic conference. Sudden death in a young woman with sickle cell anemia. *Am J Med* 1992;**92**:556–60.

28 Collins FS, Orringer EP. Pulmonary hypertension and cor pulmonale in the sickle hemoglobinopathies. *Am J Med* 1982;**73**:814–21.

29 Rubin JL. Primary pulmonary hypertension. *Chest* 1993;**104**:236–50.

30 Aessopos A, Stamatelos G, Skoumas V *et al*. Pulmonary hypertension and right heart failure in patients with β-thalassemia intermedia. *Chest* 1995;**107**:50–3.

●31 Aessopos A, Farmakis D, Karagiorga M *et al*. Cardiac involvement in thalassemia intermedia: a multicenter study. *Blood* 2001;**97**:3411–16.

32 Rich S, Dantzker DR, Ayres SM *et al*. Primary pulmonary hypertension. A national prospective study. *Ann Intern Med* 1987;**107**:216–23.

33 Giaid A, Saleh D. Reduced expression of endothelial nitric oxide synthase in the lungs of patients with pulmonary hypertension. *N Engl J Med* 1995;**333**:214–21.

34 Barst RJ, Rubin LJ, Long WA *et al*. Primary Pulmonary Hypertension Group: a comparison of continuous intravenous epoprostenol (prostacyclin) with conventional therapy for primary pulmonary hypertension. *N Engl J Med* 1996;**334**:296–301.

35 McLaughlin V, Genthner DE, Panella MM *et al*. Compassionate use of continuous prostacyclin in the management of secondary pulmonary hypertension: a case series. *Ann Intern Med* 1999;**130**:740–3.

36 Kaur K, Brown B, Lombardo F. Prostacyclin for secondary pulmonary hypertension. [Correspondence] *Ann Intern Med* 2000;**132**:165.

37 Badesch DB, Tapson VF, McGoon MD *et al*. Continuous intravenous epoprostenol for pulmonary hypertension due to the scleroderma spectrum of disease. A randomized, controlled trial. *Ann Intern Med* 2000;**132**:425–34.

38 Claster S, Hammer M, Hagar W *et al*. Treatment of pulmonary hypertension in sickle cell disease with transfusion. *Blood* 1999;**94**(Suppl 1):420a.

39 Morris CR, Morris SM Jr, Hagar W *et al*. Arginine therapy: a new treatment for pulmonary hypertension in sickle cell disease? *Am J Respir Crit Care Med* 2003;**168**:63–9.

●40 Castro O, Hoque M, Brown BD. Pulmonary hypertension in sickle cell disease: cardiac catheterization results and survival. *Blood* 2003;**101**:1257–61.

41 Simonneau G, Barst RJ, Galie N *et al*. with the Treprostinil Study Group. Continuous subcutaneous infusion of treprostinil, a prostacyclin analogue, in patients with pulmonary arterial hypertension. *Am J Respir Crit Care Med* 2002;**165**:800–4.

42 Hoeper MM, Schwarze M, Ehlerding S *et al*. Long-term treatment of primary pulmonary hypertension with aerosolized iloprost, a prostacyclin analogue. *N Engl J Med* 2000;**342**:1866–70.

43 Machherndl S, Kneussl M, Baumgartner H *et al*. Long-term treatment of pulmonary hypertension with aerosolized iloprost. *Eur Resp J* 2001;**17**:8–13.

44 Channick RN, Simonneau G, Sitbon O *et al*. Effects of the dual endothelin-receptor antagonist bosentan in patients

with pulmonary hypertension: a randomized-placebo controlled study. *Lancet* 2001;**358**:1119–23.

45 Graido-Gonzalez E, Doherty JC, Bergreen EW *et al.* Plasma endothelin-1, cytokine, and prostaglandin E2 levels in sickle cell disease and acute vaso-occlusive sickle crisis. *Blood* 1998;**92**:2551–5.

46 Hammerman SI, Kourembanas S, Conca TJ *et al.* Endothelin-1 production during the acute chest syndrome in sickle cell disease. *Am J Respir Crit Care Med* 1997;**156**:280–5.

47 Zakynthinos E, Vassilakopoulos T, Kaltsas P *et al.* Pulmonary hypertension, interstitial lung fibrosis, and lung iron deposition in thalassaemia major. *Thorax* 2001;**56**:737–9.

48 Kremastinos DT, Tsetsos GA, Tsiapras DP *et al.* Heart failure in beta thalassemia: a 5-year follow-up study. *Am J Med* 2001;**111**:349–54.

49 Sonakul D, Pacharee P, Laohapand T *et al.* Pulmonary artery obstruction in thalassaemia. *Southeast Asian J Trop Med Public Health* 1980;**11**:516–23.

50 Jootar P, Fucharoen S. Cardiac involvement in beta-thalassemia/hemoglobin E disease: clinical and hemodynamic findings. *Southeast Asian J Trop Med Public Health* 1990;**21**:269–73.

51 Grisaru D, Rachmilewitz EA, Mosseri M *et al.* Cardiopulmonary assessment in beta-thalassemia major. *Chest* 1990;**98**:1138–42.

52 Olivieri NF, Weatherall DJ. Clinical aspects of β-thalassemia. In: Steinberg MH, Forget BG, Higgs DR *et al.* (eds), *Disorders of hemoglobin. Genetics, pathophysiology, and clinical management.* Cambridge, UK: Cambridge University Press, 2001;277–341.

◆53 Hoppe CC, Walters MC. Bone marrow transplantation in sickle cell anemia. *Curr Opin Oncol* 2001;**13**:85–90.

◆54 Giardini C, Lucarelli G. Bone marrow transplantation for beta-thalassemia. *Hematol Oncol Clin North Am* 1999;**13**:1059–64.

Conventional medical therapies

NAZZARENO GALIÈ, ALESSANDRA MANES AND ANGELO BRANZI

INTRODUCTION

Pulmonary arterial hypertension (PAH) is defined, according to the 1998 World Health Organization classification,[1] as a group of diseases characterized by a progressive increase of pulmonary vascular resistance leading to right ventricular failure and death.[2,3] PAH includes primary pulmonary hypertension (PPH) and pulmonary hypertension associated with various conditions such as collagen vascular diseases, congenital systemic-to-pulmonary shunts, portal hypertension and HIV infection. The severity of PAH is testified by the mean survival of 2.5 years of patients with PPH treated with 'conventional' medical therapies, before the introduction of prostacyclin.[4]

The definition of 'conventional' medical therapies derives from the history of the therapeutic approach to PAH and not from clear pharmacological or pathophysiological reasons. In fact, conventional therapies can be defined as the treatment options available before the introduction of continuous intravenous administration of prostacyclin in the 1990s (Table 13K.1). Conventional medical treatments include anticoagulants, calcium channel antagonists, inotropic agents, diuretics, supplemental oxygen and general measures.

The progress in the treatment of PAH has been substantially slow in the past decades: the initial therapeutic approaches started just after the first modern description of the disease in the 1950s by Dresdale[5] and Wood[6] with empiric attempts to reduce pulmonary artery pressure by various vasodilators used both in acute testing and as long-term treatment. In the 1980s, the results of uncontrolled studies on the effects of oral anticoagulant treatment[7] and calcium channel antagonists in PAH[8] were published. In the same period, the therapeutic option of heart/lung or lung transplantation became available even if the shortage of organ donation has limited the number of patients that could benefit from this treatment. The 1990s have witnessed the development of the continuous intravenous prostacyclin treatment, the efficacy of which has been positively tested in several controlled clinical trials.[9,10] This form of therapy was defined as 'non-conventional' for the cumbersome modality of administration that requires a tunnelized catheter and portable infusion pumps.[11] An interventional procedure, the balloon atrial septostomy, was also proposed in this period and small series of treated patients have been published, showing favorable results.[12] Finally, the new millennium has started with the completion of different controlled clinical trials with new compounds such as

Table 13K.1 *Chronology of treatments for pulmonary arterial hypertension*

Year	Treatment
1950–1980	Empiric/various vasodilators
1980 …	Oral anticoagulants
	Calcium channel antagonists
	Lung, heart/lung transplantation
1990 …	Intravenous epoprostenol (PGI_2)
	Balloon atrial septostomy
2000 …	New compounds

Table 13K.2 *Conventional medical therapies at baseline in controlled clinical trials in patients with pulmonary arterial hypertension*

Trial	Epoprostenol[9]	Epoprostenol[10]	Terbogrel[13]	Treprostinil[14]	BREATHE-1 oral bosentan[18]	ALPHABET oral beraprost[15]	AIR[16]
Etiology	PPH	Scleroderma	PPH	PPH, CTD, CHD	PPH, CTD	PPH, CTD, CHD, HIV, portal-PH	PPH, CTD, CTEPH
NYHA functional class	III–IV	III–IV	II–III	II–III–IV	III–IV	II–III	III–IV
Treatment at inclusion (%)							
Anticoagulants	86	51	58	66	71	73	84
Diuretics	66	70	49	57	52	53	65
Calcium channel blockers	N/A	60	54	42	48	22	38
Vasodilators*	67		N/A	N/A	N/A	N/A	N/A
Digoxin	53	29	18	25	20	19	20
Oxygen	46	72	17	35	30	9	44

*In some trials the data on vasodilator use rather than on calcium channel antagonists were collected. However, the authors affirm that in the great majority of the cases vasodilators were represented by calcium channel antagonist drugs. CHD, congenital heart disease; CTD, connective tissue disease; CTEPH, chronic thromboembolic pulmonary hypertension; HIV, human immunodeficiency virus; N/A, not available; portal-PH, portopulmonary hypertension; PPH, primary pulmonary hypertension.

the thromboxane inhibitor terbogrel,[13] the prostacyclin analogs treprostinil (subcutaneous),[14] beraprost (oral)[15] and iloprost (inhaled)[16] and the endothelin receptor antagonist bosentan.[17,18]

A common characteristic of conventional treatments is that the evidence for their efficacy and safety has not been tested by controlled trials but it is based on the clinical experience and/or on retrospective analysis and uncontrolled studies.[19] Nevertheless, conventional therapies are largely used in PAH patients as demonstrated by the baseline treatment of PAH patients included in the controlled clinical trials completed up to the time of writing (Table 13K.2). Even if the results of the trials with new compounds have substantially changed the current algorithms of treatment of PAH,[20] the role of conventional treatments has not yet been challenged. In fact, it can be argued that the efficacy of the new compounds has been demonstrated when added to the conventional treatments (including anticoagulants and diuretics) and no information is available if the investigational treatments were used alone.

The purpose of this chapter is to discuss the conventional treatments of PAH and to analyze the rationale, the evidence and the clinical implications for their utilization.

ANTICOAGULANTS

Rationale

The rationale for the use of oral anticoagulant treatment in patients with PAH is based on the presence of traditional risk factors for venous thromboembolism, such as heart failure and sedentary lifestyle, as well as on the demonstration of thrombophilic predisposition[21–23] and of thrombotic changes in the pulmonary microcirculation[24,25] and in the elastic pulmonary arteries.[26]

Venous thromboembolism may be particular ominous in PAH patients because even a small additional embolic obstruction in a severely compromised pulmonary circulation may lead to acute irreversible right heart failure.

The thrombophilic predisposition is shown by an increase of fibrinopeptide A levels and thromboxane metabolites in patients with PPH.[21,22] In addition, markers of endothelial cell injury and abnormalities of platelet aggregation function have also been demonstrated in these patients.[23] It is not clear if the presence of microthrombotic lesions in the small pulmonary arteries[24,25] represents the consequence of, or the cause for, pulmonary hypertension but, in any case, the thrombotic changes likely contribute to the progression of the disease. Mural thrombi has been shown in central elastic pulmonary arteries of patients with primary pulmonary hypertension[26] as a consequence of several factors, including prothrombotic abnormalities, vessel dilatation, atherosclerotic intimal lesions and low cardiac output. It is possible that the peripheral embolization from proximal thrombi may favor the progression of the obstructive changes in smaller vessels.

Evidence

The evidence for favorable effects of oral anticoagulant treatment in patients with PPH or PAH associated with anorexigens is based on retrospective analysis of single-center studies.[7,8,27] The survival of anticoagulated patients, selected on the basis of clinical judgment, was improved compared to a concurrent population that was not treated with oral anticoagulants. Three-year survival improved from 21% to 49% in the series reported by Fuster et al.[7] and from 31% to 47% in the series of Rich et al.[8] Interestingly, in this second report the survival improvement was observed either in the presence or in the absence of a concomitant treatment with calcium channel antagonists. The design of these studies was not randomized and one can argue that the lower survival of the control groups could be related to co-morbidities that prevented the use of anticoagulation in the untreated patients. In addition, only PPH and anorexigen-related PAH patients were included in the studies. Nevertheless, the uniformity of the results in all series and the strong rationale discussed above have convinced the experts to indicate the oral anticoagulant treatment in PPH patients in the absence of clear contraindications.[1] In recent clinical trials, oral anticoagulant treatment was present at inclusion in a fraction of patients ranging from 51% to 86% (Table 13K.2). Interestingly, the highest prevalence of oral anticoagulant treatment was shown in the trials involving mainly PPH patients in NYHA classes III and IV while the lowest prevalence was present in the trial on patients with scleroderma. It should be emphasized that there is no evidence of different efficacy of oral anticoagulant therapy according to functional class severity.

Clinical implications

Even if oral anticoagulant treatments are one of the main components of the conventional treatment of PAH, different clinical issues need to be determined, including the optimal range of oral anticoagulation, the indication in associated conditions and in children and the use of antiplatelet agents or heparin.

Doses of oral anticoagulants are adjusted according to the levels of international normalized ratio (INR) and the therapeutic range varies in different cardiovascular conditions.[28] Increased risk for thrombosis is present if the INR consistently falls below 2 while there is no detectable increase of risk for bleeding as long as the INR remains below 3. Accordingly, the appropriate INR therapeutic range in most conditions is between 2 and 3. No studies give clear evidence for the optimal INR therapeutic range in PPH patients even if some experts recommend a target INR of 2 or even between 1.5 and 2. It is reasonable in PPH patients to maintain the traditional INR therapeutic range of 2–3 in the absence of bleeding risk factors such as low platelet count, liver function or gastrointestinal abnormalities, frequent haemoptysis, etc. A lower level of anticoagulation (INR of 1.5–2.0) may be more appropriate in these last circumstances.

The rationale discussed above for the use of anticoagulation also includes the PAH conditions different from PPH even if no evidence of clinical efficacy has been provided by specific trials. In the largest controlled trial performed in 447 PAH patients,[14] anticoagulation treatment was performed at baseline in 80% of PPH patients compared to 66% of patients with connective tissue diseases and 65% of patients with congenital heart diseases. The prevalence of anticoagulant treatment in the trial on scleroderma patients treated with intravenous prostacyclin was 51%. It is possible that the potential risk for bleeding complications such as haemoptysis in congenital heart disease patients and gastrointestinal bleeding in patients with scleroderma has induced physicians to a more restrictive use of anticoagulation in these cases. In patients with PAH associated with portal hypertension or HIV infection, the risk-to-benefit ratio of anticoagulant treatment is increased by the frequent concomitant coagulation abnormalities and/or low platelet count.

It is reasonable to adopt anticoagulant treatment in PAH-associated conditions in the absence of all traditional bleeding risk factors and in particular in the presence of thrombotic predisposition (e.g. heart failure, central venous catheters, high hematocrit, etc.) to minimize the incidence of adverse events and increase the likelihood of favorable results. The same strategy can be adopted in children with PAH, in which no studies on the effects of anticoagulation are available.

No data are provided for the use of antiplatelet agents or heparin in patients with PAH. The antiproliferative action on smooth muscle cells exerted by low molecular weight heparins represents a rationale for their use but deserves further clinical investigation.

CALCIUM CHANNEL ANTAGONISTS

Rationale

The evidence for medial hypertrophy in the small pulmonary arteries together with the reduction of pulmonary vascular resistance obtained by vasodilator drugs led Paul Wood many years ago[6] to elaborate the 'vasoconstrictive' hypothesis as the basis for understanding the pathogenesis and the pathophysiology of PPH. He suggested that the active vasoconstriction of small muscular pulmonary arteries and arterioles was the main determinant of the hemodynamics and subsequent evolution of PPH. Since then, many attempts to reduce pulmonary vascular resistance and improve symptoms have been performed in small series of PAH patients in both acute and long-term studies. A variety of vasodilators have been used, including tolazoline, acetylcholine, diazoxide, hydralazine, phentolamine, isoproterenol, nitrates, verapamil, nifedipine and diltiazem.[5,6,8,29–33]

It soon became clear that only a minority of patients with PPH could obtain a meaningful reduction of pulmonary artery pressure associated with a reduction of pulmonary vascular resistance on acute vasoreactivity tests. In addition, the favorable results of long-term treatments were confirmed in larger scale trials with only calcium channel antagonists, namely nifedipine and diltiazem.[8,33]

Therefore, the aim of vasoreactivity tests is to detect the residual properties of vasodilatation of small pulmonary arteries and arterioles and to differentiate this reversible component from fixed obstructive changes. Patients in which an acute response of pulmonary vasodilatation is demonstrable are likely to benefit from chronic administration of oral calcium channel antagonists.[34] The sustained reduction of right ventricular afterload obtained by these drugs produces substantial improvement of right ventricular function and of exercise capacity. For non-responders to vasoreactivity tests, chronic calcium channel antagonist therapy has failed to demonstrate efficacy.[8,33]

Vasoreactivity tests

Vasoreactivity tests are performed under hemodynamic monitoring in intensive care units or catheterization laboratories by the use of short-acting compounds that share selective pulmonary vasodilator properties. The most used substances[34–40] are adenosine and prostacyclin, administered intravenously, or nitric oxide and the prostacyclin analog iloprost that are administered by inhalation. Half-lives, dose ranges, increments and duration of administration of these substances are shown in Table 13K.3. The most selective are the inhaled compounds that barely influence the systemic circulation.[40] Hypotension is the more ominous side effect of the intravenous substances that may result in circulatory shock and cardiac arrest if the administration is not promptly stopped. Even if severe reactions are uncommon, it is advisable to perform these procedures only in reference centers where

there is extensive experience. In the registry on primary pulmonary hypertension of the National Institutes of Health,[4] the incidence of hypotension requiring treatment during acute vasoreactivity tests was 6% and 2% of deaths were attributable to vasodilators.[32]

Multiple administration of short-acting pulmonary vasodilators are useless and should be avoided. In some centers, patients vasoreactive to short-acting compounds are tested also by the acute administration of calcium channel antagonists to identify the rare cases that respond only to the short-acting substances and would not benefit from chronic treatment.[41]

There is no consensus on the definition of vasodilator responsiveness according to the hemodynamic changes.[34] A minimum acceptable response is a reduction in mean pulmonary artery pressure of 15–20% and of at least 10 mmHg from baseline, associated with either no change or an increase in cardiac output.[1] Based on this definition, only about 20% of PPH adult patients[8] and about 40% of children[33] are considered acute responders to vasoreactivity tests. Usually, patients with the greater reduction of mean pulmonary artery pressure in response to the vasoreactivity tests present a more predictable clinical benefit from the chronic administration of calcium channel antagonists and a better prognosis. It is obvious that any definition of acute responsiveness is somewhat artificial and the clinical benefit of long-term treatment with calcium channel antagonists needs to be confirmed by an appropriate follow-up. In fact, usually only half of the 20% acute responders benefit from sustained treatment.

Currently, after the demonstration of clinical efficacy of oral, subcutaneous and inhaled prostanoids and of endothelin-receptor antagonists, some experts argue for the need to continue to perform vasoreactivity tests.[42] In recent trials, both populations were enrolled – the vasoreactive patients treated with calcium channel antagonists and the non-vasoreactive patients – and the investigational compounds were added to the current treatments.[14–16,18] As a stratified randomization based on the vasoreactivity test was not performed, any inference on the effect in the single groups is difficult. On the other hand, we do not have demonstration of efficacy of the

Table 13K.3 *Route of administration, half-lives, dose ranges, increments and duration of administration of the most used substances for pulmonary vasoreactivity tests*

Drug	Route	Half-life	Dose range*	Increments[†]	Duration[‡] (min)
Prostacyclin	Intravenous	3 min	2–16 ng/kg·min	2 ng/kg·min	10
Adenosine	Intravenous	5–10 s	50–200 ng/kg·min	20 ng/kg·min	2
Nitric oxide	Inhaled	15–30 s	10–60** p.p.m.	not needed	5–10
Iloprost	Inhaled	30 min	8–10 μg	not needed	10

*Initial dose and maximal dose suggested.
[†] Increments of dose by each step.
[‡] Duration of administration on each step.
**Safe limit.

new treatments in vasoreactive patients not treated with calcium channel antagonists. The opinion of the writers is that the identification of the subgroup of vasoreactive patients that present a good prognosis on a simple and low-cost treatment is still an advisable strategy. In addition, the effectiveness of the new compounds in vasoreactive patients has been tested on top of calcium channel antagonist treatment and the same approach should be followed in clinical practice.

Evidence

The demonstration of a favorable prognostic effect of calcium channel antagonist in vasoreactive patients with PPH has been shown in a single-center, non-randomized, non-controlled study.[8] In this case, the control group was represented by non-vasoreactive patients that have a spontaneous worst prognosis compared to vasoreactive ones.[37] Therefore, the favorable prognostic effect of calcium channel antagonist treatment shown in the study could have been exaggerated by an inappropriate comparison. The randomization of vasoreactive patients in treated and untreated groups would have given a more reliable demonstration of the positive effect of calcium channel antagonists. On the other hand, the demonstration of a consistent reduction of pulmonary artery pressure by acute pharmacological test, as observed in vasoreactive patients, raises ethical questions on the opportunity to give placebo instead of calcium channel antagonist in these subjects. Unfortunately, the results of this study have been extended, in clinical practice, also to a fraction of the non-vasoreactive patients or to patients not acutely tested. In fact, in recent clinical trials on new compounds, the patients treated with calcium channel antagonists at inclusion ranged from 22% to 60% (mean 44%) (Table 13K.2). Interestingly, the highest incidence of calcium channel antagonist treatment was observed in the scleroderma trial,[10] where probably some patients were treated with these compounds for Raynaud's phenomenon and not for PPH. On the other hand, the unrestricted use of calcium channel antagonist treatment in PPH patients may reduce its global beneficial impact due to frequent and sometimes severe side effects of these drugs when administered in non-vasoreactive subjects.[34] Favorable results of long-term administration of calcium channel antagonists have been shown also in children with PPH.[33] Conversely, the effects of this treatment on associated PAH forms have not been clearly demonstrated.[43]

Clinical implications

The calcium channel antagonists that have been proved effective in long-term trials in PPH patients are nifedipine

and diltiazem. Recommended doses for these compounds in PPH are definitely higher than those used in the treatment of systemic hypertension. In fact, the doses that were utilized in studies are up to 240 mg/day for nifedipine and 900 mg/day for diltiazem.[8,44] It is advisable, in vasoreactive patients, to start with reduced doses (e.g. 30 mg of extended release nifedipine b.i.d. or 60 mg of diltiazem t.i.d.) to be increased progressively in the subsequent weeks to the maximal tolerated regimen. Limiting factors for dose increase are usually systemic hypotension and lower limb peripheral edema. In some cases, the addition of digoxin and/or diuretics can improve the calcium channel antagonists side effects.[44] More pronounced side effects usually identify patients with poor clinical response. It is a common experience that, among the 20% responders to acute vasoreactivity tests, only half will obtain a consistent clinical benefit from the long-term administration of calcium channel antagonists.

Experience with the new generation of calcium channel antagonists is scarce and also the optimal doses in PPH are unknown. The empiric use of these drugs has probably to be discouraged in the absence of more consistent data.

INOTROPIC AGENTS

Rationale

The importance of the progression of right heart failure on the outcome of PPH patients is reinforced by the prognostic impact of right atrial pressure, cardiac index and pulmonary artery pressure,[4] three main determinants of right ventricular pump function. Since the depression of myocardial contractility seems to be one of the primary events in the progression of heart failure, the drugs that increase the force of contraction of myocytes, defined as inotropic agents, have been considered as a logical approach to the treatment of this condition. However, in patients with precapillary pulmonary hypertension, excessive afterload seem to be the leading determinant of heart failure. In fact, its removal as after successful pulmonary thromboendoarterectomy or lung transplantation[45] leads almost invariably to a sustained recovery of right ventricular function. On the other hand, changes in the adrenergic pathways of right ventricular myocytes leading to reduced contractility have been shown in PPH patients.[46] Thus, the use of inotropic drugs should be considered in selected situations.

Evidence

The effects of adrenergic inotropic drugs on the failing right ventricle have received little attention by investigators.

From theoretical points of view and from some experimental studies,[47] it emerges that the inotropic stimulation of these compounds is similar on the right and left ventricular myocardium. Data on humans are available mostly for the prevalent β_2-adrenergic receptor agonist isoproterenol[48] that was administered to PPH patients for its supposed effects of vasodilatation on the pulmonary circulation.[29,49] Isoproterenol induced increase of cardiac output and heart rate and in some cases reduction of blood pressure.

Dobutamine[48] is a prevalent β_1-adrenergic receptor agonist that exerts inotropic and vasodilator effects comparable to isoproterenol, but it has a less pronounced chronotropic activity. Dobutamine is widely used in the acute deterioration of patients with chronic biventricular failure. No data are available on the acute and long-term administration of dobutamine in PAH patients but it is likely that its effects are comparable to those of isoproterenol.

Dopamine[48] is a β-, α- and dopaminergic-receptor agonist and its profile of action may present some advantages over the prevalent β-receptor agonists. In fact, the α-adrenergic activity allows blood pressure levels to be preserved and even increased. The stimulation of β_1-adrenergic receptors induces a consistent increase of cardiac output while the dopaminergic stimulation increases the renal blood flow, facilitating diuresis. The dopaminergic effect is present at low doses ($2\,\mu g/kg\cdot min$) while the stimulation of β_1-adrenergic receptors increases progressively up to $10\text{--}15\,\mu g/kg\cdot min$ and a consistent α-adrenergic effect is detectable at high doses ($10\text{--}20\,\mu g/kg\cdot min$). A possible effect of pulmonary vasoconstriction seems not to be present at doses $<20\,\mu g/kg\cdot min$.

Even if digoxin increases indices of right ventricular contractility,[50] its clinical impact in PAH patients is still unknown. The effects of digoxin have been analyzed in patients with cor pulmonale secondary to chronic airflow obstruction[51–53] and in this setting no consistent results have been obtained. In fact, some investigators claimed a reduction in right-sided filling pressures and an increase of cardiac output after the administration of digitalis[33,34] while others did not confirm these findings.[53] Moreover, the acute administration of digoxin may induce pulmonary vasoconstriction[54] and the presence of hypoxia and electrolyte imbalance could increase the incidence of digitalis toxicity. On the other hand, short-term intravenous administration of digoxin in PPH patients induces a modest increase of cardiac output and a significant reduction in circulating norepinephrine.[55] In chronic 'biventricular' heart failure patients, digoxin treatment has no influence on mortality but it reduces the rate of hospitalization for acute decompensation.[56] For all those reasons, the use of digitalis in PAH patients is based mostly upon the personal experience and 'feelings'

of the expert rather than on clear scientific evidence of efficacy.

In PAH clinical trials (Table 13K.2) digoxin was administered at entry to a proportion of patients, varying from 18% to 53%. Interestingly, in the oldest study,[9] the incidence of digoxin treatment was the highest (53%), while in the more recent studies the incidence was around 20%.

Clinical implications

In severe, decompensated right heart failure, the use of intravenous adrenergic support may help the recovery of blood pressure and renal function. The absence of systemic hypotensive effects together with the renal blood flow increase suggest the use of dopamine alone or in combination with dobutamine as the inotropic strategy of choice in PAH patients. In critical cases, dopamine can be used together with intravenous prostanoids for its synergistic activity on cardiac output and its antagonistic effect on blood pressure decrease.

Empirically, digitalis could be used in PPH patients with evidence of right ventricular failure, especially in the presence of increased heart rate. In fact, one of the possible favorable effects of digoxin is its antiadrenergic activity[55,57] that can allow a reduction of the metabolic demands of the right ventricle. Digitalis is indicated also in the rare cases of PPH patients with atrial fibrillation or flutter, to reduce the ventricular rate. Finally, some investigators suggest the use of digoxin in patients treated with calcium channel blockers to antagonize the negative inotropic effects of these compounds.[44]

DIURETICS

Rationale

Patients with decompensated right heart failure develop fluid retention that leads to increased central venous pressure, abdominal organ congestion and peripheral edema.[58] Increased intra- and extra-vascular volumes can markedly impair symptoms and exercise capacity. In advanced cases, hepatic congestion and, occasionally, ascites may reduce diaphragmatic respiratory dynamics compromising lung volumes. In addition, increases of right ventricular preload and volumes may induce marked ventricular septal displacement, contributing to the reduced left ventricle dimensions. Parameters related to salt and water retention, such as right atrial pressure and pericardial effusion size, are prognostic determinants in PPH patients. The goal of proper diuretic treatment is to correct excessive fluid expansion and improve symptoms without reducing inappropriately right ventricular preload.

Evidence

The clear symptomatic and clinical benefits of diuretic treatment in cases of right heart failure prevent the need for controlled trials to show efficacy in PAH patients. In the recent clinical trials of new treatments, 49–70% of patients were treated with diuretics (Table 13K.2). On the other hand, it is quite surprising that about one-third of patients enrolled in trials on NYHA class III and IV patients were without diuretic treatment. PAH patients tend to have low blood pressure and it is a common experience that diuretic treatment tends to favor hypotension; it is possible that these problems have prevented the use of diuretics in some patients. Nevertheless, a further reduction of blood pressure can be avoided by an appropriate titration of the diuretic dose and by clinical monitoring of fluid balance. However, the lack of specific trials on diuretics in PAH patients and the individual variability leave to the direct experience of the physician the choice on the type and dose of drug to be used in individual cases.

Clinical implications

The need for diuretic treatment in PAH patients is usually based on the presence of symptoms and clinical signs of fluid retention, such as abdominal tension, increased jugular venous pressure, hepatomegaly, ankle edema, increased body weight and occasionally ascites. The appropriate diuretic dose is strictly individual and theoretically should be the lower dose that is able to maintain the ideal body weight and reduce symptoms. The reasons for variation in diuretic requirement include varying salt intake, hormonal profile, ventricular performance and different bioavailability.[58,59] Proper fluid balance can be facilitated by a controlled salt and water intake. Loop diuretics are generally used and furosemide oral doses may vary from 20 to 25 mg/day up to 500 mg/day. Loop diuretics with better bioavailability may present some advantages.[59] Intravenous administration is temporary, and is preferred in cases of important extravascular fluid expansion to overcome reduced intestinal absorption. Care is required to avoid hypokalemia and hyponatremia by selected supplementation. The combination of loop diuretics with anti-aldosteronic drugs can help in the preservation of electrolyte plasma levels.

The combination of loop diuretics with thiazides may be temporarily used in selected cases with refractory edema for the synergistic effects of the two compounds. The protracted combination of these two types of diuretics increases the incidence of severe hyponatremia and hypokalemia.

SUPPLEMENTAL OXYGEN

Rationale

The oxygen content of arterial blood and oxygen delivery to tissues are generally not reduced unless the PaO_2 falls <60 mmHg.[60] Most patients with chronic respiratory insufficiency are hypoxemic because of altered ventilation/perfusion matching.[61] By contrast, most patients with PAH (except those with associated congenital heart disease) present with only mild degrees of arterial hypoxemia at rest. The pathophysiological mechanisms in this case include a low mixed venous oxygen saturation caused by low cardiac output and only minimally altered ventilation/perfusion matching. In some patients with profound hypoxemia, a secondary opening of a patent foramen ovale can be found. In patients with PAH associated with congenital cardiac defects, hypoxemia is related to reversal of left-to-right shunting. Shunt-induced hypoxemia is refractory to increased inspired oxygen.

Evidence

Oxygen therapy improves quality of life and decreases mortality in patients with pulmonary hypertension related to chronic respiratory insufficiency[62,63] and it is currently indicated in patients with chronic lung disease and arterial oxygen pressure repeatedly measured below 55–60 mmHg, or in patients with sleep-associated or exercised-induced hypoxemia.[64]

No consistent data are currently available on the effect of long-term oxygen treatment in patients with PAH. Even if acute administration of 100% oxygen seems to reduce pulmonary vascular resistance and increase cardiac output in PAH patients,[65] the potential adverse effects of long-term administration of high levels of inhaled oxygen are not known. Although improvement in pulmonary hypertension with low-flow supplemental oxygen has been reported in some PAH patients, this has not been confirmed in controlled studies. In a controlled study on Eisenmenger syndrome patients, nocturnal oxygen therapy had no effect on hematology variables, quality of life and survival.[66]

Clinical implications

Supplemental low-flow oxygen is currently indicated in patients with chronic parenchymal lung disease and arterial oxygen pressure repeatedly measured below 55–60 mmHg, or in patients with sleep-associated or exercised-induced hypoxemia.[64]

If the same strategy has to be performed also in patients with PAH, it is unknown. Patients who have severe right heart failure and resting hypoxemia caused by low cardiac output and low mixed venous oxygen saturation may benefit from continuous oxygen therapy. The symptomatic improvement related to the use of portable oxygen equipment should be confirmed in clinical practice by objective assessment of functional capacity. In fact, psychological dependency and mobility limitations related to these devices may overcome the benefits of supplemental oxygen.

There is little rationale to treat with long-term oxygen therapy patients with hypoxemia predominantly due to right-to-left shunt through a patent foramen ovale, atrial or ventricular septal defects or patent ductus arteriosus.

GENERAL MEASURES

General measures include strategies devoted to limit the deleterious impact of some circumstances and external agents on patient with PAH.

Physical activity

It is unclear whether physical activity may have a negative impact on the evolution of PAH. Nevertheless, potentially dangerous symptoms such as severe dyspnea, syncope and chest pain should be avoided. Exercise should be limited to a symptom-free level in order to maintain adequate skeletal muscle conditioning. Physical activity after meals or in extreme temperatures should be avoided. Appropriate adjustments of daily activities may improve the quality of life and reduce the frequency of symptoms.

Travel/altitude

Hypoxia may aggravate vasoconstriction in PAH patients and it is advisable to avoid also mild degrees of hypobaric hypoxia that starts at altitudes between 1500 and 2000 meters. Commercial airplanes are pressurized to an equivalent altitude of 2400 meters and supplemental oxygen in PAH patients should be considered. Before planning travel, information on the nearest pulmonary hypertension clinics should be obtained.

Prevention of infections

Patients with PAH are susceptible to develop pneumonia, which is the cause of death in 7% of cases.

Pulmonary infections are poorly tolerated and need to be promptly recognized and treated. Vaccine strategies are also recommended. Any persistent fever in patients with an intravenous catheter for continuous administration of prostacyclin should raise the suspicion of catheter infection.

Pregnancy, birth control and postmenopausal hormonal therapy

Pregnancy and delivery in PAH patients are associated with an increased rate of deterioration and death.[67] Even if successful pregnancies have been reported in PPH patients,[68] an appropriate method of birth control is highly recommended in women with childbearing potential. Currently, there is no consensus among experts on the more appropriate birth control method in these subjects. The safety of hormonal contraception is questioned for its influence on prothrombotic changes. However, the current availability of low-estrogen-dose products and the concomitant oral anticoagulant treatment may limit the risk of these agents. In addition, recent studies of large numbers of patients failed to reveal any relationship between intake of hormonal contraceptive agents and PAH.[69] Some experts suggest the use of estrogen-free products or surgical sterilization or barrier contraceptives.

It is not clear whether the use of hormonal therapy in postmenopausal women with PAH is advisable. Probably it could be suggested only in cases of intolerable menopausal symptoms and in conjunction with anticoagulation.

Haemoglobin levels

Patients with PAH are highly sensitive to reduction of hemoglobin levels. Any kind of anemia, even of milder degrees, should be promptly treated. On the other hand, patients with longstanding hypoxemia such as those with right-to-left shunts tend to develop erythrocytosis with elevated levels of hematocrit. In these circumstances, to reduce hyperviscosity side effects, venesections are indicated if the hematocrit is above 65%.

Concomitant medications

Care is needed to avoid drugs that interfere with oral anticoagulants or increase the risk for gastrointestinal bleeding. Even if non-steroidal anti-inflammatory drugs seem not to be associated with PAH in a case–control study,[69] their use may further reduce glomerular filtration rate in patients with low cardiac output and pre-renal azotemia. Anorexigens that have been linked to the development of PAH are no longer marketed. The effects of the new generation serotonin-related anorexigens are unknown, but no reports of pulmonary-related side effects are available to date. The efficacy of current treatments for chronic 'biventricular' heart failure, such as ace inhibitors and β-blockers has not been tested in patients with PAH. On the other hand, the empiric use of these treatments, even at low doses, may result in severe side effects such as hypotension and right heart failure and should be discouraged.

Psychological assistance

Patients with PAH have a median age of about 40 years and exercise limitation may interfere considerably with their previous lifestyle. In addition, information on the severity of the disease may be collected from many sources that may not be updated or may be confusing or inappropriately explicit. Also, for these reasons, many PAH patients are affected by a variable degree of anxiety and/or depression that can have a profound impact on their quality of life. The role of the PAH expert is important in supporting patients with adequate information and in referring them to psychologists or psychiatrists when needed. In addition, support groups of patients led or not by psychologists or psychiatrists are useful in improving the understanding and the acceptance of the disease condition.

Elective surgery

Even if appropriate studies are lacking, it is expected that elective surgery has an increased risk in patients with PAH. In addition, the risk should increase with the severity of NYHA functional class and in cases of thoracic and abdominal interventions. It is not clear which type of anesthesia is advisable, but probably epidural is better tolerated than general. General anesthesia should be performed by experienced anesthesiologists with the support of pulmonary hypertension experts for deciding the most appropriate treatment in case of complications. Patients on intravenous and subcutaneous prostacyclin treatment should have fewer problems compared to subjects on oral or inhaled treatments who may suffer from temporary obstacles to drug administration such as fasting, general anesthesia and assisted ventilation. In cases when a prolonged period of withdrawal is foreseen (more than 12–24 hours), provisional shifting to intravenous treatments is advisable, reverting to the original therapy subsequently. Anticoagulant treatment should be interrupted for the shortest possible time and deep venous thrombosis prophylaxis should be performed.

KEY POINTS

- Conventional treatments are used in virtually all patients with PAH.
- Oral anticoagulant treatment seems to be required in any PAH patient unless contraindicated.
- Calcium channel antagonists are indicated only in vasoreactive patients (20% of cases).
- The use of inotropic agents is based on empiric evidence.
- Diuretic treatment is very important in maintaining stability in patients with right heart failure.
- The usefulness of supplemental oxygen in PAH patients is controversial.
- General measures such as physical activity adjustments and psychological assistance are required.

REFERENCES

◆1 Rich S (ed.) Executive summary. Primary Pulmonary Hypertension: The World Symposium-Primary Pulmonary Hypertension 1998, 25–7. World Health Organization http://www.who.int/ncd/cvd/pph.html.

2 Rubin LJ. Primary pulmonary hypertension. *N Engl J Med* 1997;**336**:111–17.

3 Galiè N, Manes A, Uguccioni L *et al.* Primary pulmonary hypertension: insights into pathogenesis from epidemiology. *Chest* 1998;**114**(3 Suppl):184S–94S.

●4 D'Alonzo GE, Barst RJ, Ayres SM *et al.* Survival in patients with primary pulmonary hypertension. Results from a national prospective registry. *Ann Intern Med* 1991;**115**:343–9.

5 Dresdale DT, Schultz M, Michtom RJ. Primary pulmonary hypertension. I. Clinical and hemodynamic study. *Am J Med* 1951;**11**:686–705.

6 Wood P. Primary pulmonary hypertension, with special reference to the vasoconstrictive factor. *Br Heart J* 1958;**20**:557–65.

7 Fuster V, Steele PM, Edwards WD *et al.* Primary pulmonary hypertension: natural history and the importance of thrombosis. *Circulation* 1984;**70**:580–7.

●8 Rich S, Kaufmann E, Levy PS. The effect of high doses of calcium-channel blockers on survival in primary pulmonary hypertension [see comments]. *N Engl J Med* 1992;**327**:76–81.

●9 Barst RJ, Rubin LJ, Long WA *et al.* A comparison of continuous intravenous epoprostenol (prostacyclin) with conventional therapy for primary pulmonary hypertension. The Primary Pulmonary Hypertension Study Group [see comments]. *N Engl J Med* 1996;**334**:296–302.

10 Badesch DB, Tapson VF, McGoon MD *et al.* Continuous intravenous epoprostenol for pulmonary hypertension due to the scleroderma spectrum of disease. A randomized,

controlled trial [see comments]. *Ann Intern Med* 2000;**132**:425–34.

11 Galiè N, Manes A, Branzi A. Medical therapy of pulmonary hypertension. The prostacyclins. *Clin Chest Med* 2001;**22**:529–37, x.

12 Sandoval J, Gaspar J, Pulido T *et al.* Graded balloon dilation atrial septostomy in severe primary pulmonary hypertension. A therapeutic alternative for patients nonresponsive to vasodilator treatment. *J Am Coll Cardiol* 1998;**32**:297–304.

13 Langleben D, Christman W, Barst R *et al.* Effects of the thromboxane synthetase inhibitor and receptor antagonist, terbogrel, in patients with primary pulmonary hypertension. *Am Heart J* 2002;**143**:E4.

●14 Simonneau G, Barst RJ, Galiè N *et al.* Continuous subcutaneous infusion of treprostinil, a prostacyclin analogue, in patients with pulmonary arterial hypertension. A double-blind, randomized, placebo-controlled trial. *Am J Respir Crit Care Med* 2002;**165**:800–4.

●15 Galiè N, Humbert M, Vachiery JL *et al.* Effects of beraprost sodium, an oral prostacyclin analogue, in patients with pulmonary arterial hypertension: a randomized, double-blind placebo-controlled trial. *J Am Coll Cardiol* 2002;**39**:1496–502.

●16 Olschewski H, Simonneau G, Galiè N *et al.* Inhaled iloprost for severe pulmonary hypertension. *N Engl J Med* 2002;**347**:322–9.

17 Channick RN, Simonneau G, Sitbon O *et al.* Effects of the dual endothelin-receptor antagonist bosentan in patients with pulmonary hypertension: a randomised placebo-controlled study. *Lancet* 2001;**358**:1119–23.

●18 Rubin LJ, Badesch DB, Barst RJ *et al.* Bosentan therapy for pulmonary arterial hypertension. *N Engl J Med* 2002;**346**:896–903.

19 Galiè N. Do we need controlled clinical trials in pulmonary arterial hypertension? *Eur Respir J* 2001;**17**:1–3.

◆20 Hoeper M, Galiè N, Simonneau G *et al.* New treatments for pulmonary arterial hypertension. *Am J Respir Crit Care Med* 2002;**165**:1209–16.

21 Eisenberg PR, Lucore C, Kaufman L *et al.* Fibrinopeptide A levels indicative of pulmonary vascular thrombosis in patients with primary pulmonary hypertension. *Circulation* 1990;**82**:841–7.

22 Christman BW, McPherson CD, Newman JH *et al.* An imbalance between the excretion of thromboxane and prostacyclin metabolites in pulmonary hypertension [see comments]. *N Engl J Med* 1992;**327**:70–5.

23 Friedman R, Mears JG, Barst RJ. Continuous infusion of prostacyclin normalizes plasma markers of endothelial cell injury and platelet aggregation in primary pulmonary hypertension. *Circulation* 1997;**96**:2782–4.

24 Pietra GG, Edwards WD, Kay JM *et al.* Histopathology of primary pulmonary hypertension. A qualitative and quantitative study of pulmonary blood vessels from 58 patients in the National Heart, Lung, and Blood Institute, Primary Pulmonary Hypertension Registry [see comments]. *Circulation* 1989;**80**:1198–206.

25 Wagenvoort CA, Mulder PG. Thrombotic lesions in primary plexogenic arteriopathy. Similar pathogenesis or complication? [see comments] *Chest* 1993;**103**:844–9.

26 Moser KM, Fedullo PF, Finkbeiner WE *et al.* Do patients with primary pulmonary hypertension develop extensive central thrombi? *Circulation* 1995;**91**:741–5.

27 Frank H, Mlczoch J, Huber K *et al.* The effect of anticoagulant therapy in primary and anorectic drug-induced pulmonary hypertension. *Chest* 1997;**112**:714–21.

28 Ansell J, Hirsh J, Dalen J *et al.* Managing oral anticoagulant therapy. *Chest* 2001;**119**(1 Suppl):22S–38S.

29 Shettigar UR, Hultgren HN, Specter M *et al.* Primary pulmonary hypertension favorable effect of isoproterenol. *N Engl J Med* 1976;**295**:1414–15.

30 Rubin LJ, Peter RH. Oral hydralazine therapy for primary pulmonary hypertension. *N Engl J Med* 1980;**302**:69–73.

31 Reeves JT, Groves BM, Turkevich D. The case for treatment of selected patients with primary pulmonary hypertension. *Am Rev Respir Dis* 1986;**134**:342–6.

32 Weir EK, Rubin LJ, Ayres SM *et al.* The acute administration of vasodilators in primary pulmonary hypertension. Experience from the National Institutes of Health Registry on Primary Pulmonary Hypertension. *Am Rev Respir Dis* 1989;**140**:1623–30.

33 Barst RJ, Maislin G, Fishman AP. Vasodilator therapy for primary pulmonary hypertension in children. *Circulation* 1999;**99**:1197–208.

34 Galiè N, Ussia G, Passarelli P *et al.* Role of pharmacologic tests in the treatment of primary pulmonary hypertension. *Am J Cardiol* 1995;**75**:55A–62A.

35 Rubin LJ, Groves BM, Reeves JT *et al.* Prostacyclin-induced acute pulmonary vasodilation in primary pulmonary hypertension. *Circulation* 1982;**66**:334–8.

36 Morgan JM, McCormack DG, Griffiths MJ *et al.* Adenosine as a vasodilator in primary pulmonary hypertension [see comments]. *Circulation* 1991;**84**:1145–9.

37 Raffy O, Azarian R, Brenot F *et al.* Clinical significance of the pulmonary vasodilator response during short-term infusion of prostacyclin in primary pulmonary hypertension. *Circulation* 1996;**93**:484–8.

●38 Sitbon O, Humbert M, Jagot JL *et al.* Inhaled nitric oxide as a screening agent for safely identifying responders to oral calcium-channel blockers in primary pulmonary hypertension [see comments]. *Eur Respir J* 1998;**12**:265–70.

39 Ricciardi MJ, Knight BP, Martinez FJ *et al.* Inhaled nitric oxide in primary pulmonary hypertension: a safe and effective agent for predicting response to nifedipine. *J Am Coll Cardiol* 1998;**32**:1068–73.

40 Hoeper MM, Olschewski H, Ghofrani HA *et al.* A comparison of the acute hemodynamic effects of inhaled nitric oxide and aerosolized iloprost in primary pulmonary hypertension. German PPH study group. *J Am Coll Cardiol* 2000;**35**:176–82.

41 Ricciardi MJ, Bossone E, Bach DS *et al.* Echocardiographic predictors of an adverse response to a nifedipine trial in primary pulmonary hypertension: diminished left ventricular size and leftward ventricular septal bowing [see comments]. *Chest* 1999;**116**:1218–23.

◆42 Galiè N, Torbicki A. Pulmonary arterial hypertension: new ideas and perspectives. *Heart* 2001;**85**:475–80.

43 Nootens M, Kaufmann E, Rich S. Short-term effectiveness of nifedipine in secondary pulmonary hypertension. *Am J Cardiol* 1993;**71**:1475–6.

44 Rich S, Kaufmann E. High dose titration of calcium channel blocking agents for primary pulmonary hypertension: guidelines for short-term drug testing. *J Am Coll Cardiol* 1991;**18**:1323–7.

45 Ritchie M, Waggoner AD, Dávila R *et al.* Echocardiographic characterization of the improvement in right ventricular function in patients with severe pulmonary hypertension after single-lung transplantation. *J Am Coll Cardiol* 1993;**22**:1170–4.

46 Bristow MR, Minobe W, Rasmussen R *et al.* Beta-adrenergic neuroeffector abnormalities in the failing human heart are produced by local rather than systemic mechanisms. *J Clin Invest* 1992;**89**:803–15.

47 Schmidt HD, Hoppe H, Hedenreich L. Direct effects of dopamine, orciprenaline and norepinephrine on the right and left ventricle of isolated canine hearts. *Cardiology* 1979;**64**:133–48.

48 Leier CV. Acute inotropic support. In: Leier CV (ed.), *Cardiotonic drugs.* New York: Marcel Dekker, 1986;49–84.

49 Pietro DA, LaBresh KA, Shulman RM *et al.* Sustained improvement in primary pulmonary hypertension during six years of treatment with sublingual isoproterenol. *N Engl J Med* 1984;**310**:1032–4.

50 Green L, Smith T. The use of digitalis in patients with pulmonary disease. *Ann Intern Med* 1977;**87**:459–65.

51 Gray FD, Williams MH, Gray FG. The circulatory and ventilatory changes in chronic pulmonary disease as affected by lanatoside C. *Am Heart J* 1952;**44**:517–30.

52 Ferrer MI, Harvey RM, Cathcart RT *et al.* Some effects of digoxin in chronic cor pulmonale. *Circulation* 1950;**1**:161–86.

53 Berglund E, Widminsky J, Malmberg R. Lack of effect of digitalis in patients with pulmonary disease with and without heart failure. *Am J Cardiol* 1963;**11**:447.

54 Kim YS, Aviado DM. Digitalis and the pulmonary circulation. *Am Heart J* 1961;**62**:680–6.

55 Rich S, Seidlitz M, Dodin E *et al.* The short-term effects of digoxin in patients with right ventricular dysfunction from pulmonary hypertension. *Chest* 1998;**114**:787–92.

56 The Digitalis Investigation Group. The effects of digoxin on mortality and morbidity in patients with heart failure. *N Engl J Med* 1997;**336**:533.

57 Newton GE, Tong JH, Schofield AM *et al.* Digoxin reduces cardiac sympathetic activity in severe congestive heart failure. *J Am Coll Cardiol* 1996;**28**:155–61.

58 Cohn JN. Optimal diuretic therapy for heart failure. *Am J Med* 2001;**111**:577.

59 Murray MD, Deer MM, Ferguson JA *et al.* Open-label randomized trial of torsemide compared with furosemide therapy for patients with heart failure. *Am J Med* 2001;**111**:513–20.

60 Hales CA. The site and mechanisms of oxygen sensing for the pulmonary vessels. *Circulation* 1985;**88**:235s–40s.

61 West JB. Ventilation/perfusion relationships. *Am Rev Respir Dis* 1977;**116**:919–43.

●62 Long term domiciliary oxygen therapy in chronic hypoxic cor pulmonale complicating chronic bronchitis and emphysema. Report of the Medical Research Council Working Party. *Lancet* 1981;**i**:681–6.

●63 Continuous or nocturnal oxygen therapy in hypoxemic chronic obstructive lung disease: a clinical trial. Nocturnal Oxygen Therapy Trial Group. *Ann Intern Med* 1980;**93**:391–8.

64 Tarpy SP, Celli BR. Long-term oxygen therapy. *N Engl J Med* 1995;**333**:710–14.

65 Roberts DH, Lepore JJ, Maroo A *et al.* Oxygen therapy improves cardiac index and pulmonary vascular resistance in patients with pulmonary hypertension. *Chest* 2001;**120**:1547–55.

66 Sandoval J, Aguirre JS, Pulido T *et al.* Nocturnal oxygen therapy in patients with the Eisenmenger syndrome. *Am J Respir Crit Care Med* 2001;**164**:1682–7.

67 Nelson DM, Main E, Crafford W *et al.* Peripartum heart failure due to primary pulmonary hypertension. *Obstet Gynecol* 1983;**62**(3 Suppl):58s–63s.

68 Nootens M, Rich S. Successful management of labor and delivery in primary pulmonary hypertension. *Am J Cardiol* 1993;**71**:1124–5.

69 Abenhaim L, Moride Y, Brenot F *et al.* Appetite-suppressant drugs and the risk of primary pulmonary hypertension. International Primary Pulmonary Hypertension Study Group [see comments]. *N Engl J Med* 1996;**335**:609–16.

Intravenous prostacyclin for pulmonary arterial hypertension

TERRY A FORTIN AND VICTOR F TAPSON

INTRODUCTION

Over the past decade, continuous intravenous prostacyclin therapy has revolutionized the treatment of pulmonary arterial hypertension (PAH) and remains the most effective pharmacological approach for patients with advanced disease. The effectiveness of intravenous prostacyclin, a vasodilator and inhibitor of platelet aggregation, reflects the mechanisms believed to contribute substantially to the development of PAH. Early observations of the beneficial acute hemodynamic changes in patients with PAH led to clinical applications for chronic usage.[1,2] Subsequently, the prognosis and well-being of patients with PAH was definitively shown to improve when compared with placebo[3] as well as with historic controls.[4] Early use as a bridge to lung or heart/lung transplantation evolved as it became clear that long-term survival on prostacyclin was possible in some patients. The clinical use of long-term prostacyclin expanded from limited use in primary pulmonary hypertension (PPH) to secondary causes of PAH, particularly that due to underlying collagen vascular disease, but also to other forms of PAH.

THE PATHOPHYSIOLOGICAL BASIS FOR PROSTACYCLIN USE

Initially described in 1976 by Moncada and Vane, prostacyclin (epoprostenol, PGI_2, PGX) is a member of the prostaglandin family produced by vascular endothelial cells.[5,6] It is the major metabolite of arachadonic acid in vascular tissue and is formed via the cyclooxygenase pathway. It is a powerful direct vasodilator of both the pulmonary and systemic vascular beds, as well as an inhibitor of platelet aggregation.[5,6] There is growing evidence that it also acts chronically as an antiproliferative factor. Prostacyclin analogs have been shown *in vitro* to inhibit smooth muscle cell growth.[7] The mechanism by which it mediates vasodilation is via ligand binding to a G-protein-coupled receptor with subsequent signal transduction inducing relaxation of vascular smooth muscle. Signal transduction via adenylate cyclase increases intracellular cyclic adenosine monophosphate (cAMP). Intracellular levels of cAMP are also increased in platelets exposed to prostacyclin.[2] In addition to vasodilation, prostacyclin has positive inotropic effects. In a group of 19 patients with pulmonary hypertension secondary to heart failure, contractile element maximal velocity, as estimated from cardiac catheterization, was shown to reflect this positive inotropy.[8] It was not clear, however, whether or not this represented an indirect action related to activation of the sympathetic nervous system. With low doses of intravenous prostacyclin, there may be bradycardia, but in response to vasodilation at higher doses, a reflex tachycardia usually results.

The pathogenesis of PAH is multifactorial. Endothelial and smooth muscle cell dysfunction, pulmonary vasoconstriction[9] and *in situ* thrombosis as well as vascular wall remodeling all potentially contribute to the onset and progression of PAH. Diminished production of vasodilator and antiproliferative factors such as prostacyclin and nitric oxide versus an imbalance in the normal ratio of these to thromboxane and/or endothelin also contribute to the perpetuation of PAH.[10,11] Circulating levels of prostacyclin are reduced in patients with PPH.[10] Moreover, prostacyclin synthase expression has been shown to be reduced in the pulmonary arteries of patients with PPH.[12] Initiation of prostacyclin in patients with PPH has been shown to result in an increased amount of nitric oxide exhaled after 24 hours.[13] Of note, at baseline, PPH patients exhaled significantly less nitric oxide than controls. Other studies have shown increased levels of thromboxane metabolites in the urine of those with pulmonary hypertension.[10,11]

Several studies suggest that long-term prostacyclin therapy in PPH results in remodeling of the pulmonary vascular bed.[14,15] Histological studies reveal increased tissue levels of endothelin-1 production, and a net reduction in the pulmonary clearance of this powerful vasoconstrictor and smooth muscle mitogen has been demonstrated in PPH.[14] Normally, about 60–70% of endothelin is cleared in the lungs with a normal arterial/venous ratio of less than one. After 12 weeks of prostacyclin therapy, 82% of treated patients had normalized ratios compared with only 29% of conventional therapy patients.[14] Mikhail *et al.* also measured elevated levels of endothelin in eight patients, although decreased clearance was not found.[11] Alterations in the coagulation system may contribute to the pathogenesis of PPH; the normalization of endothelial markers concomitant with improvement in hemodynamic parameters with long-term prostacyclin suggests that long-term therapy remodels the pulmonary vascular bed, with subsequent decreases in endothelial cell injury and hypercoagulability.[15,16] These data support the hypothesis that endothelial cell injury and dysfunction initiate and/or exacerbate the pulmonary vascular disease in PPH. There is evidence derived from prostacyclin receptor knockout mice indicating that prostacyclin and its receptor play a role in regulation of the remodeling found in PAH.[17] Patients with severe PAH also have reduced expression of prostacyclin receptors in the remodeled areas.[18] These prostacyclin effects may in part,

explain the antiproliferative effect on smooth muscle and, particularly in patients with little or no acute vasodilator response, may be responsible for long-term therapeutic effects.[2] Thus, the effect of the drug appears related to its effect as a vasodilator, as well as its effects on vascular growth, remodeling, and/or platelet function.

THE CLINICAL USE OF INTRAVENOUS PROSTACYCLIN (EPOPROSTENOL): PRIMARY PULMONARY HYPERTENSION

From 1981 to 1985, a National Institutes of Health (NIH) registry for PPH enrolled and characterized 187 patients.[4,19] The median survival from diagnosis was 2.8 years and the diagnosis was made an average of 2 years after the onset of symptoms.[4] The survival rate was 68% at 1 year, 48% at 3 years, and 34% at 5 years. Importantly, variables associated with poor prognosis included New York Heart Association (NYHA) functional class III or IV, elevated mean right atrial and pulmonary artery pressures, and decreased cardiac index. Median survival for class I or II patients was 58.6 months compared with 31.5 months for class III and 6 months for class IV. Only 20% of patients had hemodynamic and clinical responses to oral vasodilators. A prediction formula based upon variables of mean pulmonary artery pressure, mean right atrial pressure and cardiac index was developed. In this registry, only 19% of patients were receiving long-term therapy consisting of oral vasodilators, warfarin, diuretics and digitalis.[19] The poor outcome and inadequate response to available therapies necessitated the development of new treatment modalities such as intravenous prostacyclin.

In 1976, while looking for the enzyme that generates the unstable prostanoid thromboxane A_2 from arachadonic acid, Moncada and Vane discovered PGI_2 and renamed it 'prostacyclin'.[5,6] The impact of this drug on PAH was suggested shortly thereafter. In 1982, Rubin and colleagues[1] studied seven patients with PPH, examining the acute hemodynamic effects of prostacyclin. Infusions from 2 to 12 ng/kg·min resulted in hemodynamic benefit. Mean pulmonary artery pressure was reduced from 62 ± 15 to 55 ± 16 mmHg (P < 0.05) and cardiac output increased from 4.22 ± 1.64 to 6.57 ± 2.04 L/min (P < 0.01). Three patients who received a continuous infusion for 24–48 hours had sustained reductions in pulmonary vascular resistance during the infusion period. The first experience with long-term use of prostacyclin in a PPH patient was described by Higenbottam *et al.* in 1984.[20] A young woman experienced an impressive hemodynamic response coupled by improved exercise tolerance enabling discharge home to await transplantation. Higenbottam's group treated a series of 10 patients with PPH unresponsive to oral vasodilators with continuous intravenous epoprostenol, all of whom were referred for heart/lung transplantation. Short-term hemodynamic improvement was proven and functional status and maximum oxygen consumption were noted to improve for periods up to 25 months of therapy.[21] Patients without an acute vasodilator response were still noted to improve on chronic therapy. Compared with historical controls, exercise capacity and survival improved.[4,19–21]

These early trials ultimately led to larger, prospective, randomized trials, in patients with PPH. In these studies, hemodynamics and exercise capacity were the primary end points. Based upon animal data and a few human case reports of successful responses to prostacyclin, patients were treated with continuous intravenous prostacyclin (epoprostenol sodium) and this therapy potentially served as a bridge to lung transplantation.

In 1990, the first randomized trial involving 25 patients with PPH treated with continuous intravenous epoprostenol compared with conventional therapy (oral vasodilators, diuretics, digoxin, and oxygen) was reported by Rubin et al.[22] A sustained reduction in pulmonary artery pressure and increase in cardiac output were documented after only 2 months of therapy in the epoprostenol group. Barst et al.[23] then reported sustained improvement in the 18 survivors of that study by continued treatment with epoprostenol. Complications were noted in some patients and were attributed to the portable infusion system. Walk distance was improved at 6 months and at 18 months and hemodynamics were improved at 6 months and at 12 months. Interestingly, demonstration of an acute hemodynamic response was not a prerequisite for long-term clinical improvement. This early study helped to better characterize the potential adverse effects of intravenous epoprostenol as well as the potential for infectious complications and pump malfunction. Survival in these 18 patients was compared with a stratified sample of historical controls from the NIH Registry using a Kaplan–Meier proportional hazards regression model analysis. The patients were followed for up to 69 months. The survival rates at 1, 3 and 5 years for the epoprostenol patients and historical controls were 87, 63, 54 versus 77, 41 and 27%, respectively. Although this study was uncontrolled, supporting evidence to confirm this survival benefit in prospective, randomized, controlled trials subsequently followed.

The landmark study definitively proving the efficacy of epoprostenol in PPH was reported in the *New England Journal of Medicine* in 1996.[3] This prospective, randomized study of 81 patients with NYHA class III or IV PPH compared prostacyclin plus conventional therapy with conventional therapy alone over a 12-week period. Baseline characteristics were similar between the groups. The primary objective was exercise capacity as measured by change in distance walked on a standardized 6-minute walk test. The treated group improved by 31 meters while the controls **decreased** by 29 meters for a statistically

significant change. The secondary end points of hemodynamics, symptoms and mortality were all significantly improved with epoprostenol. Cardiac index increased significantly while mean pulmonary artery pressure and pulmonary vascular resistance trended toward improvement. Functional class improved in 40% of epoprostenol patients and in only 3% of the conventional therapy group. A total of three patients were transplanted, one being from the epoprostenol group.[3] Importantly, there was a survival benefit noted even at 12 weeks. Of the 40 patients in the conventional therapy group, eight died compared with none in the epoprostenol group. This was statistically significant (P < 0.003). These results led to Federal Drug Administration (FDA) approval of continuous intravenous epoprostenol (Flolan) therapy for PPH. Furthermore, it became increasingly clear that while a marked initial reduction in the total pulmonary resistance index from a short-term infusion of epoprostenol may improve prognosis when compared with a lesser response,[24] long-term survival was not dependent on such a response.

Long-term survival on epoprostenol was analyzed in a prospective cohort of 69 PPH patients with NYHA class III and IV symptoms at baseline with follow-up data being obtained at 330–770 days.[25] A gradual and sustained trend toward reduction in right ventricular pressure gradient, improved cardiac output and survival was demonstrated. Survival was 80% at 1 year, 76% at 2 years, and 49% at 3 years. Kaplan–Meier survival curves revealed significant improvement compared with the NIH Registry data. McLaughlin and colleagues[26] assessed 27 consecutive patients on epoprostenol for over 1 year with PPH. Twenty-six had improvement in functional class over a mean of 16 months. At baseline, 63% had functional class III symptoms, with the remainder being class IV. At the end of the study, 22% were class I, 72% class II, and the remainder class III. The duration of exercise increased by 142%, the mean pulmonary artery pressure decreased by 22%, and cardiac output increased by 67%.

More recently, the same group published survival data in 162 consecutive patients diagnosed with PPH and treated with continuous intravenous epoprostenol.[27] These patients were followed for a mean of 36.3 months. Observed survival with epoprostenol therapy at 1, 2 and 3 years was 87.8%, 76.3% and 62.8%, and again was significantly greater than historical survival of 58.9%, 46.3% and 35.4%. Exercise performance has also been tested in patients on intravenous epoprostenol using bicycle ergometry. Sixteen patients with PPH on epoprostenol were tested at regular intervals over an average of 19.5 months.[28] At baseline, 6-minute walk performance was 130 meters and increased by 8 meters over time. Peak work on cycle ergometry was 35% of predicted at baseline and subsequently improved to 58% of predicted. There was a positive correlation between peak oxygen consumption and peak 6-minute walk test of 0.6 (P < 0.005). Notably, cases of PAH associated with appetite-suppressant drugs are typically considered PPH as the pathological processes are similar.[29] While most of the clinical studies described involve adult patients, there is substantial experience treating children with this disease. A recent extensive review comparing children in the pre-epoprostenol era with subsequent treatment indicates that continuous intravenous epo-prostenol improves survival.[30]

Based upon the above early studies, and reinforced by the subsequent survival data, as well as by extensive clinical experience, continuous intravenous epoprostenol became standard therapy for PPH patients with advanced NYHA (now termed World Health Organization, WHO) functional class III or class IV symptoms. This treatment is not simply viewed as a bridge to more definitive therapy such as lung or heart/lung transplantation, but has served as long-term definitive treatment for many of these patients. Patients are sometimes removed from active lung transplantation listing as they improve on intravenous epoprostenol.

EPOPROSTENOL FOR PULMONARY ARTERIAL HYPERTENSION FROM COLLAGEN VASCULAR DISEASE

Because of pathological similarities between PPH and PAH secondary to collagen vascular disease, it appeared quite possible that patients with scleroderma or CREST would potentially respond to continuous intravenous epoprostenol. Small studies suggested not only that these patients would respond, but that they would potentially respond for extended periods.[31,32] Based upon the promising improvement in small series of patients with diffuse scleroderma and CREST, as well as the use of epoprostenol for Raynaud's phenomenon often associated with scleroderma, a prospective, multicenter, randomized trial of 111 patients with PAH due to the scleroderma spectrum of diseases was initiated.[33] Exercise capacity and hemodynamics were examined in patients receiving epoprostenol plus conventional therapy versus conventional therapy alone. The design was very similar to the prospective trial described above that led to FDA approval of epoprostenol for PPH.[3] Patients with a significant degree of interstitial lung disease from diffuse scleroderma were excluded. Although there was not blinding of patients and physicians, exercise tests were performed by blinded observers. As in PPH, exercise capacity improved in the epoprostenol group and continued to decline in the conventional therapy group. The median increase was 46 meters in the former group with a 48 meter decrease in the latter (P < 0.001). There was significant improvement in hemodynamic variables on epoprostenol with a tendency for these to progressively worsen in the conventionally treated

group. Functional WHO class improved in 38% of the epoprostenol group compared with none in the conventional group. Survival over this short period was not different; there were four deaths in the treated group and five in the conventional therapy group. Survivors tended to have had a shorter duration of scleroderma but not of pulmonary hypertension. One patient died from sepsis related to the pump infusion system.[33] Based upon this clinical trial, the FDA approved the use of intravenous epoprostenol for patients with PAH secondary to the scleroderma spectrum of diseases.

Pulmonary arterial hypertension due to collagen vascular disease is likely multifactorial in etiology with pulmonary arteriopathy (sometimes responsive to vasodilators) as well as parenchymal destruction and left-sided heart dysfunction. Strange and associates[31] performed right heart catheterization on nine patients with scleroderma, six of whom had concomitant interstitial lung disease. During the acute infusion, eight of nine demonstrated a reduction in pulmonary vascular resistance of >20%, suggesting that even in those with interstitial lung disease there is potential for response to epoprostenol. As in patients with PPH, some of the potential reduction in PVR appears related to improved inotropy and thus cardiac output.[3,8]

While patients with PAH associated with systemic lupus erythematosus may also experience improved symptoms, exercise tolerance and hemodynamics on intravenous epoprostenol, these patients have been studied in smaller numbers. A non-randomized case series of six patients with severe PAH related to lupus maintained on epoprostenol for 3 months to 2.5 years revealed clinical improvement in all six from WHO class III or IV to class I or II.[34] At baseline, none had evidence of thromboembolic disease and none was responsive to an acute vasodilator challenge. Four had hemodynamics measured during right heart catheterization before and after therapy. A decrease in the mean pulmonary artery pressure (baseline of 57 mmHg) of 38% and in the pulmonary vascular resistance of 58% was demonstrated. The other two patients had evidence of decreased estimated pulmonary artery pressure, by echo, of 20 and 35 mmHg. It has been suggested, however, that the risk of death related to severe thrombocytopenia (due to lupus and/or epoprostenol) may outweigh the potential for benefit in some of these patients.[35]

EPOPROSTENOL FOR OTHER FORMS OF PULMONARY ARTERIAL HYPERTENSION

There are data supporting the efficacy of chronic continuous intravenous epoprostenol in PAH in the setting of other underlying diseases, although large, prospective randomized trials have not been performed. Most large pulmonary hypertension centers follow such individuals. Patients with advanced WHO class III or class IV symptoms due to human immunodeficiency virus (HIV), inhalation of cocaine or other toxins, congenital heart disease, portopulmonary syndromes, sarcoidosis, chronic thromboembolic pulmonary hypertension, and persistent pulmonary hypertension of the newborn may respond to this therapy. In addition, patients with obstructive sleep apnea, chronic obstructive pulmonary disease, or interstitial lung disease with pulmonary hypertension that is disproportionate to the degree of parenchymal lung disease, may also sometimes respond. A series of 33 consecutive patients with PAH (14 with collagen vascular disease, seven with congenital heart disease, two with sarcoidosis, three with thromboembolic pulmonary hypertension, and seven with portopulmonary hypertension) was recently reported.[36] Significant improvement in exercise capacity as well as in hemodynamics was demonstrated. The mean dose of epoprostenol was 31 ng/kg·min. The mean pulmonary artery pressure improved by 23%, cardiac output increased by 62%, and PVR decreased by 50%. The patients with portopulmonary hypertension and congenital heart disease responded as well as those with collagen vascular disease.

Pulmonary arterial hypertension associated with HIV has been described as histologically similar to PPH with evidence of plexogenic pulmonary arteriopathy.[37] Outcome in 20 such patients was comparable to a cohort of 93 similar PAH patients without HIV.[37] Overall survival was not different with 46% survival at 2 years from diagnosis of PH. There was a significant history of intravenous drug use in 12 of 20 of the patients and in the three in whom lung pathology was available, the findings were typical of PPH without foreign body granulomas. Aguilar and Farber[38] treated six patients with HIV and showed an acute response to epoprostenol with a reduction in pulmonary artery pressure and PVR of 16% and 32%, respectively. There was incremental improvement in these variables after 1 year of continuous therapy. The WHO class also improved in all patients.

Continuous intravenous epoprostenol has been utilized in patients with significant pulmonary hypertension due to congenital heart disease. Pulmonary vascular resistance, cardiac index and pulmonary artery pressure all improved in a case series of 20 such patients at Columbia University in whom there was no acute response to epoprostenol.[39] All previously failed appropriate conventional therapy including surgical repair of defects in 11 patients. Sixteen had catheterization data repeated 1 year after the initiation of therapy. Mean pulmonary artery pressure decreased by 21% (from 77 to 61 mmHg). Cardiac index increased by 69% and pulmonary vascular resistance by 52%. There was objective improvement in exercise tolerance by 6-minute walk and improvement in WHO class in 14 patients. One

patient died at 4 months. The sample size was too small to elicit any mortality benefit. It should be noted that a severely elevated pulmonary artery pressure associated with Eisenmenger's syndrome is common and in the absence of right ventricular failure, does not generally have the same poor prognosis as with PPH. Among the reasons for this include the opportunity for significant right ventricular hypertrophy to develop in congenital heart disease. However, when these patients develop severe PAH with progressive symptoms and evidence of right ventricular failure, they should be considered for intravenous epoprostenol. The most experience has been with patients with atrial and ventricular septal defects.

Patients with portopulmonary hypertension, including those awaiting orthotopic liver transplantation in the pre-, peri- and postoperative periods, have been treated with intravenous epoprostenol.[40–42] A case series revealed that five of six patients with mean pulmonary artery pressures of greater than 35 mmHg were successfully treated with a combination of inhaled nitric oxide and infusion of epoprostenol until pressures decreased and there was echocardiographic evidence normalization of right ventricular function.[40] They were successfully transplanted and quickly weaned off of epoprostenol. One patient had progressively increased right-sided pressures and died on day 6 postoperatively. Kuo et al.[41] reported four patients awaiting liver transplantation treated with epoprostenol resulting in a 29–46% decrease in mean pulmonary artery pressure as well as an increase in cardiac output of 25–75%. The duration of therapy was 6–14 months. Mean pulmonary artery pressure decreased 29–46%, and cardiac output increased 25–75% with a resultant reduction in pulmonary vascular resistance of 22–71%. In another series, two of four patients underwent liver transplantation after the drug was initiated and remained on it 8 and 15 months after surgery.[42] A third patient died during surgery and a fourth died on epoprostenol and was not transplanted. It is appropriate in selected patients to consider this medication in an attempt to reduce the pretransplant pulmonary artery pressure, or in patients in whom transplantation is otherwise contraindicated.

Patients with sarcoidosis are among those that may have severe pulmonary hypertension that may be disproportionally severe when compared with the extent of parenchymal disease documented by radiographic studies or by pulmonary function testing. Potential mechanisms of disease in these cases may involve fibrosis and destruction of pulmonary vessels, encroachment upon the vasculature by non-caseating granulomatous inflammation, and extrinsic compression by enlarged lymph nodes.[43,44] Vasoconstrictor mechanisms could conceivably be involved as well. Acute vasodilation in response to nitric oxide has been demonstrated in patients with sarcoidosis,[45] and clinical benefit from intravenous epoprostenol has also been demonstrated.[46]

Other difficult scenarios meriting aggressive treatment include chronic thromboembolic pulmonary hypertension, PAH associated with pregnancy, and right ventricular failure in the setting of cardiac transplantation. While outcome has not been determined in large numbers of patients and while randomized studies have not been conducted, the available literature would suggest that this drug may offer benefit in these settings. Maternal mortality associated with pregnancy and pulmonary hypertension is as high as 30–50%.[47] Epoprostenol therapy has been utilized successfully during pregnancy. In one case report, a patient presented with symptoms at week 26 and the drug was initiated at 32 weeks. Caesarian section was performed for failure of labor to progress after membrane rupture at 36 weeks. Although the child also survived and was healthy at 2-year follow-up, the potential for adverse effects to the fetus are unknown.[48] Most large pulmonary hypertension centers have experience with this setting and pregnant women who choose to continue pregnancy with PAH need extremely close monitoring and a very low threshold for initiating epoprostenol.

Epoprostenol has compared favorably with other vasodilators in the postoperative treatment of right-sided heart failure following cardiac transplantation. In some cases, it has proven more effective than nitric oxide, nitroprusside and nitroglycerin, with higher stroke volumes and cardiac indices and lower resulting pulmonary vascular resistance.[49] The drug has been initiated in both the pre- and post-operative periods with good results.[50] In other rarer settings involving pulmonary hypertension, such as Gaucher's disease, epoprostenol has been utilized. However, neither large numbers nor long-term follow-up has been reported.[51]

CRITERIA FOR INITIATING EPOPROSTENOL

Epoprostenol should be prescribed in the setting of advanced PAH that has either failed traditional therapy or, if the latter has not yet been initiated, is too advanced to wait for possible benefit. It is generally agreed by most pulmonary hypertension specialists that the decision to begin continuous intravenous epoprostenol as well as long-term follow-up should involve a pulmonary hypertension center with experience treating large numbers of patients. In addition to criteria for severity, patients must be assessed for their willingness and ability to accept and undertake this form of therapy. Our experience is that while many do not easily accept a chronic intravenous infusion, the realization of the lack of simple options in the setting of a fatal disease enhances patient acceptance.

The decision to initiate this therapy in an individual patient is based upon a number of factors, including the severity of symptoms and signs, exercise tolerance,

echocardiography, hemodynamics, and the rate of progression. Most patients have WHO class III symptoms at presentation but this still represents a broad range of severity. Stable class III patients may not require intravenous epoprostenol, but progression to advanced class III with dyspnea with very minimal exertion would indicate the need for the drug. Syncope is an ominous sign and epoprostenol is usually indicated. Near-syncope, severe chest discomfort, and edema or ascites refractory to aggressive diuresis as well as severe right ventricular failure by physical examination suggests that an extremely low threshold for epoprostenol is warranted. Objective information should be used together with the evaluation of symptoms. Progressive evidence of declining performance on the 6-minute walk test or other assessment of exercise capacity with evidence of desaturation despite oxygen and other conventional therapy merits consideration of initiation. In general, the 6-minute walk distance does correlate with severity of hemodynamics.[52] Symptoms and exercise tolerance may vary to some degree from day to day and this should be considered. Echocardiographic evidence of a severely enlarged and hypocontractile right ventricle indicates advanced disease. Unless already very recently performed, right heart catheterization is preferred with a concomitant trial of epoprostenol to ascertain precise severity of PAH as well as tolerance of the drug prior to chronic initiation.[53] A significantly elevated right atrial pressure, and/or markedly reduced cardiac index ($<2.0\,$L/min$\cdot$m^2) should prompt initiation. The NIH registry indicated that prognosis was most closely related to mean right atrial pressure, mean pulmonary artery pressure, and decreased cardiac index.[4] In patients with congenital heart disease and Eisenmenger's syndrome, the magnitude of the pulmonary artery pressure alone does not predict the need for continuous intravenous epoprostenol. In general, if patients are severe enough to be considered for epoprostenol, they should be considered for listing for lung or heart/lung transplantation; criteria for initiating this therapy are outlined in Table 13L.1.

Most patients with advanced symptoms are already on ancillary PAH therapy including anticoagulation, oxygen, calcium channel blockers (if appropriate) and, with increasing frequency, the endothelin antagonist, bosentan.[54,55] If bosentan has not yet been instituted in the setting of very advanced disease, it may be considered prior to epoprostenol, but this would depend on the severity of disease and results of a very meticulous evaluation. Subcutaneous treprostinil is an alternative choice in severe disease but there is less experience with extremely ill patients.[56] The aerosolized prostacyclin analog, iloprost, has proven to be effective therapy in patients with selected forms of PAH and chronic thromboembolic pulmonary hypertension.[57,58] However, since intravenous epoprostenol has been shown to improve survival among the most severely ill patients with PPH, randomized trials

Table 13L.1 *Indications for continuous intravenous epoprostenol**

- **Symptoms and signs of severe pulmonary hypertension/right ventricular failure**
  - WHO class III (advanced) or class IV symptoms
  - Syncope or near syncope
  - Refractory edema and/or ascites
- **Echocardiographic evidence of right ventricular failure**
  - Severe right ventricular enlargement
  - Severely reduced right ventricular contractility
- **Progressive or marked reduction in exercise capacity by:**
  - 6-minute walk test[†]
  - Naughton treadmill test
  - Bicycle ergometry
- **Severely abnormal oxygenation**
- **Severely abnormal hemodynamics[‡]**
  - Cardiac index $<2.0 \, L/min/m^2$
  - Right atrial pressure $\geq 20 \, mmHg$
  - Mean pulmonary artery pressure $>85 \, mmHg$
  - Markedly reduced mixed venous oxygen saturation

*These criteria are most relevant for primary pulmonary hypertension (PPH) and pulmonary arterial hypertension (PAH) related to the scleroderma spectrum of diseases but can be considered for other PAH etiologies.
[†] When epoprostenol was compared with conventional therapy, eight of 40 patients expired by the 12-week time point. The mean 6-minute walk distance in these eight patients was $195 \pm 63 \, m$ compared with $305 \pm 14 \, m$ in the survivors from both groups.[3]
[‡] The hemodynamic data were determined from the NIH registry.[4] A reduced mixed venous saturation ($<63\%$) was shown to be associated with a 3-year survival rate of $<20\%$ for patients with PPH.[75]

comparing these two drugs with a survival end point have not been deemed ethical. In one report of three patients with PAH, inhaled iloprost was used in an attempt to replace continuous intravenous epoprostenol. While the iloprost was very effective acutely, right ventricular failure developed in all three patients; immediately after weaning in one, during weaning in the second, and after 2 weeks in the third.[59] In contrast, there are limited data suggesting the acute improvement of pulmonary hemodynamics with inhaled iloprost in patients already receiving chronic epoprostenol. Significant changes in mean pulmonary artery pressure, and cardiac index without further decline in systemic arterial pressure have been demonstrated.[60] While iloprost is appropriate in certain patients with advanced disease, continuous intravenous epoprostenol remains the first choice for the most advanced patients in countries in which it is available. An inordinate delay instituting this drug may be fatal.

PHARMACOKINETICS, INITIATION AND DOSING

The *in vitro* half-life of epoprostenol in human blood at 37°C and pH 7.4 is approximately 6 minutes and the *in vivo* half-life is expected to be no greater than this. Because of this, the drug must be given intravenously. It is rapidly hydrolyzed to two active and 14 inactive metabolites. The vast majority of these are cleared via the urine. There is a high clearance (93 mL/min/kg) and a small volume of distribution (357 mL/kg) based upon animal studies. Epoprostenol is listed as category B for pregnancy, but there are no well-controlled studies in pregnant women.

Patients are generally hospitalized for initiation of epoprostenol.[2,53] Because the drug is expensive, with high-dose chronic infusions costing as much as US$100 000 annually, insurance approval should be obtained prior to initiation except in emergencies. This also enables the distributors of the drug and supplies to mobilize their resources quickly and effectively. The initial dose is generally about 2 ng/kg·min. If this is initiated during cardiac catheterization, the dose may be increased by 2 ng every 15 minutes for acute vasodilator testing. To avoid bothersome or significant adverse effects, including hypotension, and to hasten acute vasodilator testing, nitric oxide is often used instead for acute testing and the dose of epoprostenol is increased more slowly after the procedure. Initially, during acute dosing, the drug may be administered via a peripheral line (or preferably a peripherally inserted central line) to be certain the patient will be able to tolerate the infused medication prior to dedicated central line placement. It is extremely unusual for the medication to require discontinuation due to adverse effects.

Because of the need to maintain an uninterrupted infusion and because of the high pH (10.2–10.8) after reconstitution, long-term infusion is established and maintained via a tunneled, cuffed central venous access device.[2,53] This is typically a single-lumen and usually a subclavian access line, and it is placed during the initial hospitalization. The long-term administration of high doses of the drug by peripheral access is potentially risky, as the abrupt discontinuation of therapy may be associated with rebound pulmonary hypertension and even death.

The drug is initially increased by approximately 1 ng increments one to three times per day, with the rate of increase being determined by the severity of the PAH and by the severity of side effects to the drug. Prostacyclin is administered continuously by a portable, battery-operated infusion pump. The pump (and carrying case) is generally worn on the belt. It has low-battery, end-of-infusion, and occlusion alarms, and is positive-pressure driven, with intervals between pulses not exceeding 3 minutes to deliver the prescribed medication rate.

The initiation of therapy is monitored closely in the acute care setting. Extensive teaching regarding the infusion pump, reconstitution of the drug, and central intravenous catheter care, are undertaken prior to discharge. This teaching must be performed by trained nursing personnel and pharmacists, and is methodical and

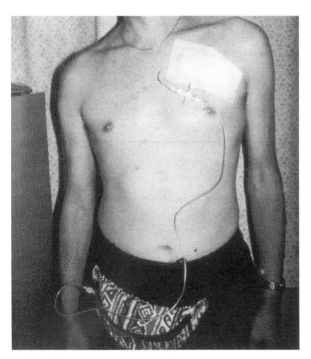

Figure 13L.1 *A patient is pictured on continuous intravenous epoprostenol. The pump and carrying case are shown.* Reproduced with permission from Jackson G, Difficult concepts in cardiology. *London: Martin Dunitz, 1994.*

Table 13L.2 *Steps for initiation of continuous intravenous epoprostenol*

- Patient screened for disease type and severity and deemed appropriate
- Insurance approval obtained
- Patient advised of potential side effects of epoprostenol
- Drug initiated at a dose of approximately 2 ng/kg·min via peripheral intravenous line
- Monitoring of blood pressure/adverse effects
- Dose increased by approximately 1 ng/kg·min increments, every 12–24 hours*
- Patient (and family member) teaching initiated with regard to:
  - Infusion pump operation
  - Drug reconstitution/aseptic technique
  - Self-administration of medication
- Long-term central venous (usually subclavian) line placed
- Teaching of central venous access maintenance, sterile dressing changes
- Back-up systems (secondary infusion equipment and supplies) made available
- Emergency numbers for resource personnel provided
- Discharge after 3–5 or more days if stable

*In more severely ill patients, more rapid increases are appropriate.

comprehensive. Once the patient adapts and adjusts to the medication induction, central line placement is obtained. The infusion pump delivery system, programming, maintenance and equipment care are reviewed until the patient and at least one family member are fully cognizant of all features of self-administration. Introduction of medication, aseptic technique, admixture procedure and self-administration of epoprostenol then follow. Emergency numbers, resource personnel and emergency preparedness protocols are provided. Self-care regarding central venous access device maintenance, sterile dressing changes, tubing changes, disposal of expended equipment and supplies, and procedures for reordering equipment are addressed. Back-up systems (secondary infusion equipment and supplies) must always be available should pump failure occur, with the patient aware that an interruption in drug delivery could be life-threatening. Stable patients are discharged after approximately 3–5 days. A patient on continuous intravenous epoprostenol is shown in Figure 13L.1.

After discharge, the dose of epoprostenol is generally increased only once to twice per week initially and then, based upon symptoms, less frequently. Epoprostenol is titrated based upon PAH symptoms and severity of side effects. During long-term therapy, there appears to be tolerance or tachyphylaxis[23,53] and the dose is generally increased at regular intervals for at least 6 months to 1 year to optimize results. The mechanism of this tolerance is not known but may be related to enhanced degradation, down-regulation of receptors or neurohormonal activation. Activation of the neurohormonal system may also play a role in the deleterious events that follow abrupt discontinuation.[2] In spite of initial tolerance, a stable dose is usually ultimately reached at which point further increases exacerbate adverse effects without further benefit. The procedures for initiating continuous intravenous epoprostenol are outlined in Table 13L.2.

ASSESSMENT OF THERAPY AND LONG-TERM MANAGEMENT

The effects of epoprostenol have traditionally been monitored by changes in hemodynamics observed acutely and over time, as assessed by direct measures taken during right heart catheterization.[1] While an acute vasodilator challenge should be performed if calcium channel blockers are to be considered, it is widely accepted that patients may clinically improve on epoprostenol **without** a significant acute vasodilator response.[1] Expected responses to acute infusion include a decrease in both systemic and pulmonary vascular resistance and increased cardiac index. The frequency of repeat right heart catheterization depends on the specific patient as well as on the practice of the pulmonary hypertension center. Many centers repeat the procedure every 1–2 years while others perform it only when deemed necessary based upon the clinical status. Surrogate objective data from echocardiography with an exercise test is often performed every 3–6 months to assess efficacy. Estimates of right ventricular pressure as well as its size and contractile function in conjunction with symptomatic scores and exercise data are practical, effective methods of monitoring patient progress.

In the prospective, randomized, multicenter trial comparing epoprostenol with conventional therapy PPH,[3] echocardiography was assessed over a 36-month follow-up period.[61] Right atrial enlargement, pericardial effusion and septal displacement as calculated by eccentricity index were predictors of adverse outcome. Baseline characteristics of these same patients revealed an association between poor exercise capacity and greater degree of RV dilatation, larger pericardial effusions, degree of septal displacement and increased severity of tricuspid regurgitation.[61] The echocardiograms reflected changes in heart structure and function that correlated to hemodynamic measures and exercise capacity. Importantly, Doppler underestimated the pressure measured at catheterization by about 11 mmHg. In 30% of patients, there was a difference of more than 20 mmHg. It was demonstrated that 12 weeks of epoprostenol infusion in this randomized sample resulted in beneficial effects on RV size, septal curvature and maximum tricuspid regurgitation jet velocity. Other echocardiographic parameters have been evaluated before and after epoprostenol initiation. Right ventricular function, as measured by the myocardial performance index (a reproducible Doppler-derived parameter used for evaluating global ventricular function), has been shown to improve after therapy with intravenous epoprostenol.[62] In summary, long-term hemodynamic improvement as assessed by cardiac catheterization and by echocardiographic parameters, as well as by exercise tolerance is common after the initiation of continuous intravenous epoprostenol. While the available data are strongly supportive in PPH and PAH due to underlying collagen vascular disease, it is also accumulating in other forms of PAH.

Among the more difficult decisions in patients with severe PAH on epoprostenol who are listed for lung or heart/lung transplantation is when to actually proceed to transplantation. While earlier transplantation, prior to extremely disabling right ventricular failure, would appear to be advantageous, the relatively poor overall survival for PAH patients with transplantation is sometimes inclined to influence clinicians to simply continue intravenous epoprostenol and delay surgery. This decision is complex and must be made by the pulmonary hypertension and transplant team on an individual patient basis.

The long-term management of patients on continuous intravenous epoprostenol involves a coordinated effort between a patient's local physician (generally cardiologist or pulmonologist) and the pulmonary hypertension center. At large centers, nurse coordinators are intimately involved with teaching about epoprostenol, preparing patients for hospital discharge and frequently telephoning patients after discharge. These individuals, together with the pulmonary hypertension physician, coordinate dose changes and monitor progress and adverse effects. A large pulmonary hypertension center cannot function effectively without intensive nursing coordinator involvement.

CONTRAINDICATIONS TO EPOPROSTENOL

Epoprostenol is indicated for advanced PAH. This drug is not indicated for secondary pulmonary hypertension related to left-sided heart disease. The Flolan International Randomized Survival Trial (FIRST), a randomized study evaluating the use of chronic epoprostenol for class IIIB and IV left-sided congestive heart failure, was terminated early because of a trend toward excess mortality in the prostacyclin-treated group.[63] Potential concerns were the deleterious effects of positive inotropy in congestive heart failure, and the possibility of vasodilator-activated deleterious neurohormone effects. During acute dosing in pulmonary veno-occlusive disease, fulminant pulmonary edema and death has been reported.[64] This may be related to acute vasodilation with increased vascular permeability and inotropy, but with inability to move blood through the pulmonary veins and into the left side of the heart. Pulmonary edema related to this drug has also been reported in pulmonary capillary hemangiomatosis.[65]

ADVERSE EFFECTS AND COMPLICATIONS

The most common early side effects include jaw pain, diarrhea, flushing, rash, nausea, headache, photosensitivity and systemic hypotension. Jaw pain is often the first symptom. It is nearly universal and often occurs at meals during the first few bites of food. These side effects are more prominent if the dose is increased rapidly. At low doses, vagally mediated bradycardia may develop, with subsequent reflex tachycardia. Development of ascites unrelated to progressive right heart failure may also occur in a minority of patients, and appears to be an effect of the drug itself. The ascites fluid is generally transudative. The incidence of these side effects varies in reported clinical trials and case series. Drug information provided by the manufacturer of epoprostenol sodium suggests that during acute dosing, flushing occurs in 50% of patients, headache in 49% and nausea or vomiting in about 32%. Hypotension, anxiety, chest pain and dizziness occur in about 10%. The side effects associated with acute dosing can be present intermittently long-term and tend to occur as the dose is increased. These side effects are tolerable and rarely result in discontinuation of the infusion. Chronic use of medication to decrease intestinal

Table 13L.3 *Potential adverse effects of epoprostenol*

Acute and chronic*
– Jaw pain
– Headache
– Flushing/erythema
– Nausea
– Diarrhea
– Anorexia
– Anxiety
– Lightheadedness/dizziness
– Hypotension
– Ascites
– Pulmonary edema[†]

Chronic[†]
– Leg and foot pain
– Alopecia
– Leukocytoclastic vasculitis and severe erythroderma
– High cardiac output failure
– Anemia
– Thrombocytopenia
– Pancytopenia
– Weight loss

Related to infusion system
– Catheter-related infection/sepsis
– Catheter-related thrombosis
– Pump failure
– Rebound symptoms due to sudden discontinuation

*These effects generally occur over the first few days to weeks but may persist, and be present long term. Some may be more prominent immediately after a dose increase.
[†] This is rare in PPH and may be more common in pulmonary veno-occlusive disease or left heart dysfunction.
[†] These effects occur after months or longer, and may be due to high and sometimes excessive dosing.

Table 13L.4 *Potential reasons for infusion pump malfunction*

• Pump not turned on
• Battery failure
• Use of improper battery
• Line obstruction/interrupted delivery
• Improperly attached cassette/bag
• Incorrect pump programming

cytoplasmic antibodies (pANCA) were borderline positive at 1:20. There was no other evidence of autoimmune disease. Treatment with prednisone and azathioprine were unsuccessful. This clinical problem appears to be exceedingly rare, and may be entirely unrelated to the drug. As the duration of therapy increases, other long-term adverse effects may be noted.

Serious complications related to the continuous intravenous and pump delivery system include local catheter infections, bacteremia, sepsis and catheter-related thrombosis. Because of the continuous infusion and chronic anticoagulation in most patients, thrombosis is relatively unusual. Of the 81 patients studied over 12 weeks in the randomized trial reported in 1996 by Barst *et al.*, four episodes of non-fatal catheter-related sepsis developed. In addition, there were seven local catheter infections, and catheter site bleeding in four patients.[3] The expected local central line infection rate is 0.22–0.68 per patient-year and that of sepsis 0–0.39 per patient-year.[3,26,36] Symptoms of severe pulmonary hypertension may recur after abrupt discontinuation of the infusion, and this can be fatal. Expected interactions with other agents include hypotension with antihypertensives and diuretics, and bleeding risk with antiplatelet agents and warfarin. Pump or catheter malfunction has been reported at up to 2.53 events per patient-year.[3] Potential reasons for infusion pump failure are listed in Table 13L.4.

DISCONTINUING EPOPROSTENOL

In the early intravenous epoprostenol era, patients with PAH were informed that they would require this drug for life, or until transplantation. This might still appear to be the case in the majority of patients, but because of the dramatic clinical and hemodynamic responses in individuals, most pulmonary hypertension centers have successfully weaned at least a few patients off the drug on to other forms of therapy. With the advent of newer therapies such as subcutaneous treprostinil and the endothelin antagonist bosentan, such weaning may be even more feasible. While there are no clear published guidelines for weaning epoprostenol, it would be advisable to utilize hemodynamic measurements, echocardiographic parameters and exercise capacity, together with carefully monitoring of symptoms, if weaning is to be considered.

motility is sometimes required. Erythema is often worse in the lower extremities and sometimes manifests as leukocytoclastic vasculitis.[66] Severe erythroderma requiring hospitalization has been reported.[67] Certain effects not generally present early may develop over time. One of the more prominent is leg and foot pain, which may be severe. The approach to this symptom involves pain-control measures including tricyclic antidepressants, gabapentin and sometimes narcotics. Decreasing the dose or reducing the frequency of dose escalation will often decrease or alleviate side effects. Potential adverse effects are listed in Table 13L.3.

Rarer complications of epoprostenol may include anemia, thrombocytopenia, or pancytopenia. Some patients with PAH have underlying autoimmune disease and may be more susceptible to these complications.[35] Non-specific interstitial pneumonitis was reported 5 years into successful therapy with epoprostenol in one patient with apparent PPH.[68] A lung biopsy revealed the pneumonitis as well as mild medial hypertrophy of the muscular pulmonary arteries, but did not reveal plexiform lesions. Notably, antinuclear antibody (ANA) testing was positive at a titer of 1:1280 and perinuclear antineutrophil

FUTURE DIRECTIONS OF THERAPY

The direction of current investigations and future therapy are reflections of the various mechanisms involved in the pathogenesis of PAH. It is likely that continuous intravenous epoprostenol will remain a major therapeutic approach in advanced PAH patients, although the endothelin antagonist bosentan (Tracleer) and subcutaneous prostacyclin (treprostinil, Remodulin) are now FDA approved for use in PAH and may have an impact upon the frequency with which intravenous epoprostenol is implemented.[54–56] The aerosolized prostacyclin, iloprost, is available in Europe, and will likely have impact.[57,58] Oral prostacyclin analogs have also been studied in prospective trials but are not, at present, available for use in the US.[69] The phosphodiesterase-5 inhibitor sildenafil has been shown to reduce pulmonary artery pressure in PAH[70] and is currently being studied in a prospective, multicenter, global trial.

Combination therapy is increasing[71–73] and allows the possibility of impacting upon different potential targets contributing to the development and progression of PAH. Combinations of continuous intravenous epoprostenol with newer agents that involve different mechanisms with possible synergy are likely to be the mainstay of therapy in the near future. The use of inhaled iloprost may be beneficial in patients already receiving chronic epoprostenol.[60] It is also feasible that pretreatment with intravenous epoprostenol may enable recovery of lung vasculature such that there is adequate response to other vasodilators.

Seven patients that initially had no response to inhaled nitric oxide were treated for a mean of 18 months with epoprostenol. Upon restudy, they had significant improvement in mean pulmonary artery pressure and cardiac index following nitric oxide.[74] Thus, epoprostenol may promote enough healing or recovery of smooth muscle or endothelial function to permit response to other vasodilators. Continuous intravenous epoprostenol has revolutionized the care of patients with advanced PAH. Future trials will determine optimal combinations of agents with this drug and whether it can be replaced with regimens that are less cumbersome to deliver.

KEY POINTS

- Labeled indications for continuous intravenous epoprostenol therapy include the long-term treatment of PPH and PAH associated with the scleroderma spectrum of diseases. The drug is indicated for use in patients who have advanced class III or class IV disease that has not responded adequately to conventional therapy.
- A careful evaluation including the severity of symptoms, physical signs, echocardiographic data, cardiac catheterizaton data and exercise data is used to determine the need for epoprostenol.
- The dose of epoprostenol is progressively increased and a balance is sought between relief of symptoms and minimizing adverse effects.
- Patients may respond long term even in the absence of an acute vasodilator response.
- Exercise tolerance and hemodynamics have been shown to improve with this therapy.
- Mortality benefit has been demonstrated in PPH when compared with conventional therapy.
- Patients on this therapy should be followed periodically at centers with experience with PAH. Extensive teaching must be undertaken when this drug is initiated.

REFERENCES

●1 Rubin LJ, Groves BM, Reeves JT et al. Prostacyclin-induced acute pulmonary vasodilation in primary pulmonary hypertension. *Circulation* 1982;**66**:334–8.

2 Galie N, Manes A, Branzi A. Medical therapy of pulmonary hypertension, the prostacyclins. *Clin Chest Med* 2001;**22**:529–37.

●3 Barst RJ, Rubin LJ, Long WA et al. A comparison of continuous intravenous epoprostenol (prostacyclin) with conventional therapy for primary pulmonary hypertension. *N Engl J Med* 1996;**334**:296–301.

●4 D'Alonzo GE, Barst RJ, Ayres SM et al. Survival in patients with primary pulmonary hypertension: results from a national prospective registry. *Ann Intern Med* 1991;**115**:343–9.

●5 Moncada S, Gryglewski R, Bunting S et al. An enzyme isolated from arteries transforms prostaglandin endoperoxides to an unstable substance that inhibits platelet aggregation. *Nature* 1976;**263**:663–5.

●6 Moncada S, Vane JR. Arachidonic acid metabolites and the interactions between platelets and blood-vessel walls. *N Engl J Med* 1979;**300**:1142–7.

7 Clapp LH, Finney P, Turcato S et al. Differential effects of stable prostacyclin analogs on smooth muscle cell proliferation and cyclic AMP generation in human pulmonary artery. *Am J Respir Cell Mol Biol* 2002;**26**:194–201.

8 Montalescot G, Drobinski G, Meurin P et al. Effects of prostacyclin on the pulmonary vascular tone and cardiac contractility of patients with pulmonary hypertension secondary to end-stage heart failure. *Am J Cardiol* 1998;**82**:749–55.

●9 Wood P. Pulmonary hypertension with special reference to the vasoconstrictive factor. *Br Heart J* 1959;**21**:557–70.

●10 Christman BW, McPherson CD, Newman JH et al. An imbalance between the excretion of thromboxane and prostacyclin metabolites in pulmonary hypertension. *N Engl J Med* 1992;**327**:70–5.

11 Mikhail G, Chester AH, Gibbs J *et al.* Role of vasoactive mediators in primary and secondary pulmonary hypertension. *Am J Cardiol* 1998;**82**:254–5.

12 Tuder RM, Cool CD, Geraci MW *et al.* Prostacyclin synthase expression is decreased in lungs from patients with severe pulmonary hypertension. *Am J Respir Crit Care Med* 1999;**159**:1925–32.

13 Ozkan M, Dweik RA, Laskowski D *et al.* High levels of nitric oxide in individuals with pulmonary hypertension receiving epoprostenol therapy. *Lung* 2001;**179**:233–43.

14 Langleben D, Barst RJ, Badesch D *et al.* Continuous infusion of epoprostenol improves the net balance between pulmonary endothelin-1 clearance and release in primary pulmonary hypertension. *Circulation* 1999;**99**:3266–71.

15 Boyer-Neumann C, Brenot F, Wolf M *et al.* Continuous infusion of prostacyclin decreases plasma levels of t-PA and PAI-1 in primary pulmonary hypertension. *Thromb Haemost* 1995;**73**:727–38.

16 Friedman R, Mears JG, Barst RJ. Continuous infusion of prostacyclin normalizes markers of endothelial cell injury and platelet aggregation in primary pulmonary hypertension. *Circulation* 1997;**96**:2782–4.

17 Hoshikawa Y, Voelkel NF, Gesell TL *et al.* Prostacyclin receptor-dependent modulation of pulmonary vascular remodeling. *Am J Respir Crit Care Med* 2001;**164**:314–18.

18 Mason NA, Bishop AE, Yacoub MH *et al.* Reduced expression of prostacyclin receptor protein on remodeled vessels in pulmonary hypertension. *Am J Respir Crit Care Med* 1999;**159**:A166.

●19 Rich S, Dantzker DR, Ayres SM *et al.* Primary pulmonary hypertension: a national prospective study. *Ann Intern Med* 1987;**107**:216–23.

●20 Higgenbottam TW, Wheeldon D, Wells FC *et al.* Long-term treatment of primary pulmonary hypertension with continuous intravenous epoprostenol (prostacyclin). *Lancet* 1984;**1**:1046–7.

●21 Jones DK, Higenbottam TW *et al.* Treatment of primary pulmonary hypertension with intravenous epoprostenol (prostacyclin). *Br Heart J* 1987;**57**:270–8.

●22 Rubin LJ, Mendoza J, Hood M *et al.* Treatment of primary pulmonary hypertension with continuous intravenous prostacyclin (epoprostenol). Results of a randomized trial. *Ann Intern Med* 1990;**112**:485–91.

●23 Barst RJ, Rubin LJ, McGoon MD *et al.* Survival in primary pulmonary hypertension with long-term continuous intravenous prostacyclin. *Ann Intern Med* 1994;**121**:409–15.

24 Raffy O, Azarian R, Brenot F *et al.* Clinical significance of the pulmonary vasodilator response during short-term infusion of prostacyclin in primary pulmonary hypertension. *Circulation* 1996;**93**:484–8.

25 Shapiro SM, Oudiz RJ, Cao T *et al.* Primary pulmonary hypertension: improved long-term effects and survival with continuous intravenous epoprostenol infusion. *J Am Coll Cardiol* 1997;**30**:343–9.

●26 McLaughlin VV, Genthner DE, Panella MM *et al.* Reduction in pulmonary vascular resistance with long-term epoprostenol (prostacyclin) therapy in primary pulmonary hypertension. *N Engl J Med* 1998;**338**:273–7.

●27 McLaughlin VV, Shillington A, Rich S. Survival in primary pulmonary hypertension. The impact of epoprostenol therapy. *Circulation* 2002;**106**:1477–82.

28 Wax D, Garofano R, Barst RJ. Effects of long term infusion of prostacyclin on exercise performance in patients with primary pulmonary hypertension. *Chest* 1999;**116**:914–20.

29 Abenhaim L, Moride Y, Brenot F *et al.* Appetite-suppressant drugs and the risk of primary pulmonary hypertension. *N Engl J Med* 1996;**335**:609–16.

30 Barst RJ, Maislin G, Fishman AP. Vasodilator therapy for primary pulmonary hypertension in children. *Circulation* 1999;**99**:1197–208.

31 Strange C, Bolster M, Mazur J *et al.* Hemodynamic effects of epoprostenol in patients with systemic sclerosis and pulmonary hypertension. *Chest* 2000;**118**:1077–82.

32 Klings ES, Hill NS, Leong MH *et al.* Systemic sclerosis-associated pulmonary hypertension: short- and long-term effects of epoprostenol (prostacyclin). *Arthritis Rheum* 1999;**42**:2638–45.

●33 Badesch DB, Tapson VF, McGoon MD *et al.* Continuous intravenous epoprostenol for pulmonary hypertension due to the scleroderma spectrum of disease: a randomized, controlled trial. *Ann Intern Med* 2001;**32**:425–34.

34 Robbins IM, Gaine SP, Schilz R *et al.* Epoprostenol for treatment of pulmonary hypertension in patients with systemic lupus erythematosus. *Chest* 2000;**117**:14–18.

35 Horn EM, Barst RJ, Poon M. Epoprostenol for treatment of pulmonary hypertension in patients with systemic lupus erythematosus. *Chest* 2000;**118**:1229–30.

36 McLaughlin VV, Genthner DE, Panella MM *et al.* Compassionate use of continuous prostacyclin in the management of secondary pulmonary hypertension: a case series. *Ann Intern Med* 1999;**130**:740–3.

37 Petitpretz P, Brenot F, Azarian R *et al.* Pulmonary hypertension in patients with human immunodeficiency virus infection: comparison with primary pulmonary hypertension. *Circulation* 1994;**89**:2772–7.

38 Aguilar RV, Farber HW. Epoprostenol (prostacyclin) therapy in HIV-associated pulmonary hypertension. *Am J Respir Crit Care Med* 2000;**162**:1846–50.

39 Rosenzweig EB, Kerstein D, Barst RJ. Long-term prostacyclin for pulmonary hypertension with associated congenital heart defects. *Circulation* 1999;**99**:1858–65.

40 Molmenti EP, Ramsay M, Ramsay K *et al.* Epoprostenol and nitric oxide therapy for severe pulmonary hypertension in liver transplantation. *Transplant Proc* 2001;**33**:1332.

41 Kuo PC, Johnson LB, Plotkin JS *et al.* Continuous intravenous infusion of epoprostenol for the treatment of portopulmonary hypertension. *Transplantation* 1997;**63**:604–6.

42 Doria C, Murali S, Alvarez R *et al.* Epoprostenol is not a panacea for the treatment of portopulmonary hypertension. *Transplantation* 1999;**67**:S194.

43 Smith LJ, Lawrence JB, Katzenstein AA. Vascular sarcoidosis: a rare cause of pulmonary hypertension. *Am J Med Sci* 1983;**285**:38–44.

44 Barst RJ, Ratner SJ. Sarcoidosis and reactive pulmonary hypertension. *Arch Intern Med* 1985;**145**:2112–14.

45 Preston IR, Klinger JR, Landzberg MJ *et al.* Vasoresponsiveness of sarcoidosis-associated pulmonary hypertension. *Chest* 2001;**120**:866–72.

46 Tso E, Rafanan A, Hague K *et al*. Epoprostenol therapy for pulmonary hypertension in sarcoidosis. *Chest* 2000;**118**:114S.

47 McCaffrey RN, Dunn LJ. Primary pulmonary hypertension in pregnancy. *Obstet Gynecol Surv* 1964;**19**:567–91.

48 Stewart R, Tuazon D, Olson G *et al*. Pregnancy and primary pulmonary hypertension: successful outcome with epoprostenol therapy. *Chest* 2001;**119**:973–5.

•49 Higenbottam T, Butt AY, McMahon A *et al*. Long-term Intravenous prostaglandin (epoprostenol or iloprost) for treatment of severe pulmonary hypertension. *Heart* 1998;**80**:151–5.

50 Stobierska-Dzierzek B, Awad H, Michler RE. The evolving management of acute right-sided heart failure in cardiac transplant recipients. *J Am Coll Cardiol* 2001;**38**:923–31.

51 Bakst AE, Gaine SP, Rubin LJ. Continuous intravenous epoprostenol therapy for pulmonary hypertension in Gaucher's disease. *Chest* 1999;**116**:1127–9.

52 Paciocco G, Bossone E, Aramu S *et al*. Correlation between hemodynamic parameters and the six-minute walk in primary pulmonary hypertension. *Chest* 2000;**118**:135S.

◆53 Rubin LJ. Current Concepts: primary pulmonary hypertension. *N Engl J Med* 1997;**336**:111–17.

54 Channick RN, Simonneau G, Sitbon O *et al*. Effects of the dual endothelin-receptor antagonist bosentan in patients with pulmonary hypertension: a randomized, placebo-controlled study. *Lancet* 2001;**358**:1119–23.

•55 Rubin LJ, Badesch DB, Barst RJ *et al*. Bosentan therapy for pulmonary arterial hypertension *N Engl J Med* 2002;**346**:896–903.

•56 Simonneau G, Barst RJ, Galie N *et al*. Continuous subcutaneous infusion of treprostinil, a prostacyclin analogue, in patients with pulmonary arterial hypertension: a double-blind, randomized, placebo-controlled trial. *Am J Resp Crit Care Med* 2002;**165**:800–4.

57 Scott JP, Higenbottam T, Wallwork J. The acute effect of the synthetic prostacyclin analogue iloprost in primary pulmonary hypertension. *Br J Clin Pract* 1990;**44**:231–4.

•58 Olschewski H, Simonneau G, Galie N *et al*. Inhaled iloprost for severe pulmonary hypertension. *N Engl J Med* 2002;**347**:322–9.

59 Schenk P, Petkov V, Ventzislav MD *et al*. Aerosolized iloprost could not replace long-term IV epoprostenol (prostacyclin) administration in severe pulmonary hypertension. *Chest* 2001;**119**:296–300.

60 Petkov V, Ziesche R, Mosgoeller W *et al*. Aerosolised iloprost improves pulmonary hemodynamics in patients with primary pulmonary hypertension receiving continuous epoprostenol treatment. *Thorax* 2001;**56**:734–6.

61 Hinderliter AL, Willis PW, Barst RJ *et al*. Effects of long-term infusion of prostacyclin on echocardiographic measures of right ventricular structure and function in primary pulmonary hypertension. *Circulation* 1997;**95**:1479–86.

62 Sebbag I, Rudski LG, Therrien J *et al*. Effect of chronic infusion of epoprostenol on echocardiographic right ventricular myocardial performance index and its relation to clinical outcome in patients with primary pulmonary hypertension. *Am J Cardiol* 2001;**88**:1060–3.

63 Califf RM, Adams KF, McKenna WJ *et al*. A randomized controlled trial of epoprostenol (prostacyclin) therapy for severe congestive heart failure: the Flolan international randomized survival trial (FIRST). *Am Heart J* 1997;**134**:44.

64 Palmer SM, Robinson LJ, Wang A *et al*. Massive pulmonary edema and death after prostacyclin infusion in a patient with pulmonary veno-occlusive disease. *Chest* 1998;**113**:237–40.

65 Humbert M, Maitre S, Capron F *et al*. Pulmonary edema complicating continuous intravenous prostacyclin in pulmonary capillary hemangiomatosis. *Am J Respir Crit Care Med* 1998;**157**:1681–5.

66 Ahearn G, Myers S, Tapson VF. Leukocytoclastic vasculitis is commonly associated with chronic epoprostenol therapy. *Chest* (in press).

67 Ahearn GS, Selim M, Angelica MD *et al*. Severe erythroderma as a complication of continuous epoprostenol therapy. *Chest* 2002;**122**:378–80.

68 Kesten S, Dainauskas J, McLaughlin V *et al*. Development of nonspecific interstitial pneumonitis associated with long-term treatment of primary pulmonary hypertension with prostacyclin. *Chest* 1999;**116**:566–9.

69 Nagaya N, Uematsu M, Okano Y *et al*. Effect of orally active prostacyclin analogue on survival of outpatients with primary pulmonary hypertension. *J Am Coll Cardiol* 1999;**34**:1188–92.

70 Michelakis E, Tymchak W, Lien D *et al*. Oral sildenafil is an effective and specific pulmonary vasodilator in patients with pulmonary arterial hypertension: comparison with inhaled nitric oxide. *Circulation* 2002;**105**:2398–403.

71 Channick RN, Rubin LJ. Combination therapy for pulmonary hypertension: a glimpse into the future? *Crit Care Med* 2000;**28**:896–7.

72 Wilkens H, Guth A, Konig J *et al*. Effect of inhaled iloprost plus oral sildenafil in patients with primary pulmonary hypertension. *Circulation* 2001;**104**:1218–22.

73 Ghofrani HA, Wiedemann R, Rose F *et al*. Combination therapy with oral sildenafil and inhaled iloprost for severe pulmonary hypertension. *Ann Intern Med* 2002;**136**:515–22.

74 Ziesche R, Petkov V, Wittman K *et al*. Treatment with epoprostenol reverts nitric oxide non-responsiveness in patients with primary pulmonary hypertension. *Heart* 2000;**83**:406–9.

75 Fuster V, Steele PM, Edwards WD *et al*. Primary pulmonary hypertension: natural history and the importance of thrombosis. *Circulation* 1984;**70**:580–7.

Inhaled iloprost

HORST OLSCHEWSKI AND WERNER SEEGER

BACKGROUND

Potent vasodilators, e.g. high-dose calcium channel blockers, may be highly valuable in those patients who present with a type of pulmonary vasoconstriction that is acutely reversible to a short-acting vasodilator.[1] However, these patients represent only a small subset of PPH patients. For the majority, this therapy is potentially dangerous and may be life-threatening (Figure 13M.1) due to the decrease in systemic pressure, reduced coronary perfusion and compression of the left ventricle by the overloaded right ventricle. This balance between pulmonary and systemic vasodilatory effects is crucial for all non-selective vasodilators but an imbalance towards systemic vasodilatation is most dangerous in the case of the calcium channel blockers because of their negative inotropic effect on the right ventricle. For those patients suffering from a pre-existing perfusion/ventilation mismatch, there is an additional drawback with non-selective vasodilators: hypoxic pulmonary vasoconstriction (HPV), adapting local perfusion to local ventilation is impaired, resulting in hypoxemia.[2] Hypoxemia then may additionally impair organ function and prognosis.

Compared with calcium channel blockers, the hemodynamic effects of prostacyclin have a clear advantage as this substance is not negative inotropic to the heart. On

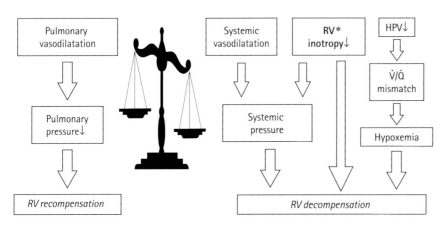

Figure 13M.1 *Balance between beneficial and adverse effects of non-selective vasodilators. HPV, hypoxic pulmonary vasoconstriction; RV, right ventricle. *If calcium channel blockers are used, the negative inotropic properties must be considered.*

the other hand, prostacyclin impairs HPV very potently and thereby increases pulmonary shunt blood flow.[3,4] Systemic pressure drop can be prevented by increasing the dose very gradually. In emergencies with right ventricular failure, however, low systemic pressure may become a serious problem.[5]

The main mechanism responsible for the beneficial clinical long-term effects of prostacyclin is not known. Probably the antithrombotic and antiproliferative effects play a major role as well as its antagonism to the endothelin system.[6] Iloprost, a stable analog of prostacyclin, has very similar biologic properties, but a longer half-life. It has been approved in Europe for use in different indications of arterial occlusive diseases and it has been used as an alternative to prostacyclin for continuous intravenous infusion for therapy of pulmonary arterial hypertension.[7,8] Recently, intravenous iloprost was approved for therapy of primary and secondary pulmonary hypertension in New Zealand. The equivalent dose compared with prostacyclin has not been defined in a controlled study. There was a suggestion of factor 2–3,[9] but this may underestimate the true relation because of the much longer half-life of iloprost, compared with prostacyclin. On clinical grounds, the relative potency of iloprost can be assumed to be in the order of 5:1 as the normal starting dose of intravenous iloprost is around 0.5 ng/kg·min, and the highest reported doses after some years of therapy are around 10 ng/kg·min (comparable to about 50 ng/kg·min of prostacyclin). The effects of inhalation with iloprost using a concentration of 10 μg/mL were almost identical to those observed with prostacyclin at a concentration of 50 μg/mL.[10] This would

also suggest a relative potency of 5:1. Compared with prostacyclin, the continuous iloprost infusion has some practical advantages as the solution is much more stable and does not necessitate cooling. Moreover, in case of discontinuation of the infusion, there is more time to re-establish the infusion, before right ventricular failure occurs.

The major drawbacks of prostacyclin and iloprost infusion are the risk of complications and the systemic side effects. These are due to the intravenous line and the non-selective action of the drugs to all organs and the non-selective action within the lungs.

How to reach the precapillary vessels with an inhaled drug

The anatomy of the lungs allows direct access to the small pulmonary vessels using the airways. The proximity of the pulmonary resistance vessels to the alveoli and the juxtapositioning of the terminal bronchiolus with a pulmonary artery make it possible to selectively target these vessels with vasodilatory agents. This is also the principle behind the inhaled administration of nitric oxide (NO) and NO donors. However, NO has some serious drawbacks when compared with prostacyclin. It is a potentially toxic substance[11] that is very short-acting and prone to serious rebound phenomena.[12,13] It also has a considerably weaker effect on the pulmonary vessels in PPH than prostacyclin.[14] The advantages of the pulmonary selectivity of prostacyclin and its stable analog

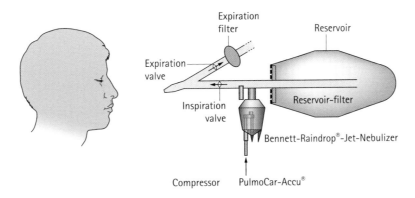

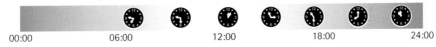

Figure 13M.2 *Application of inhaled iloprost. Iloprost is nebulized at a concentration of 5–10 μg/mL over 4–10 minutes, depending on the device. The inhaled target dose is 3–5 μg per inhalation. To achieve this, between 4 and 15 μg of iloprost must be nebulized. Inhalation devices must be physically characterized in order to assess the inhaled dose. The inhalation procedure is repeated six to nine times a day. During the night, the device is dismantled and cleaned.*

iloprost can be combined with the benefit of the very potent vasodilatory effects of prostanoids and their antiproliferative and anti-inflammatory properties.

DEVELOPMENT OF INHALED PROSTANOID THERAPY

The use of inhaled prostacyclin or iloprost is an alternative to the NO approach. The distance between the alveolar surface and smooth muscle cells of the pulmonary arteries is 10 μm at the most. The real barrier to uptake is the vascular adventitia itself. The proof of principle was first documented by our study group for patients with ARDS in 1993 and described in animal experiments by Welte *et al.*[15] in the same year. The clinical development of this approach for the treatment of primary and secondary pulmonary hypertension is the subject of the following paragraphs. Since then, inhaled prostanoids have been used by various study groups[16–20] in diseases in which pulmonary hypertension is the limiting factor, for

example, perioperatively in heart transplantation[21,22] and in persistent pulmonary hypertension of the newborn.[23–25]

PPH

The first use of inhaled iloprost for therapy of severe pulmonary hypertension was started in 1994.[10] During nebulization, there is a decrease in pulmonary artery pressure and resistance within a few minutes. The temporal progress of the hemodynamic effects and the effects on gas exchange can be clearly seen in the example shown in Figure 13M.3. Identical hemodynamic profiles were reproducible with repeated application of inhaled prostanoids.

The hemodynamic profile is characterized by a considerable drop in pulmonary pressure combined with a significant rise in cardiac output without notable effects on systemic pressure.[10] The decrease in pulmonary resistance is equal to that of a maximum tolerable intravenous dose of prostacyclin. In this latter case, however, the systemic resistance decreases considerably, thereby activating the arterial

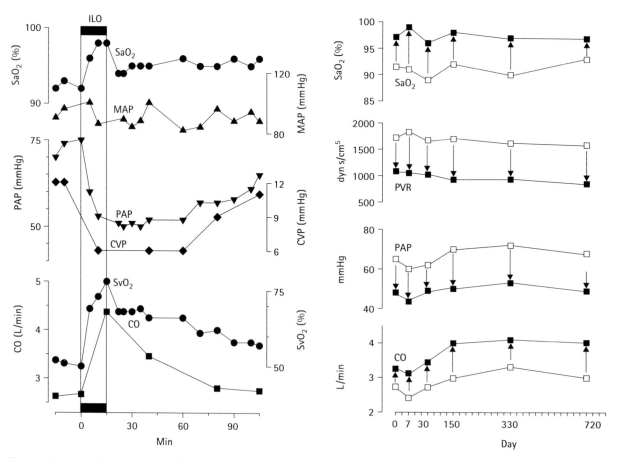

Figure 13M.3 *Top: Hemodynamic profile of inhaled iloprost in severe pulmonary hypertension. Left: During minutes 0–15, 10 μg of iloprost is nebulized, of which about 3 μg is inhaled. During and after the inhalation there are considerable hemodynamic responses, which were nearly identical during subsequent catheter investigations during continued therapy with inhaled iloprost. Reprinted from reference 10.*

baroreflex. This is indicated by increased heart rate and an overshooting rise in cardiac output. A comparison of the hemodynamics of both inhaled and intravenous application shows that selective pulmonary vasodilatation occurs with inhaled prostacyclin and thus cannot be explained by a systemic recirculation of the substance into the pulmonary arteries.

COMPARISON OF INHALED ILOPROST WITH INHALED NO

The effects of inhaled NO and aerosolized iloprost in PPH patients were directly and intra-individually compared.[14] At baseline, mean pulmonary pressure was markedly increased to 59 mmHg, and pulmonary resistance was increased to approximately 1350 dyn s/cm^5. During NO inhalation, mean pulmonary pressure decreased by 4.3 mmHg whereas it decreased by 10.3 mmHg during iloprost inhalation. The same difference in the magnitude of vasodilatory response was evident in the pulmonary resistance, which decreased by about 200 dyn s/cm^5 with NO compared with 450 dyn s/cm^5 with inhaled iloprost (a decrease of 34%). Thus, inhaled iloprost was significantly more effective than NO, especially in the patients with a moderate acute response. About 90% of patients responded better to inhaled iloprost than they did to NO.

ARDS

The first description of the successful inhalation of prostacyclin was done in ARDS patients who were mechanically ventilated.[3] In these patients, pulmonary pressure is increased while systemic resistance is decreased and there is excess low $\dot{V}/\dot{Q}$ and shunt perfusion in the lungs due to non-ventilated edematous and atelectatic areas (Plate 13M.1). If systemic prostacyclin is applied at this point in order to relieve strain on the right ventricle, the pulmonary shunt flow increases and systemic resistance further decreases. In contrast, the inhalation of aerosolized prostacyclin caused selective pulmonary vasodilatation in the ventilated areas, combining a drop in pulmonary pressure and resistance with a redistribution of pulmonary blood flow from non-ventilated to ventilated areas. This caused a significant increase in the oxygenation index.[3] Our experience with ARDS was later applied in cases of severe pneumonia where mechanical ventilation was required.[26] With a direct comparison between inhaled prostacyclin and inhaled NO, it was possible to demonstrate that both approaches had almost identical pulmonary vasodilatory potency and demonstrated the same amount of pulmonary selectivity.[27]

Interstitial lung disease

Chronically progressive cor pulmonale is one of the most common causes of death in patients with lung fibrosis of any etiology. Intravenous prostacyclin has been used in some of these patients but the deleterious effects on gas exchange limit the use in this indication. In an acute pharmacological testing, intravenous prostacyclin, inhaled NO and inhaled prostacyclin were applied to patients who suffered from both severe lung fibrosis and pulmonary hypertension.[4] It was shown that an application of inhaled prostacyclin significantly lowered pulmonary pressure and resistance and significantly increased cardiac output without deterioration of gas exchange or increase in pulmonary shunt blood flow, as assessed by multiple inert gas elimination technique (MIGET).[28]

As in PPH patients, the pulmonary-to-systemic resistance ratio decreased significantly with NO and inhaled prostacyclin but not with systemic prostacyclin, demonstrating that prostacyclin has no pulmonary selectivity of its own.[4] Intravenous prostacyclin resulted in a threefold increase in pulmonary shunt flow whereas neither inhaled prostacyclin nor inhaled NO significantly increased the shunt flow. This shows that inhalation with prostacyclin is an extremely viable therapeutic option for patients suffering from interstitial pulmonary diseases.

Chronic thromboembolic pulmonary hypertension (CETPH)

Perfusion is inhomogeneous in chronic pulmonary embolism, which can be explained by the fact that some of the pulmonary arteries are blocked and some are overperfused. In analyzing the $\dot{V}/\dot{Q}$ matching by means of the MIGET, these overperfused areas are particularly easy to recognize. They cause a 'shoulder' in the perfusion distribution curve in the low $\dot{V}/\dot{Q}$ areas. With chronic pulmonary embolism, there is much higher perfusion resistance than is to be expected from the extent of the initial vascular obstruction.[29] Remodeling or progressive active vasoconstriction of the primarily non-obstructed vessels could be the reason for this secondary increase in resistance. We administered intravenous prostacyclin as a vasodilatory agent to patients suffering from chronic thromboembolic pulmonary hypertension[30] and compared the response with that demonstrated by patients with PPH and lung fibrosis. The MIGET analysis showed that patients with chronic pulmonary embolism responded to intravenous prostacyclin with a significant drop in pulmonary pressure and resistance, but with a worsening of gas exchange due to a very characteristically increased perfusion of low $\dot{V}/\dot{Q}$ areas corresponding to a vasodilatation of primarily overperfused vessels. This is consistent with the hypothesis that in CTEPH, an active

Table 13M.1 *Hemodynamics and gas exchange in pulmonary hypertension associated with lung fibrosis*

	CO (L/min)	PAP (mmHg)	PVR (dyn s/cm^5)	RVEF (%)	CVP (mmHg)	HR (beats/min)	MAP (mmHg)	PaO$_2$ (mmHg)	Shunt (%)
Pre-NO	2.1	65	2243	7	18	113	110	69.4	3.6
During NO	5.0	44	774	15	10	90	120	88.6	6.3
Pre-PGI$_2$ i.v.	2.4	59	1789	9	19	111	121	71.9	5.1
During PGI$_2$ i.v.	6.0	42	470	20	10	102	105	62	23.1
Pre-PGI$_2$ aero	2.5	65	2179	7	18	113	112	74.6	2.4
During PGI$_2$ aero	4.7	45	644	20.5	9.5	93	113	81.5	5.6

Female patient, 27 years old, with mixed connective tissue disease resulting in severe lung fibrosis and pulmonary hypertension. With intravenous prostacyclin (PGI$_2$ i.v.) there was a large increase in pulmonary perfusion but at the same time the intrapulmonary shunt flow increased to 23% of the cardiac output (CO). With inhaled prostacyclin (PGI$_2$ aero), however, pulmonary vasodilatation occurred without an increase in shunt flow. This effect was similar to that of inhaled NO.[4]

CO, cardiac output; PAP, pulmonary artery pressure; PVR, pulmonary vascular resistance; RVEF, right ventricular ejection fraction; CVP, central venous pressure; HR, heart rate; MAP, mitogen activated protein; PaO$_2$, arterial partial pressure of oxygen.

vasoconstrictive process in the primarily non-obstructed vessels causes the secondary long-term increase in vascular resistance. Blocking this vasoconstrictive mechanism with potent vasodilators worsens the existing mismatch and therefore also affects oxygenation. However, right-ventricular strain is simultaneously reduced, which counteracts cardiac decompensation. Compared with intravenous prostacyclin, in the same trial, both inhaled NO and inhaled iloprost had pulmonary vasodilatory effects but caused less $\dot{V}/\dot{Q}$ mismatch.[30]

Finally, because non-operable patients with chronic thromboembolic pulmonary hypertension were included in the controlled long-term trials (see below), and clinically did not respond differently from PPH patients, they can be considered for long-term therapy with inhaled iloprost.

AEROSOLIZATION TECHNOLOGY

The inhalation device that is used to administer inhaled iloprost plays a decisive role in the effectiveness, the side-effect profile, and the patient's acceptance of the therapy. For example, an important issue is whether the aerosol is deposited mostly in the alveoli as required or mostly in the mucous membranes of the respiratory tract. This is very much dependent on the size of the droplets and the ventilation pattern. The best results are obtained with a slow deep inspiration and a faster expiration. Important criteria for new devices include generation of droplets with an average diameter of approximately 3 μm and a small standard deviation in the droplet size distribution, alveolar targeting, safety, robustness, and easy handling including hygienic cleaning. It should provide inhalations independent of mains and should be light and small. The device should be absolutely tight for aerosol and the complete expiration should go into the device to ensure that there is no contamination of the surrounding atmosphere.

Jet nebulizers

Three different types of jet nebulizer have been compared in a crossover design with hemodynamic measurement;[31] they were using different methods of alveolar targeting (spacer versus Venturi effects versus computer-assisted pulsed delivery, see pharmacokinetics). If an inhaled dose (mouth dose of 5 μg) was applied with each device, the hemodynamic effects were the same. As a general disadvantage, these devices need a noisy portable compressor and only about 20–40% of the drug filled into the device reaches the patient. These devices can be described as suitable but by no means ideal.

Ultrasonic devices

Specialized ultrasonic devices have been developed without any valve between the nebulizer and the mouthpiece. They deliver the aerosol to the lungs with less loss of drug. In addition, the inhalation time can be shortened to about 4 minutes without loss of pulmonary selectivity.[32] Information on new devices for iloprost is available from http://www.med.uni-giessen.de/med2/pph.

PHARMACOKINETICS AND PHARMACO-DYNAMICS OF INHALED ILOPROST

We investigated the pharmacokinetics and the pharmacodynamic effects of a standardized iloprost aerosol dose (5 μg; nebulized within approximately 10 minutes), delivered by three different jet nebulizers in a crossover design.[30] The pharmacodynamic and pharmacokinetic profiles of iloprost inhalation with these devices were superimposable. The pulmonary vascular resistance (baseline approximately 1250 dyn s/cm^5) decreased significantly (−35.5 to −38.0%), as well as mean pulmonary artery pressure (baseline approximately 58 mmHg, decline −18.4 to −21.8%), whereas the systemic arterial pressure was largely unaffected. Cardiac output, mixed venous and arterial oxygen saturation increased significantly. Moreover, rapid entry of iloprost into the systemic circulation was noted, peaking immediately after termination of the inhalation maneuver, with maximum plasma concentrations of about 155 pg/mL and half-lives of disappearance of about 7 minutes. Interestingly, the 'half-life' of the pharmacodynamic effects in the pulmonary vasculature (e.g. decrease in PVR, ranging between 21 and 25 minutes) clearly outlasted the plasma-level-based pharmacokinetic half-life. This supports the hypothesis that local drug deposition largely contributes to the preferential pulmonary vasodilation in response to inhaled iloprost.

LONG-TERM THERAPY WITH INHALED ILOPROST

There have been many documented cases concerning practical clinical experience with inhaled iloprost therapy in European countries and Australia, Argentina, and Israel. Since 1994, inhaled iloprost has become the therapy of first choice for severe pulmonary hypertension in Germany.

DECOMPENSATED PULMONARY HYPERTENSION

We successfully applied inhaled iloprost in patients who were in an emergency situation due to right ventricular failure and did not tolerate intravenous prostacyclin due to systemic hypotension[5] or to shunting.[4] In comparison, inhalation with aerosolized iloprost was well tolerated and led to a marked decrease in pulmonary pressure and resistance and an increase in pulmonary and systemic O$_2$ saturation. In an uncontrolled study of 19 patients presenting with right ventricular decompensation defined by clinical and hemodynamic measures, inhaled iloprost was used as the first-line therapy. Twelve of these patients were suffering from primary pulmonary hypertension, three had underlying CREST syndrome, two were suffering from lung fibrosis, and two had non-operable chronic thromboembolic disease.[33] The patients' initial hemodynamic situation was very poor. Mean pulmonary pressure was 66 mmHg, the heart index was reduced to 1.6 L/min·m^2, and the PVR was increased to approximately 1800 dyn s/cm^5. Mean central venous O$_2$ saturation was severely reduced to below 50% and confirmed the extremely unfavorable prognosis of the collective. The average 6-minute walking distance was only 89 meters, due to the fact that nine of the patients were initially confined to bed or were only able to walk a distance of a few meters.

Long-term therapy with inhaled iloprost was initiated following acute tests. The daily used dose was between 100 and 200 µg/day, translating into an inhaled dose of about 25–60 µg. In the first 3 months of treatment, 21% of the patients died, despite trying intravenous prostacyclin or iloprost in most cases, but 43% improved in NYHA class during inhaled iloprost treatment. The average walking distance more than doubled to 192 meters (P < 0.05). The hemodynamics were also significantly improved with a decrease in pulmonary artery pressure, an increase in cardiac output, a reduction in pulmonary vascular resistance, and a reduction in central venous pressure. Interestingly, systemic pressure and resistance did not decrease in the course of 3 months so that there was a 17% improvement in the pulmonary/systemic vascular resistance (PVR/SVR) ratio over the 3-month period.

Table 13M.2 *Hemodynamic effects of inhaled iloprost in decompensated right heart failure*

	Weeks of therapy			
	0		12	
	Before	After	Before	After
Iloprost inhalation, inhaled dose (pg)		3		3
PAP (mmHg)	66	33	56	22
PVIR (dyn s/cm^5)	2444	657	1449	289
RVEF (%)	5	18	17	27
CVP (mmHg)	19	10	3	0
CO (L/min)	1.98	3.35	2.87	4.98
HR (/min)	83	54	61	55
PVIR/SVIR	1.01	0.372	0.675	0.234
6-minute walk (m)	0	0	380	426

Following the 3-month trial phase, all the surviving patients received further treatment with inhaled iloprost. After 1 year, 42% of the initial population were still successfully treated with inhaled iloprost, whereas 21% had undergone lung transplantation and 16% had died. One patient was switched to intravenous iloprost after 1.5 years of inhalation therapy.[33] Similar findings were published from a large German transplant center where 40% of patients who started iloprost inhalation after referral for lung transplantation completed at least 1 year of therapy whereas 25% were switched to intravenous iloprost or prostacyclin therapy.[34]

These data show that a majority of very sick patients can be stabilized or improved with inhaled iloprost for at least 3 months and about 40% for more than a year, making intravenous therapy dispensable or at least postponing its use. There is also some experience with the combination of inhaled and intravenous iloprost. The acute effect of inhalation adds to the effect of the intravenous infusion with few side effects,[35] allowing effective intravenous therapy with minimal side effects. According to our current experience, severely ill patients who were treated with this combination for at least 6 months needed an intravenous iloprost dose of only 1.5 ng/kg·min after 3 months and 2 ng/kg·min after 1 year of combined therapy (mean inhaled dose 0.25 ng/kg·min).

The effect of therapy on mortality rate in these decompensated patients cannot be directly assessed, as it is unethical to use a placebo control in such a clinical situation. The experience, however, strongly suggests a beneficial effect on mortality, similar to the effect of intravenous prostacyclin. Furthermore, the long-term effect on hemodynamics is reminiscent of long-term prostacyclin effects.[36]

CLINICAL TRIALS WITH INHALED ILOPROST

One phase II study and two phase III studies, a long-term surveillance study and a pivotal study were conducted for approval of inhaled iloprost in the indication pulmonary hypertension.

In the long-term surveillance study, a total of 63 patients suffering from severe primary or secondary pulmonary hypertension were included in a German multicenter, randomized, controlled trial. Patients with severe primary and secondary pulmonary hypertension despite maximum conservative therapy were included except for patients with chronic obstructive lung disease, pulmonary venous hypertension, and an increased risk of hemorrhage. Chronic thromboembolic patients who were suitable for pulmonary thromboendarterectomy were also excluded. Following a random controlled phase lasting 3 months, the trial patients were given inhaled iloprost over a period of 2 years. During the controlled phase there was a difference in NYHA class, the Mahler dyspnea index and a quality of life measure in favor of iloprost and during the open label phase there was a stabilization of hemodynamics along with an improvement in physical capacity. The preliminary results showed an excellent tolerability and safety with hardly any tachyphylaxis.[37,38]

The Aerosolized Iloprost Randomized Study (AIR Study) in primary and non-primary pulmonary hypertension was designed as a European pivotal trial to show the efficacy of inhaled iloprost on a clinical end point that is hard to reach. It consisted of an improvement by at least one NYHA class combined with an improvement by at least 10% in the 6-minute walk distance and no deterioration or death.[39] In this large, randomized, double-blind, placebo-controlled multicenter study, 37 expert centers participated and enrolled 203 patients with primary pulmonary hypertension (50%) or other forms of pulmonary hypertension (non-primary pulmonary hypertension, 50%), including appetite suppressant (5%), collagen vascular disease-associated (17%) and non-operable thromboembolic pulmonary hypertension (28%). Patients were in NYHA class III (59%) or IV (41%). The primary end point was assessed at week 12. Iloprost inhalations were administered six or nine times a day with a standard nebulizer. The inhaled single dose was 2.5 or 5 μg iloprost per 5–10 minute inhalation session. The median daily dose was 30 μg, corresponding to a mean dose of 0.37 ng/kg·min. Baseline parameters were not different between the iloprost and placebo group. The combined clinical end point was reached by 17% of patients in the iloprost group but only 5% in the placebo group ($P = 0.007$). The clinical benefit became apparent for all subgroups. In the 6-minute walking test, the treatment effect was 36.4 meters in favor of iloprost ($P < 0.01$). Quality of life assessments showed improvement in the EuroQoL visual analog scale ($P < 0.05$) and in the Mahler Dyspnoea Transition Index ($P < 0.05$). Hemodynamics significantly deteriorated in the placebo group, whereas in the iloprost group pre-inhalation values were largely unchanged compared with baseline and post-inhalation values were significantly improved. There was no indication of tachyphylaxis. Defined criteria of deterioration were met less frequently in iloprost versus placebo patients. Death rate was lower in the iloprost-treated group with one (iloprost) versus four patients (placebo). Overall, the therapy was well tolerated. Cough occurred more frequently in the iloprost compared with the placebo group (38.6 versus 25.5%) as well as headache (29.7 versus 19.6%) and flush (26.7 versus 8.8%). These adverse events were mild and mostly transient. Syncopes occurring in the iloprost group, although not occurring more frequently, were rated as more severe than in the placebo group, but were commonly not associated with clinical deterioration.[40]

DISADVANTAGES USING INHALED PROSTANOID THERAPY

Local intolerance

A small number of patients demonstrated local intolerance with dry coughing during inhalation. To date, only two documented patients were forced to discontinue therapy with inhaled iloprost because of these side effects. However, there was no evidence of damage to the pulmonary or bronchial areas. Antitussive drugs may be helpful to overcome a period of increased coughing.

Systemic side effects

The systemic side effects are usually mild and include jaw pain, flushing, systemic hypotension, and headache that persists for 5–15 minutes after inhalation. If inhalation-associated headache newly develops in a patient who has been inhaling without complaints, this points to acute sinusitis or swelling of the mucosa.

Short half–life and nocturnal intervals

Therapy with inhaled iloprost is applied discontinuously in six to nine inhalations a day and up to 12 in isolated cases. Some patients feel that the very necessity of having to inhale every 2–3 hours limits their freedom of movement, although the modern ultrasonic inhalation devices allow battery-driven inhalation sessions without noise. This is particularly true of the younger patients. There are recurrent increases in the pulmonary pressure and resistance in the intervals between inhalations that lead to strain on the right ventricle. Some patients experience this as a worsening of exercise tolerance and breathing difficulties on performing even light tasks. For that reason, some patients prefer shorter inhalation intervals of 60–90 minutes, for example. The nocturnal pause may be a problem for a few patients but mostly it is well tolerated. Less than 10% of patients need additional inhalation during the night. These patients often have a distinctive vasoconstrictive component relating to the disease that reacts well to inhaled iloprost but for which effectiveness is short-lived. Once these patients are recompensated, they may tolerate an oral calcium channel blocker before sleep, ameliorating the problem.

INHALED ILOPROST IN COMBINATION WITH OTHER MEDICAL APPROACHES

Inhaled iloprost can easily be combined with other therapies, e.g. with intravenous iloprost. An alternative combination avoiding the intravenous line is an orally or subcutaneous prostanoid. Of particular advantage is the combination with phosphodiesterase inhibitors, which can prolong the effects of inhalation even if given at sub-threshold doses that do not exert hemodynamic effects of their own.[41,42] This could be demonstrated in patients with severe pulmonary hypertension using the potent phosphodiesterase type 5 (PDE5) inhibitor sildenafil.[43,44] In addition to its acute effects, sildenafil possesses considerable potency to improve hemodynamics and exercise tolerance in the long run when added to inhaled iloprost.[45]

FUTURE DIRECTIONS

Current technology pertaining to the inhaled application of prostanoids is entirely suitable for testing and therapy on a long-term basis, although there is considerable room for improvement. The main clinical aims are the prolongation of the inhalation intervals, a reduction of the inhalation period, a scaling down of the inhalation device, and a reduction in drug waste inside the device.

Using specific nebulizers, it is possible to administer an entire target dose of inhaled iloprost within 4 minutes. However, increased systemic and local side effects can limit the use of shorter inhalation times.

Prolonging the duration of the hemodynamic effect of an inhalation represents the biggest challenge for future development. A reasonable technical solution would be the application of an inhaled 'retarded aerosol'. This could be realized by cross-linking the agent with long-chain sugar residues that are cleaved slowly to yield active drug molecules within the alveolar space. Another possibility would be to apply the inhaled drug in nanoparticles from which the drug is slowly released. Developments along these lines are under way.

PLACE OF INHALED ILOPROST IN THE TREATMENT OF DISORDERS OF THE PULMONARY CIRCULATION

In addition to the well established therapies with high-dose calcium channel blockers and continuous intravenous prostacyclin, new effective drugs have been developed, particularly stable prostacyclin analogs and the endothelin receptor antagonist bosentan. New drugs (potent PDE inhibitors) are on the horizon. Inhaled iloprost is unique due to the combination of the beneficial effects of prostacyclin with pulmonary and intrapulmonary selectivity. This makes it suitable as first-line therapy in moderate and severe PPH as well as secondary pulmonary hypertension. It combines effectiveness and fast onset of effects with safety and tolerability. By this means it allows therapy of right ventricular decompensation even with severe pre-existing ventilation/perfusion mismatch, in patients who may not tolerate other therapies. In addition, it can easily be combined with other drugs, e.g. if these are dose limited due to systemic side effects, toxic effects or unfavorable effects on gas exchange.

KEY POINTS

- This balance between pulmonary and systemic vasodilatory effects is crucial for all non-selective vasodilators but an imbalance towards systemic vasodilatation is most dangerous in the case of the calcium channel blockers because of their negative inotropic effect on the right ventricle.
- The inhalation of aerosolized prostacyclin causes selective pulmonary vasodilatation in ventilated areas, combining a drop in pulmonary pressure and resistance with a redistribution of pulmonary blood flow from non-ventilated to ventilated areas. Local drug deposition contributes to the preferential pulmonary vasodilation in response to inhaled iloprost.
- The Aerosolized Iloprost Randomized Study (AIR Study) in primary and non-primary pulmonary hypertension, a European pivotal trial, showed the efficacy of inhaled iloprost.
- Prolonging the duration of the hemodynamic effect of an inhalation represents the biggest challenge for future development.

REFERENCES

●1 Rich S, Kaufmann E, Levy PS. The effect of high doses of calcium-channel blockers on survival in primary pulmonary hypertension. *N Engl J Med* 1992;**327**:76–81.

2 Agusti AG, Rodriguez-Roisin R. Effect of pulmonary hypertension on gas exchange. *Eur Respir J* 1993;**6**:1371–7.

●3 Walmrath D, Schneider T, Pilch J *et al.* Aerosolised prostacyclin in adult respiratory distress syndrome. *Lancet* 1993;**342**:961–2.

●4 Olschewski H, Ghofrani HA, Walmrath D *et al.* Inhaled prostacyclin and iloprost in severe pulmonary hypertension secondary to lung fibrosis. *Am J Respir Crit Care Med* 1999;**160**:600–7.

●5 Olschewski H, Ghofrani HA, Walmrath D *et al.* Recovery from circulatory shock in severe primary pulmonary hypertension (PPH) with aerosolization of iloprost. *Intens Care Med* 1998;**24**:631–4.

6 Davie N, Haleen SJ, Upton PD *et al.* ET(A) and ET(B) receptors modulate the proliferation of human pulmonary artery smooth muscle cells. *Am J Respir Crit Care Med* 2002;**165**:398–405.

7 Higenbottam T, Butt AY, McMahon A *et al.* Long-term intravenous prostaglandin (epoprostenol or iloprost) for treatment of severe pulmonary hypertension. *Heart* 1998; **80**:151–5.

8 Higenbottam TW, Butt AY, Dinh-Xaun AT *et al.* Treatment of pulmonary hypertension with the continuous infusion of a prostacyclin analogue, iloprost. *Heart* 1998;**79**:175–9.

9 Scott JP, Higenbottam T, Wallwork J. The acute effect of the synthetic prostacyclin analogue iloprost in primary pulmonary hypertension. *Br J Clin Pract* 1990;**44**:231–4.

●10 Olschewski H, Walmrath D, Schermuly R *et al.* Aerosolized prostacyclin and iloprost in severe pulmonary hypertension. *Ann Intern Med* 1996;**124**:820–4.

11 Warren JB, Higenbottam T. Caution with use of inhaled nitric oxide. *Lancet* 1996;**348**:629–30.

12 Cueto E, Lopez-Herce J, Sanchez A *et al.* Life-threatening effects of discontinuing inhaled nitric oxide in children. *Acta Paediatr* 1997;**86**:1337–9.

13 Miller OI, Tang SF, Keech A *et al.* Rebound pulmonary hypertension on withdrawal from inhaled nitric oxide. *Lancet* 1995;**346**:51–2.

●14 Hoeper MM, Olschewski H, Ghofrani HA *et al.* A comparison of the acute hemodynamic effects of inhaled nitric oxide and aerosolized iloprost in primary pulmonary hypertension. German PPH study group. *J Am Coll Cardiol* 2000;**35**:176–82.

15 Welte M, Zwissler B, Habazettl H *et al.* PGI2 aerosol versus nitric oxide for selective pulmonary vasodilation in hypoxic pulmonary vasoconstriction. *Eur Surg Res* 1993;**25**:329–40.

16 Eichelbronner O, Reinelt H, Wiedeck H *et al.* Aerosolized prostacyclin and inhaled nitric oxide in septic shock – different effects on splanchnic oxygenation? *Intens Care Med* 1996;**22**:880–7.

17 Kleen M, Habler O, Hofstetter C *et al.* Efficacy of inhaled prostanoids in experimental pulmonary hypertension. *Crit Care Med* 1998;**26**:1103–9.

18 Mikhail G, Gibbs J, Richardson M *et al.* An evaluation of nebulized prostacyclin in patients with primary and secondary pulmonary hypertension. *Eur Heart J* 1997;**18**: 1499–504.

19 Putensen C, Hormann C, Kleinsasser A *et al.* Cardiopulmonary effects of aerosolized prostaglandin E1 and nitric oxide inhalation in patients with acute respiratory distress syndrome. *Am J Respir Crit Care Med* 1998;**157**(6 Pt 1):1743–7.

20 Zobel G, Dacar D, Rodl S *et al.* Inhaled nitric oxide versus inhaled prostacyclin and intravenous versus inhaled prostacyclin in acute respiratory failure with pulmonary hypertension in piglets. *Pediatr Res* 1995;**38**:198–204.

21 Haraldsson A, Kieler-Jensen N, Nathorst-Westfelt U *et al.* Comparison of inhaled nitric oxide and inhaled aerosolized prostacyclin in the evaluation of heart transplant candidates with elevated pulmonary vascular resistance. *Chest* 1998;**114**:780–6.

22 Schulze-Neick I, Uhlemann F, Nurnberg JH *et al.* [Aerosolized prostacyclin for preoperative evaluation and post-cardiosurgical treatment of patients with pulmonary hypertension.] *Z Kardiol* 1997;**86**:71–80.

23 De Jaegere AP, van den Anker JN. Endotracheal instillation of prostacyclin in preterm infants with persistent pulmonary hypertension. *Eur Respir J* 1998;**12**:932–4.

24 Santak B, Schreiber M, Kuen P *et al.* Prostacyclin aerosol in an infant with pulmonary hypertension. *Eur J Pediatr* 1995; **154**:233–5.

25 Soditt V, Aring C, Groneck P. Improvement of oxygenation induced by aerosolized prostacyclin in a preterm infant with persistent pulmonary hypertension of the newborn. *Intens Care Med* 1997;**23**:1275–8.

26 Walmrath D, Schneider T, Pilch J *et al.* Effects of aerosolized prostacyclin in severe pneumonia. Impact of fibrosis. *Am J Respir Crit Care Med* 1995;**151**(3 Pt 1):724–30.

●27 Walmrath D, Schneider T, Schermuly R *et al.* Direct comparison of inhaled nitric oxide and aerosolized prostacyclin in acute respiratory distress syndrome. *Am J Respir Crit Care Med* 1996;**153**(3):991–6.

28 Wagner PD, Saltzman HA, West JB. Measurement of continuous distributions of ventilation–perfusion ratios: theory. *J Appl Physiol* 1974;**36**:588–99.

29 Azarian R, Wartski M, Collignon MA *et al.* Lung perfusion scans and hemodynamics in acute and chronic pulmonary embolism. *J Nucl Med* 1997;**38**:980–3.

30 Ghofrani H, Schermuly R, Wiedemann R *et al.* Ventilation/perfusion patterns in primary and secondary pulmonary hypertension during nonselective and selective vasodilatation. *Am J Respir Crit Care Med* 1998;**157**:A592.

●31 Olschewski H, Rohde B, Behr J *et al.* Pharmacodynamics and pharmacokinetics of inhaled iloprost, aerosolized by three different devices, in severe pulmonary hypertension. *Chest* 2003;**124**(4):1294–304.

●32 Gessler T, Schmehl T, Hoeper MM *et al.* Ultrasonic versus jet nebulization of iloprost in severe pulmonary hypertension. *Eur Respir J* 2001;**17**:14–19.

●33 Olschewski H, Ghofrani HA, Schmehl T *et al.* Inhaled iloprost to treat severe pulmonary hypertension. An uncontrolled trial. German PPH Study Group. *Ann Intern Med* 2000;**132**:435–43.

34 Ewert R, Opitz C, Wensel R *et al.* [Iloprost as inhalational and intravenous long-term treatment of patients with primary pulmonary hypertension. Register of the Berlin Study Group for Pulmonary Hypertension.] *Z Kardiol* 2000;**89**:987–99.

35 Petkov V, Ziesche R, Mosgoeller W *et al.* Aerosolised iloprost improves pulmonary haemodynamics in patients with primary pulmonary hypertension receiving continuous epoprostenol treatment. *Thorax* 2001;**56**:734–6.

●36 Hoeper MM, Schwarze M, Ehlerding S *et al.* Long-term treatment of primary pulmonary hypertension with aerosolized iloprost, a prostacyclin analogue. *N Engl J Med* 2000;**342**:1866–70.

37 Nikkho S, Seeger W, Baumgartner R *et al.* One-year observation of iloprost therapy in patients with pulmonary hypertension. *Eur Respir J* 2001;**18**(Suppl 33):324s.

38 Behr J, Baumgartner R, Borst M *et al.* Consistency of the acute hemodynamic response to inhaled iloprost in pulmonary hypertension patients treated long-term with iloprost aerosol. *Eur Respir J* 2001;**18**(Suppl 33):324s.

●39 Olschewski H, Simonneau G, Galie N *et al.* Inhaled iloprost for severe pulmonary hypertension. *N Engl J Med* 2002; **347**:322–9.

●40 Schermuly RT, Krupnik E, Tenor H *et al.* Coaerosolization of phosphodiesterase inhibitors markedly enhances the pulmonary vasodilatory response to inhaled iloprost in experimental pulmonary hypertension. Maintenance of lung selectivity. *Am J Respir Crit Care Med* 2001;**164**:1694–700.

41 Schermuly RT, Roehl A, Weissmann N *et al.* Combination of nonspecific PDE inhibitors with inhaled prostacyclin in experimental pulmonary hypertension. *Am J Physiol Lung Cell Mol Physiol* 2001;**281**:L1361–8.

42 Schermuly RT, Leuchte H, Ghofrani HA *et al.* Zardaverine and aerosolized iloprost in a model of acute respiratory failure. *Eur Respir J* 2003;**22**(2):342–7.

●43 Wilkens H, Guth A, Konig J *et al.* Effect of inhaled iloprost plus oral sildenafil in patients with primary pulmonary hypertension. *Circulation* 2001;**104**:1218–22.

●44 Ghofrani HA, Wiedemann R, Rose F *et al.* Combination therapy with oral sildenafil and inhaled iloprost for severe pulmonary hypertension. *Ann Intern Med* 2002;**136**:515–22.

●45 Ghofrani HA, Rose F, Schermuly RT *et al.* Oral sildenafil as long-term adjunct therapy to inhaled iloprost in severe pulmonary arterial hypertension. *J Am Coll Cardiol* 2003;**42**(1):158–64.

Oral and subcutaneous prostacyclin analogs

VALLERIE V McLAUGHLIN

In the 1990s, epoprostenol therapy revolutionized the treatment of pulmonary arterial hypertension (PAH).[1-3] Patients realized an improvement in quality of life, hemodynamics and survival, and this therapy even offered hope to patients with advanced disease.[1,4] However, these attributes must be balanced against the complicated nature of the intravenous delivery system. Infections may range in severity from local exit site infections easily treated with oral antibiotics to life-threatening sepsis. Because of the short half-life of epoprostenol, interruptions in therapy related to catheter displacement or pump malfunction may be life-threatening. Rare adverse events associated with the delivery system include pneumothorax, deep venous thrombosis, and paradoxical embolus. Additionally, the patient's life is forever changed by the need to mix the medication on a daily basis, store the drug under refrigerated conditions, and use the continuous ambulatory drug delivery (CADD) pump. The success of epoprostenol coupled with these limitations of the delivery system has been the motivation to develop prostacyclin analogs with alternative routes of delivery. The analog iloprost was discussed in a previous chapter. This chapter focuses on the analogs beraprost and treprostinil.

BERAPROST

Beraprost sodium is an orally active prostacyclin analog with a stable structure due to its cyclopentabenzofuranyl skeleton.[5] Beraprost is rapidly absorbed in the fasting condition with peak plasma concentrations reached after 30 minutes and elimination half-life of 35–40 minutes after a single oral administration.[6] When administered with a meal, peak concentration is lower and the half-life is prolonged to approximately 3–3.5 hours. Like other prostacyclin analogs, beraprost induces vasodilatation, inhibition of platelet aggregation, and *in vitro* inhibition of smooth muscle cell proliferation.[7,8] Beraprost has been shown to exert a protective effect against the development of monocrotaline-induced pulmonary hypertension in the rat.[9] High doses of beraprost have been demonstrated to exert a positive inotropic and chronotropic effect on isolated guinea pig myocardium.[10] Beraprost has also been studied for the treatment of peripheral vascular disease and Raynaud's phenomenon and digital necrosis in systemic sclerosis.[11] Enthusiasm for the treatment of pulmonary arterial hypertension with beraprost arose from the initial experiences in Japan and subsequently in Europe.

The short-term hemodynamic effects of beraprost were reported by Saji and colleagues in 1996.[12] They studied seven patients with PAH, four with primary pulmonary hypertension (PPH) and three with PAH associated with congenital heart disease. Patients underwent cardiac catheterization, with baseline measurements obtained at rest and then every 15 minutes after the administration of various doses of oral beraprost. In the four patients with PPH, there was a $24 \pm 20\%$ reduction in pulmonary vascular resistance. The cardiac index increased by $20 \pm 18\%$. The maximal changes in the hemodynamic parameters occurred at the 15–30 minute intervals after oral administration. There was a similar reduction of $24 \pm 14\%$ in pulmonary vascular resistance in the patients with PAH associated with congenital heart disease. Importantly, there were no serious complications observed during this short-term study.

In 1997, Okano *et al.* described a group of 12 patients with PPH treated with beraprost.[13] All patients were unresponsive to oral calcium channel blockers and inhaled nitric oxide. Hemodynamics were obtained before and after patients received a daily dose of 80–180 μg for an average of 2 months. Pulmonary vascular resistance fell by 26%, from 19.3 ± 4.8 to 14.3 ± 3.3 Wood units. The pulmonary artery pressure was reduced by 12% from 66 ± 7 mmHg to 58 ± 9 mmHg. Statistical analysis was not reported. There was no control group.

In 1999, Nagaya and colleagues reported the effect of beraprost on survival in patients with PPH.[14] They studied 58 consecutive patients who could safely be discharged from the hospital after their first diagnostic cardiac catheterization for PPH between 1981 and 1997. The 34 patients diagnosed before December 1992 were treated with conventional therapy alone, which consisted of calcium channel blockers, nitrates, digitalis, and diuretics. The calcium channel blockers were used only in patients who demonstrated more than a 20% reduction in total pulmonary resistance with short-term oral administration of nifedipine. The 24 patients diagnosed after January 1993 were treated with beraprost in addition to conventional therapy. Oral beraprost was initiated at a rate of 60 μg/day and increased by increments of 60 μg/day over 1–2 weeks until the highest tolerated dose. The daily dose was split into three or four doses. Survival was estimated from the date of initial diagnosis until the conclusion of the study in November 1998. Of the 34 patients in the conventional therapy group, 27 patients died of cardiopulmonary causes after a mean follow-up of 44 ± 45 months. By contrast, four of the patients in the beraprost group died of cardiopulmonary causes during a mean follow-up of 30 ± 20 months. One patient in the conventional therapy group underwent lung transplantation and one received intravenous epoprostenol during the follow-up period. Four patients in the beraprost group received epoprostenol during the follow-up period. Kaplan–Meier survival curves demonstrated the 1-, 2- and 3-year survival rates in the beraprost group to be 96%, 86% and 76%, respectively, compared to the 77%, 47% and 44% survival, respectively, in the conventional therapy group. This was statistically significant by the log-rank test with a P value <0.05. A subgroup of 15 patients treated with beraprost underwent repeat cardiac catheterization after a mean of 53 days on therapy. There was a reduction in mean pulmonary artery pressure of 13% and a reduction in total pulmonary resistance of 25%. The cardiac output increased by 17%. Sixty-seven per cent of the patients treated with beraprost reported an improvement in New York Heart Association (NYHA) functional class. Although this study suggested an improvement in survival with beraprost therapy, there were several limitations. The study was small and retrospective in nature. Other medical therapies were not controlled and there was a significant difference in the use of calcium channel blockers and digitalis between the conventional therapy group and the beraprost group. The mean follow-up was substantially

longer in the conventional therapy group than the beraprost group. In addition, a larger proportion of the patients in the beraprost group went on to treatment with intravenous epoprostenol.

More recently, Vizza and colleagues reported their results of long-term treatment of PAH with beraprost.[15] They studied 13 patients, nine of whom had PPH, three of whom had thromboembolic pulmonary hypertension, and one who had PAH related to congenital heart disease. The mean daily dose of beraprost was 116 ± 24 μg after the first month of treatment and 193 ± 74 μg at the end of 12 months. One patient died at 40 days and one patient was lost to follow-up. Follow-up data at 12 months was therefore achieved in 11 of the patients. Patients demonstrated an improvement in NYHA functional class from 3.4 ± 0.7 at baseline to 2.9 ± 0.7 at the end of 1 month (P < 0.016). No further improvement was noted after a full year of therapy. The 6-minute walk distance increased by 63 ± 47 meters from a baseline of 213 ± 64 meters. This improvement occurred at 1 month and was maintained over the 12-month period. They also noted a decrease in systolic pulmonary artery pressure, as measured by echocardiogram. This prospective uncontrolled trial suggested that beraprost improved symptoms, functional class and exercise capacity in patients with pulmonary hypertension.

A prospective, double-blind, placebo-controlled, randomized study of beraprost in the study of PAH has recently been completed in Europe.[16] Galiè and colleagues studied 130 patients with PAH, including PPH and PAH associated with collagen vascular disease, congenital heart disease, portal hypertension and HIV infection. Patients were randomized to the maximal tolerated dose of beraprost or placebo for 12 weeks. The primary end point of distance walked in 6 minutes improved by 25.1 meters (P = 0.036) in the active treatment group. They also noted an improvement in symptoms, as measured by the Borg dyspnea index, which decreased by 0.94 in the active beraprost group (P = 0.009). Subgroup analysis demonstrated that patients with PPH realized the most substantial improvement with a mean change of 6-minute walk distance of 46.1 meters. They noted no statistically significant differences in cardiopulmonary hemodynamics or NYHA functional class. The median dose of beraprost in the study was 80 μg four times per day. A double-blind placebo-controlled trial in PAH was also conducted in the US.[17] While there were improvements in excercise tolerance as measured by six minute walk distance at three and six months, the improvement was not sustained at nine and twelve months.

The most common side effects of beraprost reported in the above-cited studies include headache, flushing, jaw pain, diarrhea, leg pain and nausea. Side effects can be minimized when the drug is taken with a meal. Beraprost is currently available in Japan and may become available in Europe. A placebo-controlled trial with beraprost in the USA was terminated prematurely and this drug will not likely become commercially available in the USA. Presumably, the early termination was because of a lack of efficacy estimation by the Data and Safety Monitoring Board.

TREPROSTINIL

Treprostinil is a prostacyclin analog with a half-life of 3 hours. The drug is stable at room temperature. Animal studies have suggested that the hemodynamic effects of treprostinil are similar to those of epoprostenol.[18,19] To test this hypothesis in humans, we studied 14 patients with PPH acutely with intravenous epoprostenol and then intravenous treprostinil.[20] Both drugs had similar effects on hemodynamics. There was a 22% reduction in pulmonary vascular resistance with epoprostenol versus a 20% reduction in pulmonary vascular resistance with treprostinil. To then test the alternative subcutaneous delivery method, we compared the effects of intravenous treprostinil in 25 patients with PPH followed by subcutaneous treprostinil in the same patients.[20] In the intravenous treprostinil and subcutaneous treprostinil groups, there was a 6% and 13% decline in mean pulmonary artery pressure and a 23% and 28% decline in pulmonary vascular resistance, respectively. Dose-limiting side effects for subcutaneous treprostinil were similar to intravenous treprostinil and included nausea, vomiting, headache, dizziness and anxiety. Having demonstrated that the drug favorably effects cardiopulmonary hemodynamics when given subcutaneously acutely, we embarked on an 8-week, placebo-controlled, 2:1, randomized trial of subcutaneous treprostinil.[20] Twenty-six patients with PPH were enrolled. Two patients in the treprostinil group did not complete the study owing to intolerable side effects. The remaining patients 15 were on a mean dose of 13.0 ± 3.1 ng/kg·min of treprostinil while the nine patients receiving placebo were on 38.9 ± 6.7 ng/kg·min at the end of the 8-week period. There was an improvement of 37 ± 17 meters in the 6-minute walk distance in patients receiving the active therapy (from 373 meters to 411 meters) compared to a 6 ± 28 meter reduction in those receiving placebo (379 meters versus 384 meters), a non-statistically significant trend. There was also a favorable trend in hemodynamics with a 20% reduction in pulmonary vascular resistance index over the 8-week period in the group receiving active treprostinil. Adverse events including headache, diarrhea, flushing, jaw pain and foot pain were common in the treprostinil group as they are with epoprostenol. An unexpected adverse effect was related to pain, which was occasionally severe, erythema, and induration at the site of the subcutaneous infusion. Eighty-eight per cent of patients experienced infusion site pain while 94% experienced

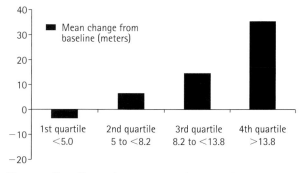

Figure 13N.1 *Change in exercise as a function of dose.*

infusion site erythema in the active treprostinil group. By contrast, only 22% of patients in the placebo group complained of such effects. However, this proof of concept trial demonstrated that this novel subcutaneous agent could be given safely and effectively on an outpatient basis and paved the way for the larger, pivotal trial.

The largest placebo-controlled randomized study for PAH was an international trial assessing the efficacy of subcutaneously delivered treprostinil in patients with PAH, either primary or associated with connective tissue disease or congenital systemic-to-pulmonary shunts.[21] Patients were enrolled between November 1998 and October 1999 in 24 centers in North America and 16 centers in Europe, Australia and Israel. A total of 470 patients were randomly assigned to receive either continuous subcutaneous infusion of treprostinil plus conventional therapy or continuous infusion of placebo (vehicle solution without treprostinil) plus conventional therapy. Randomization was based on a permuted block design stratified on the basis of baseline exercise capacity and type of pulmonary hypertension. Because of the adverse effects of the infusion site pain and reaction that occurred in the proof-of-concept trial, the dosing strategy called for lower doses at initiation with a maximal allowable dose at the end of 12 weeks of 22.5 ng/kg·min. The primary end point of this trial was exercise capacity as measured by the 6-minute walk distance, which improved in the treprostinil group and was unchanged with placebo. The median between treatment group difference was 16 meters (P = 0.006). This effect on exercise tolerance appeared to be dose related. The patients in the lowest two quartiles of dosing experienced little improvement in 6-minute walk distance while patients in the highest quartile of dosing (greater than 13.8 ng/kg·min) demonstrated an improvement of 36 meters in 6-minute walk distance (Figure 13N.1). Other indices of wellbeing, including the dyspnea fatigue rating and the Borg dyspnea scale, confirmed an improvement with treprostinil therapy. Treprostinil also demonstrated a significant improvement in the hemodynamic parameters of mean right atrial pressure, mean pulmonary artery pressure, cardiac index, pulmonary vascular resistance and mixed venous oxygen saturation (Table 13N.1). Common

Table 13N.1 *Hemodynamic response to subcutaneous treprostinil*

	Treprostinil	Placebo	P value
Mean right atrial pressure (mmHg)	−0.5 ± 0.4	1.4 ± 0.3	0.0002
Mean pulmonary artery pressure (mmHg)	−2.3 ± 0.5	0.7 ± 0.6	0.0003
Cardiac index (L/min·m^2)	0.12 ± 0.04	−0.06 ± 0.04	0.0001
Pulmonary vascular resistance (index units/m^2)	−3.5 ± 0.6	1.2 ± 0.6	0.0001
Mixed venous oxygen saturation (%)	2.0 ± 0.8	−1.4 ± 0.7	0.0001

Adapted from reference 21.

Table 13N.2 *Subgroup analysis of treprostinil trial*

Parameter	Treatment effect*
NYHA class	
II	+2 m
III	+17 m
IV	+54 m
Baseline walk	
50–150 m	+51 m
151–250 m	+33 m
251–350 m	+16 m
351–450 m	−2 m
Disease	
PPH	+13.0
CTD	+10.4
CHD	−1.0

CHD, congenital heart disease; CTD , connective tissue disease; PPH, primary pulmonary hypertension.
*Treatment effect refers to primary end point of 6-minute walk distance.

side effects included headache, diarrhea, nausea, rash and jaw pain. Side effects related to the infusion site were common. Eighty-five per cent of patients complained of infusion site pain and 83% had erythema or induration at the infusion site.

Although statistically significant, the 16-meter improvement in 6-minute walk distance was relatively modest, and less than the improvements demonstrated in the trials with intravenous epoprostenol for both PPH and PAH related to the scleroderma spectrum of diseases, which demonstrated treatment effects of 47 meters and 99 meters, respectively.[1,3] The reasons for this are multifactorial. The entry criteria for the treprostinil trial were much broader than for either of the epoprostenol trials. Key subgroup analyses are listed in Table 13N.2. The epoprostenol trials included only patients who were NYHA functional classes III and IV. Fifty-three patients who were functional class II were enrolled into the treprostinil trial. Their treatment effect in the 6-minute walk distance was only 2 meters compared to 17 meters for the 382 patients who were functional class III and 54 meters for the 34 patients who were functional class IV. The baseline 6-minute walk distance in the treprostinil study was 326 ± 5 meters in the active treprostinil group and 327 ± 6 meters in the placebo group. In comparison, the baseline 6-minute walk distance in the PPH epoprostenol trial was 315 meters in the epoprostenol plus conventional therapy group versus 270 meters in the conventional therapy group alone.[1] In the scleroderma epoprostenol trial the baseline 6-minute walk distance was 272 meters in the epoprostenol plus conventional therapy group and 240 meters in the conventional therapy group alone.[3] This demonstrates that the patient population was less ill in the treprostinil trial and may have contributed to the less impressive treatment effect.

The treatment effect was related to the baseline walk in the treprostinil trial (Table 13N.2). Patients who were able to walk between 351 and 450 meters did not demonstrate a treatment effect at all, whereas those patients who were able to walk in the lowest category of 50–150 meters demonstrated a treatment effect of 51 meters. The etiology of PAH was also broader in the treprostinil trial. In addition to the inclusion of PPH patients and PAH associated with the scleroderma spectrum of diseases, PAH associated with congenital heart disease was also included. This group had been untested in the past and in the treprostinil study did not demonstrate any treatment effect at all. This may in part be related to their longstanding disease and the difficulty of making an impact on such a process over a short 12-week period.

The nemesis of subcutaneous treprostinil has been pain and erythema at the infusion site (Plate 13N.1). A variety of therapies have been attempted to control this adverse effect although none has emerged as uniformly successful. Local remedies such as topical hot and cold packs and topical analgesics and anti-inflammatory agents were variably effective. Some patients also responded to oral analgesics such as non-steroidal anti-inflammatory drugs. A common observation was that the site pain and erythema improved after several months of therapy. Some patients found that moving the infusion site every 3 days as opposed to every day was useful. The infusion site most commonly used is the subcutaneous abdominal fat, although some patients were able to use the outer hips and thighs and underside of the upper arm with some success. Because of the longer half-life of treprostinil, interruptions of the drug due to dislodgment of the catheter or pump malfunction were less serious. In such instances, the catheter could either be replaced or the pump could be switched with the individual's back-up pump without any serious consequences. The Mini-Med pump used to administer treprostinil is smaller than the CADD pump used to administer epoprostenol and is about the size of a pager. The drug comes in a premixed-prefilled syringe and therefore the patient needs only to place the syringe in the pump and does not have to mix the medication in a sterile fashion on a daily basis.

The Food and Drug Administration has recently issued an approval letter for subcutaneous treprostinil pending agreement on the design of a phase IV study. The drug is now commercially available in the USA.

KEY POINTS

- Oral beraprost improves exercise tolerance in some patients with PAH; it is most effective in those with PPH.
- Subcutaneous treprostinil improves exercise tolerance and hemodynamics in patients with PAH, although these effects were modest in a randomized clinical trial.
- Optimal use of treprostinil is difficult and must include optimal dosing and adequate control of pain associated with the subcutaneous infusion.

REFERENCES

●1 Barst R, Rubin L, Long W et al. A comparison of continuous intravenous epoprostenol (prostacyclin) with conventional therapy for primary pulmonary hypertension. N Engl J Med 1996;**334**:296–301.

2 McLaughlin V, Genthner D, Panella M et al. Reduction in pulmonary vascular resistance with long-term epoprostenol (prostacyclin) therapy in primary pulmonary hypertension. N Engl J Med 1998;**338**:273–7.

●3 Badesch D, Tapson V, McGoon M et al. Continuous intravenous epoprostenol for pulmonary hypertension due to the scleroderma spectrum of disease. Ann Intern Med 2000; **132**:425–34.

4 Shapiro S, Oudiz R, Cao T et al. Primary pulmonary hypertension: improved long-term effects and survival with continuous intravenous epoprostenol infusion. J Am Coll Cardiol 1997;**30**:343–9.

5 Sim AK, McCraw AP, Cleland ME et al. Effects of a stable prostacyclin analogue on platelet function and experimentally-induced thrombosis in the microcirculation. Arzneim-Forsch 1985;**35**:1816–18.

6 Yuge T, Hamasaki T, Hase T et al. Pharmacokinetics and biotransformation of beraprost sodium 2: absorption, distribution and excretion after single administration of beraprost sodium in rat. Xenobio Metabol Dispos 1989; **4**:101–16.

7 Murata T, Murai T, Kanai T et al. General pharmacology of beraprost sodium, second communications: effects on the autonomic, cardiovascular and gastrointestinal systems, and other effects. Arzneim-Forsch 1989;**39**:867–76.

8 Clapp LH, Finney P, Turcato S et al. Differential effects of stable prostacyclin analogs on smooth muscle proliferation and cyclic AMP generation in human pulmonary artery. Am J Respir Cell Mol Biol 2002;**26**:194–201.

9 Miyata M, Ueno Y, Sekine H et al. Protective effect of beraprost sodium, a stable prostacyclin analogue, in development of monocrotaline-induced pulmonary hypertension. J Cardiovasc Pharmacol 1996;**27**:20–6.

10 Ueno Y, Okazaki S, Isogaya M et al. Positive inotropic and chronotropic effects of beraprost sodium, a stable analogue of prostacyclin, in isolated guinea pig myocardium. Gen Pharmacol 1996;**27**:101–3.

11 Lievre M, Morand S, Besse B et al. Oral beraprost sodium, a prostaglandin I(2) analogue, for intermittent claudication: a double-blind, randomized, multicenter controlled trial. Beraprost et Claudication Intermittente (BERCI) Research Group. Circulation 2000;**102**:426–31.

12 Saji T, Ozawa Y, Ishikita T et al. Short-term hemodynamic effect of a new oral PGI$_2$ analogue, beraprost, in primary and secondary pulmonary hypertension. Am J Cardiol 1996; **78**:244–7.

13 Okano Y, Yoshioka T, Shimouchi A et al. Orally active prostacyclin analogue in primary pulmonary hypertension. Lancet 1997;**349**:1365.

14 Nagaya N, Uematsu M, Okano Y et al. Effect of orally active prostacyclin analogue on survival of outpatients with primary pulmonary hypertension. J Am Coll Cardiol 1999;**34**:1188–92.

15 Vizza CD, Sciomer S, Morelli S et al. Long term treatment of pulmonary arterial hypertension with beraprost, an oral prostacyclin analogue. Heart 2001;**86**:661–5.

●16 Galiè N, Humbert M, Vachiery J-L et al. Effects of beraprost sodium, an oral prostacyclin analogue, in patients with pulmonary arterial hypertension: a randomised, double-blind, placebo-controlled trial. J Am Coll Cardiol 2002;**39**: 1496–502.

17 Barst RJ, McGoon M, McLaughlin V et al. Beraprost therapy for pulmonary arterial hypertension. J Am Coll Cardiol 2003;**41**:2119–25.

18 Steffen RP, de la Mata M. The effects of 15AU81, a chemically stable prostacyclin analog, on the cardiovascular and renin-angiotensin systems of anesthetized dogs. Prostaglandins Leukot Essent Fatty Acids 1991;**43**:277–86.

19 McNulty MJ, Sailstad JM, Steffen RP. The pharmacokinetics and pharmacodynamics of the prostacyclin analog 15AU81 in the anesthetized beagle dog. Prostaglandins Leukot Essent Fatty Acids 1993;**48**:159–66.

20 McLaughlin VV, Gaine SP, Barst RJ et al. Efficacy and safety of treprostinil: an epoprostenol analogue for primary pulmonary hypertension. J Cardiovasc Pharmacol 2003; **41**:293–9.

●21 Simonneau G, Barst RJ, Galie N et al. Continuous subcutaneous infusion of treprostinil, a prostacyclin analogue, in patients with pulmonary arterial hypertension. Am J Respir Crit Care Med 2002;**165**:800–4.

Inhaled nitric oxide

JOANNA PEPKE-ZABA AND KEITH McNEIL

INTRODUCTION

Following the identification of nitric oxide (NO) in 1986 as 'endothelium-derived relaxing factor', the explosive growth in understanding of the physiological role of NO has led to a Nobel Prize and its being named as 'molecule of the decade'.[1] Considerable research has been devoted to understanding the role of this molecule in vascular biology in general, and the pulmonary vascular system in particular.

NO is an unstable radical with a low blood-gas partition coefficient. It readily enters the gas phase, but can be dissolved. For decades NO was thought of as an environmental contaminant produced by bacteria and internal combustion engines. Considered highly toxic, it appeared an unlikely candidate for a major role as a biological mediator. However, within the last decade and a half, it has become clear that endogenously produced NO is ubiquitous in mammalian systems, playing an important role in the regulation of blood pressure and flow, inflammatory responses and neurotransmission in both health and disease states. Insight into these physiological roles has translated into its use as a therapeutic agent in a number of clinical settings. The role of this unique gas in the physiology and pathology of the pulmonary circulation, and its clinical applications are discussed in the following sections.

APPLIED CHEMISTRY AND PHYSICAL PROPERTIES OF NO

Among the various mediators released by the endothelium, NO is of major importance. In the lungs, one important molecule with which NO reacts is oxyhemoglobin (HbO_2). The affinity of HbO_2 for NO is 10^6 times greater than its affinity for O_2.[2] The rate constant for the reaction of NO with HbO_2 in solution is 3×10^7 mol/L·s and unlike O_2 there is little backward reaction.[3] Recent estimates of the half-life of NO in blood range from 0.05 to 1.8 ms.[4]

Oxidative reactions of NO with hemoglobin limit the effects of inhaled NO predominantly to the pulmonary vasculature. However, there are reports of peripheral vascular effects of high-concentration exogenous NO observed when local endothelial NO synthesis is blocked, suggesting that at least a portion of introduced NO survives for long enough to reach tissue remote from the lungs.[5]

Nitric oxide is a lipophilic, freely diffusible gas, more soluble in aqueous solutions than the other principal ligands of hemoglobin, namely oxygen (O_2) and carbon monoxide (CO). However, it is much less soluble than carbon dioxide (CO_2). On the basis of its solubility characteristics, it can be predicted that most of the NO produced in the lungs will rapidly redistribute to the gas phase.[6] This means the level of NO in exhaled air should be related to endogenous production.

The major immediate breakdown products of NO in human plasma are inactive nitroxides, such as nitrite (NO_2^-). The rate of this reaction increases exponentially with the concentration of both O_2 and NO.[7] This has several consequences. First, low NO concentrations or oxygen-free environments permit relatively long-term persistence of NO. Second, therapeutic efficacy of inhaled NO may not rise dramatically with increased doses as the more NO given, the faster it is oxidized.[8] In fact, higher doses of NO result in a relatively greater proportion of toxic products with little incremental yield of intact NO. Third, the rapid inactivation of inhaled NO in an O_2-rich environment is what makes NO a selective pulmonary vasodilator.

PHYSIOLOGICAL GENERATION OF NO

Because of its short half-life, NO must be generated continuously to be effective. The rate of NO production is determined by a variety of chemical and physical stimuli (Figure 130.1). Among physical stimuli, the shear stress exerted by blood flow on the arterial wall is one of the main factors regulating local NO release. Several neurohormonal mediators cause the release of NO through activation of specific endothelial receptors (Figure 130.1).

NO SYNTHASE (NOS) PATHWAY

The production of NO by the endothelium is dependent on the cellular conversion of L-arginine to L-citrulline[9] catalyzed by a group of enzymes, the NO synthases (NOS).[10] These enzymes can be broadly divided into two main families, namely the constitutive and the inducible forms.[11] One of the constitutive isoforms is present in endothelial cells, whereas the other is found in the nerve tissue. The endothelial constitutive NOS plays a key role in the modulation of vascular tone. The inducible isoforms are known to mediate cytotoxic activity of activated

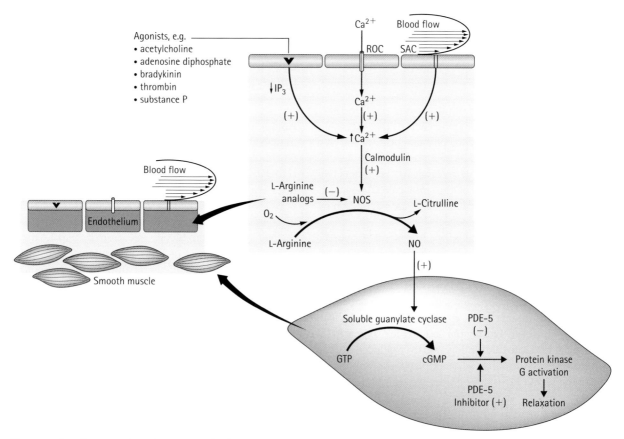

Figure 130.1 *The regulation of nitric oxide (NO) production and control of the vascular smooth muscle tone by endothelium. Receptor agonists and GTP-dependent protein (G protein) couples to the receptor generating a cytosolic messenger, inositol triphosphate (IP₃). NOS, nitric oxide synthase; PDE-5, phosphodiesterase type 5; ROC, receptor-operated non-selective cation channel. SAC, stretch-activated cation channel. See text for details.*

macrophages against numerous pathogens and intracellular micro-organisms.[12] In sepsis, induction of these isoforms leads to the pathological release of large amounts of NO, resulting in the profound systemic hypotension characteristic of septic shock.

The location of the human NOS genes have been assigned to chromosomes 7 and 12 for the endothelial and neuronal constitutive isoforms, respectively.[13] Polyclonal antibodies against various isoforms of the NO synthases have been purified and used for localization of the enzymes in tissues and organs. There is evidence that several cell types, including vascular endothelial cells, contain both the constitutive and inducible NO synthases.[14]

VASORELAXATION

In vascular smooth muscle, the molecular target of NO is the cytosolic enzyme guanylate cyclase.[12] Stimulation of the latter by NO increases the level of the second messenger cyclic guanosine monophosphate (cGMP) within vascular smooth muscle, promoting vasorelaxation through the protein kinase G (PKG) mechanism. cGMP is rapidly hydrolyzed within smooth muscle cells by cyclic nucleotide phosphodiesterases (PDE). In the lung, inhibition of PDE5 potentiates the vasorelaxant effect of NO. Administration of PDE5 inhibitors thus allows the use of much lower inhaled concentrations.[15] Along similar lines, angiotensin converting enzyme (ACE) inhibitors also prevent the breakdown of bradykinin, which stimulates the synthesis of NO. ACE inhibitors enhance the production of NO in endothelial cells, and treatment of animals with NOS inhibitors reduces the antihypertensive effect of ACE inhibitors in the systemic circulation.[16] Similar results have been reported in the hypoxic pulmonary hypertensive mouse model.[14]

The rise in intracellular level of cGMP also mediates many of the neural and other cardiovascular actions of NO. In addition, the NO-cGMP transduction system inhibits smooth muscle cell and fibroblast proliferation, platelet aggregation, and the nuclear transcription of leukocyte-binding adhesion molecules in endothelium[17] (see below also). This further highlights the pivotal role played by NO in the general homeostatic control of the vasculature.

PHYSIOLOGICAL ROLE OF NO IN THE PULMONARY CIRCULATION

Basal NO activity in normoxia

The demonstration of a basal release of NO in the pulmonary circulation is important because it likely explains the normal low pulmonary vascular tone under normoxic conditions. Studies of infusion of L-LMMA directly into the pulmonary circulation of the adults[18] and infants[19] found that inhibition of NO by an L-arginine analog significantly increased pulmonary vascular resistance and decreased pulmonary blood flow velocity in both adults and infants with normal pulmonary artery pressure at rest.

NO activity in response to acute hypoxia

Direct measurement of NO in cultured cells[20] or in expired air[21,22] has been shown to be decreased during acute hypoxia. However, the endothelial NOS knockout mouse does display increased susceptibility to hypoxia-induced pulmonary hypertension.[23] Therefore, despite some controversial results from early research, it appears that acute hypoxia-induced pulmonary hypertension leads to increased production of NO by the pulmonary endothelium, which serves to limit the rise in tone or pressure.

NO activity in experimental chronic hypoxia

In both human[24] and rat[25,26] lungs, basal release of NO seems to be preserved in chronic hypoxia. This conclusion comes from the observation of a raised basal pulmonary vascular tone after inhibition of either NO activity by methylene blue[24] or NO synthesis by various L-arginine analogs,[25,26] In addition, increased NOS expression was found in the lungs of rats exposed to chronic hypoxia. These results suggest that background NO activity is increased in the pulmonary circulation of chronically hypoxic rats, and that NO participates in a critical manner in the modulation of pulmonary vascular tone in both acute and chronic hypoxic pulmonary hypertension.

DOES NO CONTRIBUTE TO THE PATHO-PHYSIOLOGY OF PULMONARY VASCULAR DISEASES?

Human studies[27] of pre-contracted pulmonary artery rings from patients with COPD show full relaxation with the endothelium-independent agent, sodium nitroprusside, but only partial relaxation was achieved with endothelium-dependent vasodilators such as acetylcholine, adenosine diphosphate and the calcium ionophore A23187. Dinh-Xuan et al.[27] have shown that in patients with chronic hypoxic pulmonary hypertension, the more hypoxic the patients, the less the endothelium-dependent relaxation of pulmonary arterial rings. O_2 tension probably accounts for the reduced NO release in chronic hypoxic pulmonary hypertension. A likely explanation is that a long-term fall in O_2 tension affects expression of the gene encoding for constitutive endothelial enzyme NOS. Such regulatory mechanisms of gene expression by O_2 tension occur in other cellular processes.[28]

There remains some controversy between those reporting general reduction of expression of endothelial NOS in the pulmonary circulation of patients with primary pulmonary hypertension compared with control subjects,[29] and those suggesting normal expression.[30] Recently, an explanation has been found that in diseased lungs there is a patchy distribution of NOS compared with normal subjects. It is interesting to note that there is enhanced expression of endothelial NOS in the plexiform lesions of the PPH patient's lungs.[31] The suggestion is that diseased arteries lose endothelial NOS expression, while the plexiform lesions have enhanced expression. Similar controversies are around lung NO production. This may or may not reflect pulmonary vascular NO production. Some report enhanced[32] or preserved[33] NO generation in these patients. Similarly, patients with primary pulmonary hypertension have higher urinary cGMP concentrations than controls[34] and this parameter is inversely correlated with cardiac index and mixed venous oxygen saturation. These observations suggest that the pulmonary circulation responds to pulmonary hypertension by increasing synthesis of NO in an attempt to restore normal tone.

The effects of inhaled NO are thought to be restricted to the pulmonary vasculature because of its rapid inactivation by hemoglobin to form methemoglobin and nitrate. Recent animal studies, however, have shown that after infusion of a NOS inhibitor, inhaled NO does have effects on the systemic vasculature. This was shown by reduced systemic vascular resistance, increased kidney filtration rates, increased aortic cGMP levels, and restoration of blood flow to the intestine.[35] In humans, altered tubular salt and water reabsorption was observed in response to NO inhalation.[36] Cannon examined the contribution of blood-transported NO to regional vascular tone in humans before and during NO inhalation. Results of this study indicated that inhaled NO can supply intravascular NO to sites remote from the lungs, and thus contribute to the maintenance of normal vascular function.[5] This suggests that at least a portion of the NO introduced to the lungs via the inhaled route can be stabilized and transported in blood and is available peripherally to modulate blood flow.

THERAPEUTIC USES OF NO

Pepke-Zaba et al. reported the first clinical use of NO in 1991.[37] Inhaled NO therapy has subsequently been tried (with variable success) in a variety of disease states. These clinical situations have in common, either abnormalities of gas exchange based on low ventilation/perfusion ($\dot{V}/\dot{Q}$) ratios, and/or some form of pulmonary vascular endothelial dysfunction manifesting as increased pulmonary vascular resistance and right ventricular dysfunction.

The most widely recognized therapeutic application of NO is in the setting of pulmonary hypertension. As detailed above, NO acts as a direct smooth muscle relaxant via activation of the guanylate cyclase system. As such, it plays a pivotal role in endothelial-dependent control of vascular tone. By the same mechanism, NO contributes to regulation of bronchial smooth muscle tone, where, in addition, it acts as a neurotransmitter in non-adrenergic, non-cholinergic (NANC) bronchodilator nerves.[38]

Directly related to its vasodilating properties is the application of inhaled NO therapy in conditions complicated by gas exchange abnormalities. Because of its very short therapeutic half-life (seconds),[4] inhaled NO will predominantly vasodilate blood vessels in ventilated lung units only, thus maximizing $\dot{V}/\dot{Q}$ matching and improving gas exchange. This is in contrast to pulmonary vasodilators such as prostacyclin, which, administered systemically, have the potential to vasodilate the entire pulmonary vascular bed with the prospect of actually worsening $\dot{V}/\dot{Q}$ matching and gas exchange.

In many cases, pulmonary vascular disease and gas exchange problems coexist. Hypoxemia itself is a potent cause of pulmonary hypertension and the therapeutic target in this situation is improvement of $\dot{V}/\dot{Q}$ matching. NO in these situations is of benefit in both ameliorating the hypoxemia and lowering the PVR by direct pulmonary vasodilatation.

Therapeutic uses of NO in pulmonary arterial hypertension

The main indications in this setting have been primary pulmonary hypertension, congenital heart disease and persistent pulmonary hypertension of the newborn. NO has also been applied in the setting of pulmonary hypertension complicating conditions such as acute lung injury (also known as ARDS) and cardiac transplantation.

In addition to its therapeutic potential, NO can also be used to assess vasodilator responsiveness of the pulmonary circulation in patients with pulmonary arterial disease. In patients with PPH, it has been shown to be equivalent to prostacyclin in this respect.[39–41] Doses of 20–40 p.p.m. are conventionally used; however, additional responses in some patients have been demonstrated with doses of 80 p.p.m.[42]

A recent study compared the acute hemodynamic effects of inhaled NO and inhaled iloprost in 35 patients with PPH.[43] At the doses used (40 p.p.m. and 14–17 μg, respectively), iloprost was the more potent agent in improving the hemodynamic abnormalities, causing a significantly greater decline in pulmonary artery pressure (PAP) and pulmonary vascular resistance (PVR). In addition, inhaled iloprost was also associated with a beneficial effect on arterial oxygenation, reflecting its more potent effect on the pulmonary vasculature (improved $\dot{V}/\dot{Q}$ matching). The iloprost was, however, associated with systemic side effects in a number of patients attributable to systemic vasodilatation, much the same as is seen with intravenous prostacyclin.

This study also highlighted another issue with six of the 35 (17%) patients studied showing an increase in PVR. A similar finding was reported by Sitbon et al.[39] with 11 out of 35 (31%) showing an increase in PVR. The mechanism underlying this observation remains unclear; however, it has been shown that under certain (experimental) circumstances, NO can behave as a pulmonary vasoconstrictor.[44]

Use of NO in primary pulmonary hypertension (PPH)

The efficacy of long-term prostacyclin therapy in PPH has been firmly established. The need for continuous intravenous administration of this agent, however, has led to the search for alternative treatment options and inhaled NO offers several advantages in this setting. It is both a potent and selective pulmonary vasodilator[37] and because of its rapid inactivation by hemoglobin, it has none of the systemic (side) effects associated with systemically administered agents.[4]

A number of groups have reported the longer-term use of inhaled NO in patients with severe pulmonary hypertension.[44–47] Channick and Yung[45] reported the feasibility of using pulsed NO therapy delivered via a nasal cannula, as outpatient treatment for patients with PPH. Snell et al.[47] reported the use of inhaled NO as a bridge to lung transplantation in a patient with end-stage pulmonary hypertension. Currently, chronic use of NO in the ambulatory setting is limited by delivery systems, and there are as yet no long-term data for survival.

In addition to its direct vasodilator effect, NO has further potential benefits in pulmonary hypertension. It has been shown that NO is a potent inhibitor of smooth muscle cell migration, proliferation and matrix production,[17,42] probably via alteration in the gene expression for growth factors such as EGF (endothelial growth factor) and PDGF (platelet-derived growth factor).[48] This is clearly important in the treatment of a disease such as PPH, characterized by pulmonary vascular remodeling involving smooth muscle hyperplasia. In addition, NO inhibits platelet aggregation, again a potentially important action in a disease group where in situ thrombosis may play a role in the pathogenesis and progression of the condition.[49]

Eisenmenger's syndrome and congenital heart disease

There are few data available on the effect or use of NO in the setting of the established severe pulmonary hypertension characteristic of Eisenmenger's syndrome. Significant changes in the NO-cGMP axis are present in patients with pulmonary hypertension with alterations in nitric NOS activity demonstrated in remodeled pulmonary arteries.[29] Reduced endothelial NO production/release has been reported in children with congenital heart disease and associated pulmonary hypertension,[50] raising the possibility of using NO therapeutically in this group of patients.[51]

In children with congenital heart disease associated with a significant left-to-right shunt, inhaled NO has been used post-corrective surgery to reduce pulmonary artery pressure and improve gas exchange.[52–54] Although inhaled NO has been shown to be effective in reducing pulmonary pressures in this setting, the available data should be interpreted with caution. At least one case series showed no survival benefit where inhaled NO was used in the setting of severe postoperative pulmonary hypertension.[53]

In adults with Eisenmenger's syndrome, it has been shown that inhaled NO produces a dose-dependent increase in cGMP concentrations, associated with pulmonary vasodilatation in 29% of patients.[54] No response was seen in those with predominant right-to-left shunting, probably reflecting the fixed remodeling characteristic of more advanced disease.

Persistent pulmonary hypertension of the newborn (PPHN)

In this condition, elevated pulmonary vascular resistance results from persistence of the fetal circulation, with right-to-left shunting through the patent ductus arteriosus and foramen ovale. The resulting severe hypoxemia causes a vicious cycle, which if not reversed, is fatal.[55] In the era prior to inhaled NO therapy, PPHN was often refractory to therapy and no treatment was clearly associated with a reduction in mortality.[56] Inhaled NO therapy, however, has been reported to improve systemic oxygenation and outcome in this condition.[52,57–59]

Following the successful use in PPHN, inhaled NO has been used in a wide variety of pediatric conditions associated with lung disorders. Inhaled NO has been successful, but not equally effective, in many cases.[60]

Other pulmonary arteriopathy

There are no published data on the use of inhaled NO as a long-term therapy for the pulmonary vasculopathy associated with connective tissue diseases (such as scleroderma and systemic lupus erythematosus, etc.) or sarcoidosis.

NO has, however, been shown to be effective as a vasodilator challenge agent in these disorders, with short-term responsiveness equal to that seen with prostacyclin.[61,62] Prostacyclin therapy is an established treatment of the secondary pulmonary hypertension associated with these disorders,[61] and our own experience with these conditions suggests that the pulmonary vascular abnormalities respond to therapy in a very similar way to PPH.

THERAPEUTIC USE OF INHALED NO IN THE OPERATIVE SETTING

There are four main postoperative settings where inhaled NO is used to reduce pulmonary vascular resistance (PVR) and/or improve oxygenation. Its use postoperatively in children with congenital heart disease has been discussed above. The other three operative indications are pulmonary endarterectomy, heart transplantation and lung transplantation.

Pulmonary endarterectomy

Pulmonary endarterectomy is the treatment of choice in selected cases of chronic thromboembolic pulmonary hypertension.[63,64] In the immediate postoperative period, the PVR often remains elevated with a steady fall over the ensuing 24–48 hours. In the setting of chronic right ventricular dysfunction characteristic of this condition, any postoperative pulmonary hypertension is poorly tolerated. Pulmonary endarterectomy also results in pulmonary vascular endothelial dysfunction, manifesting in the first 12–24 hours post-procedure as reperfusion injury. This phenomenon results in non-cardiogenic pulmonary edema due to breakdown of the normal alveolar/capillary endothelial barrier. As a consequence, gas exchange is impaired and severe hypoxemia can result. This in turn stimulates an increase in the PVR (thus increasing RV afterload), as well as necessitating more intensive ventilatory support with the potential for barotrauma.

Strategies to support the RV include the use of inhaled NO to reduce the right ventricular afterload and improve gas exchange by optimizing $\dot{V}/\dot{Q}$ matching. Several cases reports[65,66] as well as one small crossover study (seven patients)[67] describe the efficacy of inhaled NO in this situation.

Heart transplantation

Chronic left ventricular dysfunction leads to an increase in the pulmonary vascular resistance. If significant, this is a contraindication to heart transplantation as it leads to graft (right ventricular) failure post-transplant.[68,69] If heart allograft (right ventricular) dysfunction does manifest post-transplant, any degree of pulmonary hypertension will exacerbate the problem and delay recovery of right ventricular function. Pre-transplant, the PVR of all potential recipients is assessed. Inhaled NO can be used in this situation to assess reversibility of pulmonary hypertension.

Strategies to support the struggling RV in the early post-heart-transplant period include the use of inhaled NO to reduce PVR.[70–73] Significant RV dysfunction will usually be evident with difficulty weaning from cardiopulmonary bypass. NO is used to aid weaning from bypass usually in conjunction with intra-aortic balloon counterpulsation and inotrope support (preferably with a phosphodiesterase inhibitor such as enoximone or milrinone). Inhaled NO can be continued in the ICU setting whilst the patient remains ventilated. If significant RV dysfunction persists after extubation, strategies to replace NO include inhaled iloprost or intravenous prostacyclin.

Use in lung transplantation

NO has been used in lung transplantation for a number of different indications. Reduced gene expression and activity of NO synthase has been demonstrated in a rat model of lung transplantation.[74]

In the presence of ischemia-reperfusion injury, inhaled NO has the potential to improve gas exchange via optimization of $\dot{V}/\dot{Q}$ matching. This reduces the need for high inspiratory and end-expiratory (PEEP) ventilator pressures, with a consequent reduction in the risk of barotrauma.

Ischemia-reperfusion injury results from a complex of pathophysiological processes.[75] Injury is initiated by ischemic endothelial damage, and augmented by the reperfusion response characterized by neutrophil activation and adherence to the damaged endothelium. NO may reduce the severity of this response by a number of mechanisms related to anti-inflammatory activity[76,77] (see also section on acute lung injury, below). There are now a number of publications reporting the clinical use of inhaled NO in the treatment of early allograft dysfunction,[78,79] but there are no controlled trials of this therapeutic application.

The third potential use for inhaled NO post-lung-transplant is in the setting of single or bilateral lung transplantation performed for severe pulmonary hypertension. If the ischemia-reperfusion injury is severe, the resulting hypoxemia and endothelial dysfunction results in pulmonary hypertension. A chronically stressed right ventricle, particularly following the cardioplegic arrest necessary for cardiopulmonary bypass, tolerates elevated pulmonary vascular resistance very poorly. Frank RV failure can occur, resulting in either an inability to wean from bypass or marked hemodynamic instability in the immediate postoperative period. NO can improve this situation both by directly reducing PVR, and improving gas exchange.

The donor lung has also become a target for NO therapy. It is postulated that by maintenance of endothelial integrity, leukocyte and platelet activation can be minimized with the potential to reduce subsequent reperfusion damage. In a porcine model of lung transplantation (non-heart-beating donors), the use of inhaled NO in the donors led to lower post-transplant PVR and lung injury scores.[80] In a rat model of isolated lung perfusion, pre- (but not post-) treatment with 10–50 p.p.m. of inhaled NO significantly reduced the microvascular leak associated with ischemia-reperfusion injury.[81] Several other studies using either inhaled NO or NO donors, support this contention.[82–84]

THERAPEUTIC USE OF NO IN ACUTE LUNG INJURY

Acute lung injury (ALI) or adult respiratory distress syndrome (ARDS) results from a variety of clinical situations including infection/sepsis, multiple trauma, cardiopulmonary bypass, etc. These all have in common an inflammatory insult to the lung, often in the setting of a systemic inflammatory response syndrome (SIRS), resulting in impaired gas exchange, reduced lung compliance, and in many cases, pulmonary hypertension with associated RV dysfunction.

Inhaled NO has been shown to reduce pulmonary hypertension and improve oxygenation in patients with ARDS.[85] Improvements in gas exchange occur in a high percentage of these patients with two-thirds showing a 20% improvement in oxygenation above baseline.

Levels of NO required to improve gas exchange are generally lower than those required to reduce pulmonary artery pressure. Physiologically inhaled NO (produced endogenously in the upper airways) corresponds to alveolar concentrations. The effects of exogenously administered NO may therefore simply be to replace the NO normally produced and inhaled from the upper airways, which are bypassed in intubated patients.[86]

NO may also be helpful in ARDS via a variety of anti-inflammatory effects. In rat models of lung injury, NO has been shown to reduce IL-1-induced neutrophil accumulation,[76] and damage caused by reactive oxygen species.[77] Inhaled NO was associated with a reduction in leukocyte-mediated mesenteric dysfunction,[87] a significant observation for two reasons. First, this effect was observed despite the rapid reaction of NO with heme groups, which is thought to limit downstream bioactivity (see above). Second, in the context of SIRS, the gut is thought to lose its natural antibacterial barrier function, with subsequent transudation of bacteria and toxins into the bloodstream. Protection of this function is therefore potentially of great significance in these situations.

Despite all the theoretical attractiveness and promise suggested by observational and retrospective studies using inhaled NO in ARDS,[85,86] randomized trials have produced disappointing results. Dellinger et al.[89] reported a placebo-controlled (nitrogen gas) trial of 177 patients with ARDS, using inhaled NO at concentrations from 1.25 to 80 p.p.m. After 28 days, mortality and duration of ventilation were the same between the two groups. Observed improvements in oxygenation and pulmonary hemodynamics were only temporary. In a more recent French study,[90] 203 patients with ARDS randomized to either inhaled NO 10 p.p.m. or placebo (nitrogen) showed again no difference in duration of ventilation or mortality.

CHRONIC OBSTRUCTIVE PULMONARY DISEASE

Pulmonary hypertension associated with COPD is a major cause of morbidity and mortality. Conventionally, this is treated with long-term oxygen therapy, with demonstrated improvements in survival. Inhaled NO has also been used in this setting.[91] In addition, a recent study (unpublished) looked at the safety and effectiveness of the combined use of oxygen and inhaled (pulsed) NO administered for 3 months to patients with pulmonary hypertension secondary to COPD. When compared with oxygen alone, the combined therapy was more effective in decreasing PVR and increasing cardiac output, with no increase in toxic reaction products of NO and oxygen (personal communication). The longer-term effectiveness of such strategies is not yet known.

HIGH–ALTITUDE PULMONARY EDEMA

In this situation, extreme alveolar hypoxia results in pulmonary hypertension and in susceptible individuals, HAPE. The effects of inhaled NO were studied in a high-altitude laboratory in 18 mountaineers known to be susceptible to the development of HAPE.[92] Pulmonary hypertension was attenuated by inhalation of NO. In addition, in those subjects who developed radiographic evidence of pulmonary edema, arterial oxygenation was improved by inhaling NO. It is likely that these beneficial effects reflect improved blood distribution ($\dot{V}/\dot{Q}$ matching) in the lungs.

TOXICITY OF INHALED NO

The practical issues of using NO therapeutically reflect the formation of nitrogen dioxide in the inhaled gases.

For this reason, continuous monitoring of NO, O_2 and NO_2 levels is important for anything other than very short-term therapy. In our experience, with modern delivery and monitoring systems, the use of NO for days to weeks is not associated with the production of significant levels of NO_2, and under normal circumstances the administration of inhaled NO to ventilated patients can be done very safely. In all cases, however, the lowest effective dose should be used.

Chronic ambulatory therapy, however, is a different situation. Delivery devices for this form of therapy are not as well developed as those designed for use in conjunction with a mechanical ventilator. In addition, it is very difficult to accurately monitor the dose delivered and NO_2 produced. Additionally, continuous monitoring of the inhaled and exhaled gases is impractical.

NO_2 can cause pulmonary edema and it may also be associated with histological changes in the lung. These changes are not seen with the very low levels normally associated with the clinical use of NO, requiring concentrations of NO_2 >2 p.p.m. for these changes to manifest. Low levels (as little as 0.4 p.p.m.) of NO_2 have, however, been associated with an increase in pro-inflammatory cytokine expression.[93]

In addition to NO_2, other oxidizing agents such as peroxynitrite can form when NO and O_2 interact. This compound has effects on surfactant, lipid peroxidation and induction of apoptosis. In one study, inhaled NO actually worsened reperfusion injury in rat lungs, ameliorated by the administration of superoxide dismutase concurrently with NO.[93] In addition, this effect could also be reduced by delaying administration of NO for the first 10 minutes of reperfusion.

NO therapy is associated with the development of methemoglobinemia. This occurs with the binding of NO to deoxyhemoglobin, the subsequent reduction to nitrate and nitrite, and conversion of hemoglobin iron from the ferrous to ferric state (methemoglobin). At normal clinical doses (up to 80 p.p.m.), however, this is not usually a problem, but it does require that the delivered NO concentration is accurately measured.

The final problem associated with the clinical use of inhaled NO, is the possibility of rebound pulmonary hypertension on withdrawal. This has been reported in a number of situations where an acute and potentially life-threatening rise in PVR was observed on withdrawal of inhaled NO.[94,95] This rebound phenomenon has been seen after only hours of therapy and is independent of initial response to NO – patients showing no pulmonary vasodilatation can show rebound pulmonary vasoconstriction on withdrawal. Our own experience, and that of others,[86] suggests that this rebound effect can be modified by slow weaning of the inhaled NO as opposed to sudden cessation of therapy.

It has been shown that inhaled NO decreases NOS activity[96,97] and increases plasma endothelin-1 (ET-1) concentrations.[98] In humans, the increased plasma ET-1 levels can remain elevated for up to 24 hours after discontinuation of inhaled NO.[99]

In anesthetized mechanically ventilated piglets with pulmonary hypertension, inhaled NO (short exposure, c. 30 minutes) was also associated with increased lung tissue expression as well as increased plasma concentrations of ET-1. Withdrawal of inhaled NO caused a rebound increase in pulmonary artery pressure and a further increase in plasma ET-1 levels.[100] Furthermore, recent data suggest that the reduced NOS activity involves endothelin (ET_A) receptor-mediated superoxide production and it appears that in this setting, endogenous NOS activity can be preserved with endothelin (ET_A) receptor antagonism, which prevents rebound pulmonary hypertension on withdrawal of NO.[101]

Results of current studies suggest that up-regulation of ET-1 and down-regulation of NOS activity contribute to the rebound reaction to withdrawal of inhaled NO, and this might be prevented by ET_A receptor antagonism.

KEY POINTS

- The pulmonary endothelial NO production and activity plays a pivotal role in the physiology of the pulmonary vasculature.
- NO participates in a critical manner in the modulation of pulmonary vascular tone in both acute and chronic pulmonary hypertension.
- The recent body of evidence suggests that in patients with primary pulmonary hypertension, endothelial expression has patchy distribution; diseased arteries show reduced expression while the plexiform lesions have enhanced expression of NOS in an attempt to restore normal tone.
- Inhaled NO is useful in many clinical circumstances, and properly administered there are very few disadvantages in trying it in clinical situations where pulmonary hypertension and/or hypoxemia is a problem. However, it is important that the limitations and potential hazards of this therapy are recognized.
- Most experience of the therapy has been gathered in the use of inhaled NO with mechanical ventilation. The use of inhaled NO in the chronic ambulatory setting is being investigated, with the major limitations at present being the delivery device and monitoring systems necessary to ensure accurate dosing.

REFERENCES

◆1 www.nobel.se/medicine/laureats/1998.

●2 Carlsen E, Comroe JH Jr. The rate of uptake of carbon monoxide and of nitric oxide by normal human erythrocytes and experimentally produced spherocytes. *J Gen Physiol* 1958;**42**: 83–107.

●3 Olson JS. Stopped-flow, rapid mixing measurement of ligand binding to haemoglobin and red cells. *Methods Enzymol* 1981;**76**:631–704.

●4 Borland C. Endothelium in control. *Br Heart J* 1991;**66**:405.

◆5 Cannon RO III, Schechter AN, Panza JA *et al.* Effects of inhaled nitric oxide on regional blood flow are consistent with intravenous nitric oxide delivery. *J Clin Invest* 2001;**108**: 279–87.

◆6 Glasstone S. *Textbook of physical chemistry.* London: Macmillan, 1940;686.

◆7 Ford PC, Wink DA, Standbury DM. Autoxidation kinetics of aqueous nitric oxide. *FEBS Lett* 1993;**326**:1–3.

◆8 Kinsella JP, Neish SR, Shaffer E *et al.* Low-dose inhalational nitric oxide in persistent pulmonary hypertension of the newborn. *Lancet* 1992;**340**:819–20.

◆9 Palmer RMJ, Ashton DS, Moncada S. Vascular endothelial cells synthesize nitric oxide from L-arginine. *Nature* 1988;**333**:664–6.

◆10 Palmer RMJ, Moncada S. A novel citrulline-forming enzyme implicated in the formation of nitric oxide by vascular endothelial cells. *Biochem Biophys Res Commun* 1989;**158**:348–52.

◆11 Forstermann U, Schmidt HHHW, Pollock JS *et al.* Isoforms of nitric oxide synthase: characterization and purification from different cell types. *Biochem Pharmacol* 1991; **10**:1849–57.

●12 Moncada S, Palmer RMJ, Higgs EA. Nitric oxide: physiology, pathophysiology and pharmacology. *Pharmacol Rev* 1991;**43**:109–42.

◆13 Robinson LJ, Weremowicz S, Morton CC *et al.* Isolation and chromosomal localization of the human endothelial nitric oxide synthase (*NOS3*) gene. *Genomics* 1994;**19**:350–7.

●14 Morrell NW, Morris KG, Stenmark KR. Role of angiotensin converting enzyme and angiotensin II in the development of the hypoxic pulmonary hypertension. *Am J Physiol* 1995;**269**:H1186–94.

●15 Ichinose F, Adrie C, Hurford WE *et al.* Prolonged pulmonary vasodilator action of inhaled nitric oxide by Zaprinast in awake lambs. *J Appl Physiol* 1995;**78**:1288–95.

●16 Cachofeiro V, Sakakibara T, Nasjletti A. Kinins, nitric oxide and the hypotensive effect of captopril and ramiprilat in hypertension. *Hypertension* 1992;**19**:138–45.

◆17 Ignaro LJ, Cirino G, Casini A *et al.* Nitric oxide as a signalling molecule in the vascular system: overview. *J Cardiovasc Pharmacol* 1999;**34**:8779–886.

●18 Stamler JS, Loh E, Roddy M-A *et al.* Nitric oxide regulates basal systemic and pulmonary vascular resistance in healthy humans. *Circulation* 1994;**89**:2035–40.

●19 Celermajer DS, Dollery C, Burch M *et al.* Role of endothelium in the maintenance of low pulmonary vascular tone in normal children. *Circulation* 1994;**89**:2041–4.

●20 Warren JB, Maltby NH, MacCormac D *et al.* Pulmonary endothelium-derived relaxing factor is impaired in hypoxia. *Clin Sci Lond* 1989;**77**:671–6.

●21 Cremona G, Higenbottam TW, Takao M *et al.* Exhaled nitric oxide in isolated pig lungs. *J Appl Physiol* 1995;**78**: 59–63.

●22 Gustafsson LE, Leone AM, Persson MG *et al.* Endogenous nitric oxide is present in the exhaled air of rabbits, guinea pigs and humans. *Biochem Biophys Res Commun* 1991;**181**:852–7.

●23 Fagan KA, Fouty BW, Tyler RC *et al.* The pulmonary circulation of homozygous and heterozygous eNOS-null mice is hyperresponsive to mild hypoxia. *J Clin Invest* 1999;**103**:991–9.

●24 Cremona G, Higenbottam TW, Dinh-Xuan AT *et al.* Inhibitors of endothelium-derived relaxing factor increase pulmonary vascular resistance in isolated perfused human lungs. Abstract *Eur Respir J* 1991;Suppl 14:336s.

●25 Zhao L, Crawley DE, Hughes JM *et al.* Endothelium-derived relaxing factor activity in rat lung during hypoxic pulmonary vascular remodelling. *J Appl Physiol* 1993;**74**:1061–5.

●26 Isaacson TC, Hampl V, Weir EK *et al.* Increased endothelium-derived NO in hypertensive pulmonary circulation of chronically hypoxic rats. *J Appl Physiol* 1994;**76**:933–40.

●27 Dinh-Xuan AT, Higenbottam TW, Clelland CA *et al.* Impairment of endothelium-dependent pulmonary artery relaxation in chronic obstructive lung disease. *N Engl J Med* 1991;**324**:1539–47.

●28 Fanburg BL, Massaro DJ, Gerutti PA *et al.* Regulation of gene expression by O_2 tension. *Am J Physiol* 1992;**262**:L235–41.

●29 Giad A, Saleh D. Reduced expression of endothelial nitric oxide synthase in the lungs of patients with pulmonary hypertension. *N Engl J Med* 1995;**333**:214–21.

●30 Xue C, Johns RA. Endothelial nitric oxide synthase in the lungs of patients with pulmonary hypertension [letter]. *N Engl J Med* 1995;**333**:1642–4.

●31 Springall DR, Mason NA, Burke M *et al.* Endothelial (Type III) nitric-oxide synthase is highly expressed in plexiform lesions in pulmonary hypertension. *J Pathol* 1996;**179**:A7.

●32 Archer SL, Djaballah K, Humbert M *et al.* Nitric oxide deficiency in fenfluoramine and dexfenfluoramine-induced pulmonary hypertension. *Am J Respir Crit Care Med* 1998;**158**:1061–7.

●33 Forrest IA, Small T, Corris PA. Effect of nebulised epoprostenol on exhaled nitric oxide in patients with pulmonary hypertension due to congenital heart disease and in normal controls. *Clin Sci* 1999;**97**:99–102.

●34 Bogdan M, Humbert M, Francoual J *et al.* Urinary cGMP concentrations in severe primary pulmonary hypertension. *Thorax* 1998;**53**:1049–62.

●35 Kielbasa WB, Fung HL. Systemic biochemical effects of inhaled NO in rats: increased expression of NOS III, nitrotirosine and phosphotyrosine-immunoreactive proteins in liver and kidney tissues. *Nitric Oxide* 2001;**5**:587–94.

●36 Wright WM, Young JD. Renal effects of inhaled nitric oxide in humans. *Br J Anaesth* 2001;**86**:267–9.

●37 Pepke-Zaba J, Higenbottam TW, Dinh-Xuan AT *et al.* Inhaled nitric oxide as a cause of selective pulmonary vasodilatation in pulmonary hypertension. *Lancet* 1991;**338**:1173–4.

●38 Dwelk RA, Comhair SAA, Gaston B *et al.* Nitric oxide chemical events in the human airway during the immediate and late antigen-induced asthmatic response. *Proc Natl Acad Sci USA* 2001;**98**:2622–7.

●39 Sitbon O, Brenot F, Denjean A *et al.* Inhaled nitric oxide as a screening vasodilator agent in primary pulmonary hypertension. A dose–response study and comparison with prostacyclin. *Am J Respir Crit Care Med* 1995;**151**:384–9.

●40 Jolliet P, Bulpa P, Thorens JB *et al.* Nitric oxide and prostacyclin as test agents of vasoreactivity in severe precapillary pulmonary hypertension: predictive ability and consequences on haemodynamics and gas exchange. *Thorax* 1997;**52**:369–72.

●41 Ricciardi MJ, Knight BP, Martinez FJ *et al.* Inhaled nitric oxide in primary pulmonary hypertension: a safe and effective agent for predicting response to nifedipine. *J Am Coll Cardiol* 1998;**32**:1068–73.

●42 Ignarro LJ, Buga GM, Wood KS *et al.* Endothelium-derived relaxing factor produced and released from artery and vein in nitric oxide. *Proc Natl Acad Sci USA* 1987;**84**:9265–9.

●43 Hoeper MM, Olschewski H, Hossein AG *et al.* A comparison of the acute hemodynamic effects of inhaled nitric oxide and aerosolized iloprost in primary pulmonary hypertension. *J Am Coll Cardiol* 2000;**35**:176–82.

●44 Voekel NF, Lobel K, Westcott JY *et al.* Nitric oxide-related vasoconstriction in lungs perfused with red cell lysate. *FASEB J* 1995;**5**:379–86.

●45 Channick RN, Yung GL. Long-term use of inhaled nitric oxide for pulmonary hypertension. *Respir Care* 1999;**44**:212–19.

●46 Koh E, Niimura J, Nakamura T *et al.* Long-term inhalation of nitric oxide for a patient with primary pulmonary hypertension. *Jpn Circ J* 1998;**62**:940–2.

●47 Snell GI, Salamonsen RF, Bergin P *et al.* Inhaled nitric oxide used as a bridge to heart-lung transplantation in a patient with end-stage pulmonary hypertension. *Am J Respir Crit Care Med* 1995;**151**:1263–6.

●48 Dweik RA. The promise and reality of nitric oxide in the diagnosis and treatment of lung disease. *Cleveland Clin J Med* 2001;**68**:486–93.

●49 Singh S, Evans TW. Nitric oxide, the biological mediator of the decade: fact or fiction? *Eur Respir J* 1997;**10**:699–707.

●50 Celermajer DS, Cullen S, Deanfield JE. Impairment of endothelium-dependent pulmonary artery relaxation in children with congenital heart disease and abnormal pulmonary haemodynamics. *Circulation* 1993;**87**:440–6.

●51 Atz AM, Adatia I, Jonas RA *et al.* Inhaled nitric oxide in children with pulmonary hypertension and congenital mitral stenosis. *Am J Cardiol* 1996;**77**:316–19.

●52 Journois D, Pouard P, Mauriat P *et al.* Inhaled nitric oxide as a therapy for pulmonary hypertension after operations for congenital heart defects. *J Thorac Cardiovasc Surg* 1994;**107**:1129–35.

●53 Sharma R, Raizada N, Choudhary SK *et al.* Does inhaled nitric oxide improve survival in operated congenital disease with severe pulmonary hypertension? *Indian Heart J* 2001;**53**:48–55.

●54 Budts W, Van Pelt N, Gillyns H *et al.* Residual pulmonary vasoreactivity to inhaled nitric oxide in patients with severe obstructive pulmonary hypertension and Eisenmenger syndrome. *Heart* 2001;**86**:553–8.

●55 Fox WW, Duara S. Persistent pulmonary hypertension in the neonate: diagnosis and management. *J Pediatr* 1983; **103**:505–14.

∗56 Walsh-Sukys MC, Tyson JE, Wright LL *et al.* Persistent pulmonary hypertension of the newborn in the era before nitric oxide: practice variation and outcomes. *Pediatrics* 2000;**105**:14–20.

∗57 Davidson D, Barefield ES, Kattwinkel J *et al.* Inhaled nitric oxide for the early treatment of persistent pulmonary hypertension of the term newborn: a randomized, double-masked, placebo-controlled, dose-response, multicenter study. *Pediatrics* 1998;**101**:325–34.

●58 Chen JY, Su PH, Chen FL *et al.* Inhaled nitric oxide in the management of persistent pulmonary hypertension of term infants. *J Formosan Med Assoc* 2001;**100**:703–6.

●59 Clark RH, Kueser T, Walker MW *et al.* Low-dose nitric oxide therapy for persistent pulmonary hypertension of the newborn. *N Engl J Med* 2000;**342**:469–74.

∗60 The Neonatal Inhaled Nitric Oxide Study Group. Inhaled nitric oxide in full-term and nearly full-term infants with hypoxic respiratory failure. *N Engl J Med* 1997;**336**:597–604.

●61 Jones K, Higenbottam T, Wallwork J. Pulmonary vasodilatation with prostacyclin in primary and secondary pulmonary hypertension. *Chest* 1989;**96**:784–9.

●62 Preston IR, Klinger JR, Landzberg MJ *et al.* Vasoresponsive-ness of sarcoidosis-associated pulmonary hypertension. *Chest* 2001;**120**:866–72.

◆63 Jamieson SW. Pulmonary thromboendarterectomy. *Heart* 1998;**79**:118–20.

◆64 Dunning J, McNeil KD. Pulmonary thromboendarterectomy for chronic thromboembolic pulmonary hypertension. *Thorax* 1999;**54**:755–8.

●65 Pinelli G, Mertes PM, Carteaux JP *et al.* Inhaled nitric oxide as an adjunct to pulmonary thromboendarterectomy. *Ann Thorac Surg* 1996;**61**:227–9.

●66 Gardeback M, Larsen FF, Radegran K. Nitric oxide improves hypoxaemia following reperfusion oedema after pulmonary thromboendarterectomy. *Br J Anaesth* 1995;**75**:798–800.

●67 Imanaka H, Miyano H, Takeuchi M *et al.* Effects of nitric oxide inhalation after pulmonary thromboendarterectomy for chronic pulmonary thromboembolism. *Chest* 2000; **118**:39–46.

◆68 Kirklin JK, Naftel DC, McGiffin DC *et al.* Analysis of morbid events and risk factors for death after cardiac transplantation. *J Am Coll Cardiol* 1988;**11**:917–24.

◆69 Kirklin JK, Naftel DC, Kirklin JW *et al.* Pulmonary vascular resistance and the risk of heart transplantation. *J Heart Transplant* 1988;**7**:331–6.

∗70 Stobierska-Dzierzek B, Awad H, Michler RE. The evolving management of acute right-sided heart failure in cardiac transplant recipients. *J Am Coll Cardiol* 2001;**38**:923–31.

●71 Ardehali A, Hughes K, Sadeghi A *et al.* Inhaled nitric oxide for pulmonary hypertension after heart transplantation. *Transplantation* 2001;**72**:638–41.

●72 Auler Junior JO, Carmona MJ, Bocchi EA *et al.* Low doses of inhaled nitric oxide in heart transplant recipients. *J Heart Lung Transplant* 1996;**15**:443–50.

∗73 Fullerton DA, McIntyre RC Jr. Inhaled nitric oxide: therapeutic applications in cardiothoracic surgery. *Ann Thorac Surg* 1996;**61**:1856–64.

●74 Luh SP, Tsai CC, Shau WY *et al*. The effects of inhaled nitric oxide, gabexate mesilate, and retrograde flush in the lung graft from non-heart beating minipig donors. *Transplantation* 2000;**69**:2019–27.

●75 Heffner JE. Mechanisms underlying ischemia/reperfusion injury of the lung. *Pulmon Edema* 1998;**116**:379–412.

●76 Guidot DM, Hybertson BM, Kitlowski RP *et al*. Inhaled NO prevents IL-1-induced neutrophil accumulation and associated acute edema in isolated rat lungs. *Am J Physiol* 1996;**271**:L225–9.

●77 Guidot DM, Repine MJ, Hybertson BM *et al*. Inhaled nitric oxide prevents neutrophil-mediated, oxygen radical-dependent leak in isolated rat lungs. *Am J Physiol* 1995;**269**:L2–5.

●78 Date H, Triantafillou AN, Trulock EP *et al*. Inhaled nitric oxide reduces human lung allograft dysfunction. *J Thorac Cardiovasc Surg* 1996;**111**:913–19.

●79 Kemming GI, Merkel MJ, Schallerer A *et al*. Inhaled nitric oxide (NO) for the treatment of early allograft failure after lung transplantation. *Intens Care Med* 1998;**24**:1173–80.

●80 Liu M, Tremblay L, Cassivi SD *et al*. Alterations of nitric oxide synthase expression and activity during rat lung transplantation. *Am J Physiol* 2000;**278**:L1071–81.

●81 Chetham PM, Sefton WD, Bridges JP *et al*. Inhaled nitric oxide pretreatment but not posttreatment attenuates ischemia-reperfusion-induced pulmonary microvascular leak. *Anesthesiology* 1997;**86**:895–902.

●82 Sunose Y, Takeyoshi I, Ohwada S *et al*. The effect of FK409 – a nitric oxide donor – on canine lung transplantation. *J Heart Lung Transplant* 2000;**19**:298–309.

●83 Fujino S, Nagahiro I, Yamashita M *et al*. Preharvest nitroprusside flush improves post-transplantation lung function. *J Heart Lung Transplant* 1997;**16**:1073–80.

●84 Fujino S, Nagahiro I, Triantafillou AN *et al*. Inhaled nitric oxide at the time of harvest improves early lung allograft function. *Ann Thorac Surg* 1997;**63**:1383–9.

●85 Rossaint R, Falke KJ, Lopez F *et al*. Inhaled nitric oxide for the adult respiratory distress syndrome. *N Engl J Med* 1993;**328**:399–405.

∗86 Braschi A, Iannuzzi M, Melliato M *et al*. Therapeutic use of nitric oxide in critical settings. *Monaldi Arch Chest Dis* 2001;**56**:177–9.

●87 Fox-Robichaud A, Payne D, Hasan SU *et al*. Inhaled NO as a viable antiadhesive therapy for ischemia/reperfusion injury of distal microvascular beds. *J Clin Invest* 1998;**101**:2497–505.

●88 Rossaint R, Gerlach H, Schmidt-Ruhnke H *et al*. Efficacy of inhaled nitric oxide in patients with severe ARDS. *Chest* 1995;**107**:1107–15.

∗89 Dellinger RP, Zimmerman JL, Taylor RW *et al*. Effects of Inhaled nitric oxide in patients with acute respiratory distress syndrome: results of a randomized phase II trial. *Crit Care Med* 1998;**26**:15–23.

∗90 Payden D, Vallet B. The Genoa Group. Results of the French prospective multicentre randomised double-blind placebo controlled trial on inhaled nitric oxide in ARDS. *Intens Care Med* 1999;**25**:S166.

●91 Katayama Y, Higenbottam TW, Diaz de Atauri MJ *et al*. Inhaled nitric oxide and arterial oxygen tension in patients with chronic obstructive pulmonary disease and severe pulmonary hypertension. *Thorax* 1997;**52**:20–4.

●92 Scherrer U, Vollenweider L, Delabays A *et al*. Inhaled nitric oxide for high-altitude pulmonary edema. *N Engl J Med* 1996;**334**:624–9.

●93 Eppinger MJ, Ward PA, Jones ML *et al*. Disparate effects of nitric oxide on lung ischemia-reperfusion inury. *Ann Thorac Surg* 1995;**60**:1169–75.

●94 Atz A, Adatia I, Wessel D. Rebound pulmonary hypertension after inhalation of nitric oxide. *Ann Thorac Surg* 1996;**62**:1759–64.

●95 Miller OI, Tang SF, Keech A *et al*. Rebound pulmonary hypertension on withdrawal from inhaled nitric oxide. *Lancet* 1995;**346**:51–2.

●96 Black SM, Heidersbach RS, McMullan DM *et al*. Inhaled nitric oxide inhibits NOS activity in lambs: a potential mechanism for rebound pulmonary hypertension. *Am J Physiol* 1999;**277**:H1849–56.

●97 Sheehy AM, Burson MA, Black SM. Nitric oxide exposure inhibits endothelial NOS activity but not gene expression: a role for superoxide. *Am J Physiol* 1998;**274**:L833–41.

●98 McMullan DM, Bekker JM, Johengen MJ *et al*. Inhaled nitric oxide-induced rebound pulmonary hypertension: a role for endothelin-1. *Am J Physiol* 2001;**280**:H777–85.

●99 Pearl JM, Nelson DP, Raake JL *et al*. Inhaled nitric oxide increases endothelin-1 levels: a potential cause of rebound pulmonary hypertension. *Crit Care Med* 2002;**30**:89–93.

●100 Chen L, He H, Femandez Mondejar E *et al*. Endothelin-1 and nitric oxide synthase in short rebound reaction to short exposure to inhaled nitric oxide. *Am J Physiol Heart Circ Physiol* 2001;**281**:H124–31.

●101 Wedgwood S, McMullan DM, Bekker JM *et al*. Role for endothelin-1-induced superoxide and peroxynitrite production in rebound pulmonary hypertension associated with inhaled nitric oxide. *Circ Res* 2001;**89**:357–64.

Endothelin receptor antagonists

DOUGLAS HELMERSEN, RICHARD N CHANNICK AND LEWIS J RUBIN

INTRODUCTION

The endothelins are a family of 21-amino acid peptides that play a key role in the regulation of vascular tone. The first member of this family identified was endothelin-1 (ET-1), a 2492 Dalton peptide with potent vasoconstrictor properties, isolated by Yanagisawa and colleagues in 1988.[1] Two additional endothelin isopeptides, endothelin-2 (ET-2) and endothelin-3 (ET-3), were subsequently discovered.[2] All three of these proteins share a high degree of amino acid homology. They also bear structural similarity to a family of peptides labeled sarafotoxins which are isolated from the venom of the snake *Atractaspis engaddensis*, suggesting a possible shared evolutionary origin.[3]

Vascular endothelial cells are the major source of endothelins in humans. However, genes encoding the endothelin peptides are also found in a wide range of additional cell types including bronchial epithelium, macrophages, cardiac myocytes, glomerular mesangium and glial cells, to name but a few.[4–7]

The 15 years following the discovery of endothelins have seen an explosion of basic research into these compounds.[8] This has led clinicians to postulate numerous potential applications to the manipulation of the endothelin system, including the treatment of renal diseases, systemic hypertension and cerebral vasospasm.[8,9]

It is in the therapy of pulmonary vascular disease, however, that endothelin biology has, thus far, shown its greatest penetration into the clinical arena. This chapter reviews the current understanding of the role of endothelins in the physiology and pathophysiology of the pulmonary circulation, as well as the clinical experiences gained from the use of endothelin receptor antagonists in the treatment of pulmonary arterial hypertension.

PHYSIOLOGY

Although marked structural similarity amongst the endothelins results in significant areas of overlapping biological function, these compounds are not as similar as they first may appear. The human genes for ET-1, ET-2 and ET-3 are each located on different chromosomes.[8] Furthermore, the distribution of the three endothelin proteins throughout different tissues appears to be quite heterogeneous. Endothelial cells, including those of the pulmonary circulation, predominantly generate ET-1. Kidney cells appear to express higher levels of ET-2.[10] ET-3 has been found in high concentrations in the intestine and brain[11,12] Each of these three compounds seem to have distinct physiological roles that guide their site(s) of expression. Our understanding of these unique yet overlapping roles remains incomplete.

Investigators have focused in particular on the physiology of ET-1, due to its prominent role in vascular control. The molecular mechanisms of ET-1 activity merit review (even in a clinical text), not only because of their emerging clinical relevance but also because they represent novel pathways in the regulation of the pulmonary circulation.

Endothelin-1 production

The human ET-1 gene is located on the telomeric region of chromosome 6p.[8] The ET-1 gene includes five exons that

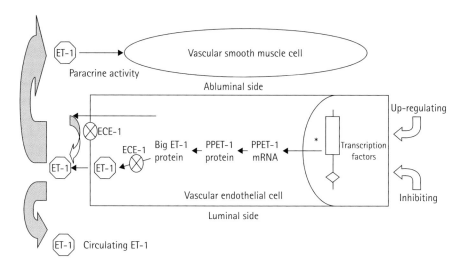

Figure 13P.1 *Schematic illustration of production of endothelin-1 (ET-1) by pulmonary artery endothelial cells. PPET-1, preproendothelin-1; mRNA, messenger ribonucleic acid; ECE-1, endothelin-1 converting enzyme; *rate-limiting step.*

Table 13P.1 *Transcriptional regulation of endothelin-1 production*

Up-regulating factors
Angiotensin II[65]
Norepinephrine[12]
Vasopressin[65]
TGF-β[66]
TNF-α[67]
Thrombin[68]
Interleukin-1[69]
Bradykinin[70]
Low shear stress[71]
Oxidated low density lipoproteins[72]
Hypoxia[12]

Inhibiting factors
Nitric oxide[12]
Atrial natriuretic peptide[73]
Brain natriuretic peptide[73]
Prostacyclin[12]
Prostaglandin E_2[2]
Endothelin-3[12]

TGF-β, transforming growth factor β; TNF, tumor necrosis factor.

encode mRNA for a large precursor protein: prepro-endothelin-1 (PPET-1). The intermediate steps between transcription of PPET-1 and release of ET-1 from the endothelial cell are summarized in Figure 13P.1.

Unlike some other proteins, ET-1 is not kept in secretory granules[13] within cells. The rate-limiting step in the biosynthesis of ET-1 occurs at the level of transcription.[1] Many stimuli that regulate ET-1 production have evolved through direct action upon transcription factors (Table 13P.1). It appears that vascular endothelial cells are able to rapidly increase or inhibit ET-1 production to regulate vascular tone.[14]

The majority of ET-1 secreted from cultured endothelial cells occurs from the abluminal side of the cells towards the adjacent vascular smooth muscle cells, which contain specific endothelin receptors.[15] Thus, it is important to note that although circulating ET-1 can be detected in the plasma, and may have important clinical correlations with pulmonary vascular disease, these plasma levels may not necessarily reflect the paracrine action of ET-1 on adjacent smooth muscle cells.

Endothelin receptors

There are two distinct receptors for the endothelin family of peptides, endothelin receptor A (ET_A) and endothelin receptor B (ET_B). The endothelin receptors belong to the family of receptors connected to guanine nucleotide-binding (G) proteins.[16] The two receptors have unique locations[17] and binding affinities[10] for the endothelin peptides. ET_A receptors are expressed on pulmonary vascular smooth muscle cells, and have high affinity for ET-1 and ET-2, with lower affinity for ET-3. ET_B receptors are located on both pulmonary vascular endothelial cells and smooth muscle cells. ET_B receptors bind all three endothelin isoforms with nearly equal affinity.

When activated, the ET_A receptor located in pulmonary vascular smooth muscle cells mediates vasoconstriction. The mechanism is thought to occur via G-protein-induced phospholipase C activation, 1,4,5-inositol triphosphate (IP_3) formation, and the consequent release of Ca^{2+} from intracellular stores.[16] There is some evidence that ET_A receptor may also increase intracellular calcium by activating non-selective calcium channels on the surface of the smooth muscle cell.[18] The vasoconstriction induced by ET_A has been shown to persist even after ET-1 is removed from the receptor, likely due to persistently elevated concentrations of intracellular Ca^{2+}.[19]

In addition to its powerful vasoconstricting effects, ET-1 is known to be a potent mitogen, with the ability to induce cell proliferation in a number of cell types, including vascular smooth muscle cells.[20] It has been shown that the mitogenic actions of ET-1 are mediated by both the ET_A[21] and ET_B[22] receptors.

In the pulmonary vasculature, ET_B receptors are predominantly expressed on endothelial cells.[23,24] ET_B receptors on endothelial cells mediate vasodilation via increased production of nitric oxide and prostacyclin.[24–26] Nitric oxide and prostacyclin also negatively feedback on ET-1 activity by inhibition of PPET-1 transcription (see Figure 13P.1).

ET_B receptors contribute to the clearance of circulating ET-1, likely owing to internalization of the ET-1/ET_B receptor complex into the cell after binding.[27]

It has been observed that the normal human lung removes roughly 50% of circulating ET-1, and that it releases a similar quantity, resulting in the lack of an arterial-to-venous ET-1 gradient across the pulmonary vasculature in the normal state.[28]

There are data suggesting that the ET_B receptor does not exclusively mediate pulmonary vasodilation. Under some circumstances it may actually contribute to pulmonary vasoconstriction, through a population of ET_B receptors located on vascular smooth muscle cells.[29] The vasoconstrictive actions of ET_B receptor may become more pronounced in the pathological setting of pulmonary hypertension[30] than in the normal pulmonary vasculature. It has been postulated that this action may result from down-regulation of ET_A receptors in states of pulmonary hypertension, possibly as an adaptive response to high levels of circulating ET-1.[31]

The vasoconstrictive actions of the ET_B receptor may confer a therapeutic advantage to the strategy of dual ET_A/ET_B receptor blockade over selective ET_A receptor blockade in the treatment of pulmonary arterial hypertension.

PATHOPHYSIOLOGY

The endothelins are thought to participate in the pathophysiology of a spectrum of pulmonary vascular diseases. The extent to which the endothelin system is involved in each disease affecting the pulmonary circulation is not completely understood; however, similarities in the pathogenesis of this family of disorders suggest that endothelin biology has broad applicability. The evidence for the role of the endothelin system in the pathophysiology of several individual pulmonary vascular diseases is reviewed here.

Primary pulmonary hypertension

Patients with primary pulmonary hypertension (PPH) demonstrate higher serum levels of ET-1 and higher arterial-to-venous ratios of ET-1 than healthy controls.[32] This phenomenon may represent increased production of ET-1 by the lung, reduced clearance by the lung, or a combination of these processes. Lung specimens from patients with PPH, when compared to those from patients without pulmonary hypertension, exhibit increased ET-1 staining of the muscular pulmonary arteries and increased expression of PPET-1 in the endothelial cells of the same vessels.[33] There is, furthermore, a correlation between the intensity of staining for ET-1 and the patients' hemodynamic measurements of pulmonary vascular resistance. Recent studies have shown increased endothelin-1 converting enzyme (ECE-1) in the pulmonary vascular endothelial cells of PPH patients[34] and increased net pulmonary clearance of ET-1 in patients with PPH treated with continuous intravenous epoprostenol.[35]

Other pulmonary vascular diseases

PULMONARY HYPERTENSION FROM CHRONIC HYPOXIA

Pulmonary hypertension from chronic hypoxia has been shown in animal models to be associated with increased ET-1 and ET_A expression.[36,37] In these models, it is also notable that dual ET_A/ET_B receptor blockade resulted in amelioration of pulmonary hypertensive changes.[38] Interestingly, rat models have also demonstrated regional differences in endothelin expression throughout the lung, leading some authors to suggest that heterogeneity of the endothelin system may help to regulate local responses to hypoxia in the pulmonary circulation.[39,40] Detailed human investigations into the role of the endothelin system in chronic hypoxemia have not been reported to date.

PULMONARY HYPERTENSION FROM CONGENITAL CARDIAC DISEASE

Pulmonary hypertension from congenital cardiac disease has been shown in human investigations to correlate with high levels ET_A receptor density and circulating ET-1, which in some instances decreased following surgical correction of the cardiac lesions.[41–43] The development of hypoxemia in patients with congenital shunts may be an additional factor which magnifies the detrimental effects of ET-1.[44]

CHRONIC THROMBOEMBOLIC PULMONARY HYPERTENSION

Chronic thromboembolic pulmonary hypertension (CTEPH) has been associated with increased activity of the ET-1 system in both animal[45,46] and human[47] pathological studies. Pulmonary hypertensive changes were attenuated in the presence of dual ET_A/ET_B receptor blockade in a canine model of CTEPH.[45] It is known that many patients with CTEPH have a concomitant small vessel vasculopathy which can limit the hemodynamic improvement following pulmonary thromboendarterectomy. These data suggest that endothelin may play a role in this process.

PERSISTENT PULMONARY HYPERTENSION OF THE NEWBORN

Persistent pulmonary hypertension of the newborn (PPHN) has been associated with increased ET-1 expression and ETA receptor activity in a number of animal studies, involving several different models of PPHN.[48–51] Clinical studies of human babies with PPHN[52–55] have also revealed elevated levels of circulating ET-1, which appear to correlate with other markers of disease severity.

CLINICAL USE OF ENDOTHELIN RECEPTOR ANTAGONISTS

Selective ET$_A$ receptor antagonists

The compound sitaxsentan possesses high selective affinity for the ET$_A$ receptor. Barst and colleagues[56] studied sitaxsentan in a small open-label 12-week study in patients with PAH. The population consisted of three patients with PPH, two with associated connective tissue disorders, and nine with congenital heart defects. There was a trend in this study population towards improved 6-minute walk testing (6MWT), mean pulmonary artery pressure, cardiac index and pulmonary vascular resistance. Adverse effects attributed to sitaxsentan in this study, as well as another study in which the drug was used for chronic congestive heart failure,[57] included elevated liver function tests, other gastrointestinal symptoms, nasal congestion and flushing.

There have been no placebo-controlled trials of ET$_A$ receptor antagonists in PAH to date. Clinical comparisons of ET$_A$ receptor antagonists and dual ET$_A$/ET$_B$ antagonists have not been performed in humans.

Dual ET$_A$/ET$_B$ receptor antagonists

A number of dual endothelin receptor antagonists have been developed in the laboratory. The majority of clinical experience is with the compound bosentan (Ro 47-0203, Tracleer), which was recently approved for clinical use by the federal drug administration in the USA. Bosentan is an antagonist of both the ET$_A$ and ET$_B$ receptors, with only slightly higher *in vitro* affinity for the ET$_A$ receptor.

BOSENTAN – PRE-CLINICAL STUDY

An acute study[58] of bosentan in humans involved intravenous infusions of the drug to seven patients with PAH (five PPH, two with associated scleroderma). The hemodynamic response was a dose-dependent fall in the mean

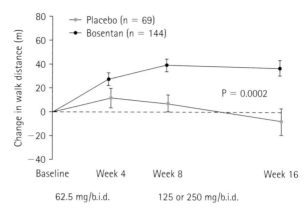

Figure 13P.2 *Six-minute walk test improvement in patients receiving bosentan for 12 weeks compared to placebo in a pilot study of 32 patients. (Reproduced with permission from Channick R, Simonneau G, Sitbon O et al. Effects of the dual endothelin-receptor antagonist bosentan in patients with pulmonary hypertension: a randomized placebo controlled study. Lancet 2001;358:1119–23.)*

pulmonary artery pressure but also in the mean arterial pressure. This study prompted the question of whether chronic doses of Bosentan were required for a significant and selective pulmonary vascular effect.

BOSENTAN – CLINICAL TRIALS

The first multicenter, randomized, placebo-controlled study of chronic oral bosentan was performed in 32 patients with pulmonary arterial hypertension due to PPH (n = 27) or associated with scleroderma (n = 5).[59] Recruited patients were all WHO functional class III. Mean baseline pulmonary artery pressures were approximately 55 mmHg. There was 2:1 randomization to the bosentan group in relation to placebo. Patients in the bosentan group received the drug at a dose of 62.5 mg twice daily for 4 weeks followed by 125 mg twice daily. Concurrent therapy with digoxin, anticoagulants, diuretics and calcium channel blockers was permitted; however, patients receiving epoprostenol were excluded. The primary endoint was exercise capacity, as measured by 6MWT, and secondary end points included hemodynamic improvement by right heart catheterization, change in functional class, and time to clinical worsening – all measured at 12 weeks. The intention-to-treat analysis demonstrated statistically significant improvements in the bosentan group compared to placebo in 6MWT (Figure 13P.2) and pulmonary hemodynamics (cardiac output, pulmonary vascular resistance, mean pulmonary arterial pressure).

A subsequent larger double-blind, placebo-controlled study of bosentan in PAH[60] enrolled 213 patients with PAH due to PPH (n = 150), scleroderma (n = 47), and systemic lupus erythematosus (n = 16). All patients belonged to WHO III or IV functional class. Baseline parameters

Figure 13P.3 *Six-minute walk improvement in patients on bosentan in a pivotal study. Patients receiving placebo had a decline in 6-minute walk distance. (Reproduced with permission from Rubin LJ, Badesch DB, Barst RJ et al. Bosentan therapy for pulmonary arterial hypertension. N Engl J Med 2002;346:896–903.)*

included mean 6MWT of approximately 330 metres, and mean pulmonary artery pressures of approximately 55 mmHg. Patients randomized to the bosentan group received 62.5 mg twice daily for 4 weeks, then either 125 mg twice daily (n = 74) or 250 mg twice daily (n = 70) for an additional 12 weeks, compared to placebo (n = 69). The primary end point was functional status as measured by the 6MWT at 16 weeks. The results in this trial (intention to treat) also showed a statistically significant improvement in 6MWT in both bosentan groups compared to placebo (Figure 13P.3). Analysis of secondary measures of efficacy revealed a trend in the bosentan groups towards lower Borg dyspnea indices and improved functional class. There was also a statistically significant increase in the bosentan groups in time to clinical worsening, as measured by the composite end point of time to death, lung transplantation, hospitalization, or study dropout because of worsening pulmonary hypertension, need for epoprostenol therapy, or atrial septostomy.

BOSENTAN – SAFETY

Bosentan is a highly substituted pyrimidine derivative that is primarily eliminated by hepatic metabolism through the P450 enzyme systems CYP2C9 and CYP3A4. Steady-state levels are usually achieved after 3–5 days with twice daily dosing. Upon reaching steady state, the elimination half-life becomes constant. One metabolite of bosentan (Ro 48-5033) is pharmacologically active but is thought to contribute less than 20% of the clinical response to bosentan. Renal clearance of bosentan appears to be negligible.

There is clinical evidence to suggest that bosentan administration can precipitate hepatocellular injury, particularly at higher doses. Combined data from existing clinical trials reveals greater than threefold elevations

of the aminotransferases in 11% of bosentan patients (n = 658) compared with 2% of patients given placebo (n = 280). This effect was observed both early and late in treatment. The more severe elevations in aminotransferases were observed in the patients receiving 250 mg twice daily or higher. The liver abnormalities were often asymptomatic and all resolved with dose reduction or cessation. In some patients, reintroduction of bosentan did not lead to recurrent hepatic enzyme elevations. Studies in rats have revealed that bosentan-induced liver injury is likely mediated by drug-induced inhibition of the hepatocanalicular bile-salt export pump.[61]

A treatment regimen including bosentan must include monitoring of alanine aminotransferase (ALT) and aspartate aminotransferase (AST) prior to drug initiation and monthly thereafter. Patients with significant baseline elevations of the aminotransferases should not be given bosentan. In patients with hepatic congestion from right heart failure, aggressive diuresis may correct abnormal aminotransferases occurring solely on this basis, and consequently requalify these patients for bosentan.

Bosentan is contraindicated in pregnancy. Animal models reveal that the endothelin peptides appear to play an important role in fetal development. ET-1 has been implicated in the closure of the ductus arteriosus at birth.[62] Mice with ET-1 deficiency[63] and those given bosentan (product monograph, Actelion Pharmaceuticals USA, Inc.) as fetuses develop severe craniofacial abnormalities. Pregnancy must be excluded prior to therapy with bosentan and prevented thereafter with reliable contraception. Hormonal forms of contraception may not be reliable in the setting of bosentan therapy, and thus should not be the sole form of contraception in females of childbearing potential. Other common side effects observed with bosentan include a dose-related decrease in hemoglobin of unknown etiology, headaches and flushing.

A number of drugs have been shown to interact with bosentan through the P450 system. Glyburide and cyclosporin A are contraindicated with concurrent bosentan therapy. Although a small study has shown that humans given bosentan 500 mg twice daily have reduced the effect of warfarin,[64] no influence on warfarin activity has been seen in the clinical trials using the 125 mg and 250 mg twice daily doses of bosentan.

BOSENTAN – ROLE IN THE CONTEXT OF EXISTING TREATMENTS FOR PAH

Bosentan received approval in 2001/2002 by a number of regulatory agencies, including those in Canada and the USA. The approved indications are PAH, functional class III or IV. As with all new medical therapies, there remains much to learn about the precise role of bosentan in the existing medical regime for PAH. For WHO functional class III and possibly early class IV patients who are not acutely vasoreactive or who have failed calcium channel blocker therapy, bosentan should be considered the initial treatment of choice, based on the available clinical trials. For patients with significant hemodynamic decline, or those who progress to WHO functional class IV, epoprostenol (Flolan) remains the initial therapy of choice.

The addition of bosentan to epoprostenol is a potentially attractive approach, as the two agents work through different and possibly complementary mechanisms. A randomized controlled trial of combined epoprostenol-bosentan has recently been completed.

Future directions

The next steps in the research of endothelin receptor antagonists for the therapy of PAH appear to have great promise. Questions which remain to be answered include the role of endothelin receptor antagonists in:

- early PAH, including WHO classes I and II;
- upfront combination therapies, for example with epoprostenol or sildenafil;
- additive therapy to existing epoprostenol patients; and
- expanded disease indications, such as CTEPH or fibrotic lung disease.

The ease of oral administration and relatively well tolerated side effect profile of endothelin receptor antagonists will likely allow them to provide continued advances in the therapy of a range of diseases of the pulmonary circulation.

KEY POINTS

- Endothelin-1 is produced by pulmonary vascular endothelial cells.
- Endothelin receptor A is located on pulmonary vascular smooth muscle cells, and mediates vasoconstriction.
- Endothelin receptor B is located on both the endothelial and smooth muscle cells, and can mediate either vasoconstriction or vasodilation.
- The endothelins play a role in the pathophysiology of a variety of pulmonary vascular diseases.
- The dual endothelin receptor antagonist bosentan has been shown in two clinical trials to have efficacy in PAH patients with WHO class III functional status.
- Bosentan can precipitate hepatocellular injury at higher doses; its use requires monthly monitoring of liver tests.

REFERENCES

●1 Yanagisawa M, Kurihara H, Kimura S et al. A novel potent vasoconstrictor peptide produced by vascular endothelial cells. Nature 1988;**332**:411–15.

2 Inoue A, Yanagisawa M, Kimura S et al. The human endothelin family: three structurally and pharmacologically distinct isopeptides predicted by three separate genes. Proc Natl Acad Sci USA 1989;**86**:2863–7.

3 Takasaki C, Tamiya N, Bdolah A et al. Sarafotoxins S6: several isotoxins from Atractaspis engaddensis (burrowing asp) venom that affect the heart. Toxicon 1988;**26**:543–8.

4 Mattoli S, Mezzetti M, Riva G et al. Specific binding of endothelin on human bronchial smooth muscle cells in culture and secretion of endothelin-like material from bronchial epithelial cells. Am J Respir Cell Mol Biol 1990;**3**:145–51.

5 Yu J, Davenport A. Secretion of endothelin-1 and endothelin-3 by human cultured vascular smooth muscle cells. Br J Pharmacol 1995;**114**:551–7.

6 Ehrenreich H, Anderson RW, Fox CH et al. Endothelins, peptides with potent vasoactive properties, are produced by human macrophages. J Exp Med 1990;**172**:1741–8.

◆7 Miyauchi T, Masaki T. Pathophysiology of endothelin in the cardiovascular system. Ann Rev Physiol 1999;**61**:391–415.

◆8 Michael J, Markewitz B. Endothelins and the lung. Am J Respir Crit Care Med 1996;**154**:555–81.

9 Benigni A, Remuzzi G. Endothelin antagonists. Lancet 1999;**353**:133–8.

10 Masaki T. The discovery of endothelins. Cardiovasc Res 1998;**39**:530–3.

11 Shinmi O, Kimura S, Sawamura T et al. Endothelin-3 is a novel neuropeptide: isolation and sequence determination of endothelin-1 and endothlin-3 in porcine brain. Biochem Biophys Res Commun 1989;**164**:587–93.

◆12 Levin E. Endothelins. N Engl J Med 1995;**333**:356–63.

13 Nakamura S, Naruse M, Naruse K et al. Immunocytochemical localization of endothelin in cultured bovine endothelial cells. Histochemistry 1990;**94**:475–7.

14 Inoue A, Yanagisawa M, Takuwa Y et al. The human preproendothelin-1 gene. Complete nucleotide sequence and regulation of expression. J Biol Chem 1989; **264**:14954–9.

15 Yoshimoto S, Ishizaki Y, Sasaki T et al. Effect of carbon dioxide and oxygen on endothelin production by cultured porcine cerebral endothelial cells. Stroke 1991;**22**:378–83.

16 Takuwa Y, Kasuya Y, Takuwa N et al. Endothelin receptor is coupled to phospholipase C via pertussis toxin insensitive guanine nucleotide binding regulatory protein in vascular smooth muscle cells. J Clin Invest 1990;**85**:653–8.

17 Benigni A. Defining the role of endothelins in renal pathophysiology on the basis of selective and unselective endothelin receptor antagonist studies. Curr Opin Nephrol Hypertens 1995;**4**:349–53.

18 Iwamuro Y, Miwa S, Zhang XF et al. Activation of three types of voltage-independent Ca^{2+} channel in A7r5 cells by endothelin-1 as revealed by a novel Ca^{2+} channel blocker LOE 908. Br J Pharmacol 1999;**126**:1107–14.

19 Clarke J, Benjamin N, Larkin SW *et al*. Endothelin is a potent long-lasting vasoconstrictor in men. *Am J Physiol* 1989;**257**:H2033–5.

20 Chua BH, Krebs CJ, Chua CC *et al*. Endothelin stimulates protein synthesis in smooth muscle cells. *Am J Physiol* 1992;**262**:E412–16.

21 Davie N, Haleen SJ, Upton PD *et al*. ET_A and ET_B receptors modulate the proliferation of human pulmonary artery smooth muscle cells. *Am J Respir Crit Care Med* 2002;**165**:398–405.

22 Sugawara F, Ninomiya H, Okamoto Y *et al*. Endothelin-1-induced mitogenic responses of Chinese hamster ovary cells expressing human endothelin A: the role of a wortmannin-sensitive signalling pathway. *Mol Pharmacol* 1996;**49**:447–57.

●23 Sakurai T, Yanagisawa M, Takuwa Y *et al*. Cloning of a cDNA encoding a non-isopeptide-selective subtype of the endothelin receptor. *Nature* 1990;**348**:732–5.

24 Hirata Y, Emori T, Eguchi S. Endothelin receptor subtype B mediates synthesis of nitric oxide by cultured bovine endothelial cells. *J Clin Invest* 1993;**91**:1367–73.

25 De Nucci G, Thomas R, D'Orleans-Juste P *et al*. Pressor effects of circulating endothelin are limited by its removal in the pulmonary circulation and by the release of prostacyclin and endothelium-derived relaxing factor. *Proc Natl Acad Sci USA* 1988;**85**:9797–800.

26 Filep JG, Herman F, Battistini B *et al*. Antiaggregatory and hypotensive effects of endothelin-1 in beagle dogs: role for prostacyclin. *J Cardiovasc Pharmacol* 1991;**17** (Suppl 7):S216–18.

27 Dupuis J, Goresky C, Fournier A. Pulmonary clearance of circulating endothelin-1 in dogs *in vivo*: exclusive role of ET_B receptors. *J Appl Physiol* 1996;**81**:1510–15.

28 Dupuis J, Stewart DJ, Cernacek P *et al*. Human pulmonary circulation is an important site for both clearance and procuction of endothelin-1. *Circulation* 1996;**94**:1578–84.

◆29 Masaki T. Possible role of endothelin in endothelial regulation of vascular tone. *Annu Rev Pharmacol Toxicol* 1995;**35**:235–55.

30 Dupuis J, Jasmin JF, Prie S *et al*. Importance of local production of endothelin-1 and of the ET_B receptor in the regulation of pulmonary vascular tone. *Pulmon Pharmacol Ther* 2000;**13**:135–40.

31 Kuc R, Davenport A. Endothelin-A-receptors in human aorta and pulmonary arteries are downregulated in patients with cardiovascular disease: an adaptive response to increased levels of endothelin-1? *J Cardiovasc Pharmacol* 2000; **36**(Suppl 1):S377–9.

32 Stewart D, Levy RD, Cernacek P *et al*. Increased plasma endothelin-1 in pulmonary hypertension: marker or mediator of disease? *Ann Intern Med* 1991;**114**:464–9.

●33 Giaid A, Michel RP, Stewart DJ *et al*. Expression of endothelin-1 in the lungs of patients with pulmonary hypertension. *N Engl J Med* 1993;**328**:1732–9.

34 Giaid A. Nitric oxide and endothelin-1 in pulmonary hypertension. *Chest* 1998;**114**:S208–12.

35 Langleben D, Barst RJ, Badesch D *et al*. Continuous infusion of epoprostenol improves the net balance between pulmonary endothelin-1 clearance and release in primary pulmonary hypertension. *Circulation* 1999;**99**:3266–71.

36 Chen Y, Oparil S. Endothelin and pulmonary hypertension. *J Cardiovasc Pharmacol* 2000;**35**(Suppl 2):S49–53.

37 Chen SJ, Chen YF, Opgenorth TJ *et al*. The orally active nonpeptide endothelin A-receptor antagonist A-127722 prevents and reverses hypoxia-induced pulmonary hypertension and pulmonary vascular remodelling in Sprague-Dawley rats. *J Cardiovasc Pharmacol* 1997;**29**:713–25.

38 Eddahibi S, Raffestin B, Clozel M *et al*. Protection from pulmonary hypertension with an orally active endothelin receptor antagonist in hypoxic rats. *Am J Physiol* 1995;**268**:H828–35.

39 Takahashi H, Soma S, Muramatsu M *et al*. Upregulation of ET-1 and its receptors and remodelling in small pulmonary veins under hypoxic conditions. *Am J Physiol Lung Cell Mol Physiol* 2001;**280**:L1104–14.

40 Takahashi H, Soma S, Muramatsu M *et al*. Discrepant distribution of big endothelin (ET)-1 and ET receptors in the pulmonary artery. *Eur Respir J* 2001;**18**:5–14.

41 Bando K, Vijayaraghavan P, Turrentine MW *et al*. Dynamic changes of endothelin-1, nitric oxide, and cyclic GMP in patients with congenital heart disease. *Circulation* 1997;**96**(Suppl II):II 346–51.

42 Ishikawa S, Miyauchi T, Sakai S *et al*. Elevated levels of plasma endothelin-1 in young patients with pulmonary hypertension caused by congenital heart disease are decreased after successful surgical repair. *J Thorac Cardiovasc Surg* 1995;**110**:271–3.

43 Lutz J, Gorenflo M, Habighorst M *et al*. Endothelin-1- and endothelin-receptors in lung biopsies of patients with pulmonary hypertension due to congenital heart disease. *Clin Chem Lab Med* 1999;**37**:423–8.

44 Allen SW, Chatfield BA, Koppenhafer SA *et al*. Circulating immunoreactive endothelin-1 in children with pulmonary hypertension. Association with acute hypoxic pulmonary vasoreactivity. *Am Rev Respir Dis* 1993;**148**:519–22.

45 Kim H, Yung GL, Marsh JJ *et al*. Endothelin mediates pulmonary vascular remodelling in a canine model of chronic embolic pulmonary hypertension. *Eur Respir J* 2000;**15**:640–8.

46 Kim H, Yung GL, Marsh JJ *et al*. Pulmonary vascular remodeling distal to pulmonary artery ligation is accompanied by upregulation of endothelin receptors and nitric oxide synthase. *Exp Lung Res* 2000;**26**:287–301.

47 Bauer M, Wilkens H, Langer F *et al*. Selective upregulation of endothelin B receptor gene expression in severe pulmonary hypertension. *Circulation* 2002;**105**:1034–6.

48 Ivy DD, Le Cras TD, Horan MP *et al*. Increased lung preproET-1 and decreased ET_B receptor gene expression in fetal pulmonary hypertension. *Am J Physiol* 1998;**274**:L535–41.

49 Ivy D, Kinsella J, Abman S. Physiologic characterization of endothelin A and B receptor activity in the ovine fetal pulmonary circulation. *J Clin Invest* 1994;**93**:2141–8.

50 Okazaki T, Sharma HS, McCune SK *et al*. Pulmonary vascular balance in congenital diaphragmatic hernia: enhanced endothelin-1 gene expression as a possible cause of pulmonary vasoconstriction. *J Pediatr Surg* 1998;**33**:81–4.

51 Shima H, Oue T, Taira Y *et al*. Antenatal dexamethasone enhances endothelin receptor B expression in hypoplastic

lung in nitrofen-induced diaphragmatic hernia in rats. *J Pediatr Surg* 2000;**35**:203–7.

52 Christou H, Adatia I, Van Marter LJ *et al.* Effect of inhaled nitric oxide on endothelin-1 and cyclic guanosine 5′-monophosphate plasma concentrations in newborn infants with persistent pulmonary hypertension. *J Pediatr* 1997;**130**:603–11.

53 Kumar P, Kazzi N, Shankaran S. Plasma immunoreactive endothelin-1 concentrations in infants with persistent pulmonary hypertension of the newborn. *Am J Perinatol* 1996;**13**:335–41.

54 MacDonald P, Paton Rd, Logan RW *et al.* Endothelin-1 levels in infants with pulmonary hypertension receiving extracorporeal membrane oxygenation. *J Perinat Med* 1999;**27**:216–20.

55 Rosenberg AA, Kennaugh J, Koppenhafer SL *et al.* Elevated immunoreactive endothelin-1 levels in newborn infants with persistent pulmonary hypertension. *J Pediatr* 1993;**123**:109–14.

56 Barst R *et al.* Efficacy and safety of chronic treatment with the oral selective endothelin-A receptor blocker sitaxsentan in pulmonary arterial hypertension. *Circulation* 2000;**102**(Suppl II):II-427.

57 Givertz M, Colucci WS, LeJemtel TH *et al.* Acute endothelin A receptor blockade causes selective pulmonary vasodilation in patients with chronic heart failure. *Circulation* 2000;**101**:2922–7.

58 Williamson DJ, Wallmen LL, Jones R *et al.* Hemodynamic effects of bosentan, an endothelin receptor antagonist, in patients with pulmonary hypertension. *Circulation* 2000;**102**:411–18.

●59 Channick R, Simonneau G, Sitbon O *et al.* Effects of the dual endothelin-receptor antagonist bosentan in patients with pulmonary hypertension: a randomized placebo controlled study. *Lancet* 2001;**358**:1119–23.

●60 Rubin LJ, Badesch DB, Barst RJ *et al.* Bosentan therapy for pulmonary arterial hypertension. *N Engl J Med* 2002;**346**:896–903.

61 Fattinger K, Funk C, Pantze M *et al.* The endothelin antagonist bosentan inhibits the canalicular bile salt export pump: a potential mechanism for hepatic adverse reactions. *Clin Pharmacol Ther* 2001;**69**:223–31.

62 Coceani F, Kelsey L. Endothelin-1 release from lamb ductus arteriosus: relevance to postnatal closure of the vessel. *Can J Physiol Pharmacol* 1991;**69**:218–21.

63 Kurihara Y, Kurchara H, Suzuki H *et al.* Elevated blood pressure and craniofacial abnormalities in mice deficient in endothelin-1. *Nature* 1994;**368**:703–10.

64 Weber C, Banken L, Birnboeck H *et al.* Effect of the endothelin-receptor antagonist bosentan on the pharmacokinetics and pharmacodynamics of warfarin. *J Clin Pharmacol* 1999;**39**:847–54.

65 Imai T, Hirato Y, Emori T *et al.* Induction of endothelin-1 gene by angiotensin and vasopressin in endothelial cells. *Hypertension* 1992;**19**:753–7.

66 Kurihara H, Yoshizumi M, Sugiyama T *et al.* Transforming growth factor beta stimulates the expression of endothelin mRNA from vascular endothelial cells. *Biochem Biophys Res Commun* 1989;**159**:1435–40.

67 Marsden P, Brenner B. Transcriptional regulation of the endothelin-1 gene by TNF alpha. *Am J Physiol* 1992;**262**:C854–61.

68 Emori T, Hirata Y, Imai T *et al.* Cellular mechanisms of thrombin on endothelin-1 biosynthesis and release in bovine endothelial cell. *Biochem Pharmacol* 1992;**44**:2409–11.

69 Maemura K, Kurihara H, Morita T *et al.* Production of endothelin-1 in vascular endothelial cells is regulated by factors associated with vascular injury. *Gerontology* 1992;**38**(Suppl 1):29–35.

70 Marsden PA, Dorfman DM, Collins T *et al.* Regulated expression of endothelin 1 in glomerular capillary endothelial cells. *Am J Physiol* 1991;**261**:F117–25.

71 Yoshizumi M, Kurihara H, Sugiyama T *et al.* Hemodynamic shear stress stimulates endothelin production by cultured endothelial cells. *Biochem Biophys Res Commun* 1989;**161**:859–64.

72 Masaki T, Miwa S, Sawamura T *et al.* Subcellular mechanisms of endothelin action in vascular system. *Eur J Pharmacol* 1999;**375**:133–8.

73 Emori T, Hirata Y, Imai T *et al.* Cellular mechanism of natriuretic peptides induced inhibition of endothelin-1 biosynthesis in rat endothelial cells. *Endocrinology* 1993;**133**:2474–80.

13Q

Novel medical approaches – growth inhibitors

MARLENE RABINOVITCH

INTRODUCTION

In trying to prevent and reverse the pathophysiological processes leading to pulmonary hypertension, there has been a focus on targeting the mechanisms that cause heightened endothelial, smooth muscle cell (SMC) and fibroblast proliferation and migration, and the associated increase in the production of extracellular matrix proteins. This chapter addresses the basis for thinking that aberrant growth leads to obliterative pulmonary vascular disease, and describes the growth factors implicated, the mechanisms of their regulation and action, and the therapies that have been developed to inhibit this process.

GROWTH AND GROWTH FACTORS

Smooth muscle cells

Aberrant proliferation of smooth muscle cells is a prominent feature of pulmonary arterial changes that are observed both in the clinical setting and in experimental animals that develop pulmonary vascular disease (reviewed in reference 1). With the discovery of growth factors that could induce this response, a profusion of studies tried to analyze which specific ones might be involved.

Transforming growth factor-β (TGF-β)

In the search for growth factors that could mediate both the increase in connective tissue synthesis and accumulation as well as the smooth muscle cell proliferative response, TGF-β was an ideal candidate. Indeed, heightened immunoreactivity for TGF-β was observed in the neointima of occluded pulmonary arteries in patients with primary pulmonary hypertension (PPH) and secondary pulmonary hypertension (SPH) (Plate 13Q.1).[2] The increase in the expression of growth factors is likely coupled to mechanisms which facilitate their signaling mechanism. This could result from an increase in the number and type of receptors, in their affinity for the ligand (growth factor) or in the state of their activation related to signaling complexes. For example, when SMCs from patients with PPH are harvested and exposed to TGF-β, proliferation is observed whereas normal smooth muscle cells show a growth inhibitory response to TGF-β.[3]

This concept is supported by genetic studies suggesting that the propensity for TGF-β to act as a growth stimulatory or inhibitory factor is dependent on the availability of specific receptors on the cell surface. That is, a mutation in one of the members of the TGF-β family of receptors, bone morphogenetic protein receptor II, has been identified in both familial and sporadic primary pulmonary hypertension[4–6] and a mutation in *ALK1*, another receptor for TGF-β, is observed in patients who have both telangiectasia and pulmonary hypertension.[7]

When a TGF-β receptor is engaged by a ligand, signaling molecules called SMADs are activated and translocate to the nucleus.[8] Although the exact mechanisms remain to be worked out, it appears that certain members of the SMAD family can couple with other transcription factors and either repress or induce their transactivating activity.[8] Thus, normal TGF-β receptor signaling produces the interaction of transcription factors in the nucleus that suppress the proliferative response whereas abnormalities in the expression of this family of receptors 'sets the cell up' to respond to TGF-β signaling by inducing genes associated with proliferation.

In experimental studies, increased expression of TGF-β was observed in rats after injection of the toxin monocrotaline[9] and in association with air embolization in sheep, which also causes pulmonary hypertension,[10,11] although not in association with the remodeling that occurs in neonatal calves in response to hypoxia-mediated pulmonary hypertension.[12] The distribution of TGF-β in the hypertrophied pulmonary arteries following monocrotaline-induced pulmonary hypertension would suggest that it may also be linked to elastin rather than collagen synthesis.[13] Of interest are studies in cultured smooth muscle cells suggesting that, in association with pulmonary hypertension, increased TGF-β may regulate production of the vasoconstrictor and smooth muscle cell mitogen, endothelin.[14] The excess endothelin production in hypoxia-induced pulmonary hypertension is, however, thought to be related to increased production by endothelial cells.

Endothelin

Whether the production of endothelin is related to endothelial or smooth muscle cells, or both, it has been shown that endothelin receptor blockade prevents hypoxia-induced pulmonary hypertension.[15] While the mitogenic effect of endothelin is thought to involve engagement of both A and B receptors,[16] in experimental animals prolonged selective blockade of endothelin receptor B causes pulmonary hypertension in the ovine fetus.[17] This is presumably related to the loss of dilator properties of endothelin through the B receptor. Recent clinical trials in patients with primary pulmonary hypertension, however, have reported success in improving cardiac function and symptomatology with bosentan, a dual endothelin receptor antagonist.[18] Endothelin is processed from preproendothelin by endothelin converting enzyme and by activity of an endogenous chymase enzyme, which recent data show is also elevated in experimental pulmonary hypertension (our unpublished observations).

Other growth factors and growth inhibitors

In addition to TGF-β, other growth factors including platelet-derived growth factor,[19,20] fibroblast growth factor-2[21] and insulin-like growth factor[22,23] have been implicated in the pathophysiology of the smooth muscle cell proliferative response in models of pulmonary hypertension. Epidermal growth factor[24] has also been implicated. The mechanisms causing proliferation have been related to enhanced intracellular calcium resulting from inhibition of voltage-gated K channels,[25] Na/H exchange,[26]

suppression of p27kip (the cell cycle inhibitor)[27] and activation of protein kinase C.[28] Nitric oxide and cyclic GMP, however, appear to be negative regulators of SMC growth.[29,30] This is in keeping with the potential efficacy of sildenafil in preventing the progression of pulmonary vascular disease in patients.[31]

Endothelial cell growth factors

The endothelial cell proliferative response is noted in advanced lesions, i.e. plexiform complexes in patients with both primary and secondary pulmonary hypertension. In the former, the mechanism appears to be related to a monoclonal proliferative response. The endothelial proliferative response has been attributed to increased VEGF expression[32,33] and microsatellite instability in the receptor for TGF-β receptor II resulting in its reduced expression and function in proliferating endothelial cells.[34] Altered patterns of homeobox gene expression which may regulate VEGF expression[35] have also been described and recently gene array technology has been applied and a profile of genes related to apoptosis has been identified.[33] In experimental models, loss of VEGF signaling may underlie the loss of small vessels associated with endothelial cell apoptosis. This is in keeping with studies showing cell cycle arrest in endothelial cells from rats in which pulmonary hypertension is induced by monocrotaline. That is, blockade of VEGF receptors worsens chronic hypoxia-induced pulmonary hypertension[36] and VEGF adenoviral gene therapy[37] protects against hypoxia-induced pulmonary hypertension as does cell-based gene therapy with VEGF for monocrotaline-induced pulmonary hypertension[38] (Plate 13Q.2). Thus, the pathophysiology of pulmonary hypertension may be characterized by early loss of expression of VEGF, associated with loss of small vessels via apoptosis. This is followed much later by induction of VEGF that does not induce the return of arteries, but rather the plexiform lesion characterized by endothelial cell proliferation in advanced lesions.

Adventitial fibroblast

Less well studied is the proliferative response of the adventitial fibroblast first identified in the studies on hypoxic newborn calves.[39] These cells would be expected to be responsive to the same growth factors identified in smooth muscle cells and may play a role in the migration that is observed in the formation of the occlusive neointima.

RELEASE AND FUNCTION OF GROWTH FACTORS

Our laboratory has shown that increased activity of elastase is related both to the release of growth factors from the extracellular matrix and to the responsivity of the cells to their proliferative action. Ultrastructural study of lung biopsy tissue from patients with congenital heart defects first suggested that an elastolytic enzyme might be important in the pathophysiology of pulmonary vascular disease. Fragmentation of elastin was apparent in the pulmonary arteries of children with pulmonary hypertension in association with congenital heart defects[40] and in rats in which injection of the toxin, monocrotaline was used to experimentally induce pulmonary hypertension.[41]

The structural observations were supported by biochemical studies revealing high elastin turnover in pulmonary arteries from rats with monocrotaline-induced pulmonary hypertension suggesting neosynthesis as well as degradation, and direct enzymatic assay confirmed increased activity of a serine elastase.[41,42] We also showed that we could suppress the development of pulmonary hypertension associated with a smooth muscle cell proliferative response in three different experimental rat models by concomitant administration of elastase inhibitors.[41–43]

Cell culture studies were carried out to determine how an increase in elastase might occur and how it might cause proliferative and obliterative changes, which occur in association with progressive pulmonary hypertension. We hypothesized that in response to a perturbing stimulus, structural and functional alterations in endothelium would lead to loss of barrier properties and, as a consequence, a serum factor would accumulate in the subendothelium inducing activity of the endogenous vascular elastase (EVE) in vascular smooth muscle cells (Figure 13Q.1). We showed, in cultured pulmonary artery smooth muscle cells, that both serum and endothelial factors can induce smooth muscle cell elastase activity.[44] The factor(s) adhere to elastin and to the cell surface and induce binding of the elastin to the elastin binding protein.[45] An elastin-binding serum factor shown to have elastase-inducing properties was purified from the serum and N-terminal sequence analysis indicated that it was apolipoprotein A1.[45] As a consequence of binding of elastin to cell surfaces via serum components, a signal transduction mechanism associated with increased tyrosine kinase activity, phosphorylation of focal adhesion kinase (FAK) and members of the MAP kinase family (ERK1 or extracellular regulated kinase-1)[46] was observed. We identified the transcription factor AML1 as a target of ERK1 phosphorylation and as the candidate transcription factor for the vascular elastase gene.[47,48] Nitric oxide can repress elastase activity in vascular smooth muscle cells through a cGMP-dependent pathway which prevents ERK phosphorylation and the associated expression of AML1 in nuclear extracts,[46] thus biologically linking reduction in pulmonary artery pressure with suppression of vascular remodeling. As has

been shown for other serine proteinases, expression of EVE activity leads to the release of smooth muscle cell mitogens from storage sites in the extracellular matrix.[46,48] For example, both human leukocyte elastase and EVE can liberate fibroblast growth factor-2 (FGF-2) from the extracellular matrices of smooth muscle cells.

For cells to respond optimally to growth factors, however, their receptors must be available and in some way 'primed'. This occurs also as a result of elastase activity. Smooth muscle cells activate metalloproteinases, which depolymerize collagen, revealing cryptic RGD peptide sites. These peptides bind the smooth muscle cells through the α v β_3-integrin receptor.[49] As a result of this interaction, ERK phosphorylation occurs and tenascin-C is induced (Figure 13Q.2) by a transcriptional mechanism[50] related to Prx.[51] Tenascin co-distributes with proliferating smooth muscle cells and its increased expression correlates with the severity of the vascular lesion (Plate 13Q.3). The examination of lung biopsy tissue from patients with pulmonary hypertension showed progressive deposition of tenascin in the media and neointima in association with proliferating smooth muscle cells as judged by positive immunoreactivity with an antibody that recognizes the proliferating cell nuclear antigen.[52]

When rat pulmonary artery smooth muscle cells are cultured on collagen gels supplemented with tenascin-C, they increase their proliferative response to fibroblast growth factor and only when the collagen gels are supplemented with tenascin-C do pulmonary artery smooth muscle cells proliferate in response to epidermal growth factor (Figure 13Q.3).[53] The mechanism of tenascin-C 'priming' is related to the change in cell shape that occurs as a result of clustering of β_3-integrins since this leads to the reorganization of the actin cytoskeleton into focal contacts which, in turn, causes clustering of growth factor receptors which rapidly phosphorylate, transmitting a nuclear signal which is reflected in cell growth (Figure 13Q.2).[49]

THE DARK SIDE OF CELL GROWTH – CELL DEATH

The reverse process, i.e. inhibition of elastase, results not only in suppression of cell proliferation, but also in programmed cell death. That is, suppression of elastase leads to reduction in matrix metalloproteinase activity, down-regulation of tenascin-C, unclustering of β_3-integrins and unclustering of EGF receptors.[49] When this happens, apoptosis of smooth muscle cells occurs. In organ culture we could reproduce this phenomenon and, in fact, showed that hypertrophied pulmonary arteries could be

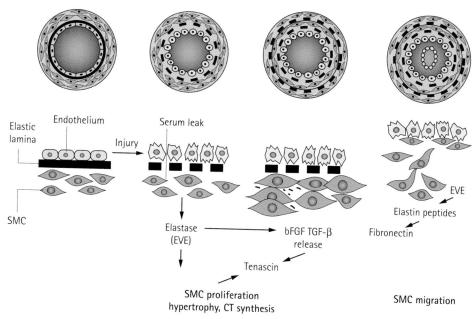

Figure 13Q.1 *The author has speculated as to how a stimulus could induce activity of an elastolytic enzyme and how this might stimulate the remodeling process. The process of progressive pulmonary hypertension involves a series of switches in the smooth muscle cell phenotype (i.e. differentiation of muscle from non-muscle precursor cells, smooth muscle cell hypertrophy and proliferation accounting for medial hypertrophy, and smooth muscle cell migration resulting in neointimal formation). In response to a stimulus, such as high flow and pressure, the first 'casualty' is the endothelial cell. As a result of structural and functional alterations in endothelial cells, some of the barrier function would be lost, allowing a leak into the subendothelium of a serum factor normally excluded from the region. The serum factor could induce activity of an endogenous vascular elastase (EVE). This enzyme released from precursor or mature smooth muscles cells would activate growth factors normally stored in the extracellular matrix in an inactive form, such as basic fibroblast growth factor and transforming growth factor-β, which are known to induce smooth muscle hypertrophy and proliferation and increases in connective tissue protein (e.g. collagen and elastin) synthesis. Basic fibroblast growth factor (bFGF) also induces tenascin, a matrix glycoprotein that amplifies the proliferation response as described in the text. This amplification results in the differentiation of precursor cells to mature smooth muscle related to the muscularization of normally non-muscular small peripheral arteries. In the muscular arteries, the release of growth factors would result in hypertrophy of the vessel wall. Continued elastase activity would cause migration of smooth muscle cells in several ways. The elastin peptides or degradation products of elastin can stimulate fibronectin, a glycoprotein that is pivotal in altering smooth muscle cell shapes and switches them from the contractile to motile phenotype. (Reproduced with permission from Rabinovitch M. It all begins with EVE. Israeli J Med Sci 1996;32:803–8.)*

made to regress by 'stress unloading'[54] or by incubating them with either a matrix metalloproteinase or a serine elastase inhibitor; we documented, in all cases, reduced tenascin-C expression and regression of medial hypertrophy associated with SMC apoptosis and resorption of excess extracellular matrix (elastin and collagen).[55] We subsequently showed that this phenomenon could be reproduced in the whole animal by treatment of rats with severe (near fatal) pulmonary hypertension with elastase inhibitors. All the untreated animals died within a few weeks but the treated rats nearly all survived and by 2 weeks they were demonstrating a return to normal levels of pulmonary artery pressure in association with reversal of structural changes in their pulmonary arteries (Plate 13Q.4). It is of interest that neither in normal vessels in organ culture nor in the control animal was there an adverse effect from elastase inhibitor treatment. Moreover, there was some restoration in the number of peripheral vessels that were initially lost following injection of monocrotaline.

CONCLUSION

New understanding of cell biology and genetics is unraveling the mechanisms by which growth factors and their intracellular pathways cause pulmonary vascular disease. This knowledge should lead to improved understanding of the benefits and limitations of current therapies and the design of novel approaches to prevent progression and induce regression of pulmonary vascular disease and other systemic vasculopathies.

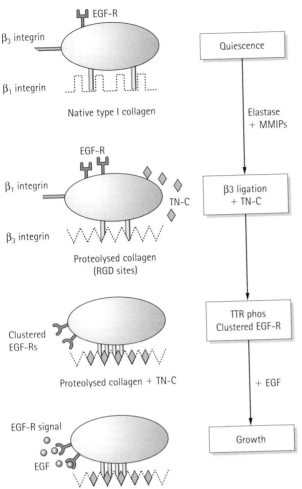

Figure 13Q.2 *A hypothetical model for the regulation and function of tenascin-C (TN-C) in vascular smooth muscle cells. (a) Vascular smooth muscle cells attach and spread on native type I collagen using β_1-integrins. Under serum-free conditions, the cells withdraw from the cell cycle and become quiescent. (b) Degradation of naive type I collagen by elastase and matrix metalloproteinases (MMPs) leads to exposure of cryptic arginine glycine aspartic acid (RGD) sites that preferentially bind β_3 subunit-containing integrins. In turn, occupancy and activation of β_3 integrins signal the production of TN-C. (c) Incorporation of multivalent TN-C protein into the underlying substrate leads to further aggregation and activation of β_3-containing integrins ($\alpha\beta_3$) and to the accumulation of tyrosine-phosphorylated (Tyr-P) signaling molecules and actin into a focal adhesion complex. Note that even in the absence of the epidermal growth factor (EGF) ligand, the TN-C dependent reorganization of the cytoskeleton leads to clustering of actin-associated EGF-Rs. Addition of EGF ligand to clustered EGF-Rs results in rapid and substantial tyrosine phosphorylation of the EGF-R and activation of downstream pathways culminating in the generation of nuclear signals leading to cell proliferation.*

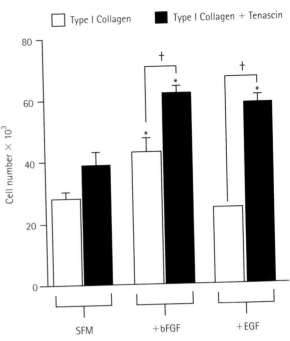

Figure 13Q.3 *Effect of exogenous tenascin (15 μg/mL) on pulmonary artery smooth muscle and growth factor-dependent proliferation. Smooth muscle cell growth in serum-free medium (SFM) was unaffected by addition of exogenous tenascin. By contrast, addition of basic fibroblast growth factor (bFGF) or EGF to tenascin-treated cultures resulted in a significant increase in cell number. Values represent mean $\pm$ SEM; $P < 0.05$. *Difference from SFM level whereas † denotes difference related to tenascin. (From Jones PL, Rabinovitch M. Tenascin-C is induced with progressive pulmonary vascular disease in rats and is functionally related to increased smooth muscle cell proliferation.* Circ Res 1996;**79**:1131–42.)

KEY POINTS

- Normal TGF-β receptor signaling produces the interaction of transcription factors in the nucleus that suppresses the proliferative response, whereas abnormalities in the expression of this family of receptors 'sets the cell up' to respond to TGF-β signaling by inducing genes associated with proliferation.
- The pathophysiology of pulmonary hypertension may be characterized by early loss of expression of VEGF, associated with loss of small vessels via apoptosis. This is followed much later by induction of VEGF that induces the formation of the plexiform lesion, characterized by endothelial cell proliferation in advanced lesions.
- The development of pulmonary hypertension associated with a smooth muscle cell proliferative

response can be suppressed in experimental rat models by concomitant administration of elastase inhibitors, suggesting a pathogenic role for the elastase system: suppression of elastase leads to reduction in matrix metalloproteinase activity, down-regulation of tenascin-C, unclustering of β_3-integrins and unclustering of EGF receptors.

REFERENCES

◆1 Rabinovitch M. Pathophysiology of pulmonary hypertension. In: Allen HD, Gutgesell HP, Driscoll DJ (eds), *Heart disease in infants, children and adolescents.* Philadelphia: Lippincott, Williams and Wilkins, 2000;1311–46.

●2 Botney MD, Bahadori L, Gold LI. Vascular remodeling in primary pulmonary hypertension. Potential role for transforming growth factor-beta. *Am J Pathol* 1994;**144**:286–95.

●3 Morrell NW, Yang X, Upton PD *et al.* Altered growth responses of pulmonary artery smooth muscle cells from patients with primary pulmonary hypertension to transforming growth factor-beta(1) and bone morphogenetic proteins. *Circulation* 2001;**104**:790–5.

●4 Deng Z, Morse JH, Slager SL *et al.* Familial primary pulmonary hypertension (gene *PPH1*) is caused by mutations in the bone morphogenetic protein receptor-II gene. *Am J Hum Genet* 2000;**67**:737–44.

●5 Lane KB, Machado RD, Pauciulo MW *et al.* Heterozygous germline mutations in BMPR2, encoding a TGF-beta receptor, cause familial primary pulmonary hypertension. *Nat Genet* 2000;**26**:81–4.

●6 Newman JH, Wheeler L, Lane KB *et al.* Mutation in the gene for bone morphogenetic protein receptor II as a cause of primary pulmonary hypertension in a large kindred. *N Engl J Med* 2001;**345**:319–24.

●7 Trembath RC, Thomson JR, Machado RD *et al.* Clinical and molecular genetic features of pulmonary hypertension in patients with hereditary hemorrhagic telangiectasia. *N Engl J Med* 2001;**345**:325–34.

●8 Attisano L, Wrana JL. Signal transduction by the TGF-beta superfamily. *Science* 2002;**296**:1646–7.

●9 Arcot SS, Lipke DW, Gillespie MN *et al.* Alterations of growth factor transcripts in rat lungs during development of monocrotaline-induced pulmonary hypertension. *Biochem Pharmacol* 1993;**46**:1086–91.

●10 Perkett EA, Pelton RW, Meyrick B *et al.* Expression of transforming growth factor-beta mRNAs and proteins in pulmonary vascular remodeling in the sheep air embolization model of pulmonary hypertension. *Am J Respir Cell Mol Biol* 1994;**11**:16–24.

●11 Perkett EA, Lyons RM, Moses HL *et al.* Transforming growth factor β activity in sheep lung lymph during the development of pulmonary hypertension. *J Clin Invest* 1990;**86**:1459–64.

●12 Botney MD, Parks WC, Crouch EC *et al.* Transforming growth factor-beta 1 is decreased in remodeling hypertensive bovine pulmonary arteries. *J Clin Invest* 1992;**89**:1629–35.

●13 Tanaka Y, Bernstein ML, Mecham RP *et al.* Site-specific responses to monocrotaline-induced vascular injury: evidence for two distinct mechanisms of remodeling. *Am J Respir Cell Mol Biol* 1996;**15**:390–7.

●14 Markewitz BA, Farrukh IS, Chen Y *et al.* Regulation of endothelin-1 synthesis in human pulmonary arterial smooth muscle cells. Effects of transforming growth factor-beta and hypoxia. *Cardiovasc Res* 2001;**49**:200–6.

●15 Chen YF, Oparil S. Endothelin and pulmonary hypertension. *J Cardiovasc Pharmacol* 2000;**35**:S49–53.

●16 Davie N, Haleen SJ, Upton PD *et al.* ET(A) and ET(B) receptors modulate the proliferation of human pulmonary artery smooth muscle cells. *Am J Respir Crit Care Med* 2002;**165**:398–405.

●17 Ivy DD, Parker TA, Abman SH. Prolonged endothelin B receptor blockade causes pulmonary hypertension in the ovine fetus. *Am J Physiol Lung Cell Mol Physiol* 2000;**279**:L758–65.

◆18 Rubin LJ, Roux S. Bosentan: a dual endothelin receptor antagonist. *Expert Opin Investig Drugs* 2002;**11**:991–1002.

●19 Katayose D, Ohe M, Yamauchi K *et al.* Increased expression of PDGF A- and B-chain genes in rat lungs with hypoxic pulmonary hypertension. *Am J Physiol* 1993;**264**:L100–6.

●20 Berg JT, Breen EC, Fu Z *et al.* Alveolar hypoxia increases gene expression of extracellular matrix proteins and platelet-derived growth factor-B in lung parenchyma. *Am J Respir Crit Care Med* 1998;**158**:1920–8.

●21 Arcot SS, Fagerland JA, Lipke DW *et al.* Basic fibroblast growth factor alterations during development of monocrotaline-induced pulmonary hypertension in rats. *Growth Factors* 1995;**12**:121–30.

●22 Perkett EA, Badesch DB, Roessler MK *et al.* Insulin-like growth factor I and pulmonary hypertension induced by continuous air embolization in sheep. *Am J Respir Cell Mol Biol* 1992;**6**:82–7.

●23 Badesch DB, Lee PD, Parks WD *et al.* Insulin-like growth factor I stimulates elastin synthesis by bovine pulmonary arterial smooth muscle cells. *Biochem Biophys Res Commun* 1989;**160**:382–7.

●24 Powell PP, Klagsbrun M, Abraham JA *et al.* Eosinophils expressing heparin-binding EGF-like growth factor mRNA localize around lung microvessels in pulmonary hypertension. *Am J Pathol* 1993;**143**:784–93.

●25 Golovina VA, Platoshyn O, Bailey CL *et al.* Upregulated TRP and enhanced capacitative Ca^{2+} entry in human pulmonary artery myocytes during proliferation. *Am J Physiol Heart Circ Physiol* 2001;**280**:H746–55.

●26 Quinn DA, Dahlberg CG, Bonventre JP *et al.* The role of Na^+/H^+ exchange and growth factors in pulmonary artery smooth muscle cell proliferation. *Am J Respir Cell Mol Biol* 1996;**14**:139–45.

●27 Fouty BW, Grimison B, Fagan KA *et al.* p27(Kip1) is important in modulating pulmonary artery smooth muscle cell proliferation. *Am J Respir Cell Mol Biol* 2001;**25**:652–8.

●28 Dempsey EC, Frid MG, Aldashev AA *et al.* Heterogeneity in the proliferative response of bovine pulmonary artery smooth muscle cells to mitogens and hypoxia: importance of protein kinase C. *Can J Physiol Pharmacol* 1997;**75**:936–44.

●29 Ambalavanan N, Mariani G, Bulger A *et al.* Role of nitric oxide in regulating neonatal porcine pulmonary artery smooth muscle cell proliferation. *Biol Neonate* 1999;**76**:291–300.

●30 Roberts JD, Jr, Chiche JD, Weimann J et al. Nitric oxide inhalation decreases pulmonary artery remodeling in the injured lungs of rat pups. Circ Res 2000;87:140–5.

●31 Michelakis E, Tymchak W, Lien D et al. Oral sildenafil is an effective and specific pulmonary vasodilator in patients with pulmonary arterial hypertension: comparison with inhaled nitric oxide. Circulation 2002;105:2398–403.

●32 Geiger R, Berger RM, Hess J et al. Enhanced expression of vascular endothelial growth factor in pulmonary plexogenic arteriopathy due to congenital heart disease. J Pathol 2000;191:202–7.

●33 Yeager ME, Halley GR, Golpon HA et al. Microsatellite instability of endothelial cell growth and apoptosis genes within plexiform lesions in primary pulmonary hypertension. Circ Res 2001;88:E2–11.

●34 Geraci MW, Moore M, Gesell T et al. Gene expression patterns in the lungs of patients with primary pulmonary hypertension: a gene microarray analysis. Circ Res 2001;88:555–62.

●35 Golpon HA, Geraci MW, Moore MD et al. HOX genes in human lung: altered expression in primary pulmonary hypertension and emphysema. Am J Pathol 2001;158:955–66.

●36 Le Cras TD, Markham NE, Tuder RM et al. Treatment of newborn rats with a VEGF receptor inhibitor causes pulmonary hypertension and abnormal lung structure. Am J Physiol Lung Cell Mol Physiol 2002;283:L555–62.

●37 Partovian C, Adnot S, Raffestin B et al. Adenovirus-mediated lung vascular endothelial growth factor overexpression protects against hypoxic pulmonary hypertension in rats. Am J Respir Cell Mol Biol 2000;23:762–71.

●38 Campbell AI, Zhao Y, Sandhu R et al. Cell-based gene transfer of vascular endothelial growth factor attenuates monocrotaline-induced pulmonary hypertension. Circulation 2001;104:2242–8.

●39 Stenmark KR, Fasules J, Hyde DM et al. Severe pulmonary hypertension and arterial adventitial changes in newborn calves at 4,300 m. J Appl Physiol 1987;62:821–30.

●40 Rabinovitch M, Bothwell T, Hayakawa BN et al. Pulmonary artery endothelial abnormalities in patients with congenital heart defects and pulmonary hypertension: a correlation of light with scanning electron microscopy and transmission electron microscopy. Lab Invest 1986;55:632–53.

●41 Ye C, Rabinovitch M. Inhibition of elastolysis by SC-37698 reduces development and progression of monocrotaline pulmonary hypertension. Am J Physiol 1991;261:H1255–67.

●42 Maruyama K, Ye C, Woo M et al. Chronic hypoxic pulmonary hypertension in rats and increased elastolytic activity. Am J Physiol 1991;261:H1716–26.

●43 Koppel R, Han RN, Cox D et al. Alpha 1-antitrypsin protects neonatal rats from pulmonary vascular and parenchymal effects of oxygen toxicity. Pediatr Res 1994;36:763–70.

●44 Kobayashi J, Wigle D, Childs T et al. Serum-induced vascular smooth muscle cell elastolytic activity through tyrosine kinase intracellular signalling. J Cell Physiol 1994; 160:121–31.

●45 Thompson K, Kobayashi J, Childs T et al. Endothelial and serum factors which include apolipoprotein A1 tether elastin to smooth muscle cells inducing serine elastase activity via tyrosine kinase-mediated transcription and translation. J Cell Physiol 1998;174:78–89.

●46 Mitani Y, Zaidi SHE, Dufourcq P et al. Nitric oxide reduces vascular smooth muscle cell elastase activity through cGMP-mediated suppression of ERK phosphorylation and AML1B nuclear partitioning. FASEB J 2000;14:805–14.

●47 Wigle DA, Thompson KE, Yablonsky S et al. AML1-like transcription factor induces serine elastase activity in ovine pulmonary artery smooth muscle cells. Circ Res 1998;83:252–63.

●48 Thompson K, Rabinovitch M. Exogenous leukocyte and endogenous elastases can mediate mitogenic activity in pulmonary artery smooth muscle cells by release of extracellular matrix-bound basic fibroblast growth factor. J Cell Physiol 1996;166:495–505.

●49 Jones PL, Crack J, Rabinovitch M. Regulation of Tenascin-C, a vascular smooth muscle cell survival factor that interacts with the alpha v beta 3 integrin to promote epidermal growth factor receptor phosphorylation and growth. J Cell Biol 1997;139:279–93.

●50 Jones PL, Jones FS, Zhou B et al. Induction of vascular smooth muscle cell tenascin-C gene expression by denatured type I collagen is dependent upon a beta3 integrin-mediated mitogen-activated protein kinase pathway and a 122-base pair promoter element. J Cell Sci 1999;112:435–45.

●51 Jones FS, Meech R, Edelman DB et al. Prx1 controls vascular smooth muscle cell proliferation and tenascin-C expression and is upregulated with Prx2 in pulmonary vascular disease. Circ Res 2001;89:131–8.

●52 Jones PL, Cowan KN, Rabinovitch M. Tenascin-C, proliferation and subendothelial fibronectin in progressive pulmonary vascular disease. Am J Pathol 1997;150:1349–60.

●53 Jones PL, Rabinovitch M. Tenascin-C is induced with progressive pulmonary vascular disease in rats and is functionally related to increased smooth muscle cell proliferation. Circ Res 1996;79:1131–42.

●54 Cowan KN, Jones PL, Rabinovitch M. Regression of hypertrophied rat pulmonary arteries in organ culture is associated with suppression of proteolytic activity, inhibition of tenascin-C and smooth muscle cell apoptosis. Circ Res 1999;84:1223–33.

●55 Cowan K, Jones P, Rabinovitch M. Elastase and matrix metalloproteinase inhibitors induce regression, and tenascin-C antisense prevents progression of vascular disease. J Clin Invest 2000;105:21–34.

●56 Cowan KN, Heilbut A, Humpl T et al. Complete reversal of fatal pulmonary hypertension in rats by a serine elastase inhibitor. Nat Med 2000;6:698–702.

Lung transplantation

PAUL A CORRIS

INTRODUCTION

Lung transplantation for pulmonary vascular disease began in 1981 when workers at Stanford introduced combined transplantation for heart and lungs (HLT).[1] The indications for HLT were subsequently widened to include pulmonary parenchymal and airway diseases.[2] Survival rates were good, and in marked contrast to the universal failures reported after single lung transplantation (SLT) in the preceding 25 years.[3] It was realized, however, that many patients undergoing HLT received a new heart unnecessarily. After a period of research, clinical success with SLT in fibrosing lung disease was reported by the Toronto group in 1986.[4]

In 1988, double lung transplantation (DLT) with a tracheal anastomosis was introduced by Patterson and colleagues.[5] However, this procedure was accompanied by more frequent problems with airway healing than HLT.[6] In addition, the operation was more complex than HLT and the extensive mediastinal dissection led frequently to denervation of the recipient's native heart. Bleeding was at least as great a problem as for HLT, and by 1989 the procedure, as originally described, had been largely abandoned.

Noirclerc et al.[7] provided the solution to the problem of airway healing by performing two separate anastomoses, since, as in SLT, the donor bronchus is better vascularized initially if the anastomosis is close to the lung parenchyma. This concept was further developed by Pasque et al.[8] with the bilateral sequential single lung transplant (BLT). A previous study in hypoxic patients with idiopathic pulmonary fibrosis and pulmonary hypertension demonstrate sustained improvements in right ventricular function and falls in pulmonary artery pressure (PAP) following SLT.[9] This led to the successful application of isolated pulmonary transplantation in primary pulmonary hypertension in selected cases (Table 13R.1).[10,11] Transplant centers, however, not only have a choice of transplant operations to offer patients with pulmonary vascular disease, but should also consider pulmonary thromboendarterectomy for patients presenting with severe pulmonary arterial hypertension (PAH) due to chronic massive thrombotic obstruction of the central pulmonary arteries.

Investigations of all patients presenting with severe unexplained pulmonary hypertension should include radionuclide ventilation/perfusion imaging and a minority will show evidence of multilobar or segmental non-matched perfusion defects. Such defects provide an

Table 13R.1 *Changes in hemodynamic data in seven patients undergoing single lung transplantation (SLT) for primary pulmonary hypertension*

	Pre–SLT	Post–SLT	P
Mean PAP	64 ± 18 mmHg	18 ± 5 mmHg	0.001
Mean RAP	10 ± 6 mmHg	1 ± 2 mmHg	0.02
Cardiac index	2.54 ± 0.98 L/min·m^2	3.54 ± 0.7 L/min·m^2	0.065

PAP, pulmonary artery pressure; RAP, right atrial pressure. Adapted from reference 10.

indication for pulmonary angiography (including contrast CT) in order to define the anatomy of vascular obstruction with particular reference to the presence of chronic massive thromboemboli in central vessels. Many of these patients will benefit from thromboendarterectomy[12] rather than transplantation.

CRITERIA AND INDICATIONS FOR TRANSPLANT ASSESSMENT

See Table 13R.2 for guidelines on transplantation for pulmonary hypertension.

Choice of transplant operation

There are three operative procedures currently used in patients with PAH and each procedure has its own advocates,[13] including single lung,[14–18] bilateral lung[19] and heart/lung[21–23] transplantation.

Proponents of SLT have argued that it is technically an easier procedure to perform, has less morbidity and mortality when compared to BLT and HLT and allows more patients to receive lung transplants. Opponents have argued that patients transplanted with a single lung are more at risk not only for developing severe postoperative pulmonary edema,[14,24] but also for severe ventilation/perfusion mismatches in case of acute or chronic rejection,[25,26] both adversely affecting early and late survival and functional outcome. Any dysfunction that changes the compliance in the allograft can lead to rapid and sometimes marked hypoxemia in the recipient due to further shifting of ventilation from the allograft to the native lung. Early graft dysfunction due to reperfusion injury may be extremely difficult to manage, leading to severe hypoxemia and hemodynamic instability. Diffuse alveolar damage may result and is often associated with infection.[14] Single lung transplantation is a very satisfactory procedure in patients with PAH secondary to pulmonary parenchymal diseases with no differences in outcome when compared to a same group of patients without PAH.[27]

Proponents of BLT have argued that this procedure results in fewer ventilation/perfusion mismatches and as a result, patients are easier to look after in the immediate postoperative period. Moreover, this allows more marginal donor lungs to be utilized and hence makes best of the rare resource of donor lungs. Patients also have better pulmonary function and better long-term survival. According to a recent survey, this type of transplant procedure was preferred by 83% of responding centres.[4] Interestingly, 100% of the North American centers respond that double lung transplantation was their preferred type of procedure compared to only 29% in Europe and Israel where heart/lung transplant remains the first choice.

Table 13R.2 *Guidelines for transplant in pulmonary hypertension*

Age limits
Heart/lung transplant – 55 years
Double/bilateral lung transplant – 60 years
Single lung transplant – 65 years
NYHA class III or IV despite trial of epoprostenol for 3 months

Useful hemodynamic parameters
Cardiac index <2 L/min·m^2
Mean right atrial pressure >15 mmHg
Mean pulmonary artery pressure >55 mmHg
6-Minute walk test <332 m
Major hemoptysis

Relative contraindications
Symptomatic osteoporosis
Severe musculoskeletal disease of the thorax
Current use of corticosteroids >20 mg/day
Nutritional issues $<70\%$ or $>130\%$ of ideal body weight
Tobacco and/or substance abuse
Untreated/unresolved psychosocial problems
Requirement for invasive ventilator support
Colonization with fungi or atypical mycobacterium
Systemic diseases with multi-end-organ damage

Contraindications
Creatinine clearance <50 mg/mL·min
Infection with human immunodeficiency virus
Active malignancy within 2 years with exceptions
Hepatitis B antigen positivity
Hepatitis C with biopsy proven liver disease

Heart/lung transplantation historically was the first and only procedure in these patients.[1] Advocates of this procedure argue that this operation is not only technically more straight forward and thus associated with fewer postoperative complications, but also that obliterative bronchiolitis responsible for late death seems to occur less frequently with this type of procedure.[21] Opponents of this procedure argue that isolated lung transplantation alone will result in immediate and long-term normalization of pulmonary vascular resistance and right ventricular ejection fraction.[16,17,28,29] The donor heart can be used for isolated cardiac transplantation. Patients subjected to HLT are also at risk for accelerated graft coronary disease, although the incidence in the series from Stanford University was only 8% at 5 years following the transplant.[21] For all these reasons, many authors have pointed out that HLT should be reserved for special indications such as patients with Eisenmenger's syndrome caused by complex congenital heart disease[20,30,31] or children.

COMPARATIVE STUDIES

No prospective randomized studies are available to relieve the uncertainty as to the best lung transplant procedure for patients with PAH.

Four single centers have reported the outcomes between different transplant types for both primary and secondary hypertension. Chapelier and his colleagues reported on the results of HLT, BLT and SLT for PAH from the Paris-Sud University Lung Transplant Group.[32] There was a similar improvement in early and late right-sided hemodynamic function, pulmonary function and 2-year and 4-year survival between HLT and BLT recipients. The sole patient who received a single lung developed severe pulmonary edema, left ventricular failure, persistent desaturation and an important ventilation/perfusion mismatch. They concluded that HLT and BLT are equally effective but single lung transplantation should be avoided.

The Pittsburgh group reported on their experience in two studies. In the first study published in 1994 by Bando et al.,[33] pulmonary artery pressures decreased in all three allograft groups, but those in the single lung recipients remains significantly higher than in the two other groups. A significant ventilation/perfusion mismatch occurred in the SLT recipients but not in the others because of preferential blood flow to the allograft. Graft-related mortality was significantly higher and overall functional recovery was significantly lower at 1 year in the single compared to BLT and HLT recipients. The authors concluded that bilateral lung transplantation is a more satisfactory option for patients with pulmonary hypertension and that heart/lung transplantation should be preserved for recipients with complex congenital heart diseases or left ventricular dysfunction. In the second study from this group reported by Gammie et al. in 1998, SLT was compared to BLT with primary or secondary pulmonary hypertension.[34] There was no difference in median duration of intubation, length of stay in the intensive care unit, hospital stay, 1-month, 1-year and 4-year survival and late functional status between both groups. During this study period, 58 patients with PAH died awaiting transplantation. The authors therefore concluded that SLT could be preferentially applied for patients on the waiting list. The group from Ann Arbor compared the outcome of SLT and simultaneous intracardiac repair versus HLT for patients with pulmonary hypertension secondary to congenital cardiac anomalies.[30] One SLT recipient died perioperatively. Three of the four remaining patients surviving the first year died during the second year. The two HLT recipients were doing well 15 and 18 months after the operation. The authors concluded that SLT and simultaneous repair of intracardiac defects may have good early results, but that long-term results are considerably less favorable.

Finally, the group at Johns Hopkins Hospital in Baltimore recently reported their results in 57 recipients with primary and secondary pulmonary hypertension.[35] The survival up to 4 years in patients with primary pulmonary hypertension was superior in BLT compared to SLT recipients (100% versus 67%; P = 0.02). There was no clear advantage to SLT versus BLT for secondary pulmonary hypertension, although 4-year survival was better in single lung recipients if pulmonary artery pressure was ≤40 mmHg (91% versus 75%; P = 0.11) and it was better in bilateral lung recipients if this value was ≥40 mmHg (88% versus 62%; P = 0.19). The authors concluded that bilateral lung transplantation is the procedure of choice for patients with primary pulmonary hypertension and also with secondary hypertension with pulmonary artery pressures ≥40 mmHg.

No true consensus exists for the optimal lung transplant procedure for pulmonary hypertension and likely never will. The choice will largely depend upon the local situation regarding organ donors and experience of the transplant team.

Timing of transplantation

There has been considerable change in the approach to the assessment and listing of patients with severe PAH since the development of prostanoid therapy. Until the 1990s. medical treatment had focused on chronic vasodilator therapy based on calcium channel blockade, anticoagulation and use of diuretics, digoxin and oxygen. In the NIH Registry of 1991,[36] the median survival was 2.8 years and hence patients were generally referred for consideration of transplantation when they had reached New York Heart Association (NYHA) class III or class IV. A better comprehension of the pathogenesis of PAH has changed the focus of medical treatments to evaluate drugs that may reverse the vasoproliferative effects resulting in pulmonary vascular remodeling. The first drug shown to be effect was epoprostenol (PGI_2) given by a continuous intravenous infusion. In a pivotal study by Barst and colleagues,[37] 81 patients were randomized to receive epoprostenol or conventional therapy. The survival was significantly improved at 5 years from 27% to 54% in the epoprostenol-treated group. More recent studies suggest that median survival may be approaching 6 years and exercise performance and quality of life are also significantly improved (for review see Chapter 13L). This has clearly impacted greatly on the timing of transplant listing and, moreover, two studies have now demonstrated that 60–70% of patients who had previously been listed for transplantation on pre-epoprostenol criteria can be de-listed because of clinical improvement.[38,39] The most recent survival data for the ISHLT Registry suggests a 5-year survival of approximately 40–50% following heart/ lung or bilateral lung transplantation; however, PAH is one of the major risk factors for both early and late mortality with an odds ratio of 1.52.[40]

It is in this setting that pulmonary hypertension and transplant centers must decide whom to refer for listing and the timing of such a referral. A recent study[41] has surveyed current practices in a wide variety of transplant centers throughout North America, Europe and Australia. Forty per cent of centers felt all NYHA class III patients should be referred to transplant centers. By contrast, 57% of centers limited referral to those NYHA class III and IV patients who had failed to show benefit after an average of 3 months of epoprostenol therapy. A recent single-center report has demonstrated the value of assessment after 3 months of epoprostenol therapy. An improvement in NYHA to class II and a decrease in PVR of 30% or more is associated with a survival of 90% at 5 years.

Only 40% of centers use one or more hemodynamic criteria for listing. These include a mean right atrial pressure of more than 15 mmHg, PVR of 4–15 Wood units, a mixed venous oxygen saturation of less than 63% and a cardiac index of less than 2 L/min.[42,43] The vast majority of centers use some form of exercise testing and echocardiography to help determine functional status referral and listing.[44] No single measurement on echocardiogram has emerged as most useful. The evidence suggests, however, that exercise testing can be more helpful. A 6-minute walking test of more than 332 metres is associated with a good prognosis and this simple exercise test is both reproducible and correlates reasonably well with hemodynamics. It is also very sensitive in the detection of improvements related to therapy. A more formal exercise test with measurement of metabolic gas exchange is utilized by approximately 25% of centers with a mean oxygen consumption of less than 10 mL/kg·min used as an indicator for listing.

Overall, the results show that major pulmonary hypertension and transplant centers vary considerably regarding patterns of referral, listing and transplantation of patients and it is only with continued carefully collected registry data that guidelines for best practice will be refined. One important issue relates to the potential delay, for a NYHA class IV patient who fails to respond to intravenous epoprostenol over 3 months, in listing for transplantation and the effect this has on his or her overall chances of receiving a graft.

Patients who remain in a stable clinical state at NYHA class III will also prove a potentially difficult group and it is suggested that careful note is taken of the patients' informed views in this situation.

Patients who are experiencing problems with exertional syncope but who otherwise seem to have a good quality of life should be considered for atrial septostomy in addition to receiving prostenoid therapy.

Finally, potentially life-threatening hemoptysis should also be considered an indication for listing for transplant patients. A suggested guideline for transplant listing is shown in Table 13R.2.

General issues

AGE

There is a shortfall in suitable donor lungs and this has led most centers to impose an upper age limit of 50 years for transplantation of heart and lungs or both lungs alone, and an upper age limit of 60 years for SLT. The higher the age limit for SLT reflects the increased availability of suitable single lungs. The lower age limit for HLT or BLT is also influenced by data showing an increased 1-year mortality for these procedures in patients over the age of 40 years and 50 years, respectively. Patients who develop end-stage pulmonary vascular disease unresponsive to conventional medical therapy may be considered for transplantation provided that they conform to other criteria below.

DISEASE IN OTHER ORGANS

The presence of uncontrolled systemic disease in addition in respiratory failure precludes lung transplantation. Good renal function is essential in view of cyclosporin toxicity and a creatinine clearance of more than 50 mL/min is required. Only minor abnormalities of liver function are acceptable with no abnormalities of coagulation. A raised hepatic alkaline phosphatase with minimal elevation of transaminases requires investigation, but does not preclude assessment. Pulmonary hypertension is seen occasionally in patients with cirrhosis[45] and hence it is important to exclude the presence of this in patients with pulmonary hypertension and abnormal liver function tests. Severe hepatic congestion may occur in patients with terminal pulmonary hypertension. Patients with severe pulmonary hypertension due to systemic disease, such as systemic sclerosis, may be suitable transplant recipients provided that there is no evidence of active vasculitis affecting other organs.

SEPSIS

The presence of localized sepsis may lead to severe systemic infection postoperatively because of the need for immunosuppressive therapy. Persistent extrapulmonary sepsis therefore reduces the chance of successful transplantation. Oral hygiene is important and all patients should have any dental sepsis eradicated preoperatively. The presence of an aspergilloma colonizing an old pulmonary infarct is a contraindication to any form of lung transplant. Experience has shown that removal of a lung containing and aspergilloma results in seeding of the pleural space with *Aspergillus*, leading to fungal empyema. Removal of the contralateral lung in a patient otherwise suitable for single lung transplantation leaves the aspergilloma *in situ* and subsequent immunosuppression leads to an unacceptably high risk of disseminated *Aspergillus* infection.

PREVIOUS SURGERY

There is a risk of life-threatening hemorrhage when the native lungs are removed if there are extensive pleural adhesions. Clearly, there is a graduation of risk from scarring due to previous open lung biopsy via a limited thoracotomy to previous total pleurectomy, and the latter is regarded as a contraindication for HLT. The use of the antifibrinolytic aprotinin during transplant surgery reduces bleeding in patients who have undergone previous thoracotomy[46] and the recent development of single sequential lung transplantation (SSLT) via a transverse bilateral thoracotomy allows the surgeon much better access to the pleural space than is afforded by a sternotomy. In this regard the SSLT has advantages over the original HLT.

PSYCHOLOGICAL FACTORS

Any potential recipient must be well motivated and want a lung transplant, be able to cope and have demonstrated a willingness to comply. A supportive family or circle of close friends is essential. Underlying psychiatric illness and abuse of alcohol or drugs including cigarettes are contraindications.

Matching donor to recipients

Donor matching is based on ABO compatibility alone, and HLA is not possible except in the small group of patients who receive organs from living related donors. Size matching is achieved by calculating the predicted total lung capacity (TLC) of both donor and recipient using height, age and sex. No direct measurement of donor lung TLC is available. A screening lymphocytotoxic cross-match, using recipient serum and a banked pool of lymphocytes, is carried out in all potential recipients accepted for transplantation to exclude the presence of preformed antibodies. Direct cross-match with lymphocytes from a potential donor is only carried out prospectively when this screening test is positive. Wherever possible, donor and recipient are matched for cytomegalovirus (CMV) status. If a CMV-negative recipient receives a CMV-positive organ, serious CMV infection can be ameliorated by giving prophylactic CMV hyperimmunoglobulin,[47] ganciclovir, or both.

POSTOPERATIVE MANAGEMENT

Most patients can be extubated 12–24 hours after surgery and then begin an active program of mobilization. Fluid intake is restricted in the early postoperative period and diuresis encouraged to avoid accumulation of fluid in the lungs. The current methods of donor lung preservation all result in a degree of pulmonary vascular injury typified by the development of protein-rich edema fluid and

neutrophil accumulation.[48] Prophylactic antibiotics, such as flucloxacillin and metronidazole, are given for the first 5 days.

Routine immunosuppression

Initial immunosuppression comprises azathioprine or mycophenolate mofetil, rabbit antithymocyte globulin, methylprednisolone, cyclosporin or tacrolimus. Antithymocyte globulin is stopped after 3 days and methylprednisolone substituted by oral prednisolone at a rapidly reducing dose to a maintenance of 0.1 g/kg. If patients have no evidence of lung rejection at 6 months' maintenance, steroids are commonly withdrawn. Currently, patients remain on azathioprine or mycophenolate (MMF) and cyclosporin or tacrolimus indefinitely. Rejection episodes are treated with pulsed methylprednisolone 10 mg/kg i.v. for 3 days followed by increased oral prednisolone for 1 month. Rejection episodes resistant to increased steroids may be treated by intravenous murine monoclonal T-cell antibody (OKT-3) or total lymphoid irradiation.

Acute pulmonary rejection

A diagnosis of rejection currently is based on transbronchial lung biopsy using alligator forceps under radiological screening.[49] The principal morphological changes found in acute rejection are perivascular lymphocytic infiltrates which may extend into alveolar septa at the later stages of rejection. Additionally, airways may show a lymphocytic infiltrate. It is usual to carry out three or four biopsies from each lobe of one lung, since rejection may be patchy and multiple biopsies from different lobes afford a greater chance of positive diagnosis. There have been many studies trying to establish reliable, less invasive methods of diagnosing rejection on blood or bronchoalveolar lavage cells and fluid. To date, none has proven to be sufficiently sensitive and specific for routine clinical use, although the Pittsburgh group have reported some success using the donor-specific primed lymphocyte response of bronchoalveolar lavage cells in the diagnosis of lung allograft rejection.[50]

Acute pulmonary rejection is now graded according to consensus guidelines reported by the International Society of Heart and Lung Transplantation.[51] The classification is based on transbronchial lung biopsy specimens carried out during fiberoptic bronchoscopy and relates to the intensity of lymphocytic infiltrate (see Table 13R.3). Many groups have encouraged home monitoring of FEV_1 by patients, using a hand-held spirometer, in an attempt to identify at an early stage those patients who are developing complications. More recent studies have demonstrated that if routine surveillance biopsies

Table 13R.3 *Histological grading system for acute vascular pulmonary rejection*

Grade	Description
Normal (A0)	No significant abnormality
Minimal acute rejection (A1)	Infrequent perivascular infiltrates
Mild acute rejection (A2)	Frequent perivascular infiltrates around venules and arterioles
Moderate acute rejection (A3)	Dense perivascular infiltrates with extension into alveolar septa
Severe acute rejection (A4)	Diffuse perivascular, interstitial and air–space infiltrates; alveolar pneumocyte damage; possibly parenchymal necrosis, infarction or necrotizing vasculitis

are carried out at intervals during the first 6 months after transplantation, 20–25% show evidence of significant acute vascular rejection in the absence of clinical or functional deterioration.

Chronic pulmonary rejection

Obliterative bronchiolitis is a form of chronic allograft rejection associated with both an increased frequency and persistence of acute lung rejection. Accordingly, the prompt identification and treatment of occult lung rejection may ultimately lead to a reduction in the frequency of obliterative bronchiolitis, which currently affects up to 30% of lung transplant recipients.

Infection

The principal cause of early postoperative death is infection. Bacterial pneumonia is common in the early postoperative period, affecting up to 35% of patients, and is the major infectious complication in the intermediate and late postoperative periods.[52] The factors that influence the development of pneumonia include both immunosuppression and alterations in the natural defence mechanisms, such as depressed cough reflex and reduced clearance due to depressed ciliary beat frequency.[53] In the late postoperative period, the presence of obliterative bronchiolitis is often associated with colonization of the lungs by Gram-negative organisms.

CMV infection may cause problems, particularly 4–8 weeks post-surgery. It is a particular problem if CMV-negative recipients receive organs from CMV-positive donors without receiving prophylaxis. The prognosis of CMV pneumonia has been dramatically improved following the introduction of ganciclovir, a guanine derivative. Herpes pneumonia was reported in early series of lung transplants but has been largely eliminated by the use of prophylactic aciclovir over the first 6 weeks after transplantation. Finally, fungal pneumonia should always be considered and *Candida*, in particular, may complicate the early postoperative period in part due to the high frequency of colonization in the airways of donor lungs. *Aspergillus* may also be a problem post-transplantation, and may present as fungal 'bronchitis', invasive pneumonia or disseminated aspergillosis.

Prior to the application of prophylaxis, lung transplant recipients were also particularly prone to developing symptomatic infection with *Pneumocystis carinii*. Regular oral treatment with trimethoprim/sulfamethoxazole on 3 days each week provides extremely effective prophylaxis.

Results

The International Society for Heart and Lung Transplantation Registry shows a 1-year survival of 70% with a 5-year survival of 50% following lung transplantation. The most important complications leading to death are opportunist infections and the development of obliterative bronchiolitis (OB). Functional results in survivors measured in terms of both FEV_1 and exercise performance are good with patients returning to NYHA class I from their preoperative level of class III or IV. Recipients can expect to attain their normal predicted FEV_1 and VC by 1 year in the absence of complications if they receive two new lungs, although the diffusing capacity usually remains reduced. All patients should expect restoration of normal lifestyle with little or no functional restriction during normal activities of daily living. Exercise data comparing the 6-minute walking distances and maximum oxygen consumption during an incremental symptom-limited exercise test show that recipients of successful transplants, irrespective of the operation, return to a normal 6-minute walking distance of 600 meters or greater by 1 year with no evidence of desaturation on exercise. The maximum oxygen consumption is significantly greater in HLT and BLT compared to SLT alone. However, maximum oxygen consumption during a symptom-limited test remains at around 50% predicted for a given subject in the first year, in part due to decompensation on account of the pre-transplant disability. Nevertheless, the functional results allow restoration of a comfortable lifestyle.

Lung function, computed tomographic scans and transbronchial lung biopsies have been normal in patients more than 5 years after transplantation, indicating the potential for prolonged survival in patients who do not develop OB. PAH, unfortunately, is one of the major risk factors for early and late mortality in lung transplant recipients with an odds ratio of 1.52 (95% CI: 1.25–1.85; $P < 0.0001$).[13] Primary pulmonary hypertension has also been identified as an individual risk factor for the development of OB in transplanted patients.[54]

Long-term complications

OBLITERATIVE BRONCHIOLITIS

This process may be defined functionally by the development of progressive irreversible airflow obstruction unresponsive to steroids.[55] Functional evidence of OB leads to the clinical diagnosis of obliterative bronchiolitis (OB) syndrome. Pathology shows obliteration of bronchioles by organizing fibrin associated with fibroblasts and mononuclear cells. Immunohistology shows that the walls of the bronchioles are infiltrated by CD8 lymphocytes.[56] The small bronchioles are left as fibrous bands extending out to the pleura with associated dilatation and bronchiectasis of proximal airways. Vascular sclerosis affecting both pulmonary arteries and veins may be seen in conjunction with OB. Current evidence suggests that OB is a feature of chronic rejection.

Usually, OB results in a progressive loss of function due to airflow obstruction over a period of 6–12 months, leading to respiratory failure and death (Figure 13R.1). However, a few patients appear to 'stabilize' with evidence of inactive OB on biopsy and an attenuation of the loss in FEV_1. Some patients with OB have demonstrated a clinical response to increased immunosuppression.[57] Most transplant units switch patients from cyclosporin- to tacrolimus-based immunosuppression when OB is diagnosed. Research seems to identify those patients at risk of this most important complication at an early stage, when augmented immunosuppression might be successful in preventing irreversible bronchiolar obliteration.

LYMPHOPROLIFERATIVE DISORDERS

An association between immunosuppression and lymphoproliferative disorders is well recognized, B-cell non-Hodgkin's lymphoma being the most common. These lymphomas are usually associated with the Epstein–Barr virus and may involve any organ. The lymphoma usually responds to a reduction in the level of immunosuppression and the administration of high-dose aciclovir. If disseminated, however, it may require more formal chemotherapy

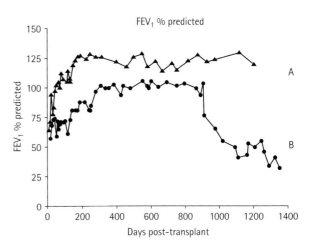

Figure 13R.1 *A plot of forced expiratory volume in 1 second (FEV₁) against time in two patients following heart/lung transplantation showing typical time course of improvement to a normal FEV₁. Patient A remains free of obliterative bronchiolitis, but patient B shows a typical deterioration in FEV₁ due to the onset of this complication.*

or use of a monoclonal antibody directed against the surface marker called CD20.

DISEASE RECURRENCE

There has been great interest in the study of lungs after successful lung transplantation to see if the acquired lung disease will recur in the allografts. To date, there is no evidence of primary pulmonary hypertension returning in lung grafts. Vascular sclerosis of pulmonary vessels is seen in all patients who have obliterative bronchiolitis.

CONSEQUENCES OF DENERVATION

The surgery involved in lung transplantation severs all vagal supply to and from the lung. To date, there is no evidence of reinnervation with time after human lung transplantation. As a consequence of the denervation, the cough reflex is depressed, but the pattern of breathing during wakefulness and sleep remains normal. Most studies have demonstrated a normal ventilation response to hypercapnia. The pattern of increased ventilation on exercise has been reported as showing a faster rise in tidal volume and slower rise in rate compared to controls.[58] Early reports suggest that the lungs of patients following HLT show evidence of denervation hypersensitivity to the muscarinic agonist methacholine.[59] However, more recent *in vivo* studies have failed to confirm this convincingly, and *in vitro* studies of bronchial muscle from the lungs of transplant recipients have not demonstrated denervation hypersensitivity.

CONCLUSIONS

Lung transplantation now offers an effective therapy for patients with end-stage pulmonary vascular disease. Debate continues as to which transplant operation should be performed for such patients. The major practical problem facing lung transplantation at this time is a shortfall in suitable donor organs compared with the number of potential recipients. The shortfall in donor organs has led to a renewed interest in xenotransplantation. However, this is not likely to be feasible within the next 5 years. Children or small adults may be considered for living donor lobar transplantation. In the early postoperative period, opportunist infection and graft rejection remain major problems and, in the long term, obliterative bronchiolitis affects approximately 30% of patients, leading to graft failure. Much current research is aimed at reducing this figure. Patients who have received lung transplants and remain free of this complication enjoy an excellent standard of life with normal or near-normal restoration of activities and good prospects for prolonged survival.

KEY POINTS

- No prospective randomized studies are available to relieve the uncertainty as to the best lung transplant procedure for patients with PAH.
- There has been considerable change in the approach to the assessment and listing of patients with severe PAH since the development of prostanoid therapy.
- Overall the results show that major pulmonary hypertension and transplant centers vary considerably regarding patterns of referral, listing and transplantation of patients, and it is only with continued carefully collected registry data that guidelines for best practice will be refined.
- The International Society for Heart and Lung Transplantation Registry shows a 1-year survival of 70% with a 5-year survival of 50% following lung transplantation.
- Primary pulmonary hypertension has also been identified as an individual risk factor to the development of obliterative bronchiolitis in transplanted patients.

REFERENCES

●1 Reitz BA, Wallwork J, Hunt SA *et al.* Heart-lung transplantation: a successful therapy for patients with pulmonary vascular disease. *N Engl J Med* 1982;**306**:557–63.

2 Penketh A, Higenbottam T, Hakim M *et al.* Heart and lung transplantation in patients with end stage lung disease. *Br Med J* 1987;**295**:311–14.

3 Wildevuuer CRH, Benfield JR. A review of 23 lung transplantations by 20 surgeons. *Ann Thorac Surg* 1979;**9**:489–515.

●4 Toronto Lung Transplant Group. Unilateral transplant for pulmonary fibrosis. *N Engl J Med* 1986;**314**:1140–5.

●5 Patterson GA, Cooper JD, Goldman B *et al.* Technique of successful clinical double lung transplantation. *Ann Thorac Cardiovasc Surg* 1988;**45**:626–33.

6 Patterson GA, Todd TR, Cooper JD *et al.* Airway complications after double lung transplantation. Toronto Lung Transplant Group. *J Thorac Cardiovasc Surg* 1990;**99**:14–20.

7 Noirclerc MJ, Metras D, Vaillant A *et al.* Bilateral bronchial anastomosis in double lung and heart lung transplantations. *Eur J Cardiothorac Surg* 1990;**4**:314–17.

8 Pasque ML, Cooper JD, Kaiser LR *et al.* Improved technique for bilateral lung transplantations: rationale and initial clinical experience. *Ann Thorac Surg* 1990;**48**:785–91.

9 Doig JC, Richens D, Corris PA *et al.* Resolution of pulmonary hypertension after single lung transplantation. *Br Heart J* 1991;**66**:431–4.

10 Pasque MK, Kaiser LR, Dresler CM *et al.* Single lung transplantation for pulmonary hypertension. *J Thorac Cardiovasc Surg* 1992;**103**:475–82.

●11 Levine SM, Gibbons WJ, Dresler CM *et al.* Single lung transplantation for primary pulmonary hypertension. *Chest* 1990;**98**:1107–15.

12 Moser KM, Daily PA, Peterson K *et al.* Thromboendarterectomy for chronic major-vessel thromboembolic pulmonary hypertension. Immediate and long-term results in 42 patients. *Ann Intern Med* 1987;**107**:560–5.

13 Hosenpud JD, Bennet LE, Keck BM *et al.* The Registry of the International Society for Heart and Lung transplantation: eighteenth official report 2001. *J Heart Lung Transplant* 2001;**20**:805–15.

14 Bando K, Keenan RJ, Paradis IL *et al.* Impact of pulmonary hypertension on outcome after single lung transplantation. *Ann Thorac Surg* 1994;**58**:1336–42.

15 McCarthy PM, Rosenkranz ER, White RD *et al.* Single lung transplantation with atrial septal defect repair for Eisenmenger's syndrome. *Ann Thorac Surg* 1991;**52**:300–3.

16 Pasque MK, Trulock EP, Kaiser LR *et al.* Single lung transplantation for pulmonary hypertension: three month haemodynamic follow up. *Circulation* 1991;**84**:2275–9.

17 Pasque MK, Trulock EP, Cooper JD, *et al.* Single lung transplantation for pulmonary hypertension: single institution experience in 34 patients. *Circulation* 1995;**92**:2252–8.

18 Starnes VA, Stinson EB, Oyer PE *et al.* Single lung transplantation: a new therapeutic option for patients with pulmonary hypertension. *Transplant Proc* 1991;**23**:1209–10.

19 Ueno T, Smith JA, Snell GI *et al.* Bilateral sequential single lung transplantation for pulmonary hypertension and Eisenmenger's syndrome. *Ann Thorac Surg* 2000;**69**:381–7.

20 Birsan T, Zuckermann Z, Artemiou O, *et al.* Bilateral lung transplantation for pulmonary hypertension. *Transplant Proc* 1997;**29**:2892–4.

21 White RI, Robbins RC, Altinger J et al. Heart-lung transplantation for primary pulmonary hypertension. Ann Thorac Surg 1999;**67**:937–42.

22 Mikhail G, Al-Kattan K, Banner N et al. Long term results of heart lung transplantation for pulmonary hypertension. Transplant Proc 1997;**29**:633.

23 Stoica SC, McNeil KD, Perreas K et al. Heart lung transplantation for Eisenmenger syndrome: early and long term results. Ann Thorac Surg 2001;**72**:1887–91.

24 Boujoukos AJ, Martich GD, Vega JD et al. Reperfusion injury in single lung transplant recipients with pulmonary hypertension and emphysema. J Heart Lung Transplant 1997;**16**:440–8.

25 Kramer MR, Marshall SE, McDougall IR et al. The distribution of ventilation and perfusion after single lung transplantation in patients with pulmonary fibrosis and pulmonary hypertension. Transplant Proc 1991;**23**:1215–16.

26 Levine SM, Jenkinson SG, Bryan CL et al. Ventilation-perfusion inequalities during graft rejection in patients undergoing single lung transplantation for primary pulmonary hypertension. Chest 1992;**101**: 401–5.

27 Huerd SS, Hodges TN, Grover FL et al. Secondary pulmonary hypertension does not adversely affect outcome after single lung transplantation. J Thorac Cardiovasc Surg 2000;**119**:458–65.

28 Kramer MR, Valantine HA, Marshall SE et al. Recovery of the right ventricle after single lung transplantation. Am J Cardiol 1994;**73**:494–500.

29 Shulman LR, Leibowitz DW, Anadarangam T et al. Variability of right ventricular functional recovery after lung transplantation. Transplantation 1996;**62**:622–5.

30 Lupinetti FM, Bolling SF, Bove EL et al. Selective lung or heart lung transplantation for pulmonary hypertension associated with congenital cardiac anomalies. Ann Thorac Surg 1994;**57**:1545–9.

31 Waddell TK, Bennett LW, Kennedy R et al. Lung or heart lung transplantation for Eisenmenger's syndrome: Analysis of the ISHLT/UNOS joint thoracic registry (abstract). J Heart Lung Transplant 2000;**19**:57.

32 Chapelier A, Vouhe P, Macchiarini P et al. Comparative outcome of heart lung and lung transplantation for pulmonary hypertension. J Thorac Cardiovac Surg 1993;**106**:299–307.

●33 Bando K, Armitage JM, Paradis IL et al. Indications for, and results of, single, bilateral and heart lung transplantation for pulmonary hypertension. J Thorac Cardiovasc Surg 1994;**108**:1056–65.

34 Gammie JS, Keenan RJ, Pham SM et al. Single versus double lung transplantation for pulmonary hypertension. J Thorac Cardiovasc Surg 1998;**115**:397–403.

35 Conte JV, Borja MJ, Patel CB et al. Lung transplantation for primary and secondary pulmonary hypertension. Ann Thorac Surg 2001;**72**:1673–80.

36 D'Alonzo GE, Barst RJ, Ayers SM et al. Survival in patients with primary pulmonary hypertension. Ann Intern Med 1991;**115**:343–9.

37 Barst RJ, Rubin LJ, Long WA et al. A comparison of continuous intravenous epoprostenol (prostacyclin) with conventional therapy for primary pulmonary hypertension. N Engl J Med 1996;**334**:296–301.

38 Robbins IM, Christman BW, Newman JH et al. A survey of diagnostic practices and the use of epoprostenol in patients with primary pulmonary hypertension. Chest 1998;**114**:1269–75.

39 Conte JV, Gaine SP, Orens JB et al. The influence of continuous intravenous prostacyclin therapy for primary pulmonary hypertension on the timing and outcome of transplantation. J Heart Lung Transplant 1998;**17**:679–85.

40 Hosenpud JD, Bennett LE, Keck BM et al. The registry of the International Society for Heart and Lung Transplantation: seventeenth official report. J Heart Lung Transplant 2000;**19**:909–31.

41 Pielsticker EJ, Martinex FJ, Rubenfire M. Lung and heart lung transplant practice patterns in pulmonary hypertension centres. J Heart Lung Transplant 2001;**20**:1297–304.

42 Rich S, Levy PS. Characteristics of surviving and non-surviving patients with primary pulmonary hypertension. Am J Med 1984;**76**:573–8.

43 Glanville AR, Burke CM, Theodore J et al. Primary pulmonary hypertension: length of survival of patients referred for heart and lung transplantation. Chest 1987;**91**:675–81.

44 Eysmann SB, Palevsky HI, Reichek N et al. Two dimensional echocardiography and cardiac catheterisation correlates of survival in primary pulmonary hypertension. Circulation 1989;**79**:353–60.

45 Morrison EB, Gaffrey FA, Eigenbrodt EH et al. Severe pulmonary hypertension associated with macronodular (post-necrotic) cirrhosis and auto-immune pneumonia. Am J Med 1980;**69**:513–19.

46 Bidstrup BP, Royston D, Supsfold RW et al. Reduction in blood loss and blood use after cardiopulmonary bypass with high dose aprotinin. J Thorac Cardiovasc Surg 1989;**93**:364–72.

47 Gould FK, Freeman R, Taylor CE et al. Prophylaxis and management of cytomegalovirus pneumonitis following pulmonary transplantation. J Heart Lung Transplant 1993;**12**:695–9.

48 Corris PA, Odom NJ, Jackson G et al. Reimplantation injury after lung transplantation in a rat model. J Heart Transplant 1987;**6**:234–7.

49 Higenbottam T, Stuart S, Penketh A et al. Transbronchial lung biopsy for the diagnosis of rejection in heart lung transplant recipients. Transplantation 1988;**46**:532–9.

50 Rabinowich H, Zeevi A, Paradis IL et al. Proliferative responses of bronchoalveolar lavage lymphocytes from heart lung transplant patients. Transplantation 1990;**49**:115–21.

51 Yousem SA, Berry GJ, Brunt EM et al. A working formulation for the standardisation of nomenclature in the diagnosis of heart and lung rejection: Lung Rejection Study Group. J Heart Transplant 1990;**9**:593–601.

52 Dauber JH, Paradis IL, Drummer JE et al. Allograft recipients. Clin Chest Med 1990;**11**:291–308.

53 Veale D, Glasper P, Gascoigne AD et al. Ciliary beat frequency in transplanted lungs. Thorax 1992;**48**:629–31.

54 Kshetty VR, Kroshus TJ, Savik K *et al.* Primary pulmonary hypertension as a risk factor for he development of obliterative bronchiolitis in lung allograft recipients. *Chest* 1996;**110**:704–9.

55 Scott JP, Higenbottam TW, Sharples C *et al.* Risk factors for obliterative bronchiolitis in heart lung transplant recipients. *Transplantation* 1991;**51**:813–17.

56 Milne DS, Gascoigne AD, Wilkes J *et al.* The immuno-histological features of obliterative bronchiolitis following lung transplantation. *Transplantation* 1992;**54**:748–50.

57 Glanville AR, Baldwin JC, Burke CM *et al.* Obliterative bronchiolitis after heart lung transplantation. Apparent arrest by augmented immunosuppression. *Ann Intern Med* 1987;**107**:300–4.

58 Sciurba FC, Owens GR, Sanders MH *et al.* Evidence of an altered pattern of breathing during exercise in recipients of heart lung transplants. *N Engl J Med* 1988;**319**:1186–92.

59 Glanville AR, Burke CM, Theodore J *et al.* Bronchial hyper-responsiveness after human cardiopulmonary transplantation. *Clin Sci* 1987;**73**:299–303.

13S

Atrial septostomy

JULIO SANDOVAL AND JORGE GASPAR

INTRODUCTION

Right ventricular (RV) function is an important determinant of natural history in primary pulmonary hypertension (PPH):[1–3] hemodynamic parameters that reflect RV dysfunction, such as an elevated mean right atrial pressure (RAP), a low cardiac output (CO), and low pulmonary arterial oxygen saturation are associated with poor prognosis.[1–3] This chapter reviews the pathophysiology of right ventricular dysfunction and provides a perspective regarding the mechanisms of RVF in the setting of PPH. The role of atrial septostomy, an intervention specifically oriented to the relief of RVF, in the treatment scheme of PPH is then discussed.

MECHANISMS OF RIGHT VENTRICULAR DYSFUNCTION

Because the characteristics of the right ventricle make it difficult to assess its function, the precise nature of right ventricular dysfunction (RVD) in most of clinical situations remains unknown. In general, there are three types of right ventricular dysfunction:[4]

- volume overload (i.e. atrial septal defect, tricuspid insufficiency);
- ischemia (i.e. atherosclerotic-related ischemic heart disease affecting the RV); and
- pressure overload (i.e. all forms of pulmonary arterial hypertension).

It is likely that a combination of these factors is necessary to produce RVF.

In contrast to volume overload, pressure overload is poorly tolerated by the right ventricle due to its intrinsic functional characteristics.[4,5] Acute elevations in RV afterload such as occur in patients with massive pulmonary embolism (PE) preclude the compensatory development of RV hypertrophy and geometric alterations.[4,6] RV ischemia combined with increased RV afterload contributes to the development of RVF in the setting of acute PE.[6]

Chronic RV pressure overload is better tolerated than acute RV pressure overload, since all the compensatory mechanisms (i.e. increased preload, geometric alteration and RV hypertrophy) can be called upon.[4,5] Even chronicity, however, does not abolish the often inadequate RV response to pure pressure overload occurring in variety of situations such as pulmonic stenosis, congenital transposition of the great arteries, chronic PE and PPH.[4,5] These patients demonstrate reduced right ventricular ejection fraction (RVEF) and abnormal RV Frank–Starling curves, with marked right atrial pressure elevations, particularly during exercise.[4,7]

THE RIGHT VENTRICLE IN PPH

In PPH, gradual increases in afterload are well tolerated because the RV has time to assemble new sarcomeres in parallel to increase wall thickness (appropriate RV hypertrophic response) in order to minimize wall stress via the La Place relationship.[5] In severe PPH, however,

RV volume and size are typically markedly increased in both systole and diastole.[5,8] The increase in RV diastolic dimension is the result of chamber remodeling due to an increase in cardiac myocyte length,[9] secondary to the new synthesis of sarcomeres assembled in series, thus allowing the pressure-overloaded RV to produce a larger stroke volume and to maintain cardiac output. The increase in systolic volume is secondary to the marked and longstanding increase in systolic wall stress and possibly to the presence of intrinsic systolic contractile dysfunction.[5]

There is great variability in the tendency of PPH patients to develop RVF. Despite similar levels of pulmonary artery pressure, some individuals sustain an adequate RV function and live for a long period of time while others develop RVF and die sooner. It appears that factors other than simply pressure overload are necessary to explain RVF in PPH. Hypotheses for the development of RVF from chronic pressure overload in the setting of PPH include:

- RV ischemia
- sympathetic nervous system overdrive
- altered cardiac gene expression in PPH
- volume overload (Figure 13S.1).

Right ventricular ischemia

The importance of RV ischemia in the genesis of RVF has been clearly demonstrated in the setting of acute pressure overload.[6] The possibility also exists that cardiac ischemia, resulting from anomalies in RV microcirculation, may lead to RVF in chronic pressure overload.

Chronic pressure overload generates RV wall hypertrophy in order to overcome systolic wall stress. In the presence of severe RV systolic hypertension, transmural and coronary perfusion pressures increase accordingly. This phenomenon limits RV coronary flow to diastole only.[10] Compensatory epicardial arterial enlargement occurs but it is not proportional to wall hypertrophy,[11] neither is it observed at a capillary level,[12] making the muscle fibers more susceptible to ischemia.

In animal models,[13,14] it has been demonstrated that the subendocardial to subepicardial blood flow ratio is diminished at rest and after the injection of adenosine. This generates a loss of coronary reserve due to an increase in the basal flow, making the RV more susceptible to ischemia. These RV microcirculatory abnormalities in blood flow supply are present in a moment when the hypertrophied right heart increases its metabolic oxygen demands as a result of chamber dilation and increased wall stress.[6,14]

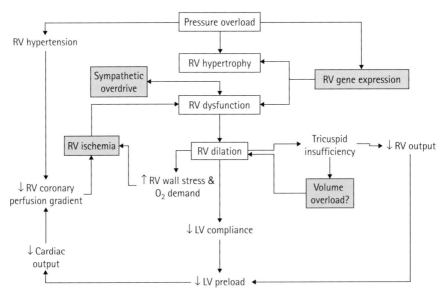

Figure 13S.1 *Mechanistic hypotheses for the development of right ventricular (RV) failure (RVF) from severe chronic pressure overload. RVF is mainly the result of pressure overload. Other factors, such as RV ischemia, excessive sympathetic overdrive, RV volume overload and altered RV gene expression, may contribute to modulate the response of the right ventricle and play a role in the pathogenesis of RVF. Changes in gene expression may dictate the response to either an appropriate RV hypertrophy or to RV dysfunction. RV dysfunction may elicit a sympathetic overdrive response, which in turn contributes to RV damage and dysfunction. RV dilation and dysfunction produces a reduction in left ventricular (LV) preload by both a reduction in LV compliance and a reduction in RV output due to tricuspid insufficiency and possibly to a deficit in RV systolic function. Tricuspid insufficiency might contribute to volume overload. As a result of low cardiac output and RV hypertension, the RV coronary perfusion gradient diminishes, which along with an increase in RV wall stress and oxygen demand produces RV ischemia, which contributes to RV dysfunction and failure. See text.*

In a group of patients with PPH, we have recently shown[15] that RV ischemia, as assessed by stress myocardial scintigraphy, was present in nine of 23 patients. In these patients, a significant correlation was found between RV ischemia and elevation of right ventricular end-diastolic pressure, right atrial pressure, and a decrease in mixed venous oxygen saturation. Patients without RV ischemia in this study did not show hemodynamic evidence of RVF.

Sympathetic nervous system overdrive

In patients with PPH, there is growing evidence that excessive adrenergic stimulation, as seen in other forms of heart failure, may impair RV function. Studying failing, hypertrophied RV from patients with PPH, Bristow et al.[16] described a decrease in the gene and protein expression of β_1-adrenergic receptors (down-regulation) and adenylyl cyclase that contributes to β_1-adrenergic receptor pathway desensitization, which is produced in response to locally increased adrenergic activity. These effects compromise myocardial reserve of the RV and may also reduce intrinsic contractile function.[17]

Biochemical evidence of neurohormonal activation, as assessed by increased levels of norepinephrine, has been demonstrated in patients with right heart failure from pulmonary hypertension.[18,19] The increased levels of norepinephrine correlated with the degree of hemodynamic abnormality found in these patients,[18] and a significant reduction in circulating norepinephrine after digoxin administration has also been reported.[19]

There are other indirect pieces of evidence of excessive adrenergic stimulation in PPH. Through the use of spectral analysis of heart rate variability (HRV), our group[20] has been able to demonstrate that an autonomic cardiac disturbance is present in Eisenmenger's syndrome and to a greater extent in PPH patients. The circadian rhythm of HRV in these patients is lost mainly due to an increase in sympathetic tone. Moreover, sympathetic denervation of the RV, as assessed by a scan of myocardial sympathetic function ([^{123}I]MIBG), has been demonstrated in a patient with pulmonary hypertension and Eisenmenger reaction.[21] Interestingly, RV denervation in this case occurred prior to the impairments in RV perfusion and free fatty acid metabolism (i.e. viability).

Together, these studies suggest that excessive adrenergic stimulation exists in the setting of severe pulmonary hypertension. This may lead to sympathetic denervation of the RV and it may play a significant role in the genesis of RVF from pulmonary hypertension. Studies in this direction may be useful not only in elucidating the mechanisms of RVF, arrhythmias and sudden death seen in these patients, but also in opening the potential for therapeutic selective β-blockade.

Altered gene expression

One interesting hypothesis regarding the mechanisms of RVF, advanced by Bristow and colleagues,[5] is that chronically elevated wall stress leads to changes in gene expression that produce contractile dysfunction and perhaps other deleterious biological phenomena such as programmed cell death (apoptosis). In this model, the variability of the patients in their tendency to develop RVF is explained by gene polymorphisms that influence the ability to reduce wall stress by modifying the concentric hypertrophic response (i.e. myocardial compensation occurs in subjects who have increased RV wall thickness because of a reduction in wall stress).

One suspected molecular variant is the angiotensin converting enzyme (ACE) gene, a form of which (DD genotype) is associated with increased circulating and cardiac tissue ACE activity.[22] In this study, PPH patients with DD genotype (prevalence of 50%) had lower levels of right atrial pressure and higher levels of cardiac output than those without this genotype (non-DD), despite similar levels of mean pulmonary artery pressure. In our population of PPH patients, the prevalence of DD genotype is lower (about 33%) and is also associated with a relatively better preserved RV function, although significant overlap exists.[23]

Other changes in gene expression occurring in the pressure-overloaded right ventricle[5] that may be relevant in the genesis of intrinsic contractile systolic dysfunction include:

- the already mentioned decrease in the gene and protein expression of β_1-adrenergic receptors and adenylyl cyclase that occurs in response to locally increased adrenergic activity;
- a decrease in type 1 angiotensin II (AT1) receptor density;
- an increase in β_2-adrenergic receptor mRNA and protein expression in the early stage and an attenuation in the advanced stage of RVF;
- an increase in the expression of atrial natriuretic peptide (ANP), a non-specific marker of myocyte hypertrophy; and
- a change in the isoform distribution of myosin heavy chain isogenes (i.e. down-regulation in the gene expression of the fast myosin adenosine triphosphatase activity α-isoform and up-regulation in the slow-activity β-isoform), which, in addition to a reduction in adrenergic signal transduction proteins that mediate support to the failing heart, is a candidate for the molecular basis of systolic dysfunction in the pressure-overloaded RV. Further studies need to test this hypothesis as the basis for RV systolic dysfunction and RVF in PPH.[5]

Volume overload

The role of volume overload as a causative factor of RV dysfunction in PPH has not been fully appreciated. Volume overload, however, by increasing diastolic wall stress, is likely to be a major stimulus for remodeling and changes in gene expression that lead to contractile dysfunction.[5] Volume overload in the setting of PPH may occur either as a result of the activation of the adrenergic pathway and its interaction with the renin–angiotensin–aldosterone system[5,22,24] or as a consequence of associated tricuspid insufficiency. Experimental animal models combining pressure and volume overload have underlined the importance of tricuspid insufficiency in the genesis of pure RVF.[25,26] Similarly, in a recent clinical study involving the use of a right ventricular ejection fraction thermodilution catheter, and MRI studies to evaluate right ventricular performance in patients with pulmonary arterial hypertension, the severity of tricuspid insufficiency was the major determinant of cardiac output in these patients.[8] Accordingly, the real contribution of tricuspid insufficiency to RVF, either as a result of RV dilation or as a consequence of dysfunction of the subvalvular apparatus (i.e. ischemia), should be addressed in future studies.

In summary, despite its importance as a determinant of survival, the pathophysiology of RVF is incompletely understood. Although excessive and longstanding RV afterload plays the main causative role, there is now growing evidence of the potential participation of RV ischemia, excessive sympathetic overdrive, volume overload, and altered gene expression (Figure 13S.1). Participation or absence of each of these factors in a given patient may explain the highly variable presentation of RVF in the setting of PPH. A better knowledge of the intrinsic pathophysiological factors involved in the genesis of RV failure may increase our therapeutic options in PPH.

MEDICAL TREATMENT OF RVF IN PPH

As discussed above, RV dysfunction and failure are mainly the result of increased, longstanding, pressure overload in PAH. Accordingly, any intervention capable of reducing pulmonary vascular resistance and pressure is a logical and effective approach to treatment. It is not valid, however, to extrapolate from what has been learned from global (left and right) ventricular failure to the management of RVF.

Contemporary treatment of PPH attempts to alleviate pulmonary microvascular obstruction,[27–30] and is reviewed elsewhere in this book. These interventions have proved useful in improving quality of life and survival in PPH. There is evidence that partial reversal of remodeling in the RV occurs in patients responding to pharmacological interventions such as calcium channel blockers[31] and prostacyclin therapy.[32] Although not completely defined, this effect is likely related to reduced afterload, since it also occurs in PPH patients after lung transplantation, where RV function recovers after normalization of afterload.[33]

Other pharmacological interventions for RVF in PPH may be indicated. Diuretics are used to prevent fluid overload and to treat edema and passive liver congestion.[24,27,28] Increased RV filling pressures and upstream venous congestion lead to salt and water retention because of activation of the sympathetic nervous system and the renin–angiotensin–aldosterone axis.[24] Although diuretics may exert a beneficial effect by decreasing right-sided filling pressures, tricuspid regurgitation, chamber dilation, and thus, diastolic wall stress,[5] a high-normal jugular venous pressure (increased preload) is necessary to maintain cardiac output in the setting of increased afterload.[7,24,27,28] Similarly, both excessive diuretic and vasodilator use may decrease systemic arterial pressure, increase the risk of RV ischemia, and consequently aggravate RV dysfunction.[24,27] Accordingly, cautious use of diuretics is highly recommended to avoid excessive preload reduction, systemic arterial hypotension, renal dysfunction and electrolyte imbalance.

Inotropic support for the failing RV may be also necessary. Both dobutamine and dopamine, alone or combined with norepinephrine, are helpful when decompensation occurs.[24] Digoxin may have a place in the treatment of RVF from PPH, not only for its mild inotropic properties but also for its antiarrhythmogenic and mild anti-adrenergic effects.[5,19,24,27,28] Careful monitoring is also advised to avoid digoxin toxicity.

The potential benefit of other pharmacological interventions such as ACE inhibitors and, in particular, selective β-blockade, has not been explored in PPH. It is possible that future treatments would reverse not only pulmonary vascular remodeling but also myocardial remodeling and the changes in myocardial gene expression that cause contractile dysfunction.[5]

Although there is no question that all the above-mentioned interventions are useful in the treatment of RVF from PPH, it is also true that their effectiveness is not universal. A beneficial long-term response to oral vasodilators in PPH is achieved in fewer than 25% of patients.[34,35] On the other hand, for the larger group of patients with severe disease, interventions such as the long-term infusion of prostacyclin and lung transplantation have been beneficial,[34,36–38] but their worldwide application is limited by technical difficulties and cost. Furthermore, despite intravenous prostacyclin infusion, RV dysfunction may recur or progress. Given the ominous prognostic implications of RVF in the setting of PPH, the use of alternatives specifically oriented for the relief of RVF, such as atrial septostomy, may be indicated.

ATRIAL SEPTOSTOMY IN THE TREATMENT OF RIGHT VENTRICULAR FAILURE FROM PRIMARY PULMONARY HYPERTENSION

Background and rationale

The use of atrial septostomy (AS) in PPH is supported by the fact that survival in PPH is largely influenced by the functional status of the right ventricle; right ventricular failure and recurrent syncope are associated with a poor short-term prognosis.[1-3] Second, several experimental and clinical observations have suggested that an inter-atrial defect might be of benefit in severe pulmonary hypertension. Early animal studies by Austen et al.[39] showed that an inter-atrial communication allowed decompression of a hypertensive right ventricle and augmentation of systemic blood flow, particularly during exercise. In addition, clinical studies showed that patients with PPH who had a patent foramen ovale lived longer than those without intracardiac shunting.[40,41] Similarly, patients with Eisenmenger syndrome appear to live longer and have heart failure less frequently than patients with PPH.[42,43] Taken together, these studies have suggested that deterioration in symptoms, right heart failure, and death in PPH are associated with obstruction to systemic flow and failure of the right ventricle. The presence of an atrial septal defect in this setting would allow right-to-left shunting to increase systemic output that, in spite of the fall in systemic arterial oxygen saturation, will produce an increase in systemic oxygen transport. Furthermore, the shunt at the atrial level would allow decompression of the right atrium and right ventricle, alleviating signs and symptoms of right heart failure.

Blade balloon atrial septostomy (BBAS) as a palliative therapy for refractory PPH was first reported by Rich and Lam in 1983.[44] Subsequent studies, particularly those of Nihill et al.[45] and Kerstein et al.[46] have shown that BBAS can be successfully performed in patients with advanced PPH and can bring about significant clinical and hemodynamic improvement. In addition to symptomatic improvement, there seems to be a trend toward improved survival in patients with severe PPH who have undergone successful BBAS. Similar results have been obtained with the use of graded balloon dilation atrial septostomy (BDAS), a variant of BBAS described recently.[47,48]

Worldwide experience with atrial septostomy in pulmonary hypertension

The precise role of AS in the treatment of PPH remains uncertain because most of the knowledge regarding its use comes from small series or case reports and there have been no randomized trials. The potential beneficial effects and risks of AS have been recently addressed in a review[49] derived from a collective analysis of 64 cases from the literature.[44-48,50-57] Important issues derived from this review were discussed and debated at the World Symposium–Primary Pulmonary Hypertension 1998 in Evian, France.[58,59] Information derived from this review regarding the role of AS in the setting of PPH is presented in this chapter.

Patients

Severe PPH has been the main indication (84%) for AS.[49] Other indications have included PAH associated to surgically corrected congenital heart disease (12.5%) and peripheral chronic thromboembolic pulmonary hypertension (3.5%). The procedure has been performed mainly in young women. Patients from the worldwide collective experience had a mean age of 25 ± 13 years (range 0.33–51 years) and 80% were women. Most patients who have undergone AS have had severe PPH unresponsive to conventional treatment (which included oral vasodilators, if clinically indicated, but excluded chronic intravenous prostacyclin), with severe exercise-related dyspnea (83%), syncope or near syncope (51%) and evidence of right heart failure (60%). In some of the patients the procedure was performed on an emergency basis; in others it was performed electively for severe pulmonary hypertension and functional limitation.[49]

The baseline hemodynamic profile of these patients was in support of the severity of their pulmonary hypertension. The mean pulmonary artery pressure (mPAP) was 66 ± 19 mmHg, the mean cardiac index (CI) was 2.07 ± 0.54 L/min·m^2 and the calculated pulmonary vascular resistance (PVR) index was 30 ± 14 u/m^2. Right ventricular dysfunction in most of these patients was also evident by an elevated mean right atrial pressure (mRAP) of 13 ± 8 mmHg.[49]

Procedure

Two types of atrial septostomy, BBAS and BDAS, have been used in the treatment of PPH. The basic difference between the two procedures is that, in contrast to BBAS, in BDAS, the Park blade septostomy catheter is not used and the inter-atrial orifice is created by puncture with a Brockenbrough needle and use of progressively larger balloon catheters in a step-by-step fashion. Both procedures follow a similar protocol, that is, standard right and left heart catheterization performed under conscious sedation, and hemodynamic monitoring in the cardiac catheterization laboratory. In the collective worldwide experience,[49] a combined procedure of BBAS[45,46] was performed in 35 (55%) of the 64 patients, and BDAS[47,48,53] was performed in the remainder. A prospective evaluation of potential differences between the two procedures with regard to hemodynamic results and risk of complications has not been done.

EVALUATION AND PREPARATION FOR BDAS

To ensure preservation of systemic O_2 transport once a right-to-left shunt is created, patients in whom BDAS is being considered should have a resting arterial O_2 saturation of at least 90% and a hematocrit level greater than 35%. In addition, in order to avoid the LV volume overload imposed by the shunt, LV function should be preserved,[28] as evidenced by the absence of clinically apparent left heart failure and an ejection fraction by echocardiography greater than 0.45. If LV function is adequate, atrial septostomy can be attempted in the critically ill patient with the graded dilatation procedure. Finally, it should be emphasized the procedure should be performed only in centers experienced in both interventional cardiology and pulmonary hypertension.[28,29,50]

BDAS TECHNIQUE

Whenever possible, the procedure is performed without supplemental oxygen in order to adequately gauge the shunt-induced changes in arterial O_2 saturation, which are of utmost importance in determining the final (optimal) size of the inter-atrial orifice. Mild conscious sedation may be used (i.e. midazolam 0.02–0.03 mg/kg), otherwise we prefer to avoid sedation in order to minimize its respiratory depressant effects.

A 6F introducer is placed in the right femoral artery for left heart catheterization using a 6F pigtail catheter. Two introducers are placed in the right femoral vein, with the punctures at least 2 cm apart. The most proximal puncture is for the trans-septal procedure and in the distal puncture a conventional introducer is placed for right heart catheterization using a balloon flow-directed catheter or a Cournand catheter. Anticoagulation is not initiated prior to the trans-septal puncture but frequent and thorough flushing of the catheters and sheaths, with heparinized saline (1000 U heparin in 1 liter of saline), is performed.

Right and left heart baseline pressures are recorded simultaneously and cardiac output is calculated through the indirect Fick principle using assumed oxygen consumption values. The finding of a large gradient between the right and left atria, which is considered a contraindication for blade atrial septostomy,[50] is not considered a contraindication for the graded balloon technique. On the other hand, it is recommended that patients with a baseline LVEDP above 12 mmHg should not undergo atrial septostomy.

Trans-septal puncture is performed with the Mullins introducer (without the sheath) and Brockenbrough needle using standard techniques.[60] We have always found the 2.5 cm Mullins catheter curve to be adequate but in patients with a markedly dilated right atrium a

3.0 cm curve would allow an easier approach to the out-bulging inter-atrial septum. The adequacy of the intended puncture site can be mapped by a tiny contrast staining of the septum through the Mullins introducer before puncturing with the needle (Figure 13S.2). As opposed to the situation where trans-septal puncture is done to perform percutaneous mitral commisurotomy (the most frequent current indication for trans-septal catheterization in adults), in the PPH population left atrial pressure is comparatively low and a brisk inspiration by the patient carries the theoretical risk of inadvertently allowing air to be suctioned into the left atrium. For this reason, once the correct and stable position of the Mullins introducer in the left atrium is confirmed, the needle is withdrawn and the catheter hub immediately occluded with a fingertip followed by a careful double flush. At this point heparin is administered (70 U/kg) and left atrial pressure is recorded. In our hospital we use the Inoue circular-end guidewire (Toray Industries, Inc., catalog number GMS-1) to maintain access in the left atrium because the rigidity of its shaft greatly facilitates balloon catheter trackability and the 4.5 cm diameter of its distal circled end, with a very soft tip, sits nicely and safely in the left atrium, providing great stability (Figure 13S.3). This guidewire has a diameter of 0.025 inch and the length of the straight segment is 150 cm (total length 175 cm) and therefore adequate for the majority of the current peripheral balloons. An alternative is to use a 0.035 inch extra support exchange guidewire, which should be advanced deeply into the left inferior pulmonary vein for adequate tracking support.

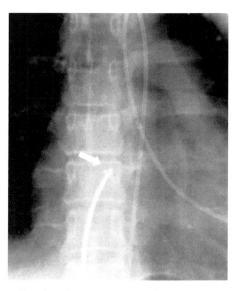

Figure 13S.2 *Anterio-posterior view of the Mullins dilator with the Brocken-brough needle at its tip. A small contrast injection (white arrow) is done to map the intended puncture site, which can then be seen in different projections to determine its correct location.*

Septostomy dilatation is then done in a graded step-by-step approach, beginning at 4 mm diameter with the Inoue septostomy dilator or at 3.7 mm with the dilator of a long 80 cm 11F introducer (Super-Arrow-Flex, Arrow International, Inc.) and followed by successive balloon diameters of 8, 12 and 16 mm as shown in Figure 13S.4 (if an 11 F dilator is used, its sheath can accommodate current low-profile peripheral balloons up to 18 mm diameter). After each step, a 3-minute waiting period is allowed to achieve steady state, followed by the careful measurement of LVEDP and arterial O_2 saturation. The final size of the defect is individualized for each patient and is determined when either of the following occurs:

- a LVEDP approaching 18 mmHg,
- an arterial oxygen saturation reduction near 80%, or
- when a 16 mm diameter dilatation has been achieved.

With the above criteria we have sought to decrease both the risk of excessive left ventricular volume overload that may lead to pulmonary edema and an excessive unwanted arterial oxygen desaturation, which have been identified as the causes of the high (25%) procedure-related death rate in earlier publications.[50] Using this incremental dilation protocol, we have reported one procedure-related death in a total of 22 procedures performed in 15 patients.[53] Also, this approach allows performing atrial septostomy even in the setting of a high-pressure gradient between right and left atria, which should probably not be attempted with the blade septostomy technique as the size of the defect, and, therefore, the shunted volume cannot be adequately controlled with this approach (Figure 13S.5). Using the described step-by-step approach some investigators have successfully dilated to 22 mm without complications (R Naeije, personal communication).

After achieving the final septostomy dilatation, complete right and left heart pressure recording (Figure 13S.6) and cardiac output determination are repeated and the patient is started on supplementary oxygen. The sheaths are removed 2 hours after the procedure.

The patients are monitored in an intensive care setting during the first 48 hours after the procedure in a 30–45° upright position, with continuous supplementary

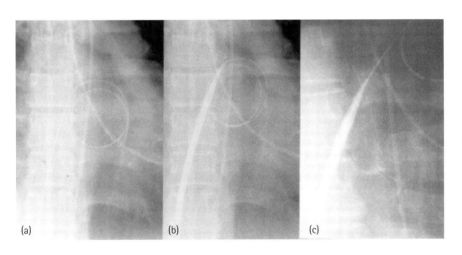

Figure 13S.3 *The Inoue circular-end guidewire is shown positioned in the left atrium (a). A 4 mm initial dilation of the atrial septum is achieved with the Inoue dilator (b) and concluded with a 8 mm balloon (c).*

(a) (b) (c)

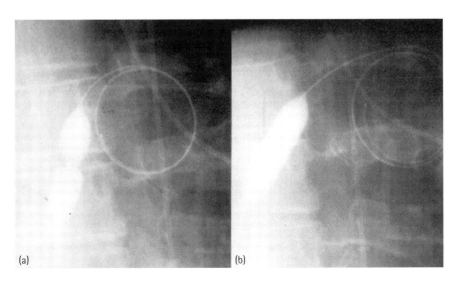

Figure 13S.4 *Dilation of the atrial septum can occasionally offer moderate resistance as shown in (a), but it has been always opened successfully with hand inflation (b), which has been measured to reach 4–6 ATM. Inflation is increased just enough to eliminate balloon waist and is repeated at least twice to counter elastic recoil.*

(a) (b)

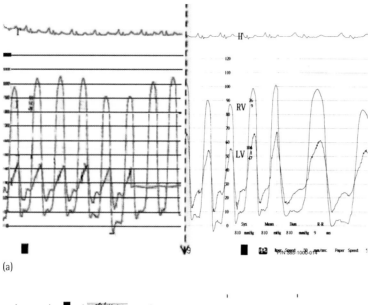

(a)

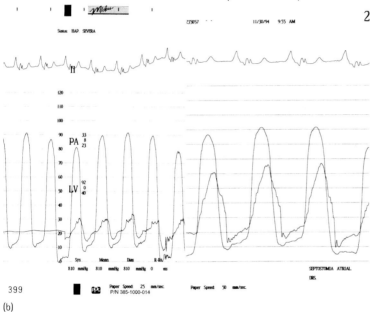

399

(b)

Figure 13S.5 *(a) Pressure recordings before atrial septostomy show, on the left panel, a mean right atrial pressure (mRAP) of 28 mmHg and a left ventricular (LV) end-diastolic pressure (LVEDP) of 9 mmHg; the inter-atrial gradient was 18 mmHg. Note the giant right atrial c-v waves peaking at 43 mmHg due to severe tricuspid regurgitation. Right ventricular end-diastolic pressure (RVEDP) was 27 mmHg (right panel). (b) After atrial septostomy, mRAP falls to 21 mmHg and c-v waves to 30 mmHg, whilst LVEDP has increased to 15 mmHg (left panel). The right panel shows a decrease of RVEDP to 20 mmHg. Usually, pulmonary artery pressure does not change significantly during the procedure, as can be seen by the systolic right ventricular (RV) pressure which is still around 65 mmHg as it was in the right panel of (a).*

oxygen administration. Echocardiography is useful to monitor for evidence of LV volume overload and is also useful in determining the baseline inter-atrial orifice diameter, which should be approximately 20% smaller than the maximal balloon diameter used due to tissue recoil (Figure 13S.7).

Immediate outcome after atrial septostomy

Atrial septostomy has been performed only in the setting of severe pulmonary hypertension, in patients who have been considered terminally ill. Accordingly, there is an inherent risk of complications and death during the procedure.

In the worldwide experience,[49] there were 10 procedure-related deaths, defined as death occurring within 1 month after the procedure, giving an overall procedure-related mortality of 16%. Patients who died during the procedure were in severe right ventricular failure, evidenced by a high mRAP (22 ± 9.6 mmHg) and a low CI (1.6 ± 0.69 L/min·m^2). In most patients who died immediately after the procedure, severe and refractory arterial hypoxemia (due to a large intracardiac shunting) was the cause of death. Severe pulmonary edema has also been described.[44] By univariate analysis, a baseline mRAP greater than 20 mmHg, PVR index greater than 55 u/m^2, and a predicted 1-year survival expectancy (using the equation of a multicenter National Institutes of Health study[1]) lower than 40% were all associated

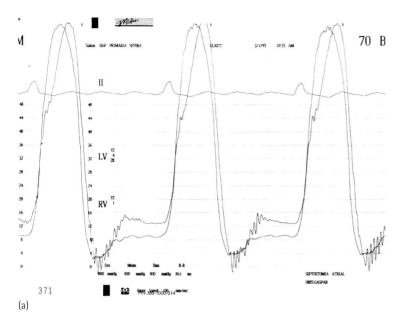

(a)

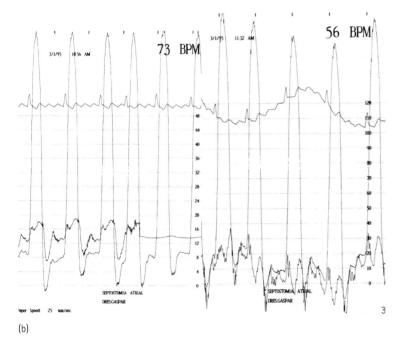

(b)

Figure 13S.6 *(a) Before atrial septostomy, right ventricular (RV) pressure tracing shows a sharp diastolic rise to a right ventricular end-diastolic pressure (RVEDP) of 13 mmHg while left ventricular (LV) diastolic pressure rises at a normal rate with a left ventricular end-diastolic pressure (LVEDP) of 9 mmHg. (b) Also before atrial septostomy, the left panel shows a LVEDP of 9 mmHg and a mean right atrial (RA) pressure of 14 mmHg with characteristic sharp y descent. The right panel shows a normal left atrial pressure and waveform; mean left atrial (LA) pressure was 8 mmHg.*

significantly with periprocedural death (P < 0.0001). Table 13S.1 shows the 1998 World Symposium recommendations to reduce the risk of death during the procedure.[58,59]

In most patients, symptoms and signs of RVF, including systemic venous congestion and syncope, are improved immediately after AS. In the worldwide experience,[49] the clinical status after septostomy improved in 47 out of 50 patients (94%) and was unchanged in three. Exercise endurance, assessed by the 6-minute walk, improved in most of the patients after septostomy.[53]

Immediate hemodynamic effects

With the exception of the decrease in systemic arterial oxygen saturation ($SaO_2\%$), most of the changes in hemodynamic variables after septostomy, while statistically significant, are only of modest magnitude.[49] The mRAP decreased by 3 mmHg (from 13 ± 7.8 to 10 ± 5.6 mmHg), equivalent to the concomitant increase in mean left atrial pressure (mLAP) from 5.2 ± 2.6 to 8.2 ± 3.1 mmHg. Cardiac index increased about 0.7 L/min·m^2, which resulted in an increase in systemic oxygen transport

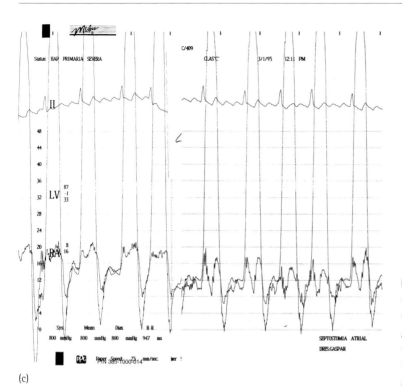

(c)

Figure 13S.6 (c) After atrial septostomy, the diastolic gradient between the left ventricle (LV) and right atrium (RA) has disappeared (left panel) mostly due to a left ventricular end-diastolic pressure increase to 14 mmHg. The right panel shows the concomitant left atrial (LA) pressure rise.

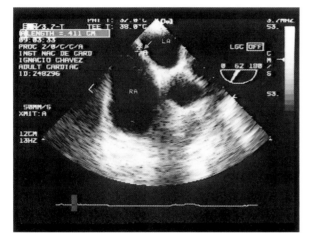

Figure 13S.7 Two-dimensional transesophageal approach in longitudinal plane (62°). The arrow shows the created inter-atrial defect. The diameter of septostomy is 4.1 mm.

(from 407 ± 117 to 461 ± 123 mL/min·m^2) despite a drop in SaO$_2$ from 93.4 ± 4.7 to $82 \pm 10.5\%$. There were no significant changes in mPAP or mean systemic artery pressures after the procedure.

The magnitude of hemodynamic changes after septostomy is not the same for all patients. Significant negative correlations were found between baseline mRAP and the change in mRAP after septostomy ($r = -0.66$; $P < 0.01$) and between baseline inter-atrial gradient and the change in inter-atrial gradient after septostomy ($r = -0.76$; $P < 0.01$), indicating that patients with

higher baseline mRAP and inter-atrial gradient had greater change in these variables after the procedure. Similarly, a significant positive correlation was found between the change in inter-atrial gradient after septostomy and the increase in cardiac index after the procedure ($r = 0.60$; $P < 0.01$), indicating that the increase in CI after septostomy was higher in patients who had a greater decrease in inter-atrial gradient after the procedure.[49] Moreover, when these patients were analyzed separately according to baseline mRAP as less than 10 mmHg, between 10 and 20 mmHg, or more than 20 mmHg, a different hemodynamic response to the procedure became evident (Table 13S.2). There was almost no change in the hemodynamic variables after septostomy in patients with a baseline mRAP less than 10 mmHg, whereas a large hemodynamic change occurred in patients with a baseline mRAP greater than 20 mmHg. Patients with a baseline mRAP between 10 and 20 mmHg had an intermediate, although significant, change after the procedure. It appears then, that the beneficial hemodynamic effects after septostomy (i.e. an increase in cardiac index and systemic oxygen transport) are more pronounced in patients with a more compromised baseline hemodynamic profile, a finding previously reported.[50] It is important to stress, however, that it is in this group, with a baseline mRAP greater than 20 mmHg, in which procedure-related deaths occurred.

Although the hemodynamic changes after septostomy seem only moderate, these measurements represent only the resting state. The hemodynamic impact of septostomy is likely to manifest further during exercise, as shown in

Table 13S.1 *Recommendations to minimize the risk of procedure-related mortality of atrial septostomy[49]*

- Atrial septostomy should be attempted only by those institutions with an established track record in the treatment of advanced pulmonary hypertension where atrial septostomy is performed with low morbidity.

- Atrial septostomy should not be performed in the patient with impending death and severe right ventricular failure on maximal cardiorespiratory support. An mRAP >20 mmHg, a PVR >55 U/m^2 and a predicted 1-year survival $<40\%$ are all significant predictors of procedure-related death.

- Before cardiac catheterization, it is important to confirm an acceptable baseline systemic oxygen saturation ($>90\%$ in room air) as well as to optimize cardiac function (adequate right heart filling pressure, additional inotropic support if needed).

- During cardiac catheterization the following are mandatory:
  - supplemental oxygen
  - mild and appropriate sedation to prevent anxiety
  - careful monitoring of variables (LAP, SaO$_2$% and mRAP)
  - to attempt a step-by-step procedure.

- After atrial septostomy, it is important to optimize oxygen delivery. Transfusion of packed red blood cells or erithropoietin (prior to and following the procedure if needed) may be necessary to increase oxygen content.

LAP, left atrial pressure; mRAP, mean right atrial pressure; PVRI, pulmonary vascular resistance index; SaO$_2$%, systemic arterial oxygen saturation.

Table 13S.2 *Hemodynamic effects after atrial septostomy according to the baseline right atrial pressure[49]*

Group	% Change in mRAP	% Change in CI	% Change in SaO$_2$	% Change in SOT
mRAP $<$ 10 mmHg (n = 15)	-5.5 ± 47	13 ± 14	-4.4 ± 4.3	8 ± 13
mRAP 10–20 mmHg (n = 18)	-31 ± 22	39 ± 27	-14 ± 7	19 ± 22
mRAP $>$ 20 mmHg (n = 6)	-32 ± 20	69 ± 49	-17 ± 15	34 ± 22

CI, cardiac index; mRAP, mean right atrial pressure; SaO$_2$, systemic arterial oxygen saturation; SOT, systemic oxygen transport.

dogs with right ventricular hypertension.[39] Serial transesophageal echocardiograms performed in some of the patients at rest and during mild supine exercise support the concept that the decompression and shunting effects of atrial septostomy become more pronounced during exercise[53] (see Plate 13S.1).

Long-term hemodynamic effects

The long-term hemodynamic effects of atrial septostomy in PPH have been reported:[46] right ventricular function improved over time after septostomy, with a further decrease in mRAP and a further increase in CI and systemic oxygen transport in the eight of 15 patients who underwent evaluation 7–27 months after septostomy. These results are in agreement with the improvement in right ventricular function by echocardiography after septostomy in PPH.[61]

Effects on right heart structure and function

Echocardiography performed before and after septostomy in patients with PPH by our group[61] suggest that AS may also exert beneficial effects on right heart structure and function. We found significantly decreased right atrial and ventricular systolic and diastolic areas after septostomy, reflecting less right heart dilation. RV systolic function, assessed by mean percentage change in area and the changes in global RV wall motion, also improved, particularly in the patients with a severely depressed systolic function prior to the procedure. The easiest way to explain the beneficial effects of AS on RV function is that the simple decompression effect (decrease in radius) reduces wall stress and improves performance via the La Place relationship;[5] relief of RV wall tension and ischemia, mediated by decompression itself might also have contributed.[6] The effects of AS on other potential mechanisms of failure such as sympathetic overdrive, volume overload and alterations in gene expression remain to be elucidated. Interestingly, neither RV wall thickness nor the bulging of atrial and ventricular septa toward the left chambers were affected by the procedure.[61]

Compared with other therapeutic interventions such as calcium channel blockers,[31] intravenous infusion of prostacyclin,[32] pulmonary thromboendarterectomy[62] and lung transplantation,[33] the effects of AS on RV structure and function are less dramatic. This is probably due to a more direct and pronounced effect of those interventions on RV afterload (i.e. decrease in PVR).

Table 13S.3 *Comparison of selected hemodynamic variables before and after atrial septostomy as a function of clinical outcome*

Variable	Improved clinically (n = 34)				Not improved clinically (n = 7)			
	Before	After	% Change	P <	Before	After	% Change	P <
mRAP (mmHg)	13.7 ± 7.9	10.1 ± 6.4	26.8	0.001	14.6 ± 9.4	12.3 ± 7.9	16	0.056
SaO$_2$ (%)	93.3 ± 4.4	84.1 ± 9.1	9.2	0.001	97 ± 1.4	90.1 ± 5.0	6.9	0.009
CI (L/min·m^2)	2.0 ± 0.6	2.7 ± 0.7	35	0.001	2.2 ± 0.6	2.3 ± 0.4	4.5	0.3
SOT (mL/min·m^2)	393 ± 126	457 ± 123	16.5	0.001	368 ± 125	370 ± 116	0.5	0.9

CI, cardiac index; mRAP, mean right atrial pressure; SaO$_2$ (%), systemic arterial oxygen saturation; SOT, systemic oxygen transport. Data from references 46, 51, 53 and 62.

Long-term outcome and survival after septostomy

Not all patients have clinical improvement after the procedure. In a recent article, Rothman *et al.*[63] showed that long-term clinical outcome after septostomy is dependent on the immediate hemodynamic response to the procedure, particularly the changes in CI and systemic oxygen transport (SO$_2$T). In an attempt to extend this observation, we combined the series of the Rothman,[63] Kerstein,[46] Sobrino[51] and Sandoval groups.[53] Patients included for this analysis were those in whom follow-up information on clinical status and a complete set of hemodynamic variables were available. Procedure-related deaths were excluded from analysis. From a total of 41 patients, 34 were reported as improved and seven as unchanged after AS. At baseline, both groups were comparable in terms of age (30.4 ± 11 versus 32.6 ± 12 years, respectively; P = NS), and hemodynamic variables. As can be seen in Table 13S.3, compared with patients with no clinical improvement after the procedure, those with significant clinical benefit had a higher baseline and significant increases after AS in CI and SO$_2$T. The decrease in mRAP and arterial oxygen saturation was also greater in this group.

Among the 54 patients who survived the procedure in the worldwide experience,[49] there were eight late deaths; in at least five the cause of death was progression of disease. The remaining patients were alive at the time of their report and four of them survived to receive lung transplantation. Figure 13S.8 shows the Kaplan–Meier survival estimates in the 54 patients who survived AS. The median survival was 19.5 months (range 2–96 months). In this figure, a predicted survival curve constructed with mean values of the survival estimates predicted by the equation of the NIH study[1] (for patients on conventional therapy alone, excluding chronic intravenous infusion of prostacyclin) is also plotted for comparison. Although no formal statistics are applied, there seems to be an improvement in the survival of patients with severe PPH after septostomy.

The duration of this initial beneficial effect on survival seems to be limited by late deaths, primarily due to

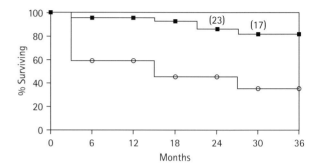

Figure 13S.8 *Kaplan–Meier survival curve in 54 patients from the worldwide collective experience[49] who had a successful atrial septostomy (squares) compared with their estimated survival derived from the National Institutes of Health study[1] (circles).*

disease progression. By updating the survival estimates of a series of patients reported previously,[53] we found that the survival of patients diminished considerably at 3 years of follow-up.[49] Progression of pulmonary vascular disease is often manifested by the reappearance of dyspnea and cyanosis as a result of an increase in right-to-left shunt.

Possible mechanisms of improvement after atrial septostomy

Our understanding of the physiological changes occurring after AS is incomplete, but several mechanisms seem to be involved. In PPH with right ventricular dysfunction (i.e. a marked increase in baseline mRAP), a decompression effect of the right heart chambers occurs (see above). For those with less severe right ventricular dysfunction at baseline and only mild to moderate hemodynamic changes after septostomy, the benefit of the procedure may be more likely to manifest during exercise by preventing further right ventricular dilation and dysfunction and by allowing right-to-left shunting to increase cardiac output. Finally, an increase in SO$_2$T also may produce beneficial effects on peripheral oxygen use,[46] particularly during exercise, and be responsible for the improvement in functional class and exercise tolerance.

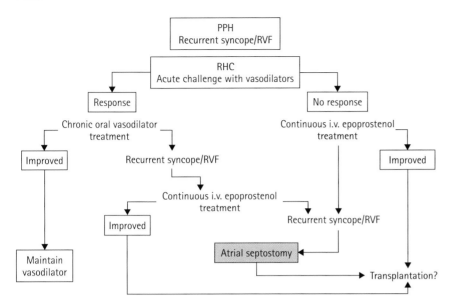

Figure 13S.9 *Atrial septostomy in the management of primary pulmonary hypertension. The procedure should be considered after short-term failure of maximal medical therapy. PPH, primary pulmonary hypertension; RVF, right ventricular failure; RHC, right heart catheterization. Adapted from reference 66.*

COMBINED THERAPY

Although there was initial concern that the administration of systemic vasodilators would be dangerous in patients with a right-to-left shunt because drug would be diverted away from the pulmonary circulation into the systemic vascular bed, intravenous epoprostenol[63,64] and subcutaneous trepostinil[65] may be used safely and have beneficial effects in pulmonary hypertension and associated congenital heart disease and in patients with AS. This combination may prove useful in patients with severe PPH who are unresponsive to epoprostenol alone.

SUMMARY

Atrial septostomy represents an additional, promising strategy in the treatment of severe PPH. Experience with this procedure is still limited; however, based on analyses of the worldwide experience, several general conclusions can be made.[27,49]

KEY POINTS

- Atrial septostomy can be performed successfully in selected patients with advanced pulmonary vascular disease.
- Patients with primary pulmonary hypertension who have undergone successful AS have shown:
  - a significant clinical improvement
  - beneficial and long-lasting hemodynamic effects at rest
  - a trend toward improved survival.

- The procedure-related mortality of the worldwide collective experience is high (16%). Several recommendations to minimize the risk are listed in Table 13S.1.
- Because the disease process in PPH is unaffected by the procedure (late deaths), the long-term effects of an AS must be considered to be palliative.
- Despite its risk, AS may represent a viable alternative for selected patients with severe PPH. Indications for the procedure may include:
  - recurrent syncope or right ventricular failure, despite maximal medical therapy, including oral calcium-channel blockers or continuous intravenous prostacyclin (Figure 13S.9);
  - intervention to keep patient alive until transplantation;
  - when no other option exists.

REFERENCES

- 1 D'Alonso GE, Barst RJ, Ayres SM *et al.* Survival in patients with primary pulmonary hypertension. Results of a national prospective study. *Ann Intern Med* 1991;**115**:343–9.
- 2 Kanemoto N. Natural history of pulmonary hemodynamics in primary pulmonary hypertension. *Am Heart J* 1987;**114**:407–13.
- 3 Sandoval J, Bauerle O, Palomar A *et al.* Survival in primary pulmonary hypertension: validation of a prognostic equation. *Circulation* 1994;**89**:1733–44.
- 4 Barnard D, Alpert JS. Right ventricular function in health and disease. *Curr Probl Cardiol* 1987;**12**:417–49.
- 5 Bristow MR, Zisman LS, Lances BD *et al.* The pressure-overloaded right ventricle in pulmonary hypertension. *Chest* 1998;**114**(Suppl):101S–6S.

●6 Vlahakes GJ, Turley K, Hoffman JIE. The pathophysiology of
    failure in acute right ventricular hypertension: hemodynamic
    and biochemical correlations. *Circulation* 1981;**63**:87–95.
 7 Sylvester JT, Goldberg HS, Permutt S. The role of the
    vasculature in the regulation of cardiac output. *Clin Chest
    Med* 1983;**4**:111–26.
 8 Hoeper MM, Tangers J, Leppert A *et al*. Evaluation of right
    ventricular performance with right ventricular ejection
    fraction thermodilution catheter and MRI in patients with
    pulmonary hypertension. *Chest* 2001;**120**:502–7.
 9 Werchan PM, Summer WR, Gerdes AM *et al*. Right
    ventricular performance after monocrotaline-induced
    pulmonary hypertension. *Am J Physiol* 1989;**256**:111325–36.
10 Bache R. Effects of hypertrophy on the coronary circulation.
    Prog Cardiovasc Dis 1988;**31**:403–40.
11 Lowensohn HS, Khouri EM, Gregg DE *et al*. Phasic right
    coronary artery flow in conscious dogs with normal and
    elevated right ventricular pressures. *Circ Res* 1976;**39**:760.
12 Pereira N, Klutz W, Fox R *et al*. Identification of severe right
    ventricular dysfunction by technetium-99 m-sestamibi gated
    SPECT imaging. *J Nucl Med* 1997;**38**:254–6.
13 Murray PA, Vatner SF. Reduction of maximal coronary
    vasodilator capacity in conscious dogs with severe right
    ventricular hypertrophy. *Circ Res* 1981;**48**:25–33.
14 Kusachi S, Nishiyama O, Yasuhara K *et al*. Right and left
    ventricular oxygen metabolism in open-chest dogs. *Heart
    Circ Physiol* 1982;**12**:H761–6.
●15 Gómez A, Bialostozky D, Zajarias A *et al*. Right ventricular
    ischemia in patients with primary pulmonary hypertension.
    J Am Coll Cardiol 2001;**38**:1137–42.
16 Bristow MR, Minobe W, Rasmussen R *et al*. β-Adrenergic
    neuroeffector abnormalities in the failing human heart are
    produced by local, rather than systemic mechanisms. *J Clin
    Invest* 1992;**89**:803–15.
17 Bristow MR. Mechanism of action of beta-blocking
    agents in heart failure. *Am J Cardiol* 1997;**80**:26L–40L.
●18 Nootens M, Kaufmann E, Rector T *et al*. Neurohormonal
    activation in patients with right ventricular failure from
    pulmonary hypertension: relation to hemodynamic variables
    and endothelin levels. *J Am Coll Cardiol* 1995;**26**:1581–5.
●19 Rich S, Seidlitz M, Dodin E *et al*. The short-term effects of
    digoxin in patients with right ventricular dysfunction from
    pulmonary hypertension. *Chest* 1998;**114**:782–92.
20 Rosas M, Kuri J, Hermosillo JA *et al*. Circadian regulation of
    heart rate variability in primary pulmonary hypertension: an
    unappreciated risk marker? [Abstract] *J Am Coll Cardiol*
    1999;**33**(Suppl):120A.
21 Hirose Y, Ishida Y, Hayashida K *et al*. Viable but denervated
    right ventricular myocardium: a case of Eisenmenger
    reaction. *Cardiology* 1997;**88**:609–12.
●22 Abraham WT, Raynolds MV, Gottschall V *et al*. Importance of
    angiotensin-converting enzyme in pulmonary hypertension.
    Cardiology 1995;**86**(Suppl I):9–15.
23 Pulido T, Massó LF, Bautista E *et al*. The angiotensin-
    converting enzyme (ACE) DD genotype in Hispanic patients
    with primary pulmonary hypertension. [Abstract] *Am J
    Respir Crit Care Med* 2002;**165**:A99.
24 Naeije R, Vachiery JL. Medical therapy of pulmonary
    hypertension. Conventional therapies. *Clin Chest Med*
    2001;**22**:517–27.

●25 Barger AC, Roe BB, Richardson GS. Relation of valvular
    lesions and of exercise to auricular pressure, work tolerance,
    and to development of chronic congestive failure in dogs.
    Am J Physiol 1952;**169**:384–99.
●26 Higgins CB, Pavelec R, Vatner SF. Modified technique for
    production of experimental right sided congestive failure.
    Cardiovasc Res 1973;**7**:870–4.
27 Barst RJ. Medical therapy for pulmonary hypertension.
    An overview of treatment and goals. *Clin Chest Med*
    2001;**22**:509–15.
*28 British Cardiac Society Guidelines and Medical Practice
    Committee. Recommendations on the management of
    pulmonary hypertension in clinical practice. *Heart*
    2001;**86**(Suppl I):i1–13.
29 Galié N. Pulmonary arterial hypertension: new ideas and
    perspectives. *Heart* 2001;**85**:475–80.
30 Channick RN, Rubin LJ. New and experimental therapies
    for pulmonary hypertension. *Clin Chest Med* 2001;**22**:
    539–45.
31 Rich S, Brundage BH. High dose calcium channel blocking
    therapy for primary pulmonary hypertension: evidence for
    long-term reduction in pulmonary artery pressure and
    regression of right ventricular hypertrophy. *Circulation*
    1987;**76**:135–41.
32 Hinderliter AL, Willis W, Barst RJ *et al*. Effects of long-term
    infusion of prostacyclin (epoprostenol) on echocardiographic
    measures of right ventricular structure and function in
    primary pulmonary hypertension. *Circulation*
    1997;**95**:1479–86.
33 Ritchie M, Waggoner A, Dávila-Roman VG *et al*.
    Echocardiographic characterization of the improvement in
    right ventricular failure in patients with severe pulmonary
    hypertension after single lung transplantation. *J Am Coll
    Cardiol* 1993;**22**:1170–4.
34 Rubin LJ. Primary pulmonary hypertension. *N Engl J Med*
    1977;**336**:111–17.
●35 Rich S, Kaufmann E, Levy PS. The effect of high doses of
    calcium-channel blockers on survival in primary pulmonary
    hypertension. *N Engl J Med* 1992;**327**:76–81.
●36 Barst RJ, Rubin LJ, Long WA *et al*. A comparison of
    continuous intravenous epoprostenol (prostacyclin) with
    conventional therapy for primary pulmonary hypertension.
    N Engl J Med 1996;**334**:296–301.
37 Higenbottam TW, Spiegelhalter D, Scott JP *et al*. Prostacyclin
    (epoprostenol) and heart-lung transplantation as treatments
    for severe pulmonary hypertension. *Br Heart J*
    1993;**70**:366–70.
●38 Pasque MK, Trulock EP, Cooper JD *et al*. Single lung
    transplantation for pulmonary hypertension. Single
    institution experience in 34 patients. *Circulation*
    1995;**92**:2252–8.
●39 Austen WG, Morrow AG, Berry WB. Experimental studies of
    the surgical treatment of primary pulmonary hypertension.
    J Thorac Cardiovasc Surg 1964;**48**:448–55.
●40 Rozkovec A, Montanes P, Oakley CM. Factors that influence
    the outcome of primary pulmonary hypertension. *Br Heart J*
    1986;**55**:449–58.
41 Glanville AR, Burke CM, Theodore J *et al*. Primary pulmonary
    hypertension. Length of survival in patients referred for
    heart-lung transplantation. *Chest* 1987;**91**:675–81.

42 Young D, Mark H. Fate of the patient with Eisenmenger syndrome. *Am J Cardiol* 1971;**28**:655–69.

●43 Hopkins WE, Ochoa LL, Richardson GW *et al.* Comparison of the hemodynamics and survival of adults with severe primary pulmonary hypertension or Eisenmenger syndrome. *J Heart Lung Transplant* 1996;**15**:100–5.

●44 Rich S, Lam W. Atrial septostomy as palliative therapy for refractory primary pulmonary hypertension. *Am J Cardiol* 1983;**51**:1560–1.

●45 Nihill MR, O'Laughlin MP, Mullins CE. Effects of atrial septostomy in patients with terminal cor pulmonale due to pulmonary vascular disease. *Cathet Cardiovasc Diagn* 1991;**24**:166–72.

●46 Kerstein D, Levy PS, Hsu DT *et al.* Blade balloon atrial septostomy in patients with severe primary pulmonary hypertension. *Circulation* 1995;**91**:2028–35.

●47 Hausknecht MJ, Sims RE, Nihill MR *et al.* Successful palliation of primary pulmonary hypertension by atrial septostomy. *Am J Cardiol* 1990;**65**:1045–6.

●48 Rothman A, Beltran D, Kriett JM *et al.* Graded balloon dilation atrial septostomy as a bridge to transplantation in primary pulmonary hypertension. *Am Heart J* 1993;**125**:1763–6.

◆*49 Sandoval J, Rothman A, Pulido T. Atrial septostomy for pulmonary hypertension. *Clin Chest Med* 2001;**22**:547–60.

*50 Rich S, Dodin E, McLaughlin W. Usefulness of atrial septostomy as a treatment for primary pulmonary hypertension and guidelines for its application. *Am J Cardiol* 1997;**80**:69–71.

51 Sobrino N, Frutos A, Calvo L *et al.* Septostomía interatrial paliativa en la hipertensión pulmonar severa. *Rev Esp Cardiol* 1993;**46**:125–8.

52 Thanopoulos BD, Georgakopoulos D, Tsaousis GS *et al.* Percutaneous balloon dilation of the atrial septum: immediate and midterm results. *Heart* 1996;**76**:502–6.

●53 Sandoval J, Gaspar J, Pulido T *et al.* Graded balloon dilation atrial septostomy in severe primary pulmonary hypertension. A therapeutic alternative for patients non-responsive to vasodilator treatment. *J Am Coll Cardiol* 1998;**32**:297–304.

54 Collins TJ, Moore JW, Kirby WC. Atrial septostomy for pulmonary hypertension. *Am Heart J* 1988; **116**:873–4.

55 Unger P, Stoupel E, Vachiery JL *et al.* Atrial septostomy under transesophageal guidance in a patient with primary pulmonary hypertension and absent right superior vena cava. *Intens Care Med* 1996;**22**:1410–11.

56 Fulwani M, Nabar A, Iyer R *et al.* Palliative blade-balloon atrial septostomy in primary pulmonary hypertension. *Indian Heart J* 1997;**49**:185–6.

57 Takigiku K, Shibata T, Yasui K *et al.* Successful blade atrial septostomy in a patient with severe primary pulmonary hypertension – a case report. *Jpn Circ J* 1997;**61**:877–81.

*58 Rich S. Primary pulmonary hypertension: Executive Summary from the World Symposium on PPH 1998. http://www. Who.int/ncd/cvd/pph.html.

*59 Sandoval J, Barst RJ, Rich S *et al.* Atrial septostomy for pulmonary hypertension. In: Rich S (ed.), PPH: Executive Summary from the World Symposium on PPH 1998. http://www. Who.int/ncd/cvd/pph.html.

60 Baim DS. Percutaneous approach, including and transseptal and apical puncture. In: Baim DS, Grossman W (eds), *Grossman's cardiac catheterization, angiography, and intervention*, 6th edn. Philadelphia: Lippincott, Williams and Wilkins, 2000;69–100.

61 Espínola-Zavaleta N, Vargas-Barrón J, Tazar JI *et al.* Echocardiographic evaluation of patients with pulmonary hypertension before and after atrial septostomy. *Echocardiography* 1999;**16**:625.

62 Dittrich HC, Nicod PH, Chow LC *et al.* Early changes of right heart geometry after pulmonary thromboendarterectomy. *J Am Coll Cardiol* 1988;**11**:937–43.

●63 Rothman A, Slansky MS, Lucas VW *et al.* Atrial septostomy as a bridge to lung transplantation in patients with severe pulmonary hypertension. *Am J Cardiol* 1999;**84**:682–6.

●64 Rosenzweig EB, Kerstein D, Barst RJ. Long-term prostacyclin for pulmonary hypertension with associated congenital heart defects. *Circulation* 1999;**99**:1858–65.

65 Galié N, Manes A, Branzi A. Medical therapy of pulmonary hypertension. The prostacyclins. *Clin Chest Med* 2001;**22**:529–37.

66 Barst, RJ. Role of atrial septostomy in the treatment of pulmonary vascular disease. *Thorax* 2000; **55**: 95–6.

An integrated approach to the treatment of pulmonary arterial hypertension

MARC HUMBERT, OLIVIER SITBON AND GÉRALD SIMONNEAU

It is widely assumed that a vasoconstrictive factor is involved in pulmonary arterial hypertension.[1] However, the vast majority of patients have little or no effect of pure vasodilators, presumably because the pulmonary arteriopathy includes fibrotic and proliferative changes that predominate over vasoconstriction.[1–3] The evolution of therapy from vasodilators to antiproliferative agents is one of the most important issues in the field.[3]

Endothelial dysfunction is a hallmark of pulmonary arterial hypertension, and is accompanied by exaggerated vasoconstriction and impaired vasodilation (Figure 13T.1). Chronically impaired production of vasodilators such as nitric oxide and prostacyclin, along with prolonged over-expression of vasoconstrictors such as endothelin-1 not only affect vascular tone but also promote vascular remodeling and therefore represent a logical target for therapeutic manipulation.[4–7] Medical advances over the last decade, and particularly disease-targeted therapies (prostaglandins and endothelin receptor antagonists) have both vasodilator and antiproliferative properties and the long-term effects of treatment may therefore extend beyond simple acute vasodilator activity.[3,8–10] This chapter attempts to provide an evidence-based integrated approach to the treatment of pulmonary arterial hypertension in 2003.

CONVENTIONAL MEDICAL THERAPY

Patients with pulmonary arterial hypertension have a restricted pulmonary circulation, and any increase in cardiac output can exacerbate pulmonary hypertension and right heart failure. Physical activity should therefore be restricted and guided by symptoms. Diuretics and supplemental oxygen are indicated for peripheral edema and hypoxemia.[11] Patients may receive digoxin, particularly in case of intermittent or chronic atrial fibrillation.[12] Immunization against influenza and pneumococcus is also recommended. Pregnancy is contraindicated and a safe and effective method of contraception, typically an intrauterine device or surgical sterilization, is always recommended in women of childbearing age.

Results from two observational studies suggest that oral anticoagulant therapy may be beneficial in pulmonary arterial hypertension.[13,14] Warfarin is the most widely used anticoagulant, with the recommended dose adjusted to achieve an International Normalized Ratio around 2.0.[11]

CALCIUM CHANNEL BLOCKERS

Vasoconstriction of pulmonary arteries contributes to the pathogenesis of pulmonary arterial hypertension.[14] Pure vasodilators reverse this component of the disease with little or no effect on the fibrotic and proliferative changes that predominate over vasoconstriction in many cases.[3]

Uncontrolled studies have indicated that long-term administration of calcium channel blockers may prolong survival in the rare subset of responsive patients compared with unresponsive patients.[14] Patients who benefit

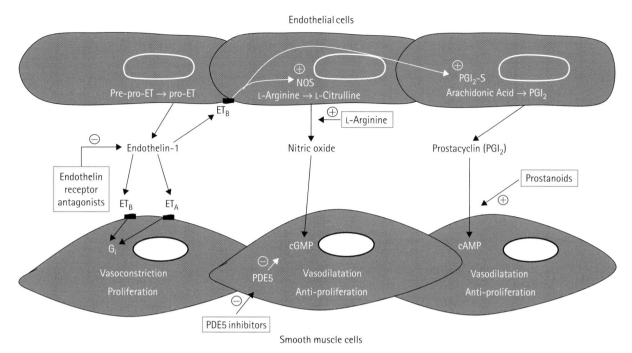

Figure 13T.1 *Pathophysiology of pulmonary arterial hypertension: targets for current or emerging therapies. cAMP, cyclic adenosine monophosphate; cGMP, cyclic guanosine monophosphate; ET, endothelin; ET_A, endothelin receptor A; ET_B, endothelin receptor B; NOS, nitric oxide synthase; PDE5, phosphodiesterase type 5; PGI_2, prostaglandin I_2 (prostacyclin); PGI_2-S, prostacyclin synthase.*

from long-term calcium channel blockers could be identified by an acute vasodilator challenge.[2,14] This challenge must be performed during right heart catheterization in specialized pulmonary vascular units. The magnitude of acute vasodilator response that predicts a favorable outcome on long-term calcium channel blocker therapy remains poorly defined.[2] In our experience, retrospective analysis of 557 consecutive patients with primary pulmonary hypertension showed that only 7% had a sustained benefit of calcium channel blocker therapy [defined as patients being in New York Heart Association (NYHA) functional class I or II with near-normal hemodynamics after at least 1 year follow-up].[15] During acute vasodilator challenge, these rare patients almost normalize their pulmonary hemodynamics with a mean pulmonary artery pressure <35–40 mmHg, associated with a normal or high cardiac output.[14,15] A major issue concerns the possible occurrence of severe side effects during acute vasodilator challenge with calcium channel blockers.[2] Therefore, the most widely used drugs for testing vasoreactivity are intravenous prostacyclin, adenosine, or inhaled nitric oxide rather than calcium channel blockers.[11]

CONTINUOUS INTRAVENOUS EPOPROSTENOL (PROSTACYCLIN)

Prostaglandin I_2 (prostacyclin) is a potent systemic and pulmonary vasodilator and a powerful inhibitor of

platelet aggregation.[16] Epoprostenol therapy also protects against pulmonary vascular remodeling[10] and improves exercise tolerance by decreasing the slope of the pressure/flow relationship in the pulmonary circulation.[17]

Intravenous prostacyclin (epoprostenol) was first used to treat primary pulmonary hypertension in the early 1980s (see Chapter 13L).[18] Since then it has proved to be life-saving in a large number of patients with pulmonary arterial hypertension.[8,19–21] Interestingly, it was apparent from an early stage that the absence of an acute hemodynamic response to intravenous epoprostenol did not preclude improvement with long-term therapy.[16] A prospective, randomized open trial was conducted in 81 patients with primary pulmonary hypertension of NYHA functional class III or IV and who were randomly assigned to receive either conventional therapy alone or with intravenous epoprostenol infusion.[8] After 12 weeks of therapy there was a functional improvement with epoprostenol, as demonstrated by the increase in the 6-minute walk distance (an increase of 32 meters in the epoprostenol group compared with a decrease of 15 meters in the conventional therapy group).[8] During the same period of time, an improvement in hemodynamics was shown in the epoprostenol-treated group (mean pulmonary artery pressure was reduced by 5 mmHg on epoprostenol whereas it increased by 2 mmHg on conventional therapy; cardiac index increased by 0.3 L/min·m² in the epoprostenol group whereas it decreased by 0.2 L/min·m² in the conventional therapy group).[8] A significant improvement in survival

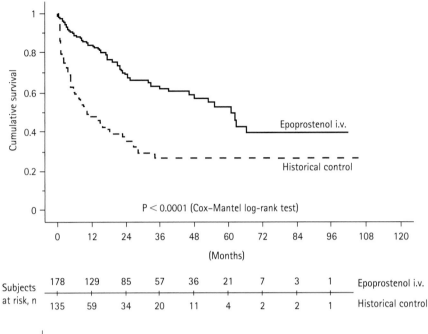

Figure 13T.2 *Kaplan–Meier survival estimates in 178 patients with primary pulmonary hypertension (PPH) from the initiation of epoprostenol therapy.[20] For comparison, survival data are also shown for a historical group of 135 PPH patients matched for New York Heart Association functional class, and who never received epoprostenol therapy. In the population of patients treated with epoprostenol (solid line), overall survival rates at 1, 2, 3 and 5 years are 85%, 70%, 63% and 55%, respectively, compared with 58%, 43%, 33% and 28% in the historical control group (dashed line).*

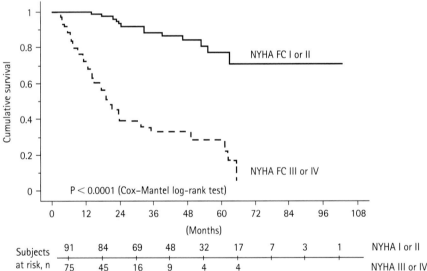

Figure 13T.3 *Survival in primary pulmonary hypertension (PPH) patients according to New York Heart Association (NYHA) functional class after 3 months of treatment with intravenous epoprostenol.[20] Survival rates for patients reclassified as NYHA functional class I or II (solid line) were 100%, 93% and 88% at 1, 2 and 3 years, respectively, compared with 77%, 46% and 33% for patients persisting in NYHA class III or IV (dashed line).*

with epoprostenol treatment was also demonstrated (eight patients in the conventional therapy group died during the study whereas no death was reported on epoprostenol).[8] Epoprostenol is approved in North America and in some European countries since 1995 and 1997, respectively.

There is no long-term randomized trial with epoprostenol in pulmonary arterial hypertension. Nevertheless, analysis of cohorts of patients on continuous intravenous prostacyclin compared with historical control groups on conventional therapy clearly demonstrated clinical benefits in patients of NYHA functional classes III and IV.[20,21] In our cohort of 178 patients with primary pulmonary hypertension, intravenous epoprostenol improved exercise tolerance, hemodynamics and long-term survival compared with a historical group on medical supportive therapy. Survival rates at 1, 2, 3 and 5 years were 85%, 70%, 63% and 55%, respectively, compared with 58%, 43%, 33% and 28% in the historical control group ($P < 0.0001$)[20] (Figure 13T.2). Survival was mainly related to simple baseline clinical parameters such as a history of right heart failure, emphasizing the fact that death can result from delays in diagnosis and treatment.[20,21] In addition, prognosis was clearly related to clinical and hemodynamic responses to long-term epoprostenol therapy.[20,21] Patients whose symptoms had improved such that they could be reclassified in NYHA functional class I or II after 3 months on epoprostenol had a markedly improved probability of survival compared with patients persisting in functional class III or IV[20] (Figure 13T.3). Similar results were recently reported in

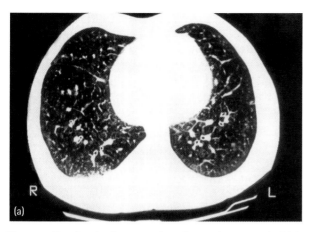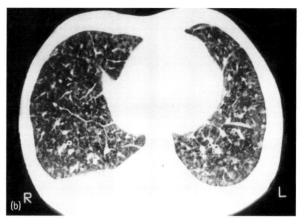

Figure 13T.4 *Fatal pulmonary edema in a patient treated with long-term intravenous epoprostenol infusion. Postmortem examination revealed pulmonary capillary hemangiomatosis (a) before continuous intravenous epoprostenol therapy; (b) after 1 month of continuous intravenous epoprostenol therapy.*

North America.[21] In addition, regarding exercise tolerance, the most important prognostic factor was the absolute value of the 6-minute walking distance after 3 months of epoprostenol therapy (>380 m) rather than the improvement from baseline.[20]

Initially proposed as a bridge to lung transplantation, intravenous epoprostenol is now considered as a first-line therapy and an alternative to lung transplantation in patients with severe disease.[11] In a survey collected from 19 centers in the USA, it was shown that more than two-thirds of patients treated with long-term epoprostenol were sufficiently improved to be removed from the lung transplantation list.[22] However, eligible patients who remain in NYHA functional class III or IV after 3 months of epoprostenol therapy should still be considered for lung transplantation.[20]

Epoprostenol can only be administered by continuous intravenous infusion because of its short half-life in circulation (3 minutes) and it is inactivated at low pH.[8] Epoprostenol is infused continuously with the use of a portable infusion pump connected to a permanent tunneled catheter inserted into a subclavian vein.[8] During initial hospitalization, patients are trained in pump programming, drug preparation, sterile technique and catheter care. The optimal dosing of epoprostenol remains undefined and varies among patients.[20,21] Epoprostenol therapy is progressively increased during initial hospitalization to a dose around 10 ng/kg·min before patients are discharged. Dose adjustments are subsequently made according to clinical symptoms, adverse events, the 6-minute walk test and hemodynamic measurements.[20]

Despite favorable outcomes, continuous intravenous epoprostenol infusion is a far from ideal treatment of severe pulmonary arterial hypertension because it is complicated, uncomfortable for patients and very costly, especially in Europe. Common side effects attributable to

epoprostenol include jaw pain, headache, diarrhea, flushing, leg pain, nausea and vomiting.[8,20,21] These side effects are generally mild and dose-related.[20] More serious complications are generally related to the delivery system (mainly catheter-relater infections or thrombosis).[20] The incidence of catheter-related sepsis has been reported to range from 0.1 to 0.6 per patient-year.[22] Pump failure or dislocation of the central venous catheter leading to interruption in drug infusion may be life-threatening.[20] Severe pulmonary edema may occur in pulmonary hypertension with prominent pulmonary vein involvement (pulmonary veno-occlusive disease and pulmonary capillary hemangiomatosis)[11,23] (Figure 13T.4).

Continuous intravenous infusion of epoprostenol markedly improved exercise capacity and hemodynamics in patients with pulmonary arterial hypertension related to the scleroderma spectrum of diseases, although there was no effect on mortality.[24] Uncontrolled studies with intravenous epoprostenol therapy also suggest improvement in patients with pulmonary arterial hypertension associated with systemic-to-pulmonary congenital cardiac shunts,[25] portal hypertension[26] and human immunodeficiency virus infection.[27,28]

NOVEL MEDICAL THERAPIES

End points in controlled studies

Development of novel therapeutic agents in pulmonary arterial hypertension has generated intense research and several placebo-controlled trials have been completed in the last 3 years worldwide.[29] The question of the most relevant end points in such trials has generated intense discussion. Since continuous epoprostenol infusion has been shown to improve survival in severe pulmonary arterial hypertension, NYHA functional class IV patients in unstable condition should not be included in placebo-controlled studies for ethical reasons. Therefore, survival cannot be regarded as an acceptable primary end point in short-term (less than 16 weeks) placebo-controlled studies. Hemodynamics only marginally improve, even in patients with excellent clinical results, emphasizing the fact that improvements obtained with these drugs were only partly related to hemodynamic modifications.[8,9,20,21] NYHA functional class is an important parameter, but there are too many discrepancies between investigators to use it widely as a primary end point. The 6-minute walk test is a submaximal exercise test that can be performed even by a patient with heart failure not tolerating maximal exercise testing.[30] This test is very simple, requires inexpensive equipment, and is highly reproducible. In addition, it is considered safe because patients are self-limited during exercise. This test is conducted in a corridor and requires the patient to walk for as far as they can manage in 6 minutes. In primary pulmonary hypertension, the distance walked in 6 minutes has a strong, independent association with mortality.[8,20,21,30] The 6-minute walk test therefore appears to be a valuable surrogate end point that predicts clinical benefit.

Prostacyclin analogs

CONTINUOUS SUBCUTANEOUS TREPROSTINIL

The potential complications related to the central venous catheter required for intravenous prostacyclin have led to the development of treprostinil (see Chapter 13N), a stable prostacyclin analog, for continuous subcutaneous infusion by minipump systems that have been used extensively in the treatment of diabetes mellitus.[31] Treprostinil has a half-life of 27 minutes when administered intravenously and 58–83 minutes when delivered subcutaneously.[29] The efficacy of treprostinil has been tested in a 12-week multicenter, randomized, placebo-controlled trial in 470 patients with primary pulmonary hypertension, and pulmonary arterial hypertension associated with congenital systemic-to-pulmonary shunts or connective tissue diseases in NYHA functional classes II, III and IV.[31] The modest but significant treatment effect (between treatment group difference) in median 6-minute walking distance was 16 meters in the overall population and 19 meters in primary pulmonary hypertension.[31] Concomitantly, treprostinil significantly improved indices of dyspnea, signs and symptoms of pulmonary hypertension and hemodynamics. The best exercise improvement was observed in patients who could tolerate the highest doses (increase in median 6-minute walking distance was 36 meters in patients with a dose >13.8 ng/kg·min).[31] Local pain and inflammation at the infusion site was a significant side effect occurring in 85% of the patients. It precluded

dose increase in a significant proportion of patients and led to discontinuation in 8% of cases.[31] Interestingly, patients with pulmonary arterial hypertension who presented with life-threatening complications of intravenous epoprostenol have been safely transitioned to subcutaneous treprostinil.[32] Treprostinil has been an approved therapy for pulmonary arterial hypertension in the USA since 2002.

ORALLY ACTIVE BERAPROST

Beraprost sodium is the first chemically stable and orally active prostacyclin analog (see Chapter 13N).[33] It is absorbed rapidly in fasting conditions, peak concentration is reached after 30 minutes and elimination half-life is 35–40 minutes.[29] A 12-week double blind, randomized, placebo-controlled trial has been performed in 130 NYHA functional class II and III patients with pulmonary arterial hypertension of various etiologies (primary pulmonary hypertension, connective tissue diseases, congenital systemic-to-pulmonary shunts, portal hypertension and human immunodeficiency virus infection).[34] Beraprost, at a median dose of 80 μg administered four times a day, improved the 6-minute walking distance by 25 meters in the overall population. In fact, the treatment effect was 45 meters in primary pulmonary hypertension, whereas no significant changes were observed in the exercise capacity of subjects with the associated conditions.[34] Hemodynamics had no statistically significant changes.[34] Side effects linked to systemic vasodilatation were frequent, mainly in the initial titration period.[34] Tolerance may affect the long-term effects of this drug. A 12-month double-blind, randomized, placebo-controlled trial confirmed that beraprost-treated patients in NYHA functional classes II and III had improved 6-minute walk distance at 3 months and 6 months compared with placebo, but not at either 9 or 12 months.[35] Therefore, the beneficial effects of beraprost may attenuate with time.[35] Beraprost is an approved therapy for pulmonary arterial hypertension in Japan and is currently under evaluation by the European Agency for the Evaluation of Medicinal Products.

INHALED ILOPROST

Iloprost is a chemically stable prostacyclin analog that may be safely delivered by inhalation in patients with pulmonary arterial hypertension (see Chapter 13M).[36] It is crucial that the delivery system produces aerosol particles of appropriate size (optimal mass median diameter 0.5–3.0 μm) to ensure alveolar deposition improving pulmonary selectivity.[37] The relatively short duration of action is a major disadvantage of this form of treatment that may require 6–12 inhalations a day.[36,38] A 12-week multicenter, randomized, placebo-controlled trial in 207 NYHA functional class III and IV patients has recently been reported.[38] Subjects with primary pulmonary hypertension, pulmonary arterial hypertension associated with connective tissue diseases and inoperable chronic thromboembolic pulmonary hypertension were included. The combined end point of a 10% improvement of 6-minute walk distance and NYHA functional class improvement in the absence of deterioration in the clinical condition has been observed in 17% of treated patients compared with 4% on placebo.[38] The treatment effect on the 6-minute walking distance was 36 meters in the overall population and 57 meters in primary pulmonary hypertension.[38] Compared with baseline values, hemodynamic values were significantly improved at 12 weeks when measured after iloprost inhalation, were largely unchanged when measured before inhalation, and were significantly worse in the placebo group.[38] Side effects include cough and symptoms linked to systemic vasodilatation.[38] In addition, syncope was more frequent in the iloprost group.[38] Although uncontrolled data are encouraging,[36] long-term efficacy of inhaled iloprost remains to be established. Iloprost has been an approved therapy for primary pulmonary hypertension in Europe since 2003.

Orally active endothelin receptor antagonists

Endothelin-1 mediates its effects through ET_A and ET_B receptors (see Chapter 13P).[39–41] Bosentan is an orally available dual (ET_A and ET_B) endothelin receptor antagonist.[9,42] Two double-blind, randomized, placebo-controlled trials have tested the efficacy of oral bosentan in patients with pulmonary arterial hypertension (primary or associated with scleroderma).[9,42] In the first pilot study, 33 NYHA functional class III patients were randomly assigned to placebo or bosentan (62.5 mg b.i.d. for 4 weeks then 125 mg b.i.d. for at least 12 weeks).[9] In patients given bosentan, a treatment effect of 76 meters in the 6-minute walking distance was observed, as well as significant improvements in pulmonary artery pressure and cardiac output.[9] In a subsequent larger study, 213 NYHA functional class III and IV patients were randomized to placebo or bosentan (62.5 mg b.i.d. for 4 weeks then 125 mg or 250 mg b.i.d. for at least 12 weeks).[42] Treatment effect on the 6-minute walking distance was 44 meters in the overall population and 52 meters in primary pulmonary hypertension.[9] Bosentan-treated individuals also showed improvements in time to clinical worsening (defined as death, lung transplantation, hospitalization for pulmonary hypertension, lack of clinical improvement or worsening leading to discontinuation, need for epoprostenol therapy, or atrial septostomy).[9] No dose response for efficacy could be ascertained whereas abnormal hepatic function was dose-dependent.[9] Increases in hepatic aminotransferase levels to more than eight times the upper limit of normal occurred in 3% and 7% of patients receiving 125 mg and

250 mg bosentan b.i.d., respectively.[9] An echocardiography substudy on 85 patients demonstrated that bosentan improved cardiac index, right ventricular systolic function and left ventricular early diastolic filling, leading to decrease in right ventricular dilatation and increase in left ventricular size.[43] Although a recent study provided some preliminary evidence for sustained efficacy at 12 months of therapy, the long-term effects of bosentan require further evaluation.[44] Bosentan at a dose of 125 mg administered twice daily has been an approved therapy for pulmonary arterial hypertension in North America and Europe since 2001 and 2002, respectively.

Selective ET_A blockers such as sitaxsentan and ambrisentan are currently being tested.[45] Cases of acute hepatitis have been described with selective ET_A blockers (fatal in one patient), emphasizing the importance of liver function monitoring.[45]

Orally active phosphodiesterase inhibitors

The contractile cells of the pulmonary arteries contain predominantly phosphodiesterase types 3, 4, and 5. Phosphodiesterase type 5 is specific for cyclic guanosine monophosphate and can be inhibited.[46] Phosphodiesterase type 5 inhibitors have a pulmonary vasodilator effect, as demonstrated in acute vasodilator challenge in patients with pulmonary hypertension secondary to pulmonary fibrosis.[46] Case reports have suggested a beneficial effect of phosphodiesterase type 5 inhibitor sildenafil in long-term treatment of primary pulmonary hypertension.[47] The experiences with sildenafil are still preliminary and controlled studies are ongoing to determine efficacy and safety of this drug for treatment of pulmonary arterial hypertension.

Orally active thromboxane synthase inhibitor and receptor antagonist

Thromboxane A_2 is a vasoconstrictor, platelet aggregant and smooth muscle mitogen which may contribute to the pathogenesis of pulmonary arterial hypertension.[4] A randomized, double-blind, placebo-controlled study has evaluated the effects of terbogrel, an orally active thromboxane synthase inhibitor and receptor antagonist, in primary pulmonary hypertension.[48] The study was halted prematurely because of the occurrence of severe leg pain confounding the primary end point of 6-minute walking distance.[48]

L–Arginine

There have been observational reports that L-arginine, the substrate of nitric oxide synthase, may reduce pulmonary artery pressure and increase exercise tolerance in pulmonary arterial hypertension.[49] A placebo-controlled study is currently underway to evaluate the effects of L-arginine in this patient population.

NON–MEDICAL THERAPIES

Non-medical therapies include atrial septostomy and lung transplantation. Blade balloon atrial septostomy in refractory pulmonary arterial hypertension has been successfully applied in several studies.[50,51] Unfortunately, the procedure-related mortality remains high, especially if patients already have a low arterial oxygen saturation or evidence of right ventricular failure.[50,51]

Atrial septostomy may be an interesting alternative for selected patients with severe disease, particularly if a transplantation candidate deteriorates despite maximal medical therapy (see Chapter 13S).[52]

Lung transplantation is the ultimate alternative for severe pulmonary arterial hypertension cases who cannot be managed medically.[53–55] Long-term survival and quality of life are limited by the high prevalence of chronic allograft rejection.[55] The optimal timing to make the initial referral to a transplant center is the crucial initial step in the transplantation process, and the long waiting time before transplantation due to the shortage of organ donors must be integrated into this decision (see Chapter 13R).

PRESENT AND FUTURE APPROACH TO THE TREATMENT OF PULMONARY ARTERIAL HYPERTENSION

Despite recent major improvements, all current treatments of pulmonary arterial hypertension do not achieve a cure of this devastating condition. However, in fewer than 20 years these patients have gone from a state of no hope to one where prolonged survival and improvements in quality of life can be achieved. Several treatments of pulmonary arterial hypertension are now approved in North America (epoprostenol, treprostinil, bosentan) and Europe (epoprostenol, iloprost, bosentan), whilst beraprost is currently under evaluation by European regulatory agencies (Table 13T.1). Except for recent data from patients receiving prolonged epoprostenol therapy, the long-term effects of novel treatments are still unknown.[20,21] There is therefore a substantial need for long-term observational studies evaluating the different treatments in terms of survival, side effects, quality of life and costs. As head-to-head comparisons of currently approved therapies are not available, the choice of treatment will depend on local experiences and administrative regulations, as well as on the clinical context and patient preference. Most experts recommend that severe NYHA functional class IV patients in unstable condition should receive continuous intravenous epoprostenol. Aside from this dramatic situation, first-line therapy may include oral bosentan, inhaled iloprost or subcutaneous treprostinil or continuous i.v. epoprostenol on careful observation in a pulmonary vascular center (Table 13T.1). Little information is currently available regarding early stages of pulmonary arterial hypertension. There is no approved drug for patients in NYHA functional class I and the only approved drug for patients in NYHA functional class II is treprostinil in the USA (Table 13T.1). In the near future other novel therapies, including beraprost, selective ET_A blockers and sildenafil, could play a role in the management of pulmonary arterial hypertension on the basis of placebo-controlled studies and regulatory agencies approval. An algorithm for the management of pulmonary arterial hypertension is shown in Figure 13T.5.

Another important issue is represented by the possibility to combine different targeted drugs with distinct mechanisms of action in order to maximize clinical benefits. Preliminary results from combined therapies have

Table 13T.1 *Disease-targeted therapies for pulmonary arterial hypertension (drugs with efficacy demonstrated in at least one published randomized control trial)*

Drug	Delivery system	Frequency of administration	Serious drawbacks	FDA/EMEA approval (year)	Indication
Epoprostenol	Intravenous infusion	Continuous	Catheter-related infections and thrombosis	FDA (1995); EMEA (1997)	PPH and CTD-PAH; NYHA III–IV
Bosentan	Tablets	b.i.d.	Elevation of liver enzymes	FDA (2001); EMEA (2002)	PAH; NYHA III–IV*
Treprostinil	Subcutaneous infusion	Continuous	Painful infusion sites	FDA (2002)	PAH; NYHA II, III, IV
Iloprost	Nebulized solution	6–12 times daily	Cough; syncope	EMEA (2003)	PPH; NYHA III
Beraprost	Tablets	q.i.d.	Headache, flush, diarrhea	–	–

FDA, Food and Drug Administration; EMEA: European Agency for the Evaluation of Medicinal Products; NYHA, New York Heart Association; PPH, primary pulmonary hypertension; CTD-PAH, connective tissue disease-associated pulmonary arterial hypertension; PAH, pulmonary arterial hypertension.
*Only NYHA functional class III for EMEA.

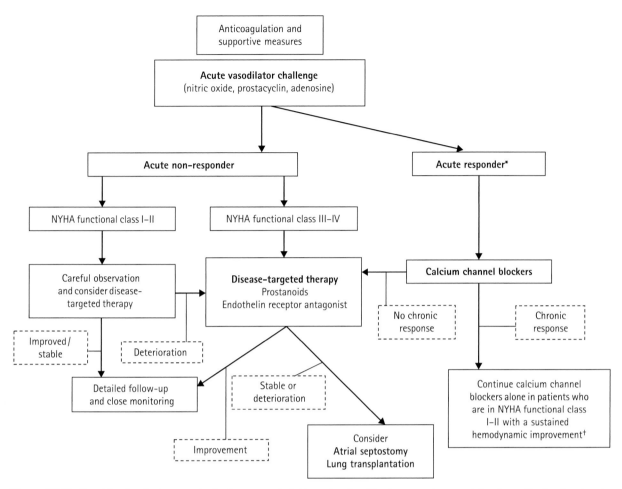

Figure 13T.5 *Algorithm for the treatment of pulmonary arterial hypertension. *Acute responders are defined as patients who almost normalize their pulmonary hemodynamics during acute vasodilator challenge (mean pulmonary artery pressure <35–40 mmHg, associated with a normal or high cardiac output). †There is no approved drug for patients in New York Heart Association (NYHA) functional class I and the only approved drug for patients in NYHA functional class II is trepostinil in the USA.*

recently been reported with encouraging results. First, oral phosphodiesterase type 5 inhibitor sildenafil increases and prolongs the vasodilatory action of inhaled nitric oxide and aerosolized iloprost.[56,57] Second, subthreshold dual-selective phosphodiesterase types 3 and 4 inhibition amplifies the lung vasodilatory response to inhaled iloprost.[58] Last, in a 16-week controlled study, bosentan plus epoprostenol was well tolerated, with a trend for a greater improvement in total pulmonary resistance compared with placebo plus epoprostenol.[59] Whether combined therapy will provide additional clinical benefits to patients with severe pulmonary arterial hypertension warrants further investigation.

The coming years are likely to witness a major step forward in the treatment of pulmonary arterial hypertension. The better understanding of the pathogenesis of this condition should eventually lead to the development of novel approaches focusing directly on the abnormal proliferation of vascular endothelial and smooth muscle cells. Signaling pathways involving bone morphogenetic protein receptor 2 and angiopoietin-1 constitute specific molecular targets for therapeutic intervention in pulmonary arterial hypertension.[59–64]

KEY POINTS

- Chronically impaired production of vasodilators such as nitric oxide and prostacyclin along with prolonged overexpression of vasoconstrictors such as endothelin-1 not only affect vascular tone but also promote vascular remodeling and therefore represent a logical target for therapeutic manipulation in pulmonary arterial hypertension.
- Despite recent major improvements, all current treatments of pulmonary arterial hypertension do not achieve a cure of this devastating condition.
- The rare patients who may have a sustained benefit of calcium channel blocker therapy can be

detected during acute vasodilator challenge with nitric oxide, prostacyclin or adenosine.

- Continuous intravenous prostacyclin (epoprostenol) has proved to be life-saving in a large number of patients with pulmonary arterial hypertension.
- Several treatments of pulmonary arterial hypertension are now approved in North America (epoprostenol, treprostinil, bosentan) and Europe (epoprostenol, iloprost, bosentan) while beraprost is currently under evaluation by European regulatory agencies.
- There is a substantial need for long-term observational studies evaluating the different treatments in terms of survival, side effects, quality of life and costs. As head-to-head comparisons of currently approved therapies are not available, the choice of treatment will depend on local experiences and administrative regulations, as well as on the clinical context and patient preference.
- Combining different targeted drugs with distinct mechanism of action may maximize clinical benefits. Whether combined therapy will provide additional clinical benefits to patients with severe pulmonary arterial hypertension warrants further investigation.
- The better understanding of the pathogenesis of this condition should eventually lead to the development of novel approaches focusing directly on the abnormal proliferation of vascular endothelial and smooth muscle cells. Abnormal transforming growth factor-β signaling is one of the most promising therapeutic targets in pulmonary arterial hypertension.

REFERENCES

1 Palevsky HI, Schloo BL, Pietra GG et al. Primary pulmonary hypertension. Vascular structure, morphometry and responsiveness to vasodilators agents. Circulation 1989;**80**:1207–21.

2 Sitbon O, Humbert M, Jagot JL et al. Inhaled nitric oxide as a screening agent for safely identifying responders to oral calcium-channel blockers in primary pulmonary hypertension. Eur Respir J 1998;**12**:265–70.

3 Rubin LJ. Therapy of pulmonary hypertension: the evolution from vasodilators to antiproliferative agents. Am J Respir Crit Care Med 2002;**166**:1309–10.

●4 Christman BW, McPherson CD, Newman JH et al. An imbalance between the excretion of thromboxane and prostacyclin metabolites in pulmonary hypertension. N Engl J Med 1992;**327**:70–5.

●5 Giaid A, Yanagisawa M, Langleben D et al. Expression of endothelin-1 in the lungs of patients with pulmonary hypertension. N Engl J Med 1993;**328**:1732–9.

6 Giaid A, Salch D. Reduced expression of the endothelial nitric oxide synthase in the lungs of patients with pulmonary hypertension. N Engl J Med 1995;**333**:214–21.

7 Tuder RM, Cool CD, Geraci MW et al. Prostacyclin synthase expression is decreased in lungs from patients with severe pulmonary hypertension. Am J Respir Crit Care Med 1999; **159**:1925–32.

*8 Barst RJ, Rubin LJ, Long WA et al. A comparison of continuous intravenous epoprostenol (prostacyclin) with conventional therapy for primary pulmonary hypertension. N Engl J Med 1996;**334**:296–302.

*9 Rubin LJ, Badesch DB, Barst RJ et al. Bosentan therapy for pulmonary arterial hypertension. N Engl J Med 2002; **346**:896–903.

10 Clapp LH, Finney P, Turcato S et al. Differential effects of stable prostacyclin analogues on smooth muscle proliferation and cyclic AMP generation in human pulmonary artery. Am J Respir Cell Mol Biol 2002;**26**:194–201.

◆11 Rubin LJ. Primary pulmonary hypertension. N Engl J Med 1997;**336**:111–17.

12 Rich S, Seidlitz M, Dodin E et al. The short-term effects of digoxin in patients with right ventricular dysfunction from pulmonary hypertension. Chest 1998;**114**:787–92.

13 Fuster V, Steele PM, Edwards WD et al. Primary pulmonary hypertension. Natural history and the importance of thrombosis. Circulation 1984;**70**:580–7.

*14 Rich S, Kaufmann E, Levy PS. The effect of high doses of calcium-channel blockers on survival in primary pulmonary hypertension. N Engl J Med 1992;**327**:76–81.

15 Sitbon O, Humbert M, Ioos V et al. Who does benefit from long-term calcium-channel blocker therapy in primary pulmonary hypertension? [Abstract] Am J Respir Crit Care Med 2003;**167**:A440.

16 Rubin LJ, Mendoza J, Hood M et al. Treatment of primary pulmonary hypertension with continuous intravenous prostacyclin (epoprostenol). Results of a randomized trial. Ann Intern Med 1990;**112**:485–91.

17 Castelain V, Chemla D, Humbert M et al. Improvement of the pressure flow relationships of the pulmonary circulation in primary pulmonary hypertension after six weeks prostacyclin. Am J Respir Crit Care Med 2002;**165**:338–40.

●18 Higenbottam T, Wheeldon D, Wells F et al. Long-term treatment of primary pulmonary hypertension with continuous intravenous epoprostenol (prostacyclin). Lancet 1984;**1**:1046–7.

19 Shapiro SM, Oudiz RJ, Cao T et al. Primary pulmonary hypertension: improved long-term effects and survival with continuous intravenous epoprostenol infusion. J Am Coll Cardiol 1997;**30**:343–9.

●20 Sitbon O, Humbert M, Nunes H et al. Long-term intravenous epoprostenol infusion in primary pulmonary hypertension: prognostic factors and survival. J Am Coll Cardiol 2002;**40**:780–8.

●21 McLaughlin VV, Shillington A, Rich S. Survival in primary pulmonary hypertension: the impact of epoprostenol therapy. Circulation 2002;**106**:1477–82.

22 Robbins IM, Christman BW, Newman JH et al. A survey of diagnostic practices and the use of epoprostenol in patients with primary pulmonary hypertension. Chest 1998;114:1269–75.

23 Humbert M, Maitre S, Capron F et al. Pulmonary edema complicating continuous intravenous prostacyclin in pulmonary capillary hemangiomatosis. Am J Respir Crit Care Med 1998;157:1681–5.

*24 Badesch DB, Tapson VF, McGoon MD et al. Continuous intravenous epoprostenol for pulmonary hypertension due to the scleroderma spectrum of disease. Ann Intern Med 2000;132:425–34.

25 Rosenzweig EB, Kerstein D, Barst RJ. Long-term prostacyclin for pulmonary hypertension with associated congenital heart defects. Circulation 1999;99:1858–65.

26 Kuo PC, Johnson LB, Plotkin JS et al. Continuous intravenous infusion of epoprostenol for the treatment of portopulmonary hypertension. Transplantation 1997;63:604–6.

27 Aguilar RV, Farber HW. Epoprostenol (prostacyclin) therapy in HIV-associated pulmonary hypertension. Am J Respir Crit Care Med 2000;162:1846–50.

*28 Nunes H, Humbert M, Sitbon O et al. Prognostic factors for survival in HIV-associated pulmonary arterial hypertension. Am J Respir Crit Care Med 2003;167:1433–9.

29 Galiè N, Manes A, Branzi A. The new clinical trials on pharmacological treatment in pulmonary arterial hypertension. Eur Respir J 2002;20:1037–49.

30 Miyamoto S, Nagaya N, Satoh T et al. Clinical correlates and prognostic significance of six-minute walk test in patients with primary pulmonary hypertension: comparison with cardiopulmonary exercise testing. Am J Respir Crit Care Med 2000;161:487–92.

*31 Simonneau G, Barst RJ, Galiè N et al. Continuous subcutaneous infusion of treprostinil, a prostacyclin analogue, in patients with pulmonary arterial hypertension: a double-blind randomized controlled trial. Am J Respir Crit Care Med 2002;165:800–4.

32 Vachiéry JL, Hill N, Zwicke D et al. Transitioning from IV epoprostenol to subcutaneaous treprostinil in pulmonary arterial hypertension. Chest 2002;121:1561–5.

33 Okano Y, Yoshioka T, Shimouchi A et al. Orally active prostacyclin analogue in primary pulmonary hypertension. Lancet 1997;349:1365.

*34 Galiè N, Humbert M, Vachiéry JL et al. Effects of beraprost sodium, an oral prostacyclin analogue, in patients with pulmonary arterial hypertension: a randomized, double-blind placebo-controlled trial. J Am Coll Cardiol 2002;39:1496–502.

35 Barst RJ, McGoon M, McLaughlin V et al. Beraprost therapy for pulmonary arterial hypertension. J Am Coll Cardiol 2003;41:2119–25.

36 Hoeper MM, Schwarze M, Ehlerding S et al. Long-term treatment of primary pulmonary hypertension with aerosolized iloprost, a prostacyclin analogue. N Engl J Med 2000;342:1866–70.

37 Gessler T, Schmehl T, Hoeper MM et al. Ultrasonic versus jet nebulization of iloprost in severe pulmonary hypertension. Eur Respir J 2001;17:14–19.

*38 Olschewski H, Simonneau G, Galiè N et al. Inhaled iloprost in severe pulmonary hypertension. N Engl J Med 2002;347:322–7.

39 Yanisagawa M, Kurihara H, Kimura S et al. A novel potent vasoconstrictor peptide produced by vascular endothelial cells. Nature 1988;332:411–15.

40 Hirata Y, Katagi Y, Fukuda Y et al. Endothelin is a potent mitogen for rat vascular smooth muscle cells. Atherosclerosis 1989;78:225–8.

41 DiCarlo VS, Chen S-J, Meng QC et al. ETA-receptor antagonist prevents and reverses chronic hypoxia-induced pulmonary hypertension in rat. Am J Physiol 1995;269:L690–7.

42 Channick RN, Simonneau G, Sitbon O et al. Effects of the dual endothelin-receptor antagonist bosentan in patients with pulmonary hypertension: a randomised placebo-controlled study. Lancet 2001;358:1119–23.

43 Galiè N, Hinderliter AL, Torbicki A, et al. Effects of the oral endothelin-receptor antagonist bosentan on echocardiographic and doppler measures in patients with pulmonary arterial hypertension. J Am Coll Cardiol 2003;41:1380–6.

44 Sitbon O, Badesch DB, Channick RN et al. Effect of the dual endothelin receptor antagonist bosentan in patients with pulmonary arterial hypertension: a one year follow-up study. Chest 2003;124:247–54.

45 Barst RJ, Rich SA, Horn EM et al. Clinical efficacy of sitaxsentan, an endothelin-A receptor antagonist, in patients with pulmonary arterial hypertension. Chest 2002;121:1860–8.

46 Ghofrani HA, Wiedemann R, Rose F et al. Sildenafil for teatment of lung fibrosis and pulmonary hypertension: a randomised controlled trial. Lancet 2002;360:895–900.

47 Prasad S, Wilkinson J, Gatzoulis MA. Sildenafil in primary pulmonary hypertension. N Engl J Med 2000;343:1342.

48 Langleben D, Christman BW, Barst RJ et al. Effects of the thromboxane synthetase inhibitor and receptor antagonist terbogrel in patients with primary pulmonary hypertension. Am Heart J 2002;143:E4.

49 Nagaya N, Uematusu M, Oya H et al. Short-term oral administration of L-arginine improves hemodynamics and exercise capacity in patients with precapillary pulmonary hypertension. Am J Respir Crit Care Med 2001;163:887–91.

50 Kerstein D, Levy PS, Hsu DT et al. Blade balloon atrial septostomy in patients with severe primary pulmonary hypertension. Circulation 1995;91:2028–35.

51 Sandoval J, Gaspar J, Pulido T et al. Graded balloon dilation atrial septostomy in severe primary pulmonary hypertension: a therapeutic alternative for patients nonresponsive to vasodilator treatment. J Am Coll Cardiol 1998;32:297–304.

52 Rothman A, Sklanksky MS, Lucas X et al. Atrial septostomy as a bridge to lung transplantation in patients with severe pulmonary hypertension. Am J Cardiol 1999;84:682–6.

53 Mendeloff EN, Meyers BF, Sundt TM et al. Lung transplantation for pulmonary vascular disease. Ann Thorac Surg 2002;73:209–19.

54 Reitz BA, Wallwork JL, Hunt SA et al. Heart-lung transplantation: successful therapy for patients with pulmonary vascular disease. N Engl J Med 1982;306:557–64.

55 Hosenpud JD, Bennett LE, Keck BM et al. The Registry of the International Society for Heart and Lung Transplantation: eighteenth official report 2001. J Heart Lung Transplant 2001;20:805–15.

56 Bigatello LM, Hess D, Dennehy KC *et al*. Sildenafil can increase the response to inhaled nitric oxide. *Anesthesiology* 2000;**92**:1827–9.

57 Ghofrani HA, Wiedemann R, Rose F *et al*. Combination therapy with oral sildenafil and inhaled iloprost for severe pulmonary hypertension. *Ann Intern Med* 2002;**136**:515–22.

58 Ghofrani HA, Rose F, Schermuly RT *et al*. Amplification of the pulmonary vasodilatory response to inhaled iloprost by subtreshold phosphodiesterases types 3 and 4 inhibition in severe pulmonary hypertension. *Crit Care Med* 2002;**30**:2489–92.

59 Humbert M, Barst RJ, Robbins I *et al*. Safety and efficacy of bosentan in combination with epoprostenol in patients with severe pulmonary arterial hypertension. [Abstract] *Am J Respir Crit Care Med* 2003;**167**:A441.

60 Lane KB, Machado RD, Pauciulo MW *et al*. Heterozygous germline mutations in a TGFβ receptor, BMPR2, are the cause of familial primary pulmonary hypertension. *Nat Genet* 2000;**26**:81–4.

61 Deng Z, Morse JH, Slager SL *et al*. Familial primary pulmonary hypertension (gene *PPH1*) is caused by mutations in the bone morphogenetic protein receptor-II gene. *Am J Hum Genet* 2000;**67**:737–44.

62 Trembath R, Thomson JR, Machado RD *et al*. Clinical and molecular genetic features of pulmonary hypertension in patients with hereditary hemorrhagic telangiectasia. *N Engl J Med* 2001;**345**:325–34.

63 Morrell NW, Yang X, Upton P *et al*. Altered growth responses of pulmonary artery smooth muscle cells from patients with primary pulmonary hypertension to transforming growth factor β1 and bone morphogenetic proteins. *Circulation* 2001;**104**:790–5.

64 Du L, Sullivan CC, Chu D *et al*. Signaling molecules in nonfamilial pulmonary hypertension. *N Engl J Med* 2003;**348**:500–9.

14

Pulmonary venous hypertension

Diagnosis and treatment of left heart disease

J SIMON R GIBBS AND MICHAEL HENEIN

HOW DOES LEFT HEART DISEASE AFFECT THE PULMONARY CIRCULATION?

The purpose of this chapter is to examine the effects of left heart disease and its treatment on the pulmonary circulation. Pulmonary venous hypertension in left heart disease is caused by elevated left atrial pressure. This may be a direct consequence of mitral valve disease, thrombus or atrial myxoma obstructing the mitral valve, or a result of elevated left ventricular diastolic pressure with or without mitral regurgitation. The commonest cause of left heart disease with pulmonary venous hypertension is heart failure.

Prevalence and prognosis of pulmonary hypertension in heart failure

There is a paucity of good epidemiological information about pulmonary hypertension in heart failure. In patients with moderate to severe heart failure referred to transplant clinics, pulmonary hypertension with a pulmonary vascular resistance >3.5 Wood units is reported in between 19 to 35% of patients.[1,2]

Pulmonary hypertension carries a poor prognosis for patients with heart failure.[3–6] At 28 months of follow-up, the mortality rate was 57% in patients with moderate pulmonary hypertension compared with 17% in normotensive patients.[3] In another study, pulmonary artery wedge pressures of ≤16 mmHg had 1-year survival of 83 versus 38%.[5]

Hemodynamic stress and pathological changes in the pulmonary circulation

Although heart failure has hemodynamic effects throughout the circulation, early heart failure affects the pulmonary before the systemic circulation.[7] This may occur without clinical manifestation. In an animal model of heart failure where the resting cardiac output was the same as in control animals, pulmonary hypertension preceded changes in aortic hemodynamics. While pulmonary arterial pulse pressure was unchanged, pulmonary arterial pressure, lumen diameter and wall tension increased whereas blood velocity and wall shear stress decreased in comparison to normal values.[7] These hemodynamic changes were associated with increased medial cross-sectional area, thickness, smooth muscle cell number and collagen content of the pulmonary arteries.

The high compliance of the pulmonary circulation ensures that small increases in pressure enlarge lumen size much more than the systemic circulation. Increase in lumen size reduces shear stress and amplifies the increased tensile stress. Chronically, these changes affect vasomotor tone and endothelial function. In patients with chronic heart failure with normal pulmonary artery pressure, pulmonary artery endothelium may play a significant role in inhibiting vasoconstriction.[8–10]

Pulmonary arterial endothelial function is blunted in heart failure because of reduced basal nitric oxide activity while stimulated nitric oxide release is normal.[7,11,12] These changes in the endothelium are associated with increased vascular responsiveness to norepinephrine. This dissociation of basal and stimulated nitric oxide release may affect pulmonary hemodynamics at an early stage of heart failure.[12] Enhanced vascular superoxide production in heart failure inactivates nitric oxide and may contribute to the endothelial dysfunction, an effect which is reduced by spironolactone and endothelin antagonists.[13–15] In addition, pulmonary vasomotor tone may be affected by decreased expression of angiotensin converting enzyme,[16] increased levels of endothelin[17,18] and interleukin-6 production,[19] as well as other proinflammatory cytokines.

Pulmonary vascular disease associated with prolonged pulmonary venous hypertension gives rise to medial hypertrophy of the muscular pulmonary arteries, muscularization of the arterioles with intimal and adventitial fibrosis, focal hemosiderosis, and sometimes necrotizing arteritis. The alveolar wall is affected by changes in the capillary endothelial cells, the lung interstitium and the alveolar epithelial cells. The pulmonary veins develop medial hypertrophy, and intimal fibrosis.

The pulmonary venous hypertension resulting from chronic heart failure tends to be less severe than occurs in mitral stenosis, although exceptions to this are reported. In its most severe chronic form, pulmonary venous hypertension results in pulmonary interstitial fibrosis, lymphangiectasis, ossification in the alveolar spaces and microlithiasis, which render the lungs very stiff.

Hemodynamic effects of pulmonary vascular changes

The distension of pulmonary arteries and capillaries, and remodeling of the pulmonary circulation in heart failure in response to pulmonary venous hypertension causes more recruitment of pulmonary resistance vessels than at normal pulmonary venous pressure, increases pulmonary vascular resistance, low- and high-frequency impedance, and wave reflections, and reduces the pulsatile properties of pulmonary arteries. These alterations in hemodynamics contribute to reduced forward flow and increased power requirement of the right ventricle per unit forward flow,[20,21] eventually leading to right ventricular hypertrophy, dilatation and failure.[20,22] Unlike normal subjects, the perfusion of the lung apices is high at rest and this does not increase on exercise, suggesting that blood flow is maximally diverted at rest.[23]

In response to exercise, pulmonary vascular resistance tends to fall in patients with elevated resistance at rest, and rises in those with normal resistance, although these changes are relatively small.[1,24]

Determinants of pulmonary hypertension

There is a close relationship between pulmonary arterial pressure and pulmonary capillary wedge pressure both at rest and during changes induced by vasodilator therapy,[4,25] suggesting that left heart filling pressure, and hence pulmonary venous hypertension, is the main determinant of pulmonary hypertension. The degree of reduction in the pulmonary capillary wedge pressure is also predictive of survival in severe heart failure.[26]

Consistent with this finding are other studies which have identified estimates of the severity of left ventricular diastolic dysfunction but not systolic dysfunction,[25,27] the degree of mitral regurgitation[27] and left atrial function[25] as being independently related to the degree of pulmonary hypertension. Old age is also correlated closely with pulmonary hypertension.[27]

Pathophysiology of left ventricular disease

Relaxation may be impaired in the early stages of left ventricular dysfunction irrespective of whether the etiology is coronary artery disease, cardiomyopathy or aortic valve disease.[28,29] The result is prolongation of isovolumic relaxation time, reduced early diastolic filling velocity and a long deceleration time. As the dysfunction progresses, the ventricle becomes stiff, incompliant and end-diastolic pressure increases. This compromises late diastolic ventricular filling, which is overcome by a compensatory increase in left atrial pressure that augments the left atrial–left ventricular pressure gradient in early diastole.[30]

RESTRICTIVE LV PHYSIOLOGY

Raised left atrial pressure can be determined using Doppler echocardiography: isovolumic relaxation time is short and early diastolic filling is dominant with fast acceleration and deceleration (Plate 14A.1).[31] With the loss of ventricular compliance, provided that sinus rhythm is maintained, left atrial contraction causes retrograde flow in the pulmonary veins.[32] Patients presenting with this filling pattern demonstrate varying degrees of mitral regurgitation, which augments the elevated left atrial pressure.

Restrictive left ventricular filling in patients with severe left ventricular disease may also affect right ventricular physiology. This can be assessed either from the peak retrograde pressure drop across the tricuspid valve or the extent of delay of right ventricular filling with respect to end-ejection (Figure 14A.1 and 2). In addition, the increased left atrioventricular pressure gradient in early diastole directly transmitted across the ventricular septum can suppress or compromise right ventricular early diastolic filling (Figure 14A.3).[33] Successful offloading of the left atrium by vasodilators reverses these disturbances in the majority of patients. Furthermore, along with the significant symptomatic improvement with vasodilators, left ventricular filling becomes of the slow relaxation pattern, mitral regurgitation disappears and right ventricular filling delay regresses.[34]

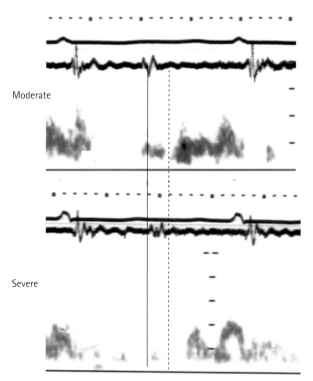

Figure 14A.2 *Right ventricular filling velocities from a patient with moderate pulmonary hypertension (top) and after developing severe pulmonary hypertension (bottom). Note the progressive delay in the onset of right ventricular filling.*

Figure 14A.1 *Forward and retrograde blood flow velocities across the tricuspid valve from a patient with pulmonary hypertension. Note the raised right ventricular − right atrial pressure drop 80 mmHg and the delayed onset of forward flow with respect to end-ejection.*

VENTRICULAR MEASUREMENTS AND PROGNOSIS

Progressive increase in left ventricular dimensions and mass[35] and reduction in ejection fraction over time can predict an objective fall in patients exercise tolerance assessed by cardiopulmonary exercise testing. Changes in peak oxygen consumption predict clinical outcome in patients with chronic left ventricular failure.[36] An isovolumic relaxation time >30 ms had a 78% cumulative 3-year survival compared to 52% survival with values <30 ms.

Right ventricular function is equally important in patients with left ventricular disease. Right ventricular free wall amplitude is a modest determinant of peak oxygen consumption and restrictive filling carries the worst clinical outcome (Plate 14A.2).[36,37] A number of studies have suggested that right ventricular ejection fraction is an independent prognostic indicator in patients with moderate to severe heart failure,[38–41] as is contractile reserve.[42] Impaired right ventricular function only appears to be an important prognostic factor when

pulmonary arterial pressure is raised:[43] impaired right ventricular function with normal pulmonary arterial pressure does not carry additional risk, and normal right ventricular function with pulmonary hypertension has a similar prognosis to patients with normal pulmonary arterial pressure.

ACTIVATION–INDUCED LV DYSFUNCTION

Severe left ventricular disease is almost always associated with delayed ventricular depolarization, i.e. broad QRS complex. Progressive prolongation of ventricular depolarization has been shown to be associated with poor clinical outcome.[44] This electrical disturbance is often associated with delayed and prolonged ventricular shortening and lengthening and hence significant incoordination.[45] The latter contributes to raised diastolic segmental wall tension resulting in presystolic mitral regurgitation. Such prolonged mitral regurgitation tends to limit the ventricular filling time at fast heart rates in patients with poor left ventricular function and reduces the stroke volume. Although these ventricles fill with a single component 'summation filling pattern', the prolonged mitral regurgitation augments the raised left atrial pressure.

This condition responds to dual chamber right heart pacing with a short atrioventricular delay or biventricular pacing.[46] The symptomatic improvement with the

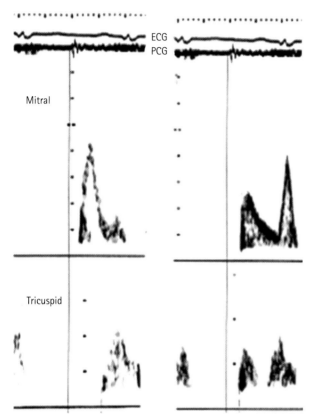

ECG
PCG

Mitral

Tricuspid

Figure 14A.3 *A composite of transmitral and transtricuspid flow velocities from a patient with restrictive left ventricular filling (left) and after successful unloading of the left atrium with angiotensin converting enzyme (ACE) inhibitors (right). Note the significant normalization of the pattern of right ventricular filling. PCG, phonocardiogram.*

optimal pacing mode is associated with shortened mitral regurgitation and prolonged ventricular filling time.

LEFT VENTRICULAR FUNCTION DURING STRESS

The symptoms of heart failure are precipitated by exercise and this makes stress echocardiography a useful investigation for the assessment of symptoms and related hemodynamic disturbances. In patients with dilated cardiomyopathy, an increase of ejection fraction by 30% with stress carries better outcome and predicts progressive improvement of ventricular performance compared to those that do not increase.[47]

While angina is the main stress end point in patients with coronary artery disease irrespective of the cavity size, exaggerated incoordination and reduction in cardiac output are the main limitations in patients with dilated cardiomyopathy and left bundle branch block, irrespective of the presence of coronary disease.

In elderly patients with basal septal hypertrophy and exertional breathlessness (Plate 14A.3), the increase in heart rate with stress precipitates their symptoms along with left ventricular outflow tract obstruction, a drop in

systolic blood pressure and mitral regurgitation.[48] The acute development of functional (dynamic) mitral regurgitation in such patients may augment pressures in the incompliant left atrium and hence worsens pulmonary venous hypertension. Differences in stress-related ventricular behavior have implications for the management of the patient groups so defined.

LEFT ATRIAL FUNCTION

Atrial function is important in determining atrioventricular pressure gradient and hence atrial pressure. In patients with mitral stenosis, left atrial compliance and mitral valve area were found to be the most sensitive predictors of left atrial pressure.[49] Reduced left atrial compliance, calculated from the ratio of effective mitral valve area to atrioventricular pressure gradient decline in early diastole, has also been found to correlate with pulmonary arterial pressure during exercise.[50] Patients with low compliance were more symptomatic and had higher pulmonary arterial pressure.

In the absence of mitral valve disease, increasing degrees of left ventricular filling impairment result in mechanical alterations of left atrial function. These are based on Starling's law and atrial pump function is enhanced according to the preloading condition of the chamber. In late left ventricular dysfunction, atrial reservoir and pump function decline and the atrium starts to function as a conduit, consistent with depressed compliance and suppressed contractile function.

Consequences for right heart hemodynamics

There are several possible mechanisms for the changes in right heart hemodynamics seen in heart failure. First, the right ventricle may be involved in the same pathological process impairing myocardial function as the left ventricle, such as myocardial ischemia or myocarditis, or an inflammatory process in common with the pulmonary arteries.

Second, where the left ventricular stroke volume is low it must be matched by the right ventricle. This is a necessary requirement of the pulmonary and systemic circulations being arranged in series.

Third, elevated left atrial pressure is transmitted via the pulmonary circulation and right atrial pressure.[8,33,51] There is an inverse relationship between pulmonary artery pressure and systolic right ventricular ejection fraction in pulmonary hypertension.[52] This is consistent with the finding that right ventricular function is afterload dependent, pulmonary artery pressure being an important component of right ventricular afterload. The importance of right ventricular function is emphasized by the correlation of right ventricular ejection fraction with maximum oxygen consumption, in contrast to the lack of correlation of left ventricular function with exercise capacity.[53]

Exceptions to the inverse relationship between pulmonary arterial pressure and right ventricular function are not uncommon in clinical practice. In the presence of pulmonary hypertension, right ventricular function may be preserved if the onset of pulmonary hypertension is slow, allowing time for right ventricular compensation, or the pulmonary vascular resistance is <3.0 Wood units.[6] In addition, right ventricular dysfunction in the absence of pulmonary hypertension may occur at a low cardiac output despite pulmonary vascular disease, or in the presence of atrial fibrillation, suggesting that this arrhythmia could play a role in the pathogenesis of right ventricular dysfunction.[43]

Where significant pulmonary hypertension is present at rest, right ventricular failure may be precipitated by exercise: this is associated with a rise in right atrial pressure but a fall in left ventricular filling pressure,[1] suggesting that a fall in cardiac output as a result of reduced left ventricular filling may occur as a consequence of pulmonary hypertension.

Volume overload and sympathetic venoconstriction increase venous return to the right atrium. Acute increases in venous return increase right heart pressures without any increase in cardiac work.[54]

In addition, increased coronary venous pressure as a result of high right atrial pressure decreases left ventricular diastolic distensibility with increasing left ventricular wall volume, resulting in higher left ventricular filling pressures.[55] This mechanism appears to act independently of diastolic ventricular interaction caused by right ventricular enlargement.

Fourth, ventricular interaction may occur, mediated via the septum or pericardium.[8,9,33,56–59] Right-sided filling abnormalities may be directly related to high early diastolic pressures in the left ventricle, the time relations suggesting ventricular interaction rather than the effect of pulmonary hypertension.[8,33] The net effect is to delay forward diastolic flow across the tricuspid valve (Figure 14A.4).

Hemodynamics and acute heart failure

In acute heart failure, patients complain of shortness of breath and this is caused by pulmonary congestion. Acutely elevated left ventricular end-diastolic pressure causes pulmonary venous hypertension. At a critical left atrial pressure of 24 mmHg (for an albumin level of 36 g/L), water crosses from the capillaries to the alveolar air spaces.[60] Pulmonary function tests show evidence of airways obstruction,[61] and this is associated with a restrictive ventilatory defect characterized by a reduced vital capacity and air trapping due to early closure of dependent airways.[62] A high intrapleural pressure is required to distend stiff lungs and this reduces tidal volume and

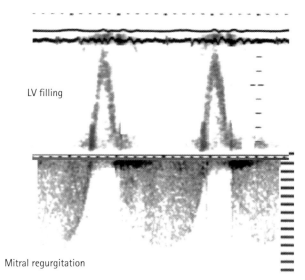

Figure 14A.4 *Transmitral forward and backward flow velocities from a patient with severe left ventricular (LV) disease showing long mitral regurgitation that is limiting filling time.*

increases respiratory rate. This may be exacerbated by the caliber of small airways being reduced by dilatation of blood vessels which increase airway resistance.[63]

As a consequence of these changes, respiratory workload is increased[64] and the efficiency of gas exchange is reduced. Ventilation/perfusion mismatch widens the alveolar − arterial oxygen difference and increases the dead space/tidal volume ratio.

In addition, sympathetic nervous system activation promotes pulmonary edema by increasing venous tone and atrial pressures, and this is associated with increased systemic vascular resistance and worsening left ventricular function.

Hemodynamics and chronic heart failure

The fundamental cause of chronic heart failure is a low cardiac output. While traditionally the symptoms of breathlessness and fatigue were believed to be related to pulmonary hemodynamics, this relationship has been challenged.

Exercise capacity is not related to resting cardiac output, resting ejection fraction or non-invasive indices of left ventricular function;[65,66] neither is there a direct relation between breathlessness and pulmonary capillary wedge pressure at rest or on exercise.[67–69] Pulmonary arterial pressure shows wide fluctuations during the day and night[70] and does not correlate with symptoms during maximal or submaximal exercise.[71]

Neither hypoxia nor hypercapnia are important in heart failure since patients retain near-normal levels of respiratory gases during exercise.[67] There is an increase in ventilation relative to carbon dioxide production. The increased ventilation is not related to pulmonary capillary wedge pressure, and exercise ventilation has been shown to be unaffected by an acute reduction in wedge pressure.[68]

An explanation for the discrepancies between cardiopulmonary function and exercise capacity may be found in changes in skeletal muscle. A full treatise on this subject is beyond the scope of this chapter.

HOW DO INTERVENTIONS FOR LEFT HEART DISEASE AFFECT THE PULMONARY CIRCULATION?

Hemodynamics and clinical outcomes in heart failure

The symptoms of acute heart failure are relieved by lowering left atrial pressure and hence improving pulmonary congestion.

In chronic heart failure, reduction in filling pressures and increased myocardial contractility have been assumed to correlate with symptomatic improvement. Randomized trials of these drugs have shown that significant hemodynamic improvements do not necessarily translate into clinical benefit in chronic heart failure. This could be a result either because central hemodynamics are not the main determinants of the disease process or because a drug exerts a deleterious effect by mechanisms not measured by hemodynamics.[72]

Phosphodiesterase inhibitors and β-agonists have a positive inotropic effect and increase mortality.[73–77] Although they increase cardiac index, their effect on pulmonary hemodynamics is varied.[78]

Vasodilators reduce hydraulic load on the ventricles. Nitrates have been shown to improve exercise duration and the maximum rate of oxygen consumption with long-term treatment[79,80] without a reliable fall in pulmonary capillary wedge pressure. For a comparable improvement in filling pressures, patients receiving hydralazine and nitrates have a higher mortality than those on angiotensin converting enzyme inhibitors.[81] Flosequinan in addition to angiotensin converting enzyme inhibitors improves hemodynamics but increased mortality.[82]

Chronic intravenous epoprostenol therapy in chronic heart failure is not associated with improvement in distance walked, quality of life, or morbid events and is associated with an increased risk of death,[83] possibly as a result of its positive inotropic effect.[84] Hemodynamically beneficial vasodilator therapy with nifedipine worsens clinical outcomes when compared to isosorbide dinitrate.[85] A similar lack of clinical benefit has been shown with minoxidil.[86] Sildenafil modestly reduces pulmonary arterial

pressure in patients with severe coronary artery disease without altering pulmonary capillary wedge pressure or pulmonary vascular resistance.[87] Furthermore, β-blockers have been shown to improve mortality and morbidity despite acute deterioration in hemodynamics.[88,89]

Conversely, intensive vasodilator and diuretic therapy in severe heart failure is associated with clinical improvement, increased exercise capacity and reduced hospital admissions.[4,5,90–93] While there appears to be a correlation between pulmonary hemodynamics and survival in these circumstances, the clinical benefits may have resulted from higher dosing of therapies proven to improve outcomes in heart failure or as part of a complex intervention.

Surgery

Symptomatic patients who are resistant to medical therapy and who do not fulfill the criteria for ventricular pacing may receive life-saving ventricular-assist devices. These are used either as a bridge to recovery or transplantation. The symptomatic improvement in patients who receive assist devices is associated with reduction in pulmonary venous pressure. The device aims to offload the left ventricle and eject blood directly into the descending aorta, thus reducing wall tension and allowing recovery of myocardial function.

Pulmonary hypertension has been shown to decrease gradually following cardiac transplantation,[94–96] implying that pulmonary vascular disease in chronic heart failure is potentially reversible. A fall in preoperative pulmonary vascular resistance in response to glyceryl trinitrate predicts an immediate postoperative fall in pulmonary pressures and pulmonary vascular resistance.[97] The time to resolution also depends on the severity of preoperative pulmonary hypertension[98] and for patients with high pressures, residual pulmonary hypertension may take years to resolve.[95] A similar pattern has been reported following surgery for mitral stenosis.[99]

KEY POINTS

- Pulmonary hypertension probably occurs in up to 35% of patients with severe heart failure.
- Pulmonary hypertension carries a poor prognosis in chronic heart failure.
- The main determinant of pulmonary hypertension in chronic heart failure is the left heart filling pressure.
- Right ventricular dysfunction is an adverse prognostic factor in the presence of pulmonary hypertension.
- The symptoms of chronic heart failure correlate poorly with pulmonary hemodynamics.

REFERENCES

1 Butler J, Chomsky DB, Wilson JR. Pulmonary hypertension and exercise intolerance in patients with heart failure. *J Am Coll Cardiol* 1999;**34**:1802–6.

2 Costard-Jackle A, Fowler MB. Influence of preoperative pulmonary artery pressure on mortality after heart transplantation: testing of potential reversibility of pulmonary hypertension with nitroprusside is useful in defining a high risk group. *J Am Coll Cardiol* 1992;**19**: 48–54.

●3 Abramson SV, Burke JF, Kelly JJ, Jr *et al.* Pulmonary hypertension predicts mortality and morbidity in patients with dilated cardiomyopathy. *Ann Intern Med* 1992;**116**:888–95.

4 Drazner MH, Hamilton MA, Fonarow G *et al.* Relationship between right and left-sided filling pressures in 1000 patients with advanced heart failure. *J Heart Lung Transplant* 1999;**18**:1126–32.

5 Stevenson LW, Tillisch JH, Hamilton M *et al.* Importance of hemodynamic response to therapy in predicting survival with ejection fraction less than or equal to 20% secondary to ischemic or nonischemic dilated cardiomyopathy. *Am J Cardiol* 1990;**66**:1348–54.

6 Cappola TP, Felker GM, Kao WH *et al.* Pulmonary hyper-tension and risk of death in cardiomyopathy: patients with myocarditis are at higher risk. *Circulation* 2002;**105**:1663–8.

7 Driss AB, Devaux C, Henrion D *et al.* Hemodynamic stresses induce endothelial dysfunction and remodeling of pulmonary artery in experimental compensated heart failure. *Circulation* 2000;**101**:2764–70.

8 Hofmann T, Keck A, van Ingen G *et al.* Simultaneous measurement of pulmonary venous flow by intravascular catheter Doppler velocimetry and transesophageal Doppler echocardiography: relation to left atrial pressure and left atrial and left ventricular function. *J Am Coll Cardiol* 1995;**26**:239–49.

9 Ohno M, Cheng CP, Little WC. Mechanism of altered patterns of left ventricular filling during the development of congestive heart failure. *Circulation* 1994;**89**:2241–50.

10 Porter TR, Taylor DO, Cycan A *et al.* Endothelium-dependent pulmonary artery responses in chronic heart failure: influence of pulmonary hypertension. *J Am Coll Cardiol* 1993;**22**:1418–24.

11 Ontkean M, Gay R, Greenberg B. Diminished endothelium-derived relaxing factor activity in an experimental model of chronic heart failure. *Circ Res* 1991;**69**:1088–96.

12 Teerlink JR, Gray GA, Clozel M *et al.* Increased vascular responsiveness to norepinephrine in rats with heart failure is endothelium dependent. Dissociation of basal and stimulated nitric oxide release. *Circulation* 1994;**89**:393–401.

13 Bauersachs J, Bouloumie A, Fraccarollo D *et al.* Endothelial dysfunction in chronic myocardial infarction despite increased vascular endothelial nitric oxide synthase and soluble guanylate cyclase expression: role of enhanced vascular superoxide production. *Circulation* 1999;**100**:292–8.

14 Bauersachs J, Fraccarollo D, Galuppo P *et al.* Endothelin-receptor blockade improves endothelial vasomotor dysfunction in heart failure. *Cardiovasc Res* 2000;**47**:142–9.

15 Bauersachs J, Heck M, Fraccarollo D *et al.* Addition of spironolactone to angiotensin-converting enzyme inhibition in heart failure improves endothelial vasomotor dysfunction: role of vascular superoxide anion formation and endothelial nitric oxide synthase expression. *J Am Coll Cardiol* 2002;**39**:351–8.

16 Huang H, Arnal JF, Llorens-Cortes C *et al.* Discrepancy between plasma and lung angiotensin-converting enzyme activity in experimental congestive heart failure. A novel aspect of endothelium dysfunction. *Circ Res* 1994;**75**:454–61.

17 Stangl K, Dschietzig T, Richter C *et al.* Pulmonary release and coronary and peripheral consumption of big endothelin and endothelin-1 in severe heart failure: acute effects of vasodilator therapy. *Circulation* 2000;**102**:1132–8.

18 Sakai S, Miyauchi T, Sakurai T *et al.* Pulmonary hypertension caused by congestive heart failure is ameliorated by long-term application of an endothelin receptor antagonist. Increased expression of endothelin-1 messenger ribonucleic acid and endothelin-1-like immunoreactivity in the lung in congestive heart failure in rats. *J Am Coll Cardiol* 1996;**28**:1580–8.

19 Mabuchi N, Tsutamoto T, Wada A *et al.* Relationship between interleukin-6 production in the lungs and pulmonary vascular resistance in patients with congestive heart failure. *Chest* 2002;**121**:1195–202.

20 Kono T, Sabbah HN, Rosman H *et al.* Left atrial contribution to ventricular filling during the course of evolving heart failure. *Circulation* 1992;**86**:1317–22.

21 Kussmaul WG, III, Altschuler JA, Matthai WH *et al.* Right ventricular-vascular interaction in congestive heart failure. Importance of low-frequency impedance. *Circulation* 1993;**88**:1010–15.

22 Kussmaul WG, III, Wieland J, Altschuler J *et al.* Pulmonary impedance and right ventricular-vascular coupling during coronary angioplasty. *J Appl Physiol* 1993;**74**: 161–9.

23 Mohsenifar Z, Amin DK, Shah PK. Regional distribution of lung perfusion and ventilation in patients with chronic congestive heart failure and its relationship to cardio-pulmonary hemodynamics. *Am Heart J* 1989;**117**:887–91.

●24 Janicki JS, Weber KT, Likoff MJ *et al.* The pressure-flow response of the pulmonary circulation in patients with heart failure and pulmonary vascular disease. *Circulation* 1985;**72**:1270–8.

25 Capomolla S, Febo O, Guazzotti G *et al.* Invasive and non-invasive determinants of pulmonary hypertension in patients with chronic heart failure. *J Heart Lung Transplant* 2000;**19**:426–38.

26 Shah MR, Stinnett SS, McNulty SE *et al.* Hemodynamics as surrogate end points for survival in advanced heart failure: an analysis from FIRST. *Am Heart J* 2001;**141**:908–14.

●27 Enriquez-Sarano M, Rossi A, Seward JB *et al.* Determinants of pulmonary hypertension in left ventricular dysfunction. *J Am Coll Cardiol* 1997;**29**:153–9.

28 Henein MY, Priestley K, Davarashvili T *et al.* Early changes in left ventricular subendocardial function after successful coronary angioplasty. *Br Heart J* 1993;**69**:501–6.

29 Henein MY, O'Sullivan CA, Ramzy IS *et al.* Electromechanical left ventricular behavior after nonsurgical septal reduction in patients with hypertrophic obstructive cardiomyopathy. *J Am Coll Cardiol* 1999;**34**:1117–22.

•30 Appleton CP, Hatle LK, Popp RL. Demonstration of restrictive ventricular physiology by Doppler echocardiography. *J Am Coll Cardiol* 1988;**11**:757–68.

31 Henein MY, Gibson DG. Abnormal subendocardial function in restrictive left ventricular disease. *Br Heart J* 1994;**72**:237–42.

32 Rossvoll O, Hatle LK. Pulmonary venous flow velocities recorded by transthoracic Doppler ultrasound: relation to left ventricular diastolic pressures. *J Am Coll Cardiol* 1993;**21**:1687–96.

33 Henein MY, O'Sullivan CA, Coats AJ *et al.* Angiotensin-converting enzyme (ACE) inhibitors revert abnormal right ventricular filling in patients with restrictive left ventricular disease. *J Am Coll Cardiol* 1998;**32**:1187–93.

34 Henein MY, Amadi A, O'Sullivan CA *et al.* ACE inhibitors unmask incoordinate diastolic wall motion in restrictive left ventricular disease. *Heart* 1996;**76**:326–31.

35 Florea VG, Henein MY, Cicoira M *et al.* Echocardiographic determinants of mortality in patients >67 years of age with chronic heart failure. *Am J Cardiol* 2000;**86**:158–61.

36 Florea VG, Henein MY, Anker SD *et al.* Prognostic value of changes over time in exercise capacity and echocardiographic measurements in patients with chronic heart failure. *Eur Heart J* 2000;**21**:146–53.

37 Webb-Peploe KM, Henein MY, Coats AJ *et al.* Echo derived variables predicting exercise tolerance in patients with dilated and poorly functioning left ventricle. *Heart* 1998;**80**:565–9.

38 de Groote P, Millaire A, Foucher-Hossein C *et al.* Right ventricular ejection fraction is an independent predictor of survival in patients with moderate heart failure. *J Am Coll Cardiol* 1998;**32**:948–54.

39 Di Salvo TG, Mathier M, Semigran MJ *et al.* Preserved right ventricular ejection fraction predicts exercise capacity and survival in advanced heart failure. *J Am Coll Cardiol* 1995;**25**:1143–53.

40 Karatasakis GT, Karagounis LA, Kalyvas PA *et al.* Prognostic significance of echocardiographically estimated right ventricular shortening in advanced heart failure. *Am J Cardiol* 1998;**82**:329–34.

41 Polak JF, Holman BL, Wynne J *et al.* Right ventricular ejection fraction: an indicator of increased mortality in patients with congestive heart failure associated with coronary artery disease. *J Am Coll Cardiol* 1983;**2**:217–24.

42 Gorcsan J, III, Murali S, Counihan PJ *et al.* Right ventricular performance and contractile reserve in patients with severe heart failure. Assessment by pressure–area relations and association with outcome. *Circulation* 1996;**94**: 3190–7.

43 Ghio S, Gavazzi A, Campana C *et al.* Independent and additive prognostic value of right ventricular systolic function and pulmonary artery pressure in patients with chronic heart failure. *J Am Coll Cardiol* 2001;**37**:183–8.

44 Shamim W, Yousufuddin M, Cicoria M *et al.* Incremental changes in QRS duration in serial ECGs over time identify high risk elderly patients with heart failure. *Heart* 2002;**88**:47–51.

45 Duncan AM, O'Sullivan CA, Gibson DG *et al.* Electromechanical interrelations during dobutamine stress in normal subjects and patients with coronary artery disease: comparison of changes in activation and inotropic state. *Heart* 2001;**85**:411–16.

46 Brecker SJ, Gibson DG. What is the role of pacing in dilated cardiomyopathy? *Eur Heart J* 1996;**17**:819–24.

47 Picano E, Lattanzi F, Sicari R *et al.* Role of stress echocardiography in risk stratification early after an acute myocardial infarction. EPIC (Echo Persantin International Cooperative) and EDIC (Echo Dobutamine International Cooperative) Study Groups. *Eur Heart J* 1997;**18**(Suppl D): D78–85.

•48 Henein MY, O'Sullivan C, Sutton GC *et al.* Stress-induced left ventricular outflow tract obstruction: a potential cause of dyspnea in the elderly. *J Am Coll Cardiol* 1997;**30**:1301–7.

49 Ko YG, Ha JW, Chung N *et al.* Effects of left atrial compliance on left atrial pressure in pure mitral stenosis. *Catheter Cardiovasc Interv* 2001;**52**:328–33.

50 Schwammenthal E, Vered Z, Agranat O *et al.* Impact of atrioventricular compliance on pulmonary artery pressure in mitral stenosis: an exercise echocardiographic study. *Circulation* 2000;**102**:2378–84.

51 Nagueh SF, Kopelen HA, Zoghbi WA. Relation of mean right atrial pressure to echocardiographic and Doppler parameters of right atrial and right ventricular function. *Circulation* 1996;**93**:1160–9.

52 Morrison D, Goldman S, Wright AL *et al.* The effect of pulmonary hypertension on systolic function of the right ventricle. *Chest* 1983;**84**:250–7.

•53 Baker BJ, Wilen MM, Boyd CM *et al.* Relation of right ventricular ejection fraction to exercise capacity in chronic left ventricular failure. *Am J Cardiol* 1984;**54**:596–9.

54 Bain RJ, Tan LB, Murray RG *et al.* Central haemodynamic changes during lower body positive pressure in patients with congestive cardiac failure. *Cardiovasc Res* 1989; **23**:833–7.

55 Watanabe J, Levine MJ, Bellotto F *et al.* Effects of coronary venous pressure on left ventricular diastolic distensibility. *Circ Res* 1990;**67**:923–32.

56 Clyne CA, Alpert JS, Benotti JR. Interdependence of the left and right ventricles in health and disease. *Am Heart J* 1989;**117**:1366–73.

•57 Taylor RR, Covell JW, Sonnenblick EH *et al.* Dependence of ventricular distensibility on filling of the opposite ventricle. *Am J Physiol* 1967;**213**:711–18.

58 Tyberg JV, Misbach GA, Glantz SA *et al.* A mechanism for shifts in the diastolic, left ventricular, pressure-volume curve: the role of the pericardium. *Eur J Cardiol* 1978;**7**(Suppl):163–75.

•59 Janicki JS, Weber KT. The pericardium and ventricular interaction, distensibility, and function. *Am J Physiol* 1980;**238**:H494–503.

60 Guyton AC, Lindsey AW. Effect of elevated left atrial pressure and decreased plasma protein concentration on the development of pulmonary edema. *Circ Res* 1959;**7**:649–57.

●61 Light RW, George RB. Serial pulmonary function in patients with acute heart failure. *Arch Intern Med* 1983;**143**:429–33.

62 Collins JV, Clark TJ, Brown DJ. Airway function in healthy subjects and patients with left heart disease. *Clin Sci Mol Med* 1975;**49**:217–28.

63 Depeursinge FB, Depeursinge CD, Boutaleb AK *et al.* Respiratory system impedance in patients with acute left ventricular failure: pathophysiology and clinical interest. *Circulation* 1986;**73**:386–95.

64 Aubier M, Trippenbach T, Roussos C. Respiratory muscle fatigue during cardiogenic shock. *J Appl Physiol* 1981;**51**:499–508.

65 Franciosa JA, Park M, Levine TB. Lack of correlation between exercise capacity and indexes of resting left ventricular performance in heart failure. *Am J Cardiol* 1981;**47**:33–9.

66 Weber KT, Kinasewitz GT, Janicki JS *et al.* Oxygen utilization and ventilation during exercise in patients with chronic cardiac failure. *Circulation* 1982;**65**:1213–23.

67 Franciosa JA, Leddy CL, Wilen M *et al.* Relation between hemodynamic and ventilatory responses in determining exercise capacity in severe congestive heart failure. *Am J Cardiol* 1984;**53**:127–34.

68 Fink LI, Wilson JR, Ferraro N. Exercise ventilation and pulmonary artery wedge pressure in chronic stable congestive heart failure. *Am J Cardiol* 1986;**57**:249–53.

69 Sullivan MJ, Higginbotham MB, Cobb FR. Increased exercise ventilation in patients with chronic heart failure: intact ventilatory control despite hemodynamic and pulmonary abnormalities. *Circulation* 1988;**77**:552–9.

70 Gibbs JS, Cunningham D, Shapiro LM *et al.* Diurnal variation of pulmonary artery pressure in chronic heart failure. *Br Heart J* 1989;**62**:30–5.

71 Gibbs JS, Keegan J, Wright C *et al.* Pulmonary artery pressure changes during exercise and daily activities in chronic heart failure. *J Am Coll Cardiol* 1990;**15**:52–61.

72 Psaty BM, Weiss NS, Furberg CD *et al.* Surrogate end points, health outcomes, and the drug-approval process for the treatment of risk factors for cardiovascular disease. *JAMA* 1999;**282**:786–90.

73 The Xamoterol in Severe Heart Failure Study Group. Xamoterol in severe heart failure. *Lancet* 1990;**336**:1–6.

74 Flosequinan withdrawn. *Lancet* 1993;**342**:235.

75 Packer M, Carver JR, Rodeheffer RJ *et al.* Effect of oral milrinone on mortality in severe chronic heart failure. The PROMISE Study Research Group. *N Engl J Med* 1991;**325**:1468–75.

76 Packer M, Narahara KA, Elkayam U *et al.* Double-blind, placebo-controlled study of the efficacy of flosequinan in patients with chronic heart failure. Principal Investigators of the REFLECT Study. *J Am Coll Cardiol* 1993;**22**:65–72.

77 Cohn JN, Goldstein SO, Greenberg BH *et al.* A dose-dependent increase in mortality with vesnarinone among patients with severe heart failure. Vesnarinone Trial Investigators. *N Engl J Med* 1998;**339**:1810–16.

78 Lowes BD, Tsvetkova T, Eichhorn EJ *et al.* Milrinone versus dobutamine in heart failure subjects treated chronically with carvedilol. *Int J Cardiol* 2001;**81**:141–9.

79 Franciosa JA, Leddy CL, Schwartz DE. Importance of venodilation during long-term vasodilator therapy of chronic left ventricular failure. *Z Kardiol* 1983;**72**(Suppl 3):168–72.

80 Leier CV, Huss P, Magorien RD *et al.* Improved exercise capacity and differing arterial and venous tolerance during chronic isosorbide dinitrate therapy for congestive heart failure. *Circulation* 1983;**67**:817–22.

81 Fonarow GC, Chelimsky-Fallick C, Stevenson LW *et al.* Effect of direct vasodilation with hydralazine versus angiotensin-converting enzyme inhibition with captopril on mortality in advanced heart failure: the Hy-C trial. *J Am Coll Cardiol* 1992;**19**:842–50.

82 Gottlieb SS, Kukin ML, Penn J *et al.* Sustained hemodynamic response to flosequinan in patients with heart failure receiving angiotensin-converting enzyme inhibitors. *J Am Coll Cardiol* 1993;**22**:963–7.

83 Califf RM, Adams KF, McKenna WJ *et al.* A randomized controlled trial of epoprostenol therapy for severe congestive heart failure: The Flolan International Randomized Survival Trial (FIRST). *Am Heart J* 1997;**134**:44–54.

84 Montalescot G, Drobinski G, Meurin P *et al.* Effects of prostacyclin on the pulmonary vascular tone and cardiac contractility of patients with pulmonary hypertension secondary to end-stage heart failure. *Am J Cardiol* 1998;**82**:749–55.

85 Elkayam U, Amin J, Mehra A *et al.* A prospective, randomized, double-blind, crossover study to compare the efficacy and safety of chronic nifedipine therapy with that of isosorbide dinitrate and their combination in the treatment of chronic congestive heart failure. *Circulation* 1990;**82**:1954–61.

86 Franciosa JA, Jordan RA, Wilen MM *et al.* Minoxidil in patients with chronic left heart failure: contrasting hemodynamic and clinical effects in a controlled trial. *Circulation* 1984;**70**:63–8.

87 Herrmann HC, Chang G, Klugherz BD *et al.* Hemodynamic effects of sildenafil in men with severe coronary artery disease. *N Engl J Med* 2000;**342**:1622–6.

88 A randomized trial of beta-blockade in heart failure. The Cardiac Insufficiency Bisoprolol Study (CIBIS). CIBIS Investigators and Committees. *Circulation* 1994;**90**: 1765–73.

89 Effect of metoprolol CR/XL in chronic heart failure: Metoprolol CR/XL Randomised Intervention Trial in Congestive Heart Failure (MERIT-HF). *Lancet* 1999;**353**:2001–7.

90 Chomsky DB, Lang CC, Rayos G *et al.* Treatment of subclinical fluid retention in patients with symptomatic heart failure: effect on exercise performance. *J Heart Lung Transplant* 1997;**16**:846–53.

91 Fonarow GC, Stevenson LW, Walden JA *et al.* Impact of a comprehensive heart failure management program on hospital readmission and functional status of patients with advanced heart failure. *J Am Coll Cardiol* 1997;**30**:725–32.

92 Johnson W, Lucas C, Stevenson LW *et al.* Effect of intensive therapy for heart failure on the vasodilator response to exercise. *J Am Coll Cardiol* 1999;**33**:743–9.

93 Lucas C, Johnson W, Hamilton MA *et al.* Freedom from congestion predicts good survival despite previous class IV symptoms of heart failure. *Am Heart J* 2000;**140**:840–7.

94 Bhatia SJ, Kirshenbaum JM, Shemin RJ *et al.* Time course of resolution of pulmonary hypertension and right ventricular remodeling after orthotopic cardiac transplantation. *Circulation* 1987;**76**:819–26.

95 Bourge RC, Kirklin JK, Naftel DC *et al*. Analysis and predictors of pulmonary vascular resistance after cardiac transplantation. *J Thorac Cardiovasc Surg* 1991;**101**:432–44.

96 Greenberg ML, Uretsky BF, Reddy PS *et al*. Long-term hemodynamic follow-up of cardiac transplant patients treated with cyclosporine and prednisone. *Circulation* 1985;**71**:487–94.

97 Bundgaard H, Boesgaard S, Mortensen SA *et al*. Effect of nitroglycerin in patients with increased pulmonary vascular resistance undergoing cardiac transplantation. *Scand Cardiovasc J* 1997;**31**:339–42.

98 Delgado JF, Gomez-Sanchez MA, Saenz dlC *et al*. Impact of mild pulmonary hypertension on mortality and pulmonary artery pressure profile after heart transplantation. *J Heart Lung Transplant* 2001;**20**:942–8.

99 Zener JC, Hancock EW, Shumway NE *et al*. Regression of extreme pulmonary hypertension after mitral valve surgery. *Am J Cardiol* 1972;**30**:820–6.

Pulmonary veno-occlusive disease

BARBARA A COCKRILL AND CHARLES A HALES

Pulmonary veno-occlusive disease (PVOD) is a rare disorder that causes pulmonary hypertension. The hallmark feature of PVOD is widespread microscopic obstruction of pulmonary venules due to intimal fibrosis and *in situ* thrombus. In the past it has been grouped with primary pulmonary hypertension (PPH). However, based on its distinctive pathology, PVOD has been now recognized as a discrete entity.[1] This distinction has been increasingly supported by important differences in response to therapy when compared with PPH.

The first case to be recognized and reported was in 1934 by Höra.[2] He described a 48-year-old baker who presented with progressive dyspnea and edema. Within a year of presentation, the patient was found to have pulmonary vascular obstruction centered in the pulmonary veins. The term pulmonary veno-occlusive disease was not proposed until 1966 in a case of a 37-year-old woman when a clear distinction was made between the pathology of PPH and PVOD.[3]

INCIDENCE

Pulmonary veno-occlusive disease has been reported in all age groups from 8 weeks of age[4] into the seventh decade,[5] although children and young adults appear to be most commonly affected. There may be a slight predilection for males, but this varies with series.

The actual incidence of PVOD is difficult to determine because, in the absence of lung biopsy, many cases may be misclassified as PPH.[6] As an example, in a review of the NHLBI registry biopsy specimens, 7 of 58 patients

thought to have PPH were found to have PVOD.[7] In a case series from the Mayo Clinic, 5 of 80 patients with PPH were found to have PVOD on histopathological review.[8] PVOD is clearly much less common than PPH, probably accounting for about 10% of cases diagnosed as PPH. Applying this figure to the incidence of PPH yields an estimated incidence of 0.1–0.2 cases per million persons in the general population.[1,6]

PATHOLOGY

Pathological findings in PVOD reflect a primary abnormality in the pulmonary venules and small veins, and the resulting 'upstream' consequences. The characteristic finding on lung biopsy is narrowing of pulmonary venules and small veins due to loose edematous connective tissue or more dense fibrotic tissue.[9] The presence of both patterns in a single patient may suggest progressive fibrosis. These lesions are usually distributed evenly throughout both lungs with no particular predilection for a specific lobe or region, although some patients with predominant upper lobe involvement have been described.[9] Veins may be so abnormal with prominent medial muscularization that they resemble arteries, leading the pathologist on first examination to consider the pathology to be in the arteries (Plate 14B.1). Movat elastin stain, which can delineate internal and external elastic laminae, is considered by some authors to be an essential tool to determine whether the affected vessels are arterial or venous.[10]

Organizing thrombi are seen and appear to be formed *in situ*.[9,10] The thrombi are usually limited to the pulmonary venules and, less commonly, are seen in the immediate precapillary circulation. The thrombi may be recanalized, most often with the formation of intraluminal fibrous septa.[11] The portion of the vein proximal to the recanalized thrombus will frequently demonstrate medial hypertrophy and arterialization of the vein.[9] The finding of organized and recanalized thrombi in the pulmonary venules is essentially universal, being found in a percentage of venules in all specimens (Plate 14B.2). However, intimal thickening is more prevalent. For example, in a series of pathological specimens from five patients with PVOD, only 11–13% of small veins exhibited evidence of thrombosis and recanalization whereas increased intimal thickening was present in essentially all small veins. This suggests that intimal thickening is the primary event that predisposes to subsequent *in situ* thrombosis.[12]

Infiltration of the venular walls by inflammatory cells has been reported,[13] but is a distinctly uncommon finding.

Parenchymal changes are much less evident, and reflect capillary and lymphatic congestion due to downstream obstruction. Areas of edema and hemorrhage are seen. Characteristically, small nodular areas of congested and thickened alveolar walls often associated with hemorrhage and siderosis are demonstrated.[9] These focal areas may represent sites of capillary disruption caused by locally increased pressure with extravasation of blood, and subsequent healing. Dilated lymphatics and focal areas of congestion are frequent.[12]

Pulmonary arterioles are variably involved, and when changes are present they are usually less striking than venular changes. The arterial findings tend to be patchy and crecent-shaped rather than circumferential.[9] However, at times the obstruction may be equal to that seen in the pulmonary veins, possibly reflecting the stage of the disease.[11] As an example, in a case series of 26 patients, pulmonary arteries were narrowed or obliterated in approximately half of patients.[11] In seven patients, recent *in situ* thrombi were seen. However, fibrinoid necrosis, arteritis and plexiform lesions were absent. Interestingly, in this series, lung biopsies with the most prominent arterial obstruction had the least severe parenchymal hemosiderosis, suggesting that the upstream occlusion protects that pulmonary capillary from stress disruption.

Chazova and colleagues compared venous and arterial changes in PVOD with two other forms of pulmonary venous hypertension: mitral stenosis and fibrosing mediastinitis.[12] The venular abnormalities of intimal and adventitial thickening, while most striking in PVOD, were also clearly present in the other two diseases. The authors propose that the similarity of vascular changes in the three forms of pulmonary venous hypertension indicates that the increased pressure itself is one of the triggers to vascular remodeling. Increased cyclic cell stretch of the pulmonary vascular endothelium resulting from the higher intravascular pressures may play a role in both the venous and arterial remodeling.[14]

In one case, examined at biopsy and then again 6 months later at the time of lung transplantation, progression of intimal venous changes and arterialization of veins was demonstrated. Medial thickening also progressed in the pulmonary arteries, but the total number of arteries with intimal and adventitial thickening was similar.[12]

ETIOLOGY AND PATHOGENESIS

Genetic predisposition

The cause of pulmonary veno-occlusive disease is unknown. It is likely that it represents a syndrome of characteristic pathological responses to different insults – likely in the setting of a permissive genetic predisposition.

Evidence that a genetic predisposition is present is suggested by a few case reports of disease occurring in siblings. As an example, a case of two siblings was reported in which a 14-year-old boy developed effort-induced dyspnea. He had a rapid course and died. Several months later, his 13-year-old sister died of the same process. At autopsy, severe veno-occlusive disease was found in both. No common exposure could be found.[15]

PVOD has been reported in other sibling pairs, and in all of the reports, the disease onset in the siblings was within 1–2 years of each other.[9,16,17] While these cases are suggestive of a genetic predisposition, the possibility of a common exposure cannot be discounted. It is our opinion, however, that similar to the current theory on the pathogenesis of PPH,[18] it is likely that a permissive genetic milieu exists that allows a characteristic response to a toxic insult.

Infection

A preceding febrile illness resembling influenza has been described in many patients,[3,9,19,20] but is not present in all. The relationship between the febrile illness and the subsequent development of PVOD is not certain.

A viral etiology is suggested in some cases. In one case examined at autopsy, a generalized lymphadenopathy with erythrophagocytosis was found and was thought to indicate a viral origin. This patient had a preceding illness characterized by high spiking fevers.[21] In the youngest patient thus far reported with PVOD, an intrauterine viral infection was suggested as the cause. The mother had a prolonged upper respiratory tract illness in the third trimester and the infant died at the age of 8 weeks. Autopsy showed PVOD associated with a subacute myocarditis and chronic interstitial pneumonia.[4]

Two cases of PVOD associated with HIV have been reported, although both cases had confounding factors making the association with HIV uncertain. The first was in a 2-year-old child who was diagnosed with HIV at 8 months of age. Following a respiratory illness related to respiratory syncytial virus (RSV) and influenza A, he developed signs and symptoms consistent with PVOD. At autopsy 9 months later, the child was found to have pathological findings consistent with lymphocytic interstitial pneumonia and PVOD. Thus, in this child at least, three viruses may be related to the development of PVOD: RSV, influenza A and HIV.[22] The second report case was in a 27-year-old intravenous drug abuser. A preceding viral illness was not described. At open lung biopsy occasional foreign bodies were found consistent with intravenous drug abuse, but the primary pathology was concentrated in the pulmonary venules.[23] HIV disease is an accepted risk factor for the development of PPH.[24] It seems likely that more cases of PVOD in association with HIV have occurred, but been attributed to PPH.

Immune disorders

PVOD has been described in a single patient as part of a generalized venulopathy. Liang and co-workers described a 39-year-old woman who presented with facial swelling, conjunctival and periorbital edema.[25] She eventually died of severe pulmonary hypertension and cor pulmonale. Autopsy showed a generalize venulitis involving most organs. There was widespread phlebosclerosis of medium-sized venules with perivenular chronic inflammation. Pulmonary veins showed a similar pattern with marked obstruction. Thrombotic lesions within the pulmonary venules are not commented upon. Pulmonary arteries showed intimal hyperplasia and plexiform lesions – the latter is not usually described in PVOD.[25]

Immune complexes are described in some patients[26] and it has been suggested that immune complex deposition in the basement membrane formation can lead to venular injury and intraluminal thrombosis. Autoimmune phenomena targeting the pulmonary venules with subsequent thrombosis, fibrosis and obstruction would be a logical explanation for the pathology seen in PVOD. It has been associated with collagen vascular diseases, including systemic lupus erythematosis,[27] and the CREST (calcinosis cutis, Raynaud's phenomenon, esophageal dysfunction, sclerodactyly and telangiectasia) variant of progressive systemic sclerosis.[28,29] However, the association of PVOD cases with autoimmune disorders has been in the minority.[6]

Drug and chemical exposures

Chemotherapeutic agents used in treatment of various malignancies have been cited as possible causes of PVOD.[30–32] Most patients were treated with a number of agents, therefore isolating the specific agent responsible was not possible. In the cases reported, bleomycin, carmustine (BCNU) and mitomycin appear the most commonly involved agents.[33] PVOD may be more common after bone marrow transplantation, especially allogeneic transplantation, than after routine chemotherapy, but this association is uncertain.[6,33,34]

The possibility of a connection between hepatic veno-occlusive disease (HVOD) and PVOD is raised by the observations of Wingard and colleagues.[35] In a large series, 154 patients who underwent intensive cytoreductive therapy were evaluated for HVOD. Thirty-nine patients were diagnosed with HVOD. Of 15 cases with HVOD who had an autopsy, 11 were found to have coexisting PVOD.[35]

There is a single reported case of PVOD developing in association with inhaled toxins. This involved a 14-year-old boy with a 2-year history of inhaling a household cleaning product.[36]

There are case reports of PVOD in association with oral contraceptives[37] and pregnancy,[38] raising the possibility that estrogens and hypercoaguable states may play a role in the development of PVOD. Thrombosis within the venules is a frequent, but not universal pathological finding. In a series of lung tissue taken from five patients with PVOD, Chazova et al. found thrombosis and recanalization in only 11–13% of venules examined despite striking intimal thickening in essentially all veins.[12] This suggests that thickening of the intima is a primary event occurring in the absence of thrombosis. With currently available data, it cannot be concluded that in situ thrombosis or abnormalities in the clotting system are a primary factor.[6] A more likely scenario is that a primary injury occurs in the venules, which subsequently leads to in situ thrombosis and recanalization.

There is no single factor that is consistently associated with the development of PVOD. As is the case with PPH, it seems likely that the PVOD is a characteristic response to an injury in a susceptible individual, rather than due to a specific insult itself.

CLINICAL PRESENTATION AND DIAGNOSIS

Clinical findings

Clinically, it is very difficult to distinguish patients with PVOD from patients with PPH or isolated pulmonary vascular disease of other causes. Patients with PVOD invariably present with progressive dyspnea on exertion. About half will have a dry cough. Both orthopnea and paroxysmal nocturnal dyspnea are described in a minority of patients, as is a preceding viral-like illness. As with primary pulmonary hypertension, atypical chest pain and near-syncope may be present, and probably represent more severe disease. In more advanced disease, patients may present with lower extremity edema. Hemoptysis is rare. Cyanosis may be more prominent in patients with PVOD than PPH due to the underlying pulmonary edema, which is frequently present.

The physical findings of PVOD primarily reflect the presence of pulmonary hypertension. A prominent pulmonic heart sound and a murmur of tricuspid regurgitation are common. The majority of patients in the largest published series had signs of overt right heart failure. Of 11 patients, 7 had elevated neck veins, a third heart sound, a right ventricular heave and lower extremity edema at the time of presentation.[10] Clubbing was present in more than 50%. A clue to the diagnosis is the presence of bibasilar crackles suggestive of pulmonary edema in a patient whose examination presentation is otherwise characteristic of PPH. Physical findings of pulmonary edema are present in about half of patients.[10,39]

Pulmonary function tests

Pulmonary function testing typically shows normal spirometry and lung volumes with a markedly reduced diffusing capacity for carbon dioxide (DLCO).[40] However, both obstructive and restrictive patterns are also described.[10] As noted above, interstitial inflammation is not common and is mild when present. Therefore, it is likely the restrictive pattern seen on pulmonary function testing results from interstitial edema.

Blood gas analysis typically reveals a widened alveolar–arterial oxygen gradient, with varying degrees of hypoxemia, and a respiratory alkalosis.[10] In cases that are not associated with a known collagen vascular disease, the antinuclear antibody titers are occasionally weakly elevated, but other markers of collagen vascular disease are negative.

Radiographic findings

Radiographic studies often provide a clue that a patient with suspected PPH actually has PVOD. As an example, Holcomb and colleagues found that all 11 patients in their cases series had some radiological finding consistent with PVOD.

Plain films of the chest are usually non-specific but may show enlarged pulmonary arteries and diffuse ground glass opacities may be seen. Kerley lines are often present, as are pleural effusions.[10,39] However, PVOD may also be present in the absence of these findings.[3]

Computed tomography frequently shows a distinguishing pattern (Figure 14B.1). Interlobular septal thickening – both smooth and nodular – is the most characteristic pattern. Diffuse ground-glass opacities,

probably representing some pulmonary interstitial edema, are common (Figure 14B.1). The finding of mediastinal lymphadenopathy is inconsistent, being found in some cases[29] but not in others.[10,41] As an example, in one cases series of biopsy proven PVOD, seven out of eight patients had smooth interlobular septal thickening. All patients had regions of ground-glass opacity. Four of these had a mosaic pattern of lung attenuation.[41] In our anecdotal experience, chest CT scanning is the first study suggesting the diagnosis of PVOD – most often with findings of unexplained ground glass opacities, lymphadenopathy and pleural effusions (Figure 14B.2).

Results of pulmonary ventilation/perfusion scans are variable. The results have been reported as normal,[42] although more frequently there is some abnormal distribution of tracer material in the pulmonary vasculature.[43] A segmental contour pattern of V̇/Q̇ mismatch has been described.[44] High-probability V̇/Q̇ scans are described in three patients with PVOD in whom subsequent pulmonary angiography failed to demonstrated pulmonary emboli. The authors hypothesized that the downstream

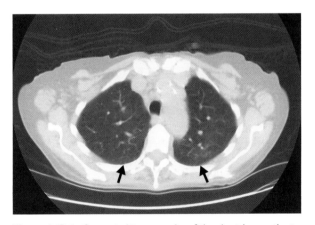

Figure 14B.1 *Computed tomography of the chest in a patient with pulmonary veno-occlusive disease. Note septal thickening and ground-glass opacities (arrows), which probably represent pulmonary edema (see text).*

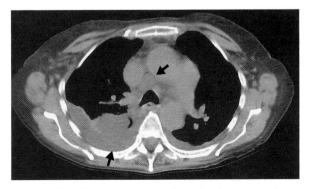

Figure 14B.2 *Computed tomography of the chest in a patient with pulmonary veno-occlusive disease. Note pleural effusion and mediastinal lymphadenopathy (arrow).*

resistance to blood flow in PVOD could account for this difference. Tracer deposition during a V̇/Q̇ scan is proportional to blood flow; therefore, the high downstream resistance would reduce the tracer deposition in the precapillary arterioles upstream from the venous resistance. Because the contrast material during a pulmonary arteriogram is performed with higher pressures, the downstream resistance may be overcome. Thus, the obstruction would not be apparent on angiogram.[45] The authors further postulated that high probability scans may be found when larger pulmonary veins are involved in contrast to the more common finding of a diffuse patchy distribution of tracer material, when smaller pulmonary veins are most involved in the process.

Intravascular ultrasound (IVUS) is a developing technology in the diagnosis of pulmonary hypertension and more data are needed.[46] Currently, there is no published information regarding the use of IVUS in PVOD. As noted above, the thickening of the pulmonary arterial wall associated with PVOD is much less prominent than is present in the pulmonary venous circulation. We hypothesize that the finding of arterial wall thickness that is **less** than would be expected for the degree of pulmonary hypertension could be a clue that PVOD is present.

Hemodynamics

Pulmonary veno-occlusive disease is associated with severe pulmonary artery hypertension and, as the process progresses, with right ventricular dysfunction.

The pulmonary artery occlusion pressure (PAOP) is most often normal. However, both elevated PAOP and measurements that vary between sites in the lung are also found. The mechanism of these findings is a source of some confusion. In order to understand how a PAOP can be normal or variable in the setting of a process that causes pulmonary edema, it is helpful to review the details of how a PAOP is measured. The pulmonary artery catheter is a flow-directed catheter that therefore is carried by blood flow into the pulmonary artery. Balloon inflation encourages migration of the catheter tip from a main pulmonary artery into a smaller caliber vessel, where it impacts and wedges. Blood flow distal to the site of impact is blocked, and a static column of blood is created beyond the inflated balloon. The pressure equilibrates between the site of balloon obstruction and the downstream junction with the next site of blood flow (the 'j' point).[47] Therefore, the pressure measured at the catheter tip is equal to the pressure at the 'j' point. The 'j' point is usually in a pulmonary vein of equal caliber to the pulmonary artery in which the balloon is lodged – in other words, a pulmonary vein **larger** than the venules that are most affected in PVOD. Thus, the PAOP measures a pressure that is distal to the site of increased resistance in the narrowed pulmonary venules in PVOD. This is unlike the typical

situation in fibrosing mediastinitis, another disease that affects the pulmonary veins and causes pulmonary edema. In fibrosing mediastinitis, large pulmonary veins are narrowed when entering the left atrium, and the PAOP will be elevated. In both PVOD and fibrosing mediastinitis, when the balloon is deflated, and blood is again flowing past the site of resistance, increased pressure will be present in the pulmonary capillaries (Figure 14B.3). In PVOD it is the increased pulmonary capillary pressure that leads to pulmonary edema.

Another reported finding is that when saline is injected through the distal port of the catheter, the pressure rises disproportionately and falls off very slowly. This is presumably due to the injected saline being trapped upstream from the site of increased venous resistance, and subsequent slow run-off.[6] Some researchers have used this technique to assess the actual pulmonary capillary pressure when blood flow is present.[48]

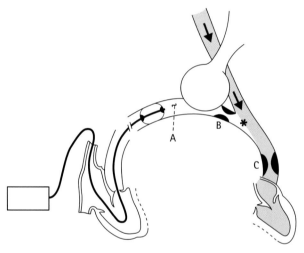

Figure 14B.3 *The definition of the pulmonary artery occlusion pressure (PAOP). Inflation of the catheter balloon, if properly done, stops blood flow through the segment of the pulmonary circulation distal to the catheter tip. The PAOP measured at point A equilibrates with the downstream pressure at the junction of static and flowing pulmonary venous blood (*). Point B, representing the pulmonary venules and small veins, is the site of increased resistance in pulmonary veno-occlusive disease (PVOD). As shown in the diagram, point B is proximal to the junction point, and therefore is not reflected in the PAOP. However, when the balloon is deflated, blood flow past point B will result in increased upstream pressure in the pulmonary capillaries. Point C represents increased resistance in the large pulmonary veins, which is usually not present in PAOP. An elevated PAOP may be recorded in PVOD if larger veins are involved, or if the catheter has migrated into a very small caliber pulmonary artery and pressure at a more proximal junction point is measured. (Reproduced with permission from Marini JJ, Wheeler AP (eds), Critical care medicine – the essentials. Baltimore: Williams & Wilkins, 1989.)*

The issue of lung biopsy in patients with suspected PVOD is a difficult one. Patients with pulmonary hypertension are at increased risk for serious complications, including hemorrhage and death. However, the diagnosis can only be definitively made by examining lung tissue. It is our practice to consider lung biopsy in those patients deemed to be acceptable surgical risks.

TREATMENT

Because PVOD is so uncommon, it is difficult to make any general statements about treatment. Supplemental oxygen and careful diuresis should be considered in all patients. There have been no controlled trials and there is no confirmed treatment for PVOD; therefore, the following discussion is based on case reports and small series.

Anticoagulants

The pathological observation of thrombosis within the venules in many cases of PVOD makes the use of anticoagulants as treatment for PVOD seem appropriate. Whether a primary or secondary event, progressive thrombus formation within the vessels would lead to clinical deterioration. There are observational data that patients with PPH have improved survival – the thinking being that *in situ* pulmonary arteriolar thrombosis contributes to progression of pulmonary hypertension. There are no trials comparing the use of anticoagulants versus withholding anticoagulants in PVOD. However, we, and many others,[6] routinely use long-term warfarin in these patients.

Immunosuppressive agents

A number of authors have reported the use of immunosuppressive agents. The information is anecdotal, and patients who appear to respond frequently have PVOD in the setting of other signs of collagen vascular disease.

Corticosteroids have been used without consistent results.[49,50] As an example, of 33 patients reported in the 1970s, seven were treated with corticosteroids. Only two of those seven patients survived more than 3 months after starting treatment.[50] By contrast, Escamilla *et al.* report a patient with HIV-associated PVOD who had a marked improvement in symptoms and pulmonary infiltrates after starting therapy with prednisone.[23] There may be a greater chance of response to corticosteroids if the PVOD is following bone marrow transplant or associated with chemotherapy.[34,51]

In one case of PVOD associated with interstitial pneumonitis, there was fatal progression of pulmonary hypertension due to PVOD despite steroid-induced remission of the interstitial pneumonitis.[49] In this case, transbronchial lung biopsies revealed prominent chronic inflammatory cell infiltration, type II cell hyperplasia, and mild interstitial fibrosis. Symptoms were improved and infiltrates resolved within 10 days of corticosteroid therapy. The patient remained stable for more than 2 years without any recognizable change in her pulmonary artery pressures. However, 27 months after starting corticosteroids, she developed a rapidly progressive right heart failure and died. At autopsy, she had a mild interstitial pneumonitis. The pulmonary veins showed intimal proliferation and medial hypertrophy. Several small veins were thrombosed with occasional recanalization. There were also some changes in the pulmonary arterioles.[49]

Azathioprine has been apparently successful in treating PVOD in the setting of severe collagen vascular disease. This patient had associated cutaneous vasculitis, myopathy and polyarteritis. She was initially treated with prednisone, with some response, and subsequently treated with azathioprine and did well for at least 2 years.[52]

Our knowledge is incomplete and we reserve the use of immunosuppressive agents for patients with either known or suspected collagen vascular disease. In this situation, we believe a therapeutic trial is indicated with careful and objective assessment for response.

Vasodilators

Vasodilator agents have been used with mixed results. Unlike in the treatment of primary pulmonary hypertension, the role of vasodilators is uncertain in PVOD at this time.

Great caution must be exercised when use of vasodilators is attempted because of the potential for causing increased pulmonary edema. The capillary bed seems to be the main exchange site for fluid between the intravascular and extravascular spaces in the lung. Increased pulmonary edema will result when there is vasodilator tone present in the pulmonary arteriolar system, but fixed disease in the pulmonary venous system. The upstream resistance in the arterial bed will fall in response to vasodilation, thus increasing pulmonary capillary pressure and flooding the parenchyma. It is suggested that there may be some vasodilator tone in the pulmonary venules in patients with PVOD. We, and others, have found that pulmonary artery pressure and pulmonary vascular resistance decrease in response to inhaled nitric oxide in PVOD.[45,53] Davis *et al.* calculated pulmonary capillary pressure in a single patient with PVOD, and suggested that post-capillary venules had vasomotor tone in this patient which required higher doses of prostacyclin to vasodilate than did the arteriolar tone.[48] In this report, calculated pulmonary capillary pressure increased at prostacyclin doses $<6\,\mathrm{ng/kg\cdot min}$ – the dose below which venular vasomotor tone was not affected. At doses 6–12 ng/kg·min, the calculated pulmonary capillary pressure was back at baseline. These findings must be confirmed by others, but if confirmed, the issue for the clinician is whether the increase in pulmonary capillary pressure (and resultant pulmonary edema) at lower doses precludes further titration of the drug to higher doses.

α–Adrenergic blockers

Two patients have been described who did well initially when treated with the α-adrenergic blocker prasozin. Both had an acute vasodilator response to this agent. One did well initially, but had progressive right heart failure and died within 2 years; the other patient maintained clinical improvement for at least 3 years after starting therapy.[54]

Calcium antagonists

Treatment with calcium channel antagonists has been attempted. Rich *et al.* report two patients who died within 48 hours of starting treatment with nifedipine, apparently with pulmonary edema.[55] The authors believed it due to an increase in cardiac output against a fixed pulmonary venous obstruction. Holcomb and colleagues report that six of 11 patients treated with calcium channel antagonists developed pulmonary edema. Only one of the episodes was during acute testing; the other episodes occurred between 3 days and 6 months after starting therapy.[10]

Scattered reports of prolonged survival during treatment with calcium channel antagonists have also been reported. The first reported case of prolonged survival was in a patient with PVOD who had a significant reduction in pulmonary vascular resistance and pulmonary artery pressure when treated with long-term nifedipine. This patient survived for more than 7 years. The authors speculate that the pulmonary artery vasodilating effect of the nifedipine allowed additional time for the PVOD to resolve before severe pulmonary arterial hypertensive changes occurred.[33] Another patient was maintained on calcium channel antagonists with sustained clinical improvement for at least 2 years.[10]

Prostacyclin

Fatal pulmonary edema during a low-dose prostacyclin infusion has been reported.[56] A 42-year-old woman was treated with 2 ng/kg·min of prostacyclin. Within 15 minutes of starting the infusion, the patient developed massive pulmonary edema. The infusion was stopped, but the patient died within 2 hours despite maximal support. Pulmonary veno-occlusive disease was confirmed at autopsy.

Two patients with PVOD were retrospectively identified at autopsy in a randomized trial designed to determine the effectiveness of prostacyclin in primary pulmonary hypertension. One patient initially responded with an improvement in symptoms but died suddenly after 2 weeks of treatment. Pulmonary congestion was found at autopsy. The second patient developed acute pulmonary edema during dose-ranging treatment with prostacyclin. The drug was discontinued and the patient was not treated further with vasodilators. This patient died 1 month after the prostacyclin trial.[57]

A recent study designed to identify radiographic predictors of epoprostenol therapy raises more concern about the use of epoprostenol in patients with PVOD.[58] Of 73 consecutive patients, 12 died within 4 months of starting epoprostenol. Radiographic findings of PVOD or pulmonary capillary hemangiomatosis (PCH), including ground-glass opacities, septal lines, pleural effusion and adenopathy, were significantly more common in the patients that died. Six of 12 patients that had died had postmortem examinations: in all six the pathology revealed PVOD or PCH. PCH is characterized by infiltration and compression of pulmonary veins by neocapillaries, and leads to 'secondary' PVOD. Therefore, the authors did not distinguish these two entities in their data analysis. The authors suggest that patients with chest CT findings suggestive of either of these diagnoses have further evaluation before starting epoprostenol.[58] Acute pulmonary edema and death has previously been described in a patient with PCH who was treated with epoprostenol.[59]

At this stage in our knowledge, it is difficult to know where, if at all, epoprostenol fits in the treatment of PVOD. On the one hand, there are numerous reports of pulmonary edema and poor outcomes when patients with PVOD are treated with epoprostenol. On the other hand, approximately 6% of all patients diagnosed with primary pulmonary hypertension actually have PVOD.[57] Some patients with PVOD have undoubtedly been treated with epoprostenol without the diagnosis having been made. In addition, there is one reported case of this very rare disease, in which the patient appears to have responded well to epoprostenol.[10]

There is one reported case of long-term clinical response to chronic inhaled nitric oxide. The patient continued to do well at 2 years after starting therapy.[45]

At the time of this writing, there is no reported experience with the use of endothelin-1 antagonists *in vitro* with pulmonary veins, let alone in patients with PVOD. However, endothelin-1 may have an important role in intimal hyperplasia in human saphenous vein grafts, and a potential therapeutic potential for the prevention of graft stenosis is suggested.[60,61]

In contrast to the treatment of primary pulmonary hypertension, the role of vasodilators in treatment of

PVOD is not certain. The mixture of apparently positive and negative results, combined with the certain risk of causing pulmonary edema in a significant number of patients, should cause the clinician to be circumspect and very cautious with these agents. However, given the dismal prognosis, we generally give most patients a careful therapeutic trial of vasodilator therapy in the intensive care unit with careful monitoring.

Lung transplantation

Lung transplantation is likely the only treatment that is consistently capable of prolonging survival in patients with PVOD.[62] To our knowledge, recurrent PVOD has not been reported in transplanted lungs. The success of transplantation is limited by the availability of organs resulting in a prolonged waiting time. Once the diagnosis is made and referral is made for lung transplantation evaluation, many patients with PVOD do not survive long enough to benefit.

The prognosis for patients with PVOD remains poor. Early reports found that the majority of patients were dead within 2 years of diagnosis.[39] In a case series of 11 patient recently reported, eight of 11 patients died within 1 year of diagnosis. Of the three surviving patients, one had a clinical reponse to oral nifedipine, one was treated with epoprostenol, and one underwent a successful lung transplantation.[10] With currently available information, no conclusions can be made regarding the medical therapy of choice in patients with PVOD. Lung transplantation appears to be the only treatment capable of significantly improving survival.

CONCLUSIONS

PVOD is a rare cause of pulmonary hypertension. The disease is characterized by widespread pulmonary venular obstruction due to intimal hyperplasia, muscularization of venular walls and *in situ* thrombosis. In some cases, retrograde histopathology is apparent in the pulmonary arterioles, but is much less prominent than the venous changes. These pathological findings are distinct from other forms of pulmonary hypertension such as PPH. The pathogenesis of the disorder is uncertain, but it is likely that PVOD represents a characteristic response to venular injury. Reported familial cases raise the possibility that an underlying genetic predisposition is present. Clinically, PVOD is difficult to differentiate from PPH. However, signs and symptoms of pulmonary hypertension and pulmonary edema in the absence of left ventricular dysfunction should raise the question of PVOD. Prognosis is poor, and treatment is largely supportive.

KEY POINTS

- The cause of PVOD is unknown, but it likely represents a syndrome of characteristic pathological responses to different insults, possibly in the setting of a permissive genetic predisposition.
- A clue to the diagnosis of PVOD is the presence of bibasilar crackles suggestive of pulmonary edema in a patient whose presentation is otherwise characteristic of PPH.
- Computed tomography frequently shows a distinctive pattern of interlobular septal thickening and diffuse ground-glass opacities, probably representing some pulmonary interstitial edema.
- The pulmonary artery occlusion pressure (PAOP) is most often normal in PVOD. However, both elevated PAOP and measurements that vary between sites in the lung are also found.
- The mixture of apparently positive and negative results with medical therapy for PVOD, combined with the risk of causing pulmonary edema in a significant number of patients, should cause the clinician to be circumspect and very cautious with vasodilator agents.
- Lung transplantation is likely the only treatment that is consistently capable of prolonging survival in patients with PVOD.

REFERENCES

◆1 Rubin LJ. Current concepts: primary pulmonary hypertension. *N Engl J Med* 1997;**336**:111–17.
●2 Höra J. Zur Histologie der klinischen 'primaren Pulmonalsklerose'. *Frankfurt Z Pathol* 1934;**47**:100–8.
●3 Heath D, Segel N, Bishop J. Pulmonary veno-occlusive disease. *Circulation* 1966;**34**:242–8.
4 Wagenvoort CA, Losekoot G, Mulder E. Pulmonary veno-occlusive disease of presumably intrauterine origin. *Thorax* 1971;**26**:429–34.
5 Glassroth J, Woodford DW, Carrington CB *et al.* Pulmonary veno-occlusive disease in the middle-aged. *Respiration* 1985;**47**:309–21.
◆6 Mandel J, Mark EJ, Hales CA. State of the art: pulmonary veno-occlusive disease. *Am J Respir Crit Care Med* 2000;**162**:1964–73.
7 Pietra GG. The pathology of primary pulmonary hypertension. In: Rubin LJ, Rich S (eds), *Primary pulmonary hypertension: lung biology in health and disease.* New York: Marcel Dekker, 1997;19–63.
8 Bjornsson J, Edwards WD. Primary pulmonary hypertension: a histopathologic study of 80 cases. *Mayo Clin Proc* 1985;**60**:16–25.

●9 Wagenvoort CA, Wagenvoort N. The pathology of pulmonary veno-occlusive disease. *Virchows Arch Pathol Anat Histol* 1974;**364**:69–79.

10 Holcomb BW, Loyd JE, Ely EW *et al.* Pulmonary veno-occlusive disease: a case series and new observations. *Chest* 2000;**118**:1671–9.

●11 Wagenvoort CA, Wagenvoort N, Takahashi T. Pulmonary veno-occlusive disease: involvement of pulmonary arteries and review of the literature. *Hum Pathol* 1985;**16**:1033–41.

12 Chazova I, Robbins I, Loyd J *et al.* Venous and arterial changes in pulmonary veno-occlusive disease, mitral stenosis and fibrosing mediastinitis. *Eur Respir* 2000;**15**:116–22.

13 Braun A, Greenberg SD, Malik S *et al.* Pulmonary veno-occlusive disease associated with pulmonary phlebitis. *Arch Pathol* 1973;**95**:67–70.

14 Matyal R, Hales CA, Quinn DA. Stretch-induced IL-8 production in human pulmonary artery endothelial cells. *Am J Crit Respir Care Med* 2000;**161**:A417.

15 Davies P, Reid L. Pulmonary veno-occlusive disease in siblings: case reports and morphometric study. *Hum Pathol* 1982;**13**:911–15.

16 Rosenthal A, Vawter G, Wagenvoort CA. Intra-pulmonary veno-occlusive disease. *Virchows Arch [Pathol Anat]* 1974;**364**:69.

17 Voordes CG, Kuipers JRG, Elema JD. Familial pulmonary veno-occlusive disease: a case report. *Thorax* 1977;**32**:763–6.

◆18 Archer S, Rich S. Primary pulmonary hypertension: a vascular biology and translational 'work in progress.' *Circulation* 2000;**102**:2871–91.

19 Carrington CB, Liebow AA. Pulmonary veno-occlusive disease. *Hum Pathol* 1970;**1**:322–4.

20 Tingelstad JB, Aterman K, Lambert EC. Pulmonary venous obstruction. Report of a case mimicking primary pulmonary artery hypertension, with a review of the literature. *Am J Dis Child* 1969;**117**:219–27.

21 McDonnell PJ, Summer WR, Hutchins GM. Pulmonary veno-occlusive disease: morphological changes suggesting a viral cause. *JAMA* 1981;**246**:667–71.

22 Ruchelli ED, Nojadera G, Rutstein RM *et al.* Pulmonary veno-occlusive disease: another vascular disorder associated with human immunodeficiency virus infection? *Arch Pathol Lab Med* 1994;**118**:664–6.

23 Escamilla R, Hermant C, Berjaud J *et al.* Pulmonary veno-occlusive disease in a HIV-infected intravenous drug abuser. *Eur Respir J* 1995;**8**:1982–4.

24 Mette SA, Palevsky HI, Pietra GG *et al.* Primary pulmonary hypertension in association with human immunodeficiency virus infection. A possible viral etiology for some forms of hypertensive pulmonary arteriopathy. *Am Rev Respir Dis* 1992;**145**:1196–200.

25 Liang MH, Stern S, Fortinn PR *et al.* Fatal pulmonary venoocclusive disease secondary to a generalized venopathy: a new syndrome presenting with facial swelling and pericardial tamponade. *Arthritis Rheum* 1991;**34**:228–33.

26 Corrin B, Spencer H, Turner-Warwick M *et al.* Pulmonary veno-occlusion – an immune complex disease? *Virchows Arch A Pathol Anat Histol* 1974;**364**:81–91.

27 Kishida Y, Kanai Y, Kuramochi S *et al.* Pulmonary venoocclusive disease in a patient with systemic lupus erythematosus. *J Rheumatol* 1993;**20**:2161–2.

28 Morassut PA, Walley VM, Smith CD. Pulmonary veno-occlusive disease and the CREST variant of scleroderma. *Can J Cardiol* 1992;**8**:1055–8.

29 Scully RE, Mark EJ, McNeely WF *et al.* Case records of the Massachusetts General Hospital: weekly clinicopathologic exercises, Case 48–1993: a 27-year-old woman with mediastinal lymphadenopathy and relentless cor pulmonale. *N Engl J Med* 1993;**329**:1720–8.

30 Joselson R, Warnock M. Pulmonary veno-occlusive disease after chemotherapy. *Hum Pathol* 1983;**14**:88–91.

31 Lombard CM, Churg A, Winokur S. Pulmonary veno-occlusive disease following therapy for malignant neoplasms. *Chest* 1987;**92**:871–6.

32 Swift GL, Gibbs A, Campbell IA *et al.* Pulmonary veno-occlusive disease and Hodgkin's lymphoma. *Eur Respir J* 1993;**6**:596–8.

33 Salzman D, Adkins DR, Craig F *et al.* Malignancy-associated pulmonary veno-occlusive disease: report of a case following autologous bone marrow transplantation and review. *Bone Marrow Transplant* 1996;**18**:755–60.

34 Hackman RC, Madtes DK, Petersen FB *et al.* Pulmonary venoocclusive disease following bone marrow transplantation. *Transplantation* 1989;**47**:989–92.

35 Wingard JR, Mellits ED, Jones RJ *et al.* Association of hepatic veno-occlusive disease with interstitial pneumonitis in bone marrow transplant recipients. *Bone Marrow Transplant* 1989;**4**:685–9.

36 Liu L, Sackler JP. A case of pulmonary veno-occlusive disease: etiological and therapeutic appraisal. *Angiology* 1973;**23**:299–304.

37 Thadani U, Burrow C, Whitaker W *et al.* Pulmonary veno-occlusive disease. *Q J Med* 1975;**64**:133–59.

38 Townend JN, Roberts DH, Jones EL *et al.* Fatal pulmonary venoocclusive disease after use of oral contraceptives. *Am Heart J* 1992;**124**:1643–4.

39 Tsou E, Waldhorn RE, Kerwin DM *et al.* Pulmonary venoocclusive disease in pregnancy. *Obstet Gynecol* 1984;**64**:281–4.

40 Elliott CG, Colby TV, Hill T *et al.* Pulmonary veno-occlusive disease associated with severe reduction of single-breath carbon monoxide diffusing capacity. *Respiration* 1988;**53**:262–6.

41 Swensen SJ, Tashjian JH, Myers JL *et al.* Pulmonary venoocclusive disease: CT findings in eight patients. *AJR Am J Roentgenol* 1996;**167**:937–40.

42 Scheibel RL, Dedeker KL, Gleason DF *et al.* Radiographic and angiographic characteristics of pulmonary veno-occlusive disease. *Radiology* 1972;**103**:47–51.

43 Rich S, Pietra GG, Kieras K *et al.* Primary pulmonary hypertension: radiographic and scintigraphic patterns of histologic subtypes. *Ann Intern Med* 1986;**105**:499–502.

44 Sola M, Garcia A, Picado C *et al.* Segmental contour pattern in a case of pulmonary venoocclusive disease. *Clin Nucl Med* 1993;**18**:679–81.

45 Shakelford GD, Sacks EJ, Mullins JD *et al.* Pulmonary venoocclusive disease: case report and review of the literature. *AJR Am J Roentgenol* 1977;**128**:643–8.

46 Bressollette E, Dupuis J, Bonan R *et al.* Intravascular ultrasound assessment of pulmonary vascular disease in

patients with pulmonary hypertension. *Chest* 2001;**120**:809–15.

47 Bailey CL, Channick RN, Auger WR *et al.* 'High probability' perfusion lung scans in pulmonary venoocclusive disease. *Am J Respir Crit Care Med* 2000;**162**:1974–8.

48 Davis LL, deBoisblanc BP, Glynn CE *et al.* Effect of prostacyclin on microvascular pressures in a patient with pulmonary veno-occlusive disease. *Chest* 1995;**108**:1754–6.

49 Gilroy RJ, Jr, Teague MW, Lloyd JE. Pulmonary veno-occlusive disease: fatal progression of pulmonary hypertension despite steroid-induced remission of interstitial pneumonitis. *Am Rev Respir Dis* 1991;**143**:1130–3.

50 Chawla SK, Kittle CF, Faber LP *et al.* Pulmonary venoocclusive disease. *Ann Thorac Surg* 1976;**22**:249–53.

51 Williams LM, Fussell S, Veith RW *et al.* Pulmonary veno-occlusive disease in an adult following bone marrow transplantation. *Chest* 1996;**109**:1388–91.

52 Sanderson JE, Spiro SG, Hendry AT *et al.* A case of pulmonary veno-occlusive disease responding to treatment with azathioprine. *Thorax* 1977;**32**:140–8.

53 Cockrill BA, Kacmarek RM, Fifer MA *et al.* Comparison of the effects of nitric oxide, nitroprusside, and nifedipine on hemodynamics and right ventricular contractility in patients with chronic pulmonary hypertension. *Chest* 2001;**119**:128–36.

*54 Palevsky HI, Pietra GG, Fishman AP. Pulmonary veno-occlusive disease and its response to vasodilator agents. *Am Rev Respir Dis* 1990;**142**:426–9.

*55 Rich S, Kaufmann E, Levy PS. The effect of high doses of calcium-channel blockers on survival in primary pulmonary hypertension. *N Engl J Med* 1992;**327**:76–81.

56 Palmer SM, Robinson LJ, Wang A *et al.* Massive pulmonary edema and death after prostacyclin infusion in a patient with pulmonary veno-occlusive disease. *Chest* 1998;**113**:237–40.

*57 Rubin LJ, Mendoza J, Hood M *et al.* Treatment of primary pulmonary hypertension with continuous intravenous prostacyclin (epoprostenol). Results of a randomized trial. *Ann Intern Med* 1990;**112**:485–91.

58 Resten A, Maitre S, Humbert M *et al.* Pulmonary arterial hypertension: thin-section CT predictors of epoprostenol therapy failure. *Radiology* 2002;**222**:782–8.

59 Humbert M, Maitre S, Capron F *et al.* Pulmonary edema complicating continuous intravenous prostacyclin in pulmonary capillary hemangiomatosis. *Am J Respir Crit Care Med* 1998;**157**:1681–5.

60 Porter KE, Olojugba DH, Masood I *et al.* Endothelin-B receptors mediate intimal hyperplasia in an organ culture of human saphenous vein. *J Vasc Surg* 1998;**28**:695–701.

61 Dumont AS, Lovren F, McNeill JH *et al.* Augmentation of endothelial function by endothelin antagonism in human saphenous vein conduits. *J Neurosurg* 2001;**94**:281–6.

62 Cassart M, Gevenois PA, Kramer M *et al.* Pulmonary veno-occlusive disease: CT findings before and after single-lung transplantation. *AJR Am J Roentgenol* 1993;**160**:759–60.

Pulmonary capillary hemangiomatosis

DAVID LANGLEBEN

INTRODUCTION

Pulmonary capillary hemangiomatosis (PCH) is a rare condition caused by an overabundance of thin-walled, capillary-like vessels in the lung. It can present as pulmonary hypertension. Little is known about its development and management, but recent advances in the understanding of vascular growth control provide hope for improved therapy in the future.

DEFINITION AND PATHOLOGY

Although clinical findings may offer clues to its presence, the definitive identification of PCH requires microscopic examination of the lung parenchyma. The classic finding is a diffuse excess of capillary-like vessels, which can infiltrate the walls of small arteries and veins, and also thicken and infiltrate the alveolar walls and space (Figures 14C.1 and 14C.2).[1,2] The major feature distinguishing PCH from other conditions causing capillary dilatation, such as left heart disease or veno-occlusive disease, is that the vessels in PCH truly infiltrate other pulmonary structures, including the walls of larger arteries and veins, intralobular fibrous septa, and bronchi.[1] Furthermore, in PCH the proliferation of capillaries within the alveolar septa and interstitium is at least two cell layers thick.[3] Secondary muscularization of proximal pulmonary arteries may also develop, as is seen with most other forms of pulmonary hypertension. The combination of pulmonary venous hypertension from infiltrated, narrowed and fibrosed

pulmonary veins, and the thin-walled nature of the abnormal infiltrating capillaries themselves, leads to extravasation of erythrocytes into the interstitium and air spaces, with subsequent macrophage engulfment and deposition of hemosiderin.[1,2] On gross examination of the lungs, multiple hemorrhagic patches, with firmer nodular areas, may be found.[4,5] Rarely, capillary proliferation has also been described in the pericardium,[6] pleura[6] and mediastinal lymph nodes.[7,8]

Several other disorders must be considered in the differential diagnosis. First, pulmonary atelectasis and congestion with capillary dilatation may be confused for PCH. However, in that condition, reticulin staining of lung sections will reveal only a single row of capillaries in the alveolar septa, and no infiltration of other structures.[3] Pulmonary veno-occlusive disease presents with many similar clinical features, and may be indistinguishable from PCH except by histological examination.[9] With veno-occlusive disease, fibrosis or sclerosis of small intrapulmonary veins is found, with secondary capillary dilatation. There is no evidence of infiltration into other structures, and only a single layer of capillaries is found within the alveolar septa.[4,10,11] Diffuse pulmonary hemangiomatosis has been described in childhood, and can present with a clinical picture of interstitial disease and pleural effusions, but the hemangiomas are larger and do not invade other structures.[12] Pulmonary lymphangioleiomyomatosis, leiomyomatosis, tuberous sclerosis, and lymphangiomatosis may have some common clinical features with PCH, but are distinct histologically.[13–15] Intravascular lymphomatosis, also termed malignant angioendotheliomatosis, is a rare lymphoma that can present with

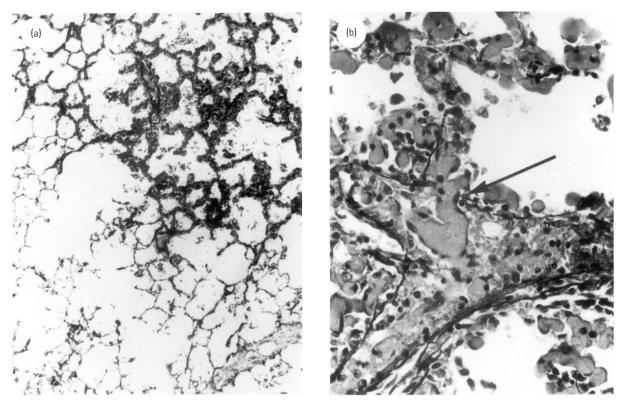

Figure 14C.1 *(a) A low-power view of a lung section showing the patchy and well-demarcated nature of the capillary proliferation within alveolar walls. Normal alveoli are present in the lower left. (b) A higher-power view of an affected area. Capillaries of various sizes proliferate along the alveolar wall and bulge into the alveolar space. Some penetrate through the elastic lamina of a pulmonary venule (arrow) and proliferate inside the vessel. (Reproduced with permission from Langleben D, Heneghan JM, Batten AP et al. Familial pulmonary capillary hemangiomatosis resulting in primary pulmonary hypertension.* Ann Intern Med *1988;109:108.)*

pulmonary hypertension, but with a different histology from PCH.[16] Sclerosing hemangioma of the lung, originally attributed to proliferation of blood vessels with subsequent fibrosis, has been shown to be epithelial in origin, rather than endothelial.[17]

INCIDENCE/EPIDEMIOLOGY

PCH seems to be an exceedingly rare condition. There have been fewer than 50 cases described in the literature.[1–4,6–9,12,18–31] Its incidence is sporadic, although familial PCH has been described in three siblings, in a fashion suggesting autosomal recessive inheritance.[18] PCH has been reported in patients ranging in age from childhood to late adulthood,[12,29,30] with most patients presenting between the ages of 20 and 40 years. It appears that some individuals without any evidence of pulmonary hypertension may have PCH-like foci in their lungs at autopsy.[3] In that series, 8 (5.7%) of 140 patients had classic histological findings of PCH.[3] It is unknown whether they would have developed clinical symptoms with time. Survival after onset of symptoms ranges from 1 to 5 years.

ETIOLOGY

There are no known causes of PCH. In the first case report of PCH in 1978, nuclear pleomorphism and hyperchromasia of the endothelial cells in the abnormal capillary-like vessels was described,[1] suggesting a neoplastic process. After the recognition of a variety of disorders characterized by excessive blood vessel proliferation, termed angiogenic diseases,[32] it was proposed that PCH represented an angiogenic disease of the lung.[18] Recently, abnormal monoclonal proliferation of endothelial cells has been described in primary pulmonary hypertension, consistent with neoplastic growth.[33] Subsequently, mutations in the gene for the bone morphogenetic protein type II receptor have been reported in familial primary pulmonary hypertension.[34,35] Bone morphogenetic protein, a member of the transforming growth factor-β superfamily, normally exercises a growth-inhibitory, proapoptotic action on cells, and loss of receptor function or signal transduction could lead to unregulated cell proliferation.[36] PCH may represent another form of unregulated endothelial growth. It might also be a *forme fruste* of primary pulmonary hypertension. It is not known whether abnormalities of TGF-β superfamily signal transduction cause PCH, but the possibility is intriguing.

A variety of secondary disorders, including collagen vascular or autoimmune disease, HIV infection, intracardiac shunts, and others, induce endothelial proliferation and plexiform lesion formation that is histologically indistinguishable from that of primary pulmonary hypertension.[37] The mechanisms by which this process develops are

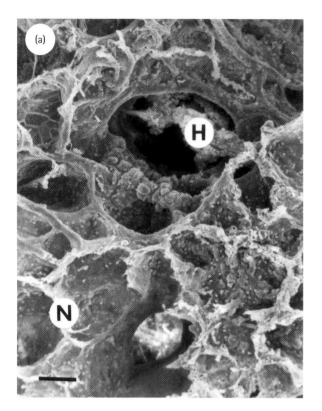

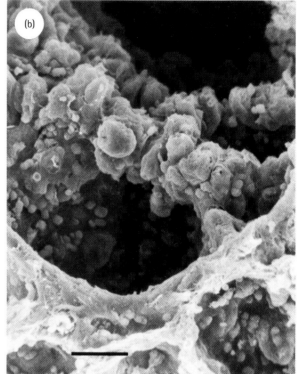

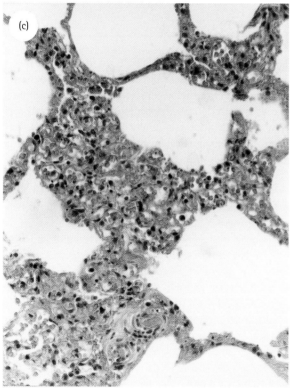

Figure 14C.2 *Scanning electron microscopy (a) of an affected lung. Capillaries are irregularly dilated and bulge into the alveolar space (H). The normal alveoli show a flat surface (N). (b) Higher magnification from area H of (a). Capillaries up to 30 μm proliferate along the edge of, and also occasionally inside, the alveolus. Small round structures in the alveolus are mononuclear cells. (c) A lung section showing marked widening of alveolar walls by the capillary proliferation and thickening of the walls of small pulmonary blood vessels (bottom). (Reproduced with permission from Langleben D, Heneghan JM, Batten AP et al. Familial pulmonary capillary hemangiomatosis resulting in primary pulmonary hypertension. Ann Intern Med 1988;109:108.)*

not fully understood, but it has been suggested that chronic inflammation or shear stress injury to the pulmonary circulation can induce gene mutations that permit uncontrolled endothelial proliferation,[38,39] similar to the phenomenon of chronic inflammatory bowel disease leading to colon cancer. PCH has been described in some patients with chronic illnesses,[26–28,40–42] although it is not known if the occurrence is coincidental. The presence of fibrous long-spacing collagen, related to chronic inflammation or infection, has been associated with angiomatosis, and has been associated with one case of PCH.[42]

CLINICAL PRESENTATION AND INVESTIGATIONS

There may be several distinct clinical presentations of PCH, depending on which pulmonary structures are infiltrated by the abnormal capillaries. Infiltration and narrowing of precapillary arterioles will cause the classic picture of primary pulmonary hypertension. Infiltration of pulmonary veins will give a picture of pulmonary venous congestion, with secondary pulmonary hypertension. Infiltration of air spaces may affect gas transfer. Any and all of these patterns can be present in an individual patient.

The most challenging diagnoses are in patients who present with what seems to be classic primary pulmonary hypertension, with clear lung fields on a chest x-ray, and a cardiac catheterization that detects pulmonary hypertension with a normal pulmonary artery wedge pressure.[25] In those patients, the diagnosis is often missed, and PCH is only recognized when the patient deteriorates on vasodilator therapy. Any sign of pulmonary venous hypertension (Kerley-B lines, interstitial markings or pleural effusion on a chest x-ray or thoracic CT scan) in a patient with unexplained pulmonary hypertension should raise the possibility of PCH.

The initial case[1] and many subsequent cases have presented with signs of pulmonary venous dysfunction, and pulmonary congestion. Pulmonary hemorrhage with hemoptysis is present in more than 30% of patients.[7,24] Bronchoalveolar lavage may reveal erythrocyte extravasation into the bronchoalveolar fluid.[8] The patients complain of dyspnea, orthopnea and cough. There may be a history of asthma. Physical examination may reveal signs of increased pulmonary arterial pressure and right heart failure. Auscultation of the lungs may detect rales at the bases, and decreased air entry at the bases from pleural effusions.

On radiography of the chest, increased interstitial markings, patchy or diffuse reticulonodular infiltrates, cardiomegaly, enlarged central pulmonary vessels, and pleural effusions are found.[6,21] Lung scintigraphy demonstrates a normal pattern of isotope distribution during inhalation of the isotope aerosol, or mildly decreased ventilation of the upper lobes, but the macroaggregated-albumin perfusion scans demonstrate non-homogeneous perfusion, with some decreased perfusion to the upper lobes.[24,43] There may be areas of enhanced perfusion, which seem to correspond to regions with particularly dense capillary proliferation.[24] The lobar or segmental perfusion defects reported in chronic pulmonary thromboembolic disease have been found in only a few cases, and may correspond to areas of pulmonary hemorrhage or infarction.[4,43] Thoracic CT scans reveal mediastinal and hilar adenopathy, enlargement of central pulmonary arteries, bilateral, diffuse intralobular septal thickening (smooth or nodular), centrilobular nodular opacities, focal areas of ground-glass opacification, and an absence of honeycombing.[9,25] In the absence of histological confirmation, the disorder may be confused for pulmonary veno-occlusive disease, even with the use of high-resolution CT scans.[9]

Most patients develop signs of pulmonary hypertension with right failure. Cardiogenic shock, uncontrollable pulmonary edema, hemoptysis or pleural effusions are frequent causes of death.

PCH has been described in association with other diseases, including systemic lupus erythematosis, scleroderma, hypertrophic cardiomyopathy, Takayasu's disease, sleep apnea and AIDS.[26–28,40–42] However, the rarity of the associations, and the finding of PCH-like foci in some clinically unaffected humans at routine autopsy, raises the possibility of coincidental occurrence.[3]

TREATMENT/MANAGEMENT

A high index of suspicion of PCH must be present in patients with seeming primary pulmonary hypertension but who have signs of pulmonary venous congestion either before or during pulmonary vasodilator therapy. If any signs of pulmonary congestion are present, vasodilator therapy should be avoided, as the increased vascular flow in the presence of venous obstruction will result in alveolar capillary hydrostatic leakage. Catastrophic pulmonary congestion has been reported with either calcium blocker therapy or epoprostenol infusions.[18,22,28]

Most cases of PCH have been diagnosed postmortem, but an increasing number are being diagnosed antemortem, offering the opportunity for therapy.[19,30] There are reports of successful treatment by orthotopic heart/lung transplantation in three cases[24] and by unilateral pneumonectomy in another case.[19] Perhaps the most encouraging advance in therapy has been the report of successful treatment of PCH with the antiangiogenic agent, interferon-α-2a.[30] The beneficial response was sustained at 14 months of therapy.

CONCLUSION

It has been proposed that PCH is not a new entity, but that it has only been recently been recognized.[44] Reticulin staining of lung sections is particularly useful in the diagnosis. There may be a wide spectrum of severity, and it is possible that many cases never become clinically relevant.[3] However, with the appearance of symptoms, the course is usually fulminant and fatal. PCH may be neoplastic in origin, a congenital abnormality, or it may result from genetic mutations caused by chronic inflammation. At the present time, attacking the process with antiangiogenic agents may be the best option for medical therapy.

KEY POINTS

- Pulmonary capillary hemangiomatosis is a rare disorder caused by proliferation of capillary-like structures in the lung, which invade larger vessels, alveoli and airways.
- The stimulus for the development of PCH is unknown, but it may represent an angiogenic disease of the lung.
- The clinical presentation most frequently mimics primary pulmonary hypertension or pulmonary veno-occlusive disease.
- Successful therapy has included lung transplantation, or the use of antiangiogenic interferon.

ACKNOWLEDGMENTS

Dr Langleben is a Chercheur-Boursier Clinicien of the Fonds de la Recherche en Sante du Quebec, and is supported in part by the Canadian Institutes for Health Research, the Quebec Lung Association, and the Bank of Montreal Center for the Study of Heart Disease in Women at the Jewish General Hospital. The author thanks Dr Robert D Schlesinger for helpful comments.

REFERENCES

●1 Wagenvoort CA, Beetstra A, Spijker J. Capillary hemangiomatosis of the lungs. *Histopathology* 1978;**2**:401–6.

2 Heath D, Reid R. Invasive pulmonary haemangiomatosis. *Br J Dis Chest* 1985;**79**:284–94.

3 Havlik DM, Massie LW, Williams WL *et al*. Pulmonary capillary hemangiomatosis-like foci. *Am J Clin Pathol* 2000;**113**:655–62.

●4 Tron V, Magee F, Wright JL *et al*. Pulmonary capillary hemangiomatosis. *Hum Pathol* 1986;**17**:1144–50.

◆5 al-Fawaz IM, al-Mobaireek KF, al-Suhaibani M *et al*. Pulmonary capillary hemangiomatosis: a case report and review of the literature. *Pediatr Pulmonol* 1995;**19**:243–8.

6 Vevaina JR, Mark EJ. Thoracic hemangiomatosis masquerading as interstitial lung disease. *Chest* 1988;**93**:657–9.

7 Whittaker JS, Pickering CAC, Heath D *et al*. Pulmonary capillary haemangiomatosis. *Diagn Histopathol* 1983;**6**:77–84.

◆8 Domingo C, Encabo B, Roig J *et al*. Pulmonary capillary hemangiomatosis: report of a case and review of the literature. *Respiration* 1992;**59**:178–80.

●9 Dufour B, Maitre S, Humbert M *et al*. High-resolution CT of the chest in four patients with pulmonary capillary hemangiomatosis or pulmonary venoocclusive disease. *Am J Roentgenol* 1998;**171**:1321–4.

10 Wagenvoort CA, Wagenvoort N. The pathology of pulmonary veno-occlusive disease. *Virchows Arch [Pathol Anat]* 1974;**364**:69–79.

11 Daroca PJ, Mansfield RE, Ichinose H. Pulmonary veno-occlusive disease: report of a case with pseudoangiomatous features. *Am J Surg Pathol* 1977;**1**:349–55.

12 Rowen M, Thompson JR, Williamson RA *et al*. Diffuse pulmonary hemangiomatosis. *Radiology* 1978;**127**:445–51.

13 Sherrier RH, Chiles C, Roggli V. Pulmonary lymphangioleio-myomatosis: CT findings. *Am J Roentgenol* 1989;**153**:937–40.

14 Wagener OE, Roncoroni AJ, Barcat JA. Severe pulmonary hypertension with diffuse smooth muscle proliferation of the lungs. *Chest* 1989;**95**:234–7.

15 Tazelaar HD, Kerr D, Yousem SA *et al*. Diffuse pulmonary lymphangiomatosis. *Hum Pathol* 1993;**24**:1313–22.

16 Snyder LS, Harmon KR, Estensen RD. Intravascular lympho-matosis (malignant angioendotheliomatosis) presenting as pulmonary hypertension. *Chest* 1989;**96**:1199–200.

17 Alvarez-Fernandez E, Carretero-Albinana L, Menarguez-Palanaca J. Sclerosing hemangioma of the lung. *Arch Pathol Lab Med* 1989;**113**:121–4.

●18 Langleben D, Heneghan JM, Batten AP *et al*. Familial pulmonary capillary hemangiomatosis resulting in primary pulmonary hypertension. *Ann Intern Med* 1988;**109**:106–9.

●19 Wagenaar SJSC, Mulder JJS, Wagenvoort CA *et al*. Pulmonary capillary hemangiomatosis diagnosed during life. *Histopathology* 1989;**14**:212–14.

20 Masur Y, Remberger K, Hoefer M. Pulmonary capillary hemangiomatosis as a rare cause of pulmonary hypertension. *Pathol Res Pract* 1996;**192**:290–5.

21 Lippert JL, White CS, Cameron EW *et al*. Pulmonary capilary hemangiomatosis: radiographic appearance. *J Thorac Imaging* 1998;**13**:49–51.

●22 Humbert M, Maitre S, Capron F *et al*. Pulmonary edema complicating continuous intravenous prostacyclin in pulmonary capillary hemangiomatosis. *Am J Respir Crit Care Med* 1998;**157**:1681–5.

◆23 Magee F, Wright JL, Kay JM *et al*. Pulmonary capillary hemangiomatosis. *Am Rev Respir Dis* 1985;**132**:922–5.

24 Faber CN, Yousem SA, Dauber JH *et al*. Pulmonary capillary hemangiomatosis. *Am Rev Respir Dis* 1989;**140**:808–13.

◆25 Eltorky MA, Headley AS, Winer-Muram H *et al*. Pulmonary capillary hemangiomatosis: a clinicopathologic review. *Ann Thorac Surg* 1994;**57**:772–6.

26 Jing X, Yokoi T, Nakamura Y *et al.* Pulmonary capillary hemangiomatosis. A unique feature of congestive vasculopathy associated with hypertrophic cardiomyopathy. *Arch Pathol Lab Med* 1998;**122**:94–6.

27 Fernandez-Alonso J, Zulueta T, Reyes-Ramirez JR *et al.* Pulmonary capillary hemangiomatosis as a cause of pulmonary hypertension in a young woman with systemic lupus erythematosus. *J Rheumatol* 1999;**26**:231–3.

28 Gugnani MK, Pierson C, Vanderheide R *et al.* Pulmonary edema complicating prostacyclin therapy in pulmonary hypertension associated with scleroderma. *Arthritis Rheum* 2000;**43**:699–703.

29 Cioffi U, De Simone M, Pavoni G *et al.* Pulmonary capillary hemangiomatosis in an asymptomatic elderly patient. *Int Surg* 1999;**84**:168–70.

●30 White CW, Sondheimer HM, Crouch EC *et al.* Treatment of pulmonary hemangiomatosis with recombinant interferon alfa-2-a. *N Engl J Med* 1989;**320**:1197–200.

31 Unterborn J, Mark EJ. Case records of the Massachusetts General Hospital: weekly clinicopathological exercises. *N Engl J Med* 2000;**343**:1788–96.

◆32 Folkman J, Klagsbrun M. Angiogenic factors. *Science* 1987;**235**:442–7.

33 Lee SD, Shroyer KR, Markham NE *et al.* Monoclonal endothelial cell proliferation is present in primary but not secondary pulmonary hypertension. *J Clin Invest* 1998;**101**:927–34.

●34 Deng Z, Morse JH, Slager SL *et al.* Familial primary pulmonary hypertension (gene *PPH1*) is caused by mutations in the bone morphogenetic protein receptor-II gene. *Am J Hum Genet* 2000;**67**:737–44.

●35 Lane KB, Machado RD, Pauciulo MW *et al.* Heterozygous germline mutations in BMPR2, encoding a TGF-beta receptor, cause familial primary pulmonary hypertension. The International PPH Consortium. *Nat Genet* 2000;**26**:81–4.

◆36 Loscalzo J. Genetic clues to the cause of primary pulmonary hypertension. *N Engl J Med* 2001;**345**:367–71.

◆37 Rich S. Executive summary from the World Symposium – Primary Pulmonary Hypertension. Available at: http://www.who.int/ncd/cvd/pph.html. 1998. Ref Type: Generic.

38 Yeager ME, Halley GR, Galphon HA *et al.* Microsatellite instability of endothelial cell growth and apoptosis genes within plexiform lesions in primary pulmonary hypertension. *Circ Res* 2001;**88**:E2–11.

◆39 Voelkel NF, Cool CD, Lee SD *et al.* Primary pulmonary hypertension between inflammation and cancer. *Chest* 1998;**114**:225S–30S.

40 Kakkar N, Vasishta RK, Banerjee AK *et al.* Pulmonary capillary hemangiomatosis as a cause of pulmonary hypertension in Takayasu's aortoarteritis. *Respiration* 1997;**64**:381–3.

41 Ahemd Q, Chung-Park M, Tomashefski JF. Cardiopulmonary pathology in patients with sleep apnea/obesity hypoventilation syndrome. *Hum Pathol* 1997;**28**:264–9.

42 Borczuk AC, Niedt G, Sablay LB *et al.* Fibrous long-spacing collagen in bacillary angiomatosis. *Ultrastruct Pathol* 1998;**22**:127–33.

43 Rush C, Langleben D, Schlesinger RD *et al.* Lung scintigraphy in pulmonary capillary hemangiomatosis. *Clin Nucl Med* 1991;**16**:913–17.

44 Thurlbeck WM. Pulmonary capillary hemangiomatosis as a rare cause of pulmonary hypertension. *Pathol Res Pract* 1996;**192**:298–9.

15

Pulmonary hypertension associated with disorders of the respiratory system and/or hypoxemia

Pulmonary hypertension due to chronic hypoxic lung disease

EMMANUEL WEITZENBLUM AND ARI CHAOUAT

INTRODUCTION

In the recent classification of pulmonary hypertension, which has been adopted following the WHO meeting held in Evian in September 1998,[1] and confirmed at the Venice meeting in 2003, Section 3 is entitled 'Pulmonary hypertension associated with disorders of the respiratory system and/or hypoxaemia'. This includes COPD, interstitial lung disease, sleep-disordered breathing, alveolar hypoventilation disorders, chronic exposure to high altitude, neonatal lung disease, alveolar capillary dysplasia. The last three conditions are considered in other chapters of this book. Pulmonary hypertension associated with sleep-disordered breathing and alveolar hypoventilation disorders is discussed in Chapter 15B of this book. The present chapter deals with pulmonary hypertension associated with chronic hypoxic lung disease, that is COPD and parenchymal lung disease (including interstitial lung disease).

Owing to its frequency, COPD is by far the most common cause of pulmonary hypertension and of cor pulmonale, more common than restrictive lung diseases, obesity-hypoventilation syndrome and pulmonary thromboembolic disease. Pulmonary hypertension may lead with time to the development of right ventricular hypertrophy (the so-called cor pulmonale[2,3]), which may result in right ventricular failure,[3,4] but it should be emphasized that pulmonary hypertension is only one among other complications of advanced COPD and that the prognosis of COPD is linked rather to the severity of respiratory insufficiency than to the occurrence of pulmonary hypertension which is essentially a 'marker' of longstanding hypoxemia.

This chapter gives an overview of pulmonary hypertension resulting from hypoxic lung disease, mainly COPD, but it also considers diffuse parenchymal lung disease (interstitial lung disease). Particular emphasis is placed on the mechanism of pulmonary hypertension and on its evolution with the possible occurrence of right heart failure.

DEFINITIONS

Pulmonary hypertension complicating chronic respiratory disease is generally defined by the presence of a resting pulmonary artery mean pressure (PAP) >20 mmHg. It must be emphasized that this is slightly different from the definition of 'primary' pulmonary hypertension

(PAP >25 mmHg).[5] In young (<50 years) healthy subjects, PAP is most often between 10 and 15 mmHg. With aging there is a slight progression of PAP, by about 1 mmHg per 10 years. A mean resting PAP >20 mmHg is always abnormal.[6]

In the 'natural history' of COPD, pulmonary hypertension is often preceded by an abnormally large increase in PAP during exercise,[7] defined by a pressure >30 mmHg for a mild level (30–40 watts) of steady-state exercise. The term 'exercising pulmonary hypertension' has been used by some authors, but we believe that the term 'pulmonary hypertension' should be reserved for resting pulmonary hypertension.

EPIDEMIOLOGY

There are in fact very few data about the incidence and prevalence of pulmonary hypertension resulting from chronic hypoxic lung disease. The main reason is that right heart catheterization cannot be performed on a large scale in patients at risk. An alternative is the use of non-invasive methods, particularly Doppler echocardiography, which is presently the best method.[8] It should soon be possible to investigate large groups of patients with COPD and other chronic lung diseases with echo Doppler within the next few years.

Another way of facing the problem is to determine the prevalence of patients at risk of developing pulmonary hypertension, that is, patients with hypoxemic lung disease. This has been done in the UK by Williams and Nicholl,[9] who have observed that in the Sheffield population aged ≥ 45 years, an estimated 0.3% had both PaO_2 <7.3 kPa (55 mmHg) and an FEV_1 $<50\%$ of the predicted value. For England and Wales this would represent 60 000 subjects at risk of pulmonary hypertension and eligible for long-term oxygen therapy. The figures provided by Williams and Nicholl are limited to COPD, whereas numerous respiratory diseases may lead to pulmonary hypertension (Table 15A.1). However, COPD is by far the major cause of respiratory insufficiency in industrialized countries and probably accounts for 90% of hypoxic pulmonary hypertension. Most patients with secondary pulmonary hypertension are over 50 years of age and about two-thirds are male.

The mortality related to secondary pulmonary hypertension is also difficult to assess. There are data about the mortality resulting from chronic lung disease (80 000/year in the USA, 15 000/year in France), but we do not know precisely the role of secondary pulmonary hypertension in this mortality. Pulmonary hypertension is a complication, among others, of advanced COPD and it is not possible to separate pulmonary hypertension from its causative diseases.

Table 15A.1 *Diseases of the respiratory system associated with pulmonary hypertension (except primary pulmonary hypertension, pulmonary thromboembolic disease and diseases of the pulmonary vascular bed)*

Obstructive lung diseases
- COPD* (chronic obstructive bronchitis, emphysema and their association)
- Asthma (with irreversible airway obstruction)
- Cystic fibrosis
- Bronchiectasis
- Bronchiolitis obliterans

Restrictive lung diseases
- Neuromuscular diseases: amyotrophic lateral sclerosis, myopathy, bilateral diaphragmatic paralysis, etc.
- Kyphoscoliosis[†]
- Thoracoplasty
- Sequelae of pulmonary tuberculosis
- Sarcoidosis
- Pneumoconiosis
- Drug-related lung diseases
- Extrinsic allergic alveolitis
- Connective tissue diseases
- Idiopathic interstitial pulmonary fibrosis[†]
- Interstitial pulmonary fibrosis of known origin

Respiratory insufficiency of 'central' origin
- Central alveolar hypoventilation
- Obesity-hypoventilation syndrome[†] (formerly 'Pickwickian syndrome')
- Sleep apnea syndrome[†]

*COPD, chronic obstructive pulmonary disease. A very frequent cause of pulmonary hypertension.
[†] Relatively frequent cause of pulmonary hypertension.

ETIOLOGY: WHICH CHRONIC LUNG DISEASE MAY LEAD TO PULMONARY HYPERTENSION?

A list of chronic respiratory diseases that may lead to pulmonary hypertension is given in Table 15A.1. Primary pulmonary hypertension, pulmonary thromboembolic disease and diseases of the pulmonary vascular bed have been excluded from that list, which is far from being exhaustive. It can be seen that there are three major groups of diseases:

- those characterized by a limitation to airflow (COPD and other causes of chronic bronchial obstruction);
- those characterized by a restriction of pulmonary volumes from extrinsic or parenchymatous origin (restrictive lung diseases); and
- those where the relatively well-preserved mechanical properties of the lungs and chest wall contrast with marked gas exchange abnormalities, which are partially explained by poor ventilatory drive (respiratory insufficiency of 'central' origin).

The last of the above is described in the next chapter of this book (Chapter 15B) and the review in this chapter is limited to obstructive and restrictive lung diseases.

COPD is the major cause of chronic respiratory insufficiency and pulmonary hypertension, since it probably accounts for 80–90% of the cases. It is presently defined as 'a disease state characterized by airflow limitation that is not fully reversible. The airflow limitation is usually both progressive and associated with an abnormal inflammatory response of the lungs to noxious particles or gases'.[10] COPD includes chronic obstructive bronchitis and emphysema, which are often associated.

Among the restrictive lung diseases, kyphoscoliosis, idiopathic pulmonary fibrosis and pneumoconiosis are the main causes of pulmonary hypertension. It must be emphasized that the mechanism of pulmonary hypertension may vary according to the causative disease even if chronic hypoxemia is a common feature. As an illustration, it is easy to understand that the mechanism of pulmonary hypertension is markedly different in kyphoscoliosis (alveolar hypoventilation) and in idiopathic pulmonary fibrosis (destruction of the pulmonary vascular bed).

MECHANISMS OF PULMONARY HYPERTENSION IN CHRONIC RESPIRATORY DISEASES

Pulmonary hypertension may result from an increased cardiac output, an increased pulmonary 'capillary' wedge pressure or an increased pulmonary vascular resistance (PVR). In chronic respiratory diseases, and particularly in COPD, the role of an elevated cardiac output and of an increase of the wedge pressure is almost negligible. An increased cardiac output may be observed during episodes of acute respiratory failure.[11] An abnormally high wedge pressure has also been noticed during such episodes[11] and during a steady-state period.[12,13] However, cardiac output and wedge pressure are generally found to be normal, and pulmonary hypertension complicating chronic lung disease is of the precapillary type,[13] almost exclusively accounted for by the increased PVR.

The factors leading to an increased PVR in chronic respiratory diseases are numerous (Table 15A.2) but in COPD alveolar hypoxia is by far the predominant factor.[4,14] Two distinct mechanisms of action of alveolar hypoxia must be considered: acute hypoxia causes pulmonary vasoconstriction and chronic longstanding hypoxia induces (with time) structural changes in the pulmonary vascular bed (pulmonary vascular remodeling).

Hypoxic pulmonary vasoconstriction

Since the historic studies on the cat in 1946 by von Euler and Liljestrand,[15] it has been known that acute hypoxia induces in humans, and in almost all species of mammals,

Table 15A.2 *Factors increasing pulmonary vascular resistance (PVR) in chronic respiratory diseases*

Anatomic factors: reduction (destruction, obstruction) of the pulmonary vascular bed
- Thromboembolic lesions
- Fibrosis
- Emphysema

Functional factors
- Alveolar hypoxia*
  - Acute hypoxia (pulmonary vasoconstriction)
  - Chronic hypoxia (remodeling of the pulmonary vascular bed)
- Acidosis, hypercapnia
- Hyperviscosity (polycythemia)
- Hypervolemia (polycythemia)
- Mechanical factors (compression of alveolar vessels)

*Most important factor.

a rise of PVR and PAP that is accounted for by hypoxic pulmonary vasoconstriction (HPV).[16,17] This vasoconstriction is localized in the small precapillary arteries. Its precise mechanism is not fully understood, but recently there has been a marked development of knowledge of the mediators involved in the regulation of the vasomotor tone, particularly nitric oxide[18] and endothelin, both of which are produced by endothelial cells.

In normal humans, the reactivity of the pulmonary circulation to acute hypoxia varies from one subject to another[19] and this inter-individual variability is also found in COPD patients.[20] This means that some patients are responders to acute hypoxia, exhibiting a marked increase of PVR and PAP during the hypoxic challenge whereas others are poor responders or even non-responders (Figure 15A.1).[20]

The clinical situations which bear the closest analogy with acute hypoxic challenges are probably exacerbations of COPD leading to acute respiratory failure and the sleep-related episodes of worsening hypoxemia (see below).

Remodeling of the pulmonary vascular bed

Pulmonary hypertension is generally observed in respiratory patients exhibiting marked chronic hypoxemia ($PaO_2 < 55$–60 mmHg). On the other hand, an almost experimental model of the effects of chronic hypoxia does exist: the pulmonary hypertension observed in healthy people living at altitudes >3500 meters, and having a PaO_2 in the range 45–60 mmHg; they have a precapillary pulmonary hypertension of mild to moderate degree[21] very similar to that observed in COPD. Morphological studies, performed in these healthy highlanders, have shown a remodeling of the pulmonary vascular bed, with

hypertrophy of the muscular media of the small pulmonary arteries, muscularization of pulmonary arterioles and intimal fibrosis.[22] This remodeling can only be explained by the effect of chronic alveolar hypoxia. The remodeling is potentially reversible since pulmonary hypertension disappears when native highlanders spend a sufficient time at sea level.[22] There is some degree of similarity between these structural changes and those observed in COPD patients with pulmonary hypertension, and it has been deduced by analogy that the latter changes were accounted for by chronic hypoxia. However, the following points should be emphasized:

- The concept of the similarity of the pulmonary vascular remodeling in healthy native highlanders and in hypoxemic COPD patients has been challenged by Wilkinson et al.[23] who have observed that vascular remodeling is not reversible under long-term oxygen therapy, but another morphological study led to different conclusions.[24]
- In COPD patients, chronic hypoxia is not the only factor. These patients have marked morphological changes of the lung parenchyma, particularly when emphysema is severe, and these changes, including mechanical distortion of the lungs,[23] could account for the increased PVR.
- Several studies have shown that remodeling of the pulmonary vessels may be observed in non-hypoxemic COPD patients with mild disease severity[25,26] and even in smokers without airflow obstruction:[27,28] the changes mainly consist of the thickening of the intimal coat of pulmonary muscular arteries and an increased proportion of muscularized small pulmonary arteries.[29,30] These structural abnormalities could be the consequence of an endothelial dysfunction of pulmonary arteries taking place early in the course of COPD, probably induced by cigarette smoke.[27,28] But it must be underlined that the COPD patients included in these studies generally had no pulmonary hypertension, and that the clinical relevance of these early abnormalities is presently unknown.

Thus, chronic hypoxia is far from being the only factor responsible for the structural changes of the pulmonary arteries and arterioles and this probably explains why the vascular remodeling is not fully reversible under long-term oxygen therapy, which is different from high altitude pulmonary hypertension.

Other functional factors

Chronic alveolar hypoxia represents the determining factor of the elevation of PVR in COPD even if there are still uncertainties about the role of chronic alveolar hypoxia in the remodeling of the pulmonary circulation. The role of

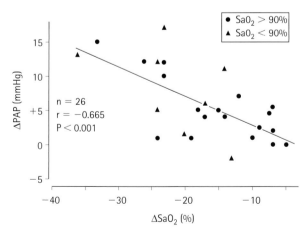

Figure 15A.1 *Variability of the pulmonary vascular response to a hypoxic challenge (fraction of inspired O_2 (FiO_2) = 0.13) in 26 chronic obstructive pulmonary disease patients. x axis: ΔSaO_2, changes in arterial oxygen saturation (SaO_2); y axis: ΔPAP, changes in pulmonary arterial pressure (PAP) during the challenge.*

other functional factors (Table 15A.2), namely hypercapnic acidosis,[31] hyperviscosity due to polycythemia[32] and mechanical factors [effects of marked respiratory swings (Figure 15A.2) on the pulmonary circulation[33]], seems small when compared to that of alveolar hypoxia.

Mechanisms of pulmonary hypertension in diseases other than COPD

In kyphoscoliosis as well as in neuromuscular restrictive lung diseases (see Table 15A.1), alveolar hypoventilation is observed at an advanced stage of disease and alveolar hypoxia is the first cause of pulmonary hypertension.

Some respiratory diseases which do not affect the bronchial and parenchymal structures may lead to pulmonary hypertension. In these diseases, which include the obesity-hypoventilation syndrome and the sleep apnea syndrome (see Chapter 15B), pulmonary hypertension is directly linked to alveolar hypoxia which probably induces, with time, structural changes of the pulmonary vascular bed.

In idiopathic pulmonary fibrosis (IPF), increased PVR, leading to pulmonary hypertension, is mainly due to anatomic factors – loss of pulmonary vascular bed or compression of arterioles and capillaries by the fibrosing process[34,35] – but the role of functional factors (alveolar hypoxia) is probably not negligible since significant correlations have been observed between PaO_2 and PVR and PAP in IPF patients.[36]

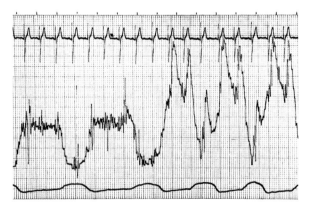

Figure 15A.2 *In chronic obstructive pulmonary disease, pulmonary hypertension is 'precapillary': the pulmonary 'capillary' wedge pressure (left part of the trace) is normal (9 mmHg) whereas pulmonary artery pressure (PAP; right part of the trace) is elevated (mean PAP = 25 mmHg) due to the elevation of pulmonary vascular resistance. This trace also shows important swings of systolic and diastolic pulmonary artery pressure from inspiration to expiration, which simply reproduce the elevated intrathoracic pressure changes.*

MAIN FEATURES OF PULMONARY HYPERTENSION IN CHRONIC RESPIRATORY DISEASE

Pulmonary artery pressures at rest

The main characteristic of pulmonary hypertension in chronic respiratory disease is probably its mild to moderate degree, resting PAP in a stable state of the disease ranging usually between 20 and 35 mmHg. This modest degree of pulmonary hypertension is well recognized in COPD.[37] but has also been observed in IPF[36] and in obstructive sleep apnea syndrome (OSAS).[38] This is very different from left heart disease, congenital heart disease, pulmonary thromboembolic disease and, in particular, primary pulmonary hypertension in which PAP is usually >40 mmHg and may exceed 80 mmHg in some patients. Table 15A.3 compares the pulmonary hemodynamic data of COPD patients with pulmonary hypertension,[37] IPF patients,[36] OSAS patients with pulmonary hypertension[38] with a large series of primary pulmonary hypertension, the American Registry.[5] It can be seen that pulmonary hypertension is severe in primary pulmonary hypertension (average PAP 60 ± 15 mmHg) whereas it is rather modest in COPD (PAP 26 ± 6 mmHg) in OSAS (PAP 26 ± 6 mmHg) and in IPF [PAP 24 ± 11 mmHg for the group as a whole and approximately 30 ± 7 mmHg in the subgroup of patients (17/31) with pulmonary hypertension]. A PAP of ≥40 mmHg is thus unusual in COPD patients except when they are investigated during an acute exacerbation[39] or when there is an associated cardiopulmonary disease (left heart disease, collagen vascular disease, etc.) and this is also true for OSAS and for most restrictive lung diseases (kyphoscoliosis, IPF, etc.).

The consequences of the modest level of pulmonary hypertension in chronic respiratory disease include the lack of stethacoustic signs of pulmonary hypertension, the absence or late occurrence of right heart failure (see below) and the frequent inability of non-invasive methods to make a diagnosis of pulmonary hypertension. Even Doppler echocardiography, which is by far the best method in this field,[8] is not as reliable in COPD[40] as it is in primary pulmonary hypertension or in left heart disease. The non-invasive diagnosis of pulmonary hypertension is particularly difficult in COPD patients who exhibit both a mild degree of pulmonary hypertension and a poor echogenicity due to hyperinflation (emphysema).

It must be emphasized that if baseline pulmonary hypertension is generally mild in COPD, it may worsen, sometimes markedly and abruptly, during exercise and sleep and during acute exacerbations of the disease.

Table 15A.3 *Comparison of pulmonary hypertension in chronic hypoxic lung disease (COPD, IPF, OSAS), to primary pulmonary hypertension*

	Primary pulmonary hypertension[5]	COPD[37]	IPF[36]	OSAS[38]
Number of patients	187	62	31	37
Number of women	110	2	8	2
Age (years)	36 ± 15	55 ± 8	58 ± 16	52 ± 11
FEV_1 (mL)		1170 ± 390	1655 ± 650	1830 ± 790
TLC (% of predicted)		110 ± 15	65 ± 20	80 ± 12
PaO_2 (mmHg)		60 ± 9	68 ± 12	64 ± 9
$PaCO_2$ (mmHg)		45 ± 6	35 ± 5	44 ± 5
PAP (mmHg)	60 ± 15	26 ± 6	$24 \pm 11^*$	26 ± 6
PCWP (mmHg)	8 ± 4	8 ± 2	7 ± 4	8 ± 3
Q $(L/mm \cdot m^2)$	2.27 ± 0.90	3.8 ± 1.1	3.4 ± 0.8	2.8 ± 0.6
PVR $(mmHg/L/min \cdot m^2)$	26 ± 14	4.8 ± 1.4	5.0 ± 3.1	3 ± 2.0

Mean values $\pm$ standard deviation.
COPD, chronic obstructive pulmonary disease; FEV_1, forced expiratory volume in 1 second; IPF, idiopathic pulmonary fibrosis; OSAS, obstructive sleep apnea syndrome; PAP, pulmonary artery mean pressure; PCWP, pulmonary capillary wedge pressure; PVR, pulmonary vascular resistance; Q, cardiac output; TLC, total lung capacity.
* $PAP = 30 \pm 7$ mmHg in the subgroup (n = 17) of patients with pulmonary hypertension.

Worsening of pulmonary hypertension during exercise, sleep and acute exacerbations

PULMONARY ARTERY PRESSURES ON EXERCISE

During steady-state exercise, PAP increases markedly in advanced COPD patients with resting pulmonary hypertension,[12,41–43] as illustrated in Figure 15A.3, which shows this in such patients (group 3). PAP rises as a mean from 26.6 ± 5.8 to 55.4 ± 11.4 mmHg during a 30-watt exercise of 7–10 minutes. Thus, a COPD patient whose baseline PAP is 25–30 mmHg may exhibit severe pulmonary hypertension (50–60 mmHg) during moderate exercise. It is of interest to observe that the behavior of PAP from rest to exercise is the same in the three groups of patients (Figure 15A.3): in the three groups PAP rises to about twice the level of its resting value. This is explained by the fact that PVR does not decrease during exercise in these advanced COPD patients,[12,41,42] whereas it does decrease in healthy subjects. As the cardiac output is doubled for this level of exercise, PAP increases by about 100% (Figure 15A.3). From a practical viewpoint, this means that daily activities such as climbing stairs or even walking can induce pronounced pulmonary hypertension.

PULMONARY ARTERY PRESSURES DURING SLEEP

Acute increases of PAP during sleep have been observed in advanced COPD patients with daytime hypoxemia and pulmonary hypertension.[44–47] They are principally observed in REM sleep during which dips of O_2 saturation are more severe, and the fall of SaO_2 from its baseline value during wakefulness may be as high as 20–30%.[48,49]

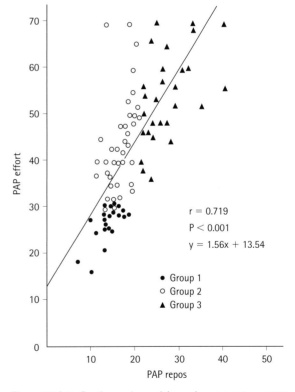

Figure 15A.3 *Resting and exercising pulmonary artery mean pressure (PAP) in a large series of chronic obstructive pulmonary disease patients (n = 92). Group 1, no resting pulmonary hypertension and exercising PAP < 30 mmHg; group 2, no resting pulmonary hypertension but exercising PAP > 30 mmHg; group 3, resting pulmonary hypertension. PAP repos, resting PAP; PAP effort, exercising PAP. Level of exercise: 30–40 watts, steady state (personal data).*

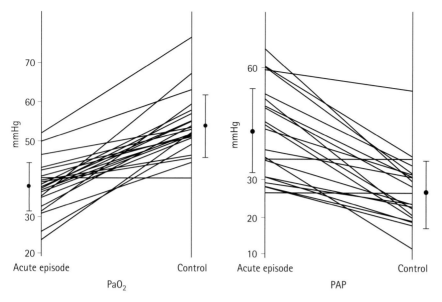

Figure 15A.4 *Changes in arterial partial pressure of O_2 (PaO_2) and pulmonary artery pressure (PAP) in 24 chronic obstructive pulmonary disease patients investigated during an episode of acute respiratory failure ('Acute episode') and after recovery ('Control'). With recovery, PaO_2 rose and PAP fell: the parallelism of these changes suggests the intervention of hypoxic vasoconstriction during acute exacerbations of chronic obstructive pulmonary disease (personal data).*

These episodes of sleep-related desaturation are not due to apneas, except if COPD is associated with an OSAS, but to alveolar hypoventilation and/or ventilation/perfusion mismatching.[50,51] These episodes are often accompanied by peaks of pulmonary hypertension.[45–47] The more profound the dips of hypoxemia, the more severe the peaks of pulmonary hypertension.[46] PAP can increase by as much as 20 mmHg from its baseline value.[44,46] There is generally a close relationship between changes in SaO_2 and PAP during sleep,[45,46] reflecting hypoxic pulmonary vasoconstriction. Sleep-related episodes of pulmonary hypertension are of short duration and PAP returns to its baseline level with morning awakening.[46]

PULMONARY ARTERY PRESSURES DURING EXACERBATIONS OF RESPIRATORY FAILURE

Episodes of acute respiratory failure are characterized, at least in COPD patients, by a worsening of hypoxemia and hypercapnia. There is simultaneously a marked increase in PAP from its baseline value.[11,52,53] PAP may increase by as much as 20 mmHg, but usually returns to its baseline after recovery.[54]

Figure 15A.4 shows personal results in 24 COPD patients investigated during an acute exacerbation and 3 weeks later following recovery. The mean baseline PAP was 27 mmHg and it increased to a mean of 44 mmHg during acute respiratory failure, exceeding 50 mmHg in some patients. There was a striking parallel between changes in PaO_2 and PAP (Figure 15A.4), suggesting the presence of hypoxic pulmonary vasoconstriction.

Thus, even though pulmonary hypertension is usually mild (20–35 mmHg) in chronic respiratory disease, and particularly in COPD patients, it may increase markedly during exercise, sleep, and exacerbations of the disease.

These acute increases of afterload can favor the development of right ventricular failure, especially during exacerbations of the disease.[39]

Longitudinal evolution of pulmonary hypertension

The progression of pulmonary hypertension is slow, at least in COPD patients, and several studies have shown that PAP may remain stable over periods of 2–5 years.[54–57] Another study[58] in which 93 COPD patients were followed for 5–12 years, with a mean of 90 months, confirmed that the changes of PAP were rather small: +0.5 mmHg/year for the group as a whole. Interestingly, the evolution of PAP was identical in patients with and without initial pulmonary hypertension. This means that in the majority of COPD patients whose PAP is initially normal (<20 mmHg), it will not exceed 20 mmHg after 3–5 years. A recent paper from our group, on the 'natural evolution' of pulmonary hemodynamics in COPD patients with an initial PAP <20 mmHg, has shown that only 33/131 patients developed pulmonary hypertension after a mean interval of 6.8 ± 2.9 years.[7] Some results of this study are given in Table 15A.4.

However, it must be emphasized that a minority (about 30%) of advanced COPD patients exhibit a marked worsening of PAP during the follow-up.[58] These patients do not differ from the others at the onset, but they are characterized by a progressive deterioration of PaO_2 and $PaCO_2$ during the evolution.[7,58] Thus, regular measurements of arterial blood gases are recommended for advanced COPD patients, particularly those with pulmonary hypertension.[58] The longitudinal evolution of pulmonary hypertension is favorably influenced by

Table 15A.4 *Long-term evolution of resting and exercising mean pulmonary artery pressure (PAP) in 131 COPD patients without resting pulmonary hypertension*

	T0	T1	P value (T0 versus T1)
Resting PAP (mmHg)			
All patients (n = 131)	15.2 ± 2.7	17.8 ± 6.6	0.001
Group 1 (n = 55)	14.1 ± 2.8	16.0 ± 5.2	0.005
Group 2 (n = 76)	16.0 ± 2.3	19.0 ± 7.3	0.001
Exercising PAP (mmHg)			
All patients (n = 79)	30.7 ± 7.3	33.3 ± 8.9	0.004
Group 1 (n = 36)	25.1 ± 4.1	30.1 ± 8.8	0.001
Group 2 (n = 43)	37.2 ± 4.3	37.2 ± 7.4	NS

Group 1, no resting or exercising pulmonary hypertension at T0; group 2, no resting but exercising pulmonary hypertension at T0; T0, time of first right heart catheterization; T1, time of second right heart catheterization. The mean interval between T0 and T1 is 6.8 ± 2.9 years. Values are mean $\pm$ SD.
Adapted from Kessler *et al.*[7]

Table 15A.5 *Evolution of functional and hemodynamic variables in 45 patients with interstitial pulmonary fibrosis who underwent repeated catheterization after an average delay of 5 years*

	1st cath.	2nd cath.	P
PAP (mmHg)	22.9 ± 6.1	25.9 ± 8.4	<0.01
PCWP (mmHg)	9.0 ± 3.5	9.8 ± 5.6	NS
$\dot{Q}$ (L/min·m^2)	3.1 ± 0.9	3.0 ± 1.1	NS
PVR (dyn s/cm^5)	213 ± 114	266 ± 183	<0.05
PaO$_2$ (mmHg)	73.5 ± 11.7	70.6 ± 9.5	NS
SaO$_2$ (%)	93.9 ± 2.4	93.0 ± 2.7	<0.05

PAP, pulmonary artery mean pressure; PCWP, pulmonary capillary wedge pressure; PVR, pulmonary vascular resistance; $\dot{Q}$, cardiac output. Values are mean $\pm$ SD.
Adapted from Jezek *et al.*[62]

long-term oxygen therapy, which allows a small improvement[59,60] or at least a stabilization[61] of PAP.

In other respiratory diseases (pneumoconioses, sarcoidosis, etc.), there have only been isolated observations dealing with small numbers of cases, with the exception of the large studies of Jezek *et al.*[62] who studied 45 patients with IPF followed for an average period of 5.3 ± 4.3 years. Some results of this study appear in Table 15A.5. The average increase in PAP, although significant, was small, 0.7 mmHg/year, which is in good agreement with the results observed in COPD.[54–58] However, IPF patients with initial PAP >30 mmHg showed a clear tendency to a further progression of pulmonary hypertension, with early death.[62]

In 44 OSAS patients treated with nasal continuous positive airway pressure (CPAP), Chaouat *et al.*[63] investigated several variables, including pulmonary hemodynamic data over the course of 5 years: PAP was stable since it was 16 ± 5 mmHg at the baseline and 17 ± 5 mmHg at the end of the study (not significant). Only 11/44 (25%) of these OSAS patients had pulmonary hypertension (PAP ≥ 20 mmHg) at the onset.

It thus appears that in most chronic respiratory patients the progression of PAP is rather slow (about 0.5 mmHg/year) but a minority of COPD (and IPF) patients clearly exhibit a marked worsening of pulmonary hypertension and it seems necessary to detect this worsening as soon as possible.

FROM PULMONARY HYPERTENSION TO RIGHT VENTRICLE ENLARGEMENT AND RIGHT HEART FAILURE

The classical view of the development of right heart failure (RHF) in chronic respiratory patients is the following:[3] pulmonary hypertension increases the work of the right ventricle, which leads more or less rapidly to right ventricular enlargement (associating hypertrophy and dilatation), which can result in right ventricular dysfunction (systolic, diastolic). Later, RHF, characterized by the presence of peripheral edema, can be observed in some COPD patients. The interval between the onset of pulmonary hypertension and the appearance of RHF is not

Table 15A.6 *Comparison of hemodynamic data in edematous and non-edematous patients with chronic obstructive pulmonary disease*

	Non-edematous (n = 8)	Edematous (n = 6)	P
PAP (mmHg)	30 ± 8	33 ± 6	NS
RAP (mmHg)	5 ± 2	9 ± 5	NS
RVEDP (mmHg)	7 ± 2	12 ± 8	NS
Q̇ (L/min·m²)	2.58 ± 0.60	3.65 ± 1.0	<0.05
RVEF (%)	0.47 ± 0.10	0.23 ± 11	<0.05
RVEDVI (mL/m²)	69 ± 26	218 ± 166	<0.05
RVESVI (mL/m²)	39 ± 21	183 ± 162	<0.05
Right ventricular elastance (mmHg/mL·m²)	1.69 ± 0.98	0.41 ± 0.27	<0.05

PAP, pulmonary artery mean pressure; Q̇, cardiac output; RAP, right atrial pressure; RVEDP, right ventricular end-diastolic pressure; RVEDVI, right ventricular end-diastolic volume index; RVEF, right ventricular ejection fraction; RVESVI, right ventricular end-systolic volume index.
Values are mean ± SD.
Adapted from MacNee et al.[69]

Table 15A.7 *Evolution of arterial blood gases and hemodynamic variables before and during an episode of peripheral edema in COPD patients*

	RVEDP (mmHg)		PAP (mmHg)		Q̇ (L/min/m²)		PaO₂ (mmHg)		PaCO₂ (mmHg)	
	T1	T2	T1	T2	T1	T2	T1	T2	T1	T2
Group 1 (n = 9)	7.5 ± 3.9	13.4 ± 1.2*	27 ± 5	40 ± 6*	3.23 ± 0.82	3.19 ± 1.07	63 ± 4	49 ± 7*	46 ± 7	59 ± 14*
Group 2 (n = 7)	5.5 ± 2.4	5.1 ± 1.5	20 ± 6	21 ± 5	3.63 ± 0.36	3.29 ± 1.32	66 ± 7	59 ± 7	42 ± 6	45 ± 6

PaCO₂, arterial partial pressure of CO₂; PaO₂, arterial partial pressure of O₂; PAP, pulmonary artery mean pressure; Q̇, cardiac output; RVEDP, right ventricular end-diastolic pressure. T1, stable state of the disease; T2, episode of edema. Group 1, patients with hemodynamic signs of right heart failure (elevated RVEDP); group 2, patients without hemodynamic signs of right heart failure.
Values are mean ± SD.
Adapted from Weitzenblum et al.[39]
*Difference between T1 and T2 statistically significant, $P < 0.001$.

known and may vary from one patient to another. Undoubtedly there is a relationship between the severity of pulmonary hypertension and the development of RHF.

Episodes of RHF are reversible under treatment, but they recur in patients with advanced disease. The occurrence of RHF was classically an indicator of poor prognosis in COPD patients,[64] but further studies have clearly shown that a prolonged survival of 10 years and more could be observed after the first episode of peripheral edema.[54] It must be underlined that the prevalence of clinical RHF has markedly decreased with the prescription of long-term oxygen therapy to the most hypoxemic COPD patients.

Peripheral edema is frequently observed in advanced COPD patients and is considered to reflect RHF, but the possible occurrence of RHF in COPD patients has been questioned,[65,66] in particular because the degree of pulmonary hypertension is most often mild in COPD (see above). Peripheral edema may simply indicate the presence of secondary hyperaldosteronism[67] induced by functional

renal insufficiency which is, in turn, a consequence of hypercapnic acidosis and/or hypoxemia.[67,68] In COPD patients, the presence of edema is not synonymous with heart failure.

The role of pressure overload in the development of RHF in these patients has also been debated. MacNee et al.[69] have found no difference in PAP between six COPD patients with marked peripheral edema and hemodynamic signs of RHF and eight other similar patients without edema and without hemodynamic signs of RHF (Table 15A.6). They concluded that RHF in these patients was probably due to causes other than pulmonary hypertension. On the other hand, some COPD patients with peripheral edema do have RHF, as illustrated in Table 15A.7, which shows data in 16 COPD patients investigated before and during an episode of marked peripheral edema.[39] In nine of 16 patients, hemodynamic signs of RHF [elevated (≥12 mmHg) right ventricular end-diastolic pressure] were present during the episode of edema and were probably accounted for by a significant worsening of pulmonary hypertension (from 27 ± 5 to 40 ± 6 mmHg, $P < 0.001$), which in turn was explained by a worsening of hypoxemia and hypercapnia.[39]

The best way of assessing right ventricular performance is to measure right ventricular contractility (end-systolic pressure/volume relationship) of the right ventricle, but indeed this cannot be done routinely. Right ventricular contractility is near normal in COPD patients with pulmonary hypertension investigated in the stable state of the disease.[70] On the other hand, right ventricular ejection fraction (RVEF) is not a good index of right ventricular contractility since a decreased RVEF is most often the consequence of an increased afterload (increased PAP or PVR or both).[71] The only circumstances where a diminished right ventricular contractility could be documented in COPD patients were the acute exacerbations with the presence of marked peripheral edema[69] (see Table 15A.6).

In summary, many patients with advanced COPD will never develop RHF and, on the other hand, at least some patients experience episodes of true RHF during exacerbations of the disease accompanied by a worsening of pulmonary hypertension.

PROGNOSIS OF PULMONARY HYPERTENSION IN CHRONIC RESPIRATORY DISEASES

The level of PAP is a good indicator of prognosis in COPD,[37,55,72] but also in various categories of chronic respiratory disease such as IPF and sequelae of pulmonary tuberculosis.[72] Prognosis is worse in patients with pulmonary hypertension when compared to patients without pulmonary hypertension (see Figure 15A.5). The prognosis is particularly poor for patients with severe degrees of pulmonary hypertension,[55] but we have seen that in COPD patients (and this also applies to most of other chronic respiratory diseases) PAP measured in the stable state of the disease is most often <35 mmHg. In most of the studies, COPD patients with a modest degree of pulmonary hypertension (20–35 mmHg) have a poor prognosis with a 5-year survival rate of about 50%.[37,55] In fact, all the patients included in the above-mentioned studies received conventional treatment but not long-term oxygen therapy (LTOT). LTOT significantly improves the survival of hypoxemic COPD patients, as demonstrated by the NOTT and MRC trials[73,74] that have included a majority of patients with pulmonary hypertension. Consequently, it can be expected that the prognosis of pulmonary hypertension will improve with LTOT, as suggested by Cooper et al.[75] who observed an overall 5-year survival rate of 62% in 72 severe COPD patients, on LTOT, whose mean initial PAP was 28 ± 10 mmHg. This improved prognosis

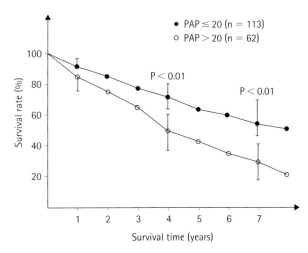

Figure 15A.5 *Survival of chronic obstructive pulmonary disease patients according to the presence or not of pulmonary hypertension. PAP, pulmonary artery pressure (personal data).*

could partly be explained by the reduction of episodes of RHF under LTOT.

Interestingly, PAP is still an excellent prognostic indicator in COPD patients treated with LTOT. Our group[76] has observed that in COPD patients under LTOT, the 5-year survival rate was 66% in those whose initial PAP was <25 mmHg, but only 36% when initial PAP was >25 mmHg ($P < 0.001$). The prognostic value of PAP can be explained by the fact that it is a good marker of both the duration and the severity of alveolar hypoxia in these patients.[76]

TREATMENT OF PULMONARY HYPERTENSION

The treatment of RHF combines diuretics (most often frusemide) and oxygen therapy. Digitalis is used only in the case of an associated left heart failure or in the case of arrhythmia. The treatment of pulmonary hypertension includes vasodilators and LTOT, both of which are considered in detail in Chapter 15C. We will just try to answer the following: Is it really necessary to treat pulmonary hypertension in chronic hypoxic lung disease? Is the treatment of the disease itself (e.g. COPD) not sufficient? As has been seen, pulmonary hypertension is generally mild to moderate in COPD and the necessity of treating such hypertension can be questioned.[77] The best argument in favor of treatment is that pulmonary hypertension, even when modest at rest and during a stable state of the disease, may worsen, particularly during acute exacerbations and exercise, and that these acute increases in PAP can contribute to the development of RHF.[77]

KEY POINTS

- Pulmonary hypertension complicating chronic respiratory disease is generally defined by the presence of a resting pulmonary artery mean pressure (PAP >20 mmHg), which is slightly different from the definition of 'primary' pulmonary hypertension (>25 mmHg).

- In the 'natural history' of chronic obstructive pulmonary disease (COPD), pulmonary hypertension is often preceded by an abnormally large increase in PAP during exercise, defined by a pressure >30 mmHg for a mild level (30–40 watts) of steady-state exercise.

- COPD is by far the major cause of chronic hypoxic pulmonary hypertension.

- In COPD, alveolar hypoxia is the first cause of pulmonary hypertension. Acute hypoxia causes pulmonary vasoconstriction and chronic longstanding hypoxia induces pulmonary vascular remodeling.

- In chronic respiratory disease, pulmonary hypertension is most often of mild to moderate degree (20–35 mmHg), but it may worsen markedly during exercise, sleep and acute exacerbations of the disease.

- The progression of pulmonary hypertension is slow in most COPD patients, with a mean yearly change of PAP of approximately +0.5 mmHg/year. However, a minority (approximately 30%) of COPD patients exhibit a marked worsening of pulmonary hemodynamics, which should be detected as soon as possible.

- Many patients with advanced COPD will never develop right heart failure, but other patients experience episodes of right heart failure during exacerbations of the disease accompanied by a worsening of pulmonary hypertension.

- The level of PAP is a good indicator of prognosis in COPD but also in various categories of chronic respiratory disease.

- Long-term oxygen therapy is at present the best treatment of pulmonary hypertension in chronic respiratory failure. In the future, the treatment may combine oxygen therapy and specific vasodilators.

REFERENCES

*1 Rich S (ed.). Primary pulmonary hypertension. Executive Summary from the World Symposium, Evian, France, September 6.10.1998. World Health Organization.

*2 Chronic cor pulmonale. Report of an expert committee. *Circulation* 1963;**27**:594–615.

◆3 MacNee W. Pathophysiology of cor pulmonale in chronic obstructive pulmonary disease. *Am J Respir Crit Care Med* 1994;**150**:833–52;1158–68.

◆4 Fishman AP. Chronic cor pulmonale. *Am Rev Respir Dis* 1978;**114**:775–94.

●5 Rich S, Dantzker DR, Ayres SM. Primary pulmonary hypertension: a national prospective study. *Ann Intern Med* 1987;**107**:216–23.

6 Tartulier M, Bourret M, Deyrieux F. Les pressions artérielles pulmonaires chez l'homme normal. Effets de l'âge et de l'exercice musculaire. *Bull Physiopathol Respir* 1972;**8**:1295–321.

7 Kessler R, Faller M, Weitzenblum E *et al*. 'Natural history' of pulmonary hypertension in a series of 131 patients with chronic obstructive lung disease. *Am J Respir Crit Care Med* 2001;**164**:219–24.

8 Naeije R, Torbicki A. More on the non-invasive diagnosis of pulmonary hypertension: doppler echocardiography revisited. *Eur Respir J* 1995;**8**:1445–9.

●9 Williams BT, Nicholl JP. Prevalence of hypoxaemic chronic obstructive lung disease with reference to long-term oxygen therapy. *Lancet* 1985;**1**:369–72.

*10 Pauwels RA, Buist AS, Calverley PM *et al*. on behalf of the GOLD Scientific Committee. Global strategy for the diagnosis, management, and prevention of chronic obstructive pulmonary disease. *Am J Respir Crit Care Med* 2001;**163**:1256–76.

11 Lockhart A, Tzareva M, Schrijen F *et al*. Etudes hémodynamiques des décompensations respiratoires aiguës des bronchopneumopathies chroniques. *Bull Physiopathol Respir* 1967;**3**:645–67.

●12 Lockhart A, Tzareva M, Nader F *et al*. Elevated pulmonary artery wedge pressure at rest and during exercise in chronic bronchitis: fact or fancy. *Clin Sci* 1969;**37**:503–17.

13 Lockhart A. Hémodynamique pulmonaire dans la bronchite chronqiue. *Bull Physiopathol Respir* 1973;**9**:1069–99.

◆14 Fishman AP. Hypoxia and its effects on the pulmonary circulation. How and where it acts. *Circ Res* 1979;**38**:221–31.

●15 von Euler US, Liljestrand G. Observations on the pulmonary arterial blood pressure in the cat. *Acta Physiol Scand* 1946;**12**:301–20.

●16 Motley HL, Cournand A, Werko L *et al*. The influence of short periods of induced acute hypoxia upon pulmonary artery pressure in man. *Am J Physiol* 1947;**150**:315–20.

●17 Fishman AP, McClement J, Himmelstein A *et al*. Effects of acute anoxia on the circulation and respiration in patients with chronic pulmonary disease studied during the steady state. *J Clin Invest* 1952;**31**:770–81.

●18 Dinh-Xuan AT, Higenbottam TW, Clelland CA *et al*. Impairment of endothelium-dependent pulmonary artery relaxation in chronic obstructive lung disease. *N Engl J Med* 1991;**324**:1539–47.

19 Grover RF. Chronic hypoxic pulmonary hypertension. In: Fishman AP (ed.), *The pulmonary circulation: normal and abnormal*. Philadelphia: University of Pensylvania Press, 1990;283–99.

20 Weitzenblum E, Schrijen F, Mohan-Kumar T *et al*. Variability of the pulmonary vascular response to acute hypoxia in chronic bronchitis. *Chest* 1988;**94**:772–8.

●21 Penaloza D, Sime F, Banchero N *et al*. Pulmonary hypertension in healthy men born and living at high altitude. *Med Thorac* 1962;**19**:449–60.

22 Harris P, Heath D. *The human pulmonary circulation*. Edinburgh: Churchill Livingstone, 1986;702 pages.

23 Wilkinson M, Langhorne CA, Heath D *et al*. A pathophysiological study of 10 cases of hypoxic cor pulmonale. *Q J Med* 1988;**66**:65–85.

24 Calverley PMA, Howatson R, Flenley DC *et al*. Clinicopathological correlations in cor pulmonale. Thorax 1992;**47**:494–8.

25 Wright JL, Lawson L, Pare PD *et al*. The structure and function of the pulmonary vasculature in mild chronic obstructive pulmonary disease. *Am Rev Respir Dis* 1983;**128**:702–7.

●26 Barbera JA, Riverola A, Roca J *et al*. Pulmonary vascular abnormalities and ventilation–perfusion relationships in mild chronic obstructive pulmonary disease. *Am J Respir Crit Care Med* 1994; **149**:423–9.

27 Hale KA, Niewoehner DE, Cosio MG. Morphologic changes in the muscular pulmonary arteries: relationship to cigarette smoking, airway disease, and emphysema. *Am Rev Respir Dis* 1980;**122**:273–8.

28 Santos S, Peinado VI, Ramirez J *et al*. Characterization of pulmonary vascular remodelling in smokers and patients with mild COPD. *Eur Respir J* 2002;**19**:632–8.

29 Peinado VI, Barbera JA, Ramirez J *et al*. Endothelial dysfunction in pulmonary arteries of patients with mild COPD. *Am J Physiol* 1998;**274**:L908–13.

30 Barbera JA, Peinado VI, Santos S. Pulmonary hypertension in COPD: old and new concepts. *Monaldi Arch Chest Dis* 1999;**55**:445–9.

●31 Enson Y, Giuntini C, Lewis ML *et al*. The influence of hydrogen ion concentration and hypoxia on the pulmonary circulation. *J Clin Invest* 1964;**43**:1146–62.

●32 Segel N, Bishop JM. The circulation in patients with chronic bronchitis and emphysema at rest and during exercise with special reference to the influence of changes in blood viscosity and blood volume on the pulmonary circulation. *J Clin Invest* 1966;**45**:1555–68.

●33 Harris P, Segel N, Green I *et al*. The influence of the airways resistance and alveolar pressure on the pulmonary vascular resistance in chronic bronchitis. *Cardiovasc Res* 1968;**2**:84–92.

34 Luchsinger CP, Moser KM, Buchlamm N *et al*. The interrelationship between cor pulmonale, capillary bed restriction and diffusion insufficiency for oxygen in the lungs. *Am Heart J* 1957;**54**:106–7.

35 Enson Y, Thomas HM, Bosken CH *et al*. Pulmonary Hypertension in interstitial lung disease: relation of vascular resistance to abnormal lung structure. *Trans Assoc Am Physicians* 1975;**88**:248–55.

36 Weitzenblum E, Ehrhart M, Rasaholinhanahary J *et al*. Pulmonary hemodynamics in idiopathic pulmonary fibrosis and other interstitial pulmonary diseases. *Respiration* 1983;**44**:118–27.

●37 Weitzenblum E, Hirth C, Ducolone A *et al*. Prognostic value of pulmonary artery pressure in chronic obstructive pulmonary disease. *Thorax* 1981;**36**:752–8.

38 Chaouat A, Weitzenblum E, Krieger J *et al*. Pulmonary hemodynamics in the obstructive sleep apnea syndrome. Results in 220 consecutive patients. *Chest* 1996;**109**:380–6.

39 Weitzenblum E, Apprill M, Oswald M *et al*. Pulmonary hemodynamics in patients with chronic obstructive pulmonary disease before and during an episode of peripheral edema. *Chest* 1994;**105**:1377–82.

40 Tramarin R, Torbicki A, Marchandise B *et al*. Doppler echocardiographic evaluation of pulmonary artery pressure in chronic obstructive pulmonary disease. A European multicentre study. *Eur Heart J* 1991;**12**:103–11.

●41 Horsfield K, Segel N, Bishop JM. The pulmonary circulation in chronic bronchitis at rest and during exercise breathing air and 80% oxygen. *Clin Sci* 1968;**43**:473–83.

42 Weitzenblum E, El Gharbi T, Vandevenne A *et al*. L'hémodynamique pulmonaire au cours de l'exercice musculaire dans la bronchite chronique non 'décompensée'. *Bull Physiopathol Respir* 1972;**8**:49–71.

43 Jezek V, Schrijen F, Sadoul P. Right ventricular function and pulmonary hemodynamics during exercise in patients with chronic obstructive bronchopulmonary disease. *Cardiology* 1973;**58**:20–31.

●44 Coccagna G, Lugaresi E. Arterial blood gases and pulmonary and systemic arterial pressure during sleep in chronic obstructive pulmonary disease. *Sleep* 1978;**1**:117–24.

45 Boysen PG, Block AJ, Wynne JW *et al*. Nocturnal pulmonary hypertension in patients with chronic obstructive pulmonary disease. *Chest* 1979;**76**:538–42.

46 Weitzenblum E, Muzet A, Ehrhart M *et al*. Variations nocturnes des gaz du sang et de la pression artérielle pulmonaire chez les bronchitiques chroniques insuffisants respiratoires. *Nouv Presse Méd* 1982;**11**:1119–22.

●47 Fletcher EC, Levin DC. Cardiopulmonary hemodynamics during sleep in subjects with chronic obstructive pulmonary disease: the effect of short and long-term oxygen. *Chest* 1984;**85**:6–14.

●48 Wynne JW, Block AJ, Hemenway J *et al*. Disordered breathing and oxygen desaturation during sleep in patients with chronic obstructive lung disease. *Am J Med* 1979; **66**:573–9.

●49 Catterall JR, Douglas NJ, Calverley PMA *et al*. Transient hypoxemia during sleep in chronic obstructive pulmonary disease is not a sleep apnea syndrome. *Am Rev Respir Dis* 1983;**128**:24–9.

50 Hudgel DW, Martin RJ, Capheart M *et al*. Contribution of hypoventilation to sleep oxygen desaturation in chronic obstructive pulmonary disease. *J Appl Physiol* 1983;**55**:669–77.

51 Flechter EC, Gray BA, Levin DC. Non-apneic mechanism of arterial oxygen desaturation during rapid-eye-movement sleep. *J Appl Physiol* 1983;**54**:632–9.

●52 Abraham AS, Cole Rb, Green ID *et al*. Factors contributing to the reversible pulmonary hypertension of patients with acute respiratory failure studied by serial observations during recovery. *Circ Res* 1969;**24**:51–60.

53 Weitzenblum E, Hirth C, Roeslin N *et al*. Les modifications hémodynamiques pulmonaires au cours de l'insuffisance respiratoire aiguë des bronchopneumopathies chroniques. *Respiration* 1971;**28**:539–54.

54 Weitzenblum E, Loiseau A, Hirth C et al. Course of pulmonary hemodynamics in patients with chronic obstructive pulmonary disease. *Chest* 1979;**75**:656–62.

55 Ourednik A, Susa Z. How long does the pulmonary hypertension last in chronic obstructive bronchopulmonary disease? In: Widimsky J (ed.), *Progress in respiration research. Pulmonary hypertension.* Basel: Karger, 1975;24–8.

56 Boushy SF, North LB. Hemodynamic changes in chronic obstructive pulmonary disease. *Chest* 1977;**72**:565–70.

57 Schrijen F, Uffholtz H, Polu JM et al. Pulmonary and systemic hemodynamic evolution in chronic bronchitis. *Am Rev Respir Dis* 1978;**117**:25–31.

●58 Weitzenblum E, Sautegeau A, Ehrhart M et al. Long-term course of pulmonary arterial pressure in chronic obstructive pulmonary disease. *Am Rev Respir Dis* 1984;**130**:993–8.

●59 Timms RM, Khaja FU, Williams GW and the Nocturnal Oxygen Therapy Trial Group. Hemodynamic response to oxygen therapy in chronic obstructive pulmonary disease. *Ann Intern Med* 1985;**102**:29–36.

●60 Weitzenblum E, Sautegeau A, Ehrhart M et al. Long term oxygen therapy can reverse the progression of pulmonary hypertension in patients with chronic obstructive pulmonary disease. *Am Rev Respir Dis* 1985;**131**:493–8.

61 Zielinski J, Tobiasz M, Hawrylkiewicz I et al. Effects of long-term oxygen therapy on pulmonary hemodynamics in COPD patients. A 6-year prospective study. *Chest* 1998;**113**:65–70.

62 Jezek V, Fucik J, Michaljanic A et al. Long-term development of pulmonary hypertension in interstitial lung fibrosis. In: *XVIe International Congress of Internal Medicine, Prague 1982*, Abstract book, p. 236.

63 Chaouat A, Weitzenblum E, Kessler R et al. Five-year effects of nasal continuous positive airway pressure in obstructive sleep apnoea syndrome. *Eur Respir J* 1997;**10**:2578–82.

64 Vandenbergh E, Clement J, Van De Woestijne KP. Course and prognosis of patients with advanced chronic obstructive pulmonary disease. *Am J Med* 1973;**55**:736–46.

65 Editorial. Edema in cor pulmonale. *Lancet* 1975;**ii**:1289–90.

66 Richens JM, Howard P. Oedema in cor pulmonale. *Clin Sci* 1982;**62**:255–9.

●67 Farber MO, Weinberger MH, Robertson GL et al. Hormonal abnormalities affecting sodium and water balance in acute respiratory failure due to chronic obstructive lung disease. *Chest* 1984;**85**:49–54.

●68 Aber GM, Bishop JM. Serial changes in renal function, arterial gas tension and the acid-base state in patients with chronic bronchitis and edema. *Clin Sci* 1965;**28**:511–25.

69 MacNee W, Wathen C, Flenley DC et al. The effects of controlled oxygen therapy on ventricular function in patients with stable and decompensated cor pulmonale. *Am Rev Respir Dis* 1988;**137**:1289–95.

70 Burghuber OC. Right ventricular contractility is preserved and preload increased in patients with chronic obstructive pulmonary disease and pulmonary artery hypertension. In: Jezek V, Morpurgo M, Tramarin R (eds), *Current topics in rehabilitation. Right ventricular hypertrophy and function in chronic lung disease.* Berlin: Springer-Verlag, 1992;135–41.

71 Brent BN, Berger HJ, Matthay RA et al. Physiologic correlates of right ventricular ejection fraction in chronic obstructive pulmonary disease: a combined radionuclide and hemodynamic study. *Am J Cardiol* 1982;**50**:255–62.

72 Bishop JM, Cross KW. Physiological variables and mortality in patients with various categories of chronic respiratory disease. *Bull Eur Physiopathol Respir* 1984;**20**:495–500.

●73 Nocturnal Oxygen Therapy Trial Group. Continuous or nocturnal oxygen therapy in hypoxemic chronic obstructive lung disease. *Ann Intern Med* 1980;**93**:391–8.

●74 Report of the Medical Research Council Working Party. Long-term domiciliary oxygen therapy in chronic hypoxic cor pulmonale complicating chronic bronchitis and emphysema. *Lancet* 1981;**1**:681–6.

75 Cooper CB, Waterhouse J, Howard P. Twelve year clinical study of patients with hypoxic cor pulmonale given long term domiciliary oxygen therapy. *Thorax* 1987;**42**:105–10.

76 Oswald-Mammosser M, Weitzenblum E, Quoix E et al. Prognostic factors in COPD patients receiving long-term oxygen therapy. *Chest* 1995;**107**:1193–8.

77 Weitzenblum E, Kessler R, Oswald M et al. Medical treatment of pulmonary hypertension in chronic lung disease. *Eur Respir J* 1994;**7**:148–52.

Pulmonary circulation in obstructive sleep apnea

JOHN STRADLING

INTRODUCTION

Obstructive sleep apnea (OSA) is an upper airway respiratory problem that has profound acute effects on the cardiovascular system, both pulmonary and systemic. Despite the surge of research work on cardiopulmonary interactions during OSA, there is still some uncertainty over the cause of both the acute changes in pulmonary artery pressure (PAP), and whether there are any significant long-term changes to the pulmonary circulation.

Obstructive sleep apnea is essentially a series of brief Mueller maneuvers (inspiration against a closed upper airway) of increasing intensity, terminated by a phase of hyperpnea. One apnea may last up to 2 minutes or so, but about 40 seconds is a common average. During these 40 seconds of apnea, there may be 10 or so frustrated inspiratory efforts of increasing strength with the initial normal efforts generating usual pleural pressures (for example, $-7\,cmH_2O$), and the final efforts (just before the apnea ends) generating pressures as low as $-50\,cmH_2O$ or even lower (Figure 15B.1). Thus the pattern is not like a classical

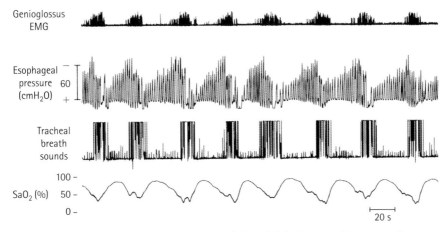

Figure 15B.1 *Five-minute tracing from a patient with sleep apnea (left to right). There are eight cycles of apnea and recovery (indicated by the alternate absence and return of tracheal breath sounds). Note the fall in arterial oxygen saturation (SaO_2) during the apneas (a little delayed due to the circulation time from the lung to the peripherally placed oximeter probe). During the actual apneas there is gradually increasing inspiratory effort that falls again once airflow resumes. EMG, electromyograph. (Reproduced with permission from Fletcher EC. Abnormalities of respiration during sleep. Orlando, FL: Grune an Stratton, 1986.)*

Mueller maneuver, where a constant inspiratory pressure is held for 30 seconds or so. Because of the absence of gas exchange during the apnea, there is a rapid fall in PaO_2 (or SaO_2, Figure 15B.1), the actual rate of fall depending on O_2 stores in the lung and the body's oxygen consumption (VO_2): apneas occur at end inspiration so that the lung volume is the functional residual capacity (FRC), and thus influenced by posture and obesity. The rate of fall of PaO_2 is usually about 8 kPa/min (60 mmHg/min).[1] In addition to the gradual and continuing PaO_2 fall, there will be a rapid rise in $PaCO_2$ to mixed venous levels, over 30 seconds or so, and then a more gradual rise [about 0.6 kPa/min (4.5 mmHg/min)] that depends on the body's carbon dioxide production (VCO_2) and buffering power of the whole body CO_2 stores.

During the apnea the 'diving reflex' is recruited due to the absence of lung expansion, the hypoxemia, and possibly pharyngeal stimulation (similar to trigeminal nerve stimulation).[2,3] This provokes a bradycardia and activation of sympathetic vasoconstriction in some vascular beds (e.g. muscle and viscera).[4]

At the termination of apnea there is an arousal with activation of the orienting reflex.[5–7] This produces sympathetic vasoconstriction in a different pattern of vascular beds, with a reduction in skin blood flow, a rise in blood pressure, and a tachycardia.

Because these apneas often recur all night (producing 300 or more cycles of altered cardiovascular variables), there is also the potential for the development of progressive changes across the night, in addition to the more acute ones.

This chapter describes what is known about the effects of OSA on the pulmonary circulation and the right ventricle, both acutely and chronically. Although there are interesting changes, there is no good evidence that they are of any prognostic importance.

ACUTE RIGHT–SIDED CHANGES IN OBSTRUCTIVE SLEEP APNEA

Early recordings of PAP during periods of OSA[8] were measured relative to atmospheric pressure and, therefore, included the large intrathoracic swings, similar to those recorded from an esophageal catheter (Figure 15B.2). However, the pressures of perhaps more interest are the transmural PAPs, obtained either by referencing the pressure to pleural, or by inspecting the tracings during passive expiration between the inspiratory efforts. This is sometimes not possible because of active expiratory efforts producing positive pleural pressure swings. Most studies have shown a gradual rise in transmural pressure during the actual apnea, with a further (steeper) rise at apnea termination, and a fall again as the hyperpnea fades away

and apnea returns. Maximum pressures reached may be as high as 100 mmHg, or even higher in those patients with severe OSA.[8] Finally, there is also a much more gradual rise in PAP over many cycles of OSA.

Various explanations have been advanced for these rises in PAP.[9–12] Possibilities include the hypoxic pulmonary vasoconstriction, reflex vasoconstriction on arousal, and the mechanical consequences of the Mueller maneuvers, that is, increased venous return and reduced left ventricular outflow.

Hypoxia

Hypoxia is clearly a potential stimulus to pulmonary arteriolar vasoconstriction. One would expect the vasoconstriction and consequent rise in PAP to lag behind the hypoxia and, although there is a small delay of a few seconds, the individual rise in PAP with each apnea is still too fast to be explicable on this basis. It would also not explain the clear biphasic nature of the PAP rise (occurring during and then again immediately after the apnea), because during each apneic cycle there is one smooth fall and rise in PaO_2. However, early studies did show a correlation between the maximum rise in PAP and the nadir in PaO_2 (or SaO_2), initially suggesting a causal relationship.[9] By contrast, careful studies in sleeping patients with OSA have been performed using added inspired oxygen (to raise PaO_2 during the apneas) that failed to influence significantly the acute apnea-to-apnea changes, or the mean nocturnal rises, in PAP.[10] A complication of this latter study, which resulted from raising the lowest PaO_2 value during OSA by about 18 mmHg, was that $PaCO_2$ also rose by about 6 mmHg, partly through the Douglas Haldane effect, and partly through apnea prolongation (on average from 25 to 30 seconds). Since $PaCO_2$ is also a stimulus to pulmonary vasoconstriction,[13] it is possible that a beneficial effect of raising the nadirs in PaO_2 by 18 mmHg was offset by a rise in PCO_2 of 6 mmHg.

In an anesthetized dog model of obstructive apneas, it was claimed that the rise in PAP during the period of obstruction could be abolished by removing the hypoxia.[14] However, alleviating the hypoxia during the fixed-length apneas also reduced, to less than half, the inspiratory effort, which could also have contributed to the reduction in PAP response (Figure 15B.3). Whether anesthesia alters the PAP responses is not known, but there are certainly differences in the response of the systemic circulation to hypoxia, depending on whether the subjects are asleep or not and, of course, arousal does not occur during anesthesia. The levels of hypoxia used in this experiment were very severe (down to 25% SaO_2) and not much change in PAP was seen until SaO_2 fell below 80%; many patients with OSA do not fall even as low as 80% SaO_2, yet experience the oscillations in pulmonary (and systemic) pressures.

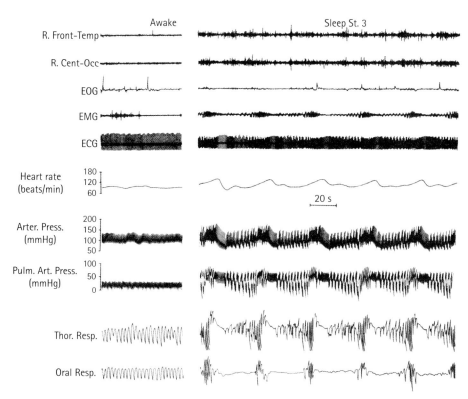

Figure 15B.2 *Recordings awake and asleep in a patient with obstructive sleep apnea (OSA) (left to right). Top two lines are the electroencephalogram; lines 3–5 are eye movements, chin muscle tone and electrocardiogram, respectively. The bottom two lines are ribcage movement and oral airflow, respectively. Note that during wakefulness, SAP (systemic arterial pressure) is fairly stable, and PAP (pulmonary arterial pressure) is about 25 mmHg systolic. While asleep, the swings in pleural pressures during the apneas are reflected in the SAP and the PAP. Transient rises in pressure on arousal are also present in both tracings. On average, PAP is considerably higher than during wakefulness, particularly obvious during the expiratory pauses. (Reproduced with permission from Coccagna G, Mantovani M, Brignani F et al. Continuous recording of the pulmonary and systemic arterial pressure during sleep in syndromes of hypersomnia with periodic breathing.* Bull Eur Physiopathol Respir *1972;8:1159–72.)*

In an attempt to separate out the possible effects of hypoxia versus the negative intrathoracic pressure swings, Marrone et al.[15] compared apneas during REM and non-REM sleep. During REM sleep there is much more profound hypoxia at any given degree of inspiratory effort and, therefore, pleural pressure swings. They found that PAP rose more during REM and ascribed it to the greater hypoxia, although once again $PaCO_2$ levels would have been slightly higher because of the longer apneas. Control of the pulmonary circulation may also be different during REM sleep, just as it is in the systemic circulation, due to changes in sympathetic/parasympathetic balance.

Thus, there is conflicting evidence as to whether hypoxia plays the dominant part in the PAP rises seen in during the actual apneic events in patients with OSA.

Mechanical effects

One of the alternative explanations for acute PAP rises in OSA centers on the effect the recurrent Mueller maneuvers themselves might have.

SYSTEMIC VENOUS RETURN

Dropping intrathoracic pressure and raising intra-abdominal pressure will tend to drive venous blood into the right atrium,[16] increasing right ventricular preload and right-sided cardiac output (CO). This would be expected to raise PAP to some extent. However, there is a limit to the effectiveness of this venous aspiration mechanism.[17] The subatmospheric intrathoracic pressures will certainly lower intrathoracic vena caval pressures relative to extrathoracic pressures. However, these intrathoracic subatmospheric pressures will tend to be transmitted, along the vena caval lumina, to just outside the boundaries of the thoracic cage.[18] This leads to 'pinching off' of the great veins at the point of entry into the thorax (Figure 15B.4) and limits the inflow of venous blood. The extent of this paradoxical effect will depend on the prevailing level of venous pressure. In the presence of a raised central venous pressure, then, the inspiratory intrathoracic falls are less likely to generate intraluminal vena caval pressures that are below the external pressures at the points of entry to the thoracic cage. Langanke et al.[19] have looked at this

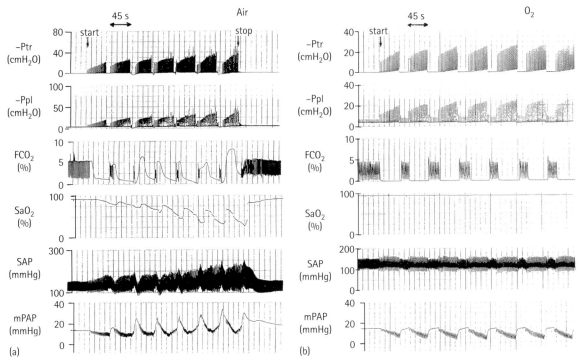

Figure 15B.3 *Two tracings (left to right) from an anesthetized dog breathing air (a) and added O_2 (b). The top two lines are the tracheal and pleural subatmospheric pressures showing the simulated periods of obstructive sleep apnea (OSA). Lines 3–6 are expired CO_2 (FCO_2%), arterial oxygen saturation (SaO_2%), systemic arterial pressure (SAP) and mean pulmonary artery pressure (mPAP), respectively. Note the changes in some of the scale ranges in (b) compared to (a). When hypoxia is allowed to develop during the apneas, then mPAP rises with each apnea (a). When hypoxia is prevented, then mPAP actually falls during the periods of obstruction (b). (Reproduced with permission from Iwase N, Kikuchi Y, Hida W et al. Effects of repetitive airway obstruction on O2 saturation and systemic and pulmonary artery pressure in anesthetized dogs. Am Rev Respir Dis 1992;**146**:1402–10).*

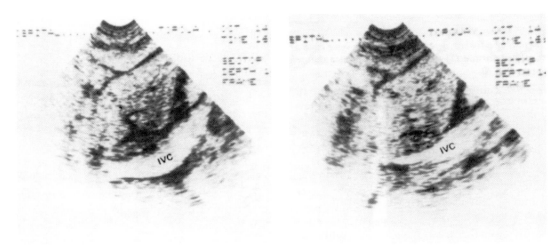

Figure 15B.4 *Real time ultrasonography views of the inferior vena cava (IVC) just below the diaphragm in a supine man. The right panel is during inspiration and demonstrates the 'pinching off' of the IVC compared to the situation during expiration (left panel). (Reproduced with permission from Gardner AMN, Fox RH. The return of blood to the heart. London: John Libbey, 1989.)*

phenomenon during OSA and shown that in some patients there remains increased flow into the right atrium down to quite considerable subatmospheric levels during the increased inspiratory efforts of a Mueller maneuver.

However, this was not true in all patients, with some demonstrating clear limitation of venous flow, which could vary through the night, perhaps due to small changes in posture, for example.

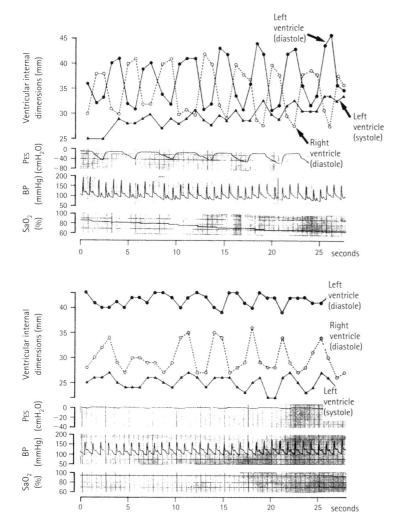

Figure 15B.5 *Measurements of internal ventricular dimensions by echocardiography (first line) in one patient with obstructive sleep apnea (OSA) (upper panel), and again while on nasal continuous positive airway pressure (CPAP) to abolish the apneas (lower panel). Lines 2–4 of each panel are esophageal pressure, systemic BP and arterial oxygen saturation (%), respectively. Note that during the obstructed inspiratory efforts (seen on the esophageal pressure tracing), the right ventricular diastolic diameter increases (from about 30 to 40 mm) and that left ventricular diastolic dimensions decrease (from about 42 to 32 mm). This could be seen to reflect a diastolic shift of the interventricular septum from right to left. The ventricular systolic dimensions gradually rise across the apnea probably reflecting the increase in left ventricular afterload during the falls in pleural pressure. (Reproduced with permission from Shiomi T, Guilleminault C, Stoohs R et al. Leftward shift of the interventricular septum and pulsus paradoxus in OSA syndrome. Chest 1991;100:894–902.)*

Supporting the idea of an increase in venous return to the right heart has been the demonstration of a leftward shift of the interventricular septum during OSA[20] (Figure 15B.5). It is extremely difficult to maintain clear echocardiographic visualization of the septum in obese patients, particularly during the obstructed inspirations when the heart tends to rotate, and such data are not regarded as totally definitive.

This increased venous return could certainly account for the small rise in PAP during the period of apneas. It is harder to ascribe the bigger rise in PAP at the end of the apnea to yet further increases in venous return, although there is, of course, a short period of marked hyperventilation and large pleural pressure swings when the apnea breaks, which would also encourage venous return.

LEFT VENTRICULAR OUTFLOW

Repetitive Mueller maneuvers also effect left ventricular function. By dropping the pressure surrounding the left ventricle, there are increases in both its preload and afterload. In particular, if the heart contracts when pleural

pressures are −50 mmHg, for example, there is a much lower head of pressure in the extrathoracic aorta to perfuse the systemic vascular beds and hence CO must fall (accompanied by a rise in end-systolic volume), although there will be some recovery possible during the expiratory periods of the apneas. Overall, across an apnea, there is a gradual fall in left-sided CO,[21,22] perhaps also contributed to by the increased right ventricular pressure shifting the interventricular septum leftward, as already mentioned. This reduction in CO will in turn raise left atrial and pulmonary venous pressure. Increases in wedge pressure have been shown to occur during OSA,[12] which may be a further factor raising PAP, although the magnitude is hard to gauge. At apnea termination, the left-sided output falls even further, despite both a sympathetically mediated tachycardia (due to arousal), and plenty of preload. In fact, there is a further rise in end-systolic volume at the arousal point.[21] It is suggested that this is due to the arousal itself, with a sympathetically mediated sudden rise in peripheral vascular resistance producing a rise in systemic BP and hence afterload. The tachycardia and continuing systemic venous return could, therefore, provoke the further rise in PAP at apnea termination, particularly when the passage of blood through the left heart has been temporarily held up yet more. It is likely that some of the apparent discrepancies in CO data during OSA[21,22] are because the left and right sides of the heart are being affected differently. Andreas *et al.*[23] looked at flow with Doppler echocardiography across all four heart valves during a conventional Mueller maneuver (-38 mmHg). If only the first few cardiac cycles were considered, so as to best simulate the inspiratory efforts during an apnea, then flow across the mitral valve decreased (-12%), and flow across the tricuspid valve increased ($+15\%$).

Schafer *et al.*[24] correlated changes in PAP with changes in SaO_2, esophageal pressure, systolic BP (as an index of left ventricular afterload) and apnea duration, during the course of apneas in six patients with OSA. On average, PAP rose 10 mmHg across an apnea. Using linear regression modeling, only the changes in SaO_2 and esophageal pressure were independently correlated with this rise in PAP. They also found that average PAP increased during the first half of the night, but not thereafter. This study thus confirms the importance of both hypoxia and mechanical influences on the acute rises in PAP during apneas.

Reflex vasoconstriction

The majority of the rise in peripheral vascular resistance and systemic BP at the termination of apnea can be accounted for by the increase in sympathetic activation on arousal. Systemic BP rises in response to any cause of arousal,[5,25] and it may be that arousal also increases pulmonary vascular resistance via a similar neurological mechanism,[26] thus contributing to the rise in PAP.

In summary, it seems likely that the overall slow rise in PAP over many cycles of OSA is due to hypoxia, when sufficiently severe. The gradual rise in PAP during the apneic cycle is likely to be caused by an increasing systemic venous return (due to aspiration of blood into the thorax) in conjunction with a reduction in left-sided output (from an increased pre- and after-load as well as interventricular shift). At apnea termination, the sharper rise in PAP is probably due to a further fall in left-sided output (increased afterload from BP rises due to systemic sympathetic vasoconstriction) and hence a rise in pulmonary venous pressure, in conjunction with continuing venous return, a tachycardia, and possibly sympathetic vasoconstriction of the pulmonary bed similar to that seen in the systemic bed (due to arousal and the orienting reflex).

CHRONIC RIGHT-SIDED CHANGES IN OBSTRUCTIVE SLEEP APNEA

Although there are clear rises in PAP during periods of OSA, it is not clear whether there is carryover into the awake hours. Despite often profound, episodic, hypoxia for 8 hours a night, most patients with OSA do not develop cor pulmonale or evidence of pulmonary hypertension.[27,28] In studies on obese patients with OSA, the prior use of appetite suppressant drugs as a potential confounder must be remembered.[29]

Experimental evidence from animal studies using intermittent hypoxia have usually shown long-term changes in the pulmonary circulation.[30,31] However, these hypoxic chamber studies have not usually perfectly mimicked the 1–2 minute cycle in patients with OSA, but have either used much longer on/off periods or allowed hypocapnia to develop. It is likely that permanent changes in the pulmonary vasculature require a certain continuous length of stimulus to be initiated. This is similar to erythropoeitin release, for example, where the transient falls in SaO_2 of OSA do not stimulate production of this hormone,[32,33] whereas an equivalent mean SaO_2 maintained for a longer period of time would. Indeed, the most recent animal study that tried to simulate the hypoxia and hypercapnia of OSA, found increases in both PAP and hematocrit.[34] Since in humans OSA very rarely raises hematocrit (except through hemoconcentration), this suggests that in some way the experimental model was different from real OSA.

The early evidence from human studies was that sustained 24-hour hypoxemia is required in patients with OSA before there are right-sided changes. The main cause of diurnal hypoxemia appears to be the coexistence of OSA and chronic lung disease, rather than just being the result of particularly severe OSA alone. The first group to establish this point looked at 46 patients with OSA and compared nine patients with pulmonary hypertension (PAP ≥ 20 mmHg) with those without.[35] The most significant difference was that the nine patients with pulmonary hypertension (mean PAP, 23.4 mmHg versus 13.7 mmHg) had worse daytime hypoxemia (61 versus 76 mmHg), worse hypercapnia (45 versus 38 mmHg) and worse airways obstruction (59 versus 73, $FEV_1/VC\%$). There were no differences in the severity of the OSA. Linear regression identified PaO_2, $PaCO_2$ and lung function as predictors of PAP, rather than OSA severity. Cardiac outputs at rest and on exercise were no different. The Toronto group found similar results using clinical evidence of right heart 'failure', rather than measurements of PAP.[36] In 50 patients with OSA they found six patients with histories of peripheral edema and raised jugular venous pressure (JVP), radiographic evidence of pulmonary artery enlargement, or ECG criteria of right ventricular hypertrophy (RVH) or right axis deviation. These six patients had similar OSA severity but worse daytime hypoxemia (52 versus 75 mmHg), worse hypercapnia (51 versus 76 mmHg), and worse airways obstruction (56 versus 76, $FEV_1/VC\%$).

Support for the concept that OSA alone, without diurnal hypoxemia, does not cause pulmonary hypertension also comes from echocardiographic data. Hanley *et al.*[37]

studied 51 snorers referred to their sleep laboratory (some with OSA), specifically excluding those with awake hypoxemia. They found no evidence of RVH using echocardiographic criteria in those with OSA compared to those without. Berman et al.,[38] in an earlier study, had found a surprisingly high prevalence of RVH by echocardiographic criteria in 50 consecutive patients referred to their sleep laboratory. In fact, 12 of the 32 found to have RVH did not have OSA at all, suggesting a rather low threshold for diagnosing RVH. The awake SaO_2 data are not given, but it is likely that this group contained some patients with baseline hypoxemia. A second study reported the echocardiographic data on 61 patients referred with loud asymptomatic snoring or suspected OSA, but no evidence of left-sided heart failure or other cardiopulmonary diseases.[39] Although left ventricular indices were not influenced by the presence or absence of OSA, there was a correlation between right ventricular wall thickness and severity of sleep apnea. This may, of course, have developed in response to the episodic rises in PAP during apneas, and is not in itself evidence for a chronically raised PAP.

More recent studies have further explored the extent to which pulmonary hypertension can occur in the absence of chronic hypoxic lung disease. For example, Bady et al.[40] performed right heart catheterization on 44 patients with OSA, but no evidence of chronic lung disease. Twenty-seven per cent had a mean PAP at rest of >20 mmHg (with a pulmonary capillary wedge pressure of <15 mmHg). There was no difference in OSA severity between those with and without a raised PAP. However, those with a raised PAP still had a significantly lower daytime PaO_2 (72 versus 85 mmHg), higher daytime $PaCO_2$ (44 versus 40 mmHg), were more obese (37.4 versus 30.3 kg/m^2), and had worse lung function tests compatible with this increased obesity (a restrictive pattern). Linear regression modeling found diurnal PaO_2 and body mass index (BMI) to be the only independent predictors of PAP.

A similar, but more detailed, study looked at 32 patients with OSA who had normal simple lung function tests.[41] PAP was measured during hyperoxia, normoxia and hypoxia, as well as during increased cardiac output (using dobutamine infusions). Eleven (34%) had a resting PAP $\geq$20 mmHg. In comparison with the normal PAP group, there were no differences in simple lung function, severity of OSA, age or obesity. There were minimal increases in small airway closure and $\dot{V}/\dot{Q}$ mismatch in the group with raised PAP. More interestingly, the group with raised PAP had a nearly threefold higher pulmonary vasoconstrictor response to hypoxia, as well as greater rises in PAP in response to increased cardiac output. It is unclear, however, whether these differences were a result of the development of a raised PAP, or represent a premorbid tendency to heightened vascular response. The absence of any relationship to OSA severity is hard to explain if OSA itself were the cause.

Looking in the reverse direction, Blankfield et al.[42] studied 20 subjects with unexplained mild bilateral leg edema who, on further investigation, had echocardiographic evidence of a raised PAP (>30 mmHg). Nine out of 15 (60%) had some OSA, although there was no matched control group, and many were obese. Again, the pulmonary function tests showed restrictive defects only, compatible with the obesity. None of the subjects apparently had daytime hypoxemia, although arterial blood gas estimations were not done, and the standard deviation of the mean oximetric awake SaO_2 (96.4%) was 1.3%, indicating that some were probably hypoxemic.

In children with OSA, there is also evidence that in some severe cases there is ECG, Doppler echocardiographic, and radionuclide evidence of right-sided changes.[43–45] Insofar as changes in right ventricular ejection fractions (RVEF) indicate abnormalities, 10 out of 27 children with sleep apnea had RVEF values below 35% that increased post-adenotonsillectomy (usually curative in children). However, without a control group, regression to the mean is a particularly significant problem with estimations of RVEF and Doppler pressure measurements of PAP, due to their significant variability on repeat estimation.

One group has explored the response of PAP to the long-term treatment of OSA.[46] Sixty-five patients with OSA treated with CPAP for approximately 5 years had two PAP measurements. There was no overall alteration in PaO_2 and a very small (1.5 mmHg) rise in $PaCO_2$ over the 5 years. Mean PAP at rest, or on exercise, did not change over this period (16–17 mmHg). In the subgroup (17%) with initial PAPs >20 mmHg, there was a small, non-significant fall. However, any study selecting subjects with an abnormally high initial value would expect to see a fall on re-examination. Without an untreated control group, which might even experience a further rises in PAP, it is difficult to assess the effects of any treatment. However, there is clearly no large improvement in PAP following treatment of OSA.

There are also other studies that have found mild pulmonary hypertension to occur in a small percentage of patients with OSA, even though they have no obvious evidence of lung disease.[47,48] One of these found left ventricular dysfunction (as measured by pulmonary capillary wedge pressure) to be an important independent predictor of PAP.[47] This suggests that any left ventricular dysfunction might be an important component of any chronic rise in PAP. The same research group have also studied RVEF in the same population,[49] and by linear regression techniques did identify (in the 20% with mildly impaired right ventricular function) that this correlated independently with the severity of OSA. Interestingly, this impairment was not correlated with raised PAP, suggesting that the two may develop independently of each other.

There are very few data on the development of pulmonary hypertension in central sleep hypoventilation or apnea. However, as with OSA, it is likely that episodic hypoxia alone will not produce sustained rises in PAP, and that this will only occur in the presence of associated diurnal ventilatory failure.

In conclusion, it is unusual for pure OSA to produce anything other than minor changes in right ventricular anatomy. For cor pulmonale, or chronically raised levels of PAP, to occur seems to require the development of diurnal hypoxemia, usually on the basis of coexisting lower airways obstruction (e.g. smoking induced or asthmatic). We have also seen the development of diurnal ventilatory failure in OSA when it was present in conjunction with extremely gross obesity and neuromuscular weakness. It has been suggested that poor ability to restore blood gases entirely to normal between each apnea (because of lung disease or weak or disadvantaged respiratory muscles), may provoke the resetting of ventilatory control mechanisms that permit diurnal ventilatory failure and subsequently cor pulmonale. It is possible that raised PAP may occur in isolation in a small subgroup with particularly high hypoxic pulmonary vasoconstrictive reflexes.

ATRIAL AND BRAIN NATRIURETIC PEPTIDE RELEASE IN OSA

Patients with OSA develop true nocturia with reversal of the usual day/night pattern of urine volumes (Figure 15B.6). Lying down during the day induces urine flow, but at night there is a mechanism that prevents this so that most people can sleep for 8 hours without having to wake to pass water. The exact mechanism during sleep that prevents the usual effect of recumbency on urine flow is, rather surprisingly, still not understood. The increased urine flow during OSA has a variety of possible explanations. It may simply be that the sleep fragmentation prevents the usually sleep-related inhibition of urinary flow. Various renally active hormones have been postulated to be important, but of interest here is a possible effect through atrial and brain natriuretic peptide (ANP, BNP) production.

ANP and BNP are released in response to a number of cardiovascular changes, but right atrial distension is certainly one of the more important.[50] As discussed earlier, there is some evidence that the frustrated inspiratory efforts during OSA (Mueller maneuvers) do aspirate more systemic venous blood into the chest, which is not immediately passed through to the systemic circulation, with consequent increases in pulmonary vascular (and presumably right atrial and ventricular) volumes. Along with rises in systemic BP, this would be expected to lead to ANP and BNP release, and thus a reduction in urine flow. In addition, hypoxemia-induced rises in PAP would also be expected to increase ANP and BNP release.

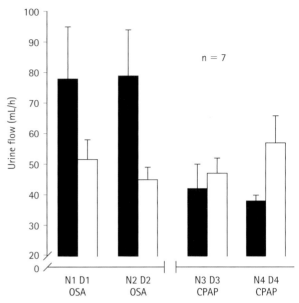

Figure 15B.6 *Urine flow during two nights (black) and days (open) in seven patients with obstructive sleep apnea (OSA) (left panel, N1&2, D1&2). N3&4 and D3&4 are two nights and days during treatment with nasal continuous positive airway pressure (CPAP) (right panel). Note the higher urine flow at night, which reverts to the normal pattern of lower nocturnal flow following successful treatment. (Reproduced with permission from Warley AR, Stradling JR. Abnormal diurnal variation in salt and water excretion in patients with OSA.* Clin Sci *1988;74:183–5.)*

Most, but not all, workers have found raised levels of ANP during sleep in patients with OSA.[51–56] In addition, there has not always been a fall in ANP when effective treatment has abolished the obstructive episodes.[53,54] For example, Krieger *et al.*[51] studied nine patients with severe OSA on and off nasal continuous positive airway pressure treatment (CPAP), which abolishes OSA instantly. In six of these patients, the levels of ANP were high and fell on CPAP. Overall ANP levels fell from 54 to 36 pg/mL, at the same time urine volume fell from 1.3 to 0.6 mL/min and sodium excretion from 0.16 to 0.08 mmol/min. There appeared to be some correlations across the night between ANP levels and both the degree of inspiratory effort and the hypoxic nadirs during the obstructions. Some of the reductions in ANP and urine production may have been due to the effects of positive pressure breathing on a congested circulation alone, rather than the abolition of obstructive apneas *per se*. Two other studies have failed to find a change in ANP levels following treatment for OSA, but can be criticized to some extent for not having sampled at the best times.[53,54] Sampling time is critical due to the short half-life of ANP.

The most recent study from Kita *et al.*[56] looked in detail at ANP and BNP levels in 14 patients with OSA. Overnight sampling demonstrated rises in BNP (and ANP) which correlated best with the systemic BP rises. Treatment of the OSA with CPAP did reduce BNP levels during sleep, and in the morning. These authors concluded that increases in systemic BP due to OSA may be the more likely explanation for increased BNP release, rather than right atrial distension from increased venous return. It will be difficult to dissect out the exact mechanisms, given the complexity of the effects of OSA on cardiovascular physiology.

The possible clinical relevance of the raised ANP and BNP levels in OSA is entirely speculative at present. It has been suggested that the extra diuresis could be beneficial in that it will tend to 'treat' any hypertension, which tends to be common in these patients, due to both the confounding variables, such as obesity, and the OSA itself.[57,58] On the other hand, ANP and BNP levels may be useful markers of cardiac 'stress' in OSA.

CONCLUSIONS

Obstructive sleep apnea clearly has profound and interesting effects on both the systemic and pulmonary circulations that are still not fully understood. The interplay and contributions to these phenomena made by hypoxia-induced, mechanical and reflex changes require further detailed work before a definitive account can be written. Long-term changes can be detected in some patients with OSA, and it is likely that in most of these individuals the sustained pulmonary hypertension develops as a result of the presence of diurnal hypoxemia due, usually, to associated lung disease. The severity of pulmonary hypertension even in these patients is usually mild and unlikely to contribute to an adverse prognosis.

KEY POINTS

- During the actual periods of obstructive apnea there is a progressive rise in PAP.
- At the moment of arousal at the end of an apnea there is a further rise in pulmonary artery pressure.
- The progressive rise during apnea is probably caused by increased venous return and decreased left ventricular outflow.
- The rise at apnea termination is probably caused by arousal-related sympathetic activity and further reductions in left ventricular outflow.
- There is a more progressive rise in pulmonary artery pressure over many apnea cycles, probably caused by the hypoxia.
- Most sustained pulmonary hypertension in obstructive apnea occurs when there is also

---

- chronic obstructive lung disease also causing diurnal hypoxia.
- Any sustained pulmonary hypertension is modest, and unlikely to adversely effect prognosis.

REFERENCES

- 1 Findley LJ, Ries AL, Tisi GM et al. Hypoxemia during apnea in normal subjects: mechanisms and impact of lung volume. *J Appl Physiol* 1983;**55**:1777–83.
- 2 Angell-James JE, DeBurgh-Daly M. Cardiovascular responses in apnoeic asphyxia: role of arterial chemoreceptors and the modification of their effects by a pulmonary inflation reflex. *J Physiol Lond* 1969;**201**:87–104.
- 3 Andreas S, Hajak G, von Breska B et al. Changes in heart rate during obstructive sleep apnoea. *Eur Respir J* 1992;**5**:853–7.
- 4 Hedner J, Ejnell H, Sellgren J et al. Is high and fluctuating muscle nerve sympathetic activity in the sleep apnoea syndrome of pathogenetic importance for the development of hypertension? *J Hypertens* 1988;**6**:S529–31.
- 5 Davies RJ, Belt PJ, Roberts SJ et al. Arterial blood pressure responses to graded transient arousal from sleep in normal humans. *J Appl Physiol* 1993;**74**:1123–30.
- 6 Ringler J, Basner RC, Shannon R et al. Hypoxemia alone does not explain blood pressure elevations after obstructive apneas. *J Appl Physiol* 1990;**69**:2143–8.
- 7 Johnson LC, Lubin A. The orienting reflex during waking and sleeping. *Electroencephalogr Clin Neurophysiol* 1967;**22**:11–21.
- 8 Coccagna G, Mantovani M, Brignani F et al. Continuous recording of the pulmonary and systemic arterial pressure during sleep in syndromes of hypersomnia with periodic breathing. *Bull Eur Physiopathol Respir* 1972;**8**:1159–72.
- 9 Marrone O, Bellia V, Ferrara G et al. Transmural pressure measurements. Importance in the assessment of pulmonary hypertension in obstructive sleep apneas. *Chest* 1989;**95**:338–42.
- 10 Marrone O, Bellia V, Pieri D et al. Acute effects of oxygen administration on transmural pulmonary artery pressure in obstructive sleep apnea. *Chest* 1992;**101**:1023–7.
- 11 Podszus T, Peter JH, Guilleminault C et al. Pulmonary artery pressure during sleep apnea. *Chest* 1990;**97**:81.
- 12 Podszus T, Feddersen O, Peter JH et al. Sleep and cardiorespiratory control. In: Gaultier C, Escourrou P, Curzi-Dascalova L (eds), *Cardiovascular risk in sleep-related breathing disorders*. Montrouge: INSERM/John Libbey Eurotext, 1991;177–85.
- 13 Emery C, Sloan P, Mohammed F et al. The action of hypercapnia during hypoxia on pulmonary vessels. *Bull Eur Physiopathol Respir* 1977;**13**:763–76.
- 14 Iwase N, Kikuchi Y, Hida W et al. Effects of repetitive airway obstruction on O_2 saturation and systemic and pulmonary artery pressure in anesthetized dogs. *Am Rev Respir Dis* 1992;**146**:1402–10.
- 15 Marrone O, Bonsignore MR, Romano S. Pulmonary artery pressure in obstructive apneas: influence of intrathoracic

pressure and hypoxia. *Am Rev Respir Dis* 1993;**147**(Part 2): 1017.

●16 Tarasiuk A, Chen L, Scharf SM. Effects of periodic obstructive apnoeas on superior and inferior venous return in dogs. *Acta Physiol Scand* 1997;**161**:187–94.

●17 Guyton AC, Lindsey AW, Abernathy B *et al.* Venous return at various right atrial pressures, and the normal venous return curve. *Am J Physiol* 1957;**189**:609–15.

●18 Gardner AMN, Fox RH. *The return of blood to the heart.* London: John Libbey, 1989;70.

●19 Langanke P, Podszus T, Penzel T *et al.* Effect of obstructive sleep apnea on preload of the right heart. *Pneumologie* 1993;**47**(Suppl 1):143–6.

●20 Shiomi T, Guilleminault C, Stoohs R *et al.* Leftward shift of the interventricular septum and pulsus paradoxus in obstructive sleep apnea syndrome. *Chest* 1991;**100**: 894–902.

●21 Garpestad E, Katayama H, Parker JA *et al.* Stroke volume and cardiac output decrease at termination of obstructive apneas *J Appl Physiol* 1992;**73**:1743–8.

●22 Guilleminault C, Motta J, Mihm F *et al.* Obstructive sleep apnea and cardiac index. *Chest* 1986;**89**:331–4.

●23 Andreas S, Werner GS, Sold G *et al.* Doppler echocardiographic analysis of cardiac flow during the Mueller manoeuver *Eur J Clin Invest* 1991;**21**:72–6.

●24 Schafer H, Hasper E, Ewig S *et al.* Pulmonary haemodynamics in obstructive sleep apnoea: time course and associated factors *Eur Respir J* 1998;**12**:679–84.

●25 Ali NJ, Davies RJ, Fleetham JA *et al.* Periodic movements of the legs during sleep associated with rises in systemic blood pressure *Sleep* 1991;**14**:163–5.

●26 Kadowitz PJ, Hyman AL. Effect of sympathetic nerve stimulation on pulmonary vascular resistance in the dog. *Circ Res* 1973;**32**:221–7.

●27 Kessler R, Chaouat A, Weitzenblum E *et al.* Pulmonary hypertension in the obstructive sleep apnoea syndrome: prevalence, causes and therapeutic consequences. *Eur Respir J* 1996;**9**:787–94.

●28 Chaouat A, Weitzenblum E, Krieger J *et al.* Pulmonary hemodynamics in the obstructive sleep apnea syndrome. Results in 220 consecutive patients. *Chest* 1996;**109**:380–6.

◆29 Sobieraj J. Appetite-suppressant drugs and primary pulmonary hypertension. *N Engl J Med* 1997;**336**:510–13.

●30 Nattie EE, Bartlett D, Johnson K. Pulmonary hypertension and right ventricular hypertrophy caused by intermittent hypoxia and hypercapnia in the rat. *Am Rev Respir Dis* 1978;**118**:653–8.

●31 McGuire M, Bradford A. Chronic intermittent hypoxia increases haematocrit and causes right ventricular hypertrophy in the rat. *Respir Physiol* 1999;**117**:53–8.

●32 Goldman JM, Ireland RM, Berthon-Jones M *et al.* Erythropoietin concentrations in obstructive sleep apnoea *Thorax* 1991;**46**:25–7.

●33 Fitzpatrick MF, Mackay T, Whyte KF *et al.* Nocturnal desaturation and serum erythropoietin: a study in patients with chronic obstructive pulmonary disease and in normal subjects. *Clin Sci* 1993;**84**:319–24.

●34 McGuire M, Bradford A. Chronic intermittent hypercapnic hypoxia increases pulmonary arterial pressure and haematocrit in rats. *Eur Respir J* 2001;**18**:279–85.

●35 Weitzenblum E, Krieger J, Apprill M *et al.* Daytime pulmonary hypertension in patients with obstructive sleep apnea syndrome *Am Rev Respir Dis* 1988;**138**:345–9.

●36 Bradley TD, Rutherford R, Grossman RF *et al.* Role of daytime hypoxemia in the pathogenesis of right heart failure in the obstructive sleep apnea syndrome. *Am Rev Respir Dis* 1985;**131**:835–9.

●37 Hanly P, Sasson Z, Zuberi N *et al.* Ventricular function in snorers and patients with obstructive sleep apnea. *Chest* 1992;**102**:100–5.

●38 Berman EJ, DiBenedetto RJ, Causey DE *et al.* Right ventricular hypertrophy detected by echocardiography in patients with newly diagnosed obstructive sleep apnea. *Chest* 1991;**100**:347–50.

●39 Davidson WR, Stauffer JL, Reeves-Hoche MK *et al.* Cardiac sequelae of sleep-disordered breathing or obstructive sleep apnea: new evidence for right ventricular dysfunction. *Am Rev Respir Dis* 1993;**147**(Part 2):A1015.

●40 Bady E, Achkar A, Pascal S *et al.* Pulmonary arterial hypertension in patients with sleep apnoea syndrome. *Thorax* 2000;**55**:934–9.

●41 Sajkov D, Cowie RJ, Thornton AT *et al.* Pulmonary hypertension and hypoxemia in obstructive sleep apnea syndrome. *Am J Respir Crit Care Med* 1994;**149**: 416–22.

●42 Blankfield RP, Hudgel DW, Tapolyai AA *et al.* Bilateral leg edema, obesity, pulmonary hypertension, and obstructive sleep apnea. *Arch Intern Med* 2000;**160**:2357–62.

●43 Wilkinson AR, McCormick MS, Freeland AP *et al.* Electrocardiographic signs of pulmonary hypertension in children who snore. *Br Med J* 1981;**282**:1579–82.

●44 Miman MC, Kirazli T, Ozyurek R. Doppler echocardiography in adenotonsillar hypertrophy. *Int J Pediatr Otorhinolaryngol* 2000;**54**:21–6.

●45 Tal A, Leiberman A, Margulis G *et al.* Ventricular dysfunction in children with obstructive sleep apnea: radionuclide assessment. *Pediatr Pulmonol* 1988;**4**:139–43.

●46 Chaouat A, Weitzenblum E, Kessler R *et al.* Five-year effects of nasal continuous positive airway pressure in obstructive sleep apnoea syndrome. *Eur Respir J* 1997;**10**:2578–82.

●47 Sanner BM, Doberauer C, Konermann M *et al.* Pulmonary hypertension in patients with obstructive sleep apnea syndrome. *Arch Intern Med* 1997;**157**:2483–7.

●48 Laks L, Lehrhaft B, Grunstein RR *et al.* Pulmonary hypertension in obstructive sleep apnoea. *Eur Respir J* 1995;**8**:537–41.

●49 Sanner BM, Konermann M, Sturm A *et al.* Right ventricular dysfunction in patients with obstructive sleep apnoea syndrome. *Eur Respir J* 1997;**10**:2079–83.

◆50 Sagnella GA, MacGregor GA. Cardiac peptides and the control of sodium excretion. *Nature* 1984;**309**:666–7.

●51 Krieger J, Follenius M, Sforza E *et al.* Effects of treatment with nasal continuous positive airway pressure on atrial natriuretic peptide and arginine vasopressin release during sleep in patients with obstructive sleep apnoea. *Clin Sci* 1991;**80**:443–9.

●52 Krieger J, Laks L, Wilcox I *et al.* Atrial natriuretic peptide release during sleep in patients with obstructive sleep apnoea before and during treatment with nasal continuous positive airway pressure. *Clin Sci* 1989;**77**:407–11.

●53 Rodenstein DO, D'Odemont JP, Pieters T *et al*. Diurnal and nocturnal diuresis and natriuresis in obstructive sleep apnea. Effects of nasal continuous positive airway pressure therapy. *Am Rev Respir Dis* 1992;**145**:1367–71.

●54 Warley ARH, Morice A, Stradling JR. Plasma levels of atrial natriuretic peptide (ANP) in obstructive sleep apnoea (OSA). *Thorax* 1988;**43**:253.

●55 Schafer H, Ehlenz K, Ewig S *et al*. Atrial natriuretic peptide levels and pulmonary artery pressure awake, at exercise and asleep in obstructive sleep apnoea syndrome. *J Sleep Res* 1999;**8**:205–10.

●56 Kita H, Ohi M, Chin K *et al*. The nocturnal secretion of cardiac natriuretic peptides during obstructive sleep apnoea and its response to therapy with nasal continuous positive airway pressure. *J Sleep Res* 1998;**7**:199–207.

●57 Davies CW, Crosby JH, Mullins RL *et al*. Case-control study of 24 hour ambulatory blood pressure in patients with obstructive sleep apnoea and normal matched control subjects. *Thorax* 2000;**55**:736–40.

●58 Pepperell JCT, Ramdassingh-Dow S, Crosthwaite N *et al*. Ambulatory blood pressure following therapeutic and sub-therapeutic nasal continuous positive airway pressure for obstructive sleep apnoea: a randomised prospective parallel trial. *Lancet* 2002;**359**:204–10.

◆59 Fletcher EC. *Abnormalities of respiration during sleep*. Orlando: Grune and Stratton, 1986.

●60 Warley AR, Stradling JR. Abnormal diurnal variation in salt and water excretion in patients with obstructive sleep apnoea. *Clin Sci* 1988;**74**:183–5.

An integrated approach to the treatment of pulmonary hypertension due to hypoxic lung disease

WILLIAM MACNEE

INTRODUCTION

The development of pulmonary hypertension is a recognized complication of hypoxic lung diseases. The chronic lung diseases which result in chronic hypoxia and lead to pulmonary hypertension are listed in Table 15C.1. The commonest causes of pulmonary hypertension amongst these diseases are chronic obstructive pulmonary disease (COPD), kyphoscoliosis, idiopathic pulmonary fibrosis and the sleep apnea/hypopnea syndrome.

This chapter focuses on the treatment of pulmonary hypertension in hypoxic lung disease, of which the commonest cause is COPD. The development of pulmonary hypertension in patients with hypoxic COPD is important, not only because it is associated with right ventricular hypertrophy and/or enlargement, so-called cor pulmonale, but because it adversely affects prognosis[1] (Figure 15C.1).

The rationale for treating pulmonary hypertension therefore is, first, that it may improve survival and second, that pulmonary hypertension may compromise right ventricular function, particularly during exercise, so reducing exercise tolerance and contributing to the symptom of breathlessness on exercise, which can significantly affect the quality of life of patients with hypoxic lung disease.

Patients with COPD who develop pulmonary hypertension usually have a forced expiratory volume in one second (FEV_1) less than 40% of the predicted value and an arterial oxygen tension (PaO_2) less than 60 mmHg. The prevalence of clinical signs of cor pulmonale increases with worsening airflow obstruction and deterioration of gas exchange. It is present in 40% of patients with an FEV_1 below 1 liter, in 70% with a FEV_1 of 0.6 liter, and it is almost universal in patients with hypoxemia, hypercapnia and polycythemia.[2,3] Other factors such as acidosis, hyperviscosity and pulmonary mechanical factors have a relatively small effect on the pulmonary arterial pressure.

In order to determine the effects which might be expected from treatments targeting the pulmonary hypertension in hypoxic lung diseases, knowledge of the pathophysiology of the pulmonary circulation is necessary.

PATHOLOGICAL CHANGES IN THE PULMONARY CIRCULATION IN COPD

The pathological changes in the pulmonary circulation in COPD are destruction of the capillaries, muscularization of pulmonary arterioles, and proliferation of longitudinal muscle in the intima of muscular arteries and larger arterioles[4–6] (Plates 15C.1a–c). A detailed description of the pathological changes is given in Chapter 15A.

Table 15C.1 *Respiratory diseases associated with pulmonary hypertension and cor pulmonale**

Obstructive pulmonary diseases
- Chronic obstructive pulmonary disease
- Cystic fibrosis
- Bronchiolitis obliterans
- Bronchiectasis

Restrictive lung diseases
- Neuromuscular diseases; myopathy, bilateral diaphragmatic paralysis, amyotropic lateral sclerosis, etc.
- Kyphoscoliosis
- Thorocoplasty
- Pulmonary tuberculosis
- Pneumoconiosis
- Sarcoidosis
- Idiopathic pulmonary fibrosis
- Connective tissue disorders
- Extrinsic allergic alveolitis
- Drug-related lung diseases

Respiratory failure of 'central' origin
- Central alveolar hypoventilation
- Obesity – hypoventilation syndrome
- Sleep apnea syndrome

Anatomic factors
- Destruction or obstruction of the pulmonary vascular bed
  - Emphysema
  - Fibrosis
  - Thromboembolism

Functional factors
- Alveolar hypoxia
  - Acute hypoxic pulmonary vasoconstriction
  - Remodeling of the pulmonary vascular bed due to chronic hypoxemia
- Hypercapnia and acidosis
- Hyperviscosity
- Hypervolemia secondary to polycythemia
- Mechanical factors – compression of alveolar vessels

*Excluding primary pulmonary hypertension, pulmonary vascular disease and pulmonary thromboembolic disease.

Hypoxia is the most potent pulmonary vasoconstricting stimulus. However, the reactivity of the pulmonary circulation to hypoxia varies in healthy subjects[7] and in patients with COPD.[8] However, the consequences of these variations in hypoxic vasoconstriction for the development of pulmonary hypertension are unknown. The underlying mechanism by which hypoxia leads to the development of pulmonary hypertension in patients with COPD has not been fully determined[9,10] (see Chapter 4). In addition to the intrinsic smooth muscle cell reactivity to hypoxia, altered endothelium-mediated relaxation of pulmonary arteries, particularly involving nitric oxide (NO), might also play a role. There is now considerable evidence that endothelium-derived nitric oxide has a modulating effect on pulmonary vascular tone.[11]

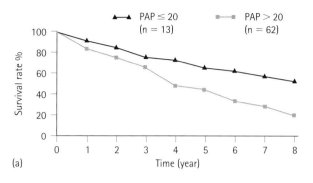

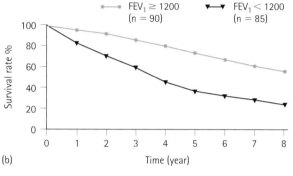

Figure 15C.1 *Effect of (a) pulmonary arterial pressure (PAP), and (b) forced expiratory volume in 1 second (FEV₁) on survival in patients with chronic obstructive pulmonary disease (COPD). (Reproduced from Weitzenblum E, Hirth C, Ducolone A et al. Prognostic value of pulmonary artery pressure in chronic obstructive pulmonary disease.* Thorax *1981;36:752–8 with permission from S. Karger AG, Basel.)*

Inhibition of NO synthesis enhances the vasoconstrictor effect of hypoxia, suggesting that NO also acts in this case as a 'chemical break' to counteract excessive hypoxic vasoconstriction.[9,12]

Endothelial cell proliferation and thickening occurs in the arterioles in response to chronic hypoxemia in patients with COPD. Endothelium-dependent dilatation is impaired in isolated pulmonary rings from patients undergoing heart/lung transplantation for end-stage COPD.[13] Furthermore, pulmonary arteries of patients with even mild COPD have impaired responses to a hypoxic stimulus.[14] Impaired endothelial-dependent vasodilatation may result from either a reduction in NO synthesis or release as a result of hypoxia.[14] These data lend further support to the hypothesis that the endothelium has a central role in regulating the pulmonary vasculature. Thus, the normal breaking mechanism that ameliorates the effect of vasoconstrictors on pulmonary vascular tone may be lacking in COPD, which may relate to the structural change in the intima that occurs in the small pulmonary arteries.

A further extension to this hypothesis is that NO may inhibit cell proliferation in the pulmonary microvasculature and may thus not only affect pulmonary vasomotor tone, but also may have an influence on the vascular remodeling which occurs in patients with hypoxic COPD.[15]

These structural and functional abnormalities in the pulmonary circulation in COPD will influence the responses to treatment.

PATHOPHYSIOLOGY

Pulmonary hemodynamics in chronic respiratory disease

Studies of pulmonary hemodynamics in patients with COPD show that pulmonary arterial pressure may be normal or only slightly elevated when measured at rest. Generally, the mean pulmonary arterial pressure is between 25 and 30 mmHg.[16] These values are generally lower than in the pulmonary hypertension which develops as a result of left ventricular failure, congenital disease, pulmonary thromboembolic disease and, in particular, those which occur in primary pulmonary hypertension, where the mean pulmonary arterial pressure is usually greater than 50 mmHg.

Before the development of significant hypoxemia and hypercapnia, patients with mild COPD have a normal or low cardiac output. The pulmonary vascular resistance is therefore normal or only slightly elevated when measured at rest. However, during steady-state exercise there is a pronounced increase in pulmonary arterial pressure, which is accounted for by an elevation in cardiac output. Patients with COPD stop exercising at a lower level of cardiac output and maximal oxygen consumption than normal subjects. However, the slope of the relationship between oxygen consumption and cardiac output is normal.[17] Thus, the limitation to exercise in patients with COPD does not appear to be cardiovascular in origin, but results from changes in pulmonary mechanics that affect ventilation.

As the airflow limitation and arterial blood gas abnormalities worsen, and with the development of chronic hypoxemia and hypercapnia, pulmonary hypertension may be present at rest and worsen further with exercise. However, the degree of pulmonary hypertension which develops in these patients at rest is relatively modest. In a study of 74 patients with severe but clinically stable COPD, who had all presented in the past with episodes of acute-on-chronic respiratory failure, and in almost half with peripheral edema, pulmonary arterial pressure was only modestly raised, with a mean value of 35 mmHg in this group[18] (Table 15C.2).

Acute changes in pulmonary arterial pressure are well documented during the oxygen desaturations that occur during rapid eye movement sleep.[19] Episodes of acute respiratory failure are accompanied by worsening hypoxemia, hypercapnia and a marked increase in pulmonary

Table 15C.2 *Hemodynamics and blood gas values in 74 patients with previous episodes of acute respiratory failure (but studied when stable) and 32 normal subjects*

Variables	COPD		Normals	
	Mean	Range	Mean	Range
PaO$_2$ (mmHg)	43	23–67	91	75–105
PaCO$_2$ (mmHg)	51	33–68	38	32–43
Q̇ (L/min·m^2)	3.8	2.3–5.8	3.6	2.6–4.5
RAP (mmHg)	3	0–21	5	2–9
PAP (mmHg)	35	15–78	13	8–20
PAWP (mmHg)	6	0–19	9	5–14
PVRI (dyn s/cm^5·m^2)	660	213–1377	58	40–200
RVSWI (g/m)	16	5–29	6	3–18

Modified from reference 19.
COPD, chronic obstructive pulmonary disease; PaCO$_2$, arterial partial pressure of CO$_2$; PaO$_2$ arterial partial pressure of O$_2$; PAP, pulmonary arterial pressure; PAWP, pulmonary arterial wedge pressure; Q̇, blood flow; PVRI, peripheral vascular resistance index; RAP, right arterial pressure; RVSWI, right ventricular systolic work index.

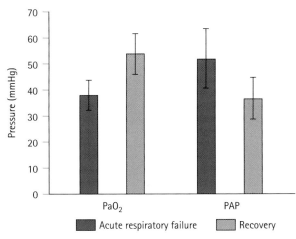

Figure 15C.2 *Changes of arterial PO$_2$ (PaO$_2$) and pulmonary arterial pressure (PAP) in 24 chronic obstructive pulmonary disease (COPD) patients investigated during an episode of acute respiratory failure and after recovery. With treatment, PaO$_2$ rose and PAP fell. (Reproduced by kind permission of S. Karger AG, Basel, from Weitzenblum E, Hirth C, Roeslin N et al. Les modifications hémodynamiques pulmonaires au cours de l'insuffisance respiratoire aigue des bronchopneumopathies chroniques. Respiration 1971;28:539–54.)*

arterial pressure from its baseline values.[20] There is a return to baseline values upon recovery from the episode of respiratory failure (Figure 15C.2).[21] Thus, during exercise, sleep and exacerbations of COPD and respiratory failure, pulmonary hypertension worsens in patients with COPD, and has the potential to increase right ventricular afterload and lead to the development of right ventricular failure.

The natural history of untreated pulmonary hypertension in patients with chronic lung disease

The progression of pulmonary hypertension in patients with COPD is slow. In a study of 93 patients with COPD followed up for 5–12 years, the hemodynamic changes were small for the group as a whole, with a change in pulmonary arterial pressure of around $+0.5$ mmHg per year.[22] Data on the progression of pulmonary arterial pressure in the British Medical Research Council Long-term Oxygen Trial showed that pulmonary arterial pressure in the untreated group rose by a mean of 3 mmHg per year, whereas there was no significant change in the treated group.[23] In the North American Nocturnal Oxygen Therapy Trial (NOTT), the pulmonary arterial pressure and pulmonary vascular resistance dropped significantly after 6 months in those patients receiving continuous oxygen therapy, but did not change in those treated with 'nocturnal oxygen therapy'.[24] A more recent study showed that long-term oxygen therapy could reverse the progression of pulmonary hypertension that had worsened before the initiation of oxygen therapy.[25] However, long-term oxygen does not normalize pulmonary arterial pressure in such patients.

Although pulmonary arterial hypertension progresses slowly in patients with COPD, its presence infers a poor prognosis. Patients with COPD and the same level of airways obstruction with a normal pulmonary arterial pressure (PAP < 20 mmHg) have a 5-year survival rate of 65%, compared with a 45% survival in those with an elevated pulmonary arterial pressure (Figure 15C.1).[1] Although the level of pulmonary arterial pressure affects survival in patients with COPD, so does the degree of airflow limitation as assessed by the FEV_1 (Figure 15C.1).[1] Other studies have shown that a number of variables correlate significantly with survival, including the PaO_2 and $PaCO_2$ and the presence of peripheral edema in COPD patients.[26]

Pulmonary hypertension remains a good predictor of mortality in COPD patients treated with long-term oxygen. In a series of 84 patients with advanced COPD treated with long-term oxygen, the 5-year survival rate was 66% in 44 patients with a mean pulmonary artery pressure below 25 mmHg, and only 36% in 40 patients with a mean pulmonary artery pressure higher than 25 mmHg.[27]

Although numerous studies have shown an association between the presence of pulmonary arterial hypertension and the prognosis in patients with COPD, pulmonary hypertension may simply be a reflection of the severity of the disease and may not have a direct effect on mortality.

RIGHT VENTRICULAR FUNCTION IN COPD

The normal right ventricle has been shown to fail, with acute dilatation and precipitous decline in cardiac output

and systemic blood pressure, when mean PAP is rapidly raised to 40–50 mmHg, that is, two to three times the upper limit of normal.[28] On the other hand, in response to chronic pressure load, the right ventricle dilates, together with an increase in wall thickness, eventually making its configuration similar to that of the left ventricle. The rate at which these changes occur in patients with COPD and pulmonary hypertension is not precisely known. However, right ventricular tolerance of mean pulmonary arterial pressure greater than 40–50 mmHg supports the view of a chronic rather than an acute pulmonary hypertensive process.

Differences exist between the two ventricles in adults and are related to the different flow/resistance conditions in the two circulations. The function of the right ventricular contraction appears to be to generate sufficient stroke volume to maintain adequate cardiac output, rather than to generate pressure. It operates, therefore, as a 'volume' rather than a 'pressure' pump.[29] In general, the thin-walled right ventricle which contracts against the low-pressure pulmonary circulation is more compliant than the thicker-walled left ventricle. The geometric configuration of the right ventricle is therefore thought to be more suited to ejecting large volumes of blood, with minimal cardiac shortening. Therefore, the right ventricle can adapt to considerable variations in systemic venous return, without producing large changes in filling pressures, because of the larger ratio of volume to surface area in the right, compared with the left ventricle. However, it is less able to cope with an acute increase in afterload. This contrasts with the left ventricle, which acts as a pressure pump in the high-pressure systemic circulation and has a small surface area relative to its intracavity volume.

Since pulmonary arterial pressures in patients with COPD and respiratory failure are not markedly elevated and the progression of pulmonary hypertension is slow, then the effect on the right ventricular configuration, mass and function in the presence of moderate pulmonary hypertension, which slowly progresses in patients with COPD, is likely to be different from the effects of acute pulmonary hypertension, such as occurs in massive pulmonary embolism. Therefore, the right ventricle has time to adapt to the modest increase in pressure load in COPD.

As pulmonary hypertension develops in patients with COPD, right ventricular stroke-work index increases on exercise owing to an increase in pressure work, as described above. However, in patients with stable COPD the relationship between the right ventricular stroke-work index and the right ventricular end-diastolic pressure suggests that although the right ventricular stroke-work index is higher in these patients, they operate on an extension of the normal right ventricular function curve.[30] The diastolic pressure in the right ventricle can be normal, even in those patients who report episodes of peripheral edema in the past and who have clinical evidence of right ventricular enlargement.[30] However, during exercise, right ventricular end-diastolic pressure is elevated in the majority of patients. The presence of a normal end-diastolic pressure at rest in patients with COPD is at least suggestive of a normal right ventricular end-diastolic volume.

The 'right ventricular hypothesis' suggests that right ventricular function is compromised in patients with cor pulmonale that influences the quality and quantity of life.[31,32] The most important factors affecting right ventricular performance are preload, afterload and contractility. As discussed earlier, cardiac output is normal in the majority of patients with COPD and in those with clinical evidence of edema. In order to assess the contractility or inotropic state of the right ventricle, rather than its global performance, it is necessary to assess a function of the ventricle that is independent of preload and afterload. The end-systolic pressure/volume relationship has been shown to be an index of contractility that is independent of the initial ventricular volume. For a given contractile state, an increase in afterload produces less complete emptying of the ventricle and an increase in end-systolic volume. However, the end-systolic pressure/volume ratio remains constant, indicating that this relationship is also independent of changes in afterload.[33]

This relationship defines the inotropic state of the left ventricle independent of loading conditions. Similar relationships have been confirmed for the right ventricle.[33] The slope of the end-systolic pressure/volume relationship describes the interaction between afterload and systolic performance and is termed 'the ventricular systolic elastance'. Measurement of the end-systolic pressure/volume relation in the right ventricle has a number of problems. The relationship may not always be linear and not entirely independent of loading conditions, since it may also be sensitive to changes in ventricular compliance. Allowing for these constraints, simultaneous measurements of stroke volume by right heart catheterization and the thermodilution technique and right ventricular ejection fraction by radionuclide ventriculography, allow quantification of right ventricular volume, which, together with simultaneous measurement of right ventricular pressure, allows measurement of the end-systolic pressure/volume relationship in patients with COPD, as an assessment of right ventricular contractility.

In a group of 20 patients with hypoxemia and variable degrees of hypercapnia, measurement of the pressure/volume relationship in the right ventricle suggested relatively well-preserved right ventricular contractility in the presence of pulmonary hypertension.[34,35] Studies on exercise in patients with pulmonary hypertension show that, despite a substantial increase in right ventricular diastolic pressure, the majority of patients did not have large changes in end-systolic volume, suggesting well-preserved right ventricular function.[34]

There has been discussion about the concept of cor pulmonale, with confusion regarding difficulties in clinical diagnosis and the concept of heart failure.[16] The debate may be clarified by the definition of heart failure proposed by Sagawa et al. as 'a state in which cardiac output cannot be maintained to meet peripheral systemic demand without an excessive use of physiological compensatory mechanisms, mainly the increase in stroke volume associated with increased preload (Frank Starling mechanism)'.[36] This definition allows the integration of normal or even high cardiac output states, as seen in patients with cor pulmonale.

Thus, in the presence of chronically increased pulmonary arterial pressures, the right ventricle dilates, with an increase in both end-diastolic and end-systolic volumes, a maintained stroke volume, and a decreased ejection fraction. Secondary hypertrophy of the right ventricular wall decreases wall tension (or afterload). The increase in right ventricular end-diastolic volume, or preload, as an adaptation to increased afterload, is enhanced by an increase in systemic venous return due to activation of sympathetic nervous and renin–angiotensin–aldosterone systems, and associated hypervolemia caused by renal salt and water retention (see below). Symptoms of right heart failure result from venous congestion secondary to upstream transmission of high right ventricular filling pressures and renal retention of salt and water in variable proportions.

Salt water and hormonal balance in COPD

Many patients with advanced COPD present with ankle edema but normal right atrial pressures. It has long been recognized that edema in advanced COPD is related to hypercapnia rather than to raised jugular pressures.[37,38] Although there is debate over the notion of right heart failure in COPD, hemodynamic studies in patients with COPD who developed edema during exacerbations of their disease, and who were studied again after recovery, have shown a consistent pattern of abnormal increase in right ventricular diastolic pressures and aggravated pulmonary hypertension, together with hypoxemia and hypercapnia.[38–41] However, it is clear that some patients present with edema without hemodynamic signs of right heart failure or significant changes in pulmonary arterial pressure from baseline.[42] In cor pulmonale secondary to chronic respiratory insufficiency, hypoxemia and hypercapnia aggravate systemic congestion by further activation of the sympathetic nervous system, already stimulated by right atrial distension, leading to a further decrease in renal plasma flow, activation of the renin–angiotensin–aldosterone system, and increased renal tubular reabsorption of bicarbonate, sodium and water.

In view of the changes in renal blood flow and activation of renin–angiotensin system, it is surprising that more patients with COPD and hypoxemia and hypercapnia do not develop edema. The reason for this is likely to lie in the fact that several factors are present which counteract the edema-promoting the factors described above.

Several studies have now shown that atrial natriuretic peptide (ANP) is elevated in patients with COPD,[43–45] particularly in those with edema. Although plasma ANP is elevated, it is clearly not effective in preventing the development of edema in some patients with COPD despite the fact that the kidney is still responsive to ANP.[43] ANP has a number of beneficial effects in opposing the neuroendocrine abnormalities that are present in patients with COPD and edema. These include natriuresis, depression of plasma renin activity, inhibition of angiotensin II-mediated aldosterone production, and pulmonary vasodilatation.

Another factor which could prevent the development of edema in patients with COPD is dopamine, which has receptors in the renal vasculature, which, when stimulated, promote natriuresis, renal vasodilatation and an increase in the glomerular filtration rate. As with ANP, dopamine has properties with the potential to protect against the development of edema. In exacerbations of COPD, renal dopamine output is maintained and, indeed, is highest in those patients who present with edema and respiratory failure and correlates with a $PaCO_2$.[46]

Thus, a complex interaction of changes in pulmonary hemodynamics and alteration in salt water and hormonal balance occurs in patients with chronic hypoxic hypercapnic respiratory failure. An imbalance between the edema protecting and edema-promoting mechanisms in favor of the latter probably accounts for the development of edema in patients with hypoxic hypercapnia in COPD. A possible sequence of events leading to the development of edema in patients with COPD is as follows: patients with COPD, who are hypoxemic but normocapnic, have normal renal hormonal function. However, with the development of hypercapnia, a salt- and water-retaining state is promoted by several factors including:

- the loss of hydrogen ions in exchange for sodium reabsorption;
- CO_2-induced peripheral vasodilatation that inactivates arterial barrier receptors, leading to a reflex increase in norepinephrine and stimulation of the renin–angiotensin system.

Renal blood flow is reduced indirectly by the increase in sympathetic activity and directly by the effects of carbon dioxide. Consequently, because of the increased renin–angiotensin activity, arginine vasopressin (AVP) is released and this affects the release of salt and water. Expanded extracellular volume, together with the presence of pulmonary arterial hypertension, leads to atrial distension and ANP release that, although largely protective against the development of edema, may be overwhelmed by the activity of the renin–angiotensin system. Furthermore, although ANP-induced pulmonary vasodilatation is potentially beneficial, it may also induce peripheral vasodilatation that may perpetuate the sequence of events described above. Intrarenal dopamine release is another mechanism that attempts to protect against the development of edema in such patients, but which also eventually fails and edema develops in some patients (Figure 15C.3).

TREATMENT

Treatment of the underlying cause

Prevention of the development of pulmonary hypertension in COPD would be best achieved by preventing the decline in lung function which is characteristic of COPD. Present therapies have, however, failed to achieve this goal. Exacerbations of COPD may be reversed with the help of bronchodilators, antibiotics and judicious use of corticosteroids.[47] Relief of hypoxemia and hyperinflation will result in decreased pulmonary vascular resistance and the strain on the right heart.

CARDIAC GLYCOSIDES

Since ventricular contractility does not appear to be compromised in patients with COPD and pulmonary hypertension, the use of an inotropic drug would not appear to be indicated in these patients. Cardiac glycosides have not been shown to be useful in the treatment of cor pulmonale due to COPD. The risk of digitalis toxicity is enhanced by hypoxemia and by diuretic-induced hypokalemia. Digitalis may be given to slow the ventricular response to atrial flutter or fibrillation in these patients.[16,38,48]

DIURETICS

Diuretics must be given with more care than usual because of the associated risk of aggravating metabolic alkalosis, leading to worsening hypercapnia, hypovolemia which compromises adequate filling of the afterloaded right ventricle, and increases blood viscosity.[16,38,48] Monitoring of plasma electrolytes is mandatory, and potassium and magnesium supplementation may be necessary. Therapy is instituted with low doses of loop diuretics, for example frusemide, 40 mg/day, increased as needed and tolerated. Some patients with severe right heart failure may require large doses of diuretics, for example frusemide 500 mg/day.

ANTICOAGULANT THERAPY

Severe pulmonary hypertension carries a risk of thromboembolism because of sedentary lifestyle, venous

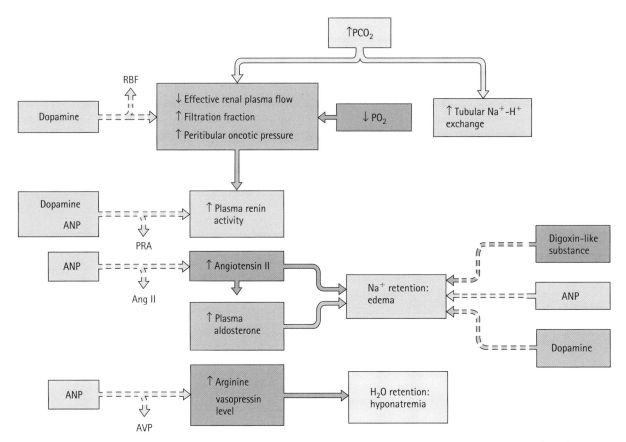

Figure 15C.3 *The mechanisms of salt and water disturbance in patients with chronic obstructive pulmonary disease (COPD). The continuous lines and boxes indicate the abnormalities in renal function and salt and water and hormonal balances. The dotted lines indicate the proposed protective mechanisms against this disturbance. Ang II, angiotensin II; ANP, atrial natriuretic peptide; AVP, arginine vasopressin; H^+, hydrogen ion; Na^+, sodium ion; PCO_2/PO_2, partial pressure of CO_2/O_2; RBF, renal blood flow.*

insufficiency, dilated right-sided heart chambers, and sluggish pulmonary blood flow.[16,38,48] Pulmonary thrombosis is frequently found at autopsy in such patients. Anticoagulation has been shown to improve survival rate in primary pulmonary hypertension.[49] Until now, no study has proved chronic anticoagulant therapy to be beneficial in cor pulmonale secondary to COPD. In these patients, it seems advisable to administer antiplatelet agents and routine prophylaxis with low molecular weight heparin during periods of hospitalization or prolonged immobilization.

Vasodilator treatment of secondary pulmonary hypertension

The major rationale for treating the pulmonary hypertension which develops in patients with COPD is that the presence of pulmonary hypertension reduces survival.[1] Pulmonary vasodilators, by decreasing right ventricular afterload and allowing cardiac output to increase, should improve oxygen transport, tissue oxygenation and perhaps survival, as well as improving symptoms in patients

with hypoxic COPD. The use of vasodilators in patients with COPD and secondary pulmonary hypertension resulted from their apparent beneficial effects in primary pulmonary hypertension.[49] This early enthusiasm has diminished because of failure to sustain the acute effects of many vasodilators. Difficulties in carrying out long-term studies include the need for repeated invasive measurements and for long-term multicenter studies of large numbers of patients to show an effect on survival and the fact that no agent, with the exception of oxygen, produces pulmonary vasodilatation without producing systemic vasodilatation. Specific pulmonary vasodilators may become available when the mechanism of the hypoxic vasoconstrictive response is elucidated. An added problem is that reversing vasoconstriction may have deleterious effects on arterial gas exchange as a result of changes in ventilation/perfusion ratios. However, the rise in cardiac output that occurs with some vasodilators may still increase oxygen delivery to the tissues.

In spite of the lack of specificity of vasodilator drugs for the pulmonary circulation, the rarity of reducing pulmonary arterial pressure to normal by vasodilators in patients with chronic lung diseases and the possible deleterious effects on gas exchange, a large number of studies have been undertaken in patients with COPD (Table 15C.3).[16]

Many vasodilators, including β_2-agonists,[35,50,51] nitrates,[52] calcium channel blockers,[53–58] angiotensin converting enzyme inhibitors,[59] theophylline,[60] α_1-receptor antagonists[61] have been repeatedly tried over the years for the treatment of cor pulmonale secondary to COPD.[16] Most studies of the acute effects of vasodilators in patients with chronic lung diseases and pulmonary hypertension have shown only a modest fall in pulmonary arterial pressure accompanied by a rise in cardiac output (Table 15C.3). The reason for the modest or lack of effect of most vasodilators in patients with pulmonary hypertension

secondary to COPD may be the remodeling of the pulmonary circulation.

In the search for the ideal drug, an optimal vasodilator response has been defined as a decrease in pulmonary arterial pressure accompanied by an increase in cardiac output with no or minimal decrease in systemic arterial pressure and arterial oxygenation. In practice, the most common response has proved to be no change in pulmonary arterial pressure, an increase in cardiac output, and mild to moderate decreases in systemic arterial pressure and arterial oxygenation.[18,38] There has been no randomized controlled trial showing benefit of long-term therapy with vasodilators in patients with cor pulmonale secondary to advanced COPD.

Most studies of the use of vasodilators in secondary pulmonary hypertension have shown a deleterious effect on gas exchange as a consequence of vasodilatation of unventilated areas in the lungs and hence worsening venous admixture and a fall in arterial PaO_2. However, this fall in arterial oxygen content has been balanced, to some extent, in some studies by the increase in cardiac output so that overall oxygen delivery may improve.

There has been recent interest in the use of nitric oxide as a vasodilator. The advantage of nitric oxide, when given by inhalation rather than systemically, is that it will affect those parts of the lung where there is good ventilation. Thus, it will vasodilate pulmonary arteries supplying well-ventilated areas in the lungs. This should have the effect of enhancing ventilation/perfusion matching and because of its vasodilator properties, will reduce pulmonary arterial pressure. Studies of the use of nitric oxide in patients with hypoxic lung disease and pulmonary

Table 15C.3 Clinical drug trials: effects on lung circulation

Drug	Duration	PAP	$\dot{Q}$	PVR	Reference
Nifedipine	6–9 weeks	↓	–	↓	59
Nifedipine	6 weeks	–	–	–	60
Nitrendipine	6 weeks	↓	↑	↓	61
Felodipine	3–5 months	–	–	–	56
Nifedipine	9 weeks	–	–	–	57
Nifedipine	18 months	–	–	–	58
Nitroglycerin	6 weeks	–	–	–	55
Isosorbide dinitrate	6 weeks	↓	–	–	55
Pirbuterol	6 weeks	–	↑	↑	38
Pirbuterol	6 months	–	–	–	53
Terbutaline	Acute	–	↑	↓	54
Prazosin	2 months	↓	↑	↓	64

PAP, pulmonary arterial pressure; PVR, pulmonary vascular resistance; $\dot{Q}$, blood flow.

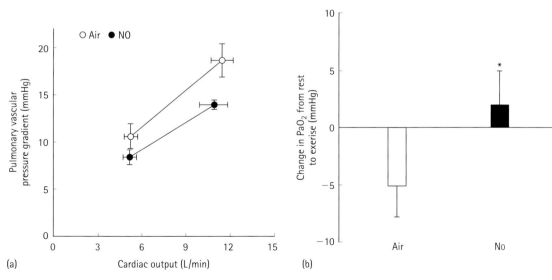

Figure 15C.4 Changes in the cardiac output and pulmonary arterial pressure gradient at rest and during exercise and the arterial partial pressure of O_2 (PaO_2) in chronic obstructive pulmonary disease (COPD) patients breathing either room air or 40 p.p.m. of nitric oxide (NO). (Reproduced with permission from Roger N, Barbera JA, Roca J et al. Nitric oxide inhalation during exercise in chronic obstructive pulmonary disease. Am J Respir Crit Care Med 1997;156:800–6.)

hypertension are contradictory. Whereas some show a lowered PAP and an improved PaO_2,[62] others, using sophisticated techniques to assess ventilation/perfusion, have shown a fall in pulmonary arterial pressure with nitric oxide, but worsening PaO_2 due to worsening ventilation/perfusion ratios[59,63,64] (Figure 15C.4). Thus inhaled nitric oxide cannot be recommended as a treatment for pulmonary hypertension secondary to COPD.

Oxygen therapy

Oxygen is the only selective vasodilator that is generally available. Two large controlled studies from the MRC and the NIH have shown that long-term oxygen therapy can reduce mortality in patients with COPD, but this improvement in survival was not clearly associated with an improvement in pulmonary hemodynamics.[23,65] In the MRC study,[23] 15 hours per day oxygen prevented the 3 mmHg per year rise in pulmonary arterial pressure in the control group, but did not lower pulmonary artery pressure. In the NOTT study,[65] those patients who were given 24 hours per day oxygen had a better survival rate than those given 12 hours per day, these patients did show a fall in pulmonary vascular resistance. Further analysis of patients in the NOTT study showed that an improvement in stroke volume, both at rest and on exercise and a decrease in pulmonary arterial pressure and pulmonary vascular resistance over the first 6 months therapy appeared to predict survival.[65] However, other studies have suggested that the acute effects of oxygen do not predict their long-term effects.[66] Other studies have shown prevention of the progression of pulmonary arterial hypertension in some patients receiving long-term oxygen therapy.[25] However, since the rise in pulmonary arterial pressure in patients with chronic lung diseases, particularly in patients with COPD, is modest and the changes in pulmonary hemodynamics with long-term oxygen therapy are small, it is unlikely these are directly responsible for the improved survival. Although the vascular remodeling in the pulmonary circulation is thought to result mainly from chronic hypoxia, the ability of long-term oxygen therapy to reverse these changes remains controversial.[4,67]

One further beneficial effect of oxygen could be to decrease the hematocrit,[68] which may improve right ventricular function by reducing pulmonary vascular resistance. Phlebotomy has been shown to reduce pulmonary arterial pressure and pulmonary vascular resistance and to increase right ventricular ejection fraction in patients with COPD and polycythemia.[68] Thus, the improvement in exercise tolerance produced by phlebotomy[69] could possibly be as a result of improvement in right ventricular function.[70] Furthermore, an important predictive factor in survival in the MRC long-term oxygen trial was the red cell mass.[23] A reduction in the red cell mass produced

by oxygen therapy could at least partially improve survival by improving the right ventricular performance. However, this is not likely to be the mechanism in most patients. Phlebotomy is at present only recommended in those patients with secondary polycythemia to maintain the heamatocrit below 50–55%.

The current recommendation is to administer at least 15 h/day of oxygen in patients with a PaO_2 below 55 mmHg, or a resting PaO_2 of 56–59 mmHg together with cor pulmonale or polycythemia (hematocrit above 55%).

In patients with COPD, administration of high inspired oxygen concentrations carry a risk of aggravation of hypercapnic acidosis. However, slight increases in the fraction of inspired oxygen will most often increase arterial PO_2 above 60 mmHg, associated with a 90% saturation of hemoglobin. Therefore, oxygen has to be given in a controlled fashion (24–28%) in these patients.

Other treatments

Since the renin–angiotensin system is activated in patients with chronic hypoxic and hypercapnia respiratory failure and the fluid retention consequent upon the respiratory failure may be in part due to salt and water retention, it was hoped that angiotensin converting enzyme (ACE) inhibitors would be of some benefit in this condition. ACE inhibition could have two beneficial effects, first by producing pulmonary vasodilation and second by preventing salt and water retention. The results of clinical trials have been disappointing and have produced neither a consistent vasodilator effect,[59,71] nor any evidence to support their use to treat the fluid retention in this condition.

TRANSPLANTATION

Single or double lung transplantation has been shown to be a suitable alternative for combined heart/lung transplantation in patients with end-stage lung disease.[72] Single lung transplantation has been reported to normalize pulmonary hemodynamics in COPD.[73] Survival rates are 60% at 1 year and 40% at 5 years, with most deaths resulting from infection, bronchiolitis obliterans and chronic rejection. Survival in patients with pulmonary vascular disease is, in general, not as good as in patients with parenchymal lung disease.

LUNG VOLUME REDUCTION SURGERY (LVRS)

Selected patients with emphysema and lung overinflation may benefit from LVRS.[73,74] Patients with moderate to severe pulmonary hypertension (pulmonary arterial pressure ≥ 35 mmHg) are not considered candidates for LVRS. Limited studies of pulmonary hemodynamics before and after LVRS[75,76] have shown conflicting results with increases in pulmonary arterial pressure post LVRS in some studies[75] but not in others.[77,78] One study has also shown significant improvements in right ventricular performance, measured as right ventricular ejection fraction, particularly during exercise.[76]

SUMMARY

The simple hypothesis that hypoxia in patients with chronic lung diseases results in pulmonary hypertension which adversely affects right ventricular function and hence increases morbidity, and decreases exercise tolerance, leading to the development of peripheral edema and increased mortality is still controversial. Whether therapeutic interventions that directly affect arterial pressure, right ventricular function or produce pulmonary vasodilatation have a significant effect on long-term survival in patients with pulmonary hypertension secondary to hypoxic lung diseases is still a matter for debate. Furthermore, whether such interventions will have an effect on symptoms or exercise tolerance remains unproven. Present therapies are limited to the correction of hypoxemia over the long term, which has been shown to have a proven benefit on survival. Further studies are required of more specific pulmonary vasodilators or of therapies aimed at improving salt and water and hormonal balance in these patients.

KEY POINTS

- The development of pulmonary hypertension in patients with COPD is associated with survival. The presence of pulmonary hypertension may reduce exercise tolerance and contribute to the symptoms on exercise of patients with COPD. The rationale for treating pulmonary hypertension in patients with COPD is to improve survival and health status.
- The pathological changes which develop in the pulmonary circulation in patients with COPD may reduce the effectiveness of therapeutic interventions to decrease pulmonary arterial pressure.
- Long-term oxygen therapy has been the only treatment which has been shown to influence pulmonary hemodynamics, over the long term, in patients with COPD. Whether these effects are causal in the improvements in survival in patients treated with long-term oxygen therapy is still unknown.
- The edema which develops in patients with cor pulmonale has a complex pathogenesis related to both right ventricular failure and salt and water

with renal and hormonal abnormalities, and therefore difficult to prevent or treat.
- The best prevention for the development of pulmonary hypertension, cor pulmonale, would be to prevent the decline in FEV_1 and associated respiratory failure.
- Many nonspecific pulmonary vasodilators have been used in patients with COPD with modest or no effects on pulmonary arterial pressure; these are usually given as short-term treatments. All these treatments have usually been associated with worsening gas exchange and have not been recommended.

REFERENCES

●1 Weitzenblum E, Hirth C, Ducolone A et al. Prognostic value of pulmonary artery pressure in chronic obstructive pulmonary disease. Thorax 1981;**36**:752–8.

●2 Renzetti AD Jr, McClement JH, Litt BD. The Veterans Administration co-operative study of pulmonary function. III Mortality in relation to respiratory function in chronic obstructive pulmonary disease. Am J Med 1966;**41**:115–19.

◆3 Mitchell RS, Vincent TN, Filley GF. Chronic obstructive bronchopulmonary disease. IV. The clinical and physiological differential of chronic bronchitis and emphysema. Am J Med Sci 1964;**247**:513–17.

●4 Wilkinson M, Langhorn CA, Heath D et al. A pathophysiological study of 10 cases of hypoxic cor pulmonale. Q J Med 1988;**66**:65–85.

●5 Hayhurst M, MacNee W, Flenley DC et al. Diagnosis of pulmonary emphysema by computerised tomography. Lancet 1984;**2**:320–2.

●6 Peinado VI, Barbera JA, Abate P et al. Inflammatory reaction in pulmonary muscular arteries of patients with mild chronic obstructive pulmonary disease. Am J Respir Crit Care Med 1999;**59**:1605–11.

◆7 Grover RF. Chronic hypoxic pulmonary hypertension. In: Fishman AP (ed.), The pulmonary circulation: normal and abnormal. Philadelphia: University of Pennsylvania, 1990;283–99.

●8 Weitzenblum E, Schrijen F, Mohan-Kumar T et al. Variability of pulmonary vascular response to acute hypoxia in chronic bronchitis. Chest 1988;**94**:772–8.

◆9 Voelkel NF. Hypoxic pulmonary vasoconstriction and hypertension. In: Peacock AJ (ed.), Pulmonary circulation. London: Chapman and Hall, 1996;71–85.

◆10 Weir EK, Archer SL. The mechanism of acute hypoxic pulmonary vasoconstriction: the tale of two channels. FASEB J 1995;**9**:183–9.

◆11 Dinh-Xuan AT. Endothelial modulation of pulmonary vascular tone. Eur Respir J 1992;**5**:757–62.

◆12 Hemple V, Cornfield DN, Huang J et al. Nitric oxide. In: Peacock AJ (ed.), Pulmonary circulation. London: Chapman and Hall, 1996;100–14.

●13 Dinh-Xuan AT, Higgenbottam TW, Clelland CA *et al.* Impairment of endothelium-dependent pulmonary-artery relaxation in chronic obstructive lung disease. *N Engl J Med* 1991;**324**:1539–47.

●14 Peinado VI, Santos S, Ramirez J *et al.* Response to hypoxia of pulmonary arteries in chronic obstructive pulmonary disease: an *in vitro* study. *Eur Respir J* 2002;**20**:332–8.

◆15 Moncada S, Palmer RMJ, Higgs EA. Prostacyclin and endothelial-derived relaxing factor : biological interactions and significance. In: Verstraete M, Verrmylen J, Lijnen RH (eds), *Thombosis and haemostasis.* Leuven: University Press Leuven, 1987;597–618.

◆16 MacNee W. State of the art: pathophysiology of cor pulmonale in chronic obstructive pulmonary disease. Part One. *Am J Respir Crit Care Med* 1994;**150**:838–52.

●17 Khaja F, Parker JO. Right and left ventricular performance in chronic obstructive lung disease. *Am Heart J* 1971;**82**:319–27.

◆18 Naeije R. Should pulmonary hypertension be treated in chronic obstructive pulmonary disease? In: Weir EK, Archer SL, Reeves JT (eds), *The diagnosis and treatment of pulmonary hypertension.* New York: Futura Publishing, 1992;209–39.

●19 Fletcher EC, Levin DC. Cardiopulmonary hemodynamics during sleep in subjects with chronic obstructive pulmonary disease: the effect of short and long-term oxygen. *Chest* 1984;**85**:6–14.

●20 Abraham AS, Cole RB, Green ID *et al.* Factors contributing to the reversible pulmonary hypertension in patients with acute respiratory failure studied by serial observations during recovery. *Circ Res* 1969;**26**:51–60.

21 Weitzenblum E, Hirth C, Roeslin N *et al.* Les modifications hemodynamiques pulmonaires au cours de l'insuffisance respiratoire aigue des bronchopneumopathies chroniques. *Respiration* 1971;**28**:539–54.

●22 Weitzenblum E, Sautageau A, Ehrihart M *et al.* Long-term course of pulmonary arterial pressure in chronic obstructive pulmonary disease. *Am Rev Respir Dis* 1984;**130**:993–8.

∗23 Medical Research Council Working Party. Long-term domiciliary oxygen therapy in chronic hypoxic cor pulmonale complicating chronic bronchitis and emphysema. *Lancet* 1981;**i**:681–6.

∗24 Timms RM, Khaja FU, Williams GW and the Nocturnal Oxygen Therapy Trial Group. Hemodynamic response to oxygen therapy in chronic obstructive pulmonary disease. *Ann Intern Med* 1985;**102**:29–36.

∗25 Weitzenblum E, Sautageau A, Ehrihart M *et al.* Long-term oxygen therapy can reverse the progression of pulmonary hypertension in patients with chronic obstructive pulmonary disease. *Am Rev Respir Dis* 1985;**131**:493–9.

●26 France AJ, Prescott RJ, Biernacki W *et al.* Does right ventricular function predict survival in patients with chronic obstructive pulmonary disease? *Thorax* 1988;**43**:621–6.

●27 Oswald-Mammosser M, Weitzenblum E, Quoix E *et al.* Prognostic factors in COPD patients receiving long-term oxygen therapy. *Chest* 1995;**107**:1193–8.

●28 Guyton AC, Lindsay AW, Gilluly J. The limits of right ventricular compensation following acute increase in pulmonary circulation resistance. *Circ Res* 1954;**2**:326–32.

◆29 Morpurgo M, Jezek V. Evaluation of right heart failure: controversies in definition and methods of evaluation. In: Jezek V, Morpurgo M, Tamarin R (eds), *Current topics in*

rehabilitation. Right ventricular hypertrophy and function in chronic lung disease. Verona: Springer-Verlag, 1992;79–95.

●30 Jezek V, Schrijen F, Sadoul P. Right ventricular function and pulmonary haemodynamics during exercise in patients with chronic obstructive broncho-pulmonary disease. *Cardiology* 1973;**58**:20–31.

◆31 Morrison DA. Pulmonary hypertension in chronic obstructive pulmonary disease. The right ventricular hypothesis. *Chest* 1987;**92**:387–9.

◆32 MacNee W. The clinical importance of right ventricular function in pulmonary hypertension. In: Weir EK, Archer SL, Reeves JT (eds), *The diagnosis and treatment of pulmonary hypertension.* New York: Futura Publishing, 1992;13–39.

◆33 Maughan WL, Oikawa PY. Right ventricular function. In: Scharf SM, Cassidy SS (eds), *Heart–lung interactions in health and disease. Lung biology in health and disease,* vol. 42. New York: Marcel Dekker, 1989;179–220.

●34 Biernacki W, Flenley DC, Muir AL *et al.* Pulmonary hypertension on right ventricular function in patients with chronic obstructive pulmonary disease. *Chest* 1988;**94**:1169–75.

∗35 MacNee W, Wathen CG, Hannan WJ *et al.* Effects of pirbuterol and sodium nitroprusside on pulmonary haemodynamics in hypoxic cor pulmonale. *Br Med J* 1983;**287**:1169–72.

◆36 Sagawa S, Maughan L, Suga H *et al. Cardiac contraction and the pressure–volume relationship.* New York: Oxford University Press, 1988.

◆37 Campbell EJM, Short DS. The cause of oedema in 'cor pulmonale'. *Lancet* 1960;**i**:1184–6.

◆38 MacNee W. State of the art: Pathophysiology of cor pulmonale in chronic obstructive pulmonary disease. Part Two. *Am J Respir Crit Care Med* 1994;**150**:1158–68.

39 Lockhart A, Tzareva M, Schrijen F *et al.* Etudes hémodynamiques des décompensations respiratoires aiguës des bronchopneumopathies chroniques. *Bull Physiopathol Respir* 1967;**3**:645–67.

●40 Weitzenblum E, Apprill M, Oswald M *et al.* Pulmonary hemodynamics in patients with chronic obstructive pulmonary disease before and during an episode of peripheral edema. *Chest* 1994;**105**:1377–82.

●41 Anand IS, Chandrasekhar Y, Ferrari R *et al.* Pathogenesis of congestive state in chronic obstructive pulmonary disease. *Circulation* 1992;**86**:12–21.

∗42 MacNee W, Wathen C, Flenley D *et al.* The effects of controlled oxygen therapy on ventricular function in acute and chronic respiratory failure. *Am Rev Respir Dis* 1988;**137**:1289–295.

∗43 Adnot S, Chabrier PE, Andrivet P *et al.* Atrial natriuretic peptide concentrations and pulmonary hemodynamics in patients with pulmonary artery hypertension. *Am Rev Respir Dis* 1987;**136**:951–6.

●44 Reihman DH, Farber MO, Weinberger MH *et al.* Effect of hypoxemia on sodium and water excretion in chronic obstructive lung disease. *Am J Med* 1985;**78**:87–94.

●45 Skwarski K, Lee M, Turnbull L *et al.* Atrial natriuretic peptide in stable and decompensated chronic obstructive pulmonary disease. *Thorax* 1993;**48**:730–5.

●46 Skwarski K, Morrison D, Sime P *et al.* Effects of hypoxia on hormonal balance in chronic obstructive lung disease (COLD). *Thorax* 1993;**48**:446.

◆47 Pauwels RA, Buist AS, Calverley PMA et al. on behalf of the GOLD Scientific Committee Global Strategy for the diagnosis, management, and prevention of chronic obstructive pulmonary disease NHLBI/WHO Global Initiative for chronic obstructive lung disease (GOLD) workshop summary. Am J Respir Crit Care Med 2001;163:1256–76.

◆48 Wiedemann HP, Matthay RA. Cor pulmonale. In: Braunwald E (ed.), Heart disease. A textbook of cardiovascular medicine, 5th edn. Philadelphia: WB Saunders Company, 1997;1604–25.

◆49 Rubin LJ. Primary pulmonary hypertension. N Engl J Med 1997;336:111–17.

∗50 Biernacki W, Prince K, Whyte K et al. The effect of six months of daily treatment with the beta-2 agonist oral pirbuterol on pulmonary hemodynamics in patients with chronic hypoxic cor pulmonale receiving long-term oxygen therapy. Am Rev Respir Dis 1989;139:492–7.

∗51 Stockley RA, Finnegan P, Bishop JM. Effects of intravenous terbutaline on arterial blood gas tensions, ventilation and pulmonary circulation in patients with chronic bronchitis and cor pulmonale. Thorax 1977;32:601–5.

∗52 Delaunois L, Jonard P, Kremer N et al. Nitroglycerin and isosorbide dinitrate in pulmonary disease. Bull Eur Physiopathol Respir 1984;20:11–18.

∗53 Bratel T, Hedenstierna G, Nyquist O et al. Long-term treatment with a new calcium antagonist, felodipine, in chronic obstructive lung disease. Eur J Respir Dis 1986;68:351–61.

∗54 Agostoni P, Doria E, Galli C et al. Nifedipine reduces pulmonary pressure and vascular tone during short- but not long-term treatment of pulmonary hypertension in patients with chronic obstructive pulmonary disease. Am Rev Respir Dis 1989;139:120–5.

∗55 Saadjian AY, Philip-Joet FF, Vestri R et al. Long-term treatment of chronic obstructive lung disease by nifedipine: an 18-month haemodynamic study. Eur Respir J 1988;1:716–20.

∗56 Sturani C, Bassein L, Schiavina M et al. Oral nifedipine in chronic cor pulmonary secondary to severe chronic obstructive pulmonary disease (COPD): short and long term hemodynamic effects. Chest 1983;84:35–42.

∗57 Mookherjee S, Ashutosh K, Dunsky M et al. Nifedipine in chronic cor pulmonale: acute and relatively long-term effects. Clin Pharmacol Ther 1988;44:289–96.

∗58 Rubin WJ, Moser K. Long-term effects of nitrendipine on hemodynamics and oxygen transport in patients with cor pulmonale. Chest 1986;89:141–5.

∗59 Burke CM, Harte M, Duncan J et al. Captopril and domiciliary oxygen in chronic airflow obstruction. Br Med J 1985;290:1251.

∗60 Matthay RA, Berger HJ, Loke J et al. Effects of aminophylline upon right and left ventricular performance in chronic obstructive pulmonary diease: noninvasive assessment by radionuclide angiocardiography. Am J Med 1978;65:903–10.

∗61 Vik-Mo H, Walde N, Jentoft H et al. Improved haemodynamics but reduced arterial blood oxygenase, at rest and during exercise after long-term oral prasozin therapy in chronic cor pulmonale. Eur Heart J 1985;6:1047–53.

∗62 Adnot S, Kouyoumdjian C, Defouilloy C et al. Haemodynamic and gas exchange responses to infusion of acetyl choline and inhalation of nitric oxide in patients with chronic obstructive lung disease and pulmonary hypertension. Am Rev Respir Dis 1993;148:310–16.

∗63 Katayama Y, Higenbottam TW, Diaz de Atauri MJ et al. Inhaled nitric oxide and arterial oxygen tension in patients with chronic obstructive pulmonary disease and severe pulmonary hypertension. Thorax 1997;52:120–4.

∗64 Roger N, Barbera JA, Roca J et al. Nitric oxide inhalation during exercise in chronic obstructive pulmonary disease. Am J Respir Crit Care Med 1997;156:800–6.

∗65 Nocturnal Oxygen Therapy Trial Group. Continuous or nocturnal oxygen therapy in hypoxemic chronic obstructive lung disease. Ann Intern Med 1980;93:391–8.

∗66 Sliwinski P, Hawrylkiewicz I, Gorecka D et al. Acute effects of oxygen on pulmonary artery pressure does not predict survival on long-term oxygen therapy in patients with chronic obstructive pulmonary disease. Am Rev Respir Dis 1992;148:665–9.

●67 Calverley PM, Howatson R, Flenley DC et al. Clinicopathological correlations in cor pulmonale. Thorax 1992;47:494–8.

∗68 Weisse AB, Moschos CB, Frank MJ et al. Hemodynamic effects of staged hematocrit reduction in patients with stable cor pulmonale and severely elevated hematocrit levels. Am J Med 1975;58:92–8.

∗69 Wedzicha JA, Rudd RM, Apps MC et al. Erythrophoresis in 7 patients with polycythemia secondary to hypoxic lung disease. Br Med J 1983;286:511–14.

∗70 Erickson AD, Golden WA, Claunch BC et al. Acute effects of phlebotomy on right ventricular size and performance in polycythemic patients with chronic obstructive pulmonary disease. Am J Cardiol 1983;53:163–6.

●71 Peacock AJ, Matthews A. Trans-pulmonary angiotensin II formation and pulmonary haemodynamics in stable hypoxic lung disease: the effect of captopril. Respir Med 1992;86:21–6.

◆72 Corris PA. Lung transplantation. In: Peacock AJ (ed.), Pulmonary circulation. A handbook for clinicians. London: Chapman and Hall, 1996;348–58.

∗73 Cooper JD, Trulock EP, Triantafillou AN et al. Bilateral pneumectomy (volume reduction) for chronic obstructive pulmonary disease. J Thorac Cardiovasc Surg 1995;109:106–16.

∗74 Sciurba FC, Robers RM, Keenan RJ et al. Improvement in pulmonary function and elastic recoil after lung-reduction surgery for diffuse emphysema. N Engl J Med 1996;334:1095–9.

●75 Weg IL, Rossoff L, McKeon K et al. Development of pulmonary hypertension after lung volume reduction surgery. Am J Respir Crit Care Med 1999;159:552–6.

∗76 Oswald-Mammosser M, Kessler R, Massard G et al. Effect of lung volume reduction surgery on gas exchange and pulmonary hemodynamics at rest and during exercise. Am J Respir Crit Care Med 1998;158:1020–5.

∗77 Kubo K, Koizumi T, Fujimoto K et al. Effects of lung volume reduction surgery on exercise pulmonary hemodynamics in severe emphysema. Chest 1998;114:1575–82.

∗78 Mineo TC, Pompeo E, Rogliani P et al. Effect of lung volume reduction surgery for severe emphysema on right ventricular function. Am J Respir Crit Care Med 2002;165:489–94.

●79 Santos S, Peinado VI, Ramirez J et al. Characterization of pulmonary vascular remodeling in smokers and patients with mild COPD. Eur Respir J 2002;19:632–8.

PART 5

Pulmonary thromboembolism and pulmonary vascular tumors

Acute pulmonary thromboembolism

Diagnosis

ARNAUD PERRIER AND HENRI BOUNAMEAUX

INTRODUCTION

Pulmonary embolism is the third most common cause of mortality due to cardiovascular disease after coronary artery disease and stroke. In Western countries, it remains the leading cause of death in the puerperium and the postoperative period. It is, therefore, a major health concern.[1] Nonetheless, pulmonary embolism is difficult to diagnose because of protean clinical manifestations and poor sensitivity and specificity of symptoms and signs. Therefore, it is still underdiagnosed and up to 80% of pulmonary emboli found at autopsy have not been suspected antemortem, a proportion which has not decreased in the last 40 years.[2,3] However, considerable progress has been made in the work-up of patients with clinically suspected pulmonary embolism with the advent of novel diagnostic instruments such as plasma D-dimer measurement,[4] lower limb venous compression ultrasonography to detect deep vein thrombosis[5] and helical CT scan,[6] and of rational and cost-effective diagnostic strategies.[7–10] Finally, deep venous thrombosis and pulmonary embolism are now considered as a single disease, venous thromboembolism, with common risk factors and treatment. Indeed, more than 90% of pulmonary emboli originate from a deep venous thrombosis of the lower limbs[11] and approximately 50% of patients with a proximal deep venous thrombosis have a silent concomitant pulmonary embolism.[12,13]

DEFINITIONS

Traditionally, pulmonary embolism was classified as massive or non-massive. However, that definition was ambiguous because the term massive could refer either to the clinical presentation of pulmonary embolism accompanied by shock, or to the radiological description of a more than 50% amputation of the pulmonary vasculature. Finally, that classification did not account for those patients who, despite absence of overt shock, have repercussions of pulmonary embolism on right ventricular function. Hence, in this text, we classify pulmonary embolism into three categories:

- massive pulmonary embolism: pulmonary embolism provoking shock or cardiorespiratory arrest;
- submassive pulmonary embolism: pulmonary embolism provoking right ventricular strain (dilatation and hypokinesis) despite normal systemic blood pressure;
- non-massive pulmonary embolism: pulmonary embolism associated with normal systemic blood pressure and normal right ventricular function.

EPIDEMIOLOGY

Several recent population-based studies have established that the incidence of venous thromboembolism is around 1 per 1000 subjects per year, with an incidence of pulmonary embolism approximately half that of deep venous thrombosis.[14,15] Venous thromboembolic recurrences account for one-third of those events. Age is an important determinant of the incidence of venous thromboembolism. Above 40 years, the incidence of venous thromboembolism doubles for every 10 additional years. Finally, the disease is slightly more common in male than in female subjects.

The case-fatality rate of treated pulmonary embolism has been a matter of debate. In the large multicenter Prospective Investigation on Pulmonary Embolism Diagnosis (PIOPED) study,[16] despite a high 15% mortality in the 3 months following the acute event, only 10% of those deaths were attributed to pulmonary embolism. By contrast, in the large International Cooperative Pulmonary Embolism Registry (ICOPER),[17] pulmonary embolism recurrence was the main cause of death in the 17.5% of patients who died during the 3-month follow-up period. In a Geneva series,[18] 3-month mortality was 8.4% and more than half the deaths that occurred during the first 15 days were due to pulmonary embolism recurrence. The much lower recurrence and case-fatality rates observed in a recent meta-analysis of randomized controlled trials on treatment of venous thromboembolism[19] are probably due to selection bias and exclusion of the sicker patients. Hence, the true recurrence rate in patients with pulmonary embolism is probably around 4% in the first 3 months,[18,20] and approximately half those events are fatal. Finally, cancer, heart failure and presence of concomitant deep vein thrombosis are significant risk factors for recurrent pulmonary embolism.[18,20]

ETIOLOGY

Venous thromboembolism is a multigenic disease with a strong influence of environmental factors. The basic pathophysiological hypothesis formulated by Virchow at the end of the nineteenth century[21] is still valid. Virchow's triad consists of venous stasis in the lower limbs, an imbalance of the hemostatic system towards thrombosis (hypercoagulable state), and direct lesions of the venous endothelium. Although the relative importance of those factors varies according to the clinical situation, venous thrombosis usually results from an interaction of those mechanisms. For instance, venous stasis and clotting activation predominate in thrombosis after surgery, but patients with more severe hypercoagulability due to cancer or a genetic thrombophilic mutation are more prone to thrombotic complications in that setting.

Genetic determinants

In recent years, several molecular markers of an increased thrombotic risk have been identified, of which the two most prevalent are the Leiden mutation of factor V, which confers a resistance to activated protein C, and the G20210A mutation of prothrombin (Table 16A.1).[22] Deficiency in protein S, protein C or antithrombin are much less prevalent.[22] Patients who are heterozygous for two of these anomalies present a much greater thrombotic risk. Conversely, certain genetic factors seem to protect from thrombosis despite the existence of a thrombophilic mutation. For instance, the O blood group appears to reduce the risk of venous thrombosis in carriers of factor V Leiden.[23] Protective factors are still largely not investigated. Factor V Leiden and prothrombin mutation are stronger risk factors for deep vein thrombosis than for pulmonary embolism, raising the question whether clot composition might be different when those anomalies are present and, therefore more adherent.[24] Finally, elevated levels of homocysteine, factors VIII, IX and XI have been identified as risk factors for venous thromboembolism, but the underlying genetic defects are yet unidentified.[25]

Environmental determinants

The main environmental risk factors for pulmonary embolism are detailed in Table 16A.2. Recent data from the Nurses' Health Study[26] and a French epidemiological study[27] have identified heavy smoking and arterial hypertension as additional risk factors. Hormone replacement therapy increases the thromboembolic risk threefold, similar to oral contraception.[28] However, the absolute incidence of venous thromboembolism is tenfold higher in women over 50 compared to women in their third decade and hormone replacement therapy may hence be responsible for a higher number of cases. Raloxifene, a new selective modulator of the estrogen receptor, is also associated with an increased risk of venous thromboembolism.[29]

Table 16A.1 *Prevalence of genetic risk factors for pulmonary embolism (PE)*

Anomaly	General population (%)	Subjects with PE (%)	Relative risk
Antithrombin deficiency	0.02	1	50
Protein C deficiency	0.2	3	15
Protein S deficiency	0.1	1–2	10–20
Factor V Leiden*	4	12	3
G20210A prothrombin mutation	4	10	2.5

*Frequency of the anomaly is very different according to the country of origin (15% in the south of Sweden versus 5% overall in Europe).

Table 16A.2 *Environmental and acquired risk factors for venous thromboembolism*

Acquired thrombophilia
- Lupus anticoagulant
- Antiphospholipid syndrome
- Acquired deficiency in coagulation inhibitors
- Hyperhomocysteinemia
Hormonal treatment
- Oral contraceptives
- Hormone replacement therapy
- Tamoxifen, raloxifen
- Pregnancy
Cancer
Surgery
Trauma
Immobilization
- Hemiplegia, paraplegia
Congestive heart failure
Myocardial infarction
Chronic inflammatory bowel disease
Nephrotic syndrome

Searching for specific etiologies

TESTING FOR THROMBOPHILIA

The opportunity of searching for a genetic thrombophilia depends on the probability of finding an anomaly in a given individual, on the feasibility of biological diagnosis and most of all on the existence of consequences on patient management.[25] Recent trials failed to report an increased recurrence rate after a first venous thromboembolic event in patients with the most frequent anomalies (heterozygous factor V Leiden or prothrombin mutation).[30] Hence, prolonged anticoagulation treatment after a first episode is not justified. By contrast, detection of thrombophilic defects may be important in particular situations. For instance, thrombotic risk is greatly increased in some thrombophilias during pregnancy, such as antithrombin deficiency, justifying prophylactic anticoagulation throughout. Common recommendations are to investigate patients with a positive family history of venous thromboembolism, recurrent idiopathic venous thrombosis or thrombosis after a trivial triggering event (travel, pregnancy, estrogen therapy), first thrombotic episode before 50 years of age, association of arterial and venous thrombosis, superficial thrombosis in a non-varicose vein, thrombosis in unusual sites, and association of thrombosis and fetal loss.[25] Nevertheless, screening decisions should be individualized according to the family and individual history, the type of suspected anomaly, patient age and consequences of a positive finding. Finally, any patient with one of the above-cited characteristics should be considered as having a clinical thrombophilia, even if the laboratory tests do not disclose a known anomaly, and given appropriate prophylaxis in at-risk situations. Since this is a rapidly moving field, specialized counseling and performance of tests in a reference laboratory should be preferred to routine testing.

SEARCHING FOR CANCER

Neoplastic cells are able to activate the clotting cascade either directly through activation of thromboplastin or indirectly by stimulating monocytes and macrophages to synthesize a variety of procoagulant molecules. Hence, cancer is a significant risk factor for venous thromboembolism and the risk of discovering a cancer during the first 6 months to a year after an acute episode venous thromboembolism is increased approximately three- to fourfold.[31,32] The prevalence of cancer may be higher in patients with idiopathic venous thromboembolism,[33] and in rare patients with bilateral deep vein thrombosis.[34] However, an extensive diagnostic work-up for cancer does not appear warranted in patients with acute venous thromboembolism. Indeed, in a recent series, most cancers were detected by clinical examination and simple tests such as a complete blood count, sedimentation rate and chest radiography,[35] and the 34-month cancer-free survival was similar in patients with a negative initial work-up and a control group without deep vein thrombosis.

CLINICAL PRESENTATION

Clinical syndromes

Symptoms of pulmonary embolism are very non-specific. In 65% of patients, pulmonary embolism is evoked because of pleuritic pain accompanied or not by dyspnea. Isolated dyspnea, usually acute but sometimes slowly progressive and without an obvious alternative cause, points towards pulmonary embolism in 20% of patients. Syncope or shock are a rare clinical presentation of pulmonary embolism (less than 10%). Pulmonary embolism is exceptionally discovered in the absence of a clinical suspicion during the investigation of a radiological infiltrate. Those clinical presentations correspond to three syndromes of different pathology and variable severity.[36]

ALVEOLAR HEMORRHAGE

The clinical hallmark of this syndrome is pleuritic pain due to irritation of the visceral pleura, and, more rarely, hemoptysis. It is due to peripheral emboli. Although it is often incorrectly referred to as 'pulmonary infarction', the histopathological correlate is in fact an alveolar hemorrhage probably provoked by the influx of blood from the high-pressure bronchial circulation in the segment obstructed by the embolus.[37] The classic radiological picture is a wedge-shaped pleural based infiltrate that affects around 20% of patients.[38] Other common chest x-ray anomalies include plate-like atelectasis and pleural effusion. Tachycardia and dyspnea are less frequent than in this clinical syndrome, reflecting the peripheral character and lesser hemodynamic repercussions of such pulmonary emboli.[36]

ISOLATED DYSPNEA

The absence of pleuritic pain in this syndrome is probably due to more proximal embolization of the pulmonary vasculature. Patients may complain of retrosternal chest pain oppressive in character evoking the differential diagnosis of angina. In fact, such pain probably reflects true myocardial ischemia due to increased right ventricular wall tension and reduced right coronary artery flow. Tachycardia, although more frequent, is still present in only 45% of patients.[36] The electrocardiogram is rarely normal, but its anomalies are often non-specific. Although dyspnea is usually of abrupt or rapid onset, in some patients it may progress over several days.

SHOCK

Syncope and/or shock are the clinical manifestations of massive pulmonary embolism causing acute severe pulmonary hypertension and right ventricular failure. It is usually caused by large central clots. Although suggestive of pulmonary embolism in patients with obvious risk factors such as recent surgery, syncope may be a misleading presentation.[39] Suspected massive pulmonary embolism with shock is a distinct situation requiring a specific diagnostic approach detailed in an appropriate section.

Laboratory tests

CHEST RADIOGRAPH

The most frequent anomalies of the chest radiograph are cardiomegaly, pleural effusion, band atelectasis and elevated hemidiaphragm.[38,40] Their presence raises the probability of pulmonary embolism, albeit modestly. Pulmonary artery enlargement and oligemia are rare and non-specific. The typical infiltrate of so-called pulmonary infarction has already been discussed. Nevertheless, the chest radiograph remains extremely useful in a patient with suspected pulmonary embolism for differential diagnosis with conditions such as left ventricular failure, pneumonia or pneumothorax.

ELECTROCARDIOGRAM

The electrocardiogram is usually normal in small peripheral pulmonary embolism. Larger pulmonary embolism

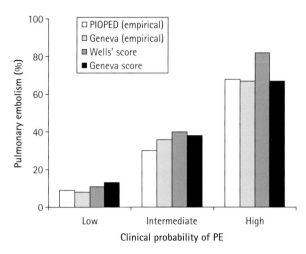

Figure 16A.1 *Predictive value of clinical evaluation. The figure shows the prevalence of pulmonary embolism (PE) according to the clinical probability category attributed either implicitly or by a prediction rule in various studies. Figures for implicit evaluation are drawn from the PIOPED study[16] and the Geneva series.[43] Figures for the Wells' and the Geneva score are drawn from a validation sample from a three-center study.[46]*

may induce modifications such as large P waves in derivations DII, DIII and atrioventricular fibrillation (AVF), the S1Q3 pattern or ST segment depression in derivations V1 to V4. A right bundle branch block or right axial deviation are also possible. When all present in a patient with a suggestive clinical presentation and risk factors for venous thromboembolism, those anomalies may be useful.

BLOOD GASES

Hypocapnia and hypoxemia are frequent in pulmonary embolism. However, approximately 20% of patients with proven pulmonary embolism have a normal arterial oxygen pressure and alveoloarterial oxygen gradient.[41,42]

Clinical probability of pulmonary embolism

Sensitivity and specificity of clinical symptoms, signs and abnormalities of blood gases, chest radiograph and electrocardiogram in suspected pulmonary embolism are low when considered singly. Nevertheless, these findings can be combined effectively by clinicians, either implicitly,[16,43] or by prediction rules.[44,45] Figure 16A.1 shows that both means of assessing clinical likelihood of pulmonary embolism allow a fairly accurate stratification of patients into three categories corresponding to a prevalence of pulmonary embolism of 10% (low clinical probability), 30–40% (intermediate clinical probability) and 67–81% (high clinical probability), respectively. The majority of patients (80–90%) have a low or intermediate clinical probability of pulmonary embolism. Those

Table 16A.3 *Clinical prediction rules for pulmonary embolism*

Score by Wicki *et al.*[45]	Points	Score by Wells *et al.*[44]	Points
Previous PE or DVT	+2	Previous PE or DVT	+1.5
Heart rate >100/min	+1	Heart rate >100/min	+1.5
Recent surgery	+3	Recent surgery or immobilization	+1.5
Age		Clinical signs of DVT	+3
60–79 years	+1	Alternative diagnosis less likely than PE	+3
≥80 years	+2	Hemoptysis	+1
$PaCO_2$		Cancer	+1
<4.8 kPa (36 mmHg)	+2		
4.8–5.19 kPa (36–39 mmHg)	+1		
PaO_2			
<6.5 kPa (49 mmHg)	+4		
6.5–7.99 kPa (49–60 mmHg)	+3		
8–9.49 kPa (60–71 mmHg)	+2		
9.5–10.99 kPa (71–82.6 mmHg)	+1		
Atelectasis	+1		
Elevated hemidiaphragm	+1		
Clinical probability		Clinical probability	
Low	0–4	Low	0–1
Intermediate	5–8	Intermediate	2–6
High	≥9	High	≥7

DVT, deep vein thrombosis; PE, pulmonary embolism.

with a low probability of pulmonary embolism can usually be investigated by entirely non-invasive algorithms, as will be discussed in a later section. Table 16A.3 shows two recently developed prediction rules. The score by Wicki *et al.*[45] has the advantage of being completely standardized, but the requirement for blood gas analysis may be a drawback in particular settings and it has been derived from an entirely outpatient population. On the other hand, the prediction rule by Wells *et al.*[44] requires subjective judgment on the probability of an alternative diagnosis, but it can be applied to both out- and in-patients. Both scores have been recently validated in a group of patients distinct from that in which they were developed (external validation).[46] Interestingly, adding implicit clinical judgment to the prediction rule appears to increase accuracy.[46] Therefore, prediction rules and implicit assessment should be viewed as complementary.

In summary, clinical evaluation of pulmonary embolism is accurate enough to be the foundation for further diagnostic evaluation.

INVESTIGATIONS

D-dimer

Plasma D-dimer is a degradation product of cross-linked fibrin and its levels increase in the plasma of patients with acute venous thromboembolism. When assayed by highly sensitive tests such as ELISA or some automated turbidimetric tests, D-dimer has been shown highly sensitive (about 99%) in acute pulmonary embolism at a cut-off value of 500 µg/L (Table 16A.4).[4,7,47] Hence, a D-dimer level below this value reasonably rules out pulmonary embolism. On the other hand, although D-dimer is very specific for fibrin, the specificity of fibrin for venous thromboembolism is poor because fibrin is produced in a wide variety of conditions, such as cancer, inflammation, infection or necrosis. Hence, a D-dimer level above 500 µg/L has a poor positive predictive value for pulmonary embolism, and cannot reliably rule in the disease. New semiquantitative latex tests based on an immunoturbidimetric method appear to be also very sensitive.[48,49] Whole-blood agglutination assays have a lower 85% sensitivity and must be combined with a low clinical probability in order to safely rule out pulmonary embolism[8,50] (Table 16A.4). Specificity of D-dimer is lower in the very elderly (9% in patients older than 80 years suspected of pulmonary embolism[51,52]) and in patients experiencing suspected pulmonary embolism during their hospital stay.[53] Hence, D-dimer measurement is unlikely to be useful in such populations. Although rapid unitary ELISA D-dimer tests have proven safe and effective to rule out venous thromboembolism in management studies,[7] their theoretical negative predictive value is lower in patients with a high clinical probability of pulmonary embolism despite their very high sensitivity. Moreover, a D-dimer level below the cut-off value appears to be rare in such patients: in a series of 918 patients,[7] 101 patients had a high clinical probability of

Table 16A.4 *Performances of diagnostic tests for non-massive pulmonary embolism*

Test	Sensitivity (%)	Specificity (%)	Likelihood ratio Positive result	Negative result
Pulmonary angiography[16,91]	97	98	48	0.03
V̇/Q̇ lung scan				
Normal[16,59,65,92]	99	–	0.02	–
Non-diagnostic[16]	–	–	0.9	–
High probability[16]	–	91	–	14
Plasma D-dimer				
Rapid ELISA[7,93]	99	41	1.7	0.02
Immunoturbidimetric[48,49]	98	40	1.6	0.05
Whole-blood agglutination[8,50]	85	68	2.7	0.2
Lower limb venous ultrasonography[5,7,51,57,59]	50	97	17	0.5
Helical CT scan[69,70]	69	89	6.3	0.3
Echocardiography[85–89]	60	90	6.0	0.4

CT, computed tomography; ELISA, enzyme-linked immunosorbent assay; V̇/Q̇, ventilation/perfusion.

venous thromboembolism, of which only 10 had a normal D-dimer level.

In summary, highly sensitive D-dimer assays allow one to exclude pulmonary embolism in outpatients with a low or intermediate clinical probability of pulmonary embolism, while whole-blood agglutination tests only rule out the disease in patients with a low clinical probability. Finally, D-dimer is unlikely to be useful in very elderly patients or in patients with suspected venous thromboembolism.

Lower limb venous compression ultrasonography

In studies using venography as the gold standard, lower limb compression venous ultrasonography, an entirely non-invasive test, has a sensitivity of 97% (95% CI 96–98%) and a specificity of 98% for symptomatic proximal deep vein thrombosis.[5,54,55] The single well-validated diagnostic criterion for deep vein thrombosis on ultrasonography is absence of full compressibility of the deep vein when applying pressure through the ultrasound probe.[56] Finding a deep vein thrombosis by ultrasonography in a patient with clinically suspected pulmonary embolism is sufficient evidence to warrant anticoagulant treatment without further testing. Compression ultrasonography shows a deep vein thrombosis in approximately 50% of patients with proven pulmonary embolism[7,57–59] (Table 16A.4). The position of ultrasonography in the diagnostic sequence for pulmonary embolism is still debated. When performed after lung scan only in patients with a non-diagnostic result, the diagnostic yield of ultrasonography is quite low (4–10%).[59,60] By contrast, given a 20–30% prevalence of pulmonary embolism, ultrasonography performed before lung scan may allow ruling in the disease

in 10–15% of all patients suspected of the disease. Whether a baseline lung scan should be systematically performed in patients with suspected pulmonary embolism and a deep vein thrombosis shown by ultrasonography is controversial. Recurrent pulmonary embolism is a rare event in treated patients, and the interpretation of a lung scan performed for a suspected recurrence is not always straightforward. In our experience, a baseline lung scan is rarely useful, and systematic lung scanning is unlikely to be cost-effective.

Ventilation/perfusion lung scintigraphy

Perfusion lung scintigraphy is a non-invasive technique allowing the visualization of pulmonary perfusion through intravenous injection of albumin macroaggregates labeled by technetium-99 m. The macroaggregates are trapped in approximately 0.1% of the pulmonary capillary vessels and may be imaged by a gamma-camera. Pulmonary hypoperfusion is not highly specific for an embolus, since any disease that narrows the airways or fills the alveoli with fluid will result in hypoxic pulmonary vasoconstriction, a protective mechanism designed to minimize the shunt effect due to poorly ventilated alveolar units. A perfusion defect corresponding to a segment or a large part of a segment is more specific for pulmonary embolism. The addition of ventilation scintigraphy (by xenon-133, krypton-81 m or aerosolized technetium-99 m) further increases specificity, a so-called mismatched defect (perfusion defect with normal ventilation), usually representing pulmonary embolism.[61] The interpretation of lung scan has long been based on criteria validated in the landmark PIOPED study,[16] and their subsequent revision (Figure 16A.2).[62,63] More recently, it has been greatly simplified and lung scan results are now classified into three

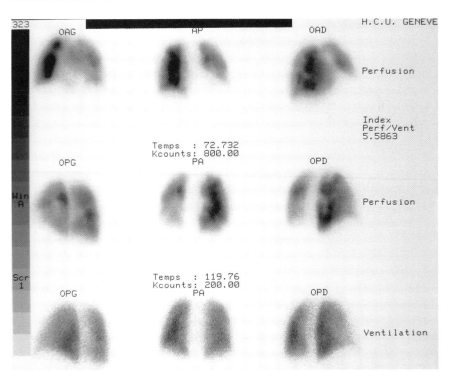

Figure 16A.2 *High probability lung scan. The six perfusion views (upper part of figure) show multiple segmental defects, mismatched compared to the three ventilation views (lower part). Such a lung scan result is highly specific for pulmonary embolism.*

Table 16A.5 *Three-month thromboembolic risk in patients left untreated according to various diagnostic criteria for ruling out pulmonary embolism*

Diagnostic criterion	No. of Patients	3-Month thromboembolic risk (%) (95% CI)	Reference
Normal pulmonary angiogram	547	1.6 (0.9–3.1)	94, 95
Normal lung scan	1031	0.7 (0.3–1.4)	59, 64, 65, 96
Plasma ELISA D-dimer level <500 µg/L and low to intermediate clinical probability of PE	444	0 (0.9–2.0)	7
Non-diagnostic lung scan and negative proximal US and low clinical probability of PE	864	2.3 (1.5–3.5)	43, 59
Normal helical CT scan and negative proximal US and low or intermediate clinical probability of PE	525	1.7 (0.9–3.2)	73

CT, computed tomography; ELISA, enzyme-linked immunosorbent assay; PE, pulmonary embolism; US, proximal lower limb venous ultrasonography.

categories: normal, high probability and non-diagnostic. Attribution of a lung scintigram to the high probability category requires two or more mismatched segmental defects or, if only one is present, the addition of two large mismatched subsegmental defects according to the revised PIOPED criteria.[62] The presence of one or more mismatched segmental defects or two or more large mismatched subsegmental defects suffices for the Canadian classification,[59] but these differences of interpretation appear to be of little clinical consequence. The high negative predictive value of a normal lung scan has been confirmed by several studies, including a large outcome study,[59,64,65] and is recognized as a valid criterion for excluding pulmonary embolism (Table 16A.4). The positive predictive value of a high probability scan is approximately 90%,[16]

and most clinicians consider such a result to rule in pulmonary embolism (Table 16A.4). Recent evidence suggests that the ventilation scan may be validly replaced by chest x-ray with an overall agreement of 88% and a positive predictive value of 86% for a scintigraphic mismatch.[66]

The proportion of diagnostic ventilation/perfusion lung scans (i.e. normal or high probability) was only 41% in the latest study by Wells *et al.*[59] and 48% in the pooled Geneva experience.[52] Hence, two large series have attempted to combine clinical probability to lung scan to increase that test's diagnostic yield. A recent analysis of a database of 1034 consecutive patients, suspected in the emergency ward of pulmonary embolism,[43] showed that the 3-month thromboembolic risk was very low (1.7%, 95% CI 0.4–4.9) in 175 suspected pulmonary embolism

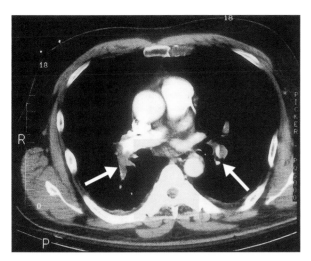

Figure 16A.3 *Helical computed tomography (CT) showing a pulmonary embolism. This CT image was taken in the same patient as the lung scan in Figure 16A.2. Bilateral thrombi in the main and lobar pulmonary artery are clearly visible (arrows).*

patients not treated on the grounds of a low empiric clinical probability and a non-diagnostic lung scan, provided that lower limb venous compression ultrasonography did not show a proximal deep vein thrombosis (Table 16A.5). This combination was found in 21% of patients, who, therefore, did not undergo an angiogram. Similarly, Wells et al.[59] withheld anticoagulant treatment in 702 of 1239 (57%) patients who had a non-diagnostic scan, a low or intermediate clinical probability of pulmonary embolism and normal serial compression ultrasonography and the 3-month thromboembolic risk was only 0.5% (95% CI 0.1–1.3).

Helical computed tomography

The rapid acquisition of high-contrast images by spiral CT scanning allows an adequate visualization of the pulmonary arteries up to at least the segmental level (Figure 16A.3).[67] Two recent systematic overviews[6,68] on the performance of helical CT in suspected pulmonary embolism reported wide variations regarding both CT sensitivity (53–100%) and specificity (73–100%). Variations in image acquisition protocols, selection bias and flaws in the design of the older studies may partly account for these differences.[6,68] Two recent studies[69,70] have shed new light on the performance of helical CT. They included a wide spectrum of patients with suspected pulmonary embolism; the diagnostic criteria for pulmonary embolism were appropriate and both helical CT and reference diagnostic tests were read in a blinded fashion. They both reported a sensitivity around 70% and a specificity of 90% (Table 16A.4). As in previous series, helical CT was technically

inadequate in 5–8% of patients because of motion artifacts or insufficient opacification of the pulmonary vessels. Sensitivity of CT is higher in central pulmonary emboli than in segmental and subsegmental arteries. Multi-detector CT, which allows both a thinner collimation (1–2 mm collimation) and a better definition without increasing image acquisition time,[71,72] will likely improve sensitivity. To what extent this will be at the expense of specificity remains to be evaluated. Indeed, in the Geneva series, the positive predictive value of helical CT decreased from 100% and 85% at the main pulmonary or lobar artery level, respectively, to 62% at the segmental level, demonstrating that specificity of CT is also dependent on the vascular level. In a recent multicenter French study,[73] performed with single-detector CT, the prevalence of isolated subsegmental pulmonary embolism was only 3% and only 3 of 12 such results were confirmed by pulmonary angiography. Moreover, the clinical significance of isolated segmental and subsegmental emboli is widely debated, and patients with no deep vein thrombosis, a negative CT scan and a low or intermediate clinical probability of pulmonary embolism left untreated may have a very low thromboembolic risk,[73] as discussed in another section.

In summary, a helical CT scan showing a thrombus up to the segmental level can be taken as adequate evidence of pulmonary embolism, whereas the necessity to treat isolated subsegmental thrombi in a patient without a deep vein thrombosis is unclear. A negative helical CT alone does not rule out pulmonary embolism. Finally, the probability of pulmonary embolism is very low in patients with a low or intermediate clinical probability, absence of proximal deep vein thrombosis and a negative helical CT.

Pulmonary angiography

Although it is considered the criterion standard for diagnosing pulmonary embolism (Figure 16A.4), pulmonary angiography is difficult to interpret, with frequent disagreement occurring even between expert readers, more often on the absence (17% of angiograms) than on the presence of pulmonary embolism (8% of angiograms).[16] It is also costly and invasive. The mortality due to pulmonary angiography was 0.2% (95% CI 0–0.3) in a pooled analysis of five series regrouping a total of 5696 patients.[74–78] The rare deaths attributable to pulmonary angiography occurred in very sick patients with hemodynamic compromise or acute respiratory failure. This should be kept in mind when discussing diagnostic strategies for suspected massive pulmonary embolism. On the other hand, complications do not appear to be more frequent in patients with pre-existing pulmonary hypertension in recent series.[78]

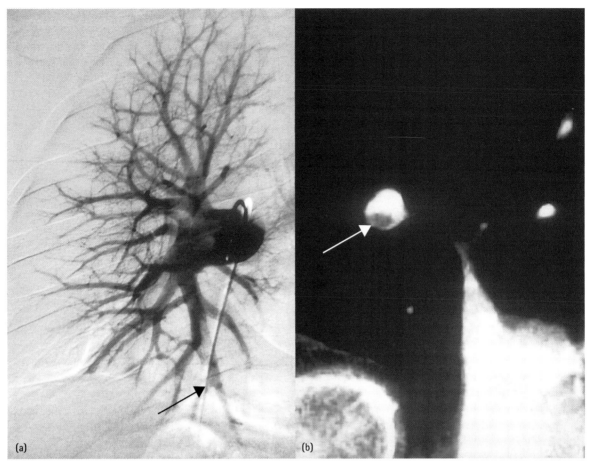

Figure 16A.4 *Helical computed tomography (CT) and corresponding pulmonary angiogram. The CT shows an isolated segmental thrombus, confirmed by a vascular filling defect in the same segmental artery on pulmonary angiography (arrows).*

Echocardiography

Doppler echocardiography has several uses in suspected pulmonary embolism and it may play a role in risk stratification. In a small subset of patients with pulmonary embolism (4% in a recent registry),[17] transthoracic echocardiography allows a direct visualization of the clot in the right heart chambers or in the right main pulmonary artery.[79,80] Direct imaging of part of the left main pulmonary artery requires transesophageal echocardiography.[81,82] However, transesophageal echocardiography is uncomfortable for patients, and its sensitivity in suspected pulmonary embolism does not appear to be significantly higher than that of transthoracic echocardiography. In fact, the most frequent echocardiographic manifestations of pulmonary embolism are indirect and reflect the hemodynamic changes caused by an acute increase in pulmonary arterial resistance and pulmonary hypertension. Pulmonary arterial pressure may be estimated in most patients by the tricuspid regurgitation velocity. A cut-off value of 2.7 m/s for the presence of pulmonary arterial hypertension was adopted in several series. Signs of right

ventricular strain include dilation of the right ventricle, right ventricular hypokinesis and, in severe cases, paradoxical motion of the interventricular septum. Several echocardiographic measurements have been proposed to quantify right ventricular dilation, of which the most standardized is the right ventricle over left ventricle diameter ratio. However, a visual estimate appears to be as accurate in the eyes of an experienced observer.[83] A particular pattern of right ventricular hypokinesis characterized by akinesia of the mid-free wall and preservation of apex motion appears to be quite specific for acute as opposed to chronic pulmonary hypertension.[84] Conversely, right ventricular hypertrophy and pulmonary artery pressures above 60 mmHg suggest chronic pulmonary hypertension. The sensitivity of these signs, which are often combined, lies between 40 and 70% in clinically suspected pulmonary embolism, and their specificity is approximately 90%,[85–89] provided that the patient does not have another disease causing chronic pulmonary hypertension (Table 16A.4). Echocardiography is the first-line test in suspected massive pulmonary embolism. Indeed, in patients with shock, it is extremely effective for differential diagnosis with tamponade and cardiogenic shock. Moreover, absence of pulmonary hypertension and/or right ventricular dilation and hypokinesis in that situation renders pulmonary embolism as the cause shock unlikely.

DIAGNOSTIC STRATEGIES

Suspected non-massive pulmonary embolism

Several diagnostic algorithms have been validated in large-scale prospective outcome studies. A sequential strategy combining clinical assessment, D-dimer, compression ultrasonography and lung scan, pulmonary angiography being performed only in case of an inconclusive non-invasive evaluation, was assessed in 444 consecutive emergency ward patients from two centers in Switzerland and Canada[7] (Figure 16A.5). An ELISA D-dimer assay was the initial test, ruling out pulmonary embolism in 36% of patients without any further testing. Compression ultrasonography was performed in patients with an elevated D-dimer result and showed a deep vein thrombosis in 11% of patients. Hence, lung scan, which was diagnostic in 18% of patients (high probability, 10%; normal or near-normal, 8%) was required in only 54% of the cohort, an interesting feature for smaller centers not equipped with nuclear medicine facilities. Twenty-one per cent of the population had a low clinical probability of pulmonary embolism, absence of deep vein thrombosis on ultrasonography, and a non-diagnostic lung scan, a constellation associated with a very low risk of pulmonary embolism,[43,59] and were not treated by anticoagulants. Pulmonary angiography was necessary in only 11% of the patients in that series and the 3-month thromboembolic risk in untreated patients was very low (0.9%, 95% CI 0.2–2.7), a figure similar to the thromboembolic risk observed in patients left untreated based on a normal pulmonary angiogram or lung scintigraphy (Table 16A.5). A similar algorithm has been validated for inpatients, but D-dimer and clinical probability were much less useful in that patient population.[53]

The strategy by Wells et al.[59] also proved highly effective in reducing the proportion of necessary angiograms in the workup of suspected pulmonary embolism. In a series of 1239 consecutive in- and out-patients from five Canadian centers, these investigators assessed an algorithm based on clinical assessment by a prediction rule, lung scan and serial ultrasonography. Patients with a non-diagnostic lung scan and a low to intermediate clinical probability of pulmonary embolism were submitted to serial compression ultrasonography. In that series, an angiogram was performed in only 4% of the patient cohort, and the 3-month thromboembolic risk in patients

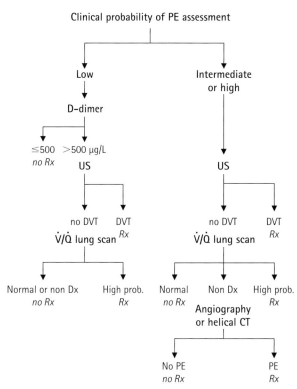

Figure 16A.5 *Algorithm for diagnostic work-up of suspected non-massive pulmonary embolism based on lung scintigraphy. Note that this scheme is only valid when using a highly sensitive D-dimer test and that D-dimer may be skipped in patients with a high clinical probability of pulmonary embolism. Preliminary evidence suggests that angiography may be substituted by helical CT. DVT, deep vein thrombosis; PE, pulmonary embolism; Rx, anticoagulant treatment; US, lower limb venous compression ultrasonography; V̇/Q̇, ventilation/perfusion.*

without pulmonary embolism and not anticoagulated was similar in patients with a non diagnostic scan, a low to moderate clinical probability of pulmonary embolism and a normal serial compression ultrasonography (0.5%, 95% CI 0.1–1.3) and those with a normal scan (0.6%, 95% CI 0.3–3.0). However, the serial ultrasonography protocol required the repetition of ultrasound on days 3, 7 and 14 in 679 patients (54% of the cohort), and a lung scan was required in every patient.

The main limitation of the diagnostic schemes described above are the persisting requirement for angiography, in around 10% of patients, and the central role of ventilation/perfusion lung scan. Indeed, lung scintigraphy is not widely available in many countries outside large teaching hospitals, in contrast to helical CT. The recently completed multicenter ESSEP study evaluated a strategy in which helical CT replaced lung scintigraphy in 1041 consecutive patients with clinically suspected pulmonary embolism.[73] All patients underwent lower limb venous compression ultrasonography and helical CT. Patients in whom either test showed a thrombus were considered as having a pulmonary embolism and treated by anticoagulants. The prevalence of pulmonary embolism was 35%. As shown formerly,[69] ultrasonography showed a deep vein thrombosis in 55 patients who had a negative helical CT (15% of the patients with pulmonary embolism), underlining the importance of combining those tests. Helical CT was inadequate in 7% of patients who must be submitted

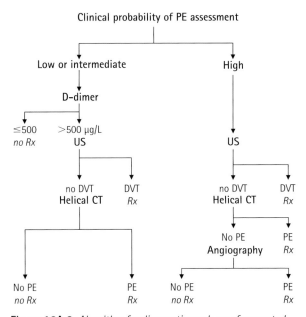

Figure 16A.6 *Algorithm for diagnostic work-up of suspected non-massive pulmonary embolism based on helical computed tomography (CT). DVT, deep vein thrombosis; PE, pulmonary embolism; Rx, anticoagulant treatment; US, lower limb venous compression ultrasonography.*

to further tests. The 525 patients with a low or intermediate clinical probability and both a negative ultrasonography and CT were left untreated and followed up during 3 months. The overall 3-month thromboembolic risk was 1.7% (0.9–3.2), which is comparable to similar outcome studies (Table 16A.5). The prevalence of pulmonary embolism was still 7% in the 76 patients with similar findings but a high clinical probability, warranting further investigation in that subgroup. These results should be confirmed by other ongoing outcome studies. Meanwhile, the algorithm depicted in Figure 16A.6 appears to be safe. Alternatively, replacing pulmonary angiography by helical CT in patients with an inconclusive non-invasive work-up including lung scan (elevated D-dimer level, negative venous ultrasound, non-diagnostic lung scan and intermediate or high clinical probability of pulmonary embolism; see Figure 16A.2) is also an acceptable use of helical CT. Table 16A.6 summarizes the accepted diagnostic criteria for pulmonary embolism according to current evidence.

Suspected massive pulmonary embolism

Patients with suspected massive pulmonary embolism have a very high mortality rate and require emergency thrombolytic treatment, in the event pulmonary embolism is confirmed. The clinical presentation evokes a differential diagnosis with other causes of shock such as pericardial tamponade or myocardial infarction and cardiogenic shock. The clot burden is usually high in that situation, and the diagnostic yield of any imaging study, whether lung scan or helical CT, is likely to be high. Therefore, the logical initial test in such patients is

Table 16A.6 *Acceptable diagnostic criteria for diagnosing pulmonary embolism (PE) according to clinical probability*

Diagnostic criterion	Clinical probability of pulmonary embolism		
	Low	Intermediate	High
Absence of pulmonary embolism			
Normal pulmonary angiogram	x	x	x
Normal lung scan	x	x	x
Plasma ELISA D-dimer level <500 µg/L*	x	x	–
Non-diagnostic lung scan and negative proximal US	x	–	–
Normal helical CT scan and negative proximal US[†]	x	x	–
Normal helical CT alone	–	–	–
Pulmonary embolism			
Pulmonary angiogram showing PE	x	x	x
High probability lung scan	x[‡]	x	x
Proximal US showing a deep venous thrombosis	x	x	x
Helical CT scan showing PE	x[‡]	x	x

*Or highly sensitive immunoturbidimetric assay.

[†] Preliminary evidence.

[‡] Lower positive predictive value in that clinical probability subgroup.

CT, computed tomography; ELISA, enzyme-linked immunosorbent assay; PE, pulmonary embolism; US, proximal lower limb venous ultrasonography.

transthoracic echocardiography. An echocardiogram showing signs of acute pulmonary hypertension and right ventricular strain in a shocked patient with a normal left ventricular contractility is a very strong argument in favor of massive pulmonary embolism. In fact, most clinicians would readily begin thrombolytic treatment in such a patient without awaiting further diagnostic information, if the patient were highly unstable. On the other hand, in a patient temporarily stabilized by vasopressive drugs (dopamine or norepinephrine), confirmation may be sought by either lung scan or helical CT, whichever is the most rapidly available. Angiography should be avoided whenever possible since it carries the highest risk in this patient population[77] and increases the risk of a major bleed at the puncture site due to thrombolytic treatment.[90]

KEY POINTS

- The incidence of pulmonary embolism is around 1/1000 per year. It is the third most common cardiovascular cause of death in Western countries.
- Pulmonary embolism is a potentially fatal complication of deep vein thrombosis. Both disorders belong to a single disease entity, venous thromboembolism.
- Venous thromboembolism is a multigenic disease with a strong environmental influence. The indication to search for genetic thrombophilic defects should be individualized.
- Clinical assessment either implicit or by a prediction rule allows an accurate classification of patients in three risk classes for pulmonary embolism (low, intermediate and high clinical probability).
- In the absence of an ideal non-invasive diagnostic test, the diagnosis of pulmonary embolism rests on strategies combining several tests (D-dimer, lower limb venous ultra-sonography, lung scan and helical CT scan) and clinical evaluation. Pulmonary angiography is still necessary in around 10% of patients in validated schemes.
- The validation of diagnostic strategies for pulmonary embolism requires outcome or management studies to identify patients who can be safely left untreated by anticoagulants.
- Massive pulmonary embolism is a distinct clinical entity with a specific diagnostic approach. Echocardiography should be the initial test in a shocked patient with suspected pulmonary embolism.

REFERENCES

1 Goldhaber SZ. Epidemiology of pulmonary embolism. In: Morpurgo M (ed.), *Pulmonary embolism*. New York: Marcel Dekker, 1994;9–16.

2 Stein PD, Henry JW. Prevalence of acute pulmonary embolism among patients in a general hospital and at autopsy. *Chest* 1995;**108**:978–81.

3 Taubman LB, Silverstone FA. Autopsy proven pulmonary embolism among the institutionalized elderly. *J Am Geriatr Soc* 1986;**34**:752–6.

◆4 Bounameaux H, de Moerloose P, Perrier A *et al*. D-dimer testing in suspected venous thromboembolism: an update. *Q J Med* 1997;**90**:437–42.

◆5 Kearon C, Ginsberg JS, Hirsh J. The role of venous ultrasonography in the diagnosis of suspected deep venous thrombosis and pulmonary embolism. *Ann Intern Med* 1998;**129**:1044–9.

◆6 Rathbun SW, Raskob GE, Whitsett TL. Sensitivity and specificity of helical computed tomography in the diagnosis of pulmonary embolism: a systematic review. *Ann Intern Med* 2000;**132**:227–32.

●7 Perrier A, Desmarais S, Miron MJ *et al*. Non-invasive diagnosis of venous thromboembolism in outpatients. *Lancet* 1999;**353**:190–5.

8 Wells PS, Anderson DR, Rodger M *et al*. Excluding pulmonary embolism at the bedside without diagnostic imaging: management of patients with suspected pulmonary embolism presenting to the emergency department by using a simple clinical model and D-dimer. *Ann Intern Med* 2001;**135**:98–107.

9 Perrier A, Buswell L, Bounameaux H *et al*. Cost-effectiveness of noninvasive diagnostic aids in suspected pulmonary embolism. *Arch Intern Med* 1997;**157**:2309–16.

◆10 Perrier A, Bounameaux H. Cost-effective diagnosis of deep vein thrombosis and pulmonary embolism. *Thromb Haemost* 2001;**86**:475–87.

11 Sevitt S, Gallagher NG. Venous thrombosis and pulmonary embolism: a clinicopathologic study in injured and burned patients. *Br J Surg* 1961;**48**:475–82.

●12 Meignan M, Rosso J, Gauthier H *et al*. Systematic lung scans reveal a high frequency of silent pulmonary embolism in patients with proximal deep venous thrombosis. *Arch Intern Med* 2000;**160**:159–64.

13 Moser KM. Venous thromboembolism. *Am Rev Respir Dis* 1990;**141**:235–49.

14 Anderson FA, Jr, Wheeler HB, Goldberg RJ *et al*. A population-based perspective of the hospital incidence and case-fatality rates of deep vein thrombosis and pulmonary embolism. *Arch Intern Med* 1991;**151**:933–8.

15 Oger E. Incidence of venous thromboembolism: a community-based study in Western France. EPI-GETBP Study Group. Groupe d'Etude de la Thrombose de Bretagne Occidentale. *Thromb Haemost* 2000;**83**:657–60.

●16 The PIOPED Investigators. Value of the ventilation-perfusion scan in acute pulmonary embolism. *JAMA* 1990;**263**:2753–9.

●17 Goldhaber SZ, Visani L, De Rosa M. Acute pulmonary embolism: clinical outcomes in the International Cooperative

Pulmonary Embolism Registry (ICOPER). *Lancet* 1999;**353**: 1386–9.

18 Wicki J, Perrier A, Perneger TV *et al.* Predicting adverse outcome in patients with acute pulmonary embolism: a risk score. *Thromb Haemost* 2000;**84**:548–52.

19 Douketis JD, Kearon C, Bates S *et al.* Risk of fatal pulmonary embolism in patients with treated venous thromboembolism. *JAMA* 1998;**279**:458–62.

20 Douketis JD, Foster GA, Crowther MA *et al.* Clinical risk factors and timing of recurrent venous thromboembolism during the initial 3 months of anticoagulant therapy. *Arch Intern Med* 2000;**160**:3431–6.

●21 von Virchow R. Weitere Untersuchungen ueber die Verstopfung der Lungenarterien und ihre Folge. In: *Traube's Beitraege exp Path u Physiol.* Berlin,1846;21–31.

◆22 Rosendaal FR. Venous thrombosis: a multicausal disease. *Lancet* 1999;**353**:1167–73.

23 Gonzalez Ordonez AJ, Medina Rodriguez JM, Martin L *et al.* The O blood group protects against venous thromboembolism in individuals with the factor V Leiden but not the prothrombin (factor II G20210A) mutation. *Blood Coagul Fibrinolysis* 1999;**10**:303–7.

◆24 Perrier A. Deep vein thrombosis and pulmonary embolism: a single disease entity with different risk factors? *Chest* 2000;**118**:1234–6.

◆25 de Moerloose P, Alhenc-Gelas M, Boehlen F *et al.* Deep venous thrombosis and thrombophilia: indications for testing and clinical implications. *Semin Vasc Med* 2001; **1**:89–95.

26 Goldhaber SZ, Grodstein F, Stampfer MJ *et al.* A prospective study of risk factors for pulmonary embolism in women. *JAMA* 1997;**277**:642–5.

27 Samama MM. An epidemiologic study of risk factors for deep vein thrombosis in medical outpatients: the Sirius study. *Arch Intern Med* 2000;**160**:3415–20.

●28 Grady D, Wenger NK, Herrington D *et al.* Postmenopausal hormone therapy increases risk for venous thromboembolic disease. The Heart and Estrogen/Progestin Replacement Study. *Ann Intern Med* 2000;**132**:689–96.

29 Cummings SR, Eckert S, Krueger KA *et al.* The effect of raloxifene on risk of breast cancer in postmenopausal women: results from the MORE randomized trial. Multiple Outcomes of Raloxifene Evaluation. *JAMA* 1999;**281**:2189–97.

30 De Stefano V, Martinelli I, Mannucci PM *et al.* The risk of recurrent deep venous thrombosis among heterozygous carriers of both factor V Leiden and the G20210A prothrombin mutation. *N Engl J Med* 1999;**341**:801–6.

31 Sorensen HT, Mellemkjaer L, Steffensen FH *et al.* The risk of a diagnosis of cancer after primary deep venous thrombosis or pulmonary embolism. *N Engl J Med* 1998;**338**:1169–73.

●32 Baron JA, Gridley G, Weiderpass E *et al.* Venous thromboembolism and cancer. *Lancet* 1998;**351**:1077–80.

33 Prandoni P, Lensing AW, Buller HR *et al.* Deep-vein thrombosis and the incidence of subsequent symptomatic cancer. *N Engl J Med* 1992;**327**:1128–33.

34 Rance A, Emmerich J, Guedj C *et al.* Occult cancer in patients with bilateral deep-vein thrombosis. *Lancet* 1997;**350**:1448–9.

●35 Cornuz J, Pearson SD, Creager MA *et al.* Importance of findings on the initial evaluation for cancer in patients with symptomatic idiopathic deep venous thrombosis. *Ann Intern Med* 1996;**125**:785–93.

●36 Stein PD, Henry JW. Clinical characteristics of patients with acute pulmonary embolism stratified according to their presenting syndromes. *Chest* 1997;**112**:974–9.

37 Dalen JE, Haffajee CI, Alpert JS *et al.* Pulmonary embolism, pulmonary hemorrhage, pulmonary infarction. *N Engl J Med* 1977;**296**:1431–5.

38 Elliott CG, Goldhaber SZ, Visani L *et al.* Chest radiographs in acute pulmonary embolism. Results from the International Cooperative Pulmonary Embolism Registry. *Chest* 2000;**118**:33–8.

39 Thames MD, Alpert JS, Dalen JE. Syncope in patients with pulmonary embolism. *JAMA* 1977;**238**:2509–11.

40 Stein PD, Terrin ML, Hales CA *et al.* Clinical, laboratory, roentgenographic, and electrocardiographic findings in patients with acute pulmonary embolism and no pre-existing cardiac or pulmonary disease. *Chest* 1991;**100**:598–603.

41 Stein PD, Goldhaber SZ, Henry JW. Alveolar-arterial oxygen gradient in the assessment of acute pulmonary embolism. *Chest* 1995;**107**:139–43.

42 Rodger MA, Carrier M, Jones GN *et al.* Diagnostic value of arterial blood gas measurement in suspected pulmonary embolism. *Am J Respir Crit Care Med* 2000;**162**:2105–8.

●43 Perrier A, Miron MJ, Desmarais S *et al.* Using clinical evaluation and lung scan to rule out suspected pulmonary embolism: is it a valid option in patients with normal results of lower-limb venous compression ultrasonography? *Arch Intern Med* 2000;**160**:512–16.

●44 Wells PS, Anderson DR, Rodger M *et al.* Derivation of a simple clinical model to categorize patients probability of pulmonary embolism: increasing the models utility with the SimpliRED D-dimer. *Thromb Haemost* 2000;**83**:416–20.

●45 Wicki J, Perneger TV, Junod A *et al.* Assessing clinical probability of pulmonary embolism in the emergency ward: a simple score. *Arch Intern Med* 2001;**161**:92–7.

46 Chagnon I, Bounameaux H, Aujesky D *et al.* Comparison of two clinical prediction rules and implicit assessment for suspected pulmonary embolism. *Am J Med* 2002;**113**:269–75.

47 Bounameaux H, de Moerloose P, Perrier A *et al.* Plasma measurement of D-dimer as diagnostic aid in suspected venous thromboembolism: an overview. *Thromb Haemost* 1994;**71**:1–6.

48 Oger E, Leroyer C, Bressollette L *et al.* Evaluation of a new, rapid, and quantitative D-dimer test in patients with suspected pulmonary embolism. *Am J Respir Crit Care Med* 1998;**158**:65–70.

49 Bates SM, Grand'Maison A, Johnston M *et al.* A latex D-dimer reliably excludes venous thromboembolism. *Arch Intern Med* 2001;**161**:447–53.

50 Ginsberg JS, Wells PS, Kearon C *et al.* Sensitivity and specificity of a rapid whole-blood assay for D-dimer in the diagnosis of pulmonary embolism. *Ann Intern Med* 1998;**129**:1006–11.

51 Perrier A, Desmarais S, Goehring C *et al.* D-dimer testing for suspected pulmonary embolism in outpatients. *Am J Respir Crit Care Med* 1997;**156**:492–6.

52 Righini M, Goehring C, Bounameaux H *et al.* Effects of age on the performance of common diagnostic tests for pulmonary embolism. *Am J Med* 2000;**109**:357–61.

53 Miron MJ, Perrier A, Bounameaux H *et al.* Contribution of noninvasive evaluation to the diagnosis of pulmonary embolism in hospitalized patients. *Eur Respir J* 1999;**13**:1365–70.

●54 Lensing AWA, Prandoni P, Brandjes D et al. Detection of deep-vein thrombosis by real-time B-mode ultrasonography. N Engl J Med 1989;**320**:342–5.

55 Becker DM, Philbrick JT, Abbitt PL. Real-time ultrasonography for the diagnosis of lower extremity deep venous thrombosis. The wave of the future? Arch Intern Med 1989;**149**:1731–4.

56 Lensing AW, Doris CI, McGrath FP et al. A comparison of compression ultrasound with color Doppler ultrasound for the diagnosis of symptomless postoperative deep vein thrombosis. Arch Intern Med 1997;**157**:765–8.

57 Turkstra F, Kuijer PMM, van Beek EJR et al. Diagnostic utility of ultrasonography of leg veins in patients suspected of having pulmonary embolism. Ann Intern Med 1997;**126**:775–81.

58 Perrier A, Bounameaux H, Morabia A et al. Diagnosis of pulmonary embolism by a decision analysis-based strategy including clinical probability, D-dimer levels, and ultrasonography: a management study. Arch Intern Med 1996;**156**:531–6.

●59 Wells PS, Ginsberg JS, Anderson DR et al. Use of a clinical model for safe management of patients with suspected pulmonary embolism. Ann Intern Med 1998;**129**:997–1005.

60 Perrier A, Bounameaux H. Ultrasonography of leg veins in patients suspected of having pulmonary embolism. Ann Intern Med 1998;**128**:243.

61 Alderson PO, Martin EC. Pulmonary embolism: diagnosis with multiple imaging modalities. Radiology 1987;**164**:297–312.

62 Gottschalk A, Sostman HD, Coleman RE et al. Ventilation-perfusion scintigraphy in the PIOPED study. Part II. Evaluation of scintigraphic criteria and interpretations. J Nucl Med 1993;**34**:1119–26.

63 Sostman HD, Coleman RE, De Long DM et al. Evaluation of revised criteria for ventilation-perfusion scintigraphy in patients with suspected pulmonary embolism. Radiology 1994;**193**:103–7.

●64 Hull RD, Raskob GE, Coates G et al. Clinical validity of a normal perfusion lung scan in patients with suspected pulmonary embolism. Chest 1990;**97**:23–6.

65 Kipper MS, Moser KM, Kortman KE et al. Longterm follow-up of patients with suspected pulmonary embolism and a normal lung scan. Chest 1982;**82**:411–15.

66 de Groot MR, Turkstra F, van Marwijk Kooy M et al. Value of chest X-ray combined with perfusion scan versus ventilation/perfusion scan in acute pulmonary embolism. Thromb Haemost 2000;**83**:412–15.

●67 Rémy-Jardin M, Rémy J, Wattinne L et al. Central pulmonary tromboembolism: diagnosis with spiral volumetric CT with the single-breath-hold technique. Comparison with pulmonary angiography. Radiology 1992;**185**:381–7.

68 Mullins MD, Becker DM, Hagspiel KD et al. The role of spiral volumetric computed tomography in the diagnosis of pulmonary embolism. Arch Intern Med 2000;**160**:293–8.

●69 Perrier A, Howarth N, Didier D et al. Performances of helical computed tomography in unselected outpatients with suspected pulmonary embolism. Ann Intern Med 2001;**135**: 88–97.

70 van Strijen MJL, de Monye W, Kieft GJ et al. Accuracy of spiral CT in the diagnosis of pulmonary embolism: a prospective multicenter cohort study of consecutive patients. The ANTELOPE Study Group. Thromb Haemost 2001;OC154.

71 Remy-Jardin M, Remy J, Baghaie F et al. Clinical value of thin collimation in the diagnostic workup of pulmonary embolism. AJR Am J Roentgenol 2000;**175**:407–11.

72 Ghaye B, Szapiro D, Mastora I et al. Peripheral pulmonary arteries: how far in the lung does multi-detector row spiral CT allow analysis? Radiology 2001;**219**:629–36.

●73 Musset D, Parent F, Meyer G et al. Diagnostic strategy for patients with suspected pulmonary embolism: a prospective multicentre outcome study. Lancet 2002;**360**:1914–20.

74 Dalen JE, Brooks HL, Johnson LW et al. Pulmonary angiography in acute pulmonary embolism: indications, techniques, and results in 367 patients. Am Heart J 1971;**81**: 175–85.

75 Mills SR, Jackson DC, Older RA et al. The incidence, etiologies, and avoidance of complications of pulmonary angiography in a large series. Radiology 1980;**136**:295–9.

76 Perlmutt LM, Braun SD, Newman GE et al. Pulmonary arteriography in the high risk patient. Radiology 1987;**162**:187–9.a

●77 Stein PD, Athanasoulis C, Alavi A et al. Complications and validity of pulmonary angiography in acute pulmonary embolism. Circulation 1992;**85**:462–8.

78 Hudson ER, Smith TP, McDermott VG et al. Pulmonary angiography performed with iopamidol: complications in 1434 patients. Radiology 1996;**198**:61–5.

79 Come PC. Echocardiographic evaluation of pulmonary embolism and its response to therapeutic interventions. Chest 1992;**101**:151S–62S.

*80 Guidelines on diagnosis and management of acute pulmonary embolism. Task Force on Pulmonary Embolism, European Society of Cardiology. Eur Heart J 2000;**21**: 1301–36.

81 Pruszczyk P, Torbicki A, Pacho R et al. Noninvasive diagnosis of suspected severe pulmonary embolism: transesophageal echocardiography vs spiral CT. Chest 1997; **112**:722–8.

82 Vieillard-Baron A, Qanadli SD, Antakly Y et al. Transesophageal echocardiography for the diagnosis of pulmonary embolism with acute cor pulmonale: a comparison with radiological procedures. Intensive Care Med 1998;**24**:429–33.

83 Jardin F, Dubourg O, Bourdarias JP. Echocardiographic pattern of acute cor pulmonale. Chest 1997;**111**:209–17.

84 McConnell MV, Solomon SD, Rayan ME et al. Regional right ventricular dysfunction detected by echocardiography in acute pulmonary embolism. Am J Cardiol 1996;**78**:469–73.

85 Perrier A, Tamm C, Unger PF et al. Diagnostic accuracy of Doppler-echocardiography in unselected patients with suspected pulmonary embolism. Int J Cardiol 1998;**65**:101–9.

86 Jackson RE, Rudoni RR, Hauser AM et al. Prospective evaluation of two-dimensional transthoracic echocardiography in emergency department patients with suspected pulmonary embolism. Acad Emerg Med 2000;**7**:994–8.

87 Nazeyrollas P, Metz D, Chapoutot L et al. Diagnostic accuracy of echocardiography-Doppler in acute pulmonary embolism. Int J Cardiol 1995;**47**:273–80.

88 Steiner P, Lund GK, Debatin JF et al. Acute pulmonary embolism: value of transthoracic and transesophageal echocardiography in comparison with helical CT. AJR Am J Roentgenol 1996;**167**:931–6.

●89 Miniati M, Monti S, Pratali L *et al.* Value of transthoracic echocardiography in the diagnosis of pulmonary embolism: results of a prospective study in unselected patients. *Am J Med* 2001;**110**:528–35.

*90 Hyers TM, Agnelli G, Hull RD *et al.* Antithrombotic therapy for venous thromboembolic disease. *Chest* 2001;**119**:176S–93S.

91 Carson JL, Kelley MA, Duff A *et al.* The clinical course of pulmonary embolism. *N Engl J Med* 1992;**326**:1240–5.

●92 Hull RD, Raskob GE, Ginsberg JS *et al.* A noninvasive strategy for the treatment of patients with suspected pulmonary embolism. *Arch Intern Med* 1994;**154**:289–97.

93 de Moerloose P, Desmarais S, Bounameaux H *et al.* Contribution of a new, rapid, individual and quantitative automated D-dimer ELISA to exclude pulmonary embolism. *Thromb Haemost* 1996;**75**:11–13.

94 Henry JW, Relyea B, Stein PD. Continuing risk of thromboemboli among patients with normal pulmonary angiograms. *Chest* 1995;**107**:1375–8.

●95 Novelline RA, Baltarowich OH, Athanasoulis CA *et al.* The clinical course of patients with suspected pulmonary embolism and a negative pulmonary arteriogram. *Radiology* 1978;**126**:561–7.

96 van Beek EJR, Kuyer PMM, Schenk BS *et al.* A normal perfusion lung scan in patients with clinically suspected pulmonary embolism. Frequency and clinical validity. *Chest* 1995;**108**:170–3.

16B

Treatment

SAMUEL Z GOLDHABER

INTRODUCTION

The adverse consequences of acute pulmonary embolism (PE) are not widely appreciated. The mortality rate is much higher than most clinicians presume, and those patients who survive are saddled with prolonged and at times lifelong physical and emotional disability. Quality of life diminishes not only as a direct result of the PE but also because of the precautions required by and frequent side effects from chronic anticoagulation. Some patients become embittered by the delay in diagnosis and by the perception, at times real and at times imagined, that those around them do not appreciate the profound impact that this illness has caused in their daily lives. They worry, justifiably, about whether they will be stricken with recurrent PE if anticoagulation is discontinued. Often, patients do not voice their silent fear that PE may affect other family members in the future and that the PE itself may be due to occult carcinoma.

When confronted with acute PE, our immediate task as clinicians is to undertake a rapid assessment of prognosis and to institute therapy guided by the degree of current and predicted severity. Ideally, anticoagulation will already have been initiated on the basis of high clinical suspicion. We must ensure that the choice of anticoagulant is appropriate, and we must determine whether additional treatment is necessary with thrombolysis or embolectomy. Those patients with absolute contraindications to anticoagulation will require inferior vena caval filters. Our challenge in that circumstance is to select an optimal filter and to manage the bleeding problem so that initiation of anticoagulation can be expedited.

After anticoagulation has been initiated, the thorny problem of deciding upon optimal duration will confront the clinician. This is the single most controversial area in the field of PE treatment. Decisions about treatment duration may depend upon etiology, with idiopathic or primary PE patients receiving more extended anticoagulant therapy than those with secondary PE from causes such as surgery or trauma.

EPIDEMIOLOGY

In the Brest district of western France, with a defined population of 342 000 inhabitants, the incidence of venous thromboembolism (VTE) was 1.8 per 1000 per year.[1] Deep venous thrombosis (DVT) without PE had an incidence of 1.2 per 1000 per year, whereas PE with or without DVT had an incidence of 0.6 per 1000 per year. The incidence of VTE increased markedly with increasing age for both men and women. For those over age 75 years, the incidence was 1 per 100 per year. VTE occurred at home in 63% of the affected population. Of those, 16% had been hospitalized within the previous 3 months.

In Olmsted County, a retrospective review of a population-based cohort found a VTE incidence of 1.2 per 1000 per year.[2] The incidence rose markedly with increasing age.

The International Cooperative Pulmonary Embolism Registry (ICOPER) enrolled 2454 consecutive PE patients from 52 participating hospitals in seven countries. The aim was to establish the 3-month all-cause mortality rate and to identify factors associated with death.[3]

Three-month follow-up was completed in 98% of the patients. The all-cause mortality rate was 11.4% during the first 2 weeks after diagnosis and 17.4% at 3 months. After exclusion of patients in whom PE was first discovered at autopsy, the mortality rate was 15.3%. Importantly, most patients that died had succumbed to PE, not to other co-morbidities such as cancer. Specifically, regarding the most common causes of death, 45% of deaths were ascribed to PE, 18% were due to cancer, 12% were sudden cardiac deaths (which undoubtedly included some undiagnosed PEs), and 12% were considered due to respiratory failure, which may also have included some deaths due to PE. Non-fatal recurrent PE occurred in 4% of patients.

Age greater than 70 years increased the likelihood of death by 60%. Six other risk factors independently increased the likelihood of mortality by a factor of two- to threefold: cancer, clinical congestive heart failure, chronic obstructive pulmonary disease, systemic arterial hypotension with a systolic blood pressure of <90 mmHg, tachypnea (defined as >20 breaths/min), and right ventricular hypokinesis on echocardiogram, an especially useful sign to identify high-risk patients who might be suitable for aggressive interventions such as thrombolysis or embolectomy.

ICOPER was a study of PE in North America and Europe. In Japan, a prospective PE registry showed remarkable similarities.[4] The in-hospital mortality rate was 14% among the 533 PE patients enrolled in the registry. Predictors of mortality included: male gender, cardiogenic shock, cancer, and prolonged immobilization.

DEFINITIONS AND TERMINOLOGY

PE is often classified as occurring due to an inherited or acquired hypercoagulable condition. When no reason for PE can be determined, it is labeled as idiopathic. However, this terminology is confusing and does not assist in deciding how to risk stratify and treat patients with PE.

I prefer to classify PE as idiopathic (synonymous with 'primary') if it occurs in the absence of surgery, trauma, or cancer. I consider all other PEs to be 'secondary'. Both primary and secondary PEs can occur in the presence of an identifiable thrombophilic condition, which can be hereditary or acquired (Table 16B.1). PEs in the setting of trauma or surgery are the least likely to recur after anticoagulation is discontinued. However, both primary and secondary PEs can range widely in severity, and both types can be fatal.

CLINICAL PRESENTATION

There are four major clinical presentations of patients with known PE:

- appears mild and is mild (about 40–50%);
- appears mild but may deteriorate with progressive right ventricular dysfunction and right ventricular myocyte injury (about 30–40%);
- appears severe and is severe, with impending or overt cardiovascular collapse (about 15%);
- appears severe, with intractable pleuritic pain, but is caused by anatomically small PE causing pulmonary infarction (about 5%).

Treatment should hinge upon accurate identification of the clinical presentation, followed by appropriate tailoring of therapy (Figure 16B.1). Those with mild PE will have excellent outcomes with anticoagulation alone. Those who appear to have mild PE but who have subclinical moderate or severe right ventricular dysfunction may lull the clinician into a conservative approach with anticoagulation alone. Such patients may deteriorate over the next few days. The best approach to achieve early recognition of an ominous prognosis is with echocardiography and

Table 16B.1 *Inherited and acquired causes of pulmonary embolism*

Inherited	Acquired
Common	
G1691A mutation in the factor V gene (factor V Leiden)	Surgery and trauma
	Prolonged immobilization
	Older age
G20210A mutation in the prothrombin (factor II) gene	
Rare	
Antithrombin deficiency	Cancer
Protein C deficiency	Pregnancy/oral contraceptives/
Protein S deficiency	hormone replacement therapy
	Antiphospholipid antibodies
	Hyperhomocysteinemia
	Air travel

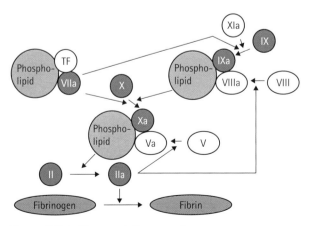

Figure 16B.1 *The coagulation cascade.*

troponin measurement. Those who have massive, severe PE require emergency mobilization of the clinical team to coordinate treatment, which will usually include thrombolysis or embolectomy. Finally, those with pulmonary infarction will do well with conservative measures, including anticoagulation, reassurance and pain control with non-steroidal anti-inflammatory agents (despite administration of concomitant anticoagulation).

MANAGEMENT

Anticoagulation with unfractionated or low molecular weight heparin

Low molecular weight heparins (LMWH) have pharmacokinetic and practical advantages over unfractionated heparin (Table 16B.2; Figure 16B.2). These compounds

Table 16B.2 *Advantages of subcutaneously administered low molecular weight heparins over continuous intravenous infusion of unfractionated heparin*

Better bioavailability
More predictable anticoagulant response
Fixed weight-adjusted dosing (in the absence of renal insufficiency or marked obesity)
No need for routine blood testing

Better bioavailability despite subcutaneous rather than intravenous dosing
Longer half-life
Permits once or twice daily dosing
Facilitates earlier hospital discharge and home treatment
Improves cost-effectiveness

Less binding to platelet factor 4
Lower risk of heparin-induced thrombocytopenia

Less binding to osteoblasts
Less osteopenia

have revolutionized the treatment of acute DVT and have converted the management of this illness from a mandatory hospitalization of at least 5 days' duration to a condition treated primarily on an outpatient basis, with an occasional overnight hospitalization. Of course, candidates for outpatient treatment must be reliable and have excellent family or community support services to ensure the success of this strategy. A meta-analysis of more than 3000 patients who participated in acute DVT trials showed that those receiving LMWH had a lower mortality rate, lower recurrence rate, and lower rate of heparin-induced thrombocytopenia than those receiving unfractionated heparin.[5] LMWH was also much more cost-effective than unfractionated heparin.[6] One pivotal study showed that the LMWH enoxaparin, administered in the dose of 1 mg/kg twice daily, decreased the average length of hospital stay from 6.5 to 1.1 days, with a trend toward fewer deaths, less recurrent DVT, and fewer major bleeding episodes.[7] The FDA has approved enoxaparin 1 mg/kg twice daily, as well as tinzaparin 175 units/kg once daily, for outpatient management of patients who present primarily with symptomatic DVT, with or without accompanying PE.

As many as half of patients with proximal DVT have concomitant asymptomatic PE.[8] However, in patients presenting with both PE and DVT, symptomatic PE confers a higher risk of adverse outcomes than symptomatic DVT with asymptomatic concomitant PE. In one study, the risk of death from a subsequent PE was 1.5% in patients who presented initially with symptoms of PE, compared with 0.4% in patients who presented with DVT.[9] A separate investigation showed that the 3-month survival was lower in patients presenting with PE compared with DVT, and this difference in survival was independent of other co-morbidities.[10] Another study showed that the risk of recurrent thromboembolism was twice as high after PE compared with DVT and that most patients with recurrence had recurrent PE, rather than DVT, if they had initially presented with PE.[11] Thus, successful outpatient

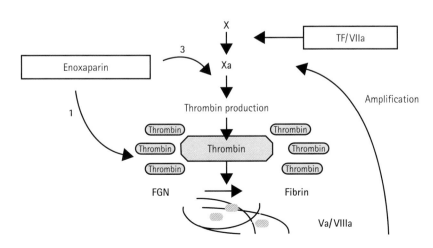

Figure 16B.2 *Mechanism of action of low molecular weight heparin. This figure shows the predominant 3:1 ratio of anticoagulant action of enoxaparin, a low molecular weight heparin, against activated coagulation factor X. FGN, fibrinogen; TF, tissue factor.*

management of DVT with LMWH cannot be presumed to ensure successful outpatient management of PE.

One large trial of 612 patients with symptomatic PE randomized subjects to once daily LMWH versus continuous intravenous unfractionated heparin as a 'bridge' to oral anticoagulation.[12] There was no difference in adverse outcomes between the two groups. However, patients receiving LMWH remained hospitalized for more than 1 week, on average, until oral anticoagulation was fully effective. This trial, as well as another large trial of 1022 patients with venous thromboembolism,[13] demonstrates that LMWH is effective and safe as a 'bridge' to oral anticoagulation in patients with PE. However, there have been no large-scale trials showing that outpatient management of PE patients is safe and effective.

A small Canadian study used LMWH for stable PE patients with a goal of early hospital discharge.[14] Dalteparin 200 units/kg once daily was utilized for at least 5 days as a 'bridge' to warfarin, with a target International Normalized Ratio (INR) of ≥2.0 for at least two consecutive days. More than 50% of patients were treated exclusively as outpatients. Recurrent PE occurred in 5.5%, major bleeds were reported in 1.9%, and fewer than 4% died, with no deaths attributed to PE.

Future treatment options include the possible use of LMWH as monotherapy without oral anticoagulation.[15] Other strategies under development include monotherapy with oral direct thrombin inhibitors, a single depot injection of a pentasaccharides as a 'bridge' to warfarin, and use of oral heparins.

Oral anticoagulation

Oral anticoagulation with warfarin or other anti-vitamin K agents remains the principal long-term therapy for patients with PE. Dosing of warfarin is adjusted according to the prothrombin time, which is standardized by reporting results as the INR. Ordinarily, the target INR for patients with PE is 2.0–3.0. However, under certain circumstances, such as patients who have suffered recurrent venous thrombosis while the INR was within the target range, the anticoagulation dosing is intensified and the target is raised to 3.0–4.0. Patients with PE ascribed to thrombophilic disorders such as the antiphospholipid antibody syndrome may also receive higher than usual doses of anticoagulation. As the INR increases, the level of anticoagulation is intensified and the likelihood of recurrence decreases. However, side effects of warfarin, most notably bleeding, will increase with higher INR levels.

Warfarin is a difficult drug to utilize because many other medications interact with it (Figure 16B.3). Most problematic are the many medications that potentiate it (Table 16B.3). Foods that contain large amounts of vitamin K, such as green leafy vegetables, result in a lower

anticoagulant effect. In addition to the common problem of hemorrhage, warfarin can also cause alopecia, rash and skin necrosis. Warfarin is not reliably effective until it has been administered for 5 days, because of the prolonged half-life of some of the vitamin K-dependent coagulation factors with which it interferes. During this period, patients are especially vulnerable to thrombosis unless concomitantly anticoagulated with heparin. Also, if warfarin is initiated as monotherapy without heparin, it will decrease the level of the anticoagulant, protein C, and will cause a paradoxical hypercoagulability that will result in a much higher rate of recurrent venous thromboembolism.[16]

The initial dose of warfarin in an average sized person without co-morbidity should be about 5 mg daily.[17,18] Most patients will not have an appreciable rise in INR for at least 3 days. However, 2–3% metabolize warfarin slowly due to an inherited genetic mutation.[19] These individuals are much more likely to have a low warfarin requirement, ≤1.5 mg daily, and because their identity as 'slow metabolizers' is not known in advance, they are predisposed to major bleeding complications. Therefore, the INR should be checked after 2 or 3 days following initiation of warfarin.

To achieve a therapeutic INR, dosing in general should be adjusted without wide day-to-day fluctuations. I try to limit dose adjustments to no more than a 20% increase or decrease. Dosing changes and INR levels should be recorded, if possible, in a software program that keeps track of when patients are due for their next blood test. Such programs will alert the clinician when patients are overdue for testing.

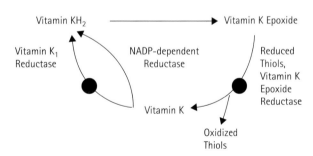

Figure 16B.3 *Mechanism of action of warfarin and other anti-vitamin K agents. These agents inhibit activated clotting factors II, VII, IX and X (●, blocked by warfarin).*

Table 16B.3 *Drugs that commonly increase the anticoagulant effect of warfarin*

Danazol
Amiodarone
Fluconazole
Ketoconazole
Metronidazole
Trimethoprim-sulfamethoxazole

When INR levels exceed 5.0, the warfarin should be held and the patient should be questioned about ongoing bruising or bleeding. Patients with bleeding may require hospitalization for observation. In most instances, however, even patients with markedly elevated INRs will be asymptomatic. The INR level can be decreased by administration of fresh frozen plasma, appropriate for patients with active bleeding, or with vitamin K, which in small doses of 2.5 mg orally will often restore a therapeutic INR level within 1–2 days.[20] Note that when vitamin K is administered subcutaneously in high doses, such as 10 mg, most patients will be resistant to warfarin anticoagulation for at least 1 week. They will consequently require therapy with concomitant heparin until the warfarin once again becomes effective.

Optimal duration of anticoagulation

The optimal duration of anticoagulation after acute PE remains controversial. Schulman and coworkers found that 6 months of oral anticoagulation halved the recurrence rate over the ensuing 2 years following cessation of anticoagulation, compared with 6 weeks of anticoagulation.[21] Consequently, 6 months of anticoagulation is the usual duration of therapy. However, other investigators have recommended either short or longer durations of treatment. Kearon and colleagues[22] studied patients with idiopathic DVT and PE. They randomized patients to either 3 months or 2 years of anticoagulation. After an average follow-up period of 10 months, there were 17 recurrences among those on 3 months of anticoagulation compared with one event among those on long-term anticoagulation. Therefore, they recommended a prolonged duration of anticoagulation that greatly exceeded 6 months.

However, prolonged anticoagulation may simply forestall but not prevent recurrent thrombosis. Furthermore, the increased bleeding with prolonged anticoagulation may negate any potential benefit of fewer recurrences. In the Warfarin Optimal Duration Italian Trial (WODIT), 267 patients with idiopathic proximal DVT were randomized to either 3 or 12 months of anticoagulation.[23] They were followed clinically for at least 2 years. The mortality and recurrence rates were the same in both groups. The average time to recurrence was 11 months among patients who received 3 months of anticoagulation, compared with 16 months in the group that received 12 months of anticoagulation. Importantly, 3% of patients receiving 12 months of anticoagulation had major non-fatal bleeding during the fourth through twelfth months of therapy. Thus, in WODIT, extending to 1 year the 3-month course of anticoagulation simply delayed the onset of recurrent venous thrombosis. Similar results were obtained in the WODIT-PE Trial.[24]

It is possible that a lower intensity of anticoagulation, after the initial phase of full-dose warfarin, might reduce bleeding complications associated with long-term therapy and yet maintain a low frequency of recurrent events. To test this hypothesis, the Prevention of Recurrent Venous Thromboembolism (PREVENT) Trial evaluated the efficacy of prolonged treatment with low-intensity warfarin to prevent recurrent events.[25] This trial was sponsored by the National Institutes of Health. Patients with a history of documented idiopathic venous thrombosis who completed a standard course of anticoagulation were enrolled in a randomized, double-blind, placebo-controlled trial comparing low-intensity anticoagulation, target INR of 1.5–2.0, with usual care without anticoagulants. The trial stopped when low-intensity warfarin reduced recurrent events by 64%, with an appreciable increase in major bleeding.

Risk stratification

Patients at high risk of an adverse outcome can be identified with risk stratification, using findings from the history, physical examination, echocardiogram and measurement of troponin.[26] Such patients, once identified, should be considered for treatment that is more aggressive than anticoagulation alone.[27] They should be screened to determine if they warrant therapy with thrombolysis or embolectomy.

The Geneva Prognostic Index permits a rapid assessment to predict death, recurrent venous thromboembolism, or major bleeding.[28] The six adverse prognostic indicators are determined from history (cancer, heart failure and prior DVT), physical examination (hypotension) and laboratory testing (hypoxemia and DVT on venous ultrasound).

ECHOCARDIOGRAPHIC FINDINGS

Right ventricular dysfunction is an independent predictor of death or recurrent PE despite adequate anticoagulation.[29,30] Qualitatively, the most important echocardiographic findings are a right ventricle that is larger than the left ventricle (on the apical four-chamber view) and hypokinesis of the right ventricular free wall.[31] Additional findings are listed in Table 16B.4.

Acute increases in right ventricular pressure can cause left ventricular dysfunction because of the anatomic juxtaposition of the two ventricles and 'ventricular interdependency'. With underfilling of the left ventricle, both systemic cardiac output and pressure decrease, potentially compromising coronary perfusion and causing myocardial ischemia.

The pulmonary arterial systolic pressure can be estimated by measuring the peak velocity of the tricuspid

Table 16B.4 *Abnormal echocardiographic findings that portend poor prognosis*

Abnormal finding	Description
Right ventricular dilatation and hypokinesis	Note leftward septal shift; an RVEDA to LVEDA ratio that exceeds 0.6
Septal flattening and paradoxical septal motion	The interventricular septum bulges toward the left ventricle
Reduced left ventricular diastolic distensibility	Doppler mitral flow exhibits a prominent A wave, much higher than the E wave
Direct visualization of pulmonary embolism	Indicates anatomically massive PE
Pulmonary arterial hypertension detected by Doppler flow velocity in the right ventricular outflow tract	Shortened acceleration time; peak velocity occurs close to onset of ejection. Mid-systolic reduction in velocity
Right ventricular hypertrophy	Wall thickness $\geq 4\,mm$
Patent foramen ovale	Right atrial pressure exceeds left atrial pressure; worsening hypoxemia and susceptibility to stroke

LVEDA, left ventricular end-diastolic area; PE, pulmonary embolism; RVEDA, right ventricular end-diastolic area.

regurgitant jet on Doppler echocardiography. The gradient across the tricuspid valve is estimated with the modified Bernoulli equation, where 'V' in the equation $P = 4V^2$ is the peak velocity of the regurgitant jet. 'P' represents the peak pressure difference between the right atrium and right ventricle.[32] The estimated right atrial pressure is added to the gradient to obtain an approximation of pulmonary arterial systolic pressure. Nonetheless, massive PE can produce right ventricular failure without substantial elevations in pulmonary artery pressure.[33]

In a case series of 139 consecutive PE patients, the presence of a patent foramen ovale was associated on multivariate analysis with more than a tenfold increase in the risk of death and a fivefold increase in the risk of major adverse events.[34] When free-floating right heart thrombi were detected on echocardiography in a separate series of 38 consecutive patients, the thrombi were usually worm-like, and almost all patients had PE with associated right ventricular dysfunction and pulmonary hypertension.[35] Their prognosis was dismal and 45% died.

Transesophageal echocardiography can diagnose PE by direct visualization of thrombus rather than by indirect signs such as right ventricular dilatation and hypokinesis.[36] The examination assesses the anatomic extent of thromboembolism as well as its surgical accessibility. The main pulmonary artery and then the right pulmonary artery are usually first visualized. The right pulmonary artery can be followed until it branches to the right lobar pulmonary arteries. The transducer is then rotated to examine the left pulmonary artery. However, interposition of the left main bronchus interferes with the ultrasound beam in the middle portion of the left pulmonary artery.[37] Therefore, PE is more difficult to detect in the left pulmonary artery.

TROPONIN LEVELS

Right ventricular microinfarction ensues from the right ventricular pressure overload caused by acute PE and can be detected by a small elevation in troponin levels,[38] often despite a normal creatine kinase-myocardial band (CK-MB), a less sensitive cardiac marker of injury. Such patients frequently have no underlying atherosclerosis of the right coronary artery, and, therefore, do not have the much more common and classic right ventricular infarction associated with inferior left ventricular infarction.

Troponin elevation in acute PE is associated with right ventricular dysfunction.[39] However, a comparison of the relative prognostic power of troponin alone, right ventricular dysfunction on echocardiogram alone, and combined troponin elevation and echocardiographic right ventricular failure remains to be elucidated. My impression is that echocardiographic right ventricular dysfunction is more sensitive than troponin elevation, but that troponin elevation confers a more ominous prognosis that the finding of mild to moderate right ventricular dysfunction.

Troponin elevations, like echocardiographic right ventricular dysfunction, help identify PE patients with an otherwise poor prognosis in whom aggressive intervention may be warranted. In a prospective study of 56 PE patients, those with elevated troponin levels were more likely to die, suffer cardiogenic shock, require inotropic agents, and need mechanical ventilation.[40] The mortality rate from PE was 44% in troponin-positive patients, compared with 3% in troponin-negative patients. Coronary angiography revealed obstructive coronary artery disease in an equal distribution of troponin-positive and troponin-negative patients.

METABOLIC ACIDOSIS

Among patients with acute cor pulmonale due to PE and consequent circulatory failure, the mortality rate is very high. In a case series from Boulogne, France, 59% of patients in this category died. Multivariate analysis showed that metabolic acidosis, defined as a base deficit $>5\,mEq/L$ was an independent predictor of mortality.[41]

Ominous prognosis: consideration of thrombolysis or embolectomy

Markers of ominous prognosis may be present even though the patient appears clinically stable. In the past, a 'watch and wait' philosophy prevailed. This dogma, now outdated, called for holding off from thrombolysis or embolectomy until patients developed overt cardiogenic shock that could not be reversed with pressors. Contemporary management takes a different approach. Using the tools of risk stratification, rapid and early identification it is now possible to predict which patients will fail conservative management. Therefore, consideration of thrombolysis and embolectomy can be accomplished while the patient remains relatively stable clinically. These more aggressive interventions can then be undertaken more safely and with better outcomes, prior to the onset of cardiovascular collapse. Ideally, patients will be assessed for thrombolysis or embolectomy as soon as they have been identified as high risk. A collaborative team comprising an interventional angiographer, vascular medicine or angiology specialist, and cardiac surgeon should make the assessment. This team should be on call round-the-clock and should have previously planned on all possible contingencies, including referral to a secondary care center for thrombolysis and a tertiary care center for embolectomy.

THROMBOLYSIS: POTENTIAL BENEFITS

Thrombolytic therapy holds the promise of rapid reversal of right ventricular failure, thereby potentially decreasing death from cardiovascular collapse.[42] By improving pulmonary capillary blood volume, thrombolysis may facilitate a more complete resolution of PE[43] with less chronic pulmonary hypertension and better preservation of the normal pulmonary vascular response to exercise.[44] The most effective and safest regimens utilize a high concentration of thrombolytic agent over a short period of time. The only contemporary regimen approved by the FDA is alteplase 100 mg as a continuous infusion over 2 hours.[45] However, other regimens are probably effective, including streptokinase 1 500 000 units over 2 hours,[46] urokinase 3 000 000 units over 2 hours, with the first 1 000 000 units administered as a 10-minute bolus,[47] and 'double bolus reteplase' in the dose of 10 units twice, separated by 30 minutes.[48]

We have demonstrated in a randomized trial of 101 hemodynamically stable patients that alteplase 100 mg/2 hours followed by anticoagulation accelerates the improvement of right ventricular function and pulmonary perfusion more rapidly than anticoagulation alone.[49] No clinical episodes of recurrent PE occurred among the alteplase patients, but there were five (two fatal and three non-fatal) clinically suspected recurrent PEs within 14 days in patients randomized to heparin alone (P = 0.06).

All five presented initially with right ventricular hypokinesis on echocardiogram, despite normal systemic arterial pressure at baseline. Thus, echocardiography identified a subgroup of patients with impending right ventricular failure at high risk of adverse outcomes if treated with heparin alone.

We subsequently showed quantitatively that most patients who receive thrombolytic therapy for PE achieve recovery of regional as well as global right ventricular function.[50] At baseline, right ventricular areas were significantly larger than normal at end-diastole and at end-systole. Diastolic and systolic right ventricular areas decreased after thrombolysis. The area of the right ventricle most severely affected (and most improved after therapy) was the mid-right ventricular free wall.

These findings provide a rationale for thrombolysis in patients with submassive PE with impending hemodynamic instability, before the onset of clinical deterioration. The FDA-approved alteplase regimen is straightforward and does not require any laboratory testing during the thrombolytic infusion, because no dosage adjustment is made. Although delay in administration of thrombolysis will attenuate efficacy, the decrement in effect is much less than with myocardial infarction thrombolysis, probably because PE patients benefit from the bronchial collateral circulation. In our registry of more than 300 patients who received thrombolysis in clinical trials, there was 0.7% less pulmonary reperfusion per additional day of symptoms. Nevertheless, thrombolysis improved pulmonary perfusion in most patients, even those who had symptoms for up to 14 days prior to drug administration.[51]

THROMBOLYSIS: POTENTIAL RISKS

Patients being considered for thrombolysis should be subjected to a meticulous evaluation for possible contraindications such as intracranial disease, recent surgery, or trauma. Registries that record 'real world' results, including bleeding complications, may be more realistic regarding limitations and complications from thrombolysis than more closely supervised clinical trials.

In ICOPER, the prospective registry of 2454 patients with PE conducted in 52 hospitals among seven countries, 304 patients received thrombolytic therapy.[3] Of patients who received thrombolysis, 3.0% suffered intracranial bleeding. Overall, 22% of those receiving thrombolysis had major bleeding and 12% required transfusions.

In our series of 312 patients receiving thrombolysis for PE in five clinical trials, there was a 1.9% risk (95% CI 0.7–4.1%) of intracranial bleeding.[52] Two of the six patients with pre-existing known intracranial disease received thrombolysis in violation of the trial protocol. Diastolic blood pressure on admission was significantly elevated in patients who developed intracranial hemorrhage compared with those who did not (90.3 versus 77.6 mmHg; P = 0.04).

In an overview of the five PE thrombolysis trials that we conducted, the mean age of patients with major bleeding was 63 years, while that of patients with no hemorrhagic complication was 56 years (P = 0.005). There was a 4% increased risk of bleeding for each additional year of age. Increasing body mass index and pulmonary angiography were also significant predictors of hemorrhage.[53]

In a registry at the Laennec Hospital in Paris, 132 consecutive patients received rt-PA for massive PE.[54] Two (1.5%) suffered intracranial bleeding, and one of the two died. Pericardial tamponade was equally problematic and occurred in two other patients (1.5%), one of whom died. Other major bleeding complications included two gastrointestinal hemorrhages, three cases of hemoptysis, and 11 hematomas at the puncture site for pulmonary angiography. In a separate registry of 64 patients treated with thrombolysis, an astounding 4.7% suffered intracranial hemorrhage.[55]

A fastidious history when considering thrombolysis may identify patients at high risk of intracranial hemorrhage. Of special concern are patients with a history of moderate or severe hypertension, head trauma or seizures. Increasing age and a high body mass index are also risk factors for bleeding and should be factored into the decision regarding thrombolysis versus alternative interventions such as embolectomy. Because intracranial hemorrhage is a devastating complication, the proper role of thrombolysis in PE treatment continues to generate controversy as a 'hot topic' and 'debatable indication'.[56] A definitive clinical trial is long overdue.[57]

EMBOLECTOMY

Transvenous catheter embolectomy in the interventional angiography laboratory provides a less invasive alternative to open surgical embolectomy (Fig. 16B.4) for patients with contraindications for thrombolysis and high likelihood of adverse outcomes if managed with anticoagulation alone. Devices designed to remove small arterial clots rather than to decompress and remove massive thrombi due to PE are widely used, and their limitations have hindered the success of this procedure.[58]

The Greenfield embolectomy device (Medi-Tech Corporation, Watertown, MA, USA) is a large and unwieldy 10F catheter. The Amplatz Thrombectomy Device (ATD; MicroVena Corporation, White Bear Lake, MN, USA) is an 8F catheter with an encapsulated impeller housed at its distal end. A drive shaft rotates the impeller at speeds exceeding 100 000 r.p.m., creating a vortex that homogenizes and macerates the thrombus to particles smaller than 13 μm. The pigtail rotational catheter (William Cook Europe, Denmark) is a 5F catheter designed

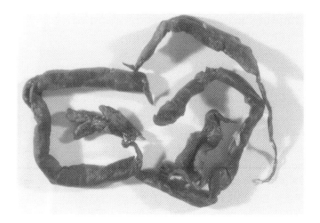

Figure 16B.4 *Thrombus removed during a successful, emergency pulmonary embolectomy.*

for manual rotation and fragmentation of thrombus. The rheolytic thrombectomy catheter (Angiojet; Possis Medical, Minneapolis, MN, USA) consists of a 5F dual lumen catheter. One lumen permits high-pressure saline delivery, and the other lumen is designed to remove the thrombotic debris. The high-pressure saline injection causes a Venturi effect, which fragments the thrombus. The Hydrolyser Thrombectomy Catheter (Hydrolyser; Cordis Europa NV, Roden, The Netherlands) also relies upon high-pressure injection of saline and the consequent Venturi effect. Most of these devices have undergone very limited formal study. At Brigham and Women's Hospital, we currently use the Angiojet more than any other embolectomy catheter. However, owing to the limitations of catheter embolectomy, we more often favor open surgical embolectomy. Nevertheless, a dedicated and skilled interventional team with round-the-clock coverage can achieve clinical improvement with combined catheter fragmentation and catheter-directed thrombolysis of massive PE.[59]

Open surgical embolectomy is the most effective procedure for emergent removal of large amounts of thrombus due to acute PE. This procedure is especially suitable for patients who have contraindications for thrombolysis and who have not yet deteriorated to the point of suffering profound cardiogenic shock or cardiac arrest.[60] At Brigham and Women's Hospital, we have organized our Thromboembolism Service so that this treatment option is available. We always have an on-call cardiac surgeon with special interest in this procedure. We have liberalized our criteria for acute pulmonary embolectomy and consider operating on patients with anatomically extensive PE and concomitant moderate to severe right ventricular dysfunction, even with preserved systemic arterial pressure. During a 2-year period, we operated on 29 patients with an 89% survival rate. The high survival rate can be attributed to improved surgical technique, rapid diagnosis and triage, and careful patient selection.[61]

Inferior vena caval filters

The two principal indications for insertion of an inferior vena caval filter are:

- massive bleeding that precludes anticoagulation
- recurrent PE despite prolonged intensive anticoagulation.

Unfortunately, filters do not halt the thrombotic process. Furthermore, they are associated with a marked increase in the frequency of subsequent DVT.[62,63] For patients with an upper extremity DVT as the source of PE, a superior vena caval filter can be placed.[64]

> - The principal indications for placement of inferior vena caval filters are major hemorrhage and recurrent PE despite intensive anticoagulation. Filters are losing popularity because of their association with an increased rate of venous thrombosis over the long-term.

KEY POINTS

- Anticoagulation is evolving from intravenous unfractionated heparin to subcutaneous low molecular weight heparin, utilized as a 'bridge' to chronic anticoagulation with warfarin or other anti-vitamin K agents.
- Due to the problems of adequately and safely dosing warfarin and other anti-vitamin K agents, there is great enthusiasm for novel anticoagulation strategies, such as low molecular weight heparin as monotherapy without warfarin and monotherapy with oral direct thrombin inhibitors. Other novel anticoagulants include weekly depot injection of pentasaccharides and oral heparins.
- For PE, after surgery or trauma, provide 6 months of therapy. Patients with idiopathic PE or those with the antiphospholipid antibody syndrome should receive indefinite duration, lifelong treatment.
- Treatment strategy must be tailored to severity of PE, which ranges widely from asymptomatic to fatal.
- Moderate or severe right ventricular dysfunction or an elevation in troponin, a cardiac marker of injury, portend an ominous prognosis with standard anticoagulation alone.
- The role of thrombolysis for patients without massive PE and hemodynamic instability remains uncertain, debatable, and highly controversial, mostly because of the high rate of intracranial hemorrhage compared with patients who receive thrombolysis for acute myocardial infarction.
- There is an improvement in techniques for catheter embolectomy as well as resurgence in interest and improved outcome with open surgical embolectomy.

REFERENCES

1 Oger E. Incidence of venous thromboembolism: a community-based study in Western France. EPI-GETBP Study Group. Groupe d'Etude de la Thrombose de Bretagne Occidentale. *Thromb Haemost* 2000;**83**:657–60.

2 Silverstein MD, Heit JA, Mohr DN *et al.* Trends in the incidence of deep vein thrombosis and pulmonary embolism: a 25-year population-based study. *Arch Intern Med* 1998;**158**:585–93.

3 Goldhaber SZ, Visani L, De Rosa M. Acute pulmonary embolism: clinical outcomes in the International Cooperative Pulmonary Embolism Registry (ICOPER). *Lancet* 1999;**353**:1386–9.

4 Nakamura M, Fujioka H, Yamada N *et al.* Clinical characteristics of acute pulmonary thromboembolism in Japan: results of a multicenter registry in the Japanese Society of Pulmonary Embolism Research. *Clin Cardiol* 2001;**24**:132–8.

5 Gould MK, Dembitzer AD, Doyle RL *et al.* Low-molecular-weight heparins compared with unfractionated heparin for treatment of acute deep venous thrombosis. A meta-analysis of randomized, controlled trials. *Ann Intern Med* 1999;**130**:800–9.

●6 Gould MK, Dembitzer AD, Sanders GD *et al.* Low-molecular-weight heparins compared with unfractionated heparin for treatment of acute deep venous thrombosis. A cost-effectiveness analysis. *Ann Intern Med* 1999;**130**:789–99.

●7 Levine M, Gent M, Hirsh J *et al.* A comparison of low-molecular-weight heparin administered primarily at home with unfractionated heparin administered in the hospital for proximal deep-vein thrombosis. *N Engl J Med* 1996;**334**:677–81.

8 Meignan M, Rosso J, Gauthier H *et al.* Systematic lung scans reveal a high frequency of silent pulmonary embolism in patients with proximal deep venous thrombosis. *Arch Intern Med* 2000;**160**:159–64.

9 Douketis JD, Kearon C, Bates S *et al.* Risk of fatal pulmonary embolism in patients with treated venous thromboembolism. *JAMA* 1998;**279**:458–62.

10 Heit JA, Silverstein MD, Mohr DN *et al.* Predictors of survival after deep vein thrombosis and pulmonary embolism: a population-based, cohort study. *Arch Intern Med* 1999;**159**:445–53.

11 Eichinger S, Schoenauer V, Minar E *et al.* The risk of recurrent venous thromboembolism in patients with symptomatic pulmonary embolism. [Abstract] *Blood* 2001;**96**:2789.

●12 Simonneau G, Sors H, Charbonnier B *et al.* A comparison of low-molecular-weight heparin with unfractionated heparin for acute pulmonary embolism. The THESEE Study Group. Tinzaparine ou Heparine Standard: Evaluations dans l'Embolie Pulmonaire. *N Engl J Med* 1997;**337**:663–9.

13 Low-molecular-weight heparin in the treatment of patients with venous thromboembolism. The Columbus Investigators. *N Engl J Med* 1997;**337**:657–62.

14 Kovacs MJ, Anderson D, Morrow B *et al.* Outpatient treatment of pulmonary embolism with dalteparin. *Thromb Haemost* 2000;**83**:209–11.

15 Beckman JA, Dunn KL, Sasahara AA *et al.* Enoxaparin monotherapy without oral anticoagulation to treat acute symptomatic pulmonary embolism. *Thromb Haemost* 2003;**89**:953–8.

●16 Brandjes DPM, Heijboer H, Buller HR *et al.* Acenocoumarol and heparin compared with acenocoumarol alone in the initial treatment of proximal-vein thrombosis. *N Engl J Med* 1992;**327**:1485–9.

17 Crowther MA, Ginsberg JB, Kearon C *et al.* A randomized trial comparing 5-mg and 10-mg warfarin loading doses. *Arch Intern Med* 1999;**159**:46–8.

18 Ageno W, Turpie AG. Exaggerated initial response to warfarin following heart valve replacement. *Am J Cardiol* 1999;**84**:905–8.

19 Aithal GP, Day CP, Kesteven PJ *et al.* Association of polymorphisms in the cytochrome P450 CYP2C9 with warfarin dose requirement and risk of bleeding complications. *Lancet* 1999;**353**:717–19.

20 Weibert RT, Le DT, Kayser SR *et al.* Correction of excessive anticoagulation with low-dose oral vitamin K1. *Ann Intern Med* 1997;**126**:959–62.

●21 Schulman S, Rhedin AS, Lindmarker P *et al.* A comparison of six weeks with six months of oral anticoagulant therapy after a first episode of venous thromboembolism. Duration of Anticoagulation Trial Study Group. *N Engl J Med* 1995;**332**:1661–5.

22 Kearon C, Gent M, Hirsh J *et al.* A comparison of three months of anticoagulation with extended anticoagulation for a first episode of idiopathic venous thromboembolism. *N Engl J Med* 1999;**340**:901–7.

●23 Agnelli G, Prandoni P, Santamaria MG *et al.* Three months versus one year of oral anticoagulant therapy for idiopathic deep venous thrombosis. Warfarin Optimal Duration Italian Trial Investigators. *N Engl J Med* 2001;**345**:165–9.

24 Agnelli G, Prandoni P, Becattini C *et al.* Extended oral anticoagulant therapy after a first episode of pulmonary embolism. *Ann Intern Med* 2003;**139**:19–25.

25 Ridker PM, Goldhaber SZ, Danielson E *et al.* Long-term low-intensity warfarin therapy for the prevention of recurrent venous thromboembolism. *N Engl J Med* 2003;**348**:1425–34.

26 Kucher N, Goldhaber SZ. Cardiac biomarkers for risk stratification of patients with acute pulmonary embolism. *Circulation* 2003;**108**:2191–4.

27 Goldhaber SZ, Elliot CG. Acute pulmonary embolism: Part II. Risk stratification treatment and prevention. *Circulation* 2003;**108**:2834–8.

28 Wicki J, Perrier A, Perneger TV *et al.* Predicting adverse outcome in patients with acute pulmonary embolism: a risk score. *Thromb Haemost* 2000;**84**:548–52.

●29 Wolfe MW, Lee RT, Feldstein ML *et al.* Prognostic significance of right ventricular hypokinesis and perfusion lung scan defects in pulmonary embolism. *Am Heart J* 1994;**127**:1371–5.

30 Grifoni S, Olivotto I, Cecchini P *et al.* Short-term clinical outcome of patients with acute pulmonary embolism, normal blood pressure, and echocardiographic right ventricular dysfunction. *Circulation* 2000;**101**:2817–22.

◆31 Goldhaber SZ. Echocardiography in the management of pulmonary embolism. *Ann Intern Med* 2002;**136**:691–700.

32 Dabestani A, Mahan G, Gardin JM *et al.* Evaluation of pulmonary artery pressure and resistance by pulsed Doppler echocardiography. *Am J Cardiol* 1987;**59**:662–8.

33 Jardin F, Dubourg O, Bourdarias JP. Echocardiographic pattern of acute cor pulmonale. *Chest* 1997;**111**:209–17.

34 Schuchlenz HW, Weihs W, Horner S *et al.* The association between the diameter of a patent foramen ovale and the risk of embolic cerebrovascular events. *Am J Med* 2000;**109**:456–62.

35 Konstantinides S, Geibel A, Kasper W *et al.* Patent foramen ovale is an important predictor of adverse outcome in patients with major pulmonary embolism. *Circulation* 1998;**97**:1946–51.

36 Pruszczyk P, Torbicki A, Kuch-Wocial A *et al.* Diagnostic value of transoesophageal echocardiography in suspected haemodynamically significant pulmonary embolism. *Heart* 2001;**85**:628–34.

37 Pruszczyk P, Torbicki A, Pacho R *et al.* Noninvasive diagnosis of suspected severe pulmonary embolism: transesophageal echocardiography vs spiral CT. *Chest* 1997;**112**:722–8.

38 Douketis JD, Crowther MA, Stanton EB *et al.* Elevated cardiac troponin levels in patients with submassive pulmonary embolism. *Arch Intern Med* 2002;**162**:79–81.

39 Meyer T, Binder L, Hruska N *et al.* Cardiac troponin I elevation in acute pulmonary embolism is associated with right ventricular dysfunction. *J Am Coll Cardiol* 2000;**36**:1632–6.

40 Giannitsis E, Muller-Bardorff M, Kurowski V *et al.* Independent prognostic value of cardiac troponin T in patients with confirmed pulmonary embolism. *Circulation* 2000;**102**:211–17.

41 Vieillard-Baron A, Page B, Augarde R *et al.* Acute cor pulmonale in massive pulmonary embolism: incidence, echocardiographic pattern, clinical implications and recovery rate. *Intensive Care Med* 2001;**27**:1481–6.

42 Jerjes-Sanchez C, Ramirez-Rivera A, de Lourdes GM *et al.* Streptokinase and heparin versus heparin alone in massive pulmonary embolism: a randomized controlled trial. *J Thromb Thrombolysis* 1995;**2**:227–9.

43 Sharma GV, Burleson VA, Sasahara AA. Effect of thrombolytic therapy on pulmonary-capillary blood volume in patients with pulmonary embolism. *N Engl J Med* 1980;**303**:842–5.

44 Sharma GV, Folland ED, McIntyre KM *et al.* Long-term benefit of thrombolytic therapy in patients with pulmonary embolism. *Vasc Med* 2000;**5**:91–5.

◆45 Goldhaber SZ, Bounameaux H. Thrombolytic therapy in pulmonary embolism. *Semin Vasc Med* 2001;**1**:213–20.

46 Meneveau N, Schiele F, Metz D *et al.* Comparative efficacy of a two-hour regimen of streptokinase versus alteplase in

acute massive pulmonary embolism: immediate clinical and hemodynamic outcome and one-year follow-up. *J Am Coll Cardiol* 1998;**31**:1057–63.

47 Goldhaber SZ, Kessler CM, Heit JA *et al*. Recombinant tissue-type plasminogen activator versus a novel dosing regimen of urokinase in acute pulmonary embolism: a randomized controlled multicenter trial. *J Am Coll Cardiol* 1992;**20**:24–30.

48 Tebbe U, Graf A, Kamke W *et al*. Hemodynamic effects of double bolus reteplase versus alteplase infusion in massive pulmonary embolism. *Am Heart J* 1999;**138**:39–44.

●49 Goldhaber SZ, Haire WD, Feldstein ML *et al*. Alteplase versus heparin in acute pulmonary embolism: randomised trial assessing right ventricular function and pulmonary perfusion. *Lancet* 1993;**341**:507–11.

50 Nass N, McConnell MV, Goldhaber SZ *et al*. Recovery of regional right ventricular function after thrombolysis for pulmonary embolism. *Am J Cardiol* 1999;**83**:804–6.

51 Daniels LB, Parker JA, Patel SR *et al*. Relation of duration of symptoms with response to thrombolytic therapy in pulmonary embolism. *Am J Cardiol* 1997;**80**:184–8.

52 Kanter DS, Mikkola KM, Patel SR *et al*. Thrombolytic therapy for pulmonary embolism. Frequency of intracranial hemorrhage and associated risk factors. *Chest* 1997;**111**:1241–5.

53 Mikkola KM, Patel SR, Parker JA *et al*. Increasing age is a major risk factor for hemorrhagic complications following pulmonary embolism thrombolysis. *Am Heart J* 1997;**134**:69–72.

54 Meyer G, Gisselbrecht M, Diehl JL *et al*. Incidence and predictors of major hemorrhagic complications from thrombolytic therapy in patients with massive pulmonary embolism. *Am J Med* 1998;**105**:472–7.

55 Hamel E, Pacouret G, Vincentelli D *et al*. Thrombolysis or heparin therapy in massive pulmonary embolism with right ventricular dilation: results from a 128-patient monocenter registry. *Chest* 2001;**120**:120–5.

56 Goldhaber SZ. Thrombolysis in pulmonary embolism: a debatable indication. *Thromb Haemost* 2001;**86**:444–51.

57 Goldhaber SZ. Thrombolysis in pulmonary embolism: a large-scale trial is overdue. *Circulation* 2001;**104**:2876–8.

58 Meyer G, Koning R, Sors H. Transvenous catheter embolectomy. *Semin Vasc Med* 2001;**1**:247–52.

59 DeGregorio MA, Gimeo MJ, Mainer A *et al*. Mechanical and enzymatic thrombolysis for massive pulmonary embolism. *J Vasc Interv Radiol* 2002;**13**:163–9.

60 Aklog L. Emergency surgical pulmonary embolectomy. *Semin Vasc Med* 2001;**1**:235–46.

●61 Aklog L, Williams CS, Byrne JG *et al*. Acute pulmonary embolectomy: a contemporary approach. *Circulation* 2002;**105**:1416–19.

62 Decousus H, Leizorovicz A, Parent F *et al*. A clinical trial of vena caval filters in the prevention of pulmonary embolism in patients with proximal deep-vein thrombosis. Prevention du Risque d'Embolie Pulmonaire par Interruption Cave Study Group. *N Engl J Med* 1998;**338**:409–15.

63 White RH, Zhou H, Kim J *et al*. A population-based study of the effectiveness of inferior vena cava filter use among patients with venous thromboembolism. *Arch Intern Med* 2000;**160**:2033–41.

64 Ascher E, Hingorani A, Tsemekhin B *et al*. Lessons learned from a 6-year clinical experience with superior vena cava Greenfield filters. *J Vasc Surg* 2000;**32**:881–7.

Chronic thromboembolic pulmonary hypertension

WILLIAM R AUGER, PETER F FEDULLO AND STUART W JAMIESON

INTRODUCTION

Chronic thromboembolic (CTE) obstruction of the main, lobar and segmental pulmonary arteries is an uncommon sequela of acute pulmonary embolism. The extent of pulmonary vascular involvement and the duration of obstruction determine the severity of pulmonary hypertension that may ensue, although the critical determinants of evolution to this stage have not been entirely elucidated. If this clinical entity is overlooked or left untreated, right ventricular decompensation and death inevitably result. However, increased physician awareness of chronic thromboembolic pulmonary hypertension (CTEPH), diagnostic advances over the past few decades, and the availability of a surgical procedure to remove thrombus from the proximal pulmonary vascular bed – pulmonary thromboendarterectomy (PTE) – have made CTEPH a potentially correctable form of pulmonary hypertension.

An expanded worldwide experience in the diagnosis and treatment of CTEPH has occurred over the past two decades.[1–16] However, numerous diagnostic and therapeutic challenges remain. As surgical techniques and clinical experience advance, defining patients with **inaccessible** chronic thromboembolic disease has become the principal diagnostic dilemma. Furthermore, a subset of patients develops residual postoperative pulmonary hypertension, which is poorly understood pathophysiologically and for which therapy is challenging. Finally, effective management of other postoperative difficulties, particularly reperfusion lung injury, continues to be a focus of investigation to further diminish morbidity and mortality.

PATHOPHYSIOLOGY OF CTEPH

Most patients with CTEPH present late in the course of their disease, and are often unable to provide symptomatic or historical clues to the events leading to their cardiopulmonary status. Although the thromboembolic basis of CTEPH has been questioned, clinical experience suggests that the failure of thromboembolic resolution following a single embolic event, or recurrent thromboembolic events, represents the inciting event in the majority of patients.[17–22]

Glimpses into the evolution of CTEPH can be derived from our understanding of the natural history of acute pulmonary embolic disease. The clinical presentation of venous thrombosis and pulmonary embolism may be subtle and easily confused with alternative diagnoses.[23–25] Accordingly, it is likely that a significant number of thromboembolic events go unrecognized and therefore untreated. Recent data would also suggest that anatomic resolution after an acute embolic event may not always be as complete as previously assumed. Wartski and colleagues reviewed follow-up lung perfusion studies in 157 patients with symptomatic, acute pulmonary embolism:[26] 104 patients (66%) demonstrated residual perfusion defects 3 months after the acute event, and 21 patients showed residual pulmonary vascular obstruction of at least 40%. Since perfusion lung scans in chronic thromboembolic disease underestimate the degree of vascular obstruction compared with angiography,[27] it is possible that perfusion scanning may also underestimate the extent of residual thromboembolic obstruction in patients recovering from an acute pulmonary embolism. Finally, recent information suggests that partial thromboembolic resolution, with mild degrees of pulmonary hypertension, may be more common following an acute embolic episode than previously suspected:[28,29] Ribeiro and colleagues[30] reported 1-year echocardiographic and 5-year clinical follow-up data in 78 patients hospitalized with acute pulmonary embolism. They found an early dynamic phase followed by a protracted stable period of pulmonary artery pressure decline after an acute thromboembolic event. The stable phase was achieved within 21 days by 90%, and in all patients by 38 days, regardless of whether the therapeutic intervention was thrombolytics or heparin. Patients with a pulmonary artery systolic pressure greater than 50 mmHg at the time of the acute event had a threefold increased risk for persistent pulmonary hypertension. Four patients developed chronic pulmonary hypertension, with three subsequently undergoing successful PTE.

Given the subtle presentation and the possibility of incomplete anatomic and hemodynamic resolution in a subset of thromboembolic patients, it is likely that CTEPH is part of the spectrum of disease associated with acute pulmonary embolism ranging from complete hemodynamic and anatomic resolution, partial resolution associated with a normal symptomatic status in most, or progression to pulmonary hypertension in a minority of patients. Although estimates vary, approximately 0.1–0.5% of survivors of an acute embolism in the USA will develop hemodynamically significant thromboembolic residua that will ultimately warrant surgical intervention.[15,31]

Most individuals with CTEPH do not have an identifiable impairment in fibrinolysis[5,32] or prothrombotic tendency. A lupus anticoagulant and/or high titer anticardiolipin antibodies can be detected in 10–24%,[33,34] whereas hereditary thrombophilias, such as protein C, protein S and antithrombin III deficiencies, are documented in less than 5% of patients. The presence of factor V Leiden has been reported in 4–6.5% of CTEPH patients,[34,35] whilst the frequency of other thrombophilic states such as factor II mutation, the prothrombin 20210 G/A gene mutation, elevated factor VIII levels, and hyperhomocystinemia are unknown.

Since most patients present late in the course of their disease, the evolution of pulmonary hypertension has been difficult to define. Progression may result from either narrowing of the proximal pulmonary vascular bed with recurrent thromboemboli or from in situ thrombosis in areas of the pulmonary vascular bed previously involved with an acute embolus. Alternatively, the gradual rise in pulmonary vascular resistance may be the result of hypertensive changes in the distal vascular bed. The poor correlation between the degree of pulmonary hypertension and the extent of central pulmonary artery obstruction or partial vascular occlusion as assessed by angiography support this concept. Moser and Bloor

demonstrated that small-vessel hypertensive arteriopathy, similar to primary pulmonary hypertension, is seen in the uninvolved vascular bed of CTEPH patients.[36] Accordingly, it is presently believed that most patients with CTEPH have suffered an acute pulmonary embolic event or events with incomplete resolution. With the loss of pulmonary vascular reserve, modest pulmonary hypertension at rest would worsen with exercise because of the loss of normal adaptive mechanisms. Over a period of time, as a result of the effects of elevated pressures and flows on the unobstructed pulmonary vascular bed, or as a result of mediator-related effects, a small-vessel arteriopathy develops, leading to a progressive cycle of worsening pulmonary hypertension, declining cardiac function and diminished exercise tolerance.

Survival of untreated patients is particularly poor and correlates with the level of pulmonary artery pressure at presentation. Riedel and colleagues reported a 50% survival rate over a 10-year period in patients presenting with a mean pulmonary artery pressure between 31 and 40 mmHg; survival rate declined to 20% over 10 years when the initial mean pulmonary artery pressure was 41–50 mmHg, and to 5% for a mean pulmonary artery pressure greater than 50 mmHg. In this last group, 2-year survival was only 20%.[29] In a group of 49 patients deemed unsuitable for surgery who were treated with anticoagulation alone, prognosis was related to the severity of pulmonary hypertension (mean PAP > 30 mmHg), the coexistence of chronic obstructive pulmonary disease, and poor exercise tolerance.[37]

CLINICAL PRESENTATION

A carefully obtained history will often provide clues suggestive of a prior acute thromboembolic event; these may be an episode of pleurisy, a lower extremity muscle strain, or a remote history of an atypical pulmonary infection. Age, co-morbid diseases, and the state of physical conditioning likely influence the time of onset and the severity of symptoms. As with other forms of pulmonary hypertension, the most common presenting complaints are exertional dyspnea and a progressive decline in exercise tolerance, which result from a reduced cardiac output along with an increase in dead-space ventilation. A nonproductive cough, atypical chest pains (usually pleuritic in character), and palpitations are also common complaints. Hemoptysis occurs infrequently. Hoarseness may result from left vocal cord dysfunction, resulting from compression of the recurrent laryngeal nerve between the aorta and an enlarged left main pulmonary artery. As right ventricular function declines, patients may experience exertion-related dizziness or syncope, resting dyspnea and exertional chest pain. The non-specific presentation of these patients, as with other forms of pulmonary hypertension, results in a delay in establishing a diagnosis of 2–3 years from the onset of cardiopulmonary symptoms.[7,16]

Physical examination

Findings on physical examination are generally similar to those in other forms of pulmonary hypertension, with one notable exception: pulmonary flow murmurs, resulting from turbulent flow across narrowed, partially obstructed large pulmonary arteries, are audible in approximately 30% of patients with chronic thromboembolic pulmonary hypertension.[38] Although these bruits are not unique to chronic thromboembolic disease and can be audible in patients with congenital branch stenoses and pulmonary arteritis, they are not heard in primary pulmonary hypertension (PPH), which is a common competing diagnosis.

DIAGNOSTIC EVALUATION

Diagnostic studies to assess exertional dyspnea or a change in exercise tolerance usually provide few clues to the presence of CTEPH. Routine hematological and blood chemistry tests are generally unremarkable early in the course of CTEPH. Longstanding hypoxemia may result in a secondary polycythemia. A modest thrombocytopenia and a prolonged activated partial thromboplastin time (in the absence of heparin anticoagulation) suggests the presence of a lupus anticoagulant. Liver function studies may be abnormal from hepatic congestion due to right ventricular failure. A reduced cardiac output and reduced renal blood flow may manifest itself by elevations in blood urea nitrogen, serum creatinine, and uric acid levels.[39] Evidence of prior venous thrombosis can be demonstrated by duplex scanning of the lower extremities in 35–47% of patients with thromboembolic pulmonary hypertension (M. Mo, personal communication).

Pulmonary function tests

Pulmonary function tests are frequently obtained to evaluate exertional dyspnea. Lung volume and airflow abnormalities attributable to CTEPH are relatively minor; therefore, these studies are most useful in excluding coexisting parenchymal or obstructive airways disease. Approximately 20% of patients demonstrate mild to moderate lung restriction due to the presence of parenchymal scarring from prior lung infarction.[40] A modest reduction in single-breath diffusing capacity for carbon monoxide (DCO) can be present in CTEPH,[41] but a normal value does not exclude the diagnosis. Severe reductions in DCO (i.e. <50% predicted) are rarely seen and should suggest a condition that affects the distal pulmonary vascular bed.[42] Resting arterial blood gases demonstrate a normal arterial oxygen level (PaO_2); with exercise, PaO_2 can decrease, with an abnormal increase in dead space ventilation. The hypoxemia is due to both ventilation/perfusion inequalities and a low mixed venous oxygen saturation resulting from a reduced cardiac output.[43] Hypoxemia at rest indicates severely compromised right heart function or right-to-left shunting through a patent foramen ovale.

Chest radiography

Depending on the stage of the disease, chest radiographic features in CTEPH can range from relatively few and subtle abnormalities to distinctive findings suggestive of the diagnosis.[44] In the absence of coexisting parenchymal lung disease, the lung fields are typically free of infiltrates, though regions of hypoperfusion or hyperperfusion, appearing as a prominent interstitial pattern, may be present. Peripheral opacities consistent with scarring from previous infarctions appear in hypoperfused lung regions, frequently accompanied by pleural thickening. Pleural effusions are uncommon unless a high right atrial pressure is present. Enlargement of the right ventricle and pulmonary outflow tract are evident on lateral films, with obliteration of the retrosternal space. Dilatation of the central pulmonary vessels is reflective of longstanding pulmonary hypertension. Unlike the symmetrical enlargement of the proximal vessels in small-vessel pulmonary hypertension, CTEPH patients often demonstrate irregularly shaped, asymmetrically enlarged pulmonary arteries.[45] The discrepancy in the size of the central pulmonary vessels may be so dramatic that agenesis of one of the main pulmonary arteries is suggested.[46] The unusual contour of the pulmonary vessels is frequently misinterpreted as adenopathy.

Echocardiography

Echocardiography is an effective, non-invasive study to screen for the presence of pulmonary hypertension[47] and is discussed in detail elsewhere in this text.

Ventilation/perfusion scan

Once the diagnosis of pulmonary hypertension has been established, or is strongly suspected, the focus of the evaluation turns to differentiating between major-vessel and small-vessel pulmonary vascular disease. In most cases, a lung ventilation/perfusion ($\dot{V}/\dot{Q}$) scan is a non-invasive means of achieving this end. Patients with major-vessel

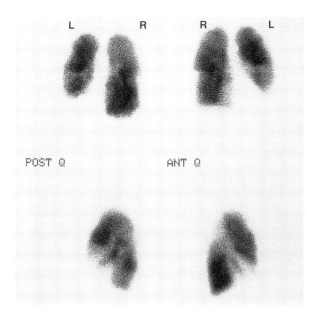

Figure 17.1 *Lung perfusion scan in a patient with chronic thromboembolic pulmonary hypertension. Ventilation study was normal.*

CTE disease will exhibit multiple segmental-sized or larger perfusion defects in lung regions with normal ventilation (Figure 17.1), in contrast to the normal or subsegmental 'mottled' perfusion pattern seen in small-vessel diseases such as primary pulmonary hypertension.[48] However, during the process of organization, proximal vessel thromboemboli may recanalize or narrow the vessel so that radiolabelled macroaggregated albumin can pass beyond the point of partial occlusion. Consequently, 'gray zones', or regions of relative hypoperfusion are frequent observed and, as a result, lung perfusion studies underestimate the degree of vascular obstruction caused by proximal vessel chronic thromboembolic disease.[27] Furthermore, mismatched segmental perfusion defects are not specific for chronic thromboembolic disease and can be seen with other disease entities that lead to occlusion of the central pulmonary arteries, such as mediastinal adenopathy or fibrosis, primary pulmonary vascular tumors, and large-vessel arteritis. Accordingly, additional imaging studies are necessary to define the pulmonary vascular anatomy and to establish a diagnosis.

Computerized tomography

The role of computerized tomography (CT) of the chest in the evaluation of patients with suspected chronic thromboembolic disease remains incompletely defined. CT features include mosaic perfusion of the lung parenchyma; pulmonary vessel enlargement with variation in the size of segmental vessels; peripheral, scar-like densities in hypoattenuated lung regions; and the presence of mediastinal collateral vessels.[49–52] Contrast enhancement may demonstrate chronic thrombus lining the larger pulmonary vessels in either a concentric or eccentric fashion (Figure 17.2).

CT imaging has considerable value in cases where alternative explanations for encroachment on the major pulmonary vessels are being considered, such as fibrosing mediastinitis;[53,54] adenopathy with parenchymal lung lesions suggestive of sarcoidosis or carcinoma;[55] and intraluminal occlusive lesions involving the pulmonary outflow tract or main pulmonary arteries characteristic of primary pulmonary vascular tumors.[54,56] CT imaging of the chest also provides useful information on the lung parenchyma when emphysema or restrictive lung disease are also present.

Chronic thromboemboli can become endothelialized, making their presence on CT angiography inapparent. Consequently, the absence of 'lining thrombus' involving the central pulmonary arteries does not exclude the diagnosis of chronic thromboembolic disease, or the possibility of surgical accessibility. Conversely, the demonstration of centrally located thrombus does not establish a diagnosis of surgically accessible chronic thromboembolic disease. Central thrombus demonstrated by CT has been described in PPH and other forms of end-stage lung disease.[57,58] Surgical endarterectomy in these cases not only presents a substantial risk, but also is unlikely to mitigate the existing pulmonary hypertension.

Pulmonary angiography

Pulmonary angiography remains the most reliable means of defining the extent and proximal location of suspected chronic thromboembolic lesions. Although performing angiography in the setting of pulmonary hypertension is often viewed with trepidation, the risks can be minimized in skilled hands and with appropriate precautions.[59,60] Pulmonary arteriography both establishes the diagnosis and provides critical information for determining surgical candidacy. The angiographic appearance of CTEPH reflects the complex pattern of organization and recanalization that occurs following an acute thromboembolic event. Consequently, chronic thromboemboli are angiographically distinct from the well-defined, intraluminal filling defects seen with acute pulmonary emboli. Several angiographic patterns have correlated with the presence of chronic thrombus: vascular webs or band-like narrowings, intimal irregularities, 'pouching defects', abrupt narrowing of major pulmonary arteries, and obstruction of pulmonary vessels, frequently at their point of origin and in the absence of an apparent intraluminal filling defect.[61] In most patients, two or more of these angiographic findings are present and are bilateral (Figure 17.3).

Alternative diagnoses can angiographically mimic CTEPH. Band-like vessel narrowing is a feature of

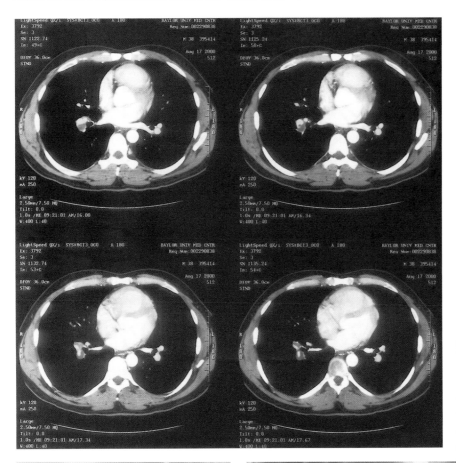

Figure 17.2 *Computerized tomography angiogram in chronic thromboembolic pulmonary hypertension patient demonstrating lining thrombus involving the right descending pulmonary artery.*

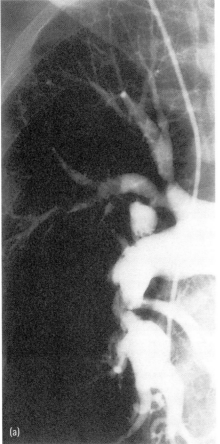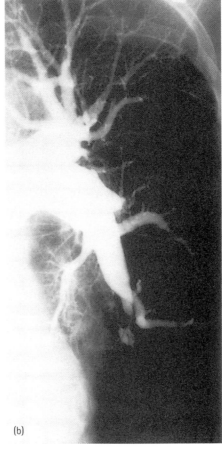

(a)   (b)

Figure 17.3 *Right (a) and left (b) pulmonary arteriogram (posterior-anterior views) of the patient whose lung scan is shown in Figure 17.1. Features of chronic thromboembolic disease include the abrupt narrowing of the right interlobar artery, a 'pouch' defect involving the proximal right descending pulmonary artery with a paucity of vessels to the right middle and lower lobes, and an enlarged, irregularly shaped right upper lobe vessel. On the left, an upper lobe artery is narrowed proximally, with occlusion of the anterior upper lobe and lingular vessels.*

medium- or large-vessel pulmonary arteritis (Takayasu's arteritis)[62,63] and is a hallmark finding in congenital stenosis of the pulmonary arteries.[64] Total or partial obstruction of the central pulmonary vessels, particularly when unilateral, may be the result of extrinsic (lymphadenopathy, carcinoma, fibrosis) or intrinsic (primary pulmonary vascular tumor) vascular disease.

Pulmonary angioscopy

Despite the utility of pulmonary angiography, a subgroup of patients exists where the diagnosis and surgical accessibility are not completely defined by angiography. In approximately 20–25% of patients, visualization of the vascular intima using pulmonary angioscopy is a useful tool.[65] This fiber-optic device is introduced into the pulmonary circulation through a central venous access, a balloon tied to the tip of the angioscope is inflated, and blood flow is briefly interrupted so that the walls of the pulmonary arteries can be visualized. The angioscopic appearance of organized thromboemboli consists of roughening or pitting of the intimal surface, 'bands' traversing the vascular lumen, irregularly shaped vessel ostia, and 'recanalization' or the presence of multiple channels where a single lumen should occur. Angioscopy is most useful in confirming operability in patients with severe pulmonary hypertension who would not have been considered surgical candidates based on angiographic findings alone, and in predicting a good hemodynamic outcome in patients with modest pulmonary hypertension in whom pulmonary angiography did not precisely define the extent of proximal disease.[66]

Defining the extent of coexisting cardiac disease is an important part of the determination of candidacy for PTE. Patients with risk factors for coronary artery disease, or those in whom echocardiography has revealed previously undetected left ventricular dysfunction or valvular heart disease, should undergo left heart catheterization and coronary arteriography.

PULMONARY THROMBOENDARTERECTOMY

Pulmonary thromboendarterectomy is the most effective treatment for properly selected patients with chronic thromboembolic pulmonary hypertension. The procedure has evolved over 100 years, from the original description by Trendelenburg of an unsuccessful acute pulmonary embolectomy in a moribund, pulseless patient.[67] Successful outcomes were reported with the early use of cardiopulmonary bypass.[68] By the late 1960s, it became clear that an endarterectomy, not an embolectomy, was required to adequately remove thromboembolic material once the process became chronic.[69–72] Several groups have subsequently modified both the surgical instruments and the techniques

for PTE, bringing it to the current state-of-the-art described below.[73–75]

Patients with suspected CTEPH undergo evaluation with the goals of:

- establishing the need for surgical intervention;
- determining the surgical accessibility of the chronic thromboemboli;
- assessing the risk of surgery.

Most patients who ultimately go to surgery have a pulmonary vascular resistance greater than 300 dyn s/cm^5. Preoperative pulmonary vascular resistance has ranged between 700 and 1100 dyn s/cm^5 at major centers.[7–14,16] With this degree of pulmonary hypertension, most patients have impairment at rest and with exercise, and prognosis is poor with conservative management.[29,37] For those with mild to moderate pulmonary pressures at rest, pulmonary hypertension can become more significant with exertion, limiting lifestyle in some patients who may elect to have surgery.

An absolute criterion for surgery is the presence of accessible chronic thrombi, assessed by pulmonary angiography or angioscopy and the experience of the surgical team. Organized thrombi in the main and lobar levels, extending to the proximal segmental vessels, are readily removable, and highly experienced surgeons are capable of removing segmental-level thrombus as well. Failure to remove sufficient thromboembolic material to reduce the pulmonary vascular resistance is associated with a greater perioperative mortality rate and poorer long-term outcome.[76,77]

The third consideration in assessing surgical candidacy is the presence of co-morbid conditions that may adversely affect perioperative mortality or morbidity. Coexisting coronary artery disease, parenchymal lung disease, renal insufficiency, hepatic dysfunction, or the presence of a hypercoagulable state may complicate postoperative management. However, the reversal of pulmonary hypertension and right ventricular dysfunction with PTE surgery may result in improved hepatic and renal function. Coronary artery bypass grafting or valve replacement can be performed at the time of thromboendarterectomy without an increase in surgical risk.[78] Accordingly, advanced age or coexistent disease are not absolute contraindications to pulmonary thromboendarterectomy, although they do impact on risk assessment and postoperative management strategies. One exception is the presence of severe parenchymal or obstructive lung disease, where prolonged ventilatory support may be needed and thromboendarterectomy often produces minimal symptomatic improvement.

Surgical procedure

Details of the surgical procedure have been described elsewhere.[15,75] Surgery is performed through a median sternotomy. Anticoagulation is achieved by administering 400 units/kg of beef-lung heparin sodium. Phenytoin sodium is administered at the onset of cardiopulmonary bypass to reduce the risk of perioperative seizure. Cardiopulmonary bypass is then initiated, following placement of an ascending aortic and two vena caval cannulae.

Once on cardiopulmonary bypass, surface cooling with a head jacket and cooling jacket is begun, and the blood is cooled to a core temperature of approximately 18–20°C. Most of the dissection of the great vessels is performed during this cooling period, which may take up to 45–60 minutes. Once the temperature reaches 20°C, the aorta is cross-clamped, and the heart is arrested by a single dose of cardioplegic solution. The superior vena cava is fully mobilized to the level of the innominate vein. With a retractor in place between the aorta and superior vena cava, the right pulmonary artery is incised and the plane of dissection is identified and raised. When blood obscures the field of vision, circulatory arrest is initiated and the patient is exsanguinated. Arrest times are typically limited to 20 minutes for each side, with more than one 20-minute period per side rarely required.

Dissection within the correct vessel plane is a critical aspect of this surgical procedure. Too deep a plane may perforate the pulmonary artery with fatal results, whilst too shallow a plane results in the inadequate removal of the chronic thromboembolic material. With attainment of the correct surgical plane, dissection is carried out distally in each of the segmental and subsegmental vessels. Each segmental vessel is followed until the specimen is freed from the wall and ends in a tail (Plate 17.1).

Once the dissection is completed, and the lumen is carefully inspected and freed of any residual debris; circulation is re-established while the arteriotomy is closed. Attention is then directed to the left pulmonary vasculature. The endarterectomy on the left is essentially analogous in all respects to that performed on the right. Once completed, circulation is restarted and warming commenced. The rewarming period is typically about 90 minutes, but varies with the patient's body mass. If there is echocardiographic (either transthoracic or transesophageal) evidence for an interatrial communication, the right atrium is opened and interatrial communications are surgically repaired.

If other cardiac procedures are required, such as coronary artery or valve surgery, they can be performed during the rewarming period.[78] Once all procedures are concluded, myocardial cooling is discontinued, de-airing maneuvers are performed, and the patient is 'weaned' from cardiopulmonary bypass. Inotropic and vasoactive medications are used as needed to maintain an acceptable hemodynamic status.

Wound closure is performed in a routine fashion once temporary atrial and ventricular epicardial pacing wires are placed. The mediastinum is drained using two large-bore chest tubes, the sternum is approximated using stainless steel wires, and the subcutaneous layers and skin are closed using absorbable sutures.

Although there may be technical differences between surgical groups,[79–81] certain principles are fundamental to the successful completion of this operation. Chronic pulmonary thromboemboli typically involves both pulmonary vascular beds, particularly when pulmonary hypertension is present. It is this concept that underscores the need to proceed through a median sternotomy, thereby achieving access to the pulmonary vasculature on both sides. Cardiopulmonary bypass is essential, not only to maintain hemodynamic stability throughout the procedure, but also to achieve deep hypothermia and hence, circulatory arrest periods. It is only during periods of circulatory arrest that a bloodless operative field is obtained, allowing a complete and effective endarterectomy. Finally, a thorough endarterectomy is only possible by identification of the correct surgical plane with extension of the dissection to the 'feathered tail' of the specimen in each of the segmental branches involved.

Postoperative problems

Several problems encountered following PTE surgery are similar to those experienced by patients undergoing other forms of cardiac surgery, and include coagulation disorders, arrhythmias, wound infections, delirium, pleural and pericardial fluid accumulation, atelectasis and nosocomial infections.[82] Table 17.1 shows the incidence of the frequent complications in 250 operated patients at the University of California, San Diego (UCSD) between 2000 and 2002.

The postoperative care of PTE patients is further complicated by the changes resulting from a redistribution of pulmonary blood flow, along with in the improved cardiac output resulting from the fall in right ventricular afterload. Following a successful endarterectomy, pulmonary artery blood flow is 'redistributed' away from heretofore

Table 17.1 *Postoperative complications in 250 pulmonary thromboendarterectomy (PTE) patients who underwent surgery at the University of California, San Diego, between January 2000 and January 2002*

Complication	No. of patients	Per cent
Reperfusion lung injury	76	30.4
Persistent pulmonary hypertension*	34	14.0
Atrial fibrillation–flutter	30	12.0
Delirium	26	10.4
Nosocomial lung infection	23	9.2
Wound infection	7	2.8

*Postoperative pulmonary vascular resistance >500 dyn s/cm^5; complete perioperative hemodynamic values available in 242 patients.

well-perfused lung regions into newly revascularized segments, resulting in a 'pulmonary vascular steal' phenomenon.[83] The duration of this 'steal' phenomenon is variable, although follow-up studies have demonstrated that it is usually reversible.[84]

Reperfusion edema is one of the most difficult and life-threatening problems following PTE surgery.[85] The mechanism responsible for this form of lung injury remains uncertain, although it has features of a localized form of high-permeability, neutrophil-mediated lung damage. The lung injury typically occurs within the first 24 hours postoperatively, but may appear up to 72 hours after surgery, and can result in mild or moderate hypoxemia or profound, and usually fatal, alveolar hemorrhage. This form of lung injury is usually limited to endarterectomized lung regions, the lung regions to which blood flow is preferentially redistributed.

The management of reperfusion lung edema is generally supportive. High-dose corticosteroids have been used to modulate the inflammatory component of the process, although their effectiveness is unpredictable. Positional changes occasionally improve ventilation/perfusion mismatching. The use of inverse ratio ventilation, a low-volume ventilatory strategy to minimize the risk of ongoing alveolar damage, or incremental levels of positive end-expiratory pressure have occasionally proved useful when conventional ventilator therapy has failed. In extreme situations, extracorporeal support (ECCO2R) has been used successfully when aggressive conventional measures have been incapable of maintaining oxygenation. In a recent study of 47 patients undergoing PTE surgery, the postoperative avoidance of positive inotropic catecholamines and vasodilators, along with a strategy of low volume (<8 mL/kg) ventilation, resulted in a lower incidence of reperfusion pulmonary edema.[86]

Persistent pulmonary hypertension following PTE surgery is a particularly difficult management problem and, like reperfusion lung injury, remains a major cause of postoperative mortality. In the immediate postoperative period, patients with residual pulmonary hypertension can experience significant hemodynamic instability. Management goals focus on minimizing systemic oxygen consumption, optimizing right ventricular preload, and providing inotropic support. Since pulmonary vascular resistance is fixed, pharmacological approaches intended to reduce right ventricular afterload are ineffectual and risk decreasing systemic vascular resistance, systemic blood pressure, and coronary artery perfusion pressure. Inhaled nitric oxide (iNO) has appeal in this setting, owing to its pulmonary vasodilatory properties and negligible systemic effects. However, experience with iNO in this setting has been disappointing. Long-term therapy with continuous intravenous epoprostenol may be considered for residual, non-thrombotic pulmonary vascular disease.[87]

OUTCOME FOLLOWING PULMONARY THROMBOENDARTERECTOMY

To date, it is estimated that over 2000 thromboendarterectomies have been performed worldwide, with more than 1500 of these having been done at the University of California, San Diego, USA.[31] In reported series of PTE patients since 1996, in-hospital mortality rates range between 5 and 24%.[7–15] In the 32-year history of PTE operations at UCSD, a trend of declining mortality rates has been noted;[77] between 1970 and 1983, the group of 17 patients undergoing PTE surgery at UCSD exhibited a 17.6% in-hospital mortality rate. From January 1984 to November 1989, the mortality rate in 171 operated patients was 15.2%. With the current medical-surgical team providing care for the PTE patients, the mortality rate between the end of 1989 and 1992 was 7.2% of 207 operated patients; since 1993, an additional 1117 patients have undergone surgery with an in-hospital mortality rate of 6.6%.

The factors determining perioperative mortality have not been completely defined. Moser and colleagues suggested that several factors appeared to influence postoperative survival:[88]

- NYHA functional class IV status preoperatively;
- age >70 years;
- morbid obesity;
- the presence of significant co-morbid diseases;
- the severity of preoperative pulmonary vascular resistance;
- the presence of right ventricular failure as manifested by high right atrial pressures; and
- 'perhaps' the duration of pulmonary hypertension.

Recently, Hartz et al. found that a preoperative pulmonary vascular resistance >1100 dyn s/cm^5 and a mean pulmonary artery pressure >50 mmHg predicted a higher operative mortality.[9] However, D'Armini and colleagues[14] failed to demonstrate a relationship between either preoperative severity of pulmonary hypertension or the degree of cardiac failure and early postoperative death. Tscholl et al. in a study of 69 PTE patients, showed that older age, increased right atrial pressure, decreased cardiac output, a higher NYHA functional class, a greater number of pulmonary segments involved, and higher pulmonary vascular resistance (>1136 dyn s/cm^5) influenced hospital mortality.[89] Mares and colleagues also demonstrated that postoperative management strategies could affect outcome.[86] Combining a low tidal volume (<8 mL/kg) ventilator strategy with the avoidance of positive inotropic catecholamines and vasodilators in the postoperative period, this group was able to achieve lower in-hospital mortality rates for their patients (9.1% versus 21.4%).

Cardiac arrest, uncontrollable mediastinal bleeding, cerebrovascular accidents, myocardial injury, massive pulmonary hemorrhage, sepsis syndrome, and multiorgan failure are among the frequently cited causes of death.[4,6,9,11–14,89] However, most postoperative deaths have resulted from reperfusion lung injury or persistent pulmonary hypertension and right ventricular failure. At UCSD, between January 1984 and November 1995, one or both of these postoperative complications accounted for 54.2% of the deaths.[78]

In the majority of CTEPH patients undergoing thromboendarterectomy, the hemodynamic and functional outcomes have been remarkable. Restoration of blood flow to previously occluded lung regions produces an immediate reduction in right ventricular afterload, resulting in a decline in pulmonary arterial pressures and an augmentation in cardiac output. This postoperative improvement in pulmonary hemodynamics has been reported by several groups;[6,9–13,80,86,90] data available from UCSD between January 2000 and January 2002 are presented in Table 17.2. Postoperative echocardiography typically demonstrates dramatic improvement in right and left heart dimensions, typically within 1–3 weeks after surgery.[91,92]

The long-term results following PTE surgery have been similarly impressive. Sustained hemodynamic improvement (>3 months postoperatively) has been reported by numerous groups, accompanied by substantial improvement in functional status.[8,14,93,94] Gas exchange improves concomitantly.[95,96]

In a large cross-sectional study, Archibald et al. examined functional status and quality-of-life issues in a cohort of 308 patients who underwent PTE surgery between 1970 and 1994.[97] At an average of 3.3 years following surgery (range 1–16 years), 93% of 306 respondents fell into NYHA class I or II. Most patients (63% of 303 respondents) reported no dyspnea walking on a level surface; 73.2% of patients noted their dyspnea to be 'much improved'; and

89.6% of 275 respondents were no longer using supplemental oxygen, with the mean duration of oxygen use post-PTE of 7.1 weeks (range 1–64 weeks). Sixty-three patients, or 20.5% of the respondents, were disabled prior to surgery and had remained disabled, and 75% were alive beyond 6 years. More than half of the post-hospital deaths were unrelated to pulmonary vascular disease; however, persistent pulmonary hypertension or recurrent pulmonary emboli contributed to 22 of the 51 deaths.

FUTURE DIRECTIONS

The fate of many patients with chronic thromboembolic pulmonary hypertension can be altered from that of progressive deterioration and death to restoration of a normal functional status and improved quality of life. However, challenges remain. Accurately defining the surgical accessibility of chronic thromboembolic lesions remains a critical diagnostic challenge. The role of CT and magnetic resonance imaging in assisting with this determination requires careful study. These imaging modalities may also prove helpful in characterizing those patients with extensive small-vessel disease who would be at risk of a poor hemodynamic outcome following PTE surgery. However, effort should also be directed in detecting CTEPH earlier in its course and, as a result, potentially limiting the extent of these secondary small-vessel changes. This may ultimately prove to be the most effective measure in decreasing the incidence of persistent postoperative pulmonary hypertension. The efficacy of chronic vasodilator therapy and catheter-based angioplasty in patients with segmental-level disease need to be more fully addressed.[98] Improved understanding of the pathophysiology of postoperative reperfusion lung injury is needed if new preventive and therapeutic strategies are to be developed. Finally, recurrence of CTEPH is seen in approximately 1% of operated patients.[99] Clarification of risk factors for recurrence, development of prevention strategies, and evaluation of the risks and benefits of repeat operation require more study.

Table 17.2 *Perioperative hemodynamics in 250 pulmonary thromboendarterectomy patients* who underwent surgery at the University of California, San Diego, between January 2000 and January 2002*

	Preoperative	Postoperative	Significance[†]
Mean PAP (mmHg)	45.9 ± 9.9	28.5 ± 10.0	P < 0.001
PASP (mmHg)	75.8 ± 16.6	47.5 ± 16.8	P < 0.001
Cardiac output (L/min)	3.61 ± 1.18	5.46 ± 1.52	P < 0.001
PVR (dyn s/cm^5)	942 ± 422	317 ± 236	P < 0.001

*Complete pre- and postoperative hemodynamic numbers available in 242 patients; postoperative values within 72 hours following surgery.
[†]Significance: two-tailed Student's *t*-test.
PAP, pulmonary artery pressure; PASP, pulmonary artery systolic pressure; PVR, pulmonary vascular resistance.

KEY POINTS

- Chronic thromboembolic pulmonary hypertension (CTEPH) is an unusual consequence of acute pulmonary embolism. Most patients with CTEPH present late in the course of their disease.
- The most common presenting complaints of patients with chronic thromboembolic disease are exertional dyspnea and a progressive decline

in exercise tolerance. A non-productive cough, atypical chest pains and palpitations are also experienced by these patients to a varying degree.

- Once pulmonary hypertension has been diagnosed, a V̇/Q̇ scan can be helpful to distinguish between major- and small-vessel pulmonary vascular disease. The role of CT imaging of the chest in diagnosing CTEPH and establishing surgical accessibility of chronic thromboembolic lesions is as yet incompletely defined.
- Pulmonary angiography remains the most reliable means of defining the extent and proximal location of suspected chronic thromboembolic lesions.
- In selected patients, pulmonary thrombo-endarterectomy (PTE) is the most effective treatment for chronic thromboembolic pulmonary hypertension.
- Post-PTE problems are similar to those experienced by patients undergoing other forms of cardiac surgery. Reperfusion lung injury is one of the most difficult and life-threatening problems following PTE surgery. Persistent pulmonary hypertension is also a difficult problem to manage.
- The majority of patients undergoing surgery experience a significant improvement in pulmonary hemodynamics postoperatively. This leads to an enhanced quality of life and improved long-term survivorship. In addition, in-hospital mortality rates in PTE patients have been declining. The factors determining perioperative mortality have not been completely defined but most postoperative deaths have resulted from reperfusion lung injury or persistent pulmonary hypertension and right ventricular failure.

REFERENCES

1 Sabiston DC, Jr, Wolfe WG, Oldham HN, Jr et al. Surgical management of chronic pulmonary embolism. *Ann Surg* 1977;**185**:699–712.

2 Utley JR, Spragg RG, Long WB et al. Pulmonary endarterectomy for chronic thromboembolic obstruction: recent surgical experience. *Surgery* 1982;**92**:1096–102.

◆3 Chitwood WR Jr, Sabiston DC, Wechsler AS. Surgical treatment of chronic unresolved pulmonary embolism. *Clin Chest Med* 1984;**5**:507–36.

●4 Moser KM, Daily PO, Peterson K et al. Thromboendarterectomy for chronic, major-vessel thromboembolic pulmonary hypertension: immediate and long-term results in 42 patients. *Ann Intern Med* 1987;**107**:560–5.

5 Rich S, Levitsky S, Brundage BH. Pulmonary hypertension from chronic pulmonary thromboembolism. *Ann Intern Med* 1988;**108**:425–34.

6 Jamieson SW, Kapelanski DP, Sakakibara N et al. Pulmonary endarterectomy: experience and lessons learned in 1500 cases. *Ann Thorac Surg* 2003;**76**:1457–64.

7 Simonneau G, Azarian R, Brenot F et al. Surgical management of unresolved pulmonary embolism: a personal series of 72 patients. *Chest* 1995;**107**:52S–5S.

8 Mayer E, Dahm M, Hake U et al. Mid-term results of pulmonary thromboendarterectomy for chronic thromboembolic pulmonary hypertension. *Ann Thorac Surg* 1996;**61**:1788–92.

9 Hartz RS, Byme JG, Levitsky S et al. Predictors of mortality in pulmonary thromboendarterectomy. *Ann Thorac Surg* 1996;**62**:1255–9.

10 Nakajima N, Masuda M, Mogi K. The surgical treatment for chronic pulmonary thromboembolism – our surgical experience and current review of the literature. *Ann Thorac Cardiovasc Surg* 1997;**3**:15–21.

11 Gilbert TB, Gaine SP, Rubin LJ et al. Short-term outcome and predictors of adverse events following pulmonary thromboendarterectomy. *World J Surg* 1998;**22**:1029–32.

12 Ando M, Okita Y, Tagusari O et al. Surgical treatment for chronic thromboembolic pulmonary hypertension under profound hypothermia and circulatory arrest in 24 patients. *J Cardiovasc Surg* 1999;**14**:377–85.

13 Rubens F, Wells P, Bencze S et al. Surgical treatment of chronic thromboembolic pulmonary hypertension. *Can Respir J* 2000;**7**:49–57.

14 D'Armini AM, Cattadori B, Monterosso C et al. Pulmonary thromboendarterectomy in patients with chronic pulmonary hypertension: hemodynamic characteristics and changes. *Eur J Cardiothorac Surg* 2000;**18**:696–702.

15 Jamieson SW, Kapelanski DP. Pulmonary endarterectomy. *Curr Probl Surg* 2000;**37**:165–252.

16 Fedullo PF, Auger WR, Channick RN et al. Chronic thromboembolic pulmonary hypertension. *Clin Chest Med* 2001;**22**:561–81.

●17 Owen WR, Thomas WA, Castleman B et al. Unrecognized emboli to the lungs with subsequent cor pulmonale. *N Engl J Med* 1953;**249**:919–26.

18 Ball KP, Goodwin JF, Harrison CV. Massive thrombotic occlusion of the large pulmonary arteries. *Circulation* 1956;**14**:766–83.

19 Carroll D. Chronic obstruction of major pulmonary arteries. *Am J Med* 1950;**9**:175–85.

20 Hollister LE, Cull VL. The syndrome of chronic thrombosis of the major pulmonary arteries. *Am J Med* 1956;**21**:312–20.

21 Egermayer P, Peacock AJ. Is pulmonary embolism a common cause of pulmonary hypertension? Limitations of the embolic hypothesis. *Eur Respir J* 2000;**15**:440–8.

22 Fedullo PF, Rubin LJ, Kerr KM et al. The natural history of acute and chronic thromboembolic disease: the search for the missing link. *Eur Respir J* 2000;**15**:435–7.

23 Karwinski B, Svendsen E. Comparison of clinical and postmortem diagnosis of pulmonary embolism. *J Clin Pathol* 1989;**42**:135–9.

●24 Meignan M, Rosso J, Gauthier H et al. Systematic lung scans reveal a high frequency of silent pulmonary embolism in patients with proximal deep venous thrombosis. *Arch Intern Med* 2000;**160**:159–64.

25 Stein PD, Terrin ML, Hales CA *et al*. Clinical, laboratory, roentgenographic, and electrocardiographic findings in patients with acute pulmonary embolism and no pre-existing cardiac or pulmonary disease. *Chest* 1991;**100**:598–603.

26 Wartski M, Collignon M-A. Incomplete recovery of lung perfusion after 3 months in patients with acute pulmonary embolism treated with antithrombolytic agents. *J Nucl Med* 2000;**41**:1043–8.

●27 Ryan KL, Fedullo PF, Davis GB *et al*. Perfusion scan findings understate the severity of angiographic and hemodynamic compromise in chronic thromboembolic pulmonary hypertension. *Chest* 1988;**93**:1180–5.

28 deSoyza NDB, Murphy ML. Persistent post-embolic pulmonary hypertension. *Chest* 1972;**62**:665–8.

29 Riedel M, Stanek V, Widimsky J *et al*. Long-term follow-up of patients with pulmonary thromboembolism: late prognosis and evolution of hemodynamic and respiratory data. *Chest* 1982;**81**:151–8.

30 Ribeiro A, Lindmarker P, Johnsson H *et al*. Pulmonary embolism. One-year follow-up with echocardiography Doppler and five-year survival analysis. *Circulation* 1999;**99**:1325–30.

◆31 Fedullo PF, Auger WR, Kerr KM *et al*. Chronic thromboembolic pulmonary hypertension. *N Engl J Med* 2001;**345**:1465–72.

32 Olman MA, Marsh JJ, Lang IM *et al*. The endogenous fibrinolytic system in chronic large-vessel thromboembolic pulmonary hypertension. *Circulation* 1992;**86**:1241–8.

33 Auger WR, Permpikul P, Moser KM. Lupus anticoagulant, heparin use, and thrombocytopenia in patients with chronic thromboembolic pulmonary hypertension: a preliminary report. *Am J Med* 1995;**99**:392–6.

34 Wolf M, Soyer-Neumann C, Parent F *et al*. Thrombotic risk factors in pulmonary hypertension. *Eur Respir J* 2000;**15**:395–9.

35 Sompradeekul S, Fedullo PF, Le DT. Congenital and acquired thrombophilias in patients with chronic thromboembolic pulmonary hypertension. [Abstract] *Am J Resp Crit Care Med* 1999;**159**:A358.

●36 Moser KM, Bloor CM. Pulmonary vascular lesions occurring in patients with chronic major vessel thromboembolic pulmonary hypertension. *Chest* 1993;**103**:685–92.

37 Lewczuk J, Piszko P, Jagas J *et al*. Prognostic factors in medically treated patients with chronic pulmonary embolism. *Chest* 2001;**119**:818–23.

38 Auger WR, Moser KM. Pulmonary flow murmurs: a distinctive physical sign found in chronic pulmonary thromboembolic disease. [Abstract] *Clin Res* 1989;**37**:145A.

39 Voelkel MA, Wynne KM, Badesch DB *et al*. Hyperuricemia in severe pulmonary hypertension. *Chest* 2000;**117**:19–24.

40 Morris TA, Auger WR, Ysrael MZ *et al*. Parenchymal scarring is associated with restrictive spirometric defects in patients with chronic thromboembolic pulmonary hypertension. *Chest* 1996;**110**:399–403.

41 Steenhuis LH, Groen HJM, Koeter GH *et al*. Diffusion capacity and haemodynamics in primary and chronic thromboembolic pulmonary hypertension. *Eur Respir J* 2000;**16**:276–81.

42 Elliott CG, Colby TV, Hill T *et al*. Pulmonary veno-occlusive disease associated with severe reduction of single-breath carbon monoxide diffusing capacity. *Respiration* 1988;**53**:262–6.

43 Kapitan KS, Buchbinder M, Wagner PD *et al*. Mechanisms of hypoxemia in chronic thromboembolic pulmonary hypertension. *Am Rev Respir Dis* 1989;**139**:1149–54.

44 Woodruff WW III, Hoeck BE, Chitwood WR Jr *et al*. Radiographic findings in pulmonary hypertension from unresolved embolism. *AJR Am J Roentgenol* 1985;**144**:681–6.

45 D'Alonzo GE, Bower JS, Dantzker DR. Differentiation of patients with primary and thromboembolic pulmonary hypertension. *Chest* 1984;**85**:457–61.

46 Moser KM, Olson LK, Schlusselberg M *et al*. Chronic thrombo-embolic occlusion in the adult can mimic pulmonary artery agenesis. *Chest* 1989;**95**:503–8.

●47 Dittrich HC, McCann HA, Blanchard DG. Cardiac structure and function in chronic thromboembolic pulmonary hypertension. *Am J Cardiac Imaging* 1994;**8**:18–27.

48 Lisbona R, Kreisman H, Novales-Diaz J *et al*. Perfusion lung scanning: Differentiation of primary from thromboembolic pulmonary hypertension. *AJR Am J Roentgenol* 1985;**144**:27–30.

49 King MA, Bergin CJ, Yeung D *et al*. Chronic pulmonary thromboembolism: detection of regional hypoperfusion with CT. *Radiology* 1994;**191**:359–63.

50 Schwickert HC, Schweden F, Schild HH *et al*. Pulmonary arteries and lung parenchyma in chronic pulmonary embolism: preoperative and postoperative CT findings. *Radiology* 1994;**191**:351–7.

51 Tardivon AA, Musset D, Maitre S *et al*. Role of CT in chronic pulmonary embolism: comparison with pulmonary angiography. *J Comput Assist Tomogr* 1993;**17**:345–52.

52 Bergin CJ. Chronic thromboembolic pulmonary hypertension: the disease, the diagnosis, and the treatment. *Semin Ultrasound CT MRI* 1997;**18**:383–91.

53 Berry PF, Buccigrossi D, Peabody J *et al*. Pulmonary vascular occlusion and fibrosing mediastinitis. *Chest* 1986;**89**:296–301.

54 Bergin CJ, Hauschildt JP, Brown MA *et al*. Identifying the cause of unilateral hypoperfusion in patients suspected to have chronic pulmonary thrombo-embolism: diagnostic accuracy of helical CT and conventional angiography. *Radiology* 1999;**213**:743–9.

55 Cho SR, Tisnado J, Cockrell CH *et al*. Angiographic evaluation of patients with unilateral massive perfusion defects on the lung scan. *RadioGraphics* 1987;**7**:729–45.

56 Anderson MB, Kriett JM, Kapelanski DP *et al*. Primary pulmonary artery sarcoma: a report of six cases. *Ann Thorac Surg* 1995;**59**:1487–90.

57 Moser KM, Fedullo PF, Finkbeiner WE *et al*. Do patients with primary pulmonary hypertension develop extensive central thrombi? *Circulation* 1995;**91**:741–5.

58 Russo A, De Luca M, Vigna C *et al*. Central pulmonary artery lesions in chronic obstructive pulmonary disease. A transesophageal echocardiographic study. *Circulation* 1999;**100**:1808–15.

59 Nicod P, Peterson K, Levine M *et al*. Pulmonary angiography in severe chronic pulmonary hypertension. *Ann Intern Med* 1987;**107**:565–8.

60 Pitton MB, Duber C, Mayer E *et al*. Hemodynamic effects of nonionic contrast bolus injection and oxygen inhalation

during pulmonary angiography in patients with chronic major-vessel thromboembolic pulmonary hypertension. *Circulation* 1996;**94**:2485–91.

●61 Auger WR, Fedullo PF, Moser KM *et al*. Chronic major-vessel thromboembolic pulmonary artery obstruction: appearance at angiography. *Radiology* 1992;**182**:393–8.

62 Yamato M, Lecky JW, Hiramatsu K *et al*. Takayasu's arteritis: radiographic and angiographic findings in 59 patients. *Radiology* 1986;**161**:329–34.

63 Kerr KM, Auger WR, Fedullo PF *et al*. Large vessel pulmonary arteritis mimicking chronic thromboembolic disease. *Am J Respir Crit Care Med* 1995;**152**:367–73.

64 D'Cruz IA, Agustsson MH, Bicoff JP *et al*. Stenotic lesions of the pulmonary arteries: clinical and hemodynamic findings in 84 cases. *Am J Cardiol* 1964;**13**:441–50.

●65 Shure D, Gregoratos G, Moser KM. Fiberoptic angioscopy: role in the diagnosis of chronic pulmonary arterial obstruction. *Ann Intern Med* 1985;**103**:844–50.

66 Sompradeekul S, Fedullo PF, Kerr KM *et al*. The role of pulmonary angioscopy in the preoperative assessment of patients with thromboembolic pulmonary hypertension (CTEPH). [Abstract] *Am J Resp Crit Care Med* 1999;**159**:A456.

67 Trendelenburg F. Uber die operative behandlung der embolie derlungarterie. *Arch Klin Chir* 1908;**86**:686–700.

68 Castleman B, McNeeley BU, Scannell G. Case records of the Massachusetts General Hospital, Case 32-1964. *N Engl J Med* 1964;**271**:40–50.

●69 Synder WA, Kent DC, Baisch BF. Successful endarterectomy of chronically occluded pulmonary artery: clinical report and physiologic studies. *J Thorac Cardiovasc Surg* 1963;**45**:482–9.

70 Moser KM, Houk VN, Jones RC *et al*. Chronic, massive thrombotic obstruction of pulmonary arteries: analysis of four operated cases. *Circulation* 1965;**32**:377–85.

71 Nash ES, Shapiro S, Landau A *et al*. Successful thromboembolectomy in long-standing thromboembolic pulmonary hypertension. *Thorax* 1966;**23**:121–30.

72 Moor GF, Sabiston DC, Jr. Embolectomy for chronic pulmonary embolism and pulmonary hypertension: case report and review of the problem. *Circulation* 1970;**41**:701–8.

73 Daily PO, Dembitsky WP, Peterson KL *et al*. Modifications of techniques and early results of pulmonary thromboendarterectomy for chronic pulmonary embolism. *J Thorac Cardiovasc Surg* 1987;**93**:221–33.

74 Daily PO, Dembitsky WP, Daily RP. Dissectors for pulmonary thromboendarterectomy. *Ann Thorac Surg* 1991;**51**:842–3.

◆75 Daily PO, Dembitsky WP, Jamieson SW. The evolution and the current state of the art of pulmonary thromboendarterectomy. *Semin Thorac Cardiovasc Surg* 1999;**11**:152–63.

76 Daily PO, Dembitsky WP, Iversen S *et al*. Risk factors for pulmonary thromboendaterectomy. *J Thorac Cardiovasc Surg* 1990;**99**:670–8.

77 Auger WR, Fedullo PF, Moser KM *et al*. In-hospital mortality has decreased for patients undergoing pulmonary thrombo-endarterectomy. [Abstract] *Am J Resp Crit Care Med* 1996;**153**:A92.

78 Thistlethwaite PA, Auger WR, Madani MM *et al*. Pulmonary thromboendarterectomy combined with other cardiac operations: indications, surgical approach, and outcome. *Ann Thorac Surg* 2001;**72**:13–19.

79 Zund G, Pretre R, Niederhauser U *et al*. Improved exposure of the pulmonary arteries for thromboendarterectomy. *Ann Thorac Surg* 1998;**66**:1821–3.

80 Dartevelle P, Fadel E, Chapelier A *et al*. Angioscopic video-assisted pulmonary endarterectomy for post-embolic pulmonary hypertension. *Eur J Cardiothorac Surg* 1999;**16**:38–43.

81 Zeebregts CJ, Dossche KM, Morshuis WJ *et al*. Surgical thromboendarterectomy for chronic thromboembolic pulmonary hypertension using circulatory arrest with selective antegrade cerebral perfusion. *Acta Chir Belg* 1998;**98**:95–7.

82 Fedullo PF, Auger WR, Dembitsky WP. Postoperative management of the patient undergoing pulmonary thromboendarterectomy. *Semin Thorac Cardiovasc Surg* 1999;**11**:172–8.

83 Olman MA, Auger WR, Fedullo PF *et al*. Pulmonary vascular steal in chronic thromboembolic pulmonary hypertension. *Chest* 1990;**98**:1430–4.

84 Moser KM, Metersky ML, Auger WR *et al*. Resolution of vascular steal after pulmonary thromboendarterectomy. *Chest* 1993;**104**:1441–4.

85 Levinson RM, Shure D, Moser KM. Reperfusion pulmonary edema after pulmonary thromboendarterectomy. *Am Rev Respir Dis* 1986;**134**:1241–5.

86 Mares P, Gilbert TB, Tschernko EM *et al*. Pulmonary artery thromboendarterectomy: A comparison of two different postoperative treatment strategies. *Anesth Analg* 2000;**90**:267–73.

87 McLaughlin V V, Genthner DE, Panella MM *et al*. Compassionate use of continuous prostacyclin in the management of secondary pulmonary hypertension: a case series. *Ann Intern Med* 1999;**130**:740–3.

88 Moser KM, Auger WR, Fedullo PF. Chronic major vessel thromboembolic pulmonary hypertension. *Circulation* 1990;**81**:1735–43.

89 Tscholl D, Langer F, Wendler O *et al*. Pulmonary thromboendarterectomy – risk factors for early survival and hemodynamic improvement. *Eur J Cardiothorac Surg* 2001;**19**:771–6.

90 Mayer E, Kramm T, Dahm M *et al*. Early results of pulmonary thrombo-endarterectomy in chronic thromboembolic pulmonary hypertension. *Z Kardiol* 1997;**86**:920–7.

91 Dittrich HC, Nicod PH, Chow LC *et al*. Early changes of right heart geometry after pulmonary thromboendarterectomy. *J Am Coll Cardiol* 1988;**11**:937–43.

92 Menzel T, Wagner S, Mohr-Kahaly S *et al*. Reversibility of changes in left and right ventricular geometry and hemodynamics in pulmonary hypertension. Echocardiographic characteristics before and after thromboendarterectomy. *Z Kardiol* 1997;**86**:928–35.

93 Moser KM, Auger WR, Fedullo PF *et al*. Chronic thromboembolic pulmonary hypertension: clinical picture and surgical treatment. *Eur Respir J* 1992;**5**:334–42.

94 Kramm T, Mayer E, Dahm M *et al*. Long-term results after thromboendarterectomy for chronic pulmonary embolism. *Eur J Cardiothorac Surg* 1999;**15**:579–84.

95 Kapitan KS, Clausen JL, Moser KM. Gas exchange in chronic thromboembolism after pulmonary thromboendarterectomy. *Chest* 1990;**98**:14–19.

96 Tanabe N, Okada O, Nakagawa Y *et al*. The efficacy of pulmonary thromboendarterectomy on long-term gas exchange. *Eur Respir J* 1997;**10**:2066–72.

●97 Archibald CJ, Auger WR, Fedullo PF *et al*. Long-term outcome after pulmonary thromboendarterectomy. *Am J Respir Crit Care Med* 1999;**160**:523–8.

●98 Feinstein FA, Goldhaber SZ, Lock JE *et al*. Balloon pulmonary angioplasty for treatment of chronic thromboembolic pulmonary hypertension. *Circulation* 2001;**103**:10–13.

99 Mo M, Kapelanski DP, Mitruka SN *et al*. Reoperative pulmonary thromboendarterectomy. *Ann Thorac Surg* 1999;**68**:1770–7.

18

Pulmonary vascular tumors

KIM M KERR

INTRODUCTION

Primary tumors of the pulmonary artery are extremely rare.[1] The majority of these tumors are malignant, sarcomatous neoplasms,[2] yet primary sarcomas of the lung represent only one in every 500 primary lung cancers. Primary soft tissue sarcomas of the lung are divided into three categories based on site of origin: parenchymal sarcomas, small-vessel sarcomas, and large-vessel sarcomas.[3] This chapter focuses on large-vessel sarcomas.

Large-vessel sarcomas are primarily intravascular tumors that arise from within the pulmonary artery. They arise proximally and spread within the lumen with multiple sites of attachment, making the origin difficult to define.[4] Symptoms result from obstruction of the pulmonary vascular bed and right ventricular failure. Patients are most likely to be incorrectly diagnosed with pulmonary embolism, with most patients not receiving the correct diagnosis until the time of autopsy.[4,5] Distant metastases are uncommon.[5] It has been postulated that the low incidence of distant metastases may be due to the vital location of the primary tumor, preventing most patients from surviving long enough to develop disseminated disease.[6] Surgery has the potential to palliate symptoms,[2] improve survival[5] and potentially cure this disease.[7,8] Hence, it is important that physicians be aware of this disease entity so that the correct diagnosis can be made and appropriate therapy instituted.

EPIDEMIOLOGY

Mandelstamm first described pulmonary artery sarcoma in 1923.[9] Because of its rarity, what is known about pulmonary artery sarcoma is based upon individual case reports and small series. A slight female predominance has been identified (1:1.3).[4] The vast majority of cases occur in adults, with an average age of 50 years;[5] however, several cases have been reported in adolescents.[10,11] The etiology remains obscure and no risk factors for the development of these tumors have been identified. On average, patients are symptomatic for 8 months before an aggressive search for an etiology is instituted.[5]

CLINICAL PRESENTATION

Patients present with symptoms related to pulmonary artery obstruction, pulmonary hypertension and right ventricular dysfunction as well as non-specific symptoms secondary to the presence of malignancy. Based upon 110 cases reported in the literature, Nonomura et al. found that the most common symptom is dyspnea (67%), followed by chest/back pain (54%), cough (43%) and hemoptysis (22%). Systemic symptoms include malaise (13%), weight loss (12%) and fever (10%).[4]

Findings on physical examination in patients with pulmonary artery sarcoma include jugular venous distension, a bruit over the pulmonary artery, a systolic flow murmur, hepatomegaly, edema, cyanosis and clubbing.[5]

Given this constellation of symptoms, it is not surprising that the most common clinical diagnosis given these patients is pulmonary thromboembolism.[4,5] However, an alternative diagnosis should be sought in patients who present with symptoms of systemic disease such as fever or weight loss. Clubbing is also not a feature of thromboembolic disease and should stimulate a search for another etiology.[12] Other preoperative or antemortem diagnoses included mediastinal tumor, lung cancer and cardiac tumor of the right ventricle.[4]

EVALUATION

Right ventricular hypertrophy is the most common electrocardiographic abnormality, occurring in up to one half of patients. The chest radiograph may be normal or demonstrate a hilar mass, prominent pulmonary artery(ies), hilar infiltrate, decreased pulmonary vascular markings, nodules, or cavities.[4,5,13] The perfusion scan demonstrates areas of decreased or absent perfusion[4,5] indistinguishable from thromboembolic disease. Perfusion defects that do not improve or that increase in size with anticoagulation suggest a diagnosis other than acute pulmonary embolism. In addition, unilateral perfusion abnormalities on scintography are rare in chronic thromboembolic disease and should prompt a search for other causes of large vessel pulmonary artery obstruction including tumor (bronchogenic carcinoma, pulmonary artery sarcoma) as well as fibrosing mediastinitis, pulmonary arteritis and congenital anomaly.[14]

Two-dimensional echocardiography may demonstrate evidence of pulmonary hypertension and may also allow for direct visualization of tumor. A pedunculated mass arising from the right ventricular outflow tract, pulmonary valve or pulmonary trunk would suggest the diagnosis of sarcoma.[8]

Whilst bronchoscopy is frequently performed to evaluate patients who present with hemoptysis or lung mass, it is likely to be non-diagnostic in pulmonary artery sarcoma cases. However, there are rare case reports of tumor eroding through the airway, allowing the diagnosis of neoplasm to be made.[15]

Pulmonary angiography typically demonstrates a proximal mass partially or totally obstructing the pulmonary artery (Figure 18.1). Sarcomas are often lobulated and polypoid,[16] but smooth gradual tapering of the pulmonary artery, indistinguishable from chronic thromboembolic disease, has also been described.[17] The mass may be fixed or pedunculated and mobile with a 'to-and-fro' movement with each cardiac cycle. Demonstration of a pressure gradient across the mass is especially helpful since such

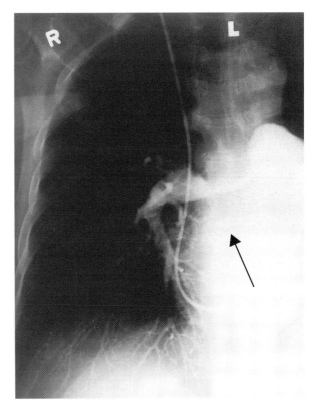

Figure 18.1 *Angiographic image of a sarcoma causing a large filling defect in the right main pulmonary artery (arrow).*

gradients are not typically seen in chronic thromboembolic disease.[18] As with scintography, vascular obstruction that increases in size on serial angiography is also very suggestive of a neoplastic process. Pulmonary angioscopy may allow for direct visualization of the tumor.[2]

Computerized tomography (CT) scanning and magnetic resonance imaging (MRI) are very useful modalities for evaluating pulmonary artery sarcomas (Figure 18.2). Both allow exclusion of some competing diagnoses such as extravascular obstruction from bronchogenic carcinoma or mediastinal fibrosis. CT and MRI are useful in assessing tumor size, degree of vascular obstruction, and the presence of extravascular invasion as well as to look for evidence of metastases. CT findings suggestive of pulmonary artery sarcoma include inhomogeneous attenuation (possibly due to hemorrhage or necrosis of tumor), contiguously soft-tissue-filled pulmonary arteries, vascular distension, and extravascular spread. These finding are more likely to occur in advanced disease.[19] Heterogenous enhancement with gadolinium-diethylenetriamine pentaacetic acid (Gd-DTPA) demonstrated by MRI is characteristic of a vascularized tumor and allows the elimination of thromboembolic disease as a diagnosis since thrombus does not enhance on T_1-weighted images after the administration of gadolinium.[8,19,20] Tumor emboli, vasculitis[20] and septic emboli[21] may also enhance

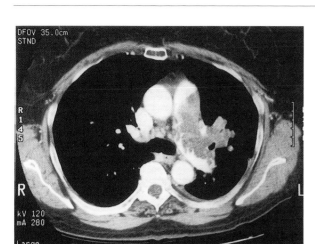

Figure 18.2 *Angiosarcoma in a 74-year-old female. Transverse computerized tomography angiogram demonstrates a large lobulated mass in the left main pulmonary artery that extends into the left upper lobe and left descending pulmonary arteries.*

with Gd-DTPA. MRI may be especially helpful in the diagnosis of recurrent or residual disease.[21]

The role of positron emission tomography in the evaluation of patients with pulmonary sarcoma remains to be defined. FDG-PET (fluorine-18-2-fluoro-2-deoxy-D-glucose positron emission tomography) tumor imaging has been reported to distinguish sarcoma from thromboembolism when the appropriate diagnosis could not be obtained from CT scanning alone.[22]

Ultimately, tissue must be obtained for a definitive diagnosis. Biopsies may be obtained via intravascular forceps during angiography,[20] transvenous catheter suction biopsy,[23] CT-guided transthoracic needle aspiration,[13] or surgical exploration. Often, patients undergo surgery for presumed thromboembolism that leads to the correct diagnosis of sarcoma. The majority of patients, however, are diagnosed at autopsy.[4,5]

PATHOLOGY

At surgery or autopsy the pulmonary trunk is distended by a multinodular yellow/tan or gray tumor which is often mixed with thrombus.[24,25] The tumors are of variable consistency ranging from myxoid to bony hard (Plate 18.1). Frequently, the sites of attachment to the pulmonary artery are multiple and the apparent origin is difficult to define.[4] On occasion, the tumor may arise from, or extend into, the right ventricle, and therefore, the broader term of right outflow tract sarcoma is used by some.[24] The pulmonary trunk is most commonly involved (80% of cases) with equal likelihood of involvement of the left (58%) and the right pulmonary arteries (57%). Both pulmonary arteries are involved in 37% of

cases, the pulmonary valve is affected in 28% and the right ventricle in 8%.[4] Some tumors remain localized to the artery, but direct extension into the lung parenchyma[24] or mediastinum is frequently present. Intrapulmonary metastases are common, occurring in 40% of cases, and are presumably embolic.[4] Nodules of metastatic tumor are usually small, but may be as large as 3 cm and may be either confined to the pulmonary vasculature or be associated with bronchial or parenchymal invasion. Pulmonary infarction may also be seen as a consequence of extensive tumor growth, tumor emboli, or thromboemboli occluding pulmonary vessels.[24] While distant metastases are less common (19%), they have been reported to involve the pericardium, heart, pleura, adrenal gland, pancreas, stomach, jejunum, brain, liver, diaphragm, skin and tongue.[4]

McGlennan *et al.*[11] summarized the pathology of 100 cases of pulmonary artery sarcoma from the literature. They found the histopathology to be heterogeneous with the sarcomatous elements most commonly described as undifferentiated (34%), consisting of cells with variations in cytological attributes. Other pathological types included myogenous (26%), fibrocytic (17%), mesenchymoma (6%), chondrosarcoma (4%), vascular (4%), osteogenic sarcoma (3%) and two were classified as malignant fibrous histiocytoma (2%).[11] With the current classifications of soft tissue sarcomas, more cases are now being diagnosed as malignant fibrous histiocytoma.[26]

TREATMENT/MANAGEMENT

Surgical resection offers palliation[2,8] and increases length of survival.[5] Aggressive surgical resection is potentially curative in patients with localized lesions. Surgical therapy depends upon tumor location, distal extension, and the presence of pulmonary metastases. Techniques include tumor and pulmonary artery resection and reconstruction, endarterectomy techniques and pneumonectomy.[2,8]

Kruger reviewed 93 cases of primary sarcoma of the pulmonary artery reported in the literature up to 1990. The tumor was resected in 27 patients; 13 underwent tumor excision from the vascular bed and 14 underwent pneumonectomy. Median survival for the 93 patients was 1.5 months from diagnosis with most patients dying from the consequences of decompensated right heart failure due to right ventricular outflow obstruction by tumor. However, despite a 22% early mortality after resection, median survival was prolonged to 10 months in those patients who underwent surgery. It is notable that 58% of patients had evidence of lung metastases at the time of diagnosis, yet no survival benefit was demonstrated for those who underwent pneumonectomy and presumed simultaneous resection of metastases versus simple tumor excision. In addition, survival was similar for both those with and without identified metastases. It appears that prognosis following successful surgery depends upon recurrence of tumor in the pulmonary artery rather than progression of metastatic disease.[5] Devendra et al. reported 16 cases of pulmonary artery sarcoma undergoing surgery at a single institution. There was no surgical mortality and the average length of hospital stay was 14 days. Hemodynamic improvement was noted following surgery with an increase in cardiac output and a decrease in mean pulmonary artery pressure. The postoperative average length of survival was 17 months and one patient remained alive 54 months following surgery.[7] Others have also reported an improvement in functional status with surgery.[2,8]

The rarity of pulmonary artery sarcomas and the histological heterogeneity of the tumors make it difficult to comment on the role of adjuvant treatment modalities. Chemotherapeutic agents such as doxorubicin, cyclophosphamide, vincristine and postoperative radiotherapy have been employed alone and in combination in the treatment of pulmonary artery sarcomas.[2,5,6,8,15] Unfortunately, there are no clinical trials to define the role of adjuvant therapy in this disease.

PULMONARY TUMOR EMBOLISM

Tumor emboli to the lungs may also present with progressive dyspnea, chest pain and evidence of pulmonary hypertension with right ventricular failure. Most patients will have an established diagnosis of malignancy, usually metastatic. The malignancies most commonly associated with tumor embolism include breast, lung, prostate, stomach and liver[27] and tend to involve smaller pulmonary arteries.[28,29] The chest radiograph is usually unremarkable. Radionuclide perfusion scanning usually demonstrates numerous small, peripheral, subsegmental perfusion defects in the presence of normal ventilation, but findings can range from normal[30] to large perfusion defects.[31] Pulmonary angiography is typically normal or demonstrates small-vessel abnormalities and is usually performed to establish or exclude the competing diagnosis of venous thromboembolic disease. Right heart catheterization in symptomatic patients will confirm the presence of pulmonary hypertension.[27] Pulmonary wedge aspiration cytology can be examined for the presence of tumor cells,[32,33] but lung biopsy is usually required to make the diagnosis of tumor embolism. It is not yet known if early diagnosis of tumor embolism changes prognosis, but it may avoid unnecessary anticoagulation.[27]

Rarely, tumor emboli may present with more proximal pulmonary artery obstruction. Distinguishing tumor emboli from venous thromboembolic disease can be difficult, but progression of disease despite adequate anticoagulation would suggest the former diagnosis. Survival following surgical resection has been reported in atrial myxoma,[34] renal cell carcinoma,[35-37] Wilms' tumor[38] and choriocarcinoma,[39] testicular cancer[40] and intravenous leiomyoma.[41]

KEY POINTS

- Primary pulmonary artery sarcomas are extremely rare.
- The diagnosis is often difficult and delayed because of symptoms that mimic more common causes of pulmonary vascular obstruction such as pulmonary embolism.
- The diagnosis should be entertained in patients who also present with systemic symptoms (weight loss, fever) or in patients who fail to improve with anticoagulation.
- CT and MRI scanning may be helpful in distinguishing sarcoma from competing diagnoses.
- The prognosis is grim without surgical intervention, with most patients dying quickly from right ventricular failure.
- Early surgical resection palliates symptoms, lengthens survival, and provides the only potential for cure.
- The role of adjuvant therapy (chemotherapy or radiotherapy) has yet to be defined.

REFERENCES

1 Colby TV. Malignancies in the lung and pleura mimicking benign processes. *Semin Diagn Pathol* 1995;**12**:30–44.

2 Anderson MB, Kriett JM, Kapelanski DP et al. Primary pulmonary artery sarcoma: a report of six cases. *Ann Thorac Surg* 1995;**59**:1487–90.

3 Miller DL, Allen MS. Rare pulmonary neoplasms. *Mayo Clin Proc* 1993;**68**:492–8.

◆4 Nonomura A, Kurumaya H, Kono N et al. Primary pulmonary artery sarcoma. Report of two autopsy cases studied by immunohistochemistry and electron microscopy, and review of 110 cases reported in the literature. *Acta Pathol Jpn* 1988;**38**:883–96.

◆5 Kruger I, Borowski A, Horst M et al. Symptoms, diagnosis, and therapy of primary sarcomas of the pulmonary artery. *Thorac Cardiovasc Surg* 1990;**38**:91–5.

6 Fer MF, Greco A, Haile KL et al. Unusual survival after pulmonary sarcoma. *South Med J* 1981;**74**:624–6.

7 Devendra G, Mo M, Kerr KM et al. Pulmonary artery sarcomas: the UCSD experience. *Am J Respir Crit Care Med* 2002;**165**:A24.

8 Mayer E, Kriegsmann J, Gaumann A *et al.* Surgical treatment of pulmonary artery sarcoma. *J Thorac Cardiovasc Surg* 2001;**121**:77–82.

•9 Mandelstamm M. Uber primäre neubildungen des herzens. *Virchows Arch (Pathol Anat)* 1923;**245**:43–54.

10 Farooki ZQ, Chang CH, Jackson WL *et al.* Primary pulmonary artery sarcoma in two children. *Pediatr Cardiol* 1988;**9**:243–51.

◆11 McGlennan RC, Manivel JC, Stanley SJ *et al.* Pulmonary artery trunk sarcoma: a clinicopathologic, ultrastructural, and immunohistochemical study of four cases. *Mod Pathol* 1989;**2**:486–94.

12 Loredo JS, Fedullo PF, Piovella F *et al.* Digital clubbing associated with pulmonary artery sarcoma. *Chest* 1996;**109**:1651–3.

13 Parish JM, Rosenow EC, Swensen SJ *et al.* Pulmonary artery sarcoma; clinical features. *Chest* 1996;**110**:1480–8.

14 Bergin CJ, Hauschildt JP, Brown MA *et al.* Identifying the cause of unilateral hypoperfusion in patients suspected to have chronic thromboembolism: diagnostic accuracy of helical CT and conventional angiography. *Radiology* 1999;**213**:743–9.

15 Nguyen GK. Exfoliative cytology of angiosarcoma of the pulmonary artery. *Acta Cytol* 1985;**29**:624–7.

16 Rafal RB, Nichols JN, Markisz J. Pulmonary artery sarcoma: diagnosis and postoperative follow-up with gadolinium-diethylenetriamine pentaacetic acid-enhanced magnetic resonance imaging. *Mayo Clin Proc* 1995;**70**:173–6.

17 Schermoly M, Overman J, Pingleton SK. Pulmonary artery sarcoma – unusual pulmonary angiographic finding – a case report. *Angiology* 1987;**38**:617–21.

18 Hynes JK, Smith HC, Holmes DR *et al.* Preoperative angiographic diagnosis of primary sarcoma of the pulmonary artery. *Circulation* 1982;**66**:672–4.

19 Kauczor HU, Schwickert HC, Mayer E *et al.* Pulmonary artery sarcoma mimicking chronic thromboembolic disease: computed tomography and magnetic resonance imaging findings. *Cardiovasc Intervent Radiol* 1994;**17**:185–9.

20 Scully RE, Mark EJ, Ebeling SH *et al.* Case records of the Massachusetts General Hospital. *N Engl J Med* 2000;**343**:493–500.

21 Kacl GM, Bruder E, Pfammatter T *et al.* Primary angiosarcoma of the pulmonary arteries: dynamic contrast-enhanced MRI. *J Comput Assist Tomogr* 1998;**22**:687–91.

22 Thurer RL, Thorsen A, Parker JA *et al.* FDG Imaging of a pulmonary artery sarcoma. *Ann Thorac Surg* 2000;**70**:1414–15.

23 Yamada N, Kamei S, Yasuda F *et al.* Primary leiomysarcoma of the pulmonary artery confirmed by catheter suction biopsy. *Chest* 1998;**113**:555–6.

24 Dail DH. Uncommon tumors. In: Dail DH, Hammar SP (eds), *Pulmonary pathology*. New York: Springer-Verlag, 1994;1279–461.

25 Corrin B. Rare pulmonary tumours. In: Corrin B (ed.), *Pathology of the lungs*. London: Churchill Livingstone, 2000;505–54.

26 Virman R, Burke A, Farb A. Tumors of great vessels. In: Virmani R, Burke A, Farb A (eds), *Atlas of cardiovascular pathology*. Philadelphia: WB Saunders, 1996;154–8.

◆27 Bassiri AG, Haghighi B, Doyle RL *et al.* Pulmonary tumor embolism. *Am J Respir Crit Care Med* 1997;**155**:2089–95.

◆28 Soares FA, Pinto APFE, Landell GA *et al.* Pulmonary tumor embolism to arterial vessels and carcinomatous lymphangitis. *Arch Pathol Lab Med* 1993;**117**:827–31.

◆29 Goldhaber SZ, Dricker E, Buring JE *et al.* Clinical suspicion of autopsy-proven thrombotic and tumor pulmonary embolism in cancer patients. *Am Heart J* 1987;**114**:1432–5.

30 Domanski MJ, Cunnion RE, Fernicola DJ *et al.* Fatal cor pulmonale caused by extensive tumor emboli in the small pulmonary arteries without emboli in the major pulmonary arteries or metastasis in the pulmonary parenchyma. *Am J Cardiol* 1993;**72**:233–4.

31 Moores LK, Burrell LM, Morse RW *et al.* Diffuse tumor microembolism. A rare cause of a high-probability perfusion scan. *Chest* 1997;**111**:1122–3.

32 Babar SI, Sobonya RE, Snyder LS. Pulmonary microvascular cytology for the diagnosis of pulmonary tumor embolism. *West J Med* 1998;**168**:47–50.

33 Bhuvaneswaran JS, Venkitachalam CG, Sandhyamani S. Pulmonary wedge aspiration cytology in the diagnosis of recurrent tumor embolism causing pulmonary arterial hypertension. *Int J Cardiol* 1993;**39**:209–12.

34 Keenan DJM, Morton P, O'Kane HO. Right atrial myxoma and pulmonary embolism: rational basis for investigation and treatment. *Br Heart J* 1982;**48**:510–21.

35 Daughtry JD, Stewart BH, Golding LAR *et al.* Pulmonary embolus presenting as the initial manifestation of renal cell carcinoma. *Ann Thorac Surg* 1977;**24**:178–81.

36 Isringhaus H, Naber M, Kopper B. Successful treatment of tumor embolism of an hypernephroma with complete occlusion of the left pulmonary artery. *Thorac Cardiovasc Surg* 1987;**35**:65–6.

37 Kubota H, Furuse A, Kotsuka Y *et al.* Successful management of massive pulmonary tumor embolism from renal cell carcinoma. *Ann Thorac Surg* 1996;**61**:708–10.

38 Bulas DI, Thompson R, Reaman G. Pulmonary emboli as a primary manifestation of Wilms tumor. *AJR Am J Roentgenol* 1991;**156**:155–6.

39 Watanabe S, Shimokawa S, Sakasegawa K *et al.* Choriocarcinoma in the pulmonary artery treated with emergency pulmonary embolectomy. *Chest* 2002;**121**:654–6.

40 Haab F, Cour F, Boutan Laroze A *et al.* Testicular neoplasm presenting as a major pulmonary embolism. *Eur Urol* 1996;**29**:494–6.

41 Marcus SG, Krauss T, Freedberg RS *et al.* Pulmonary embolectomy for intravenous uterine leiomyomatosis. *Am Heart J* 1994;**127**:1642–5.

PART 6

Pulmonary hypertension in pediatrics

19

Primary pulmonary hypertension in children

ROBYN J BARST

INTRODUCTION

Until a few years ago, the diagnosis of primary pulmonary hypertension was tantamount to a death sentence, particularly for children.[1–3] In the NIH Primary Pulmonary Hypertension (PPH) Registry,[4] the median survival for all patients was 2.8 years, and only 10 months for children less than 16 years of age. While advances in medical therapy have greatly improved the prognosis for adults with PPH,[5–8] extrapolation from adults to children is not straightforward because the anticipated life span of children is longer and children may have a more reactive pulmonary circulation, raising the prospect of greater vasodilator responsiveness.[9]

DEFINITIONS

Similar to adults, PPH in children is characterized by progressive elevation of pulmonary artery pressure that eventually leads to right ventricular failure and death. Although in both children and adults PPH continues to be referred to as unexplained or idiopathic pulmonary hypertension as first described by Romberg in 1891,[10] a revised classification of pulmonary hypertension was recommended following the 1998 WHO World Symposium[11] (Table 19.1). The inclusion of exercise hemodynamic abnormalities in the definition of PPH is important, since children with PPH often exhibit an exaggerated pulmonary vascular response to exercise. Children with a history of recurrent exertional or nocturnal syncope may have a resting mean pulmonary artery pressure of only 25 mmHg that markedly increases with exercise or with modest nocturnal systemic arterial oxygen desaturation.

The evaluation of etiology in children is similar to adults, although there are several differences (Table 19.1). For example, the pulmonary vasoconstrictor response to hypoxia or other stimuli is more profound in infants than in adults.[12–16]

The pathophysiology of persistent pulmonary hypertension of the newborn resembles PPH,[17] but differences between the two entities exist. Increased pulmonary vascular resistance, right-to-left shunting, severe hypoxemia, and pulmonary parenchymal abnormalities due to meconium aspiration, pneumonia or sepsis, characterize persistent pulmonary hypertension of the newborn. In some instances, the 'trigger' for pulmonary hypertension is unknown. Persistent pulmonary hypertension of the newborn is almost always transient;[18] by contrast, patients with PPH who respond to medical therapy appear to need treatment indefinitely.[19] Some infants with persistent pulmonary hypertension of the newborn may have a genetic predisposition to hyperreact to pulmonary vasoconstrictor stimuli, such as alveolar hypoxia. Pathological studies examining the elastic pattern of the main pulmonary artery[20,21] also suggest that PPH is present from birth in some patients, although it is acquired later in life in others.

Table 19.1 *Diagnostic classification of pulmonary hypertension*

1 *Pulmonary arterial hypertension*
  1.1 Primary pulmonary hypertension
    (a) Sporadic
    (b) Familial
  1.2 Related to
    (a) Collagen vascular disease
    (b) Congenital systemic-to-pulmonary shunts
    (c) Portal hypertension
    (d) HIV infection
    (e) Drugs/toxins
      (i) Anorexigens
      (ii) Other
    (f) Persistent pulmonary hypertension
      of the newborn
    (g) Other

2 *Pulmonary venous hypertension*
  2.1 Left-sided atrial or ventricular heart disease
  2.2 Left-sided valvular heart disease
  2.3 Extrinsic compression of central pulmonary vein
    (a) Fibrosing mediastinitis
    (b) Adenopathy/tumors
  2.4 Pulmonary veno-occlusive disease
  2.5 Other

3 *Pulmonary hypertension associated with disorders of the respiratory system and/or hypoxia*
  3.1 Chronic obstructive pulmonary disease
  3.2 Interstitial lung disease
  3.3 Sleep-disordered breathing
  3.4 Alveolar hypoventilation disorders
  3.5 Chronic exposure to high altitudes
  3.6 Neonatal lung disease
  3.7 Alveolar-capillary dysplasia

4 *Pulmonary hypertension due to chronic thrombotic and/or embolic disease*
  4.1 Thromboembolic obstruction of proximal pulmonary arteries
  4.2 Obstruction of distal pulmonary arteries
    (a) Pulmonary embolism (thrombus, ova and/or parasites, foreign material)
    (b) *In situ* thrombosis
    (c) Sickle cell disease

5 *Pulmonary hypertension due to disorders affecting the pulmonary vasculature*
  5.1 Inflammatory
    (a) Schistosomiasis
    (b) Sarcoidosis
    (c) Other
  5.2 Pulmonary capillary hemangiomatosis

Reproduced with permission from ref 11.

Whilst the definition of PPH requires the exclusion of other causes, one may find small anatomic congenital systemic-to-pulmonary shunts. Whether these represent unrelated phenomena or a genetic predisposition for PPH with a hemodynamically insignificant congenital systemic-to-pulmonary shunt 'triggering' the onset of the pulmonary vascular disease remains uncertain.[22–24] Although pulmonary vascular disease associated with congenital systemic-to-pulmonary shunts usually follows a period of increased pulmonary blood flow, it may occur in patients who never manifested a large left-to-right shunt. Support for this comes from the observation of severe, progressive pulmonary arterial hypertension following repair of atrial septal defects in two children whose mothers died from PPH.[25]

Although misalignment of pulmonary veins with alveolar capillary dysplasia is often initially diagnosed as persistent pulmonary hypertension of the newborn, it is a separate, uncommon disorder of pulmonary vascular development that is usually diagnosed only after death from fulminant pulmonary arterial hypertension.[26] Similar to PPH and pulmonary veno-occlusive disease, affected siblings (with alveolar capillary dysplasia) have variable phenotypic expression consistent with a familial predisposition.[27] This condition is associated with other non-lethal congenital malformations, delayed onset of presentation (especially after 12 hours), and severe hypoxemia refractory to medical therapy. Infants most often present with severe pulmonary arterial hypertension, with transient responses to inhaled nitric oxide or intravenous epoprostenol.

Congenital heart disease is the most common cause of pulmonary venous hypertension in children, and is due to obstructed total anomalous pulmonary venous return, left heart obstruction, or severe left ventricular failure. The lungs of those born with severe left inflow obstruction show pronounced arterial and venous wall thickening, while pulmonary veno-occlusive disease is characterized by uniform fibrotic occlusion of peripheral small venules.[28] Veno-occlusive disease may occur in early childhood and may be familial.[29] Progressive long segment pulmonary vein hypoplasia leading to pulmonary vein atresia is another uniformly fatal form of pulmonary venous hypertension presenting in infancy.

INCIDENCE/EPIDEMIOLOGY

The incidence of PPH in children remains unknown, with estimates ranging from one to two per million.[30] On occasion, infants who have died with the presumptive diagnosis of sudden infant death syndrome have had PPH diagnosed by autopsy. The gender incidence in adult patients with primary pulmonary hypertension of approximately 1.7:1 females to males[31] is similar to our experience with children, with no significant difference between younger and older children.

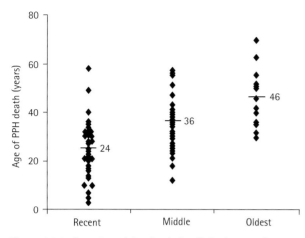

Figure 19.1 *Genetic anticipation in familial primary pulmonary hypertension (PPH), indicating the younger ages at death in subsequent generations. (Reproduced with permission from Loyd JE, Newman JH. Familial primary pulmonary hypertension. In: Rubin LJ, Rich S (eds), Primary pulmonary hypertension. New York: Marcel Dekker, 1997;99:151–62.)*

Genetics of primary pulmonary hypertension

The genetics of pulmonary hypertension are discussed in detail in Chapter 6. Familial PPH is inherited as an autosomal dominant disorder with reduced or incomplete penetrance[32] and genetic anticipation (Figure 19.1).[32–34]

Familial PPH results from mutations in the gene encoding bone morphogenetic protein receptor type II (*BMPR2*) (Figure 19.2).[35,36] Individuals in a family with familial PPH are estimated to have a 5–10% lifetime risk of developing the disease. Genetic testing remains a research endeavor, and results of genetic testing should be confidential and accompanied by appropriate genetic counseling.

Fewer males are born with PPH than in the population at large, suggesting that the PPH gene might influence fertilization or development *in utero*.[37] Our experience suggests a possible increase in fraternal twins, but this requires confirmation. Fraternal twins occur in approximately 3% in Western countries but may be as high as 16–20% in certain African nations. Seven of the first 35 familial PPH families that we studied had fraternal twins; five families had one set and two families had two sets.[38] Table 19.2 illustrates the presence of disease, results of microsatellite determinations of *PPH1* gene status and the gender of these twins. Eight of the nine sets had one or more affected twins and the ninth set had an asymptomatic gene-positive carrier. Parental gene carriers were equally divided between mothers and fathers. There were four sets of mixed gender, three with

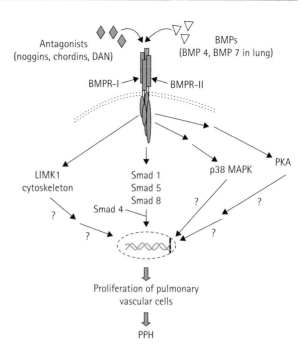

Figure 19.2 *Signaling pathways of the bone morphogenetic protein receptor type II (BMPR-II). In the extracellular space, the receptor ligands BMPs bind directly to the BMPR-II on the cell membrane. The bioavailability of BMPs is regulated by the presence of BMPR-II receptor antagonists such as noggins, chordins and DAN (differential screening-selected gene aberrative in neuroblastoma). The binding of ligands to BMPR-II leads to the recruitment of BMPR-I to form a heteromeric receptor complex at the cell surface. This results in the phosphorylation and activation of the kinase domain of BMPR-I. The activated BMPR-I subsequently phosphorylates and activates cytoplasmic signaling proteins Smads (Smad 1, 5 and 8). Phosphorylated Smads bind to the common mediator Smad 4, and the resulting Smad complex moves from the cytoplasm into the nucleus and regulates gene transcription. Other downstream signaling pathways that can be activated following the engagement of BMPR-I and BMPR-II by BMPs include cell-type-dependent activation of p38 mitogen-activated protein kinase (p38 MAPK) and protein kinase A (PKA). In addition, the cytoplasmic tail of BMPR-II has been shown to interact with the LIM motif-containing protein kinase 1 (LIMK1) that is localized in the cytoskeleton. Germline mutations of the gene encoding BMPR-II underlie primary pulmonary hypertension (PPH) that is characterized by the abnormal proliferation of pulmonary vascular cells. However, the specific cytoplasmic proteins and nuclear transcription factors that are involved in the development of PPH have not been identified. The molecular mechanism of how defects of BMPR-II leading to PPH remains to be elucidated.*

boys and two with girls. *BMPR2* mutations have been found in two of the nine families. Familial PPH family 22 had an affected boy and girl (exon 6 mutation) from each mixed gender set of twins. DNA was not available from

Table 19.2 *Fraternal twins in 35 familial primary pulmonary hypertension (FPPH) families: gender, disease and* PPH1 *gene status*

Family no.	Twins	Affected	PPH1+	Parental carrier
5	2 boys	Both (+)	Both (+)	Mother
13	2 boys	Both (−)	One (+), one (−)	Father
20	2 boys	Boy (+), boy (−)	Both (NT)	Father
	Boy/girl	Girl (+), boy (−)	Both (NT)	Mother
22	Boy/girl	Boy (+), girl (−)	Boy (+), girl (NT)	(NT)
	Boy/girl	Girl (+), boy (−)	Girl (+), boy (NT)	(NT)
25	2 girls	Both (+)	Both (+)	Father
26	Boy/girl	Girl (+), boy (−)	Both (NT)	(NT)
29	2 girls	Girl (+), girl (−)	Girl (+), girl (−)	Mother

PPH1+ by microsatellite marker analyses. NT, not tested (DNA unavailable); FPPH families no. 13 and 22 have *BMPR2* mutations; mutations not found in no. 5, 20, 25, 26 and 29. (Reproduced from *Prog in Pediatr Cardiol*, *12*, Morse JH, Knowles JA, Genetics of primary pulmonary hypertension, 271–8, © (2001), with permission from Elsevier Science.)

either unaffected twin. Family 13 had the asymptomatic gene-positive carrier (exon 3 mutation) and DNA was unavailable for his male twin. A mutation in bone morphogenetic protein 15 (BMP 15), a potential ligand of *BMPR2*, has been associated with multiple births in inbred strains of sheep.[39] Sheep with one mutant copy of BMP 15, which is expressed in the ovary, had an increased risk of having twins or triplets, via release of multiple eggs. In those with two copies of the mutation, the odds of a failed pregnancy increased. This is analogous to the deficits observed in familial PPH, where a reduction in BMP signal may lead to an increased ratio of multiple births.

Autoimmunity

Primary pulmonary hypertension is associated with autoimmune phenomena, although the nature of this relationship remains unclear. Increased frequency of Raynaud's phenomenon and positive antinuclear antibodies have been reported[31,40] and pulmonary arterial hypertension is a clinical component of many autoimmune disorders (Table 19.1). In addition, autoantibody–HLA correlations have been observed in several subsets of PPH patients,[41] suggesting that a genetically programmed and immunologically mediated component may predispose some individuals with PPH to eventually develop a connective tissue disease.

There may also be an increased association between PPH and thyroid disorders[42,43] in children, as in adults. Our experience of prevalence of hypothyroidism with PPH [12 of 132 (9%) in adults and 5 of 78 (6.5%) in children] is similar to previously published reports. The increased occurrence of hyperthyroidism in patients followed at our center treated with epoprostenol also raises the possibility that epoprostenol may be a 'trigger' to the development of thyroid disease.

As with adults, pulmonary arterial hypertension related to autoimmune phenomena also occurs with children, although the frequency appears to be lower. Although positive antinuclear antibodies occur with increased frequency in adults with PPH, this occurs less frequently in children. In our experience, 21 of 123 (17%) children with PPH had positive antinuclear antibodies at diagnosis, while 17 others (14%) seroconverted subsequently.

We have also seen an increased occurrence of positive antinuclear antibodies in mothers of children with pulmonary arterial hypertension associated with anatomically trivial congenital pulmonary-to-systemic shunts: among 41 children, eight (20%) mothers and four of the children were antinuclear antibody positive at diagnosis. An additional five children seroconverted several years later.

PATHOBIOLOGY

In young children, the pathobiology suggests failure of the neonatal vasculature to open and a striking reduction in arterial number. In older children, intimal hyperplasia and occlusive changes are found in the pulmonary arterioles. While adults with PPH often have plexiform lesions and 'fixed' pulmonary vascular changes, children with PPH have more medial hypertrophy, less intimal fibrosis, and fewer plexiform lesions. In the classic studies by Wagenvoort and Wagenvoort in 1970,[44] medial hypertrophy was severe in patients less than 15 years old, and it was usually the only change in infants. Among the 11 who were less than 1 year of age, all with severe medial hypertrophy, only three had intimal fibrosis. These studies suggested that pulmonary vasoconstriction, leading to medial hypertrophy, may occur early in the course of the disease and may precede the development of fixed pulmonary vascular changes. These observations may also provide clues to the differences in the natural history

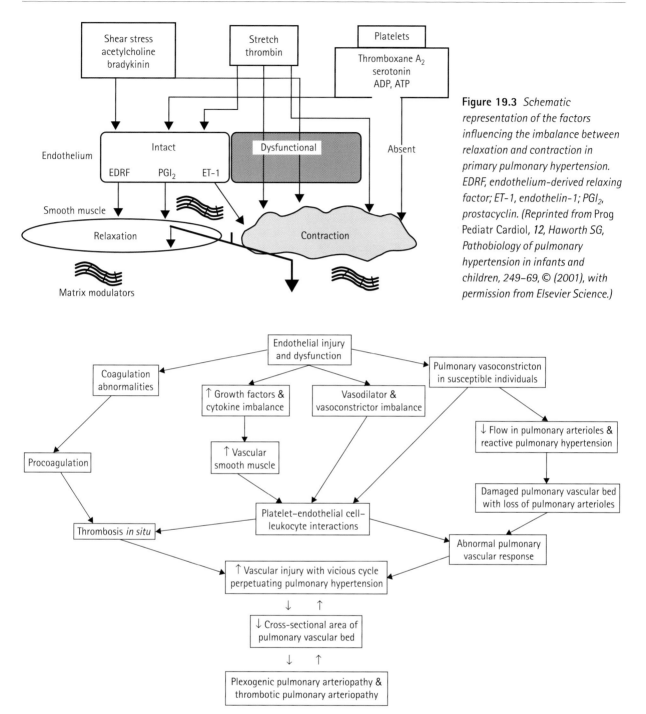

Figure 19.3 *Schematic representation of the factors influencing the imbalance between relaxation and contraction in primary pulmonary hypertension. EDRF, endothelium-derived relaxing factor; ET-1, endothelin-1; PGI$_2$, prostacyclin. (Reprinted from* Prog Pediatr Cardiol, *12, Haworth SG, Pathobiology of pulmonary hypertension in infants and children, 249–69, © (2001), with permission from Elsevier Science.)*

Figure 19.4 *Possible pathogenesis of primary pulmonary hypertension. (Reproduced with permission from Barst RJ. Medical therapy of pulmonary hypertension: an overview of treatment and goals. In: Rich S, McLaughlin VV (eds),* Clinics in chest medicine. *Philadelphia: WB Saunders, 2001;22:509–15.)*

of PPH in children compared with adults. Based on these early pathological studies, the most widely proposed mechanism for PPH until the late 1980s and early 1990s was pulmonary vasoconstriction.[45–48] Subsequent studies have identified potentially important structural and functional abnormalities, including imbalances between vasodilator/antiproliferative and vasoconstrictive/mitogenic mediators, defects in the potassium channels of pulmonary artery smooth muscle cells and increased synthesis of inflammatory mediators which promote vasoconstriction as well as enhanced cell growth (Figures 19.3–19.5).[49–56]

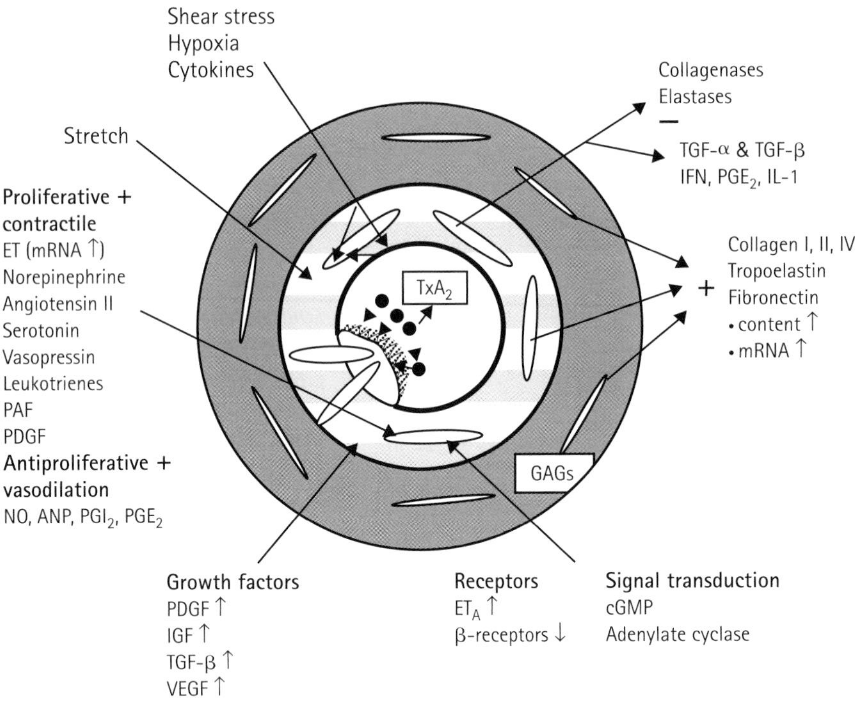

Figure 19.5 *Factors which regulate vessel wall remodeling. ANP, atrial natriuretic peptide; ET, endothelin; ET_A, endothelin A receptor; GAGs, glucosamino-glycans; IFN, interferon; IGF, insulin-like growth factor; PDGF, platelet-derived growth factor. (Reprinted from* Prog Pediatr Cardiol, *12, Haworth SG, Pathobiology of pulmonary hypertension in infants and children, 249–69, © (2001), with permission from Elsevier Science.)*

Coagulation abnormalities may also occur, initiating or further exacerbating the pulmonary vascular disease.[57,58] The interactions between the humoral and cellular elements of the blood on an injured endothelial cell surface result in remodeling of the pulmonary vascular bed and contribute to the process of pulmonary vascular injury.[59,60]

Migration of smooth muscle cells in the pulmonary arterioles occurs as a release of chemotactic agents from injured pulmonary endothelial cells.[61] Endothelial cell damage can also result in thrombosis *in situ*, transforming the pulmonary vascular bed from its usual anticoagulant state to a procoagulant state.[62] Elevated fibrinopeptide-A levels also suggest *in situ* thrombosis.[63] Further support for the role of coagulation abnormalities at the endothelial cell surface comes from the reports of improved survival in patients treated with chronic anticoagulation.[5,64,65]

PATHOPHYSIOLOGY

Although the histopathology in children is often qualitatively the same as that seen with adult patients, the clinical presentation, natural history and factors influencing survival may differ. Children also appear to have differences in their hemodynamic parameters at diagnosis compared with adult patients (Table 19.3).[66] The increased cardiac index in children may reflect an earlier diagnosis and may explain the greater frequency of an acute vasodilator response compared with adults.

Table 19.3 *Baseline hemodynamics in children versus adults with primary pulmonary hypertension**

	Children (n = 24)	Adults (n = 77)
Mean pulmonary artery pressure (mmHg)	70 ± 15[†]	55 ± 16
Mean systemic artery pressure (mmHg)	75 ± 15[†]	91 ± 12
Cardiac index (L/min/m^2)	4.3 ± 3.9[†]	2.1 ± 0.7
Pulmonary vascular resistance (units·m^2)	28 ± 18[†]	15 ± 8
Systemic vascular resistance (units·m^2)	28 ± 18	25 ± 10
Heart rate (bpm)	121 ± 29[†]	83 ± 13

*Personal communication; [†] P < 0.05 children versus adults.

DIAGNOSIS AND ASSESSMENT

The diagnosis of PPH can be made with a high degree of accuracy if care is taken to exclude all related or associated conditions. A thorough and detailed history and physical examination, as well as appropriate tests, must be performed to uncover potential causative or contributing factors, many of which may not be readily apparent. Questions should be asked about family history – pulmonary hypertension, connective tissue disorders, congenital heart disease, other congenital anomalies, and early unexplained deaths. If the family history suggests familial PPH, screening of all family members is recommended. In accordance with the WHO World Symposium on Primary Pulmonary Hypertension recommendations 1998,[11] we advocate a transthoracic echocardiogram in all first-degree relatives at baseline and every 3–5 years in asymptomatic family members. Additional issues to address include a carefully detailed birth and neonatal history, a detailed illicit drug and medication history, including psychotropic drugs and appetite suppressants, exposure to high altitude or toxic cooking oil,[67,68] travel history, and any history of frequent respiratory tract infections. The answers to these questions may offer clues to a possible 'trigger'. For example, we have seen a 6-year-old boy with pulmonary arterial hypertension who moved to New York from Spain at 1 year of age after having been exposed during infancy to rapeseed cooking oil. Another example is an 11-year-old boy from Brazil with pulmonary hypertension who had evidence at autopsy of severe pulmonary schistosomiasis.

The diagnostic evaluation in children suspected of having PPH is similar to that of adult patients (Figure 19.6) although certain conditions, e.g. chronic thromboembolic disease or obstructive sleep apnea, are uncommon. A functional assessment using the modified NYHA functional classification is also helpful (Table 19.4).[11]

Clinical presentation

The presenting symptoms in children with PPH may differ compared with adults. Infants often present with signs of low cardiac output: poor appetite, failure to thrive, lethargy, diaphoresis, tachypnea, tachycardia and irritability. In addition, infants and older children may be cyanotic with exertion, owing to right-to-left shunting through a patent foramen ovale. Children without adequate shunting through a patent foramen ovale may present with syncope, which is often effort related. After early childhood, children present with the same symptoms as adults. In older children, the most common symptoms are exertional dyspnea and, occasionally, chest pain. Right ventricular failure is rare in young children, occurring most often in children older than 10 years of age with severe and longstanding pulmonary hypertension. The interval between onset of symptoms and time of diagnosis is usually shorter in children than in adults, particularly in children who present with syncope. Some infants have crying spells, perhaps as a result of chest pain that cannot be verbalized. Children may present with seizures resulting from exertional syncope, or mild systemic arterial oxygen desaturation during sleep. Children of all ages also commonly complain of nausea

and vomiting, reflecting a reduced cardiac output. Chest pain may be the result of right ventricular ischemia.

Physical examination

Many of the physical findings in children are typical of any patient with pulmonary arterial hypertension regardless of etiology (Table 19.1). An increased pulmonic component of the second heart sound is usually audible; however, a right-sided fourth heart sound is not heard as often in children. Children may have distortion of their chest wall due to severe right ventricular hypertrophy. Tricuspid regurgitation is common, while pulmonary insufficiency is heard less often. Clinical signs of right-sided heart failure, such as hepatomegaly, peripheral edema and acrocyanosis, are rare in young children, particularly in those who present with syncope. Clubbing is not a typical feature of PPH, but it has been observed in patients with longstanding disease who develop chronic hypoxemia from right-to-left shunting via a patent foramen ovale.

Natural history

Several large survival studies of adult patients with PPH who have not undergone transplantation have reported survival rates at 1, 3 and 5 years of 68–77%, 40–56%, and 22–38%, respectively.[4,64,69,70] However, there is significant variability in the natural history of the disease in both adults and children, with some having a rapidly progressive course resulting in death within several weeks after diagnosis, while others survive for decades.

Chest radiography

Chest radiography demonstrates a large right ventricle, dilated hilar pulmonary arteries and variable peripheral lung fields depending upon the amount of pulmonary blood flow. As pulmonary blood flow decreases due to increasing pulmonary vascular resistance, the peripheral lung fields become progressively oligemic. The attenuated ('pruned') distal pulmonary vasculature, which is a common finding in adults, is rarely seen in children. If the electrocardiogram and chest radiograph are either non-diagnostic or consistent with pulmonary hypertension, further evaluation is needed (Figure 19.6).

Echocardiography

Echocardiography is extremely important in searching for congenital or acquired heart disease in the pediatric population. The typical echocardiographic appearance

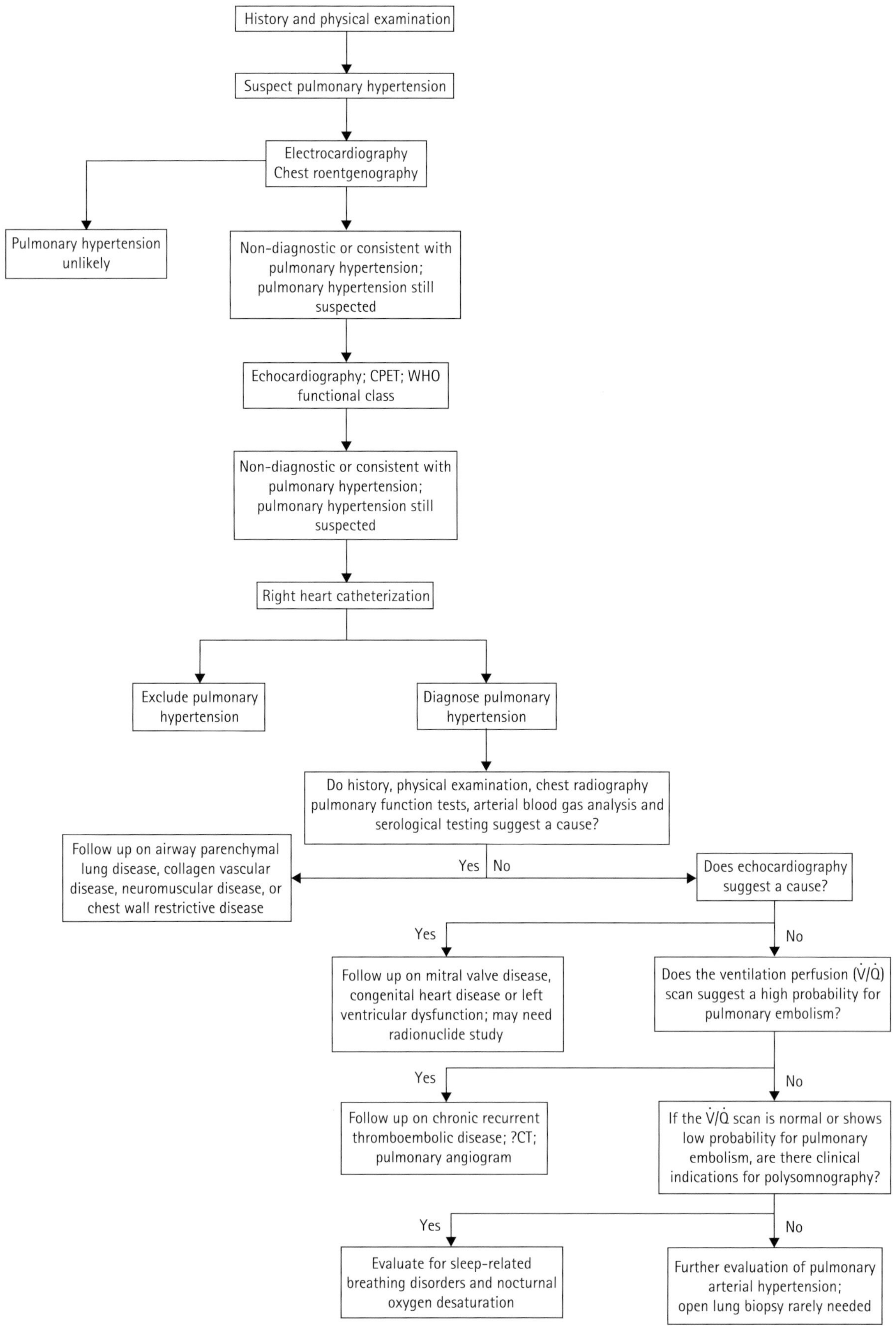

Figure 19.6 *Diagnostic evaluation in children suspected of having primary pulmonary hypertension. CPET, cardiopulmonary exercise testing; CT, computed tomography; V̇/Q̇, ventilation/perfusion; WHO, World Health Organization.*

Table 19.4 *Functional assessment*[*11]

Class I: Patients with pulmonary hypertension but without resulting limitations of physical activity. Ordinary physical activity does not cause undue dyspnea or fatigue, chest pain or near syncope.

Class II: Patients with pulmonary hypertension resulting in slight limitation of physical activity. They are comfortable at rest. Ordinary physical activity causes undue dyspnea or fatigue, chest pain or near syncope.

Class III: Patients with pulmonary hypertension resulting in marked limitation of physical activity. They are comfortable at rest. Less than ordinary activity causes undue dyspnea or fatigue, chest pain or near syncope.

Class IV: Patients with pulmonary hypertension with inability to carry out any physical activity without symptoms. These patients manifest signs of right heart failure. Dyspnea and/or fatigue may even be present at rest. Discomfort is increased by any physical activity.

*Modified after the New York Heart Association Functional Classification.

in children with PPH is similar to adult patients: right ventricular and right atrial enlargement with a normal or decreased left ventricular cavity dimension. Tricuspid or pulmonary insufficiency is detected with Doppler interrogation, and the measured velocity of the tricuspid and pulmonary regurgitant jets is useful in estimating pulmonary arterial pressures. Posterior bowing of the interventricular septum occurs with significant pulmonary hypertension, and posterior bowing of the inter-atrial septum is seen with elevated right atrial pressure. Although transesophageal echocardiography is often helpful in adult patients, it is rarely necessary with children. A contrast or bubble study during two-dimensional echocardiography can be performed to determine the presence and size of an anatomic inter-atrial septal defect or patent foramen ovale; the rate of disappearance of the bubbles is also useful as a qualitative assessment of right heart function and resting cardiac output.

Cardiopulmonary exercise testing

We reported that exercise capacity correlates with right atrial pressure, pulmonary artery pressure and cardiac index and is useful in predicting prognosis.[71] We also found that exercise capacity correlated best with right atrial pressure, one of the best predictors of survival in PPH.

Patients with severely limited exercise capacity (less than 10% of the predicted value) are at a significantly increased risk for complications during cardiac catheterization,[71] and we do not routinely perform acute vasodilator drug testing during cardiac catheterization in these patients. Conversely, an exercise capacity of more than 75% of the predicted value may identify a subgroup of

children who are capable of active pulmonary vasodilatation.[71] Serial exercise studies are also useful in monitoring disease course and in influencing timing of additional therapy, medical or surgical.[72,73] Wasserman *et al.*[74] recently reported that cardiopulmonary exercise tests may disclose the characteristic pattern of ventilatory and circulatory responses of pulmonary vascular disease in patients with unexplained dyspnea and fatigue. These abnormalities (reductions in peak O_2 uptake, anaerobic threshold, peak O_2 pulse, rate of increase in peak O_2 uptake and ventilatory efficiency) also correlated with WHO functional class. Systemic arterial oxygen desaturation during exercise, due to shunting via a patent foramen ovale or ventilation/perfusion mismatching, may also be demonstrated during cardiopulmonary exercise testing.

Pulmonary function testing

Adults with PPH have mild restrictive abnormalities, a low diffusion capacity and oxygen desaturation at rest.[31] By contrast, children with PPH most frequently exhibit small airway obstruction.[75] Reductions in the forced expiratory flow ($FEF_{25-75\%}$) may correlate with clinical disability and hemodynamic abnormalities, suggesting that pulmonary function testing may provide a non-invasive method for following disease progression. The presence of moderate or severe restrictive or obstructive impairment suggests an etiology other than PPH.

Ventilation/perfusion scintigraphy

Although we perform ventilation/perfusion scintigraphy in children with suspected PPH, we are not nearly as concerned about chronic thromboembolic disease as a cause of the elevated pulmonary artery pressure in this population compared with adults. Since chronic thromboembolic disease can occur with hemoglobinopathies, we perform hemoglobin electrophoresis with all children who present with unexplained pulmonary arterial hypertension to exclude sickle cell disease.

A coagulation assessment (including anticardiolipin antibodies, lupus anticoagulant, factor V Leiden, antithrombin III, proteins C and S, as well as factor II 201210A variant) is obtained to rule out hereditary or acquired hypercoagulable states that may be etiological or potentiating factors.[76]

Pulmonary angiography

Pulmonary angiography should be performed if the ventilation/perfusion lung scan shows more than a single segmental or multiple subsegmental defects, since chronic thromboembolic pulmonary arterial hypertension may be amenable to thromboendarterectomy.[77] Quantitative pulmonary wedge angiography using the balloon occlusion technique may give additional information on the severity of the pulmonary vascular disease. Rabinovitch *et al.* have reported the usefulness of the rate of taper, the background filling of peripheral vessels, and the pulmonary circulation time, as additional tools in evaluating disease progression.[78]

Continuous overnight oxygen saturation measurements

We recommend that all patients have a sleep evaluation, including continuous oxygen saturation monitoring to rule out airway obstruction or hypoventilation. Even modest decreases in systemic arterial oxygen saturation can significantly increase pulmonary artery pressures in children with a reactive pulmonary vascular bed. If nocturnal desaturation is observed, the patient is re-evaluated with supplemental oxygen. We perform a full sleep study when the history is suggestive of obstructive sleep apnea. Nocturnal oxygen desaturation correlates with pulmonary hemodynamics[79] and frequently resolves with effective medical treatment.

Twenty-four hour electrogram

Although significant arrhythmias rarely complicate PPH, complex ventricular or supraventricular arrhythmias requiring treatment may occur. We have occasionally seen various degrees of heart block in children with unexplained pulmonary arterial hypertension and syncope. Accordingly, our patients undergo baseline 24-hour electrocardiographic monitoring.

Radionuclide angiography and magnetic resonance imaging

These non-invasive studies can be useful in assessing right and left ventricular function prior to initiating therapy and monitoring the effects of treatment.[80,81] In addition, magnetic resonance imaging may be useful in evaluating right ventricular, right atrial and pulmonary artery morphology.

Laboratory testing

We recommend performing a battery of studies to assess multi-organ dysfunction secondary to pulmonary arterial hypertension and to exclude associated conditions. As with adults, an HIV test is performed to rule out the association of HIV infection with pulmonary arterial hypertension.[82] In addition, assays for lupus anticoagulant

and anticardiolipin antibodies are performed, since these factors predispose to secondary thromboembolic events.[83,84] We assess liver function with standard blood tests, and perform additional studies, including occasionally liver biopsy, to exclude portal hypertension[85] in selected patients when the differentiation between cirrhosis with portal-pulmonary hypertension and PPH with passive hepatic congestion cannot be made on clinical grounds alone. We measure quantitative immunoglobulins since immunoglobulin deficiencies have been reported in children and adults with PPH; patients with IgA deficiency, particularly if IgA antibodies are present, are more susceptible to potentially fatal anaphylactic or idiosyncratic reactions when receiving blood products, such as fresh frozen plasma.[86] Factor V Leiden and factor II 20210A variant may also increase the risk of thromboembolic events.[87,88] Serial determinations of coagulation studies may also be useful in evaluating the effects of therapy on endothelial dysfunction.[89] Serum protein electrophoresis is obtained to rule out plasma cell dyscrasias, which have been associated with PPH.[90]

Serial thyroid function testing is performed since there is an association between thyroid disorders and PPH in adults[42] and children.[43] Thyroid disease may occur more frequently in children receiving chronic intravenous epoprostenol than those treated with calcium channel blockers, although this may be more a reflection of disease severity or duration.

Lung biopsy

Lung biopsy, either open or thoracoscopic, is not routinely performed in children suspected of having PPH, since the risks outweigh the limited value of the information gained. Lung biopsy is reserved for the unusual case in which uncertainty exists concerning the etiology, and management could be guided by the histological information.

In most circumstances, a careful and complete non-invasive evaluation will suggest a diagnosis of pulmonary veno-occlusive disease without the need for histopathological confirmation. Since the prognosis of pulmonary veno-occlusive disease is extremely poor[91] and the response to vasodilator therapy is unpredictable,[92,93] early recognition of this disease is important in planning management, particularly transplantation.

Cardiac catheterization

Cardiac catheterization is recommended for confirmation of a diagnosis of PPH. In adults, hemodynamic values obtained at cardiac catheterization can also be used to predict survival, although this has not been validated in children. Cardiac output can be measured accurately by the thermodilution technique in patients without significant shunting through a patent foramen ovale, although the accuracy of the thermodilution method in the face of significant pulmonary or tricuspid regurgitation is controversial. We use the Fick method when concern exists regarding pulmonary or tricuspid regurgitation, or when the foramen ovale is patent. Because of the increased risk in patients with severe pulmonary vascular disease, special precautions should be taken during cardiac catheterization in children, since they are prone to acute pulmonary hypertensive crises: these include adequate sedation to minimize anxiety without depressing respiration and prevention of hypovolemia and hypoxemia. As shown in the treatment algorithm (Figure 19.7), we recommend that children undergo acute testing at the time of the initial right heart catheterization using a short-acting vasodilator to determine responsiveness. Unfortunately, there are no hemodynamic or demographic variables that accurately predict whether a child will respond to acute vasodilator testing. Although younger children are more likely to respond to acute testing, there is a wide spectrum of variability (Figure 19.8).[94] Children with symptoms for several years may manifest near-complete reversibility while others with a brief duration of symptoms may have no vasoreactivity.

The following vasodilators are recommended for acute vasodilator drug testing: intravenous epoprostenol sodium, dose range 2–12 ng/kg·min (although higher doses may be needed with children compared with adult patients), half-life 2–3 minutes; inhaled nitric oxide, dose range 10–80 p.p.m., half-life 15–30 seconds; or intravenous adenosine 50–200 ng/kg·min, half-life 5–10 seconds. Patients who are responsive with acute vasodilator testing are the most likely to have a favorable response with chronic treatment with oral calcium channel blockade,[5,94] whilst those without an acute response are unlikely to derive benefit from such therapy. Furthermore, empiric calcium channel blockade therapy may be deleterious in patients without acute vasoreactivity.[95,96]

TREATMENT

Although there is neither a cure nor a single approach that is uniformly successful for PPH, therapy has improved dramatically over the past several decades and has resulted in sustained clinical and hemodynamic improvement and prolonged survival in children with this disease.[94] An overview of our current treatment approach for children is shown in Figure 19.7.

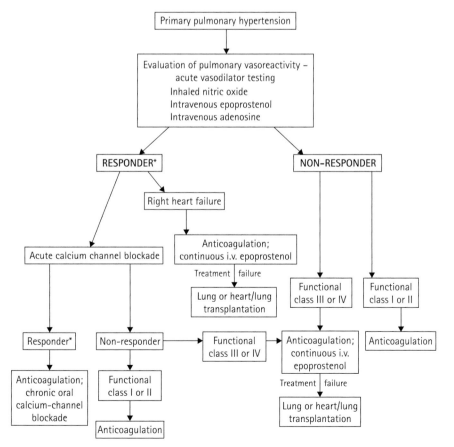

Figure 19.7 *Treatment algorithm for primary pulmonary hypertension prior to novel therapeutics. (*Responder to acute vasodilator testing defined as a significant fall in mean pulmonary arterial pressure, i.e. at least 20%, without a fall in the cardiac output.)*

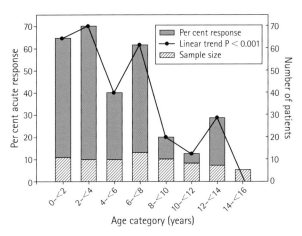

Figure 19.8 *Primary pulmonary hypertension: response to acute vasodilator drug testing by age. The younger the child at the time of testing, the greater the likelihood of eliciting acute pulmonary vasodilatation (P < 0.005). Open bar, per cent response; hatched bar, sample size; heavy line, linear trend P < 0.001. (Reproduced with permission from Barst RJ, Maislin G, Fishman AP. Vasodilator therapy for primary pulmonary hypertension in children. Circulation 1999;99:1197–208, © Lippincott Williams & Wilkins.)*

General measures

The pediatrician plays an invaluable role in the care of children with PPH. Since children often have a more reactive pulmonary vascular bed than adult patients, any respiratory tract infection that results in ventilation/perfusion mismatching and hypoxia can result in a catastrophic event if it is not treated aggressively. Influenza and pneumococcal vaccinations are recommended, unless contraindicated. We recommend hospitalization for children with pneumonia for the initiation of antibiotic therapy, and we administer antipyretics when temperatures exceed 101°F (38°C) in order to minimize the consequences of increased metabolic demands. Children may also require aggressive therapy for acute pulmonary hypertensive crises occurring with episodes of pneumonia or other infectious diseases. The acute respiratory distress syndrome may occur in children with PPH following viral infections, and require aggressive cardiopulmonary support, including inhaled nitric oxide, intravenous epoprostenol and extracorporeal membrane oxygenation. Diet or medical therapy should be used to prevent constipation, since Valsalva maneuvers transiently decrease venous return and may precipitate syncopal episodes.

Anticoagulation

The use of anticoagulants in children with PPH is an extrapolation from studies in adults.[5,64,65] Anticoagulation with warfarin was associated with improved survival in two retrospective studies and one prospective study; however, all three included only adult patients.[5,64,65]

The optimal dose of warfarin has not been addressed; most experienced clinicians use doses of warfarin that achieve an INR of 1.5–2. Certain circumstances, however, such as individuals with a lupus anticoagulant or anticardiolipin antibodies, factor V Leiden and/or factor II 20210A variant,[83,84,87,88] and those with chronic thromboembolic disease may require dose adjustment to maintain a higher INR. We anticoagulate children who have signs of right heart failure with the goal of maintaining an INR of 1.5–2.0. In children who are extremely active, particularly toddlers, we target an INR less than 1.5.

There have been no studies comparing the safety and efficacy of anticoagulation using warfarin versus heparin. However, experimental studies by Hales and colleagues *in vivo*[95] and Benitz *et al.*[96] *in vitro* suggest that the antiproliferative effects of heparin might provide additional benefit beyond its anticoagulant properties.

Calcium channel blockade

Since the degree of individual pulmonary vasoreactivity is unpredictable at diagnosis, acute vasodilator testing is routinely performed as a part of the initial assessment. Since passive distension or recruitment of pulmonary vessels can reduce pulmonary vascular resistance without necessarily indicating a decrease in pulmonary vascular tone,[97,98] and spontaneous variability in hemodynamic parameters may occur,[99] we use the following criteria to indicate acute active pulmonary vasodilatation: a decrease in mean pulmonary artery pressure of at least 20%, with no change or an increase in cardiac index. Children with a reactive pulmonary vascular bed, defined by the response to acute vasodilator testing, almost always also respond to calcium channel blockade with improved exercise capacity, hemodynamics, quality of life assessments and survival (Figure 19.9).[94] The response to acute vasodilator testing appears to be age-related (Figure 19.8), with the youngest children demonstrating the greatest degree of pulmonary vasoreactivity.[94]

Although only a minority (approximately 20%) of adult patients respond to chronic oral calcium channel blockade,[5] a significantly greater percentage of children are acute 'responders' (40%), and can be effectively treated with chronic oral calcium channel blockade.[94] While most studies have used relatively high doses of calcium channel blockers, the optimal dosing for both children and adults is uncertain.

Prostaglandins

Chronic intravenous epoprostenol improves exercise tolerance, hemodynamics and survival in PPH, although its mechanisms of action remain unclear.[6–8,100,101] The absence of an acute response to epoprostenol does not preclude long-term benefit, which appears to be due to the

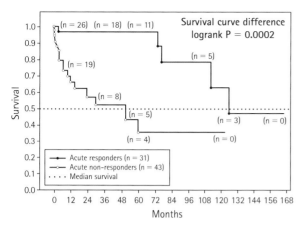

Figure 19.9 *Kaplan–Meier survival curves comparing survival on conventional therapy in responders versus non-responders: 1-, 3- and 5-year survival probabilities for 31 responders were 97%, 97% and 97%, respectively, compared with 66%, 52% and 35%, respectively, for 43 non-responders (P = 0.0002). (Reproduced with permission from Barst RJ, Maislin G, Fishman AP. Vasodilator therapy for primary pulmonary hypertension in children. Circulation 1999;99:1197–208, Lippincott Williams & Wilkins©.)*

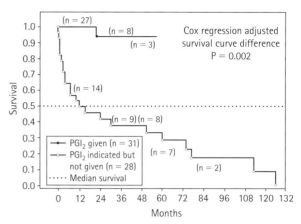

Figure 19.10 *Kaplan–Meier survival curves comparing survival on long-term chronic intravenous epoprostenol with survival of patients for whom epoprostenol was indicated but unavailable: 1-, 2, 3- and 4-year survival probabilities for the prostacyclin (PGI₂) group were 100%, 94%, 94% and 94%, respectively, compared with 50%, 43%, 38% and 38%, respectively, for patients not treated with epoprostenol (P = 0.002). (Reproduced with permission from Barst RJ, Maislin G, Fishman AP. Vasodilator therapy for primary pulmonary hypertension in children. Circulation 1999;99:1197–208, Lippincott Williams & Wilkins©.)*

antiproliferative effects of the drug (Figure 19.10).[94] The optimal dose of intravenous epoprostenol in children is unclear: similar to adult patients, we initiate epoprostenol in children at 2 ng/kg·min and increase the dose fairly rapidly during the first several months and more slowly once the child's condition has stabilized. While a typical adult patient's dose at 1 year is approximately 20–40 ng/kg·min, the average dose at 1 year in children, particularly young children, is closer to 50–80 ng/kg·min.

Prostacyclin analogues

BERAPROST

Beraprost sodium is an oral prostacyclin analogue that is chemically stable with a substantially longer half-life than epoprostenol ($t_{1/2}$ 1.11 ± 0.1 hour; peak plasma level is obtained within 2 hours, t_{max}: 1.42 ± 0.15 hours). The potency of beraprost is approximately 50% of epoprostenol. Uncontrolled studies suggest that beraprost improves hemodynamics and survival in PPH.[102,103] In addition, two double-blind, randomized, placebo-controlled trials demonstrated improved exercise capacity in patients with PPH for 3–6 months, although not at 9–12 months.[104,105] Limited data are available regarding the efficacy in children with PPH.[105]

ILOPROST

Although inhaled iloprost, a stable synthetic analogue of prostacyclin, improves hemodynamics and exercise capacity in adults with pulmonary hypertension,[106–110]

the clinical experience with children is extremely limited. The biological half-life of iloprost is 20–30 minutes.[111] The acute effects of inhaled nitric oxide and aerosolized iloprost are comparable in children with pulmonary hypertension associated with congenital heart defects.[112]

TREPROSTINIL

Treprostinil sodium is a chemically stable prostacyclin analogue that produces similar acute hemodynamic effects to intravenous epoprostenol in PPH, but treprostinil is stable at room temperature and neutral pH and has a half-life of approximately 3 hours when delivered subcutaneously.[113] Treprostinil is administered by continuous infusion subcutaneously using a portable infusion pump. A double-blind, randomized, placebo-controlled trial that included children demonstrated that treprostinil improved exercise capacity, clinical signs and symptoms and hemodynamics in pulmonary arterial hypertension.[114] The risk of central venous line infection is eliminated with treprostinil therapy. Although no serious adverse events related to treprostinil or its delivery system have been reported, side effects with this therapeutic modality are common and include pain at the infusion site.[115]

Endothelin receptor antagonists

Endothelin-1 is one of the most potent vasoconstrictors identified to date[116] and has been implicated in the pathogenesis of PPH, providing the rationale for targeting endothelin as an approach to treatment of this disease. Plasma endothelin-1 levels are increased in PPH and correlate inversely with prognosis.[117] There are at least two different receptor subtypes: ET_A receptors are localized on smooth muscle cells and mediate vasoconstriction and proliferation; ET_B receptors are found predominantly on the endothelin cells and are associated with endothelium dependent vasorelaxation through the release of vasodilators, e.g. prostacyclin and nitric oxide, clearance of endothelin, vasoconstriction (on smooth muscle cells) and bronchoconstriction (Figure 19.11). The oral combined ET_A and ET_B receptor antagonist bosentan improves exercise capacity, quality of life, as well as cardiopulmonary hemodynamics in PPH.[118,119] Although these studies were primarily performed with adult patients, the experience with bosentan in children is similar.[120] The oral selective ET_A receptor antagonist sitaxsentan also appears to improve exercise capacity and cardiopulmonary hemodynamics in PPH.[121] Similar to the bosentan experience, the studies with sitaxsentan were mostly carried out with adult patients,[121,122] although improvement appears to occur also with sitaxsentan in childern.[121,122]

Nitric oxide

Nitric oxide (NO) activates guanylate cyclase in pulmonary vascular smooth muscle and exerts selective vasodilation in the pulmonary circulation (Figure 19.12).[123] Inhaled NO is a safe and effective treatment for persistent pulmonary hypertension of the newborn.[124,125] Although there is considerable experience with the use of inhaled nitric oxide as a short-term treatment for pulmonary arterial hypertension in a variety of clinical situations, the role of inhaled nitric oxide as a chronic therapy for PPH remains under clinical investigation.[126]

Phosphodiesterase inhibitors

The pulmonary vascular effects of sildenafil, a type 5 phosphodiesterase inhibitor, are also being studied.[127,128] The rationale is that raising cyclic GMP would potentiate NO-mediated pulmonary vasodilatation and facilitate withdrawal of nitric oxide, which often results in a precipitous rise in pulmonary arterial pressure. Clinical trials are underway with particular attention paid to the potential toxicity in the pediatric population.

Elastase inhibitors

Rabinovitch and colleagues have suggested that increased activity of an elastolytic enzyme may be important in the pathophysiology of pulmonary vascular disease.[129,130] A cause and effect relationship between elastase and

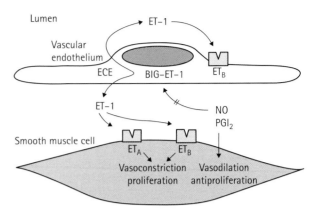

Figure 19.11 *Endothelin system in vascular disease. BIG-ET-1, proendothelin-1; ECE, endothelin-converting enzyme; ET-1, endothelin-1; NO, nitric oxide; PGI$_2$, prostacyclin. [Reproduced with permission from Elsevier Science (The Lancet 2001;358: 1113–14).]*

pulmonary vascular disease is supported by studies reporting the reversal of advanced pulmonary vascular disease induced by monocrotaline in rats. Part of the novelty of these observations is the complete regression in the treatment group even though treatment was administered in advanced disease. However, the monocrotaline model does not exhibit identical vascular pathology to the human disease.

Oxygen

Some children demonstrate modest systemic arterial oxygen desaturation with sleep, which appears to result from mild hypoventilation.[79] During these episodes, children may experience severe dyspnea, syncope and/or hypoxic seizures. Desaturation during sleep usually occurs during the early morning hours and can be eliminated by using supplemental oxygen. We also recommend that children have supplemental oxygen available at home for emergency use, even if they do not use it on a routine basis. Children should also be treated with supplemental oxygen during any significant upper respiratory tract infection if complicated by systemic arterial oxygen desaturation. Treatment in a hospital setting should be considered if more than mild oxygen desaturation occurs. When supplemental oxygen is administered to children with desaturation caused by right-to-left shunting through a patent foramen ovale, arterial oxygen saturation does not usually improve. Although survival was improved with the use of supplemental oxygen in a small study of children with Eisenmenger syndrome,[131] more recently, Sandoval et al. did not see any survival benefit in patients with Eisenmenger syndrome.[132] However, Sandoval has shown that patients with Eisenmenger syndrome do desaturate more at night, which appears to be due to change in body position with sleep.[132] Supplemental oxygen may

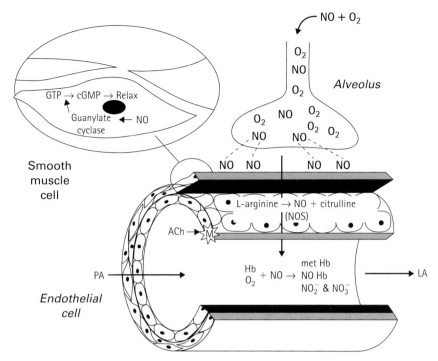

Figure 19.12 *Nitric oxide (NO) is endogenously formed from L-arginine after acetylcholine (ACh) binds to muscarinic receptors (M) on the intact endothelium and stimulates endothelial nitric oxide synthase (NOS). NO exists as a gas and can be delivered to alveoli. It diffuses across alveolar membrane to closely adjacent vessels. Constricted pulmonary vessels dilate as the result of increased intracellular cGMP production in smooth muscle cells. Nitric oxide is immediately inactivated by hemoglobin with the formation of methemoglobin (met Hb), nitrosylhemoglobin (NO Hb), nitrates (NO$_3^-$) and nitrites (NO$_2^-$), limiting its activity to the pulmonary circulation. LA, left atrium; PA, pulmonary artery. (Reprinted from* Prog Pediatr Cardiol, *12, Wessel DL, Current and future strategies in the treatment of childhood pulmonary hypertension, 289–318, © (2001), with permission from Elsevier Science.)*

also reduce polycythemia in children with right-to-left shunting via a patent foramen ovale. Similar to the experience with adults, some children experience arterial oxygen desaturation with exercise and may benefit from ambulatory supplemental oxygen. In addition, children with resting hypoxemia due to severe right ventricular failure should also be treated with continuous oxygen.

Additional pharmacotherapy

Although controversy persists regarding the value of digitalis in pulmonary hypertension.[133] we believe that children with right-sided heart failure may benefit from this drug. Diuretic therapy should be initiated cautiously, since children appear to be particularly dependent on preload to maintain optimal cardiac output.

In contrast to healthy children, in whom atrial systole is responsible for approximately 25% of the cardiac output, atrial systole in children with PPH often contributes as much as 70% of the cardiac output. Accordingly, atrial flutter or fibrillation may precipitate an abrupt decrease in cardiac output and clinical deterioration, and should be treated aggressively. We also recommend treating

significant supraventricular tachycardias or frequent episodes of non-sustained ventricular tachycardia and complex ventricular arrhythmias.

There are no studies on the usefulness of intermittent or continuous treatment with inotropic agents. We occasionally add dobutamine to continuous intravenous epoprostenol for inotropic support when severe right ventricular dysfunction develops in a child that is awaiting transplantation. By augmenting cardiac output during periods of increased metabolic demands, short-term inotropic support during acute pulmonary hypertensive crises may also be helpful.

Oral and sublingual nitrates have been used to treat children PPH, but experience with these agents is limited. Children who complain of chest discomfort that is responsive to sublingual nitroglycerin should be treated with chronic oral or sublingual nitrates.

Atrial septostomy

Children with recurrent syncope or severe right heart failure have a very poor prognosis.[4,134] Exercise-induced syncope is caused by systemic vasodilatation in the face of an inability to augment cardiac output to maintain cerebral perfusion pressure. Children with PPH and recurrent syncope are unable to adequately shunt through a patent foramen ovale.[135] If right-to-left shunting through an interatrial communication is present, cardiac output can be maintained or increased as needed. In addition, right-to-left shunting at the atrial level alleviates signs and symptoms of right heart failure by decompression of the right heart chambers. Improved survival has been reported in PPH when the foramen ovale is patent.[136] Although the worldwide experience with septostomy exceeds 100 patients, this procedure should still be considered investigational. Palliation of symptoms with atrial septostomy has been reported in several series.[137–141] In our experience, patients with PPH who have recurrent syncope and/or right heart failure significantly improve clinically and hemodynamically following atrial septostomy. Although systemic arterial oxygen desaturation decreases, cardiac output and oxygen delivery improve through right-to-left shunting at the atrial level. While atrial septostomy does not alter the underlying disease process, it may improve quality of life and represent an alternative for selected patients. Our indications for septostomy include: recurrent syncope and/or right ventricular failure despite maximal medical therapy, and as a bridge to transplantation when deterioration occurs despite maximal medical therapy (Figure 19.13). Closure of the septal defect can be performed at the time of transplantation.

Transplantation

Combined heart and lung, single lung, and bilateral lung transplantation have been performed successfully in children and adults with PPH. The 5-year survival is 40–45%.[142] The current 2-year and 5-year survival rates among pediatric lung and heart/lung recipients are 65% and 40%, respectively.[143]

The 'appropriate time' for evaluation and listing for transplantation remains problematic. Ideally, children should be listed when their probability of 2-year survival without transplantation is 50%. The availability of donor organs influences the choice of procedure, particularly in children. Early referral to a center with expertise in pediatric lung and heart/lung transplantation may decrease pretransplantation mortality and allow families to have adequate time to make an informed and thoughtful choice about this therapy. Although living related donor transplantation has been successful, experience with this procedure is limited.[144,145]

CONCLUSIONS

Although recent therapeutic advances appear to have significantly improved its natural history, PPH in children remains a devastating disease. Our experience demonstrates that chronic vasodilator therapy with calcium channel blockade in 'acute responders' to vasodilator testing, and continuous intravenous epoprostenol in 'non-responders' (as well as in 'responders' who fail to improve on calcium channel blockade) is at least as effective in children as in adults with respect to increasing survival, improving hemodynamics, and relieving symptoms.[1–3,5–8] Currently, in children[45,94] as well as in adults,[5] the selection of the vasoactive drug for long-term therapy is determined by short-term testing; those who manifest pulmonary vasodilatation in response to short-term testing can be treated with calcium channel blockade[45,94] and non-responders with long-term intravenous epoprostenol. However, in contrast to the published experience in adults,[5] although less than 20–25% of adults are responders, more than 40% of children are responders.[94] Accordingly, more children than adults can be successfully treated with chronic oral calcium channel blockade. Indeed, the acute response in children is age dependent (Figure 19.8). Although we developed a predictive model of response to acute vasodilator testing (see Appendix),[94] this model is not intended to serve as a substitute for acute vasodilator testing.

As previous studies have shown with adult PPH patients, our experience also demonstrates that right atrial pressure, cardiac index and pulmonary artery pressure are significant parameters of survival on conventional therapy, including chronic oral calcium channel blockade if indicated, i.e. not including children on chronic intravenous epoprostenol. In addition, although not shown to be survival parameters in adult patients, pulmonary vascular resistance, mixed venous saturation, response to acute vasodilator testing, age, and sex are also related to survival in children. When we re-evaluated these parameters in a multivariable model and included all factors, only age, male sex, acute response, and mixed venous saturation remained significant.[94] Furthermore, although long-term anticoagulation has been reported to improve survival in adult patients, we have been unable to determine whether anticoagulation is also an independent survival parameter in children since our experience has been with most children on an oral anticoagulant unless there was a contraindication.[94]

This is a pivotal time for the treatment of PPH as there are a number of very promising new drugs on the horizon, e.g. prostacyclin analogues, endothelin receptor antagonists, type 5 phosphodiesterase inhibitors to increase or maintain cyclic GMP activity (e.g. sildenafil), and inhaled NO. Based on distinct mechanisms of action of these various agents, a role for combination therapy may further improve the efficacy of a child's medical regimen. Furthermore, future investigations with other agents, such as type 3/4 phosphodiesterase inhibitors to increase or maintain cyclic AMP activity, substrate loading

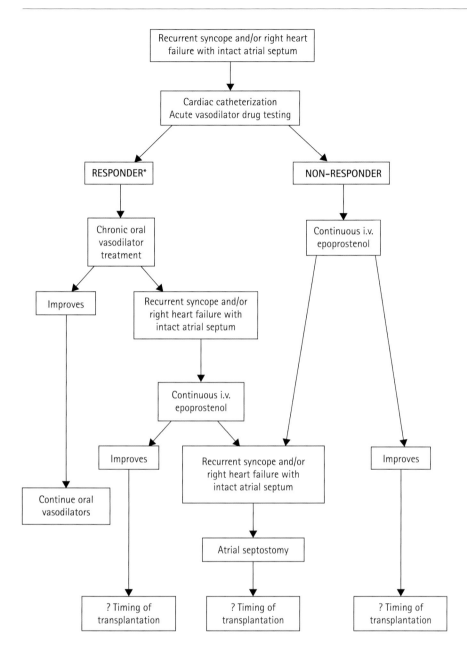

Figure 19.13 *The role of atrial septostomy in the management of primary pulmonary hypertension prior to novel therapeutics. The procedure should be considered after failure of maximal medical therapy. (*Responder to acute vasodilator testing defined as a significant fall in mean pulmonary arterial pressure, i.e. at least 20%, without a fall in the cardiac output.)*

agents (e.g. arginine to increase NO production), as well as consideration of elastase inhibitors, should further improve treatment options for children with PPH. Whether these new agents will, in fact, replace intravenous epoprostenol in selected children remains unknown.

The therapeutic algorithm that we have followed, as shown in Figure 19.7, will hopefully change as we gain more experience with the novel therapeutic agents discussed earlier in this chapter. Although at the present time we now reserve chronic oral calcium channel blockade for children who demonstrate active pulmonary vasoreactivity with acute vasodilator testing, whether some of these newer therapeutic modalities will improve the overall efficacy for these children by combining these agents with chronic oral calcium channel blockade or instead of chronic oral calcium channel blockade alone, will require further investigation. In addition, at the present time, 'non-responders' to acute vasodilator drug testing are started on chronic intravenous epoprostenol. Chronic intravenous epoprostenol is also currently being added to the medical regimen of acute 'responders' who are treated with chronic oral calcium channel blockade in whom hemodynamics fail to improve on long-term calcium channel blockade. Whether we will be able to avoid chronic intravenous epoprostenol in these children and maintain the efficacy we would anticipate with chronic epoprostenol using some of these newer agents also needs further investigation. Thus, in the future, a

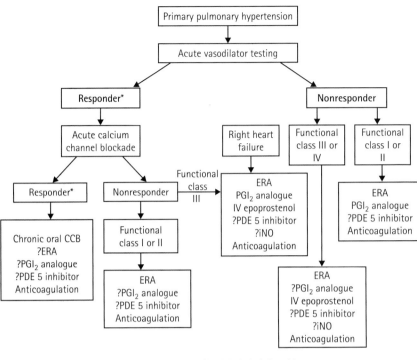

Figure 19.14 *The role of novel therapeutic agents on the treatment algorithm for primary pulmonary hypertension. (*Responder to acute vasodilator testing defined as a significant fall in mean pulmonary arterial pressure, i.e. at least 20%, without a fall in the cardiac output.)*

CCB = Calcium channel blockade
ERA = Endothelin receptor antagonist
PGI$_2$ = Prostacyclin

iNO = Inhaled nitric oxide
PDE 5 = Phosphodiesterase type 5

therapeutic algorithm for children with PPH may look something like that which is presented in Figure 19.14.

At the present time, while chronic intravenous epoprostenol remains the gold standard to treat children who do not respond to acute vasodilator testing or who are refractory to conventional agents such as treatment with chronic calcium channel blockade, chronic intravenous epoprostenol is invasive and not without risk due to its delivery system. In addition, chronic intravenous epoprostenol is a significant emotional burden to the child and his/her family. The recent attempt to compound this medication for delivery by oral, subcutaneous, and inhaled routes is a step in the right direction. However, at the present time it is too early to say if these agents will be as efficacious as chronic intravenous epoprostenol. In addition, the use of endothelin receptor antagonists also appears extremely promising. There will likely be many new developments in the next several years as trials with these novel therapeutic agents are completed.

Future developments in vascular biology will help improve our understanding of its etiology(ies) and pathobiology, as well as provide rationale for more specific medical therapies. We hope that by increasing our understanding of the pathobiology of PPH, one day we will be able to prevent or cure this disease, as opposed to only providing palliative therapy.

KEY POINTS

- The natural history of primary pulmonary hypertension in children is extremely poor, i.e. mean survival less than 1 year after diagnosis, and significantly worse than adult patients (median survival 2.8 years).
- 'Optimal' medical therapy: since the advent of long-term vasodilator/antiproliferative medical therapy, the prognosis for children has significantly improved, i.e. 5-year survival probability at least 60%.
- Current state of the art for medical therapy:
  - Chronic oral calcium channel blockade for children who demonstrate significant acute pulmonary vasoreactivity with vasodilator drug testing. Approximately 40% of children with primary pulmonary hypertension can be treated effectively with oral calcium channel blockade, compared to approximately 20% of adult patients.
  - For children who do not demonstrate significant pulmonary vasoreactivity with acute vasodilator drug testing, despite lack of a

favorable acute response, chronic intravenous epoprostenol is efficacious for these 'non-responders'; unfortunately, serious adverse events may occur due to its delivery system, i.e. central venous line.

- Although these therapies at present only provide palliative support, e.g. improve exercise capacity and hemodynamics as well as quality of life and long-term survival, future developments may allow a cure.
- Medical treatment options: chronic 'optimal' medical regimens are based on risk/benefit considerations for an individual child and, not uncommonly, change over time.
- Future:
  – Clinical investigations with novel therapeutic agents, e.g. prostacyclin analogues, endothelin receptor antagonists, phosphodiesterase inhibitors, inhaled nitric oxide, elastase inhibitors, etc., may further improve the long-term outlook for children with primary pulmonary hypertension.
  – Genetic studies to define the pathophysiological relevance of the *BMPR2* mutations may provide therapeutic pharmacogenetics, e.g. therapy tailored to the genetic findings, including gene therapy.

REFERENCES

1 Sandoval J, Bauerie O, Gomez A *et al.* Primary pulmonary hypertension in children: clinical characterization and survival. *J Am Coll Cardiol* 1995;**25**:466–74.

2 Houde C, Bohn DJ, Freedom RM *et al.* Profile of paediatric patients with pulmonary hypertension judged by responsiveness to vasodilator. *Br Heart J* 1993;**70**:461–8.

3 Clabby ML, Canter CE, Moller JH *et al.* Hemodynamic data and survival in children with pulmonary hypertension. *J Am Coll Cardiol* 1997;**30**:554–60.

◆●4 D'Alonzo GE, Barst RJ, Ayres SM *et al.* Survival in patients with primary pulmonary hypertension: results of a national prospective registry. *Ann Intern Med* 1991;**115**:343–9.

*5 Rich S, Kaufmann E, Levy PS. The effect of high doses of calcium-channel blockers on survival in primary pulmonary hypertension. *N Engl J Med* 1992;**327**:76–81.

●6 Higenbottam TW, Wells F, Wheeldon D *et al.* Treatment of primary pulmonary hypertension with continuous intravenous epoprostenol (prostacyclin). *Lancet* 1984;**i**:1046–7.

*7 Barst RJ, Rubin LJ, McGoon MD *et al.* Survival in primary pulmonary hypertension with long-term continuous intravenous prostacyclin. *Ann Intern Med* 1994;**121**:409–15.

*8 Barst RJ, Rubin LJ, Long WA *et al.* for the Primary Pulmonary Hypertension Study Group. A comparison of continuous intravenous epoprostenol (prostacyclin) with conventional therapy in primary pulmonary hypertension. *N Engl J Med* 1996;**334**:296–301.

●9 Yamaki S, Wagenvoort CA. Comparison of primary plexogenic arteriopathy in adults and children: a morphometric study in 40 patients. *Br Heart J* 1985;**54**:423–34.

●10 Romberg E. Ueber Sklerose der Lungen arterie. *Dtsch Arch Klin Med* 1891;**48**:197–206.

◆11 Rich S (ed.) Primary Pulmonary Hypertension: Executive Summary from the World Symposium – Primary Pulmonary Hypertension 1998. Available from the World Health Organization via the Internet (http://www.who.int/ncd/cvd/pph.html).

12 Grover RF, Vogel JHK, Averill KH *et al.* Pulmonary hypertension. Individual and species variability relative to vascular reactivity. *Am Heart J* 1963;**66**:1–3.

13 Grover RF, Will DH, Reeves JT *et al.* Genetic transmission of susceptibility to hypoxic pulmonary hypertension. *Prog Respir Res* 1975;**9**:112–17.

14 Vogel JHK. Importance of mild hypoxia on abnormal pulmonary vascular beds. *Adv Cardiol* 1970;**5**:159.

15 Vogel JH, McNamara DG, Blount SG, Jr. Role of hypoxia in determining pulmonary vascular resistance in infants with ventricular septal defects. *Am J Cardiol* 1967;**20**:346–9.

16 O'Neill D, Morton R, Kennedy JA. Progressive primary pulmonary hypertension in a patient born at high altitude. *Br Heart J* 1981;**45**:725–8.

●17 Gersony WM, Duc GV, Sinclair JC. 'PPC' syndrome (persistence of the fetal circulation). *Circulation* 1969;**40**(Suppl III):87.

18 Long WA. Persistent pulmonary hypertension of the newborn syndrome. In: Long WA (ed.), *Fetal and neonatal cardiology.* Philadelphia: WB Saunders, 1989;627–55.

◆19 Reeves JT, Groves BM, Turkevich D. The case for treatment of selected patients with primary pulmonary hypertension. *Am Rev Respir Dis.* 1986;**134**:342–6.

20 Heath D, Edwards JE. Configuration of elastic tissue of pulmonary trunk in idiopathic pulmonary hypertension. *Circulation* 1960;**21**:59–62.

21 Roberts WC. The histologic structure of the pulmonary trunk in patients with 'primary' pulmonary hypertension. *Am Heart J* 1963;**65**:230.

22 Bleiden LC, Moller JH. Small ventricular septal defect associated with severe pulmonary hypertension. *Br Heart J* 1984;**52**:117–18.

23 Bisset GS III, Hirschfeld SS. Severe pulmonary hypertension associated with a small ventricular septal defect. *Circulation* 1983;**67**:470–3.

24 Haworth SG. Pulmonary vascular disease in secundum atrial septal defect in childhood. *Am J Cardiol* 1983;**51**:265–72.

25 Morse JH, Barst RJ, Fotino M. Familial pulmonary hypertension: immunogenetic findings in four Caucasian kindreds. *Am Rev Respir Dis* 1992;**145**:787–92.

26 Wagenvoort CA. Misalignment of lung vessels: a syndrome causing persistent neonatal pulmonary hypertension. *Hum Pathol* 1986;**17**:727–30.

27 Boggs S, Harris MC, Hoffman DJ *et al.* Misalignment of pulmonary veins with alveolar capillary dysplasia: affected siblings and variable phenotypic expression. *J Pediatr* 1994;**124**:125–8.

28 Holcomb BW Jr, Loyd JE, Ely EW *et al.* Pulmonary Veno-occlusive disease. A case series and new observations. *Chest* 2000;**118**:1671–9.

29 Davies P, Reid L. Pulmonary veno-occlusive disease in siblings: case reports and morphometric study. *Hum Pathol* 1982;**13**:911–15.

30 Rubin LJ. Primary pulmonary hypertension. *N Engl J Med* 1997;**336**:111–17.

◆●31 Rich S, Dantzker DR, Ayres SM *et al.* Primary pulmonary hypertension: a national prospective study. *Ann Intern Med* 1987;**107**:216–23.

◆●32 Loyd JE, Primm RK, Newman JH. Familial primary pulmonary hypertension: clinical patterns. *Am Rev Respir Dis* 1984;**129**:194–7.

33 Lillienfeld DE, Rubin LJ. Mortality from primary pulmonary hypertension in the United States, 1979–1996. *Chest* 2000;**117**:796–800.

34 Langleben D. Familial primary pulmonary hypertension. *Chest* 1994;**105**:13S–16S.

●35 Deng Z, Morse JH, Slager SL *et al.* Familial primary pulmonary hypertension (gene *PPH1*) is caused by mutations in the bone morphogenetic protein receptor-II gene. *Am J Hum Genet* 2000;**67**:737–44.

●36 Lane KB, Machado RD, the International Consortium *et al.* Heterozygous germline mutation in *BMPR2*, encoding a TGF-B receptor, cause familial primary pulmonary hypertension. *Nat Genet* 2000;**26**:81–4.

37 Loyd JE, Butler MD, Foroud TM *et al.* Genetic anticipation and abnormal gender ratio at birth in familial primary pulmonary hypertension. *Am J Respir Crit Care Med* 1998;**152**:93–7.

◆38 Morse JH, Knowles JA. Genetics of primary pulmonary hypertension. *Prog Pediatr Cardiol* 2001;**12**:271–8.

39 Galloway SM, McNatty KP, Cambridge LM *et al.* Mutations in an oocyte-derived growth factor gene (BMB 15) cause increased ovulation rate and infertility in a dosage-sensitive manner. *Nat Genet* 2000;**25**:279–83.

40 Rich S, Kieras K, Hart K *et al.* Antinuclear antibodies in primary pulmonary hypertension. *J Am Coll Cardiol* 1986;**8**:1307–11.

41 Morse JH, Barst RJ, Fotino M *et al.* Primary pulmonary hypertension: immunogenetic response to HMG proteins and histone. *Clin Exp Immunol* 1996;**106**:389–95.

42 Badesch DB, Wynne KM, Bonvallet S *et al.* Hypothyroidism and primary pulmonary hypertension: an autoimmune pathogenetic link? *Ann Intern Med* 1993;**119**:44–6.

43 Ferris A, Jacobs T, Widlitz AC *et al.* Pulmonary arterial hypertension and thyroid disease. *Chest* 2001;**119**:1980–1.

●44 Wagenvoort CA, Wagenvoort N. Primary pulmonary hypertension. A pathological study of the lung vessels in 156 clinically diagnosed cases. *Circulation* 1970;**42**:1163–84.

*45 Barst RJ. Pharmacologically induced pulmonary vasodilatation in children and young adults with primary pulmonary hypertension. *Chest* 1986;**89**:497–503.

46 Edwards WD, Edwards KE. Clinical primary pulmonary hypertension: three pathologic types. *Circulation* 1977;**56**:884–8.

47 Yamaki S, Wagenvoort CA. Comparison of primary plexogenic arteriopathy in adults and children. *Br Heart J* 1985;**54**:428–34.

48 Rich S, Brundage BH. High dose calcium channel blocking therapy for primary pulmonary hypertension: evidence for long-term reduction in pulmonary arterial pressure and regression of right ventricular hypertrophy. *Circulation* 1987;**76**:135–41.

49 Barst RJ, Stalcup SA, Steeg CN *et al.* Relation of arachidonate metabolites in abnormal control of the pulmonary circulation in a child. *Am Rev Respir Dis* 1985;**131**:171–7.

●50 Christman BW, McPherson CD, Newman JH *et al.* An imbalance between the excretion of thromboxane and prostacyclin metabolites in pulmonary hypertension. *N Engl J Med* 1991;**327**:70–5.

51 Yoshibayashi M, Nishioka K, Nakao K *et al.* Plasma endothelin concentrations in patients with pulmonary hypertension associated with congenital heart defects: evidence for increased production of endothelin in pulmonary circulation. *Circulation* 1991;**84**:2280–5.

●52 Stewart DJ, Levy RD, Cernacek P *et al.* Increased plasma endothelin-1 in pulmonary hypertension: marker or mediator of disease? *Ann Intern Med* 1991;**114**:464–9.

●53 Giaid A. Nitric oxide and endothelin-1 in pulmonary hypertension. *Chest* 1998;**114**:208S–12S.

54 Christman BW. Lipid mediator disregulation in primary pulmonary hypertension. *Chest* 1998;**114**:205S–7S.

●55 Tuder RM, Cool CD, Geraci MW *et al.* Prostacyclin synthase expression is decreased in lungs from patients with severe pulmonary hypertension. *Am J Respir Crit Care Med* 1999;**159**:1925–32.

●56 Giad A, Saleh D. Reduced expression of endothelial nitric oxide synthase in the lungs of patients with pulmonary hypertension. *N Engl J Med* 1995;**333**:214–21.

57 Rabinovitch M, Andrew M, Thom H *et al.* Abnormal endothelial factor VIII associated with pulmonary hypertension and congenital heart defects. *Circulation* 1987;**76**:1043–52.

58 Geggel RL, Carvalho CA, Hoyer LW *et al.* von Willebrand factor abnormalities in primary pulmonary hypertension. *Am Rev Respir Dis* 1987;**135**:294–9.

59 Rosenberg HC, Rabinovitch M. Endothelial injury and vascular reactivity in monocrotaline pulmonary hypertension. *Am J Physiol* 1988;**255**:JH1484–91.

60 Todorovich-Hunter L, Johnson DJ, Ranger P *et al.* Altered elastin and collagen synthesis associated with progressive pulmonary hypertension induced by monocrotaline: a biochemical and ultrastructural study. *Lab Invest* 1988;**58**:184–95.

61 Smith P, Heath D, Yacoub M *et al.* The ultrastructure of plexogenic pulmonary arteriopathy. *J Pathol* 1990;**160**:111–21.

62 Ryan US. The endothelial surface and responses to injury. *Fed Proc* 1986;**45**:101–8.

63 Eisenberg PR, Lucore C, Kaufmann E *et al.* Fibrinopeptide A levels indicative of pulmonary vascular thrombosis in patients with primary pulmonary hypertension. *Circulation* 1990;**82**:841–7.

●64 Fuster V, Steele PM, Edwards WD *et al.* Primary pulmonary hypertension: natural history and the importance of thrombosis. *Circulation* 1984;**70**:580–7.

65 Frank H, Mlczoch J, Huber K *et al.* The effect of anticoagulant therapy in primary and anorectic drug-induced pulmonary hypertension. *Chest* 1997;**112**:714–21.

◆66 Barst RJ. Primary pulmonary hypertension in children. In: Rubin L J, Rich S (eds), *Primary pulmonary hypertension. (Lung biology in health and disease).* New York: Marcel Dekker, 1997;179–225.

67 Gomez-Sanchez MA, Mestre de Juan MJ, Gomez-Pajuelo C *et al.* Pulmonary hypertension due to toxic oil syndrome: a clinicopathologic study. *Chest* 1989;**95**:325–31.

68 Gomez-Sanchez MA, Saene de la Calzada C, Gomez-Pajuelo C *et al.* Clinical and pathologic manifestation of pulmonary vascular disease in the toxic oil syndrome. *J Am Coll Cardiol* 1991;**18**:1539–45.

69 Appelbaum L, Yigla M, Bendayan D *et al.* Primary pulmonary hypertension in Israel: a national survey. *Chest* 2001;**119**:1801–6.

70 Hopkins WE, Ochoa LL, Richardson GW *et al.* Comparison of the hemodynamics and survival of adults with severe primary pulmonary hypertension or Eisenmenger syndrome. *J Heart Lung Transplant* 1996;**15**:100–5.

71 Rhodes J, Barst RJ, Garafano RP *et al.* Hemodynamic correlates of exercise function in patients with primary pulmonary hypertension. *J Am Coll Cardiol* 1991;**18**:1738–44.

72 Wax D, Garafano R, Barst RJ. Effects of chronic infusion of prostacyclin on exercise performance in patients with primary pulmonary hypertension. *Chest* 1999;**116**:914–20.

73 Garofano RP, Barst RJ. Exercise testing in children with primary pulmonary hypertension: a valuable diagnostic tool. *Pediatric Cardiol* 1999;**20**:61–4.

●74 Sun XG, Hansen JE, Oudiz RJ *et al.* Exercise pathophysiology in patients with primary pulmonary hypertension. *Circulation* 2001;**104**:429–35.

75 Rastogi D, Ngai P, Barst RJ, Koumbourlic AC. Lower airway obstruction, bronchial hyperresponsiveness and primary pulmonary hypertension in children. *Pediatr Pulmonol* 2004; **37**:50–5.

76 D'Angelo A, Della Valle P, Crippa L *et al.* Autoimmune protein S deficiency in a boy with severe thromboembolic disease. *N Engl J Med* 1993;**328**:1753–7.

●77 Auger WR, Fedullo PF, Moser KM *et al.* Chronic major-vessel thromboembolic pulmonary artery obstruction: appearance at angiography. *Radiology* 1992;**182**:393–8.

78 Rabinovitch M, Keane JF, Fellows KG *et al.* Quantitative analysis of the pulmonary wedge angiogram in congenital heart defects. *Circulation* 1981;**63**:152–64.

79 Ngai P, Basner RC, Yoney AM *et al.* Nocturnal oxygen desaturation predicts poorer pulmonary hemodynamics in children with primary pulmonary hypertension. *Am J Respir Crit Care Med* 2002;**165**:A99.

80 Boxt LM, Katz J, Kolb T *et al.* Direct quantitation of right and left ventricular volumes with nuclear magnetic resonance imaging in patients with primary pulmonary hypertension. *J Am Coll Cardiol* 1992;**19**:1508–15.

81 Katz J, Whang J, Boxt LM *et al.* MRI estimation of right ventricular mass in normals and in patients with primary pulmonary hypertension. *J Am Coll Cardiol* 1993;**21**:1475–81.

82 Speich R, Jenni R, Oprvil M *et al.* Primary pulmonary hypertension in HIV infection. *Chest* 1991;**100**:1268–71.

83 Lockshin MD. Antiphospholipid antibody syndrome. *JAMA* 1992;**268**:1451–3.

84 Luchi ME, Asherson RA, Lahita RG. Primary idiopathic pulmonary hypertension complicated by pulmonary arterial thrombosis: association with antiphospholipid antibodies. *Arthritis Rheum* 1992;**35**:700–5.

85 McConnell PJ, Toye PA, Hutchins GM. Primary pulmonary hypertension and cirrhosis: are they related? *Am Rev Respir Dis* 1983;**127**:437–41.

86 Hashim SW, Kay HR, Hammond L *et al.* Noncardiac pulmonary edema after cardiopulmonary bypass. *Am J Surg* 1983;**147**:560–4.

87 Liu XY, Nelson D, Grant C *et al.* Molecular detection of a common mutation in coagulation factor V causing thrombosis via hereditary resistance to activated protein C. *Diagn Mol Pathol* 1995;**4**:191–7.

88 Poort SR, Rosendaal FR, Reitsma PH *et al.* A common genetic variation in the 3′-untranslated region of the prothrombin gene is associated with elevated plasma prothrombin levels and an increase in venous thrombosis. *Blood* 1996;**88**:3698–703.

89 Friedman R, Mears JG, Barst RJ. Continuous infusion of prostacyclin normalizes plasma markers of endothelial cell injury and platelet aggregation in primary pulmonary hypertension. *Circulation* 1997;**96**:2782–4.

◆90 Eaton AM, Serota H, Kernodle GW Jr *et al.* Pulmonary hypertension secondary to serum hyperviscosity in a patient with rheumatoid arthritis. *Am J Med* 1987;**82**:1039–45.

91 Pietra GG, Edward WD, Kay JM *et al.* Histopathology of primary pulmonary hypertension: a qualitative and quantitative study of pulmonary blood vessels from 58 patients in the National Heart, Lung, and Blood Institute Primary Pulmonary Hypertension Registry. *Circulation* 1989;**80**:1198–206.

●92 Rubin LJ, Mendoza J, Hood M *et al.* Treatment of primary pulmonary hypertension with continuous intravenous prostacyclin: results of a randomized trial. *Ann Intern Med* 1990;**112**:485–91.

93 DeVries TW, Weening JJ, Roorda RJ. Pulmonary veno-occlusive disease: a case report and a review of therapeutic possibilities. *Eur Respir J* 1991;**4**:1029–32.

●94 Barst RJ, Maislin G, Fishman AP. Vasodilator therapy for primary pulmonary hypertension in children. *Circulation* 1999;**99**:1197–208.

95 Thompson BT, Spence CR, Janssens SP *et al.* Inhibition of hypoxic pulmonary hypertension by heparins of differing antiproliferative potency. *Am J Respir Crit Care Med* 1994;**149**:1512–17.

96 Benitz WE, Lesser DS, Coulson JC *et al.* Heparin inhibits proliferation of fetal vascular smooth muscle cells in the absence of platelet derived growth factor. *J Cell Physiol* 1986;**127**:1–7.

97 Permutt S, Riley RL. Hemodynamics of collapsible vessels with tone: the vascular waterfall. *J Appl Physiol* 1963;**18**:924–32.

98 Maseri A, Caldini P, Howard P *et al.* Determinants of pulmonary vascular volume-recruitment versus distensibility. *Circ Res* 1972;**31**:218–28.

99 Rich S, D'Alonzo GE, Dantzker DR *et al.* Magnitude and implications of spontaneous hemodynamic variability in

primary pulmonary hypertension. *Am J Cardiol* 1985;**55**:159–63.

100 Shapiro SM, Oudiz RJ, Cao T *et al.* Primary pulmonary hypertension: improved long-term effects and survival with continuous intravenous epoprostenol infusion. *J Am Coll Cardiol* 1997;**30**:343–9.

101 McLaughlin VV, Genthner DE, Panella MM *et al.* Reduction in pulmonary vascular resistance with long-term epoprostenol (prostacyclin) therapy in primary pulmonary hypertension. *N Engl J Med* 1998;**338**:272–7.

102 Saji T, Ozawa Y, Ishikiata T *et al.* Short-term hemodynamic effect of a new oral prostacyclin analogue, beraprost in primary and secondary pulmonary hypertension. *Am J Cardiol* 1996;**78**:244–7.

103 Nagaya N, Uematsu M, Okano Y *et al.* Effect of orally active prostacyclin analogue on survival of outpatients with primary pulmonary hypertension. *J Am Coll Cardiol* 1999;**34**:1188–92.

104 Galie N, Humbert M, Vachiery JL *et al.* Arterial Pulmonary Hypertension and Beraprost European (ALPHABET) Study Group. Effects of beraprost sodium, an oral prostacyclin analogue, in patients with pulmonary arterial hypertension: a randomized, double-blind, placebo-controlled trial. *J Am Coll Cardiol* 2002;**39**:1496–502.

105 Barst RJ, McGoon M, McLaughlin V *et al.* for the Beraprost Study Group. Beraprost therapy for pulmonary arterial hypertension. *J Am Coll Cardiol* 2003;**41**:2119–25.

106 Hoeper MM, Schwarze M, Ehlerding S *et al.* Long-term treatment of primary pulmonary hypertension with aerosolized iloprost, a prostacyclin analogy. *N Engl J Med* 2000;**342**:1866–70.

107 Olschewski H, Ghofrani HA, Schmehl T *et al.* Inhaled iloprost to treat severe pulmonary hypertension. An uncontrolled trial. German PPH Study Group. *Ann Intern Med* 2000;**132**:435–43.

108 Higgenbottam TW, Butt AY, Dinh-Xuan AT *et al.* Treatment of pulmonary hypertension with the continuous infusion of a prostacyclin analogue, iloprost. *Heart* 1998;**79**:175–9.

109 Nikkho S, Seeger W, Baumgartner R *et al.* One-year observation of iloprost inhalation therapy in patients with pulmonary hypertension. *Eur Respir J* 2001;**16**:324.

110 Olschewski H, Simonneau G, Galie N *et al.* Aerosolized Iloprost Randomized Study Group. Inhaled iloprost for severe pulmonary hypertension. *N Engl J Med* 2002; **347**:322–9.

111 Skuballa W, Raduchel B, Borbruggen H. Chemistry of stable prostacyclin analogues: synthesis of iloprost. In: Gryglewski RS, Stock G (eds), *Prostacyclin and its stable analogue iloprost*. Berlin/Heidelberg: Springer, 1987;17–24.

112 Rimensberger PC, Spahr-Schoepfer I, Berner M *et al.* Inhaled NO *versus* aerosolized iloprost I secondary pulmonary hypertension in children with congenital heart disease. Vasodilator capacity and cellular mechanisms. *Circulation* 2001;**103**:544–8.

113 Gaine SP, Barst RJ, Rich S *et al.* Acute hemodynamic effects of subcutaneous UT-15 in primary pulmonary hypertension. *Am J Respir Crit Care Med* 1999;**159**:A161.

114 Barst RJ, Simonneau G, Rich S *et al.* for the Uniprost PAH Study Group. Efficacy and safety of chronic subcutaneous infusion of UT-15 (Uniprost) in pulmonary arterial hypertension (PAH). *Circulation* 2000;**102**(II):100–1.

115 Barst RJ, Horn EM, Widlitz AC *et al.* Efficacy of long-term subcutaneous infusion of UT-15 in primary pulmonary hypertension. *Eur Heart J* 2000;**21**(Suppl):315.

●116 Yanagisawa M, Kurihara H, Kimura S *et al.* A novel potent vasoconstrictor peptide produced by vascular endothelial cells. *Nature* 1998;**332**:411–15.

117 Galié N, Grigoni F, Bacchi-Reggiani L *et al.* Relation of endothelin-1 to survival in patients with primary pulmonary hypertension. *Eur J Clin Invest* 1996;**26**(Suppl 1):273.

●118 Channick RN, Rubin LJ, Simonneau G *et al.* Effects of the dual endothelin-receptor antagonist bosentan in patients with pulmonary hypertension: a randomised placebo-controlled study. *Lancet* 2001;**358**:1119–23.

●119 Rubin LJ, Badesch DB, Barst RJ *et al.* on behalf of the BREATHE-1 Study Group. Bosentan in patients with pulmonary arterial hypertension: BREATHE-1, a multicenter, randomized, placebo-controlled study. *N Engl J Med* 2002;**346**:896–903.

120 Barst R, Ivy D, Widlitz AW *et al.* Pharmacokinetics and safety of bosentan, an oral dual endothelin receptor antagonist in children with pulmonary arterial hypertension: BREATHE 3. *Eur Heart J* 2002;**23**(s):489.

121 Barst R, Langleben D, Frost A *et al.* Sitaxsentan therapy for pulmonary arterial hypertension. *Am J Respir Crit Care Med* 2004;**169**:441–7.

122 Barst RJ, Rich S, Widlitz A *et al.* Clinical efficacy of sitaxsentan, an endothelin a receptor antagonist, in patients with pulmonary arterial hypertension: open label pilot study. *Chest* 2002;**121**:1860–8.

123 Frostell C, Fratacci MD, Wain JC *et al.* Inhaled nitric oxide. A selective pulmonary vasodilator reversing hypoxic pulmonary vasoconstriction. *Circulation* 1991;**83**:2038–47.

124 The Neonatal Inhaled Nitric Oxide Study Group. Inhaled nitric oxide in full-term and nearly full-term infants with hypoxic respiratory failure. *N Engl J Med* 1997;**336**:597–604. [Erratum, *N Engl J Med* 1997;**337**:434].

125 Clark RH, Kueser TJ, Walker MW *et al.* Low-dose nitric oxide therapy for persistent pulmonary hypertension of the newborn. *N Engl J Med* 2000;**342**:469–74.

126 Channick RN, Newhart JW, Johnson FW *et al.* Pulsed delivery of inhaled nitric oxide to patients with primary pulmonary hypertension: an ambulatory delivery system and initial clinical tests. *Chest* 1996;**109**:1545–9.

127 Abrams D, Schulze-Neick I, Magee AG. Sildenafil is a pulmonary vasodilator in childhood primary pulmonary hypertension. *Heart* 2000;**84**:E4.

128 Prasad S, Wilkinson J, Gatzoulis M. Sildenafil in primary pulmonary hypertension. *N Engl J Med* 2000;**343**:1342.

129 Cowan KN, Heilbut A, Humpl T *et al.* Complete reversal of fatal pulmonary hypertension in rats by a serine elastase inhibitor. *Nat Med* 2000;**6**:698–702.

130 Cowan KN, Jones PL, Rabinovitch M. Elastase and matrix metalloproteinase inhibitors induce regression, and tenascin-C antisense prevents progression, of vascular disease. *J Clin Invest* 2000;**105**:21–34.

131 Sandoval J, Aguirre JS, Pulido T *et al.* Nocturnal oxygen therapy in patients with the Eisenmenger syndrome. *Am J Respir Crit Care Med* 2001;**164**:1682–7.

132 Sandoval J, Alvarado P, Martinez-Guerra ML *et al.* Effect of body position changes on pulmonary gas exchange in

Eisenmenger's syndrome. *Am J Respir Crit Care Med* 1999;**159**:1070–3.

133 Rich S, Seidlitz M, Dodin E *et al.* The short-term effects of digoxin in patients with right ventricular dysfunction from pulmonary hypertension. *Chest* 1998;**114**:787–92.

134 Thilenius OG, Nadas AS, Jockin H. Primary pulmonary vascular obstruction in children. *Pediatrics* 1965;**36**:75–87.

135 Thoele DG, Barst RJ, Gersony WM. Physiologic-based management of primary pulmonary hypertension in children and young adults. *J Am Coll Cardiol* 1990;**15**:241A.

136 Rozkovec A, Montanes P, Oakley CM. Factors that influence the outcome of primary pulmonary hypertension. *Br Heart J* 1986;**55**:449–58.

137 Rich S, Lam W. Atrial septostomy as palliative therapy for refractory primary pulmonary hypertension. *Am J Cardiol* 1983;**51**:1560–1.

138 Nihill MR, O'Laughlin MP, Mullins CE. Blade balloon atrial septostomy is effective palliation for terminal cor pulmonary. [Abstract] *Am J Cardiol* 1987;**60**(Suppl):1.

139 Hausknecht MJ, Sims RE, Nihill MR *et al.* Successful palliation of primary pulmonary hypertension by atrial septostomy. *Am J Cardiol* 1990;**65**:1045–6.

∗140 Kerstein D, Levy PS, Hsu DT *et al.* Blade balloon atrial septostomy improves survival in patients with severe primary pulmonary hypertension. *Circulation* 1995;**91**:2028–35.

◆141 Sandoval J, Gaspar J, Pulido T *et al.* Graded balloon dilation atrial septostomy in severe primary pulmonary hypertension. *J Am Coll Cardiol* 1998; **32**:297–304.

142 Pasque MK, Kaiser LR, Dresler CM *et al.* Single lung transplantation for pulmonary hypertension: technical aspects and immediate hemodynamic results. *J Thorac Cardiovasc Surg* 1992;**103**:475–82.

143 Aeba R, Griffith BP, Hardesty RL. Isolated lung transplantation for patients with Eisenmenger's syndrome. *Circulation* 1993;**88**:452–5.

144 Spray TL, Bridges ND. Lung transplantation for pediatric pulmonary hypertension. *Prog Pediatr Cardiol* 2001;**12**:319–25.

●145 Starnes VA, Brown ML, Schenkel FA *et al.* Experience with living-donor lobar transplantation for indications other than cystic fibrosis. *J Thorac Cardiovasc Surg* 1997;**114**:917–21.

APPENDIX

Prediction model of response to short–term vasodilator testing[94]

Multiple logistic regression analysis was used to develop a prediction equation for the likelihood of acute response based on age as well as hemodynamics at initial evaluation. Candidate hemodynamic variables included mean pulmonary artery pressure (mPAP), mean right atrial pressure (mRAP), cardiac index and mixed venous oxygen saturation. Both linear and non-linear relationships were considered. The best model included linear and quadratic functions of age, mPAP and mRAP. The probability of acute response is obtained using Equation 19.1 to compute a value for x and then using x in Equation 19.2 to compute the probability of acute response. For example, a 5-year-old patient with mPAP of 57 mmHg and mRAP of 4 mmHg has a predicted probability of 0.85 of a positive response to short-term vasodilator drug testing. By contrast, an 8-year-old patient with mPAP of 72 mmHg and mRAP of 5 mmHg has only an acute response predicted probability of 0.30.

$$x = 9.3046 + 0.1566 \times \text{age} - 0.0326 \times \text{age}^2 - 0.2611$$
$$\times \text{mPAP} + 0.0014 \times \text{mPAP}^2 + 0.7919 \times \text{mRAP}$$
$$- 0.0700 \times \text{mRAP}^2 \tag{19.1}$$

$$\text{Probability of response} = \frac{e^x}{(1 + e^x)} \tag{19.2}$$

Persistent pulmonary hypertension of the newborn: strategies in clinical management

STEVEN H ABMAN AND JOHN P KINSELLA

INTRODUCTION

Postnatal survival is dependent upon the ability of the fetal cardiopulmonary system to respond successfully to the sudden and harsh demands of neonatal life. Challenges to the lung at birth include the need for rapid absorption of fetal lung liquid, establishment of an air/liquid interface, initiation of spontaneous breathing with rhythmic ventilation, and closure of 'fetal vascular channels'.[1] Perhaps the most dramatic events involve the pulmonary circulation, which must undergo a marked fall from its high-resistance state *in utero* to becoming a low-resistance vasculature within minutes after delivery. This postnatal fall in pulmonary vascular resistance (PVR) allows for the eightfold increase in pulmonary blood flow that allows the lung to become an organ for gas exchange. Several mechanisms contribute to the normal fall in PVR at birth. These include increased oxygen tension, ventilation, shear stress and others.[2–5] Birth-related stimuli cause vasodilation through changes in the production of vasoactive products, including increased release of potent vasodilators, including nitric oxide (NO) and prostacyclin (PGI_2), and decreased activity of endogenous vasoconstrictors, such as endothelin-1 (ET-1)[6–13] (Table 20.1). Within minutes of this vasodilator response, high pulmonary blood flow abruptly increases shear stress and distends the vasculature, causing a 'structural reorganization' of the vascular wall, which includes flattening of the endothelium and thinning of smooth muscle cells and matrix.[14,15] Thus, the ability to accommodate this marked rise in blood flow requires rapid functional and structural adaptations to ensure the normal postnatal fall in PVR.

Some infants fail to achieve or sustain the normal decrease in PVR at birth, leading to severe respiratory distress and hypoxemia, which is referred to as persistent pulmonary hypertension of the newborn (PPHN). It is a major clinical problem, contributing significantly to high morbidity and mortality in both full-term and premature neonates.[16–19] Newborns with PPHN are at risk for severe asphyxia and its complications, including death, neurological injury and other problems. This chapter briefly reviews the normal developmental physiology of the pulmonary circulation, mechanisms underlying the pathogenesis and pathophysiology of PPHN, and clinical strategies related to the evaluation and treatment of newborns with severe PPHN.

CLINICAL DEFINITION AND INCIDENCE

The first reports of PPHN described term newborns with profound hypoxemia who lacked radiographic evidence of parenchymal lung disease and echocardiographic evidence of structural cardiac disease.[16–18,20] In these patients, hypoxemia was caused by marked elevations of PVR leading to right-to-left extrapulmonary shunting of blood

Table 20.1 *Disorders associated with neonatal pulmonary hypertension*

Pulmonary
Meconium aspiration syndrome
Respiratory distress syndrome (term and preterm newborns)
Lung hypoplasia – primary
Congenital diaphragmatic hernia
Pneumonia/sepsis
Idiopathic
Transient tachypnea of the newborn
Alveolar-capillary dysplasia
Associated abnormalities in lung development:
 – Congenital lobar emphysema (rare association)
 – Cystic adenomatoid malformation (rare association)
 – Idiopathic, with impaired distal alveolarization
 – Others

Cardiovascular
Myocardial dysfunction (asphyxia; infection; stress)
Structural cardiac diseases;
 – Mitral stenosis, cor triatriatum
 – Endocardial fibroelastosis
 – Pompe's disease
 – Aortic atresia, coarctation of the aorta, interrupted
  aortic arch
 – Transposition of the great vessels
 – Ebstein's anomaly, tricuspid atresia
Hepatic arteriovenous malformations (AVMs)
Cerebral AVMs
Total anomalous pulmonary venous return
Pulmonary vein stenosis (isolated)
Pulmonary atresia

Associations with other diseases
Neuromuscular disease
Metabolic disease
Polycythemia
Thrombocytopenia
Maternal drug use or smoking

across the patent ductus arteriosus (DA) or foramen ovale (FO) during the early postnatal period. Due to the persistence of high PVR and blood flow through these 'fetal shunts', the term 'persistent fetal circulation' was originally used to describe this group of patients.[16] Consequently, it was recognized that this physiological pattern can complicate the clinical course of neonates with diverse causes of hypoxemic respiratory failure. As a result, PPHN has been considered as a **syndrome**, and is currently applied more broadly to include neonates that have a similar physiology in association with different cardiopulmonary disorders, such as meconium aspiration, sepsis, pneumonia, asphyxia, congenital diaphragmatic hernia, respiratory distress syndrome (RDS), and others[16,17,20–23] (Table 20.2). Striking differences exist between these conditions, and mechanisms that contribute to high PVR can vary between these diseases. However, these disorders are included in the syndrome of PPHN because of common

pathophysiological features, including sustained elevation of PVR leading to hypoxemia due to right-to-left extrapulmonary shunting of blood flow across the ductus arteriosus or foramen ovale. In many clinical settings, hypoxemic respiratory failure in term newborns is often presumed to be associated with PPHN-type physiology; however, hypoxemic term newborns can lack echocardiographic findings of extrapulmonary shunting across the patent DA or patent FO.[24] Thus, PPHN should be reserved to neonates in whom **extrapulmonary shunting** contributes to hypoxemia and impaired cardiopulmonary function. Recent estimates suggest an incidence for PPHN of 1.9/1000 live births, or an estimated 7400 cases/year.[23,25]

ETIOLOGY – EXPERIMENTAL AND CLINICAL STUDIES

Diseases associated with PPHN are often classified within one of three categories:

- **maladaptation**: vessels are presumably of normal structural but have abnormal vasoreactivity;
- **excessive muscularization**: increased smooth muscle cell thickness and increased distal extension of muscle to vessels that are usually non-muscular;
- **underdevelopment**: lung hypoplasia associated with decreased pulmonary artery number.[26,27]

This designation is imprecise, however, and high PVR in most patients likely involve overlapping changes among these categories. For example, neonates with congenital diaphragmatic hernia (CDH) are primarily classified as having vascular 'underdevelopment' due to lung hypoplasia, yet lung histology of fatal cases typically shows marked muscularization of pulmonary arteries and clinically these patients can respond to vasodilator therapy. Similarly, neonates with meconium aspiration often have clinical evidence of altered vasoreactivity, but often have muscularization at autopsy.[28]

Autopsy studies of the lungs of newborns with fatal PPHN have revealed severe hypertensive structural remodeling even in newborns who die shortly after birth, suggesting that many cases of severe disease are associated with **chronic intrauterine stress**. However, the exact intrauterine events that alter pulmonary vascular reactivity and structure are poorly understood. Epidemiological studies have demonstrated strong associations between PPHN and maternal smoking and ingestion of cold remedies that include aspirin or other non-steroidal anti-inflammatory products.[29] Since these agents can induce partial constriction of the DA, it is possible that pulmonary hypertension due to DA narrowing contributes to PPHN (see below).[30–32] Other perinatal stresses, including placenta previa and abruption, and asymmetric growth

Table 20.2 *Factors that modulate pulmonary vascular resistance (PVR) in the neonatal lung*

Lowers PVR	Inreases PVR
Endogenous mediators and mechanisms	Endogenous mediators and mechanisms
Oxygen	Hypoxia
Nitric oxide	Acidosis
PGI_2, E_2, D_2	Endothelin-1
Adenosine, ATP, magnesium	Leukotrienes
Bradykinin	Thromboxanes
Atrial natriuretic factor	Platelet activating factor
Alkalosis	Ca^{2+} channel activation
K^+ channel activation	α-Adrenergic stimulation
Histamine	$PGF_{2\alpha}$
Vagal nerve stimulation	Mechanical factors
Acetylcholine	Overinflation or underinflation
β-Adrenergic stimulation	Excessive muscularization, vascular remodeling
Mechanical factors	Altered mechanical properties of smooth muscle
Lung inflation	Pulmonary hypoplasia
Vascular cell structural changes	Alveolar-capillary dysplasia
Interstitial fluid and pressure changes	Pulmonary thromboemboli
Shear stress	Main pulmonary artery distension
	Ventricular dysfunction, venous hypertension

ATP, Adenosine triphosphate; PGF_2, prostagladin F_{2a}; PGI_2, E_2, D_2, prostaglandins I_2, E_2, D_2.
Reproduced with permission from Kinsella JP, Abman SH. Recent developments in the pathophysiology and treatment of PPHN. *J Pediatr* 1995;**126**:853–64.

restriction, are associated with PPHN;[33] however, most neonates exposed to these prenatal stresses do not develop PPHN. Circulating levels of L-arginine, the substrate for NO, are decreased in some newborns with PPHN, suggesting that impaired NO production may contribute to the pathophysiology of PPHN, as observed in experimental studies.[34–36] It is possible that genetic factors increase susceptibility for pulmonary hypertension. A recent study reported strong links between PPHN and polymorphisms of the carbamoyl phosphate synthase gene.[36] However, the importance of this finding is uncertain, and further work is needed in this area. Studies of adults with idiopathic primary pulmonary hypertension have identified abnormalities of bone morphogenetic protein receptor genes;[37] whether polymorphisms of genes for the BMP or TGF-β receptors, other critical growth factors, vasoactive substances or other products increase the risk for some newborns to develop PPHN is unknown.

Several experimental models have been studied to explore the pathogenesis and pathophysiology of PPHN. Such models have included exposure to acute or chronic hypoxia after birth, chronic hypoxia *in utero*, placement of meconium into the airways of neonatal animals, sepsis and others. Although each model demonstrates interesting physiological changes that may be especially relevant to particular clinical settings, most studies examine only brief changes in the pulmonary circulation, and mechanisms underlying altered lung vascular structure and function of PPHN are poorly understood. Clinical observations that neonates with severe PPHN who die during the first

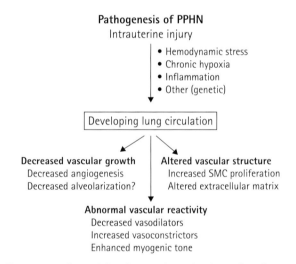

Figure 20.1 *Potential pathogenetic mechanisms of persistent pulmonary hypertension of the newborn (PPHN).*

days after birth already have pathological signs of chronic pulmonary vascular disease suggest that **intrauterine events** may play an important role in this syndrome.[15,26–28] Adverse intrauterine stimuli during late gestation, such as abnormal hemodynamics, changes in substrate or hormone delivery to the lung, hypoxia, inflammation or others, may potentially alter lung vascular function and structure, contributing to abnormalities of postnatal adaptation (Figure 20.1). Several investigators have examined the effects of chronic intrauterine stresses, such as hypoxia or hypertension, in animal models in order to attempt to mimic the clinical problem of PPHN. Whether chronic hypoxia alone can cause PPHN is controversial. A past report suggests that maternal hypoxia in rats increases pulmonary vascular smooth muscle thickening in newborns,[38] but this observation has not been reproduced in maternal rats or guinea pigs with more extensive studies.[39]

However, animal studies suggest that hypertension, due to either renal artery ligation or partial or complete closure of the ductus arteriosus, can cause structural and physiological changes that resemble features of clinical PPHN.[30–33] Pulmonary hypertension induced by early closure of the DA in fetal lambs alters lung vascular reactivity and structure, causing the failure of postnatal adaptation at delivery, and providing an experimental model of PPHN.[31,32] Over days, pulmonary artery pressure and PVR progressively increase, but flow remains low and PaO_2 is unchanged.[31] Marked right ventricular hypertrophy and structural remodeling of small pulmonary arteries develops after 8 days of hypertension. After delivery, these lambs have persistent elevation of PVR despite mechanical ventilation with high oxygen concentrations. Studies with this model show that chronic hypertension without high flow can alter fetal lung vascular structure and function. This model is further characterized by endothelial cell dysfunction and altered smooth muscle cell reactivity and growth, including findings of impaired NO production and activity due to down-regulation of lung endothelial NO synthase mRNA and protein expression.[40–44] Fetal pulmonary hypertension also impaired soluble guanylate cyclase and up-regulated cGMP-specific phosphodiesterase (type 5; PDE5) activities, suggesting further impairments in the NO-cGMP cascade.[45–47]

In addition, up-regulation of ET-1 may also contribute to the pathophysiology of PPHN. Circulating levels of ET-1, a potent vasoconstrictor and co-mitogen for vascular smooth muscle cell hyperplasia, are increased in human newborns with severe PPHN.[48] In the experimental model of PPHN due to compression of the DA in fetal sheep, lung ET-1 mRNA and protein content are markedly increased, and the balance of ET receptors are altered, favoring vasoconstriction.[49] Chronic inhibition of the ET_A receptor attenuates the severity of pulmonary hypertension, decreases pulmonary artery wall thickening, and improves the fall in PVR at birth in this model.[50] Thus, experimental studies have shown the important role of the NO-cGMP cascade and the ET-1 system in the regulation of vascular tone and reactivity of the fetal and transitional pulmonary circulation.[51,52]

CLINICAL PRESENTATION AND EVALUATION

Clinically, PPHN is most often recognized in term or near-term neonates, but clearly can also occur in premature neonates.[19,53,54] PPHN is often associated with perinatal distress, such as asphyxia, low Apgar scores, meconium staining, and other factors; however, idiopathic PPHN can lack signs of acute perinatal distress. PPHN often presents as respiratory distress and cyanosis within 6–12 hours of birth. Laboratory findings can include low glucose, hypocalcemia, hypothermia, polycythemia and thrombocytopenia. Radiographic findings are variable, depending upon the primary disease associated with PPHN. Classically, the chest x-ray in idiopathic PPHN is oligemic, may appear slightly hyperinflated, and lacks parenchymal infiltrates. In general, the degree of hypoxemia is often disproportionate to the severity of radiographic evidence of lung disease.

Not all term newborns with hypoxemic respiratory failure have PPHN-type physiology.[20,55] Hypoxemia in the newborn can be due to several mechanisms, including:

- **extrapulmonary shunt**, in which high pulmonary artery pressure at systemic levels leads to right-to-left shunting of blood flow across the PDA or PFO; and
- **intrapulmonary shunt** or **ventilation/perfusion mismatch**, in which hypoxemia results from the lack of mixing of blood with aerated lung regions due to parenchymal lung disease, without the shunting of blood flow across the patent DA and FO.

In the latter setting, hypoxemia is related to the amount of pulmonary arterial blood that perfuses non-aerated lung regions. Although PVR is often elevated in hypoxemic newborns without PPHN, high PVR does not contribute significantly to hypoxemia in these cases.

Several factors can contribute to high pulmonary artery pressure in neonates with PPHN-type physiology (Figure 20.2). Pulmonary hypertension can be caused by vasoconstriction or structural lesions that directly increase PVR. Changes in lung volume in neonates with parenchymal lung disease can also be an important determinant of PVR. PVR increases at low lung volumes due to dense parenchymal infiltrate and poor lung recruitment, or with high lung volumes due to hyperinflation associated with overdistension or gas-trapping. Cardiac disease is also associated with PPHN.[56] High pulmonary venous pressure due to left ventricular dysfunction can also elevate PAP (e.g. asphyxia, sepsis), causing right-to-left shunting, with little vasoconstriction. In this setting, enhancing cardiac performance and systemic hemodynamics may lower PAP more effectively than achieving pulmonary vasodilation. Thus, understanding the cardiopulmonary interactions are key to improving outcome in PPHN.

PPHN is characterized by hypoxemia that is poorly responsive to supplemental oxygen. In the presence of right-to-left shunting across the PDA, 'differential cyanosis' is often present, which is difficult to detect by physical examination, and is defined by a difference in

PaO$_2$ between right radial artery versus descending aorta values $\geq$10 mmHg, or an O$_2$ saturation gradient >5%. However, post-ductal desaturation can be found in ductus-dependent cardiac diseases, including hypoplastic left heart syndrome, coarctation of the aorta or interrupted aortic arch. The response to supplemental oxygen can help to distinguish PPHN from primary lung or cardiac disease.[57–59] Although supplemental oxygen traditionally increases PaO$_2$ more readily in lung disease than cyanotic heart disease or PPHN, this may not be obvious with more advanced parenchymal lung disease. Marked improvement in SaO$_2$ (increase to 100%) with supplemental oxygen suggests the presence of $\dot{V}/\dot{Q}$ mismatch due to lung disease or highly reactive PPHN. Most patients with PPHN have at least a transient improvement in oxygenation in response to interventions such as high inspired oxygen and/or mechanical ventilation. Acute respiratory alkalosis induced by hyperventilation to achieve PaCO$_2$ <30 mmHg and a pH >7.5 may increase PaO$_2$ >50 mmHg in PPHN, but rarely in cyanotic heart disease.

The echocardiogram plays an essential diagnostic role and is an essential tool for managing newborns with PPHN (Table 20.3). The initial echocardiographic evaluation is important to rule out structural heart disease causing hypoxemia (e.g. coarctation of the aorta and total anomalous pulmonary venous return). As stated above, not all term newborns with hypoxemia have PPHN physiology. Although high pulmonary artery pressure may be common, the diagnosis of PPHN is uncertain without evidence of bidirectional or predominantly right-to-left shunting across the PFO or PDA. Echocardiographic signs suggestive of pulmonary hypertension (e.g. increased right ventricular systolic time intervals and septal flattening) are less helpful. In addition to demonstrating the presence of PPHN physiology, the echocardiogram is critical for the evaluation of left ventricular function and diagnosis of anatomic heart disease, including such 'PPHN mimics' as coarctation of the aorta; total anomalous pulmonary venous return; hypoplastic left heart syndrome; and others.[60] Studies should carefully assess the predominant direction of shunting at the patent FO as well as the patent DA. Although right-to-left shunting at the patent DA and patent FO is typical for PPHN, predominant right-to-left shunting at the patent DA but left-to-right shunt at the patent FO may help to identify the important role of **left ventricular dysfunction** to the underlying pathophysiology. In the presence of severe left ventricular dysfunction with pulmonary hypertension, pulmonary vasodilation alone may be ineffective in improving oxygenation. In this setting, efforts to reduce PVR should be accompanied by targeted therapies to increase cardiac performance and decrease left ventricular afterload. Thus, careful echocardiographic assessment provides invaluable information about the underlying pathophysiology and will help guide the course of treatment.

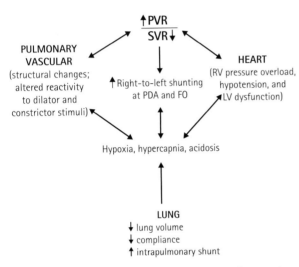

Figure 20.2 *Physiological mechanisms that contribute to the pathophysiology of persistent pulmonary hypertension of the newborn (PPHN). FO, foramen ovale; LV, left ventricle; PDA, patent ductus arteriosus; PVR, pulmonary vascular resistance; RV, right ventricle; SVR, systemic vascular resistance.*

Table 20.3 *Echocardiographic findings in persistent pulmonary hypertension of the newborn (PPHN)*

Measurement	Findings in PPHN
Assessment of cardiac anatomy	Rule out structural heart disease
Assessment of cardiac function	Determine relative role of LV dysfunction
Assess direction of PDA shunt (by pulsed and color Doppler)	Right-to-left or bidirectional PDA flow
Assess direction of atrial level shunt	Right-to-left or bidirectional PFO shunt (left-to-right shunt suggests LV dysfunction or obstruction contributes to pulmonary hypertension)
Estimate of PA pressure by Doppler study $RVSP = 4(V^2) + CVP$	Estimate PA pressure, compare with simultaneous systemic arterial pressure

CVP, central venous pressure; LV, left ventricular; PA, pulmonary artery; PDA, patent ductus arteriosus; V, peak velocity of tricuspid regurgitation jet, m/sec.

TREATMENT

In general, management of the newborn with PPHN includes:[61]

- the treatment and avoidance of hypothermia, hypoglycemia, hypocalcemia, anemia and hypovolemia;
- correction of metabolic acidosis;
- diagnostic studies for sepsis;
- serial monitoring of arterial blood pressure, pulse oximetry (pre- and post-ductal); and
- transcutaneous PCO_2, especially with the initiation of high-frequency oscillatory ventilation (HFOV).

Therapy includes aggressive management of systemic hemodynamics with volume and cardiotonic therapy (dobutamine, dopamine, and milrinone), in order to enhance cardiac output and systemic O_2 transport. In addition, increasing systemic arterial pressure can improve oxygenation in some cases by reducing right-to-left extrapulmonary shunting. Failure to respond to medical management, as evidenced by failure to sustain improvement in oxygenation with good hemodynamic function, often leads to treatment with extracorporeal membrane oxygenation (ECMO).[62] Although ECMO can be a life-saving therapy, it is costly, labor intensive, and can have severe side effects, such as intracranial hemorrhage. Since arteriovenous ECMO usually involves ligation of the carotid artery, acute and long-term central nervous system (CNS) injury remain major concerns.

The goal of mechanical ventilation is to improve oxygenation and to achieve 'optimal' lung volume to minimize the adverse effects of high or low lung volumes on PVR, while minimizing the risk for lung injury ('volutrauma'). Mechanical ventilation using inappropriate settings can produce acute lung injury (ventilator-induced lung injury; VILI), causing pulmonary edema, decreased lung compliance and promoting lung inflammation due to increased cytokine production and lung neutrophil accumulation.[63] The development of VILI is an important determinant of clinical course and eventual outcome of newborns with hypoxemic respiratory failure, and postnatal lung injury worsens the degree of pulmonary hypertension.[64] Failure to achieve adequate lung volumes (functional residual capacity) contributes to hypoxemia and high PVR in newborns with PPHN.[65] Some newborns with parenchymal lung disease with PPHN physiology improve oxygenation and decrease right-to-left extrapulmonary shunting with aggressive lung recruitment during high frequency oscillatory ventilation[65] or with an 'open lung approach' of higher positive end-expiratory pressure with low tidal volumes, as more commonly utilized in older patients with acute RDS.[66,67]

Marked controversy and variability exists between centers regarding the use of hyperventilation to achieve alkalosis in order to improve oxygenation.[25] Past studies have clearly shown that acute hyperventilation can improve PaO_2 in neonates with PPHN, providing a diagnostic test and therapeutic strategy.[57,58] However, there are many issues with the use of hypocapnic alkalosis for prolonged therapy. Depending upon the ventilator strategy and underlying lung disease, hyperventilation is likely to increase VILI, and the ability to sustain decreased PVR during prolonged hyperventilation is unproven. Experimental studies suggest that the response to alkalosis is transient, and that alkalosis may paradoxically worsen pulmonary vascular tone, reactivity and permeability edema.[59,68–72] In addition, prolonged hyperventilation reduces cerebral blood flow and oxygen delivery to the brain, potentially worsening neurodevelopmental outcome.

Additional therapies, including infusions of sodium bicarbonate, surfactant therapy and the use of intravenous vasodilator therapy, are also highly variable between centers.[25] Although surfactant may improve oxygenation in some lung diseases, such as meconium aspiration and RDS, a multicenter trial failed to show a reduction in ECMO utilization in newborns with PPHN.[73] The use of intravenous vasodilator drug therapy, with such agents as tolazoline, magnesium sulfate, prostacyclin and sodium nitroprusside, is also controversial due to the non-selective effects of these agents on the systemic circulation.[74] Systemic hypotension worsens right-to-left shunting, may impair oxygen delivery and worsen gas exchange in patients with parenchymal lung disease. In addition, the initial response to such agents as tolazoline are often transient, and can have severe adverse effects (such as gastrointestinal hemorrhage).[74,75] Endotracheal administration of vasodilators, including tolazoline and sodium nitroprusside, may cause selective pulmonary vasodilation and minimize systemic hypotension.[76] However, these data are largely limited to animal studies, and evidence is currently lacking to support the safety and efficacy of this approach in humans.

Inhaled nitric oxide (iNO) therapy at low doses (5–20 p.p.m.) improves oxygenation and decreases the need for ECMO therapy in patients with diverse causes of PPHN[77–86] (Figures 20.3 and 20.4). Multicenter clinical trials support the use of iNO in near-term (>34 weeks gestation) and term newborns, and the use of iNO in infants less than 34 weeks gestation remains investigational. Studies support the use of iNO in infants who have hypoxemic respiratory failure with evidence of PPHN, who require mechanical ventilation and high inspired oxygen concentrations. The most common criterion employed has been the oxygenation index (OI: mean airway pressure $\times$ FiO_2 $\times$ 100 $\div$ PaO_2). Although clinical trials commonly allowed for enrollment with OI levels >25, the mean OI at study entry in multicenter trials

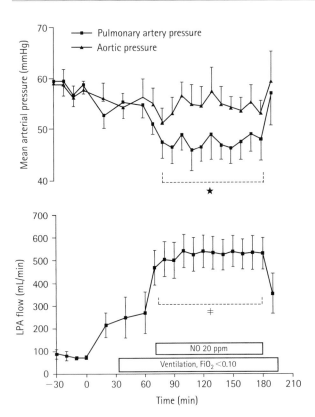

Figure 20.3 *Effects of inhaled nitric oxide (NO) in fetal lambs. As shown, inhaled NO causes selective and prolonged pulmonary vasodilation in fetal lambs during mechanical ventilation with hypoxic gas. LPA, left pulmonary artery. (Reproduced with permission from Kinsella JP, McQueston JA, Rosenberg AA et al. Effects of inhaled nitric oxide on the ovine transitional pulmonary circulation. Am J Physiol 1992;263:H875–80.)*

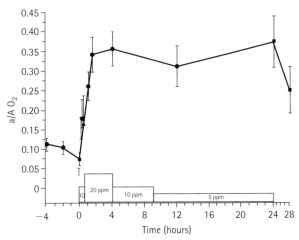

Figure 20.4 *Low doses of inhaled nitric oxide (NO) increases oxygenation, as assessed by the arterial to alveolar ratio (a/A O$_2$), in human newborns with severe persistent pulmonary hypertension of the newborn (PPHN) who met extracorporeal membrane oxygenation (ECMO) criteria. Improvement in oxygenation was sustained with continuous treatment of inhaled NO, obviating the need for ECMO in these patients. (Reproduced with permission from Kinsella JP, Neish S, Shaffer E et al. Low dose inhalational nitric oxide in persistent pulmonary hypertension of the newborn. Lancet 1992;340:819–20.)*

approximated 40. It is unclear whether infants with less severe hypoxemia would benefit from iNO therapy. The first studies of iNO treatment in term newborns reported initial doses that ranged from 80 to 6–20 p.p.m.[79,85] In the latter report, rapid improvement in PaO$_2$ was achieved at low doses (20 p.p.m.) for 4 hours, and this response was sustained with prolonged therapy at 6 p.p.m.[79] Subsequent multicenter studies confirmed the efficacy of this dosing strategy[77,82] and that increasing the dose in non-responders did not improve outcomes.[82] The available evidence, therefore, supports the use of doses of iNO beginning at 20 p.p.m. in term newborns with PPHN, since this strategy decreased ECMO utilization without an increased incidence of adverse effects. Although brief exposures to higher doses (40–80 p.p.m.) appear to be safe, sustained treatment with 80 p.p.m. NO increases the risk of methemoglobinemia.[78] In our practice, we discontinue iNO if the FiO$_2$ is <0.60 and the PaO$_2$ is >60 without evidence of 'rebound' pulmonary hypertension or an increase in FiO$_2$ >15% after iNO withdrawal. Prolonged need for inhaled NO therapy without resolution of disease should

lead to a more extensive evaluation to determine whether previously unsuspected anatomic lung or cardiovascular disease is present (for example, pulmonary venous stenosis, alveolar capillary dysplasia, severe lung hypoplasia, or others).[60,87]

In newborns with severe lung disease, HFOV is frequently used to optimize lung inflation and minimize lung injury. In clinical pilot studies using iNO, the combination of HFOV and iNO caused the greatest improvement in oxygenation in some newborns who had severe PPHN complicated by diffuse parencyhmal lung disease and underinflation (e.g. RDS, pneumonia).[55,79,80] A randomized, multicenter trial demonstrated that treatment with HFOV + iNO was often successful in patients who failed to respond to HFOV or iNO alone in severe PPHN, and differences in responses were related to the specific disease associated with the complex disorders of PPHN.[81] For patients with PPHN complicated by severe lung disease, response rates for HFOV + iNO were better than HFOV alone or iNO with conventional ventilation. By contrast, for patients without significant parenchymal lung disease, both iNO and HFOV + iNO were more effective than HFOV alone. This response to combined treatment with HFOV + iNO likely reflects both improvement in intrapulmonary shunting in patients with severe lung disease and PPHN (using a strategy designed to recruit and sustain lung volume, rather than to hyperventilate) and augmented NO delivery to its site of action. Although iNO may be an effective treatment for PPHN, it should be considered only as part of an overall clinical strategy that cautiously manages parenchymal lung disease, cardiac performance and systemic hemodynamics.

Although clinical improvement during inhaled NO therapy occurs with many disorders associated with PPHN, not all neonates with acute hypoxemic respiratory failure and pulmonary hypertension respond to iNO. Several mechanisms may explain the clinical variability in responsiveness to iNO therapy. An inability to deliver NO to the pulmonary circulation due to poor lung inflation is the major cause of poor responsiveness. In some settings, administration of NO HFOV has improved oxygenation more effectively than during conventional ventilation in the same patient.[65,81] In addition, poor NO responsiveness may be related to myocardial dysfunction or systemic hypotension, severe pulmonary vascular structural disease, and unsuspected or missed anatomic cardiovascular lesions (such as total anomalous pulmonary venous return, coarctation of the aorta, alveolar capillary dysplasia, and others). Another mechanism of poor responsiveness to inhaled NO may be altered smooth muscle cell responsiveness, and as described from animal studies and case reports, combined therapy with PDE5 inhibitors may enhance the vasodilator response to iNO in some settings.[88–90] Recent experimental studies suggest that superoxide dismutase (SOD) treatment with iNO therapy may have an additive affect on lowering PVR in lambs with pulmonary hypertension.[91] Besides administering iNO as an inhalational agent, Moya et al. have recently suggested that treatment with a unique gas, O-nitrosoethanol, may increase the endogenous pool of S-nitrosothiols in the airway and circulation, thereby providing a new treatment strategy for PPHN.[92] Whether this strategy is more effective or will improve responsiveness in neonates who fail to respond to iNO therapy is unknown.

Finally, Although newer therapies, including HFOV and inhaled NO, have led to a dramatic reduction in the need for ECMO therapy,[93–95] ECMO has been shown to be an effective rescue agent for severe PPHN.[62] Current patterns of ECMO use demonstrate persistent use in neonates with CDH and patients with severe hemodynamic instability, with less need for ECMO in meconium aspiration, RDS, idiopathic PPHN and other disorders.

COMPLICATIONS AND LONG–TERM OUTCOMES

Infants with PPHN are at high risk for death or long-term cardiopulmonary and neurological sequelae. These risks are largely due to injury caused by perinatal ischemia or asphyxia, or the results of aggressive therapies, such as

alkalosis or ECMO therapy. Major complications include cerebral palsy (11%), neurodevelopmental delays (20%) and sensorineural hearing loss (14%). In addition, chronic lung disease, as characterized by prolonged need for supplemental oxygen therapy, recurrent wheezing, and frequent hospitalizations during infancy, can occur in 10–20% of patients. Pulmonary hypertension during follow-up is rare, but infants with lung hypoplasia (especially CDH) remain at risk. Recent follow-up studies suggest, however, that iNO therapy does not increase the risk for long-term neurological, developmental or cardiopulmonary problems.[83]

CONCLUSIONS

PPHN is a clinical syndrome that is associated with diverse cardiopulmonary diseases, with pathophysiological mechanisms including pulmonary vascular, cardiac and lung disease. Experimental work on basic mechanisms of vascular regulation of the developing lung circulation and models of perinatal pulmonary hypertension has improved our therapeutic approaches to neonates with PPHN. Inhaled NO has been shown to be an effective pulmonary vasodilator for infants with PPHN, but successful clinical strategies require meticulous care of associated lung and cardiac disease. More work is needed to expand our therapeutic repertoire in order to further improve the outcome of the sick newborn with severe hypoxemia, especially in patients with lung hypoplasia and advanced structural vascular disease.

KEY POINTS

- PPHN is a clinical syndrome associated with diverse neonatal cardiopulmonary disorders that share the common pathophysiology of high PVR causing right-to-left extrapulmonary shunting of blood flow across the ductus arteriosus or foramen ovale.
- Experimental and clinical studies show that intrauterine stimuli contribute to the pathogenesis of PPHN.
- Echocardiographic studies are essential for the diagnosis and clinical management of PPHN.
- Inhaled NO is a selective and potent pulmonary vasodilator that has been proven to be effective in decreasing the need for ECMO therapy in neonates with severe PPHN.

REFERENCES

1 Dawes G, Mott JC, Widdicombe JG. Changes in the lungs of the newborn lamb. *J Physiol* 1953;**121**:141–62.

2 Heymann MA, Soifer SJ. Control of fetal and neonatal pulmonary circulation. In: Weir EK, Reeves JT (eds), *Pulmonary vascular physiology and pathophysiology.* New York: Marcel Dekker, 1989;33–50.

3 Rudolph AM, Heymann MA, Lewis AB. Physiology and pharmacology of the pulmonary circulation in the fetus and newborn. In: Hodson W (ed.), *Development of the lung.* New York: Marcel Dekker, 1977;497–523.

◆4 Rudolph AM. Fetal and neonatal pulmonary circulation. *Ann Rev Physiol* 1979;**41**:383–95.

5 Cassin S, Dawes GS, Mott JC *et al.* Vascular resistance of the foetal and newly ventilated lung of the lamb. *J Physiol* 1964;**171**:61–79.

●6 Abman SH, Chatfield BA, Rodman DM *et al.* Maturation-related changes in endothelium-dependent relaxation of ovine pulmonary arteries. *Am J Physiol* 1991;**260**:L280–5.

7 Cassin S. Role of prostaglandins, thromboxanes and leukotrienes in the control of the pulmonary circulation in the fetus and newborn. *Semin Perinatol* 1987;**11**:53–63.

8 Cornfield DN, Chatfield BA, McQueston JA *et al.* Effects of birth-related stimuli on L-arginine-dependent pulmonary vasodilation in the ovine fetus. *Am J Physiol* 1992;**262**:H1474–81.

9 Cornfield DN, Reeves HL, Tolarova S *et al.* Oxygen causes fetal pulmonary vasodilation through activation of a calcium-dependent potassium channel. *Proc Natl Acad Sci USA* 1996;**93**:8089–94.

10 Leffler CW, Hessler JR, Green RS. Mechanism of stimulation of pulmonary prostacyclin synthesis at birth. *Prostaglandins* 1984;**28**:877–87.

11 Leffler CW, Tyler TL, Cassin S. Effect of indomethacin on pulmonary vascular response to ventilation of fetal goats. *Am J Physiol* 1978;**234**:H346–51.

12 Velvis H, Moore P, Heymann MA. Prostaglandin inhibition prevents the fall in pulmonary vascular resistance as the result of rhythmic distension of the lungs in fetal lambs. *Pediatr Res* 1991;**30**:62–7.

●13 Ivy DD, Kinsella JP, Abman SH. Physiologic characterization of endothelin A and B receptor activity in the ovine fetal lung. *J Clin Invest* 1994;**93**:2141–8.

●14 Allen K, Haworth SG. Impaired adaptation of pulmonary circulation to extrauterine life in newborn pigs exposed to hypoxia. An ultrastructural study. *J Pathol* 1986; **150**:205–12.

15 Haworth SG, Reid LM. Persistent fetal circulation. Newly recognized structural features. *J Pediatr* 1976;**88**:614–20.

16 Levin DL, Heymann MA, Kitterman JA *et al.* Persistent pulmonary hypertension of the newborn. *J Pediatr* 1976;**89**:626–33.

17 Gersony WM, Duc GV, Sinclair JC. 'PFC' syundrome (persistent fetal circulation). *Circulation* 1969;**40** (Suppl 3):87.

18 Gersony WM. Neonatal pulmonary hypertension: pathophysiology, classification and etiology. *Clin Perinatol* 1984;**11**:517–24.

19 Muraskas JK, Juretschke LJ, Weiss MG *et al.* Neonatal-perinatal risk factors for the development of PPHN in preterm newborns. *Am J Perinatol* 2001;**18**:87–91.

∗20 Kinsella JP, Abman SH. Recent developments in the pathophysiology and treatment of PPHN. *J Pediatr* 1995;**126**:853–64.

◆21 Long WA. *Fetal and neonatal cardiology.* Philadelphia: WB Saunders, 1990.

◆22 Stenmark KR, Abman SH, Accurso FJ. Etiologic mechanisms of persistent pulmonary hypertension of the newborn. In: Weir EK, Reeves JT (eds), *Pulmonary vascular physiology and pathophysiology.* New York: Marcel Dekker, 1989;335.

23 Walsh MC, Stork ER. PPHN: rational therapy based on pathophysiology. *Clin Perinatol* 2001;**28**:609–27.

24 Skinner JR, Hunter S, Hey EN. Hemodynamic features at presentation in PPHN and outcome. *Arch Dis Child* 1996;**74**:F26–32.

25 Walsh-Sukys MC, Tyson JE, Wright LL *et al.* PPHN in the era before NO: practice variation and outcomes. *Pediatrics* 2000;**105**:14–20.

26 Geggel RL, Reid LM. The structural basis of persistent pulmonary hypertension of the newborn. *Clin Perinatol* 1984;**3**:525–49.

●27 Murphy JD, Rabinovitch M, Goldstein JD *et al.* The structural basis for PPHN infant. *J Pediatr* 1981;**98**:962–7.

28 Murphy JD, Vawter G, Reid LM. Pulmonary vascular disease in fatal meconium aspiration. *J Pediatr* 1984;**104**:758–62.

29 Van Marter LJ, Leviton A, Allred EN *et al.* PPHN and smoking and aspirin and nonsteroidal antiinflammatory drug consumption during pregnancy. *Pediatrics* 1996;**97**:658–63.

●30 Levin DL, Hyman AI, Heymann MA *et al.* Fetal hypertension and the development of increased pulmonary vascular smooth muscle: a possible mechanism for persistent pulmonary hypertension of the newborn infant. *J Pediatr* 1978;**92**:265–9.

●31 Abman SH, Shanley PF, Accurso FJ. Failure of postnatal adaptation of the pulmonary circulation after chronic intrauterine pulmonary hypertension in fetal lambs. *J Clin Invest* 1989;**83**:1849–58.

●32 Morin FC. Ligating the ductus arteriosus before birth causes persistent pulmonary hypertension in the newborn lamb. *Pediatr Res* 1989;**25**:245–50.

33 Williams MC, Wyble LE, O'Brien WF *et al.* PPHN and asymmetric growth restriction. *Obstet Gynecol* 1998;**91**:336–41.

34 Castillo L, DeRojas-Walker T, Yu YM *et al.* Whole body arginine metabolism and NO synthesis in newborns with persistent pulmonary hypertension. *Pediatr Res* 1995; **38**:17–24.

35 Dollberg S, Warner BW, Myatt L. Urinary nitrite and nitrate concentrations in patients with idiopathic PPHN and effect of ECMO. *Pediatr Res* 1994;**37**:31–4.

●36 Pearson DL, Dowling S, Walsh WF *et al.* Neonatal pulmonary hypertension: urea cycle intermediates, NO production and carbamoyl phosphate synthetase function. *N Engl J Med* 2001;**344**:1932–8.

37 Newman JH, Wheeler L, Lane KB *et al.* Mutation in the gene for bone morphogenetic protein receptor II as a cause of primary pulmonary hypertension in a large kindred. *N Engl J Med* 2001;**345**:367–71.

38 Goldberg SJ, Levy RA, Siassi B. The effects of maternal hypoxia and hyperoxia upon the neonatal pulmonary vasculature. *Pediatrics* 1971;**48**:528–33.

39 Murphy JD, Aronovitz MJ, Reid LM. Effects of chronic in utero hypoxia on the pulmonary vasculature of the newborn guinea pig. *Pediatr Res* 1986;**20**:292–5.

40 McQueston JA, Kinsella JP, Ivy DD *et al.* Chronic pulmonary hypertension *in utero* impairs endothelium-dependent vasodilation. *Am J Physiol* 1995;**268**:H288–94.

41 Storme L, Rairigh RL, Parker TA *et al.* Acute intrauterine pulmonary hypertension impairs endothelium-dependent vasodilation in the ovine fetus. *Pediatr Res* 1999;**45**:575–81.

42 Storme L, Parker TA, Rairhig RL *et al.* Chronic pulmonary hypertension abolishes flow-induced vasodilation and augments the myogenic response in fetal lung. *Am J Physiol* 2002;**282**:L56–66.

43 Villamor E, Le Cras TD, Horan MP *et al.* Chronic intrauterine pulmonary hypertension impairs endothelial nitric oxide synthase in the ovine fetus. *Am J Physiol* 1997; **272**:L1013–20.

44 Shaul PW, Yuhanna IS, German Z *et al.* Pulmonary endothelial NO synthase gene expression is decreased in fetal lambs with pulmonary hypertension. *Am J Physiol* 1997;**272**:L1005–12.

45 Hanson KA, Beavo JA, Abman SH *et al.* Chronic pulmonary hypertension increases fetal lung cGMP activity. *Am J Physiol* 1998;**275**:L931–41.

46 Hanson KA, Burns F, Rybalkin SD *et al.* Developmental changes in lung cGMP phosphodiesterase-5 activity, protein and message. *Am J Respir Crit Care Med* 1995;**158**:279–88.

47 Steinhorn RH, Russell JA, Morin FC. Disruption of cGMP production in pulmonary arteries isolated from fetal lambs with pulmonary hypertension. *Am J Physiol* 1995;**268**:H1483–9.

48 Rosenberg AA, Kennaugh J, Koppenhafer SL *et al.* Increased immunoreactive endothelin-1 levels in persistent pulmonary hypertension of the newborn. *J Pediatr* 1993;**123**:109–14.

49 Ivy DD, LeCras TD, Horan MP *et al.* Increased lung prepro-endothelin-1 and decreased endothelin B receptor gene expression after chronic pulmonary hypertension in the ovine fetus. *Am J Physiol* 1998;**274**:L535–41.

50 Ivy DD, Parker TA, Ziegler JW *et al.* Prolonged endothelin A receptor blockade attenuates chronic pulmonary hypertension in the ovine fetus. *J Clin Invest* 1997;**99**:1179–86.

51 Abman SH, Kinsella JP, Parker TA *et al.* Physiologic roles of NO in the perinatal pulmonary circulation. In: Weir EK, Archer SL, Reeves JT (eds), *Fetal and neonatal pulmonary circulation.* New York: Futura, 1999;239–60.

52 Ivy DD, Abman SH. Role of endothelin in perinatal pulmonary vasoregulation. In: Weir EK, Archer SL, Reeves JT (eds), *Fetal and neonatal pulmonary circulation.* New York: Futura, 1999;279–302.

53 Abman SH, Kinsella JP, Schaffer MS *et al.* Inhaled nitric oxide therapy in a premature newborn with severe respiratory distress and pulmonary hypertension. *Pediatrics* 1993;**92**:606–9.

54 Walther FJ, Bender FJ, Leighton JO. Persistent pulmonary hypertension in premature neonates with severe RDS. *Pediatrics* 1992;**90**:899–904.

55 Abman SH, Kinsella JP. Inhaled NO for PPHN: the physiology matters. *Pediatrics* 1995;**96**:1147–51.

56 Riemenschneider TA, Neilson HC, Ruttenberg HD *et al.* Disturbances of the transitional circulation: spectrum of pulmonary hypertension and myocardial dysfunction. *J Pediatr* 1976;**89**:622–5.

57 Drummond WH, Gregory G, Heymann MA *et al.* The independent effects of hyperventilation, tolazoline, and dopamine on infants with persistent pulmonary hypertension. *J Pediatr* 1981;**98**:603–11.

58 Drummond WH, Peckam GJ, Fox WW. The clinical profile of the newborn with persistent pulmonary hypertension. *Clin Pediatr* 1977;**16**:335–41.

59 Domino KB, Swenson ER, Hlastala MP. Hypocapnia-induced ventilation/perfusion mismatch: a direct CO_2 or pH mediated effect? *Am J Respir Crit Care Med* 1995;**152**:1534–9.

60 Holcomb RG, Tyson RW, Ivy DD *et al.* Congenital pulmonary venous stenosis presenting as persistent pulmonary hypertension of the newborn. *Pediatr Pulmonol* 1999;**28**:301–6.

61 Clark RH. High frequency ventilation. *J Pediatr* 1994; **124**:661–70.

●62 UK Collaborative ECMO Trial Group. UK Collaborative randomized trial of neonatal ECMO. *Lancet* 1996;**348**:75–82.

63 Tremblay L, Valenza F, Ribeiro SP *et al.* Injurious ventilator strategies increase cytokines and c-fos mRNA expression in an isolated rat lung model. *J Clin Invest* 1997;**99**:944–52.

64 Patterson K, Kapur SP, Chandra RS. PPHN: pulmonary pathologic effects. In: Rosenberg HS, Bernstein J (eds), *Cardiovascular diseases, perspectives in pediatric pathology.* Basel: Karger, 1988;**12**:139–54.

∗65 Kinsella JP, Abman SH. Clinical approach to inhaled NO therapy in the newborn. *J Pediatr* 2000;**136**:717–26.

66 Acute Respiratory Distress Syndrome Network. Ventilation with lower tidal volumes as compared with traditional tidal volumes for acute lung injury and the ARDS. *N Engl J Med* 2000;**342**:1301–8.

67 Feihl F, Perret C. Permissive hypercapnia. how permissive should we be? *Am J Respir Crit Care Med* 1994;**150**:1722–37.

68 Gordon JB, Martinez FR, Keller PA *et al.* Differing effects of acute and prolonged alkalosis on hypoxic pulmonary vasoconstriction. *Am Rev Respir Dis* 1993;**148**:1651–6.

69 Gordon JB, Rehorst-Paea LA, Hoffman GM *et al.* Pulmonary vascular responses during acute and sustained respiratory alkalosis or acidosis in intact newborn piglets. *Pediatr Res* 1999;**46**:735–41.

70 Laffey JG, Engelberts D, Kavanagh BP. Injurious effects of hypocapnic alkalosis in the isolated lung. *Am J Respir Crit Care Med* 2000;**162**:399–405.

71 Laffey JG, Kavanaugh BP. Biological effects of hypercapnia. *Intens Care Med* 2000;**26**:133–8.

72 Moreira GA, O'Donnell DC, Tod ML *et al.* Discordant effects of alkalosis on elevated PVR and vascular reactivity in lamb lungs. *Crit Care Med* 1999;**27**:1838–42.

●73 Lotze A, Mitchel BR, Bulas D *et al.* Multicenter study of surfactant (beractant) use in the treatment of term infants with severe respiratory failure. *J Pediatr* 1998;**132**:40–7.

74 Stevenson DK, Kasting DS, Darnall RA *et al.* Refractory hypoxemia associated with neonatal pulmonary disease: the use and limitations of tolazoline. *J Pediatr* 1979;**95**:595–9.

75 Abu-Osba Y, Galal O, Manasra K *et al.* Treatment of severe persistent pulmonary hypertension of the newborn with magnesium sulphate. *Arch Dis Child* 1992;**67**:31-5.

76 Curtis J, O'Neill JT, Pettett G. Endotracheal administration of tolazoline in hypoxia-induced pulmonary hypertension. *Pediatrics* 1993;**92**:403-8.

77 Clark RH, Kueser TJ, Walker MW *et al.* Low-dose inhaled NO treatment of PPHN. *N Engl J Med* 2000;**342**:469-74.

78 Davidson D, Barefield ES, Katwinkel J *et al.* Inhaled NO for the early treatment of persistent pulmonary hypertension of the term newborn: a randomized double blinded placebo-controlled dose-response multicenter study. *Pediatrics* 1998;**101**:325-34.

79 Kinsella JP, Neish S, Shaffer E *et al.* Low dose inhalational nitric oxide in persistent pulmonary hypertension of the newborn. *Lancet* 1992;**340**:819-20.

80 Kinsella JP, Neish SR, Ivy DD *et al.* Clinical responses to prolonged treatment of persistent pulmonary hypertension of the newborn. *J Pediatr* 1993;**123**:103-8.

81 Kinsella JP, Troug W, Walsh W *et al.* Randomized multicenter trial of inhaled nitric oxide and high frequency oscillatory ventilation in severe PPHN. *J Pediatr* 1997;**131**:55-62.

●82 Neonatal Inhaled NO Study Group. Inhaled NO in full-term and nearly full-term infants with hypoxic respiratory failure. *N Engl J Med* 1997;**336**:597-604.

83 Neonatal Inhaled NO Study Group. Inhaled NO in term and near-term infants: neurodevelopmental follow-up of the NINOS. *J Pediatr* 2000;**136**:611-17.

84 Roberts JD, Fineman JR, Morin FC *et al.* Inhaled NO and PPHN. *N Engl J Med* 1997;**336**:605-10.

85 Roberts JD, Polaner DM, Lang P *et al.* Inhaled nitric oxide in persistent pulmonary hypertension of the newborn. *Lancet* 1992;**340**:818-19.

86 Wessel DL, Adatia I, van Marter LJ *et al.* Improved oxygenation in a randomized trial of inhaled NO for PPHN. *Pediatrics* 1997;**100**:E7.

87 Goldman AP, Tasker RC, Haworth SG *et al.* Four patterns of response to inhaled NO for PPHN. *Pediatrics* 1996; **98**:706-13.

88 Kinsella JP, Toriella F, Ziegler JW *et al.* Dipyridamole augmentation of the response to inhaled NO. *Lancet* 1995;**346**:647-8.

89 Ziegler JW, DD Ivy, JJ Fox *et al.* Dipyridamole, a cGMP phosphodiesterase inhibitor, causes pulmonary vasodilation in the ovine fetus. *Am J Physiol* 1995;**269**:H473-9.

90 Ziegler JW, Ivy DD, Wiggins JW *et al.* Hemodynamic effects dipyridamole and inhaled NO in children with severe pulmonary hypertension. *Am J Respir Crit Care Med* 1998;**158**:1388-95.

91 Steinhorn RH, Albert G, Swartz DD *et al.* Recombinant human superoxide dismutase enhances the effect of inhaled NO in persistent pulmonary hypertension. *Am J Respir Crit Care Med* 2001;**164**:834-9.

92 Moya MP, Gow AJ, McMahon TJ *et al.* S-Nitrosothiol repletion by an inhaled gas regulates pulmonary function. *Proc Natl Acad Sci USA* 2001;**98**:5792-7.

93 Hintz SR, Suttner DM, Sheehan AM *et al.* Decreased use of neonatal ECMO: how new treatment modalities have affected ECMO utilization. *Pediatrics* 2000;**106**:1339-43.

94 Kennaugh JM, Kinsella JP, Abman SH *et al.* Impact of new treatments for neonatal pulmonary hypertension on ECMO use and outcome. *J Perinatol* 1997;**17**:366-9.

95 Rosenberg AA, Kennaugh JM, Moreland SG *et al.* Longitudinal follow-up of a cohort of newborn infants treated with inhaled NO for persistent pulmonary hypertension. *J Pediatr* 1997;**131**:70-5.

Pulmonary circulation in critical care

21

Effects of mechanical ventilation on the pulmonary circulation

MICHAEL R PINSKY

INTRODUCTION

Both spontaneous and positive-pressure ventilation can profoundly alter cardiovascular function, pulmonary blood flow and ultimately gas exchange through processes that are complex and difficult to understand by superficial bedside inspection. However, clinicians usually focus on the immediate hemodynamic effects of initiating mechanical ventilation because the cardiovascular changes often occur rapidly with the institution of mechanical ventilation and serve as the basis for specific treatment algorithms.[1]

The hemodynamic effects of positive-pressure ventilation on cardiac output have been known since positive-pressure ventilation was first introduced more than 50 years ago.[2] However, our understanding of the interactions between ventilation and pulmonary blood flow is still evolving. The boundaries of these interactions are defined by the determinants of both cardiovascular and pulmonary performance.

Positive-pressure breathing alters the pulmonary circulation by two different but related aspects of ventilation: changes in lung volume and changes in intrathoracic pressure (ITP). Changes in lung volume appear to be more important for the pulmonary circulation, whereas changes in ITP appear to be more relevant to the system circulation. The basic concepts that underpin the effects of mechanical ventilation on the pulmonary circulation are:

- whilst lung volume increases primarily during inspiration, it may be kept at a volume greater than normal with the application of increased end-expiratory airway pressure;
- the increase in ITP during inspiration produces a decrease in venous return, thereby uncoupling pulmonary blood flow changes with alveolar ventilation.

THE RELATION BETWEEN AIRWAY PRESSURE, ALVEOLAR PRESSURE, PLEURAL PRESSURES AND LUNG VOLUME DURING MECHANICAL VENTILATION

Airway and alveolar pressure

The hemodynamic effects of positive-pressure ventilation are often considered relative to changes in airway pressure (Paw).[3,4] Lung distension is a function of both increases in the transpulmonary pressure gradient, defined as the difference between alveolar pressure (P_A) and pleural pressure (Ppl), and lung compliance, which is both non-linear and non-homogeneous throughout the lung and is subject to rapid change over time. The relation between changes in Paw with changes in both Ppl and lung volume varies as ventilatory patterns, airway resistance and lung compliance change. Additionally, changes in Paw do not accurately reflect changes in pericardial pressure (Ppc), a primary determinant of transmural LV pressure. With dynamic hyperinflation, end-expiratory Paw will underestimate P_A. Even stop-flow end-expiratory Paw measures will underestimate P_A if air trapping exists. However, mean Paw is a remarkably good estimate of mean P_A under normal conditions and with acute lung injury, even when airway resistance is increased.[5] Accordingly, mean Paw is a useful parameter when determining whether a specific ventilatory pattern is causing lung volume to increase relative to end-expiratory values.

Airway pressure, lung volume and regional pleural pressures

During positive-pressure inspiration, transpulmonary pressure and lung volume increase in parallel with increasing Paw. Since changes in Paw are related to changes in lung volume through the interaction of airway resistance and both lung and chest compliances, directionally similar changes in both Paw and Ppl occur during inspiration.

Lung expansion pushes the chest wall outward, the diaphragm downward and the cardiac fossa in upon itself, increasing lateral wall, diaphragmatic, juxtacardiac Ppl, and Ppc. The degree of increase on each of these

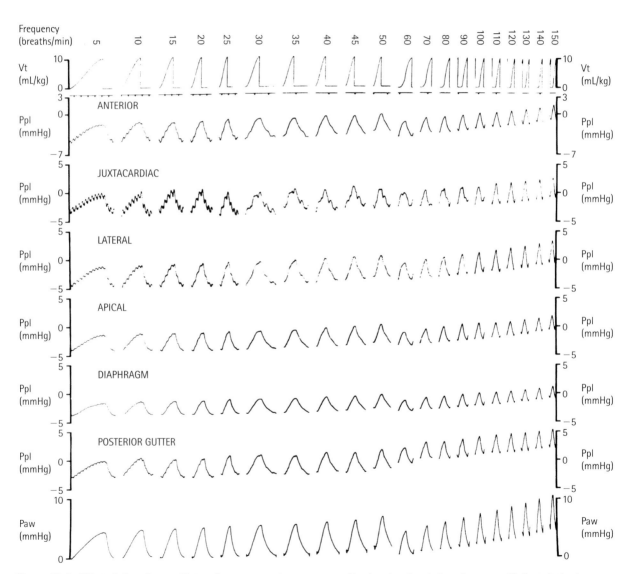

Figure 21.1 *Effect of changing ventilatory frequency on airway pressure (Paw) and regional pleural pressure (Ppl) at vital volume (Vt) = 10 mL/kg and a 50% inspiratory time for one animal. Note that end-expiratory Ppl increases in all regions as frequency increases and that the rate of increase among regions is similar despite their different baseline end-expiratory values. (Reproduced with permission from Novak RA, Matuschak GM, Pinsky MR. Effect of ventilatory frequency on regional pleural pressure. J Appl Physiol 1988;65:1314–23.)*

surfaces in response to lung expansion will be a function of the compliance and inertness of their opposing structures, specifically the chest wall, diaphragm-abdominal contents, and heart, respectively. Novak *et al.*[7] demonstrated that the changes in Ppl induced by positive-pressure ventilation are not similar in all regions of the thorax, and increase differently as inspiratory flow rate and frequency increase (Figure 21.1). Pleural pressure at the diaphragm increases least during positive-pressure inspiration, while juxtacardiac Ppl increases most. Since the diaphragm is very compliant, it seems reasonable that diaphragmatic Ppl should increase less than lateral chest wall Ppl with sudden increases in lung volume. However, if abdominal distension develops, as commonly occurs in the setting of sepsis, the diaphragm will become relatively non-compliant because of the increase in abdominal pressure. Under these conditions Paw will increase for an unchanged tidal breath, without any change in lung parenchymal compliance.[7] This distinction is important because increasing Paw to overcome chest wall stiffness should further increase Ppl, producing greater hemodynamic consequences, but would not improve gas exchange since the alveoli are not damaged, neither is the lung overdistended.

In the supine subject, apneic Ppl along the horizontal plane from apex to diaphragm are similar, whereas anterior Ppl is lower and posterior gutter Ppl is greater. This gravitational Ppl gradient is the major reason for the greater distension of non-dependent lung regions compared with dependent regions. P_A is similar in all alveoli, whereas the opposing Ppl varies along its hydrostatic gradient (Figure 21.2). Hydrostatic gradients also alter absolute PAP and PVP values. Thus, the difference between PAP and P_A decreases in non-dependent regions, and increases in dependent ones.

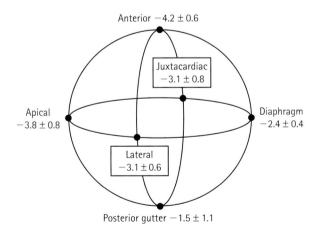

Figure 21.2 *Apneic pleural pressure (Ppl) (mean ± SE) in mmHg for six pleural regions of the right hemithorax of an intact supine canine model. Ellipses, regional measurements defining three orthogonal planes. (After Novak et al.,[7] with permission.)*

Airway pressure, regional pleural pressure and pericardial pressure

Pinsky and Guimond[8] demonstrated that the induction of heart failure was associated with a greater increase in Ppc than in juxtacardiac Ppl. With progressive increases in positive end-expiratory pressure (PEEP), juxtacardiac Ppl increased toward values similar to no PEEP Ppc levels, whereas Ppc initially remained constant. Once these two surface pressures became equal, further increases in PEEP increased both juxtacardiac Ppl and Ppc in parallel (Figure 21.3). Thus, if pericardial volume restraint exists, juxtacardiac Ppl will underestimate Ppc and have minimal effects of both pulmonary outflow (pulmonary arterial) and inflow (pulmonary venous) pressures. However, with sustained lung compression of the heart, both juxtacardiac Ppl and Ppc appear to be similar and both pulmonary arterial and venous pressure increase.

Static lung expansion occurs as Paw increases because the transpulmonary pressure (P_A relative to Ppl) increases. If lung injury induces alveolar flooding or increased pulmonary parenchyma stiffness, greater increases in Paw will be required to distend the lungs to a desired end-inspiratory volume. Romand *et al.*[9] demonstrated in an acute intact canine model that Paw increased much more during acute lung injury than in control conditions for a constant tidal volume (Vt), whereas lateral chest wall Ppl and Ppc increased similarly in both conditions (Figure 21.4). These data agree with the studies of O'Quinn *et al.*[10] and others showing that the primary determinant of the increase in Ppl and Ppc during positive-pressure ventilation is lung volume change, not the Paw, P_A or chest wall compliance. The Romand *et al.* study[9] further extended this understanding by demonstrating that the increase in Ppl induced by sustained increases in lung volume is greater than the associated increase in Ppc, because increasing lung volume also reduces ventricular filling and their size inside the cardiac fossa.

Because acute lung injury (ALI) is often non-homogeneous, the large increases in Paw often seen during mechanical ventilation should overdistend the aerated lung units.[11] Vascular structures that are distended may have a greater increase in their surrounding pressure than collapsible structures.[12] However, both Romand *et al.*[9] and Scharf and Ingram[13] demonstrated that, despite this non-homogeneous alveolar distension, Ppl increases equally if Vt is kept constant, independent of the mechanical properties of the lung. Thus, if Vt is kept constant, changes in end-inspiratory plateau and mean Paw will reflect both changes in the mechanical properties of the lungs and patient coordination, but may not reflect changes in Ppl. Similarly, these changes in Paw may not alter global cardiovascular dynamics. Pinsky *et al.*[14] showed in postoperative cardiac surgery patients that the percentage of Paw increase that will be transmitted

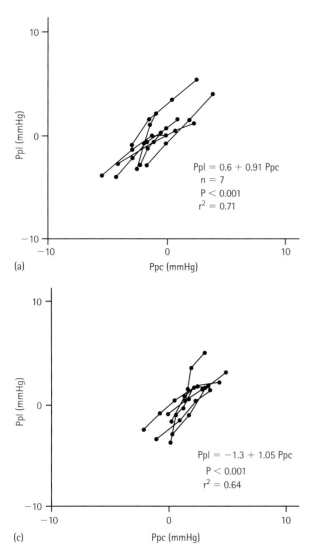

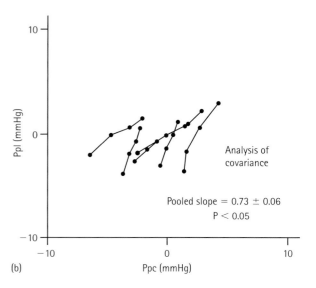

Figure 21.3 *(a) The relationship between pericardial pressure (Ppc) and juxtacardiac pleural pressure (Ppl) at 0, 5, 10 and 15 cmH$_2$O positive end-expiratory pressure in the control condition. Individual data points for the four levels of PEEP in the same dog are connected. (b) The effects of increase in PEEP on the relationship between Ppc and Ppl during acute ventricular failure. (c) The effect of increase in PEEP on the relationship between Ppc and Ppl during acute ventricular failure and lung injury. (Reproduced with permission from Pinsky MR, Guimond JG. The effects of positive end-expiratory pressure on heart-lung interactions.* J Crit Care *1991; 6:1–11.)*

to the pericardial surface is not constant as PEEP is increased (Figure 21.5).

Although it may be difficult to know the actual Ppl at end inspiration, it is possible to accurately determine the change in Ppl induced by ventilatory maneuvers. Performing either active inspiratory or expiratory maneuvers against an occluded airway (the Mueller and Valsalva maneuvers, respectively) allows one to vary ITP by an exact amount. Since lung volume does not change, transpulmonary pressure is constant so that the change in ITP is equal to the change in Paw.[15] Accordingly, a 20 mmHg increase in Paw during a Valsalva maneuver will reflect an increase in ITP of 20 mmHg; similarly, a decrease in Paw of 20 mmHg during a Mueller maneuver will reflect a 20 mmHg decrease in ITP.

Normal ventilatory efforts, either during spontaneous or positive-pressure breathing, can be used to assess the relative change in ITP in the absence of airway obstruction in a fashion similar to Mueller and Valsalva maneuvers. Since intrathoracic vascular structures sense ITP as their surrounding pressure, dynamic and rapid swings in ITP will be reflected in intrathoracic vascular pressure swings. Both right atrial and pulmonary artery diastolic pressure swings tend to closely follow Ppl changes during ventilation. The resultant 'respiratory artifacts' in the intrathoracic vascular pressure recordings induced by ventilation can be used for diagnostic purposes. For example, in the absence of LV outflow obstruction, variations in systolic arterial pressure can be used to assess swings in Ppl.

There are two limitations to the use of intrathoracic vascular and esophageal pressures to estimate Ppc. First, Ppc and ITP may not be similar or increase by similar amounts with the increasing Paw. For example, the pericardium becomes a limiting membrane in heart failure.[16,17] Operationally, this equates to Ppc exceeding juxtacardiac Ppl by the degree to which the pericardium limits biventricular dilation. Ppc is the surrounding pressure for ventricular distension such that ventricular distending pressure equals the difference between intraluminal pressure (inside the right or left ventricle) and Ppc. Thus, estimates of Ppc made by

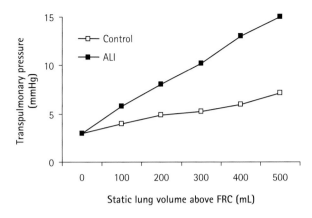

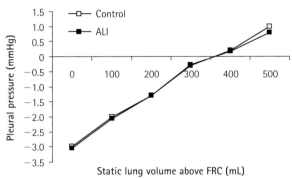

Figure 21.4 *Relation between airway pressure (Paw) and tidal volume (Vt) and between pleural pressure (Ppl) and Vt in control and oleic acid-induced acute lung injury (ALI) conditions in a canine model. Note that despite greater increases in Paw for the same Vt during ALI as compared to control conditions, Ppl and Ppc increase similarly during both control and ALI conditions for the same increase in Vt. FRC, functional residual capacity. (After Romand J et al.[9])*

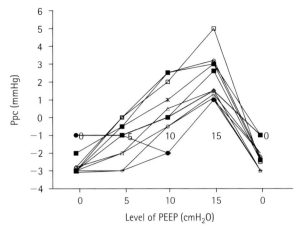

Figure 21.5 *Relation between pericardial pressure (Ppc) and airway pressure as apneic levels of positive end-expiratory pressure (PEEP) were progressively increased from zero to 15 cmH$_2$O and then back to zero in 5 cmH$_2$O increments in patients immediately following open heart surgery. Note that although Ppc increases in all subjects as PEEP is increased from 0 to 15 cmH$_2$O, the initial Ppc value and the proportional change in Ppc among incremental increases in PEEP are quite different among subject, such that no specific proportion of airway pressure transmission to the pericardial surface can be assumed to occur in all patients. (After Pinsky et al.[143])*

using ITP measures may underestimate Ppc and overestimate the increase in Ppc as Paw is increased. Second, although esophageal pressure accurately reflects negative swings in Ppl during spontaneous inspiration in upright, seated individuals[3] and in recumbent dogs in the left lateral position,[18] it underestimates both the positive swings in Ppl and the mean increase in Ppl seen with increases in lung volume during positive-pressure ventilation. During Mueller and Valsalva maneuvers, swings in esophageal pressure will accurately reflect swings in Ppl because lung volume does not change.[13]

Although lung volume increases during both spontaneous and conventional positive-pressure ventilation, ITP decreases during spontaneous ventilation and increases during positive-pressure inspiration. Thus, changes in ITP represent one of the primary determinants of the hemodynamic differences between spontaneous and positive-pressure ventilation.[19,20] The other primary difference between spontaneous and positive-pressure ventilation is the metabolic demand by exercising respiratory muscle, since spontaneous ventilation requires greater work of

breathing. The work of breathing, nominal with normal lungs, can become quite high with disease and compromise cardiovascular stability:[21] Increased work cost of breathing is associated with increases in cardiac output, pulmonary arterial pressure (PAP) and arteriovenous O$_2$ content difference, and a reduction in mixed venous O$_2$ saturation (SvO$_2$), which can augment the hypoxic pulmonary vasoconstrictor response.

HEMODYNAMIC EFFECTS OF CHANGES IN LUNG VOLUME

Changes in lung volume alter autonomic tone and its influence on pulmonary vascular resistance. Furthermore, at high lung volumes, the expanded lungs mechanically compress the heart in the cardiac fossa, limiting cardiac filling. Each of these processes is important in assessing the pulmonary vascular response to mechanical ventilation.

Autonomic tone

The lungs are richly innervated with integrated somatic and autonomic fibers that originate, traverse through, and end in the thorax. These neuronal networks mediate multiple homeostatic processes through the autonomic nervous system. They alter, for example, both instantaneous cardiovascular function, such as respiratory sinus arrhythmia, and steady-state cardiovascular status, such as antidiuretic hormone-induced fluid retention.

The most commonly described cardiovascular reflex is the inflation-chronotropic response, a vagally mediated reflex arc.[22,23] Lung inflation to normal Vt increases heart rate through withdrawal of parasympathetic tone, a process referred to as respiratory sinus arrhythmia[24] that denotes normal autonomic tone.[25] Interestingly, the reappearance of lost respiratory sinus arrhythmia precedes return of peripheral autonomic control in diabetics with peripheral neuropathy.[26] However, some degree of respiratory-associated heart rate change is intrinsic to the heart itself. Following cardiac transplantation, when the heart demonstrates no chronotropic response to atropine, a small degree of ventilation-associated heart rate changes persists.[27]

Lung inflation to larger Vt (>15 mL/kg) decreases heart rate. Minimal pulmonary vasoconstriction may also occur through vagal reflex arcs,[28] but this does not appear to result in significant hemodynamic effects. Reflex systemic arterial vasodilatation can also occur with lung hyperinflation[22,29–33] and is mediated by afferent vagal fibers since it is abolished by both selective vagotomy and atropine infusion. Blocking sympathetic afferent fibers also blocks this reflex,[31,34] presumably by withdrawing central sympathetic tone. This inflation–vasodilatation response is of minimal clinical significance under normal conditions and probably less significant for the pulmonary circulation in particular, except during high-frequency ventilation and with hyperinflation.[22,31] However, recruitment maneuvers and the use of sustained increases in end-expiratory airway pressure often induce systemic vasodilatation in subjects with acute lung injury and non-homogeneous lung collapse, and can result in clinically relevant changes in systemic blood flow (see below).

Humoral factors, including products of the cyclo-oxygenase pathway of prostaglandin synthesis,[35] are also released from the pulmonary endothelium during lung inflation. These vasodilating and bronchodilating compounds may be responsible for some of the observed decreases in airway resistance and decreased pulmonary arterial tone following lung recruitment maneuvers. However, other processes, such as withdrawal of hypoxic pulmonary vasoconstriction and stress-relaxation, are probably the primary factors determining this lung distension–vasodilatation response. Overdistension induces a depressor response by causing sympathetic withdrawal,[36–38] but, as with the vasodilatation response, these interactions do not appear to substantively alter cardiovascular status except in the setting of non-homogenous lung disease.[39] In fact, unilateral lung hyperinflation (unilateral PEEP) does not influence systemic hemodynamics or pulmonary blood flow to the opposite lung.[40]

Sustained increases in lung volume, as induced by the application of PEEP, also alters autonomic tone in a tonic fashion. The application of PEEP and the associated decline in cardiac output increases heart rate, but less than that seen when cardiac output is reduced to similar degrees by hemorrhage.[28] The reasons for this heart rate difference are not known, but may reflect diminished baroreceptor stimulation and direct increases in arterial pressure produced by PEEP.

Ventilation also alters control of intravascular fluid balance via hormonal release. Both positive-pressure ventilation and sustained hyperinflation induced by PEEP stimulate a variety of endocrinological responses that induce fluid retention via right atrial stretch receptors. Plasma norepinephrine, plasma renin activity[41,42] and atrial natriuretic peptide[43] increase during positive-pressure ventilation with or without PEEP. When subjects with congestive heart failure are exposed to continuous positive airway pressure (CPAP), however, plasma atrial natriuretic peptide activity decreases in parallel with improvements in blood flow,[44,45] suggesting that hemodynamic changes, rather than positive airway pressure ventilation *per se*, are responsible for this effect.

Pulmonary vascular resistance and hypoxic pulmonary vasoconstriction

Lung volume is a major determinant of pulmonary vascular resistance, and extrinsic processes to the lungs, such as a humoral or sympathetic tone changes, are not required to induce the changes in pulmonary vascular resistance seen with ventilation.[19,46–50] Lung inflation, independent of changes in ITP, primarily affects the pulmonary circulation by altering both pulmonary vascular resistance and the downstream pressure for pulmonary blood flow.[51]

RV afterload is the maximal RV systolic wall stress during contraction,[52] which, by the law of LaPlace, is equal to the radius of curvature of the right ventricle (a function of end-diastolic volume) and transmural pressure (a function of systolic RV pressure).[53] Changes in ITP that occur without changing lung volume, as may occur with occluded respiratory efforts, will not affect the pulmonary vascular resistance since the pressure gradients between the RV and pulmonary artery are not altered.

Since the pulmonary artery resides inside the thorax, actual RV ejection pressure and PAP reflect pulmonary arterial intraluminal pressure relative to ITP, referred to as transmural PAP. Transmural PAP can increase by one of two mechanisms:

- an increase in pulmonary arterial pressure without an increase in pulmonary vasomotor tone, as may occur with either a marked increase in blood flow (exercise) or an increases in outflow pressure (LV failure, high levels of PEEP); or

- an increase in pulmonary vascular resistance by either active changes in vasomotor tone or lung inflation.

An increase in transmural PAP during positive-pressure ventilation is due to an increase in pulmonary vascular resistance, since neither instantaneous cardiac output[54] nor LV filling[15] usually increases. However, RV ejection will be impeded if transmural PAP increases.[55] Furthermore, if RV emptying is incomplete, not only will stroke volume decrease[56] but its residual volume will increase and limit subsequent filling.[54] If RV dilation persists, RV coronary perfusion cannot be sustained across such high wall stresses, and RV free wall ischemia and infarction can develop.[57] Thus, acute cor pulmonale is associated with a profound decrease in cardiac output that is usually resistant to therapies designed to enhance venous return (e.g. fluid challenge).

The mechanisms by which pulmonary vasomotor tone varies during mechanical ventilation are complex and include the effects on hypoxic pulmonary vasoconstriction and the mechanical compression of pulmonary capillaries by lung expansion. During normal end inspiration, mild hypoxemia (PaO_2 >65 mmHg) and low levels (<7.5 cmH_2O) of PEEP have minimal effects of pulmonary vasomotor tone. If these minimal increases in transmural PAP are sustained, however, fluid retention occurs and results in an increase in RV end-diastolic volume to maintain cardiac output constant despite the increased pulmonary vasomotor tone.[53,59]

Local pulmonary vasomotor tone increases and blood flow decreases when regional alveolar PO_2 (P_AO_2) decreases below 60 mmHg.[60] Since lung volume is reduced in acute hypoxemic respiratory failure,[61,62] pulmonary vascular resistance is often increased owing to alveolar collapse and the resultant hypoxic pulmonary vasoconstriction.

Mechanical ventilation–induced changes in pulmonary vascular resistance

Mechanical ventilation opens collapsed alveolar units, refreshes alveolar gas with higher FiO_2, and reverses respiratory acidosis; as a consequence of these effects, mechanical ventilation may reduce pulmonary vasomotor tone.[64–70] These effects do not require positive-pressure breaths as much as expansion of collapsed alveoli,[71] which is usually accomplished by the addition of PEEP. The beneficial effect of PEEP on pulmonary vascular resistance is greatest in the neonate, where the vascular response to hypoxia is accentuated.

Changes in lung volume can also profoundly increase pulmonary arterial pressure by passively compressing the alveolar vessels.[61,68,69] The pulmonary circulation can be separated into two groups of blood vessels depending on the pressure that surrounds them[68] (Figure 21.6). The small pulmonary arterioles, venules, and alveolar capillaries

sense alveolar pressure as their surrounding pressure and are referred to as alveolar vessels. The large pulmonary arteries and veins, as well as the heart and intrathoracic great vessels of the systemic circulation, sense interstitial pressure or ITP as their surrounding pressure and can be called extra-alveolar vessels. Since increasing lung volume requires transpulmonary pressure to increase and vice versa, the extravascular pressure gradient between alveolar to extra-alveolar vessels varies with changes in lung volume. The radial interstitial forces of the lung[72,73] act upon the extra-alveolar vessels much as they do on the airways: as lung volume increases, the radial interstitial forces increase, increasing the diameter of both extra-alveolar vessels and airways. Thus, just as airway resistance decreases with lung distension, extra-alveolar vessels dilate,[74] causing their capacitance to increase and pooling blood in the pulmonary arteries and veins. The opposite condition occurs during deflation and with steady-state decreases in lung volume.[64,67] Accordingly, pulmonary vascular resistance is increased at small lung volumes owing to the combined effect of hypoxic pulmonary vasoconstriction and extra-alveolar vessel collapse.

Unlike the extra-alveolar vessels whose resistance decreases during lung inflation, alveolar vessels increase their resistance as lung volume progressively increases to levels above resting lung volume or functional residual capacity (FRC).[64,75] If the cross-sectional area of the pulmonary capillaries is already reduced, the addition of abnormal hyperinflation can create significant pulmonary hypertension and may precipitate acute RV failure[76] and RV ischemia.[57] Similarly, if lung volumes are reduced,

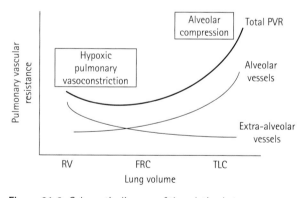

Figure 21.6 *Schematic diagram of the relation between changes in lung volume and pulmonary vascular resistance (PVR), where the extra-alveolar and alveolar vascular components are separated. Note that pulmonary vascular resistance is minimal at resting lung volume or functional residual capacity (FRC). As lung volume increases toward total lung capacity (TLC) or decreases toward residual volume (RV), pulmonary vascular resistance also increases. However, the increase in resistance with hyperinflation is caused by increased alveolar vascular resistance, whereas the increase in resistance with lung collapse is caused by increased extra-alveolar vessel tone.*

increasing lung volume back to baseline levels by the use of PEEP decreases pulmonary vascular resistance.[77]

PEEP-induced changes in pulmonary blood flow: West zones of the lung and vascular waterfalls

Increases in P_A relative to pulmonary venous pressure also influence pulmonary blood flow. West *et al.* originally described pulmonary blood flow through the alveoli as comprising at least three vascular zones, defined by hydrostatic pressure, vascular pressure and P_A (Figure 21.7).[69] When P_A exceeds PAP there can be no blood flow because downstream pressure exceeds inflow pressure (zone 1). If PAP exceeds P_A, then blood flow into that region of the lung will occur (zone 2). Conceptually, one can consider P_A to be the effective backpressure to pulmonary blood flow when P_A is greater than pulmonary venous pressure. This concept has been referred to as the 'vascular waterfall'[75] because the flow across these beds will be unaffected by downstream changes in pulmonary venous pressure. However, when pulmonary venous pressure exceeds P_A, the pressure gradient for pulmonary blood flow is defined by the difference between PAP and pulmonary venous pressure (zone 3). In the resting supine state with a PAP of 15/8 mmHg, most, if not all of the lung units are in Zone 3 conditions. However, with standing at rest, hyperinflation, or the application of PEEP, Zone 1 and 2 conditions routinely develop.[68]

Zone 1 conditions equate to areas of the lung that are ventilated but not perfused. Increasing the amount of lung in zone 1 conditions increases dead-space ventilation, increasing $PaCO_2$ for an unchanged minute ventilation and CO_2 production. This occurs when PAP decreases, as may occur in hypovolemic shock, or when P_A increases, as

would occur with the application of high levels of PEEP. Since an obligatory effect of increasing zone 1 conditions is to increase $PaCO_2$, a common finding in patients in shock on fixed minute ventilation is hypercapnia. Accordingly, fluid resuscitation by itself often reduces $PaCO_2$, if it results in an increase in pulmonary blood flow and PAP.

When P_A exceeds PVP, it becomes the outflow pressure for pulmonary blood flow. Under many clinical conditions, P_A may exceed PVP, as estimated by pulmonary artery occlusion pressure (PAOP). Since the effect of increasing PEEP on pulmonary blood flow is difficult to define in subjects being phasically ventilated and having a phasic RV ejection into the pulmonary circulation, models of isolated perfused lungs allowing one to fix lung distension as various transpulmonary pressures and P_A, as well as constant pulmonary inflow and pulmonary venous pressure levels have been used to simplify this analysis. Lopez-Muniz *et al.*[75] demonstrated in isolated canine lungs with a constant pulmonary inflow rate that increasing pulmonary venous pressure did not alter PAP until PVP exceeded P_A, regardless of the level of P_A. Once PVP exceeded P_A, increases in PVP further increased PAP (Figure 21.8). Note in Figure 21.8 that PAP is greater than PVP by an amount equal to the vascular resistance at that moment. As PVP increases further, the pressure difference between PAP and PVP decreases, as more pulmonary vascular units are recruited and pulmonary vascular resistance decreases. Thus, by increasing the outflow pressure, PEEP causes a parallel shift to the left in the pressure/flow

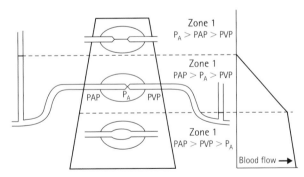

Figure 21.7 *Schematic representation of the effect of hydrostatic pressure on pulmonary blood flow. Operationally, one can define three unique situations owing to changes in alveolar pressure (P_A) relative to pulmonary artery pressure (PAP) and pulmonary venous pressure (PVP): zone 1, $P_A > PAP > PVP$; zone 2, $PAP > P_A > PVP$; zone 3, $PAP > PVP > P_A$. Since these zonal characteristics were first described by West et al., they are usually referred to as West zones, 1, 2 and 3, respectively. (After West et al.[69])*

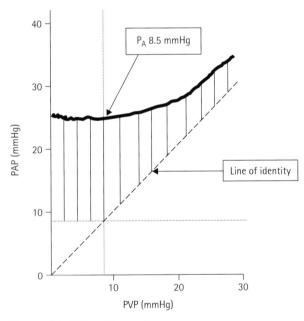

Figure 21.8 *Effect of increasing pulmonary venous pressure (PVP) on pulmonary artery pressure (PAP) at a positive end-expiratory pressure of 10 cmH₂O in an isolated perfused dog lung at a constant pulmonary flow rate. P_A, alveolar pressure. (After Lopez-Muniz et al.[75])*

relationship (Figure 21.9). Domino and Pinsky[78] found that the effects of hypoxic pulmonary vasoconstriction and PEEP were complimentary. PEEP did not alter the slope of the pressure/flow relation but shifted it leftward. Similarly, hypoxic pulmonary vasoconstriction decreased the slope of the pressure/flow relation but did not alter the zero flow intercept (Figure 21.10).

Patients with acute lung injury have complex ventilation/perfusion mismatching due to alveolar flooding, regional hyperinflation and hypoxic pulmonary vasoconstriction. By selectively increasing P_A in aerated lung units, PEEP recruits collapsed lung units by the process of alveolar interdependence. Walther et al.[79] demonstrated the application of PEEP in acute lung injury tended to restore a more uniform alveolar ventilation. These data agree with those from chest computerized tomography studies.[80]

Ventricular interdependence

Changes in RV output alter LV filling because the two ventricles are linked through the pulmonary vasculature. However, LV preload can also be indirectly altered by changes in RV end-diastolic volume. Similarly, increasing RV outflow impedance will result in a reduced RV stroke volume and RV dilation through an increase in RV end-systolic volume. If RV volume increases, LV diastolic compliance will decrease by the mechanism of ventricular interdependence.[81] Increasing RV end-diastolic volume will induce a shift of the intraventricular septum into the LV, thereby decreasing LV diastolic compliance[82] (Figure 21.11). Thus, for the same LV filling pressure, LV end-diastolic volume and cardiac output will be

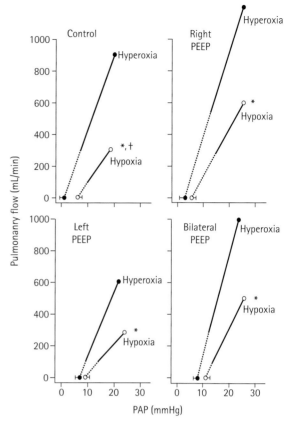

Figure 21.10 Effect of unilateral lung hypoxia and 10 cmH$_2$O positive end-expiratory pressure (PEEP) on the relation between mean PAP and pulmonary flow in the dog. (After Domino and Pinsky.[78]) * p < 0.05 slope less than hyperoxia; †p < 0.05 zero flow intercept greater than hyperoxia.

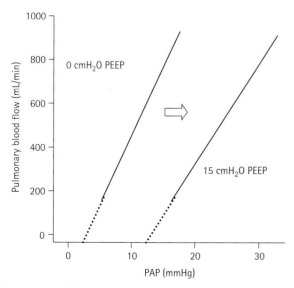

Figure 21.9 Effect of 10 cmH$_2$O positive end-expiratory pressure (PEEP) the relation between pulmonary artery pressure (PAP) and pulmonary flow as pulmonary flow is increased. (After data presented in Lopez-Muniz et al.[75])

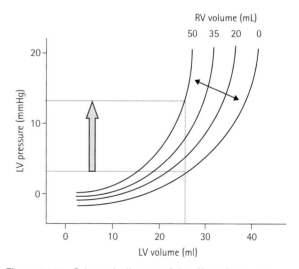

Figure 21.11 Schematic diagram of the effect of increasing right ventricular (RV) volumes on the left ventricular (LV) diastolic pressure/volume (filling) relationship. Note that increasing RV volumes decrease LV diastolic compliance, such that a higher filling pressure is required to generate a constant end-diastolic volume. (After Taylor et al.[81])

decreased. This interaction, known as pulsus paradoxus, is felt to be the major determinant of the phasic changes in arterial pulse pressure and cardiac output seen in cardiac tamponade, and can also be seen in subjects with normal cardiovascular function during loaded spontaneous inspiration. These phasic changes in LV stroke volume and arterial pulse pressure may reflect ventilation-induced changes in LV filling and can be used to predict preload responsiveness.[84]

By increasing venous return, spontaneous inspiration induces RV dilation that will decrease LV end-diastolic volume. Maintaining a relatively constant rate of venous return, either by volume resuscitation[83] or vasopressor infusion, will minimize this effect. These phasic changes in arterial pressure have also been used as a marker of functional hypovolemia during spontaneous ventilation.[1,84]

Mechanical heart/lung interactions

Increases in end-expiratory volume occur in settings of increased expiratory airway resistance such as asthma and chronic obstructive lung disease. Since mechanical ventilation can deliver breaths at almost any Vt, driving pressure and frequency, lung hyperinflation commonly occurs with profound effects on the pulmonary circulation and the heart. The heart can be compressed between the two hyperinflated lungs,[85] increasing the pressure surrounding the heart. Since the heart is confined within the cardiac fossa, juxtacardiac Ppl will increase more than lateral chest-wall or diaphragmatic Ppl.[7,17] This compressive effect of the inflated lung can be seen with either spontaneous hyperinflation[86] or positive-pressure-induced hyperinflation with PEEP.[72,73] As Ppc increases, LV distending pressure for a constant LV end-diastolic pressure also decreases. The decrease in 'apparent' LV diastolic compliance[83] was previously misinterpreted as impaired LV contractility, because LV stroke work is decreased for a given LV end-diastolic pressure or PAOP.[87,88] Numerous studies have shown that when patients are fluid resuscitated to return LV end-diastolic volume to its original level, both LV stroke work and cardiac output also return to their original levels,[48,83] despite the continued application of PEEP.[89] Takata et al.[90] proposed using the terms 'coupled' and 'uncoupled' pericardial restraint and proposed that pericardial stiffness (or elastance) over the right and left ventricles is different in constrictive pericarditis but similar in tamponade: in constrictive pericarditis, changes in venous return should selectively alter RV filling, whereas tamponade should alter both RV and LV filling. Using this theoretical framework, one may extrapolate to the dynamic effects of ventilation. Tidal increases in lung volume represent 'uncoupled' pericardial restraint because tidal breathing tends to selectively limit RV filling and not LV diastolic compliance. Hyperinflation, however, would produce a

'coupled' cardiac fossal restraint. Van den Berg et al.[91] found that the instantaneous effect of positive-pressure inspiration was to reduce RV output, whilst reductions in LV output took several beats to occur. Sustained increases in Paw induced by apneic PEEP resulted in a parallel reduction in biventricular output. Thus, hyperinflation, as occurs in severe asthma and with the use of excessive amounts of PEEP, would produce a clinical picture indistinguishable from tamponade. These findings confirmed those of Rebuck and Read[92] on the hemodynamic effects of severe asthma. Presumably, the shift from 'uncoupled' to 'coupled' cardiac fossal restraint would occur as absolute lung volume increased, biventricular volume increased, or both. Thus, if cardiac volumes are small and lung inflation does not overdistend the thoracic cage, RV filling will be primarily impeded. However, in congestive heart failure states and with marked lung overdistension, both RV and LV filling may be compromised by ventilation.

HEMODYNAMIC EFFECTS OF CHANGES IN INTRATHORACIC PRESSURE

Changes in ITP will affect the pressure gradients for both venous return to the RV and systemic outflow from the LV. Increases in ITP, by increasing right atrial pressure (RAP) and decreasing transmural LV systolic pressure, will reduce these pressure gradients and thereby decrease intrathoracic blood volume. In the extreme, these spontaneous inspiratory efforts may precipitate pulmonary edema and arterial hypoxemia. Conversely, decreases in ITP will augment venous return and impede LV ejection, thereby increasing intrathoracic blood volume. In the extreme, these positive-pressure breaths can precipitate hypovolemic cardiovascular collapse.

Systemic venous return

Systemic venous return defines RV filling and is equal to cardiac output in the steady state. As characterized by Guyton et al.,[93] venous return varies inversely with downstream RAP in a fashion described by a fixed upstream pressure. Mean circulatory filling pressure is between 7 and 12 mmHg in humans under general anesthesia.[94] Mean systemic pressure does not change rapidly during the ventilatory cycle whereas RAP does, because of the direct influence that concomitant changes in ITP have on RAP. Accordingly, variations in RAP represent the major factor determining the fluctuation in pressure gradient for systemic venous return during ventilation.[54,95] RAP increases along with increases in ITP, for example with positive-pressure ventilation or hyperinflation during mechanical ventilation. As a result, the pressure gradient for systemic venous return decreases, decelerating venous blood flow,[56] decreasing RV filling and, consequently, decreasing RV stroke volume.[54,56,96–103] During normal spontaneous inspiration, the converse occurs: RAP decreases with decreases in ITP, accelerating venous blood flow and increasing RV filling and RV stroke volume[4,20,56,98,101,104] (Figure 21.12).

The decrease in venous return during positive-pressure ventilation may be less than expected based on the above scenario. Since lung volume increase results in diaphragmatic descent, abdominal pressure also increases. Fessler et al.[105] and Takata and Robotham[106] demonstrated in dogs that PEEP-induced increase in abdominal pressure increases the pressure surrounding the intra-abdominal vasculature. Because a large proportion of venous blood

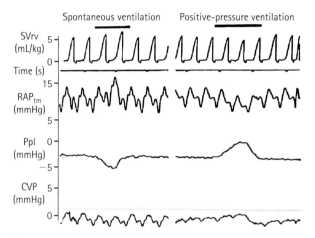

Figure 21.12 *Continuous trend recording of right ventricular stroke volume (SVrv), transmural right atrial pressure (RAP), pleural pressure (Ppl) and RAP during spontaneous ventilation (left panel) and at a similar tidal volume during positive-pressure ventilation (right panel). CVP, central venous pressure.*

is in the abdomen, the net effect of PEEP is to increase both mean systemic pressure and RAP. Accordingly, the pressure gradient for venous return may not be reduced by PEEP, particularly in patients with hypervolemia. Recently, Van den Berg et al. demonstrated that the ratio of RAP to abdominal pressure increased little with the application of up to 15 cmH$_2$O PEEP (Figure 21.13)[107] and concluded that sustained increases in Paw have minimal effects on venous return when subjects have been adequately fluid resuscitated. With exaggerated swings in ITP, as occur with obstructed inspiratory efforts, venous return behaves as if abdominal pressure is additive to mean systemic pressure in defining total venous blood flow.[108–111]

Because inverse ratio ventilation produces substantial degrees of hyperinflation, its hemodynamic effects have been the subject of concern. However, Mang et al.[112] found no hemodynamic difference between conventional ventilation and inverse ratio ventilation when total PEEP was similar.

Right ventricular filling

Under normal conditions, it is extremely difficult to document that RV filling pressures change as RV filling occurs. When RV filling pressure, defined as RAP minus Ppc, was directly measured in patients undergoing open chest operations, RV filling pressure did not change despite large changes in RV volume.[113] Although right atrial pressure increases with volume loading, Ppc also increases and RV filling pressure is unchanged. Similar results are seen when RV volumes are reduced by the application of PEEP in postoperative cardiac patients.[114] These data suggest that, under normal conditions, RV diastolic compliance is very high and most of the increase in RAP seen

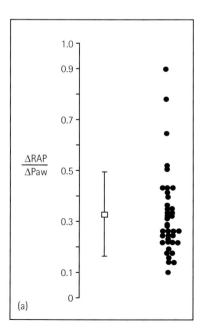

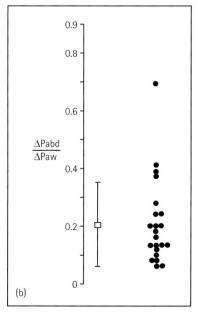

Figure 21.13 *(a) Relation between change in right atrial pressure (RAP) (ΔPra) to change in airway pressure (ΔPaw) with the application of 10 cmH$_2$O positive end-expiratory pressure (PEEP). (b) The relation between change in abdominal pressure (ΔPabd) and ΔPaw with the application of 10 cmH$_2$O PEEP. Note that although Paw increases by 10 cmH$_2$O, right atrial pressure increases by approximately 70% of that value because Pabd increases. (After data reported in Van den Berg et al.[107])*

during volume loading reflects pericardial compliance and cardiac fossa stiffness rather than changes in RV distending pressure. Presumably, conformational changes in the RV rather than wall stretch are responsible for RV enlargement.[16] However, increases in RAP may occur as a result of decreased RV diastolic compliance, increased pericardial compliance, increased end-diastolic volume, or a combination of all three. Since PEEP and, by extension, lung expansion, compresses the heart within the cardiac fossa in a fashion analogous to pericardial tamponade, it is the expanding lungs that increase ITP rather than pericardial restraint, limiting ventricular filling.[115,116]

Positive-pressure ventilation impairs normal circulatory adaptive processes operative during spontaneous ventilation. Even if one restores the coupling of RAP and RV volume by using partial ventilatory support modes of ventilation, cardiac output will increase only if the RV can convert the increased venous return to forward blood flow. During weaning from mechanical ventilation, occult RV failure, manifest by a rapid rise in RAP and a fall in cardiac output, may be exposed. Since the primary effect on normal cardiovascular function of any form of ventilation is to alter RV preload by altering venous return, the detrimental effect of positive-pressure ventilation on cardiac output can be minimized by either fluid resuscitation[4,96,108,109] or by minimizing both mean ITP and swings in lung volume. Prolonging expiratory time, decreasing tidal volume, and avoiding PEEP all minimize the decrease in systemic venous return to the RV.[2,54,98–102,117,118]

Since spontaneous inspiratory efforts increase lung volume by decreasing ITP, one sees an increase in venous return with spontaneous inspiration owing to the fall in RAP.[20,46,99–101] However, this augmentation of venous return is limited[110,111] because if ITP decreases below atmospheric pressure, venous return becomes flow-limited as the large systemic veins collapse upon entering the thorax.[93] This venous flow-limitation is a safety valve for the heart because ITP can decrease greatly with obstructive inspiratory efforts.[32] If venous return were not flow-limited, the RV could overdistend and fail.[119]

LV preload and ventricular interdependence

In the steady state, changes in venous return must eventually result in directionally similar changes in LV preload, because the two ventricles function in series.[120] However, with sustained increases in ITP, only RV output decreases because the intrathoracic blood continues to drain into the left ventricle. This phase delay in changes in output from the RV to the LV is exaggerated if Vt or respiratory rate are increased or intravascular volume is reduced.[2,49,50,83,87,88,103,117,121–125] Independent of this series interaction, direct ventricular interdependence can also occur. During positive-pressure ventilation, however, RV

volumes are usually decreased, minimizing the influence of ventricular interdependence on LV diastolic performance.[81,123–126] Jardin et al.[48,49] using transesophageal echocardiography in ventilator-dependent subjects showed that PEEP did result in some degree of right-to-left intraventricular septal shift, although the amount of this shift was small. Although increases in lung volume during positive-pressure ventilation cause some septal shift, the primary effect of increasing lung volume is to compress the two ventricles into each other, decreasing biventricular volumes.[127] Accordingly, the decrease in cardiac output during PEEP is due largely to a decrease in LV end-diastolic volume. Restoration of LV end-diastolic volume by fluid resuscitation returns cardiac output to baseline values[128,129] without any significant change in LV diastolic compliance.[83]

LV afterload

Maximal LV afterload can be equated to the maximal product of LV pressure and volume that represents maximal systolic wall tension. As for the right ventricle, maximal LV wall tension normally occurs at the end of isometric contraction, reflecting both a maximal LV radius of curvature (end-diastolic volume) and aortic pressure (diastolic pressure) product. During ejection, LV volumes decrease rapidly, decreasing LV radius of curvature and LV wall stress. Thus, under normal conditions the left ventricle unloads itself during ejection. When LV dilation exists, as in congestive heart failure, maximal LV wall stress occurs during LV ejection since the maximal product of these two variables occurs later in ejection, owing to the markedly increased radius of curvature and its minimal decrease during ejection. Accordingly, LV afterload varies in its definition depending on the baseline level of cardiac contractility and intravascular volume.

LV ejection pressure is most accurately defined as transmural LV systolic or arterial pressure. Since normal baroreceptor mechanisms tend to maintain arterial pressure, if arterial pressure were to remain constant as ITP increased, then LV wall tension would also decrease. Similarly, if transmural arterial pressure were to remain constant as ITP increased but LV end-diastolic volume were to decrease because of the decrease in systemic venous return usually seen with increases in ITP, then LV wall tension would also decrease.[130] Thus, by either mechanism, increases in ITP decrease LV afterload. Similarly, decreases in ITP with a constant arterial pressure will increase LV transmural pressure increasing LV afterload.[15,131] Decreasing ITP, a common occurrence during spontaneous inspiratory efforts, reflects an important cardiac stress during weaning from mechanical ventilation.[130–133] A similar mechanism can be proposed for the improvement in LV systolic function seen in patients with severe LV failure.[134] Interestingly, similar 'auto-end-expiratory airway pressure' effects of expiratory grunting have been reported in infants during crying[50] and in an adult with severe LV failure.[135]

Pulsus paradoxus occurs during spontaneous inspiration under conditions of marked pericardial restraint. This may occur because of pericardial limitations, such as with tamponade and constrictive pericarditis, or during loaded spontaneous ventilatory efforts when RV volumes swell and ITP decreases. In both cases, LV stroke volume decreases.[136–140] The negative swings in ITP increase LV ejection pressure (LV pressure minus ITP) increasing LV end-systolic volume.[15] Other influences on LV systolic function can also occur during loaded inspiratory efforts, including increased aortic input impedance,[141] altered synchrony of contraction of the global LV myocardium[142] and hypoxemia-induced decreased contractility and LV diastolic compliance.[143,144]

Sustained increases in ITP, for example by increasing PEEP, decrease aortic blood flow and arterial pressure due to the decrease in venous return.[15] Since normal baroreceptor-based homeostatic mechanisms tend to maintain a constant arterial pressure to maintain organ perfusion,[31] if ITP increased arterial pressure without changing transmural arterial pressure, the periphery would reflexively vasodilate to maintain a constant extrathoracic arterial pressure/flow relation.[122] Since coronary perfusion pressure reflects the intrathoracic pressure gradient for blood flow, it is not increased by ITP-induced increases in arterial pressure. However, compression of the coronaries by the expanding lungs may obstruct coronary blood flow. A decrease in coronary blood flow through these processes may induce myocardial ischemia.[145–147]

Myocardial energetics and changes in ITP

Increasing LV ejection pressure increases myocardial O_2 demand because stroke work is increased. Since negative swings in ITP increase LV ejection pressure, maneuvers that result in vigorous inspiratory efforts in the setting of airway obstruction (asthma, upper airway obstruction, vocal cord paralysis) or stiff lungs (interstitial lung disease, pulmonary edema and acute lung injury) will selectively increase LV afterload, and have been postulated to be the cause of LV failure and pulmonary edema seen in these conditions,[19,32] particularly if LV systolic function is already compromised.[148,149] Similarly, removing large negative swings in ITP by either bypassing upper airway obstruction (endotracheal intubation) or instituting mechanical ventilation will selectively reduce LV afterload without significantly decreasing either venous return or cardiac output.[4,93,121,150–152] Placing patients in cardiogenic pulmonary edema on mechanical ventilation, for example, will rapidly reverse the pulmonary edema by decreasing intrathoracic blood volume.

HEMODYNAMIC EFFECTS OF VENTILATION BASED ON CARDIOPULMONARY STATUS

Mechanical ventilatory support can be life saving for patients with markedly increased work of breathing, hypervolemia, or impaired LV pump function because of its ability to support the cardiovascular system while decreasing global O_2 demand, independent of changes in gas exchange. However, mechanical ventilation may rapidly induce cardiovascular instability by increasing pulmonary vascular resistance and impeding venous return in patients with hypovolemia or a strong tendency to develop hyperinflation. Similarly, withdrawal of ventilatory support can be an exercise stress test in patients with limited cardiovascular reserve.[148,149]

The hemodynamic differences between modes of mechanical ventilation at a constant airway pressure and PEEP can be explained solely by their differential effects on lung volume and ITP.[153] If two different modes of ventilation induce similar changes in ITP and ventilatory effort, their hemodynamic effects will also be similar despite markedly different airway waveforms. When partial ventilatory support with either intermittent mandatory ventilation (IMV) or pressure support ventilation were matched for similar Vt in 20 patients following cardiac surgery, the hemodynamic responses were similar.[154] Sternberg and Sahebjami[155] showed that switching from assist-control to either IMV and pressure-support ventilation produced similar effects on tissue oxygenation. Finally, high-frequency jet ventilation does not affect cardiac output in patients with heart failure, even if the ventilation is delivered synchronous with the cardiac cycle.[156]

Acute lung injury

Positive-pressure ventilation decreases intrathoracic blood volume in proportion to the increase in lung volume[99] and PEEP potentiates this effect[114,116] without directly altering LV contractile function.[157] Singer *et al.*[158] demonstrated that the degree of hyperinflation, not mean Paw, determined the decrease in cardiac output in critically ill patients.

Since increases in lung volume and not mean Paw are the primary determinants of the decrease in cardiac output, different ventilatory modes with similar Vt and PEEP will have similar cardiac outputs.[159,160] However, the hemodynamic effects of hyperinflation can be counterbalanced, in part, by fluid resuscitation that restores intrathoracic blood volume to pre-PEEP levels. Similarly, when LV end-diastolic volume is restored to pre-PEEP levels, as assessed by either non-invasive blood pool scanning[157] or echocardiography,[161–163] cardiac output also returns to its pre-PEEP level despite the continued application of PEEP. That the PEEP-induced decrease in cardiac output is due to a decreased pressure gradient for venous return was illustrated by Gunter et al.[164] who minimized the decrease in cardiac output in ventilator-dependent septic patients by lower body compression, increasing mean systemic pressure and restoring the pressure gradient for venous return. If cardiac output does not increase with fluid resuscitation, other processes such as cor pulmonale, increased pulmonary vascular resistance or cardiac compression, may be responsible for cardiovascular depression.[165]

Lessard et al.[166] compared volume-controlled conventional ventilation with pressure-controlled and pressure-controlled inverse-ratio ventilation in nine patients with acute lung injury. Since ventilator settings were adjusted to keep total PEEP and Vt constant between treatment arms, the changes in ITP were similar among the three therapies. Although in this study arterial pressure was slightly lower with pressure-controlled inverse-ratio ventilation compared to both volume-controlled and pressure-controlled ventilation, no significant hemodynamic effects were seen. Chan and Abraham[167] saw similar results in 10 acute lung injury patients matched for comparable Vt and total PEEP. However, when pressure control with a smaller Vt was compared to volume control, both Abraham and Yoshihara[168] and Poelaert et al.[169] found that pressure control was associated with a higher cardiac output.

Mancini et al. studied the effect of pressure-limited ventilation compared to conventional ventilation on gas exchange and hemodynamics in eight patients with acute lung injury within the first 48 hours of their time on mechanical ventilatory support.[170] They compared Vt 10–12 mL/kg 9 ± 2 cmH$_2$O PEEP (conventional ventilation) to Vt 5–7 mL/kg and PEEP 2 cmH$_2$O above the lower inflection point of the lung compliance curve, which resulted in 19 ± 4 cmH$_2$O of PEEP (pressure-limited ventilation). Pressure-limited ventilation was associated with an increase in mean Paw (18 ± 3.7 to 21 ± 4.2 cmH$_2$O), such that the associated increase in PaO$_2$ was due partially to a reduced intrapulmonary shunt (39 ± 15 to 31 ± 11%, $r^2 = 0.79$). However, hemodynamic changes also occurred that aided in improving PaO$_2$. Since increasing SvO$_2$ will increase PaO$_2$ for a constant FiO$_2$ and intrapulmonary shunt, increases in cardiac output with an unchanged O$_2$ consumption will result in increased SvO$_2$. This is the logic for paralysis and hypothermia in the management of patients with the most severe forms of acute lung injury. By simple calculation, over one-third to one-half of the increase in PaO$_2$ during pressure-limited ventilation could be explained by the hemodynamic effects alone.

One major problem with treating ALI patients with increasing levels of mean Paw is that pulmonary outflow pressure may also increase, impeding RV ejection. Schmitt et al. studied the impact of increasing PEEP on RV outflow impedance,[171] the phasic equivalent of pulmonary vasomotor tone that relates dynamic changes in pulmonary

inflow (RV stroke volume) to systolic PAP. Since increasing outflow impedance occurs when pulmonary vasomotor tone increases or greater proportions of the lung are in zone 2 conditions (increased critical closing pressure), they studied two levels of PEEP in 16 patients with acute lung injury: one level of PEEP equaled the pressure at the lower inflection point, presumably where lung recruitment started, and the other was at a higher level of PEEP associated with the highest lung compliance, presumably where most lung recruitment occurred. They demonstrated that, compared to zero end-expiratory Paw, both levels of PEEP decreased cardiac output and increased RV outflow impedance, but was significantly less when PEEP was titrated upward to the maximal lung compliance level. Thus, lung recruitment and increases in Paw play major roles in determining RV output impedance. Based on this study, it appears that increasing PEEP in subjects with acute lung injury may both increase pulmonary input impedance by overdistension of the lung and reduce it by recruiting collapsed alveolar units. Since RV input impedance is a primary determinant of cardiac output, ventilatory strategies that limit its increase would be preferred. Accordingly, pressure-limited ventilatory strategies aimed at ventilating patients from the point of their maximal lung compliance should have the least detrimental effects on hemodynamics while simultaneously improving arterial oxygenation.

Congestive heart failure

As a general rule, when PEEP increases cardiac output, hypoxic pulmonary vasoconstriction has been reversed or LV afterload has been reduced. Clinically, increases in cardiac output with the institution of positive-pressure ventilation suggest the presence of congestive heart failure.[152,172] Grace and Greenbaum[150] noted that adding PEEP to patients with heart failure either did not decrease cardiac output or actually increased cardiac output if PAOP exceeded 18 mmHg. Similarly, Calvin et al.[173] noted that PEEP did not decrease cardiac output in patients with cardiogenic pulmonary edema. Unfortunately, PEEP may be detrimental in patients with combined heart failure and acute lung injury, and can result in increased leukocyte retention in human lungs,[174] which may reflect endothelial injury[175] or the effects of stasis of pulmonary blood produced by increasing P$_A$ relative to PAP.

Rasanen et al. documented worsening ischemia in patients with myocardial ischemia and acute LV failure undergoing withdrawal of ventilatory support.[152,176] Preventing spontaneous inspiratory effort-induced negative swings in ITP could minimize this detrimental cardiac effect.[151]

The cardiovascular benefits of positive Paw can be seen by withdrawing negative swings in ITP, for example, by using increasing levels of CPAP.[173,174] Nasal CPAP can accomplish the same results in patients with obstructive sleep apnea and heart failure,[177] although the benefits do not appear to be related to changes in obstructive breathing pattern.[178] Prolonged night-time nasal CPAP can selectively improve respiratory muscle strength and LV contractile function and decrease catecholamine levels in the setting of pre-existing heart failure.[179–181]

When positive airway pressure augments LV ejection in heart failure states, systolic arterial pressure actually increases compared to spontaneous ventilation.[172] Perel et al.[182–184] suggested that the relation between ventilatory efforts and systolic arterial pressure may be used to rapidly identify patients who may benefit from cardiac assist by increases in ITP. Patients in whom systolic arterial pressure increases during ventilation relative to an apneic baseline tend to have a greater degree of volume overload[183] and heart failure.[182]

Chronic obstructive pulmonary disease

The primary hemodynamic problem seen in patients with chronic airflow obstruction is related to hyperinflation, either due to loss of lung parenchyma or dynamic hyperinflation (intrinsic PEEP) and increased work of breathing. Intrinsic PEEP alters hemodynamic function in a manner similar to extrinsic PEEP. Furthermore, matching intrinsic PEEP with externally applied PEEP has no measurable detrimental hemodynamic effect,[185–187] although it decreases the work cost of spontaneous breathing. Furthermore, like PEEP, CPAP has little detrimental effect in these patients when delivered below the intrinsic level of PEEP.[188] There is little hemodynamic difference between increasing airway pressure to generate a breath and decreasing extrathoracic pressure (iron-lung negative pressure ventilation). Ambrosino et al.[189] used negative pressure ventilation to augment ventilation in patients with chronic airflow obstruction and, not surprisingly, found no differences in hemodynamic response with similar Vt levels.

Weaning of patients with chronic airflow obstruction can tax the cardiovascular system because of the increased metabolic demand that spontaneous breathing exacts in these patients. Patients with severe chronic airflow obstruction may go into cardiogenic pulmonary edema during weaning despite adequate weaning parameters,[149] owing to both volume overload and reduced LV ejection fraction.[190] Mohsenifar et al. assessed the effect of weaning on gastric intramucosal pH (pHi), as a marker of splanchnic blood flow, in 29 ventilated patients deemed ready for weaning.[5] Patients who could not be weaned had a substantially reduced gastric pHi from 7.36 during intermittent positive-pressure ventilation to 7.09 during weaning. Patients who were successfully weaned showed no change

in pHi (7.45 to 7.46). Jubran et al.[175] examined the cardiac output and arteriovenous O_2 difference in patients with chronic airflow obstruction during weaning trials. All subjects demonstrated an increase in cardiac output, consistent with the increase metabolic demands of spontaneous ventilation. However, those who failed to wean had an associated increase in the arteriovenous O_2 difference consistent with an impaired circulatory response to the increase metabolic demand. Thus, occult cardiovascular insufficiency may play a major role in the development of failure to wean in critically ill patients.[191]

SUMMARY

Positive-pressure breathing alters the pulmonary circulation primarily by two different but related aspects of ventilation, changes in lung volume and changes in ITP. Changes in lung volume appear to be more important for the pulmonary circulation, whereas changes in ITP appear to be more relevant to the systemic circulation. Increasing lung volume increases pulmonary inflow impedance by increasing PAP. The primary cause of increasing PAP during inflation is increased alveolar collapse owing to overdistension and increased P_A relative to PAP. To the extent that recruitment decreases hypoxic pulmonary vasoconstriction, then pulmonary vascular conductance, the reciprocal of vascular resistance, will increase.

The basic concepts that underpin these physiological effects of mechanical ventilation on the pulmonary circulation are:

- that lung volume increases not only during inspiration, but may be kept at a volume greater than normal because of the application of increased end-expiratory airway pressure; and
- that positive-pressure inspiration is associated with an increase in ITP and its associated decrease in venous return, thus uncoupling pulmonary blood flow changes with alveolar ventilation.

KEY POINTS

- End-inspiratory and end-expiratory hold Paw values reflect matched ventilatory cycle P_A values, while mean Paw values reflect mean P_A values.
- It is inaccurate and potentially dangerous to assume a constant fraction of Paw transmission to the pleural surface as a means of calculating Ppl.
- Hyperinflation, as occurs in severe asthma and with the use of excessive amounts of PEEP, may

> produce a clinical picture indistinguishable from cardiac tamponade.
> - Positive-pressure ventilation, by uncoupling RAP from RV filling, impairs the normal adaptive mechanisms by which venous return is coupled to RV output.

REFERENCES

∗1 Michard F, Chemla D, Richard C et al. Clinical use of respiratory changes in arterial pulse pressure to monitor the hemodynamic effects of PEEP. Am J Respir Crit Care Med 1999;**159**:935–9.

●2 Cournaud A, Motley HL, Werko L et al. Physiologic studies of the effect of intermittent positive-pressure breathing on cardiac output in man. Am J Physiol 1948;**152**:162–74.

∗3 Milic-Emili J, Mead J, Turner JM. Improved method for assessing the validity of the esophageal balloon technique. J Appl Physiol 1964;**19**:207–11.

●4 Braunwald E, Binion JT, Morgan WL et al. Alterations in central blood volume and cardiac output induced by positive-pressure breathing and counteracted by metraminol (Aramine). Circ Res 1957;**5**:670–5.

●5 Fuhrman BR, Smith-Wright DL, Venkataraman S et al. Proximal mean airway pressure: a good estimator of mean alveolar pressure during continuous positive-pressure breathing. Crit Care Med 1989;**17**:666–70.

●6 Whittenberger JL, McGregor M, Berglund E et al. Influence of state of inflation of the lung on pulmonary vascular resistance. J Appl Physiol 1960;**15**:878–82.

7 Novak RA, Matuschak GM, Pinsky MR. Effect of ventilatory frequency on regional pleural pressure. J Appl Physiol 1988;**65**:1314–23.

8 Pinsky MR, Guimond JG. The effects of positive end-expiratory pressure on heart-lung interactions. J Crit Care 1991;**6**:1–11.

9 Romand JA, Shi W, Pinsky MR. Cardiopulmonary effects of positive-pressure ventilation during acute lung injury. Chest 1995;**108**:1041–8.

∗10 O'Quinn RJ, Marini JJ, Culver BH et al. Transmission of airway pressure to pleural pressure during lung edema and chest wall restriction. J Appl Physiol 1985;**59**:1171–7.

11 Gattinoni L, Mascheroni D, Torresin A et al. Morphological response to positive end-expiratory pressure in acute respiratory failure. Intensive Care Med 1986;**12**:137–42.

12 Globits S, Burghuber OC, Koller J et al. Effect of lung transplantation on right and left ventricular volumes and function measured by magnetic resonance imaging. Am J Respir Crit Care Med 1994;**149**:1000–4.

13 Scharf SM, Ingram Jr RH. Effects of decreasing lung compliance with oleic acid on the cardiovascular response to PEEP. Am J Physiol 1977;**233**:H635–41.

14 Pinsky MR, Vincent JL, DeSmet JM. Estimating left ventricular filling pressure during positive end-expiratory pressure in humans. Am Rev Respir Dis 1991;**143**:25–31.

●15 Buda AJ, Pinsky MR, Ingels NB et al. Effect of intrathoracic pressure on left ventricular performance. N Engl J Med 1979;**301**:453–9.

●16 Kingma I, Smiseth OA, Frais MA et al. Left ventricular external constraint: relationship between pericardial, pleural and esophageal pressures during positive end-expiratory pressure and volume loading in dogs. Ann Biomed Eng 1987;**15**:331–46.

17 Tsitlik JE, Halperin HR, Guerci AD et al. Augmentation of pressure in a vessel indenting the surface of the lung. Ann Biomed Eng 1987;**15**:259–84.

18 Marini JJ, Rodriguez RM, Lamb V. The inspiratory workload of patient-initiated mechanical ventilation. Am Rev Respir Dis 1986;**134**:902–9.

♦19 Bromberger-Barnea B. Mechanical effects of inspiration on heart functions: a review. Fed Proc 1981;**40**:2172–7.

♦20 Wise RA, Robotham JL, Summer WR. Effects of spontaneous ventilation on the circulation. Lung 1981;**159**:175–92.

♦21 Pinsky MR. Breathing as exercise: the cardiovascular response to weaning from mechanical ventilation. Intensive Care Med 2000;**26**:1164–6.

●22 Glick G, Wechsler AS, Epstein DE. Reflex cardiovascular depression produced by stimulation of pulmonary stretch receptors in the dog. J Clin Invest 1969;**48**:467–72.

23 Painal AS. Vagal sensory receptors and their reflex effects. Physiol Rev 1973;**53**:59–88.

●24 Anrep GV, Pascual W, Rossler R. Respiratory variations in the heart rate. I. The reflex mechanism of the respiratory arrhythmia. Proc R Soc Lond B Biol Sci 1936;**119**: 191–217.

25 Taha BH, Simon PM, Dempsey JA et al. Respiratory sinus arrhythmia in humans: an obligatory role for vagal feedback from the lungs. J Appl Physiol 1995;**78**:638–45.

26 Bernardi L, Calciati A, Gratarola A et al. Heart rate-respiration relationship: computerized method for early detection of cardiac autonomic damage in diabetic patients. Acta Cardiol 1986;**41**:197–206.

27 Bernardi L, Keller F, Sanders M et al. Respiratory sinus arrhythmia in the totally dennervated human heart. J Appl Physiol 1989;**67**:1447–55.

28 Persson MG, Lonnqvist PA, Gustafsson LE. Positive end-expiratory pressure ventilation elicits increases in endogenously formed nitric oxide as detected in air exhaled by rabbits. Anesthesiology 1995;**82**:969–74.

●29 Cassidy SS, Eschenbacher WI, Johnson RL Jr. Reflex cardiovascular depression during unilateral lung hyperinflation in the dog. J Clin Invest 1979;**64**:620–6.

30 Daly MB, Hazzledine JL, Ungar A. The reflex effects of alterations in lung volume on systemic vascular resistance in the dog. J Physiol (Lond) 1967;**188**:331–51.

♦31 Shepherd JT. The lungs as receptor sites for cardiovascular regulation. Circulation 1981;**63**:1–10.

●32 Stalcup SA, Mellins RB. Mechanical forces producing pulmonary edema in acute asthma. N Engl J Med 1977;**297**:592–6.

33 Vatner SF, Rutherford JD. Control of the myocardial contractile state by carotid chemo- and baroreceptor and pulmonary inflation reflexes in conscious dogs. J Clin Invest 1978;**63**:1593–601.

34 Pick RA, Handler JB, Murata GH *et al*. The cardiovascular effects of positive end-expiratory pressure. *Chest* 1982;**82**:345–50.

●35 Said SI, Kitamura S, Vreim C. Prostaglandins: release from the lung during mechanical ventilation at large tidal ventilation. *J Clin Invest* 1972;**51**:83a.

36 Bedetti C, Del Basso P, Argiolas C *et al*. Arachidonic acid and pulmonary function in a heart-lung preparation of guinea-pig. Modulation by PCO_2. *Arch Int Pharmacodyn Ther* 1987;**285**:98–116.

37 Berend N, Christopher KL, Voelkel NF. Effect of positive end-expiratory pressure on functional residual capacity: role of prostaglandin production. *Am Rev Respir Dis* 1982;**126**:641–7.

38 Pattern MY, Liebman PR, Hetchman HG. Humorally mediated decreases in cardiac output associated with positive end-expiratory pressure. *Microvasc Res* 1977;**13**:137–44.

39 Berglund JE, Halden E, Jakobson S *et al*. PEEP ventilation does not cause humorally mediated cardiac output depression in pigs. *Intensive Care Med* 1994;**20**:360–4.

40 Fuhrman BP, Everitt J, Lock JE. Cardiopulmonary effects of unilateral airway pressure changes in intact infant lambs. *J Appl Physiol* 1984;**56**:1439–48.

41 Payen DM, Brun-Buisson CJL, Carli PA *et al*. Hemodynamic, gas exchange, and hormonal consequences of LBPP during PEEP ventilation. *J Appl Physiol* 1987;**62**:61–70.

42 Frage D, de la Coussaye JE, Beloucif S *et al*. Interactions between hormonal modifications during PEEP-induced antidiuresis and antinatriuresis. *Chest* 1995;**107**:1095–100.

43 Frass M, Watschinger B, Traindl O *et al*. Atrial natriuretic peptide release in response to different positive end-expiratory pressure levels. *Crit Care Med* 1993;**21**:343–7.

44 Wilkins MA, Su XL, Palayew MD *et al*. The effects of posture change and continuous positive airway pressure on cardiac natriuretic peptides in congestive heart failure. *Chest* 1995;**107**:909–15.

45 Shirakami G, Magaribuchi T, Shingu K *et al*. Positive end-expiratory pressure ventilation decreases plasma atrial and brain natriuretic peptide levels in humans. *Anesth Analg* 1993;**77**:1116–21.

●46 Brecher GA, Hubay CA. Pulmonary blood flow and venous return during spontaneous respiration. *Circ Res* 1955;**3**:210–14.

47 Goldstein JA, Vlahakes GJ, Verrier ED. The role of right ventricular systolic dysfunction and elevated intrapericardial pressures in the genesis of low output in experimental right ventricular infarction. *Circulation* 1982;**65**:513–20.

●48 Jardin F, Farcot JC, Boisante L. Influence of positive end-expiratory pressure on left ventricular performance. *N Engl J Med* 1981;**304**:387–92.

49 Jardin FF, Farcot JC, Gueret P *et al*. Echocardiographic evaluation of ventricles during continuous positive-pressure breathing. *J Appl Physiol* 1984;**56**:619–27.

50 Prec KJ, Cassels DE. Oximeter studies in newborn infants during crying. *Pediatrics* 1952;**9**:756–61.

◆51 Luce JM. The cardiovascular effects of mechanical ventilation and positive end-expiratory pressure. *JAMA* 1984;**252**:807–11.

52 Maughan WL, Shoukas AA, Sagawa K *et al*. Instantaneous pressure-volume relationships of the canine right ventricle. *Circ Res* 1979;**44**:309–15.

53 Sibbald WJ, Driedger AA. Right ventricular function in disease states: pathophysiologic considerations. *Crit Care Med* 1983;**11**:339–45.

●54 Pinsky MR. Instantaneous venous return curves in an intact canine preparation. *J Appl Physiol* 1984;**56**:765–71.

55 Piene H, Sund T. Does pulmonary impedance constitute the optimal load for the right ventricle? *Am J Physiol* 1982;**242**:H154–60.

56 Pinsky MR. Determinants of pulmonary arterial flow variation during respiration. *J Appl Physiol* 1984;**56**:1237–45.

57 Johnston WE, Vinten-Johansen J, Shugart HE *et al*. Positive end-expiratory pressure potentates the severity of canine right ventricular ischemia-reperfusion injury. *Am J Physiol* 1992;**262**:H168–76.

◆58 Sibbald WJ, Calvin JE, Holliday RL *et al*. Concepts in the pharmacologic support of cardiovascular function in critically ill surgical patients. *Surg Clin North Am* 1983;**63**:455–66.

59 Sibbald WJ, Calvin J, Driedger AA. Right and left ventricular preload, and diastolic ventricular compliance: implications of therapy in critically ill patients. In: Shoemaker WC (ed.), *Critical care. State of the art*, vol. 3. Fullerton: Society of Critical Care, 1982.

60 Madden JA, Dawson CA, Harder DR. Hypoxia-induced activation in small isolated pulmonary arteries from the cat. *J Appl Physiol* 1985;**59**:113–18.

●61 Hakim TS, Michel RP, Chang HK. Effect of lung inflation on pulmonary vascular resistance by arterial and venous occlusion. *J Appl Physiol* 1982;**53**:1110–15.

●62 Quebbeman EJ, Dawson CA. Influence of inflation and atelectasis on the hypoxic pressure response in isolated dog lung lobes. *Cardiovasc Res* 1976;**10**:672–7.

63 Brower RG, Gottlieb J, Wise RA *et al*. Locus of hypoxic vasoconstriction in isolated ferret lungs. *J Appl Physiol* 1987;**63**:58–65.

64 Hakim TS, Michel RP, Minami H *et al*. Site of pulmonary hypoxic vasoconstriction studied with arterial and venous occlusion. *J Appl Physiol* 1983;**54**:1298–302.

●65 Marshall BE, Marshall C. A model for hypoxic constriction of the pulmonary circulation. *J Appl Physiol* 1988;**64**:68–77.

66 Marshall BE, Marshall C. Continuity of response to hypoxic pulmonary vasoconstriction. *J Appl Physiol* 1980;**49**:189–96.

67 Dawson CA, Grimm DJ, Linehan JH. Lung inflation and longitudinal distribution of pulmonary vascular resistance during hypoxia. *J Appl Physiol* 1979;**47**:532–6.

●68 Howell JBL, Permutt S, Proctor DF *et al*. Effect of inflation of the lung on different parts of the pulmonary vascular bed. *J Appl Physiol* 1961;**16**:71–6.

●69 West JB, Dollery CT, Naimark A. Distribution of blood flow in isolated lung; relation to vascular and alveolar pressures. *J Appl Physiol* 1964;**19**:713–24.

70 Fuhrman BP, Smith-Wright DL, Kulik TJ *et al.* Effects of static and fluctuating airway pressure on the intact, immature pulmonary circulation. *J Appl Physiol* 1986;**60**:114–22.

71 Thorvalson J, Ilebekk A, Kiil F. Determinants of pulmonary blood volume. Effects of acute changes in airway pressure. *Acta Physiol Scand* 1985;**125**:471–9.

●72 Hoffman EA, Ritman EL. Heart-lung interaction: effect on regional lung air content and total heart volume. *Ann Biomed Eng* 1987;**15**:241–57.

73 Olson LE, Hoffman EA. Heart-lung interactions determined by electron beam X-ray CT in laterally recumbent rabbits. *J Appl Physiol* 1995;**78**:417–27.

74 Grant BJB, Lieber BB. Compliance of the main pulmonary artery during the ventilatory cycle. *J Appl Physiol* 1992;**72**:535–42.

●75 Lopez-Muniz R, Stephens NL, Bromberger-Barnea B *et al.* Critical closure of pulmonary vessels analyzed in terms of Starling resistor model. *J Appl Physiol* 1968;**24**:625–35.

76 Block AJ, Boyson PG, Wynne JW. The origins of cor pulmonale, a hypothesis. *Chest* 1979;**75**:109–14.

77 Canada E, Benumnof JL, Tousdale FR. Pulmonary vascular resistance correlated in intact normal and abnormal canine lungs. *Crit Care Med* 1982;**10**:719–23.

78 Domino KB, Pinsky MR. Effect of positive end-expiratory pressure on hypoxic pulmonary vasoconstriction in the dog. *Am J Physiol* 1990;**259**:H697–705.

79 Walther SM, Domino KB, Glenny RW *et al.* Positive end-expiratory pressure redistributes perfusion to dependent lung regions in supine but not in prone lambs. *Crit Care Med* 1999;**27**:37–45.

◆80 Gattinoni L, Caironi P, Pelosi P *et al.* What has computed tomography taught us about the acute respiratory distress syndrome? *Am J Respir Crit Care Med* 2001;**164**:1701–11.

●81 Taylor RR, Corell JW, Sonnenblick EH *et al.* Dependence of ventricular distensibility on filling the opposite ventricle. *Am J Physiol* 1967;**213**:711–18.

82 Brinker JA, Weiss I, Lappe DL *et al.* Leftward septal displacement during right ventricular loading in man. *Circulation* 1980;**61**:626–33.

83 Marini JJ, Culver BN, Butler J. Mechanical effect of lung distention with positive-pressure on cardiac function. *Am Rev Respir Dis* 1980;**124**:382–6.

84 Michard F, Teboul JL. Using heart-lung interactions to assess fluid responsiveness during mechanical ventilation. *Crit Care* 2000;**4**:282–9.

◆85 Butler J. The heart is in good hands. *Circulation* 1983;**67**:1163–8.

86 Cassidy SS, Wead WB, Seibert GB *et al.* Changes in left ventricular geometry during spontaneous breathing. *J Appl Physiol* 1987;**63**:803–11.

87 Cassidy SS, Robertson CH, Pierce AK *et al.* Cardiovascular effects of positive end-expiratory pressure in dogs. *J Appl Physiol* 1978;**4**:743–9.

88 Conway CM. Hemodynamic effects of pulmonary ventilation. *Br J Anaesth* 1975;**47**:761–6.

89 Berglund JE, Halden E, Jakobson S *et al.* Echocardiographic analysis of cardiac function during high PEEP ventilation. *Intensive Care Med* 1994;**20**:174–80.

90 Takata M, Harasawa Y, Beloucif S *et al.* Coupled vs. Uncoupled pericardial restraint: effects on cardiac chamber interactions. *J Appl Physiol* 1997;**83**:1799–813.

91 Van den Berg P, Pinsky MR, Grimbergen CA *et al.* Positive-pressure ventilation differentially alters right and left ventricular outputs in post-operative cardiac surgery patients. *J Crit Care* 1997;**12**:56–65.

92 Rebuck AS, Read J. Assessment and management of severe asthma. *Am J Med* 1971;**51**:788–92.

●93 Guyton AC, Lindsey AW, Abernathy B *et al.* Venous return at various right atrial pressures and the normal venous return curve. *Am J Physiol* 1957;**189**:609–15.

94 Goldberg HS, Rabson J. Control of cardiac output by systemic vessels: circulatory adjustments of acute and chronic respiratory failure and the effects of therapeutic interventions. *Am J Cardiol* 1981;**47**:696–702.

95 Kilburn KH. Cardiorespiratory effects of large pneumothorax in conscious and anesthetized dogs. *J Appl Physiol* 1963;**18**:279–83.

96 Chevalier PA, Weber KC, Engle JC *et al.* Direct measurement of right and left heart outputs in Valsalva-like maneuver in dogs. *Proc Soc Exp Biol Med* 1972;**139**:1429–37.

97 Guntheroth WC, Gould R, Butler J *et al.* Pulsatile flow in pulmonary artery, capillary and vein in the dog. *Cardiovascular Res* 1974;**8**:330–7.

●98 Guntheroth WG, Morgan BC, Mullins GL. Effect of respiration on venous return and stroke volume in cardiac tamponade. Mechanism of pulsus paradoxus. *Circ Res* 1967;**20**:381–90.

◆99 Guyton AC. Effect of cardiac output by respiration, opening the chest, and cardiac tamponade. In: *Circulatory physiology: cardiac output and its regulation.* Philadelphia, PA: WB Saunders, 1963;378–86.

●100 Holt JP. The effect of positive and negative intrathoracic pressure on cardiac output and venous return in the dog. *Am J Physiol* 1944;**142**:594–603.

101 Morgan BC, Abel FL, Mullins GL *et al.* Flow patterns in cavae, pulmonary artery, pulmonary vein and aorta in intact dogs. *Am J Physiol* 1966;**210**:903–9.

●102 Morgan BC, Martin WE, Hornbein TF *et al.* Hemodynamic effects of intermittent positive-pressure respiration. *Anesthesiology* 1960;**27**:584–90.

●103 Scharf SM, Brown R, Saunders N *et al.* Hemodynamic effects of positive-pressure inflation. *J Appl Physiol* 1980;**49**:124–31.

104 Scharf SM, Brown R, Saunders N *et al.* Effects of normal and loaded spontaneous inspiration on cardiovascular function. *J Appl Physiol* 1979;**47**:582–90.

105 Fessler HE, Brower RG, Wise RA *et al.* Effects of positive end-expiratory pressure on the canine venous return curve. *Am Rev Respir Dis* 1992;**146**:4–10.

106 Takata M, Robotham JL. Effects of inspiratory diaphragmatic descent on inferior vena caval venous return. *J Appl Physiol* 1992;**72**:597–607.

∗107 Van den Berg P, Jansen JRC, Pinsky MR. The effect of positive-pressure inspiration on venous return in volume loaded post-operative cardiac surgical patients. *J Appl Physiol Respir Environ Exercise Physiol* 2002;**92**:1223–31.

*108 Magder S, Georgiadis G, Cheong T. Respiratory variation in right atrial pressure predict the response to fluid challenge. *J Crit Care* 1992;**7**:76–85.

109 Terada N, Takeuchi T. Postural changes in venous pressure gradients in anesthetized monkeys. *Am J Physiol* 1993;**264**:H21–5.

110 Scharf S, Tow DE, Miller MJ et al. Influence of posture and abdominal pressure on the hemodynamic effects of Mueller's maneuver. *J Crit Care* 1989;**4**:26–34.

111 Tarasiuk A, Scharf SM. Effects of periodic obstructive apneas on venous return in closed-chest dogs. *Am Rev Respir Dis* 1993;**148**:323–9.

112 Mang H, Kacmarek RM, Ritz R et al. Cardiorespiratory effects of volume- and pressure-controlled ventilation at various I/E ratios in an acute lung injury model. *Am J Respir Crit Care Med* 1995;**151**:731–6.

•113 Tyberg JV, Taichman GC, Smith ER et al. The relationship between pericardial pressure and right atrial pressure: an intraoperative study. *Circulation* 1986;**73**:428–32.

114 Pinsky MR, Vincent JL, DeSmet JM. Effect of positive end-expiratory pressure on right ventricular function in man. *Am Rev Respir Dis* 1992;**146**:681–7.

115 Shuey CB, Pierce AK, Johnson RL. An evaluation of exercise tests in chronic obstructive lung disease. *J Appl Physiol* 1969;**27**:256–61.

116 Jayaweera AR, Ehrlich W. Changes of phasic pleural pressure in awake dogs during exercise: potential effects on cardiac output. *Ann Biomed Eng* 1987;**15**:311–18.

117 Grenvik A. Respiratory, circulatory and metabolic effects of respiratory treatment. A clinical study in postoperative thoracic surgery patients. *Acta Anaesth Scand* 1966;**19**(Suppl):1–122.

118 Harken AH, Brennan MF, Smith N et al. The hemodynamic response to positive end-expiratory ventilation in hypovolemic patients. *Surgery* 1974;**76**:786–93.

119 Lores ME, Keagy BA, Vassiliades T et al. Cardiovascular effects of positive end-expiratory pressure (PEEP) after pneumonectomy in dogs. *Ann Thorac Surg* 1985;**40**:464–73.

•120 Sharpey-Schaffer EP. Effects of Valsalva maneuver on the normal and failing circulation. *Br Med J* 1955;**1**:693–9.

121 Peters J, Kindred MK, Robotham JL. Transient analysis of cardiopulmonary interactions II. Systolic events. *J Appl Physiol* 1988;**64**:1518–26.

•122 Pinsky MR, Matuschak GM, Klain M. Determinants of cardiac augmentation by increases in intrathoracic pressure. *J Appl Physiol* 1985;**58**:1189–98.

123 Rankin JS, Olsen CO, Arentzen CE et al. The effects of airway pressure on cardiac function in intact dogs and man. *Circulation* 1982;**66**:108–20.

124 Robotham JL, Rabson J, Permutt S et al. Left ventricular hemodynamics during respiration. *J Appl Physiol* 1979;**47**:1295–303.

125 Ruskin J, Bache RJ, Rembert JC et al. Pressure-flow studies in man: effect of respiration on left ventricular stroke volume. *Circulation* 1973;**48**:79–85.

126 Olsen CO, Tyson GS, Maier GW et al. Dynamic ventricular interaction in the conscious dog. *Circ Res* 1983;**52**:85–104.

127 Bell RC, Robotham JL, Badke FR et al. Left ventricular geometry during intermittent positive-pressure ventilation in dogs. *J Crit Care* 1987;**2**:230–44.

128 Qvist J, Pontoppidan H, Wilson RS et al. Hemodynamic responses to mechanical ventilation with PEEP: the effects of hypovolemia. *Anesthesiology* 1975;**42**:45–53.

129 Denault AY, Gorcsan III J, Deneault LG et al. Effect of positive-pressure ventilation on left ventricular pressure-volume relationship. *Anesthesiology* 1993;**79**:A315.

130 Beyar R, Goldstein Y. Model studies of the effects of the thoracic pressure on the circulation. *Ann Biomed Eng* 1987;**15**:373–83.

•131 Pinsky MR, Summer WR, Wise RA et al. Augmentation of cardiac function by elevation of intrathoracic pressure. *J Appl Physiol* 1983;**54**:950–5.

132 Cassidy SA, Wead WB, Seibert GB et al. Geometric left-ventricular responses to interactions between the lung and left ventricle: positive-pressure breathing. *Ann Biomed Eng* 1987;**15**:285–95.

133 Scharf SM, Brown R, Warner KG et al. Intrathoracic pressure and left ventricular configuration with respiratory maneuvers. *J Appl Physiol* 1989;**66**:481–91.

134 Pinsky MR, Summer WR. Cardiac augmentation by phasic high intrathoracic support (PHIPS) in man. *Chest* 1983;**84**:370–5.

135 Pinsky MR, Matuschak GM, Itzkoff JM. Respiratory augmentation of left ventricular function during spontaneous ventilation in severe left ventricular failure by grunting: an auto-EPAP effect. *Chest* 1984;**86**:267–9.

136 Blaustein AS, Risser TA, Weiss JW et al. Mechanisms of pulsus paradoxus during resistive respiratory loading and asthma. *J Am Coll Cardiol* 1986;**8**:529–36.

137 Strohl KP, Scharf SM, Brown R et al. Cardiovascular performance during bronchospasm in dogs. *Respiration* 1987;**51**:39–48.

138 Scharf SM, Graver LM, Balaban K. Cardiovascular effects of periodic occlusions of the upper airways in dogs. *Am Rev Respir Dis* 1992;**146**:321–9.

139 Viola AR, Puy RJM, Goldman E. Mechanisms of pulsus paradoxus in airway obstruction. *J Appl Physiol* 1990;**68**:1927–31.

140 Scharf SM, Graver LM, Khilnani S et al. Respiratory phasic effects of inspiratory loading on left ventricular hemodynamics in vagotomized dogs. *J Appl Physiol* 1992;**73**:995–1003.

141 Latham RD, Sipkema P, Westerhof N et al. Aortic input impedance during Mueller maneuver: an evaluation of 'effective strength'. *J Appl Physiol* 1988;**65**:1604–10.

142 Virolainen J, Ventila M, Turto H et al. Effect of negative intrathoracic pressure on left ventricular pressure dynamics and relaxation. *J Appl Physiol* 1995;**79**:455–60.

143 Garpestad E, Parker JA, Katayama H et al. Decrease in ventricular stroke volume at apnea termination is independent of oxygen desaturation. *J Appl Physiol* 1994;**77**:1602–8.

144 Gomez A, Mink S. Interaction between effects of hypoxia and hypercapnia on altering left ventricular relaxation and chamber stiffness in dogs. *Am Rev Respir Dis* 1992;**146**:313–20.

145 Abel FL, Mihailescu LS, Lader AS et al. Effects of pericardial pressure on systemic and coronary hemodynamics in dogs. *Am J Physiol* 1995;**268**:H1593–605.

146 Khilnani S, Graver LM, Balaban K et al. Effects of inspiratory loading on left ventricular myocardial blood flow and metabolism. *J Appl Physiol* 1992;**72**:1488–92.

147 Satoh S, Wtanabe J, Keitoku M et al. Influences of pressure surrounding the heart and intracardiac pressure on the diastolic coronary pressure-flow relation in excised canine heart. *Circ Res* 1988;**63**:788–97.

●148 Beach T, Millen E, Grenvik A. Hemodynamic response to discontinuance of mechanical ventilation. *Crit Care Med* 1973;**1**:85–90.

●149 Lemaire F, Teboul JL, Cinoti L et al. Acute left ventricular dysfunction during unsuccessful weaning from mechanical ventilation. *Anesthesiology* 1988;**69**:171–9.

150 Grace MP, Greenbaum DM. Cardiac performance in response to PEEP in patients with cardiac dysfunction. *Crit Care Med* 1982;**20**:358–60.

●151 Rasanen J, Nikki P, Heikkila J. Acute myocardial infarction complicated by respiratory failure. The effects of mechanical ventilation. *Chest* 1984;**85**:21–8.

152 Rasanen J, Vaisanen IT, Heikkila J et al. Acute myocardial infarction complicated by left ventricular dysfunction and respiratory failure. The effects of continuous positive airway pressure. *Chest* 1985;**87**:156–62.

153 Pinsky MR, Matuschak GM, Bernardi L et al. Hemodynamic effects of cardiac cycle-specific increases in intrathoracic pressure. *J Appl Physiol* 1986;**60**:604–12.

154 Dries DJ, Kumar P, Mathru M et al. Hemodynamic effects of pressure support ventilation in cardiac surgery patients. *Am Surg* 1991;**57**:122–5.

155 Sternberg R, Sahebjami H. Hemodynamic and oxygen transport characteristics of common ventilatory modes. *Chest* 1994;**105**:1798–803.

156 Bayly R, Sladen A, Guntapalli K et al. Synchronous versus nonsynchronous high-frequency jet ventilation: effects on cardiorespiratory variables and airway pressures in postoperative patients. *Crit Care Med* 1987;**15**:915–23.

157 Dhainaut JF, Devaux JY, Monsallier JF et al. Mechanisms of decreased left ventricular preload during continuous positive-pressure ventilation in ARDS. *Chest* 1986;**90**:74–80.

158 Singer M, Vermaat J, Hall G et al. Hemodynamic effects of manual hyperinflation in critically ill mechanically ventilated patients. *Chest* 1994;**106**:1182–7.

159 Lichtwarck-Aschoff M, Zeravik J, Pfeiffer UJ. Intrathoracic blood volume accurately reflects circulatory volume status in critically ill patients with mechanical ventilation. *Intensive Care Med* 1992;**18**:142–5.

160 Hartmann M, Rosberg B, Jonsson K. The influence of different levels of PEEP on peripheral tissue perfusion measured by subcutaneous and transcutaneous oxygen tension. *Intensive Care Med* 1992;**18**:474–8.

161 Huemer G, Kolev N, Kurz A et al. Influence of positive end-expiratory pressure on right and left ventricular performance assessed by Doppler two-dimensional echocardiography. *Chest* 1994;**106**:67–73.

◆162 Jardin F. PEEP and ventricular function. *Intensive Care Med* 1994;**20**:169–70.

163 Goertz A, Heinrich H, Winter H et al. Hemodynamic effects of different ventilatory patterns. A prospective clinical trial. *Chest* 1991;**99**:1166–71.

164 Gunter JP, deBoisblanc BP, Rust BS et al. Effect of synchronized, systolic, lower body, positive-pressure on hemodynamics in human septic shock: a pilot study. *Am J Respir Crit Care Med* 1995;**151**:719–23.

165 Schuster S, Erbel R, Weilemann LS et al. Hemodynamics during PEEP ventilation in patients with severe left ventricular failure studied by transesophageal echocardiography. *Chest* 1990;**97**:1181–9.

166 Lessard MR, Guerot E, Lorini H et al. Effects of pressure-controlled with different I:E ratios versus volume-controlled ventilation on respiratory mechanics, gas exchange and hemodynamics in patients with adult respiratory distress syndrome. *Anesthesiology* 1994;**80**:983–91.

167 Chan K, Abraham E. Effects of inverse ratio ventilation on cardiorespiratory parameters in severe respiratory failure. *Chest* 1992;**102**:1556–61.

168 Abraham E, Yoshihara G. Cardiorespiratory effects of pressure controlled ventilation in severe respiratory failure. *Chest* 1990;**98**:1445–9.

169 Poelaert JI, Visser CA, Everaert JA et al. Acute hemodynamic changes of pressure-controlled inverse ration ventilation in the adult respiratory distress syndrome. A transesophageal echocardiographic and Doppler study. *Chest* 1993;**104**:214–19.

170 Mancini M, Zavala E, Mancebo J et al. Mechanisms of pulmonary gas exchange improvement during a protective ventilatory strategy in acute respiratory distress syndrome. *Am J Respir Crit Care Med* 2001;**164**:1448–53.

171 Schmitt JM, Vieillard-Baron A, Augarde R et al. Positive end-expiratory pressure titration in acute respiratory distress syndrome patients: impact on right ventricular outflow impedance evaluated by pulmonary artery Doppler flow velocity measurements. *Crit Care Med* 2001;**29**:1154–8.

172 Abel JG, Salerno TA, Panos A et al. Cardiovascular effects of positive-pressure ventilation in humans. *Ann Thorac Surg* 1987;**43**:36–43.

173 DeHoyos A, Liu PP, Benard DC et al. Haemodynamic effects of continuous positive airway pressure in humans with normal and impaired left ventricular function. *Clin Sci Colch* 1995;**88**:173–8.

●174 Naughton MT, Rahman MA, Hara K et al. Effect of continuous positive airway pressure on intrathoracic and left ventricular transmural pressures in patients with congestive heart failure. *Circulation* 1995;**91**:1725–31.

175 Crotti S, Mascheroni D, Caironi P et al. Recruitment and derecruitment during acute respiratory failure. A clinical study. *Am J Respir Crit Care Med* 2001;**164**:131–40.

176 Rasanen J. Respiratory failure in acute myocardial infarction. *Appl Cardiopulm Pathophysiol* 1988;**2**:271–9.

177 Lin M, Yang YF, Chiang HT et al. Reappraisal of continuous positive airway pressure therapy in acute cardiogenic pulmonary edema. *Chest* 1995;**107**:1379–86.

178 Buckle P, Millar T, Kryger M. The effect of short-term nasal CPAP on Cheyne-Stokes respiration in congestive heart failure. *Chest* 1992;**102**:31–5.

179 Granton JT, Naughton MT, Benard DC et al. CPAP improves inspiratory muscle strength in patients with heart failure and central sleep apnea. *Am J Respir Crit Care Med* 1996;**153**:277–82.

180 Naughton MT, Benard DC, Liu PP *et al*. Effects of nasal CPAP on sympathetic activity in patients with heart failure and central sleep apnea. *Am J Respir Crit Care Med* 1995;**152**:473–9.

181 Yan AT, Bradley TD, Liu PP. The role of continuous positive airway pressure in the treatment of congestive heart failure. *Chest* 2001;**120**:1675–85.

182 Baeaussier M, Coriat P, Perel A *et al*. Determinants of systolic pressure variation in patients ventilated after vascular surgery. *J Cardiothorac Vasc Anesth* 1995;**9**:547–51.

183 Coriat P, Vrillon M, Perel A *et al*. A comparison of systolic blood pressure variations and echocardiographic estimates of end-diastolic left ventricular size in patients after aortic surgery. *Anesth Analg* 1994;**78**:46–53.

●184 Szold A, Pizov R, Segal E *et al*. The effect of tidal volume and intravascular volume state on systolic pressure variation in ventilated dogs. *Intensive Care Med* 1989;**15**:368–71.

185 Ranieri VM, Giuliani R, Cinnella G *et al*. Physiologic effects of positive end-expiratory pressure in patients with chronic obstructive lung disease during acute ventilatory failure and controlled mechanical ventilation. *Am Rev Respir Dis* 1993;**147**:5–13.

186 Baigorri F, De Monte A, Blanch L *et al*. Hemodynamic response to external counterbalancing of auto-positive end-expiratory pressure in mechanically ventilated patients with chronic obstructive lung disease. *Crit Care Med* 1994;**22**:1782–91.

◆187 Pinsky MR. Though the past darkly: ventilatory management of patients with chronic obstructive pulmonary disease. *Crit Care Med* 1994;**22**:1714–17.

188 Ambrosino N, Nava S, Torbicki A *et al*. Hemodynamic effects of pressure support and PEEP ventilation by nasal route in patients with stable chronic obstructive pulmonary disease. *Thorax* 1993;**48**:523–8.

189 Ambrosino N, Cobelli F, Torbicki A *et al*. Hemodynamic effects of negative-pressure ventilation in patients with COPD. *Chest* 1990;**97**:850–6.

190 Richard C, Teboul JL, Archambaud F *et al*. Left ventricular function during weaning of patients with chronic obstructive pulmonary disease. *Intensive Care Med* 1994;**20**:181–6.

191 Brochard L, Isabey D, Piquet J *et al*. Reversal of acute exacerbations of chronic obstructive lung disease by inspiratory assistance with a face mask. *N Engl J Med* 1990;**323**:1523–30.

22

Effects of lung injury on the pulmonary circulation

JULIUS H CRANSHAW AND TIMOTHY W EVANS

INTRODUCTION

The acute respiratory distress syndrome in adults (ARDS) is defined clinically by the rapid onset of non-cardiogenic pulmonary edema in association with refractory hypoxemia. Since the initial description of ARDS,[1] the defining criteria have been revised several times. The most widely used definition in current use is that of the American–European Consensus (AEC) Conference published in 1994 (Table 22.1), which also defined a less severe form of ARDS, termed acute lung injury (ALI).[2] The AEC definition is fundamentally clinical and descriptive. By contrast, basic research now suggests that ARDS represents the culmination of a process involving:[3]

- cytokine- and cell-mediated inflammation;
- endothelial, epithelial and vascular smooth muscle cell responses;
- basement membrane and interstitial matrix damage;
- abnormal coagulation and dysfunctional pulmonary surfactant.[3]

These processes have profound effects upon the pulmonary vasculature, resulting in abnormal vasomotor control leading to deficiencies in oxygenation and lung metabolic function. The multiple effects of ventilatory and pharmacological interventions may also further exacerbate the inflammatory processes involved in the pathogenesis of ARDS.

ETIOLOGY

The increased alveolar capillary permeability that characterizes ALI/ARDS is associated with many serious

Table 22.1 *The American-European Consensus Conference definitions of acute respiratory distress syndrome (ARDS) and acute lung injury (ALI)*[2]

Syndrome	Timing	Oxygenation	Chest x-ray	PAOP
ALI	Acute	$PaO_2/FiO_2 \leq 300$ mmHg regardless of PEEP	Bilateral opacities consistent with pulmonary edema	≤ 18 mm Hg if measured or no clinical evidence of left atrial hypertension
ARDS	Acute	$PaO_2/FiO_2 \leq 200$ mmHg regardless of PEEP	Bilateral opacities consistent with pulmonary edema	≤ 18 mm Hg if measured or no clinical evidence of left atrial hypertension

PAOP, pulmonary artery occlusion pressure; PaO_2/FiO_2, arterial partial pressure of oxygen/inspired oxygen fraction; PEEP, positive end-expiratory pressure.

Table 22.2 *Common precipitating causes of acute respiratory distress syndrome (ARDS)*

Direct lung injury	Indirect lung injury
Pulmonary infection	Non-pulmonary sepsis
Aspiration	Hemorrhagic shock
Pulmonary contusion	Non-thoracic trauma
Fat embolism	Multiple transfusion
Toxic gas inhalation	Acute pancreatitis
Near-drowning	Drug overdose
Oxygen toxicity	Cardiopulmonary bypass
Chemotherapy	Pneumonectomy
Radiotherapy	Pre-eclampsia
Ventilator-induced lung injury	Burns
Lung transplantation	Disseminated intravascular coagulation

medical and surgical conditions, not all of which involve the lung directly (Table 22.2). Common causes of this unique form of lung injury are listed in the table. The division of causes into direct and indirect injury to the lung is sometimes ill-defined, a well-described example being post-pneumonectomy pulmonary edema.[4]

INCIDENCE

Few data are available concerning the epidemiology and clinical significance of ALI, and the remainder of this chapter will consider only ARDS, the incidence of which in the USA and Europe is approximately 1 in 10 000 population/year.[5–7] Patients with ARDS may represent approximately 20% of those requiring mechanical ventilation in an intensive care unit at any given time,[8,9] In most studies performed over the last decade, the mortality of patients with ARDS has been approximately 40%.[5,10–12]

TREATMENT

The management of patients with ALI and ARDS is essentially supportive and directed at maintaining adequate systemic oxygen delivery and avoiding further lung injury. Mortality has been shown to be decreased significantly by employing a low tidal volume ventilatory strategy aimed at protecting the lung from excessive stretch.[12] By contrast, trials of putative therapeutic pharmacological interventions (see below) have not, to date, improved mortality, and short-term management decisions designed to alter pulmonary perfusion and ventilation favorably and achieve apparently desirable physiological values may not produce a long-term improvement.

PATHOPHYSIOLOGY OF THE PULMONARY CIRCULATION IN ARDS

Pulmonary vascular histopathological evolution in ARDS

ARDS induces changes in the pulmonary vascular tree at all anatomic levels.[13] The defining histopathological lesion of ARDS involves the alveolar–capillary complex,[14,15] which evolves through three successive phases: exudative (week 1), proliferative (weeks 2–3) and fibrotic (week 3 onwards). However, this oversimplifies the evolution of lung injury, in that phases vary in duration and may overlap, recur and resolve producing a heterogeneous pathological pattern.[14,16,17] Pulmonary vascular lesions in ARDS can be placed in a similar temporal distribution to changes in the alveoli.[18]

EXUDATIVE PHASE

Capillaries

An inflammatory milieu develops in the capillary, capable of activating endothelial cells, neutrophils and platelets. Pulmonary platelet[19,20] and neutrophil sequestration[19,21,22] occurs early in ARDS and multiple intracapillary neutrophil, platelet and fibrin microthrombi are common histological features, particularly in lung injury associated with trauma or sepsis.[18,23] Neutrophils lodge in and block capillaries because of their size and decreased deformability. Chemokines and the sequential expression of adhesion molecules may encourage neutrophil migration into the interstitium and alveoli.[24,25] Neutrophil and platelet activation can injure the endothelium and release mediators that modulate vascular tone.[26,27]

Endothelial cells may display ultrastructural changes including swelling, pinocytotic vesicle formation and inter-endothelial separation.[28,29] Such gaps explain the presence of scattered erythrocytes in alveoli, especially as necrosis with denudation of the basement membrane is rare.[30] However, such focal histological appearances do not reflect the significant molecular changes that produce the increased capillary permeability that is the hallmark of the syndrome.

The normal pulmonary capillary endothelium is comprised of a confluent layer of cells anchored at their peripheries to the basement membrane by focal adhesion complexes and linked to each other by intercellular junctions,[33] which regulate paracellular permeability[31,32] (Figure 22.1). However, transcellular transport systems also convey plasma proteins, for example albumin,[33,34] sometimes in large quantities in vesicles,[35] from the luminal plasma membrane to the abluminal side. There is also evidence of transendothelial channeling.[36] The endothelium may therefore independently regulate protein, ion and water permeability. The normal passage of electrolytes and proteins

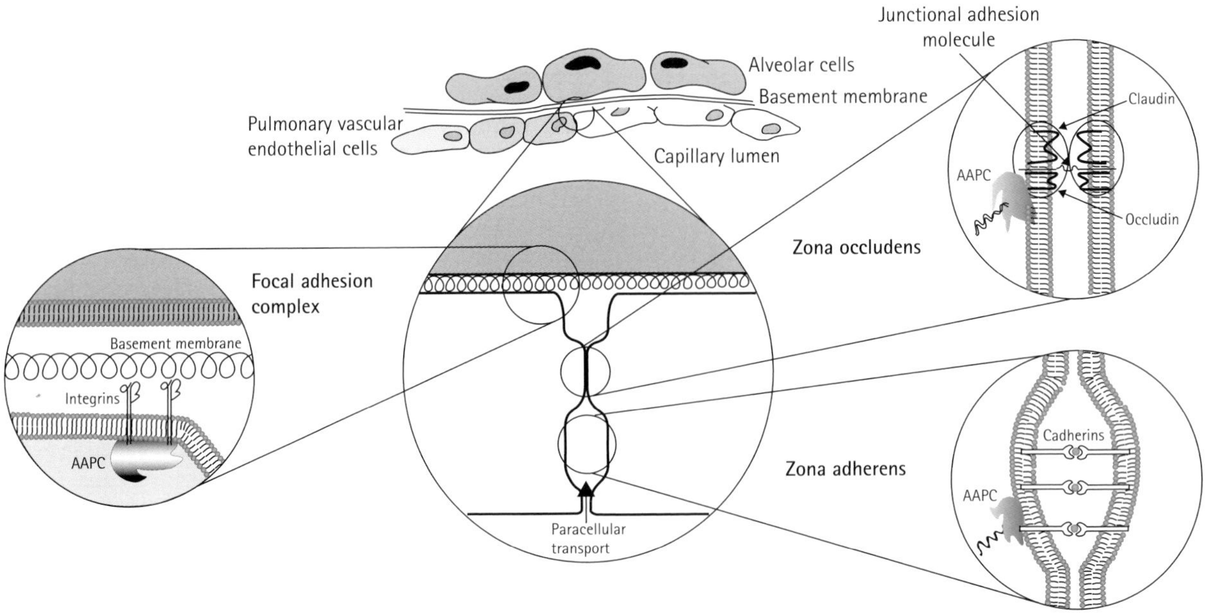

Figure 22.1 *Examples of endothelial connections modulating paracellular permeability. AAPC, adherence-associated protein complex.*

Table 22.3 *Inflammatory mediators known to modulate capillary permeability*

Cytokines	IL-1, IL-2, TNF, IFN-γ[175]
Growth factors	VEGF[1,176], TGF-beta[7,177,178]
Clotting factors	Thrombin[179]
Complement components	C3a[9,180]
Cell-derived inflammatory mediators	Prostanoids[5,11,181]
	Leukotrienes[182]
	Platelet-activating factor[183]
	Histamine[184]
Neutrophil-derived mediators	Superoxide ions
	Proteases
	Cytokines[185,186]
Bacterial-derived mediators Redox imbalance[188] Oxidative stress[189] Ischaemia-reperfusion injury[190,191]	Lipopolysaccharide[187]

IFN, interferon; IL, interleukin; TGF, transforming growth factor; TNF, tumor necrosis factor.

into the interstitium occurs at rates matched by their removal by venules, lymphatics[37] and alveolar pumps.[38]

In response to inflammatory activation (Table 22.3), endothelial cells modulate their intercellular connections and transport mechanisms leading to the passage of plasma protein-rich fluid and interstitial edema.[39] Some components of intercellular junctions are linked to the intracellular actin cytoskeleton, and relaxation of intercellular adhesion can coincide with ultrastructural changes. Although such changes are associated with inflammatory stimulation *in vitro*, to date no clear relationship has been identified between shape change and permeability.[32]

Increased pulmonary vascular permeability in patients with ARDS can be measured using a variety of techniques. Intravenously administered iodine-131-labelled albumin can be recovered from the broncho-alveolar space, demonstrating increased endothelial and epithelial permeability.[40] Larger molecules such as fibrinogen may accumulate in the lung as fast as albumin.[41] The relative accumulation of indium-113–transferrin complexes may be used to calculate an alveolar protein accumulation index (PAI).[42,43] Values may reflect the severity of lung injury, but seem to have little prognostic significance.[44] By contrast, multiple indicator dilution methods have suggested a correlation between the degree of microvascular permeability and mortality.[45]

The pulmonary transcapillary escape rate (PTCER) of gadolinium-68-transferrin complexes in patients with ARDS determined by positron emission tomography (PET) is raised tenfold above normal within the first 4 days of presentation and remains elevated (about fivefold) a week later.[46] Increases in PTCER detectable in patients with lobar pneumonia are comparable in extent with those measured in patients with ARDS;[47] and with PAI quantified in patients diagnosed with other non-pulmonary critical illnesses.[48] Increased pulmonary permeability *per se* is not therefore specific for any diagnosis, and is only an indication of generalized lung inflammation or injury. Patients with apparently localized pneumonia also have increased PTCER in radiographically unaffected lung regions, which increases as their clinical state deteriorates. Such data illustrate the probable link between a localized inflammatory lesion, a systemic inflammatory process, and generalized lung injury.

Pre-acinar arteries

Classical laminated macrothrombi occupying elastic-muscular arteries greater than 1 mm in diameter have been identified in 86% of patients with ARDS using angiography post-mortem and account for absent filling of leashes of capillaries.[18,49] The morphology of the thrombi rarely indicates if they are formed *in situ*, or represent true embolic phenomena from a distant source. Endothelial, neutrophil and platelet activation as well as procoagulant plasma protein changes favor *in situ* thrombosis.[50,51] However, specific conditions known to precipitate ARDS, including trauma, also provide sources of distal emboli.[52,53] Pulmonary vascular necrosis is a common postmortem finding in patients with ARDS even in lung regions without obvious extensive thrombosis.[54] Classical wedge-shaped infarcts localize subpleurally, possibly owing to poor collateral flow. Ischemic necrosis makes these areas attractive foci for infection, and also may account in part for the relatively high incidence of pneumothoraces in this patient population.[55]

PROLIFERATIVE PHASE

Capillaries

Ultrastructural evidence of capillary endothelial injury is more pronounced in the proliferative phase, and reduced capillary density may persist from the exudative phase.[18,56]

Pre-acinar arteries, veins and lymphatics

During the proliferative phase, fibrocellular intimal proliferation begins in small muscular arteries. These develop narrow, irregular and tortuous lumina. Equivalent changes in veins and lymphatics produce high resistance vessels that contribute to raised intracapillary pressure, edema and slow interstitial fluid drainage.[18]

FIBROPROLIFERATIVE PHASE

Capillaries

Capillary proliferation occurs in the fibrotic phase of ARDS.[18] Neovascularization may be the normal response in a post-injury environment, favoring the formation of granulation tissue. Recanalization of large thrombosed vessels may also occur by invasion of new capillaries. However, observed local increases in capillary density could actually represent apposition of vessels due to air space collapse.[57] Furthermore, fibrosis-induced traction may produce abnormal large and distorted capillaries.[18,58]

Pre-acinar arteries

Pulmonary vessels continue to remodel late in ARDS.[59] Mural fibrous infiltration and traction can produce an accordion-like appearance in large arteries. In smaller vessels, neomuscularization extends from pre-acinar arteries into intra-acinar arteries that are usually only partially muscularized, or which are non-muscular. The frequency of arteries with pathological medial hypertrophy increases with the duration of ARDS, as does the number of normally non-muscularized small arteries with muscular walls. Post-mortem angiography also demonstrates vessels splayed around dilated air spaces, and the usual anatomic arrangements or airway and vessel are lost.[18]

CLINICAL CORRELATES

Pulmonary hypertension

A persistent increase in pulmonary artery (PA) systolic pressure above 30 mmHg, or a mean greater than 25 mmHg, has been considered characteristic of early ARDS.[60] The initial degree of hypertension may reflect the severity of lung injury, but is probably not prognostic in itself.[61–64] By contrast, a rising mean PAP in the first week and beyond appears to distinguish non-survivors from survivors.[65] Right ventricular work and oxygen demand are increased. Nevertheless, with enough venous return, a normally compliant right ventricle with sufficient oxygen supply can generate an adequate cardiac output, whilst dilating in response to a threefold rise in pulmonary vascular resistance.[66] However, depressed myocardial performance may coexist with lung injury, particularly in patients with sepsis, which is the commonest cause of ARDS.[67,68] Frank right ventricular failure is a rare complication but carries a particularly poor prognosis.[62,65,69]

THE CAUSES OF PULMONARY HYPERTENSION

Hypoxic pulmonary vasoconstriction

Possible causes of pulmonary hypertension in ARDS shift as the syndrome evolves (Table 22.4). At any given stage, the relative importance of each of the causes is uncertain, as is the dominant site of vascular resistance.[70,71] In the early stages of ARDS, hypoxic pulmonary vasoconstriction (HPV) (see below) affects the pulmonary arterioles. HPV normally diverts flow from hypoxic to ventilated areas of lung, protecting ventilation/perfusion ($\dot{V}/\dot{Q}$) matching and improving arterial oxygenation. However, damaged regions of lung are extensive in patients with ARDS, and under theses circumstances the vascular resistance of the unaffected lung to the redirected flow can also be significant, thus redistributing flow to the hypoxic areas. HPV-related perfusion redistribution failure results in abnormal $\dot{V}/\dot{Q}$ and hypoxemia. HPV may also be impaired in patients with ARDS for other reasons (Table 22.5).[72]

Pulmonary venoconstriction

The density and variety of receptors on pulmonary veins,[73–76] together with their location downstream of emboli, render them prone to constriction by inflammatory mediators. Pulmonary venous hypertension raises pulmonary capillary pressure and may elevate arterial

Table 22.4 *Some possible causes of pulmonary hypertension in acute respiratory distress syndrome (ARDS)*

POSSIBLE CAUSES OF EARLY PULMONARY HYPERTENSION

Hypoxic pulmonary vasoconstriction	Alveolar hypoxia
	Mixed venous hypoxemia
	Acidosis
	Alveolar hypercarbia
	High mixed venous PCO_2
Vessel narrowing and closure	High interstitial or alveolar oedema pressure
	Alveolar collapse and low FRC
	High ventilated alveolar pressure and volume
Thromboembolism	
Pulmonary venous hypertension	
Vasodilator and constrictor imbalance	Nitric oxide
	Prostacyclin
	Endothelins
Inflammatory mediators	Thromboxane
	Prostaglandin E_2
	Platelet activating factor
	5-Hydroxytryptamine
	Superoxide ions

POSSIBLE CAUSES OF LATE PULMONARY HYPERTENSION

Vascular remodelling	General increase in vessel muscularity
	Development of muscular small vessels
	Vessel fibrosis
	Abnormal vessel tone
	Abnormal vessel reactivity
Vessel distortion	Interstitial fibrosis
	Cystic airspaces
Vessel compression	Persistently elevated interstitial pressure
Vessel obliteration	Parenchymal destruction
	Recanalization failure
Recurrent thromboembolism	

FRC, functional residual capacity; PCO_2 partial pressure of CO_2.

Table 22.5 *Factors inhibiting hypoxic pulmonary vasoconstriction in acute respiratory distress syndrome (ARDS)*

Pathological	Treatment-related
Surgery	β-adrenergic agonists
Blunt trauma	α-adrenergic antagonists
Pneumonia	Nitroprusside
Fluid overload	Nitroglycerine
High pulmonary artery pressure	Calcium channel antagonists
High pulmonary venous pressure	Prostacyclin
	Dopamine
	Low arterial PCO_2
	High pH
	High mixed venous PO_2
	Low mixed venous PCO_2

PCO_2, parial pressure of CO_2.

pressures. Although the number of pulmonary angiographic filling defects correlates with pulmonary vascular resistance,[49] physical obstruction alone is an unlikely cause of early pulmonary hypertension in ARDS as, to some extent, early hypertension is pharmacologically reversible. The comparative potency and local concentration of the transitory mediators is unknown in ARDS, but thromboxane antagonists can reduce the venous component of the rise in pulmonary vascular resistance.[77]

Imbalance between endogenous vasoconstrictors and vasodilators

Physical factors and the continuous release of mediators with opposing effects determine the overall vasomotor tone of the normal pulmonary vasculature (see above).[78,79]

However, local vascular responses depend upon the nature of the vessel, the receptors expressed and other coexistent modulating factors. The pulmonary endothelium modulates vascular tone by the release of endothelium-derived constricting factors including endothelin;[80] endothelium-derived relaxing factors including nitric oxide[81] and prostacyclin;[82,83] and putative endothelium-derived hyperpolarizing factors.[84]

Nitric oxide In health, endothelium-derived NO may be important in maintaining low basal pulmonary vascular tone.[81,85] Some pulmonary hypertensive diseases have therefore been linked with impaired NO production[86] and impaired NO release may encourage platelet- and neutrophil-endothelial adhesion in ARDS. Furthermore, endothelial denudation enhances HPV.[87] Dysfunctional endothelial modulation of smooth muscle tone might therefore contribute to pulmonary hypertension in ARDS.

However, although some animal models of pulmonary endothelial injury show early increases in vascular reactivity,[88] hyporesponsiveness to vasoconstrictors and hypoxia ensues.[89,90] This response can apparently occur simultaneously with vascular remodeling and the development of pulmonary hypertension. It is possible that part of the pulmonary vascular hyporesponsiveness is mediated by NO from inducible NO synthase that is up-regulated in endothelial and smooth muscle cells,[91] but evidence is conflicting.[92,93]

Prostacyclin The imbalance between the release and actions of vasoconstrictor and vasodilator prostanoids contributes to abnormal vascular tone in models of lung injury. Reduced prostacyclin production has been implicated in the pathogenesis of primary and secondary pulmonary hypertension,[94] but both thromboxane and prostacyclin metabolites are elevated in patients with ARDS.[95] Increased prostacyclin production might offset the vasoconstrictor effects of platelet-derived thromboxane. In some animal models, non-selective cyclooxygenase (COX) inhibitors increase HPV but patients with pneumonia show variable improvement in hypoxemia after non-selective COX inhibition[96] and there is no effect on the course or outcome of ARDS due to sepsis.[97] Lung injury induces COX-2 in endothelial and pulmonary vascular smooth muscle cells and in one animal model, selective COX-2 inhibition maintained beneficial flow redistribution attributable to HPV.[98] The effect of selective COX-2 inhibition in patients with lung injury is not known.

Endothelins Endothelins (ET) are potent vasoconstrictors and smooth muscle mitogens that are normally expressed and active in the lung.[99–101] Inflammation,[102] oxidative stress[103] and thrombin[104] can up-regulate ET-1 production, and ET-1 is elevated in the plasma of patients with ARDS.[105] ET-1 synthesis mediates late vasoconstriction in response to hypoxia,[106] making it a potentially important regulator of regional blood flow in ARDS and a stimulus for vascular remodeling. Both these phenomena are partially inhibited by endothelin receptor antagonists in animal models of hypoxic pulmonary hypertension.[107,108] However, in rodent models of sepsis, pulmonary vessels alter their responses to endothelin[109,110] and effects may be modified in patients with ARDS as well.

Reactive oxygen species There is evidence that normal vascular tone is regulated by endothelial cell-derived reactive oxygen species (ROS) including superoxide ions and hydrogen peroxide. ROS may not only modulate smooth muscle tone but are also postulated signals of cellular oxidative stress, producing adaptive or apoptotic responses.[111] Overwhelming oxidative stress with antioxidant failure leads to structural cell damage and this is also inflicted by ROS and reactive nitrogen species (RNS).[112] Patients with ARDS suffer ROS- and RNS-induced damage[113,114] and animal models of oxidative stress demonstrate that this form of injury alters pulmonary vascular tone, the most frequent response being vasoconstriction followed by hyporeactivity.[115]

Hypoxia

Several mechanisms are responsible for the refractory hypoxemia that characterizes ARDS. Lung function tests suggest impaired gas transfer, despite the presence of interstitial edema and intra-alveolar hyaline membranes, is not a principal cause,[116] although there is a reduction in accessible capillary blood volume.[117] Although alveolar injury may be widespread and even homogeneous, the distribution of the resulting atelectasis and edema within the lungs of supine patients is typically heterogeneous, as

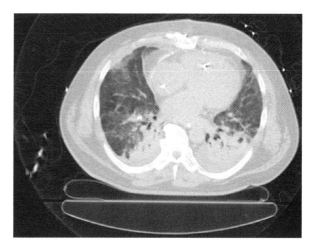

Figure 22.2 *A computed tomography scan representative of the tissue/air distribution in a patient with acute respiratory distress syndrome (ARDS).*

unequivocally demonstrated by computerized tomography (Figure 22.2).[118,119] The loss of aeration may be diffuse, patchy or lobar in distribution, but is consistently observed in the lower lobes, extending to the upper lobes in approximately two-thirds of supine patients.[120,121] The distribution of aerated and consolidated lung has profound implications for $\dot{V}/\dot{Q}$ mismatch and ventilatory strategies in patients with ARDS.

THE DISTRIBUTION OF PULMONARY PERFUSION IN PATIENTS WITH ARDS

Computed tomography (CT) (Figure 22.2) provides a radiological representation of the results of early studies of $\dot{V}/\dot{Q}$ mismatch in patients with ARDS that employed the multiple inert gas elimination technique (MIGET). This revealed a bimodal distribution of $\dot{V}/\dot{Q}$ ratios,[122,123] approximately half the pulmonary blood flow being distributed to units of normal $\dot{V}/\dot{Q}$ ratio and the other half flowing through regions of no ventilation (pure shunt), or a few units with a very low $\dot{V}/\dot{Q}$ ratio.

The effect of PEEP on the distribution of perfusion

In some patients with ARDS in studies using MIGET, the application of positive end-expiratory pressure (PEEP) at low levels alters the distribution of blood flow between units of normal and abnormal $\dot{V}/\dot{Q}$, without creating intermediate ratio units.[122,124,125] This supports the hypothesis that PEEP physically alters $\dot{V}/\dot{Q}$ relationships in a quantal fashion, anatomically represented by the opening, or 'recruitment' of collapsed alveoli. This apparently leads to a normally functioning state of gas transfer, reduces shunt and so improves arterial oxygenation.

By contrast, in other patients, PEEP causes a fall in cardiac output, the emergence of units with high $\dot{V}/\dot{Q}$ ratios and an increase in physiological dead space.[124,125] High PEEP and/or inspiratory alveolar pressure lower ventricular transmural filling pressure and potentially increase pulmonary vascular resistance[126] in areas of hyperinflated compliant lung. This resistance might interfere with the beneficial effect of HPV. In practice, arterial oxygen saturation still sometimes improves with high PEEP because shunt fraction generally decreases as cardiac output falls.[127] Improvements in arterial oxygen saturation associated with the application of high PEEP might therefore not improve oxygen delivery. However, in adequately fluid resuscitated patients the reduction in cardiac output induced by PEEP can be small,[128–131] confirming that an improvement in arterial oxygenation is produced by improving $\dot{V}/\dot{Q}$ matching.[125,132]

The effect of vasodilators on distribution of perfusion

Intravenous vasodilators have been prescribed for patients with ARDS, first, to reduce pulmonary capillary filtration pressures and thus pulmonary edema formation; and second, to reduce pulmonary vascular resistance, increase the output of the right ventricle and so improve oxygen delivery. Prostacyclin,[133] prostaglandin E$_1$,[134] nitroglycerin,[134,135] nitroprusside[54] and diltiazem[136] can raise cardiac output in patients with ARDS but oxygen delivery may fall because arterial oxygen saturation decreases. This desaturation can be attributed to inhibition of residual HPV in the damaged lung with a consequent increase in heterogeneity of $\dot{V}/\dot{Q}$ matching. Inhaled vasodilators can circumvent this problem to some extent and avoid the hypotensive side effects of vasodilators reaching the systemic circulation (see below).

The effect of the prone position

The vertical distribution of blood flow in the normal lung in the upright position is determined by the relationship between alveolar, pulmonary artery and pulmonary venous pressures.[137] Comparing transverse sections of the lung at different heights, gravity influences regional blood flows. However, flow within an individual transverse section or isogravitational plane also forms a heterogeneous pattern not predicted by a gravitational hypothesis.[138–140] One factor favoring this uneven distribution is the fractal branching architecture of the pulmonary vascular tree, which produces unequal resistances in diverging vessels.[141] Regional differences in vascular resistance related to NO synthesis have also been observed in animals.[142] The result of these effects is that perfusion to the dorsal regions of the lung is relatively preserved compared to the ventral regions in the prone position in man.[143–145]

During mechanical ventilation in the supine position, the majority of studies suggest ventral lung ventilation dominates. By contrast, in the prone position, most investigators demonstrate an even distribution of alveolar ventilation.[145] Thus, improved homogeneity in alveolar ventilation with simultaneous preservation of dorsal pulmonary blood flow in the prone position may produce a better spatial correlation of regional alveolar ventilation and pulmonary perfusion.[146] The matching of ventilation to perfusion in the prone position during mechanical ventilation explains improvements in oxygenation in some patients with ARDS turned prone.[147–149] However, prone positioning has not been shown so far to afford a survival benefit to patients with ARDS.[150]

THE EFFECT OF PULMONARY VASCULAR METABOLIC FAILURE

The pulmonary endothelium is a site of intense metabolic activity producing transpulmonary concentration differences of bioactive agents (Table 22.6).[151] The lung thus reduces recirculation of tissue-derived bioactive substances with usually brief and/or local actions. Models of lung injury demonstrate a fall in the normal pulmonary capacity to remove vasoactive substances. The effect is neither injury- nor substrate-specific. Metabolic dysfunction begins before detectable changes in endothelial permeability and ultrastructure, or the onset of hemodynamic instability.[152] A failure in metabolic function may contribute to pulmonary and systemic vasodysregulation in patients with lung injury.[153]

Catabolism of 5-hydroxytryptamine and prostaglandin E$_1$ by the lung is impaired in patients with ARDS.[154] For amines and prostaglandins, the rate-limiting metabolic step is carrier-mediated active transport, rather than enzymatic deactivation. Angiotensin converting enzyme (ACE), which activates angiotensin I and inactivates bradykinin, is present on the pulmonary endothelial surface and intracellular transport is unnecessary. ACE activity measured using

Table 22.6 *Bioactive compounds normally cleared by the pulmonary circulation*

Bioactive compound	Per cent inactivated
Amines	
5-hydroxytryptamine	65–95
Norepinephrine	25–50
Dopamine	30
Epinephrine	<10
Isoproterenol	unaffected
Histamine	unaffected
Prostaglandins	
PGE$_1$, PGE$_2$, PGF$_{2\alpha}$, PGD$_2$	65–98
Thromboxane	<10
PGA	unaffected
Peptides	
Angiotensin I	40–100
Bradykinin	75–98
Vasopressin	unaffected

PGE$_1$, prostaglandin E$_1$; PGE$_2$, prostaglandin E$_2$; PGF$_{2\alpha}$, prostaglandin F$_{2\alpha}$; PGO$_2$, prostaglandin O$_2$; PGA, prostaglandin A.

a synthetic substrate permits estimations of the perfused capillary surface area in the normal lung.[155] This activity decreases early in the course of ARDS and may correlate with severity of lung injury.[156] However, plasma angiotensin II levels may actually increase.[157]

ET-1 is both cleared from, and released into, plasma by the lung.[158] An abnormal pulmonary ET-1 clearance to production ratio develops in ARDS and could contribute to the increase in pulmonary vascular resistance.[105,159] Although ET-1 clearance normalizes as clinical state improves, the mitogenic effect of ET-1 may contribute to pulmonary vascular remodeling.

The removal of other substances, such as propranolol, is affected by lung inflation. However, a ventilatory strategy optimizing oxygenation does not improve ACE activity in a model of lung injury.[160] Equally, improving hypoxemia by turning patients with ARDS prone does not modify pulmonary angiotensin production or ET-1 clearance.[157] Although maneuvers that improve oxygenation might simultaneously improve the exposed vascular endothelial surface area available for metabolic function, this effect does not appear to be significant.

Changes in the pulmonary circulation in survivors of ARDS

Little is known about vascular remodeling in long-term survivors of ARDS.[161] Small follow-up studies have demonstrated variable residual pulmonary vascular effects.[162] Extrapolation of early investigations to those performed following publication of the AEC definition and the introduction of modern management techniques is difficult. The etiology of the ARDS, pulmonary or non-pulmonary, may influence mortality but does not alter return of lung function at 6 months.[163] Moreover, although between 40 and 80% of survivors have abnormal pulmonary function tests 12 months after recovery, the clinical significance of these results is variable and difficult to ascertain.

A low single-breath carbon monoxide diffusing capacity is a frequent finding.[164] The capillary blood volume determinant of the DLCO may be more important to reduced gas transfer than the membrane conductance.[165] The DLCO corrected for remaining alveolar volume (KCO) is also commonly reduced. Together with a raised dead space to tidal volume ratio, these results suggest a persistent loss of capillary surface area. This may be secondary to destruction and/or malperfusion of the remaining capillary bed.[165–167] CT appearances 6 months after the acute illness typically show a coarse reticular pattern with distortion of the lung parenchyma, ground-glass opacification and areas of hypoattenuation dominating the anterior zones.[168] This fibrotic appearance with cystic destruction of the lung parenchyma supports a view that collapsed and/or consolidated lung in the acute phase of ARDS is protected from alveolar overdistension during pressure-controlled inverse ratio ventilation. Because arterial and bronchial structures are paired, it is likely that the destruction of the pulmonary vascular bed in patients managed in this way is also localized anteriorly. However, while the extent of the fibrosis on CT is related to loss of lung volume on lung function testing, it is not correlated with loss of gas transfer.

Improvement in pulmonary function tests after ARDS is usually rapid during the first 3–6 months but more gradual subsequently. After 6 months, arterial blood gases at rest are often normal and a shunt fraction characteristic of active ARDS is rare. Significant oxygen desaturation may occasionally still occur on exercise.[166,169] Abnormalities persisting for greater than 1 year are unlikely to resolve.[170] In general, the relative improvement in lung volumes and restrictive and/or obstructive spirometry is greater than improvement in DLCO, suggesting more permanent destruction or slower useful remodeling of the pulmonary vasculature compared to alveolar and airway restoration. Results may be confounded by pre- and post-ARDS lung damage, most commonly caused by smoking, but the majority of the abnormalities in gas transfer are mild at 1 year.[162]

Moreover, the degree of abnormality in pulmonary function tests does not correlate with symptoms or quality of life. More than half the survivors of ARDS in some series had persistent pulmonary symptoms 1 year postdischarge, although only 12% in one study had physical limitations impairing lifestyle.[171,172] Health complaints of ARDS survivors at 1 year are not entirely related to pulmonary factors.[173] Nevertheless, compared to equally injured or ill patients without ARDS, survivors of ARDS do have health-related quality of life indices that reflect pulmonary disease-specific impairments.[174] This observation should encourage clinical practice that protects the injured lung with a view to better long-term pulmonary outcomes.

KEY POINTS

- Lung injury dramatically affects the pulmonary circulation.
- Raised capillary endothelial permeability floods the interstitium and alveoli with protein-rich exudates.
- Macroscopic and microscopic thromboemboli obstruct the circulation at all levels.
- Inflammatory mediators and endothelial dysfunction produce abnormal vasoconstriction and vasodilation.

- Pathological processes impair useful hypoxic pulmonary vasoconstriction and there is significant ventilation/perfusion mismatch.
- The clinical manifestations are profound hypoxia and moderate pulmonary hypertension.
- Treatment is supportive but should aim to protect the lung and pulmonary vasculature.
- Of the 60% who survive ARDS, the majority have minor defects in lung function tests at one year.

REFERENCES

1 Ashbaugh DG, Bigelow DB, Petty TL et al. Acute respiratory distress in adults. Lancet 1967;ii:319–23.

2 Bernard GR, Artigas A, Brigham KL et al. The American-European Consensus Conference on ARDS. Definitions, mechanisms, relevant outcomes, and clinical trial coordination. Am J Respir Crit Care Med 1994;149 (3 Pt 1):818–24.

3 Weinacker AB, Vaszar LT. Acute respiratory distress syndrome: physiology and new management strategies. Annu Rev Med 2001;52:221–37.

4 Jordan S, Mitchell JA, Quinlan GJ et al. The pathogenesis of lung injury following pulmonary resection. Eur Respir J 2000;15:790–9.

5 Luhr OR, Antonsen K, Karlsson M et al. Incidence and mortality after acute respiratory failure and acute respiratory distress syndrome in Sweden, Denmark, and Iceland. The ARF Study Group. Am J Respir Crit Care Med 1999;159:1849–61.

6 Thomsen GE, Morris AH. Incidence of the adult respiratory distress syndrome in the state of Utah. Am J Respir Crit Care Med 1995;152:965–71.

7 Lewandowski K, Metz J, Deutschmann C et al. Incidence, severity, and mortality of acute respiratory failure in Berlin, Germany. Am J Respir Crit Care Med 1995;151:1121–5.

8 Pola MD, Navarrete-Navarro P, Rivera R et al. Acute respiratory distress syndrome: resource use and outcomes in 1985 and 1995, trends in mortality and comorbidities. J Crit Care 2000;15:91–6.

9 Roupie E, Lepage E, Wysocki M et al. Prevalence, etiologies and outcome of the acute respiratory distress syndrome among hypoxemic ventilated patients. SRLF Collaborative Group on Mechanical Ventilation. Société de Réanimation de la Langue Française. Intensive Care Med 1999;25:920–9.

10 Abel SJ, Finney SJ, Brett SJ et al. Reduced mortality in association with the acute respiratory distress syndrome (ARDS). Thorax 1998;53:292–4.

11 Milberg JA, Davis DR, Steinberg KP et al. Improved survival of patients with acute respiratory distress syndrome (ARDS): 1983–1993. JAMA 1995;273:306–9.

12 ARDS Network. Ventilation with lower tidal volumes as compared with traditional tidal volumes for acute lung injury and the acute respiratory distress syndrome. N Engl J Med 2000;342:1301–8.

13 Tomashefski JF, Jr. Pulmonary pathology of acute respiratory distress syndrome. Clin Chest Med 2000;21:435–66.

14 Katzenstein AL, Bloor CM, Leibow AA. Diffuse alveolar damage – the role of oxygen, shock, and related factors. A review. Am J Pathol 1976;85:209–28.

15 Bleyl U, Rossner JA. Globular hyaline microthrombi—their nature and morphogenesis. Virchows Arch A Pathol Anat Histol 1976;370:113–28.

16 Nash G, Blennerhassett JB, Pontoppidan H. Pulmonary lesions associated with oxygen therapy and artificial ventilation. N Engl J Med 1967;276:368–74.

17 Pratt PC, Vollmer RT, Shelburne JD et al. Pulmonary morphology in a multihospital collaborative extracorporeal membrane oxygenation project. I. Light microscopy. Am J Pathol 1979;95:191–214.

18 Tomashefski JF Jr, Davies P, Boggis C et al. The pulmonary vascular lesions of the adult respiratory distress syndrome. Am J Pathol 1983;112:112–26.

19 Hechtman HB, Lonergan EA, Shepro D. Platelet and leukocyte lung interactions in patients with respiratory failure. Surgery 1978;83:155–63.

20 Spragg RG, Abraham JL, Loomis WH. Pulmonary platelet deposition accompanying acute oleic-acid-induced pulmonary injury. Am Rev Respir Dis 1982;126:553–7.

21 Warshawski FJ, Sibbald WJ, Driedger AA et al. Abnormal neutrophil-pulmonary interaction in the adult respiratory distress syndrome. Qualitative and quantitative assessment of pulmonary neutrophil kinetics in humans with in vivo [111]indium neutrophil scintigraphy. Am Rev Respir Dis 1986;133:797–804.

22 Doerschuk CM, Allard MF, Hogg JC. Neutrophil kinetics in rabbits during infusion of zymosan-activated plasma. J Appl Physiol 1989;67:88–95.

23 Eeles GH, Sevitt S. Microthrombosis in injured and burned patients. J Pathol Bacteriol 1967;93:275–93.

24 Doerschuk CM. Mechanisms of leukocyte sequestration in inflamed lungs. Microcirculation 2001;8:71–88.

25 Strieter RM, Kunkel SL, Keane MP et al. Chemokines in lung injury: Thomas A. Neff Lecture. Chest 1999; 116(Suppl 1):103S–10S.

26 Heffner JE, Sahn SA, Repine JE. The role of platelets in the adult respiratory distress syndrome. Culprits or bystanders? Am Rev Respir Dis 1987;135:482–92.

27 Patterson CE, Barnard JW, Lafuze JE et al. The role of activation of neutrophils and microvascular pressure in acute pulmonary edema. Am Rev Respir Dis 1989;140:1052–62.

28 Riede UN, Joachim H, Hassenstein J et al. The pulmonary air-blood barrier of human shock lungs (a clinical, ultrastructural and morphometric study). Pathol Res Pract 1978;162:41–72.

29 Schnells G, Voigt WH, Redl H et al. Electron-microscopic investigation of lung biopsies in patients with post-traumatic respiratory insufficiency. Acta Chir Scand Suppl 1980;499:9–20.

30 Albertine KH. Ultrastructural abnormalities in increased-permeability pulmonary edema. Clin Chest Med 1985;6:345–69.

31 Lum H, Malik AB. Regulation of vascular endothelial barrier function. Am J Physiol 1994;267(3 Pt 1):L223–41.

32 Patterson CE, Lum H. Update on pulmonary edema: the role and regulation of endothelial barrier function. *Endothelium* 2001;**8**:75–105.

33 Ghinea N, Eskenasy M, Simionescu M *et al*. Endothelial albumin binding proteins are membrane-associated components exposed on the cell surface. *J Biol Chem* 1989;**264**:4755–8.

34 Tiruppathi C, Finnegan A, Malik AB. Isolation and characterization of a cell surface albumin-binding protein from vascular endothelial cells. *Proc Natl Acad Sci USA* 1996;**93**:250–4.

35 Predescu SA, Predescu DN, Palade GE. Plasmalemmal vesicles function as transcytotic carriers for small proteins in the continuous endothelium. *Am J Physiol* 1997;**272** (2 Pt 2):H937–49.

36 Tagami M, Kubota A, Sunaga T *et al*. Increased transendothelial channel transport of cerebral capillary endothelium in stroke-prone SHR. *Stroke* 1983;**14**:591–6.

37 Taylor AE, Gibson WH, Granger HJ *et al*. The interaction between intracapillary and tissue forces in the overall regulation of interstitial fluid volume. *Lymphology* 1973;**6**:192–208.

38 Crandall ED, Matthay MA. Alveolar epithelial transport. Basic science to clinical medicine. *Am J Respir Crit Care Med* 2001;**163**:1021–9.

39 Ware LB, Matthay MA. The acute respiratory distress syndrome. *N Engl J Med* 2000;**342**:1334–49.

40 Anderson RR, Holliday RL, Driedger AA *et al*. Documentation of pulmonary capillary permeability in the adult respiratory distress syndrome accompanying human sepsis. *Am Rev Respir Dis* 1979;**119**:869–77.

41 Quinn DA, Carvalho AC, Geller E *et al*. ^{99m}Tc-fibrinogen scanning in adult respiratory distress syndrome. *Am Rev Respir Dis* 1987;**135**:100–6.

42 Gorin AB, Kohler J, DeNardo G. Noninvasive measurement of pulmonary transvascular protein flux in normal man. *J Clin Invest* 1980;**66**:869–77.

43 Hunter DN, Morgan CJ, Evans TW. The use of radionuclide techniques in the assessment of alveolar-capillary membrane permeability on the intensive care unit. *Intensive Care Med* 1990;**16**:363–71.

44 Sinclair DG, Braude S, Haslam PL *et al*. Pulmonary endothelial permeability in patients with severe lung injury. Clinical correlates and natural history. *Chest* 1994;**106**:535–9.

45 Harris TR, Bernard GR, Brigham KL *et al*. Lung microvascular transport properties measured by multiple indicator dilution methods in patients with adult respiratory distress syndrome. A comparison between patients reversing respiratory failure and those failing to reverse. *Am Rev Respir Dis* 1990;**141**: 272–80.

46 Calandrino FS, Jr, Anderson DJ, Mintun MA *et al*. Pulmonary vascular permeability during the adult respiratory distress syndrome: a positron emission tomographic study. *Am Rev Respir Dis* 1988;**138**:421–8.

47 Kaplan JD, Calandrino FS, Schuster DP. A positron emission tomographic comparison of pulmonary vascular permeability during the adult respiratory distress syndrome and pneumonia. *Am Rev Respir Dis* 1991;**143**:150–4.

48 Rocker GM, Wiseman MS, Pearson D *et al*. Diagnostic criteria for adult respiratory distress syndrome: time for reappraisal. *Lancet* 1989;**1**:120–3.

49 Greene R, Zapol WM, Snider MT *et al*. Early bedside detection of pulmonary vascular occlusion during acute respiratory failure. *Am Rev Respir Dis* 1981;**124**:593–601.

50 Carvalho A. Blood alterations in ARDS. In: Zapol WM, Falke KJ (eds), *Acute respiratory failure*. New York: Marcel Dekker, 1985;303–46.

51 Abraham E. Coagulation abnormalities in acute lung injury and sepsis. *Am J Respir Cell Mol Biol* 2000;**22**:401–4.

52 Blaisdell FW, Stallone RJ. The mechanism of pulmonary damage following traumatic shock. *Surg Gynecol Obstet* 1970;**130**:15–22.

53 Soares FA. Increased numbers of pulmonary megakaryocytes in patients with arterial pulmonary tumour embolism and with lung metastases seen at necropsy. *J Clin Pathol* 1992;**45**:140–2.

54 Zapol WM, Jones R. Vascular components of ARDS. Clinical pulmonary hemodynamics and morphology. *Am Rev Respir Dis* 1987;**136**:471–4.

55 Redline S, Tomashefski JF, Jr, Altose MD. Cavitating lung infarction after bland pulmonary thromboembolism in patients with the adult respiratory distress syndrome. *Thorax* 1985;**40**:915–19.

56 Bachofen M, Weibel ER. Alterations of the gas exchange apparatus in adult respiratory insufficiency associated with septicemia. *Am Rev Respir Dis* 1977;**116**:589–615.

57 Burkhardt A. Alveolitis and collapse in the pathogenesis of pulmonary fibrosis. *Am Rev Respir Dis* 1989;**140**:513–24.

58 Meyrick B. Pathology of the adult respiratory distress syndrome. *Crit Care Clin* 1986;**2**:405–28.

59 Snow RL, Davies P, Pontoppidan H *et al*. Pulmonary vascular remodeling in adult respiratory distress syndrome. *Am Rev Respir Dis* 1982;**126**:887–92.

60 Zapol WM, Snider MT. Pulmonary hypertension in severe acute respiratory failure. *N Engl J Med* 1977;**296**:476–80.

61 Villar J, Blazquez MA, Lubillo S *et al*. Pulmonary hypertension in acute respiratory failure. *Crit Care Med* 1989;**17**:523–6.

62 Leeman M. Pulmonary hypertension in acute respiratory distress syndrome. *Monaldi Arch Chest Dis* 1999;**54**:146–9.

63 Bone RC, Slotman G, Maunder R *et al*. Randomized double-blind, multicenter study of prostaglandin E1 in patients with the adult respiratory distress syndrome. Prostaglandin E1 Study Group. *Chest* 1989;**96**:114–19.

64 Suchyta MR, Clemmer TP, Elliott CG *et al*. The adult respiratory distress syndrome. A report of survival and modifying factors. *Chest* 1992;**101**:1074–9.

65 Sloane PJ, Gee MH, Gottlieb JE *et al*. A multicenter registry of patients with acute respiratory distress syndrome. Physiology and outcome. *Am Rev Respir Dis* 1992;**146**:419–26.

66 Rosenthal M. Hemodynamic effects of pulmonary insufficiency. *Int Anesthesiol Clin* 1986;**24**:145–58.

67 Fein AM, Calalang-Colucci MG. Acute lung injury and acute respiratory distress syndrome in sepsis and septic shock. *Crit Care Clin* 2000;**16**:289–317.

68 Kumar A, Haery C, Parrillo JE. Myocardial dysfunction in septic shock. *Crit Care Clin* 2000;**16**:251–87.

69 Naeije R. Medical treatment of pulmonary hypertension in acute lung disease. *Eur Respir J* 1993;**6**:1521–8.

70 Benzing A, Mols G, Guttmann J *et al.* Effect of different doses of inhaled nitric oxide on pulmonary capillary pressure and on longitudinal distribution of pulmonary vascular resistance in ARDS. *Br J Anaesth* 1998;**80**:440–6.

71 Nagasaka Y, Ishigaki M, Hazu R *et al.* Lung microvascular pressure profile in acute lung injury. *Tohoku J Exp Med* 1996;**179**:81–92.

72 Marshall BE, Hanson CW, Frasch F *et al.* Role of hypoxic pulmonary vasoconstriction in pulmonary gas exchange and blood flow distribution. 2. Pathophysiology. *Intensive Care Med* 1994;**20**:379–89.

73 Schellenberg RR, Foster A. Differential activity of leukotrienes upon human pulmonary vein and artery. *Prostaglandins* 1984;**27**:475–82.

74 Lippton HL, Ohlstein EH, Summer WR *et al.* Analysis of responses to endothelins in the rabbit pulmonary and systemic vascular beds. *J Appl Physiol* 1991;**70**:331–41.

75 Labat C, Ortiz JL, Norel X *et al.* A second cysteinyl leukotriene receptor in human lung. *J Pharmacol Exp Ther* 1992;**263**:800–5.

76 Walch L, de Montpreville V, Brink C *et al.* Prostanoid EP(1)- and TP-receptors involved in the contraction of human pulmonary veins. *Br J Pharmacol* 2001;**134**:1671–8.

77 Schuster DP, Kozlowski JK, Brimioulle S. Effect of thromboxane receptor blockade on pulmonary capillary hypertension in acute lung injury. *Am J Respir Crit Care Med* 2001;**163**:A820.

78 Weir EK. Does normoxic pulmonary vasodilatation rather than hypoxic vasoconstriction account for the pulmonary pressor response to hypoxia? *Lancet* 1978;**1**:476–7.

79 Luscher TF. Endothelium-derived vasoactive factors and regulation of vascular tone in human blood vessels. *Lung* 1990;**168**(Suppl):27–34.

80 Weitzberg E, Ahlborg G, Lundberg JM. Differences in vascular effects and removal of endothelin-1 in human lung, brain, and skeletal muscle. *Clin Physiol* 1993;**13**:653–62.

81 Stamler JS, Loh E, Roddy MA *et al.* Nitric oxide regulates basal systemic and pulmonary vascular resistance in healthy humans. *Circulation* 1994;**89**:2035–40.

82 Edlund A, Bomfim W, Kaijser L *et al.* Pulmonary formation of prostacyclin in man. *Prostaglandins* 1981;**22**:323–32.

83 Reeves JT, McMurtry IF, Voelkel NF. Possible role for membrane lipids in the function of the normal and ab normal pulmonary circulation. *Am Rev Respir Dis* 1987;**136**:196–9.

84 Feletou M, Vanhoutte PM. The third pathway: endothelium-dependent hyperpolarization. *J Physiol Pharmacol* 1999;**50**:525–34.

85 Greenberg B, Rhoden K, Barnes PJ. Endothelium-dependent relaxation of human pulmonary arteries. *Am J Physiol* 1987;**252**(2 Pt 2):H434–8.

86 Dinh-Xuan AT, Higenbottam TW, Clelland CA *et al.* Impairment of endothelium-dependent pulmonary-artery relaxation in chronic obstructive lung disease. *N Engl J Med* 1991;**324**:1539–47.

87 Ohe M, Ogata M, Katayose D *et al.* Hypoxic contraction of pre-stretched human pulmonary artery. *Respir Physiol* 1992;**87**:105–14.

88 Rounds S, Farber HW, Hill NS *et al.* Effects of endothelial cell injury on pulmonary vascular reactivity. *Chest* 1985;**88** (Suppl 4):213S–16S.

89 Light RB, Mink SN, Wood LD. Pathophysiology of gas exchange and pulmonary perfusion in pneumococcal lobar pneumonia in dogs. *J Appl Physiol* 1981;**50**:524–30.

90 Graham LM, Vasil A, Vasil ML *et al.* Decreased pulmonary vasoreactivity in an animal model of chronic *Pseudomonas* pneumonia. *Am Rev Respir Dis* 1990;**142**:221–9.

91 Holzmann A, Manktelow C, Taut FJ *et al.* Inhibition of nitric oxide synthase prevents hyporesponsiveness to inhaled nitric oxide in lungs from endotoxin-challenged rats. *Anesthesiology* 1999;**91**:215–21.

92 Yaghi A, Paterson NA, McCormack DG. Nitric oxide does not mediate the attenuated pulmonary vascular reactivity of chronic pneumonia. *Am J Physiol* 1993;**265**(3 Pt 2):H943–8.

93 McCormack DG. Control of vascular reactivity. *New Horiz* 1995;**3**:248–56.

94 Tuder RM, Cool CD, Geraci MW *et al.* Prostacyclin synthase expression is decreased in lungs from patients with severe pulmonary hypertension. *Am J Respir Crit Care Med* 1999;**159**:1925–32.

95 Bernard GR, Reines HD, Halushka PV *et al.* Prostacyclin and thromboxane A2 formation is increased in human sepsis syndrome. Effects of cyclooxygenase inhibition. *Am Rev Respir Dis* 1991;**144**:1095–101.

96 Hanly PJ, Roberts D, Dobson K *et al.* Effect of indomethacin on arterial oxygenation in critically ill patients with severe bacterial pneumonia. *Lancet* 1987;**i**:351–4.

97 Bernard GR, Wheeler AP, Russell JA *et al.* The effects of ibuprofen on the physiology and survival of patients with sepsis. The Ibuprofen in Sepsis Study Group. *N Engl J Med* 1997;**336**:912–18.

98 Gust R, Kozlowski JK, Stephenson AH *et al.* Role of cyclooxygenase-2 in oleic acid-induced acute lung injury. *Am J Respir Crit Care Med* 1999;**160**:1165–70.

99 La M, Reid JJ. Endothelin-1 and the regulation of vascular tone. *Clin Exp Pharmacol Physiol* 1995;**22**:315–23.

100 Giaid A, Yanagisawa M, Langleben D *et al.* Expression of endothelin-1 in the lungs of patients with pulmonary hypertension. *N Engl J Med* 1993;**328**:1732–9.

101 Dupuis J, Jasmin JF, Prie S *et al.* Importance of local production of endothelin-1 and of the ET(B)Receptor in the regulation of pulmonary vascular tone. *Pulmon Pharmacol Ther* 2000;**13**:135–40.

102 Pittet JF, Morel DR, Hemsen A *et al.* Elevated plasma endothelin-1 concentrations are associated with the severity of illness in patients with sepsis. *Ann Surg* 1991;**213**:261–4.

103 Michael JR, Markewitz BA, Kohan DE. Oxidant stress regulates basal endothelin-1 production by cultured rat pulmonary endothelial cells. *Am J Physiol* 1997;**273**(4 Pt 1): L768–74.

104 Golden CG, Nick HS, Visner GA. Thrombin regulation of endothelin-1 gene in isolated human pulmonary endothelial cells. *Chest* 1998;**114**(Suppl 1):63S–4S.

105 Langleben D, DeMarchie M, Laporta D *et al.* Endothelin-1 in acute lung injury and the adult respiratory distress syndrome. *Am Rev Respir Dis* 1993;**148**(6 Pt 1):1646–50.

106 Chen YF, Oparil S. Endothelin and pulmonary hypertension. *J Cardiovasc Pharmacol* 2000;**35**(4 Suppl 2):S49–53.

107 Chen SJ, Chen YF, Opgenorth TJ et al. The orally active nonpeptide endothelin A-receptor antagonist A-127722 prevents and reverses hypoxia-induced pulmonary hypertension and pulmonary vascular remodeling in Sprague-Dawley rats. J Cardiovasc Pharmacol 1997;29:713–25.

108 Oparil S, Chen SJ, Meng QC et al. Endothelin-A receptor antagonist prevents acute hypoxia-induced pulmonary hypertension in the rat. Am J Physiol 1995;268 (1 Pt 1):L95–100.

109 Curzen NP, Kaddoura S, Griffiths MJ et al. Endothelin-1 in rat endotoxemia: mRNA expression and vasoreactivity in pulmonary and systemic circulations. Am J Physiol 1997;272(5 Pt 2):H2353–60.

110 Guc MO, Furman BL, Parratt JR. Endotoxin-induced impairment of vasopressor and vasodepressor responses in the pithed rat. Br J Pharmacol 1990;101:913–19.

111 Vanhoutte PM. Endothelium-derived free radicals: for worse and for better. J Clin Invest 2001;107:23–5.

112 Halliwell B, Gutteridge J. Free radicals in biology and medicine, 3rd edn. Oxford: OUP, 1998.

113 Lamb NJ, Quinlan GJ, Westerman ST et al. Nitration of proteins in bronchoalveolar lavage fluid from patients with acute respiratory distress syndrome receiving inhaled nitric oxide. Am J Respir Crit Care Med 1999;160:1031–4.

114 Lamb NJ, Gutteridge JM, Baker C et al. Oxidative damage to proteins of bronchoalveolar lavage fluid in patients with acute respiratory distress syndrome: evidence for neutrophil-mediated hydroxylation, nitration, and chlorination. Crit Care Med 1999;27:1738–44.

115 Rhoades RA, Packer CS, Meiss RA. Pulmonary vascular smooth muscle contractility. Effect of free radicals. Chest 1988;93(Suppl 3):94S–5S.

116 King TK, Weber B, Okinaka A et al. Oxygen transfer in catastrophic respiratory failure. Chest 1974;65(Suppl):40S–4S.

117 Macnaughton PD, Evans TW. Measurement of lung volume and DLCO in acute respiratory failure. Am J Respir Crit Care Med 1994;150:770–5.

118 Desai SR, Wells AU, Suntharalingam G et al. Acute respiratory distress syndrome caused by pulmonary and extrapulmonary injury: a comparative CT study. Radiology 2001;218:689–93.

119 Desai SR, Hansell DM. Lung imaging in the adult respiratory distress syndrome: current practice and new insights. Intensive Care Med 1997;23:7–15.

120 Rouby JJ, Puybasset L, Cluzel P et al. Regional distribution of gas and tissue in acute respiratory distress syndrome. II. Physiological correlations and definition of an ARDS Severity Score. CT Scan ARDS Study Group. Intensive Care Med 2000;26:1046–56.

121 Puybasset L, Cluzel P, Chao N et al. A computed tomography scan assessment of regional lung volume in acute lung injury. The CT Scan ARDS Study Group. Am J Respir Crit Care Med 1998;158(5 Pt 1):1644–55.

122 Dantzker DR, Brook CJ, Dehart P et al. Ventilation-perfusion distributions in the adult respiratory distress syndrome. Am Rev Respir Dis 1979;120:1039–52.

123 Melot C. Contribution of multiple inert gas elimination technique to pulmonary medicine. 5. Ventilation-perfusion relationships in acute respiratory failure. Thorax 1994;49:1251–8.

124 Suter PM, Fairley B, Isenberg MD. Optimum end-expiratory airway pressure in patients with acute pulmonary failure. N Engl J Med 1975;292:284–9.

125 Ralph DD, Robertson HT, Weaver LJ et al. Distribution of ventilation and perfusion during positive end-expiratory pressure in the adult respiratory distress syndrome. Am Rev Respir Dis 1985;131:54–60.

126 Schmitt JM, Vieillard-Baron A, Augarde R et al. Positive end-expiratory pressure titration in acute respiratory distress syndrome patients: impact on right ventricular outflow impedance evaluated by pulmonary artery Doppler flow velocity measurements. Crit Care Med 2001;29:1154–8.

127 Dantzker DR, Lynch JP, Weg JG. Depression of cardiac output is a mechanism of shunt reduction in the therapy of acute respiratory failure. Chest 1980;77:636–42.

128 Cheatham ML, Nelson LD, Chang MC et al. Right ventricular end-diastolic volume index as a predictor of preload status in patients on positive end-expiratory pressure. Crit Care Med 1998;26:1801–6.

129 Poelaert JI, Visser CA, Everaert JA et al. Acute hemodynamic changes of pressure-controlled inverse ratio ventilation in the adult respiratory distress syndrome. A transesophageal echocardiographic and Doppler study. Chest 1993;104:214–19.

130 Abraham E, Yoshihara G. Cardiorespiratory effects of pressure controlled inverse ratio ventilation in severe respiratory failure. Chest 1989;96:1356–9.

131 Lessard MR, Guerot E, Lorino H et al. Effects of pressure-controlled with different I:E ratios versus volume- controlled ventilation on respiratory mechanics, gas exchange, and hemodynamics in patients with adult respiratory distress syndrome. Anesthesiology 1994;80:983–91.

132 Matamis D, Lemaire F, Harf A et al. Redistribution of pulmonary blood flow induced by positive end-expiratory pressure and dopamine infusion in acute respiratory failure. Am Rev Respir Dis 1984;129:39–44.

133 Radermacher P, Santak B, Wust HJ et al. Prostacyclin for the treatment of pulmonary hypertension in the adult respiratory distress syndrome: effects on pulmonary capillary pressure and ventilation-perfusion distributions. Anesthesiology 1990;72:238–44.

134 Radermacher P, Santak B, Becker H et al. Prostaglandin E1 and nitroglycerin reduce pulmonary capillary pressure but worsen ventilation-perfusion distributions in patients with adult respiratory distress syndrome. Anesthesiology 1989;70:601–6.

135 Thompson JS, Kavanagh BP, Pearl RG. Nitroglycerin does not alter pulmonary vascular permeability in isolated rabbit lungs. Anesth Analg 1997;84:359–62.

136 Melot C, Naeije R, Mols P et al. Pulmonary vascular tone improves pulmonary gas exchange in the adult respiratory distress syndrome. Am Rev Respir Dis 1987;136:1232–6.

137 West J, Dollery C, Naimark A. Distribution of blood flow in isolated lung: relation to vascular and alveolar pressures. J Appl Physiol 1964;19:713–24.

138 Beck KC, Rehder K. Differences in regional vascular conductances in isolated dog lungs. J Appl Physiol 1986;61:530–8.

139 Reed JH, Jr, Wood EH. Effect of body position on vertical distribution of pulmonary blood flow. *J Appl Physiol* 1970;**28**:303–11.

140 Hakim TS, Lisbona R, Dean GW. Gravity-independent inequality in pulmonary blood flow in humans. *J Appl Physiol* 1987;**63**:1114–21.

141 Glenny RW, Robertson HT. Fractal properties of pulmonary blood flow: characterization of spatial heterogeneity. *J Appl Physiol* 1990;**69**:532–45.

142 Pelletier N, Robinson NE, Kaiser L *et al.* Regional differences in endothelial function in horse lungs: possible role in blood flow distribution? *J Appl Physiol* 1998;**85**:537–42.

143 Nyren S, Mure M, Jacobsson H *et al.* Pulmonary perfusion is more uniform in the prone than in the supine position: scintigraphy in healthy humans. *J Appl Physiol* 1999;**86**:1135–41.

144 Jones AT, Hansell DM, Evans TW. Pulmonary perfusion in supine and prone positions: an electron-beam computed tomography study. *J Appl Physiol* 2001;**90**:1342–8.

145 Mure M, Lindahl SG. Prone position improves gas exchange – but how? *Acta Anaesthesiol Scand* 2001;**45**:150–9.

146 Sinclair SE, Albert RK. Altering ventilation-perfusion relationships in ventilated patients with acute lung injury. *Intensive Care Med* 1997;**23**:942–50.

147 Lamm WJ, Graham MM, Albert RK. Mechanism by which the prone position improves oxygenation in acute lung injury. *Am J Respir Crit Care Med* 1994;**150**:184–93.

148 Piehl MA, Brown RS. Use of extreme position changes in acute respiratory failure. *Crit Care Med* 1976;**4**:13–14.

149 Langer M, Mascheroni D, Marcolin R *et al.* The prone position in ARDS patients. A clinical study. *Chest* 1988;**94**:103–7.

150 Gattinoni L, Tognoni G, Pesenti A *et al.* Effect of prone positioning on the survival of patients with acute respiratory failure. *N Engl J Med* 2001;**345**:568–73.

151 Wiedemann HP, Gillis CN. Altered metabolic function of the pulmonary microcirculation. Early detection of lung injury and possible functional significance. *Crit Care Clin* 1986;**2**:497–509.

152 Pitt BR, Lister G. Interpretation of metabolic function of the lung. Influence of perfusion, kinetics, and injury. *Clin Chest Med* 1989;**10**:1–12.

153 Pitt BR. Metabolic functions of the lung and systemic vasoregulation. *Fed Proc* 1984;**43**:2574–7.

154 Gillis CN, Pitt BR, Wiedemann HP *et al.* Depressed prostaglandin E1 and 5-hydroxytryptamine removal in patients with adult respiratory distress syndrome. *Am Rev Respir Dis* 1986;**134**:739–44.

155 Orfanos SE, Langleben D, Khoury J *et al.* Pulmonary capillary endothelium-bound angiotensin-converting enzyme activity in humans. *Circulation* 1999;**99**:1593–9.

156 Orfanos SE, Armaganidis A, Glynos C *et al.* Pulmonary capillary endothelium-bound angiotensin-converting enzyme activity in acute lung injury. *Circulation* 2000;**102**:2011–18.

157 Wenz M, Hoffmann B, Bohlender J *et al.* Angiotensin II formation and endothelin clearance in ARDS patients in supine and prone positions. *Intensive Care Med* 2000;**26**:292–8.

158 Dupuis J, Stewart DJ, Cernacek P *et al.* Human pulmonary circulation is an important site for both clearance and production of endothelin-1. *Circulation* 1996;**94**:1578–84.

159 Druml W, Steltzer H, Waldhausl W *et al.* Endothelin-1 in adult respiratory distress syndrome. *Am Rev Respir Dis* 1993;**148**:1169–73.

160 Creamer K, McCloud L, Fisher L *et al.* Optimal positive end-expiratory pressure fails to preserve nonrespiratory lung function in acute lung injury. *Chest* 1999;**116**(Suppl 1): 16S–17S.

161 Ingbar DH. Mechanisms of repair and remodeling following acute lung injury. *Clin Chest Med* 2000;**21**:589–616.

162 Hert R, Albert RK. Sequelae of the adult respiratory distress syndrome. *Thorax* 1994;**49**:8–13.

163 Suntharalingam G, Regan K, Keogh BF *et al.* Influence of direct and indirect etiology on acute outcome and 6-month functional recovery in acute respiratory distress syndrome. *Crit Care Med* 2001;**29**:562–6.

164 Luhr O, Aardal S, Nathorst-Westfelt U *et al.* Pulmonary function in adult survivors of severe acute lung injury treated with inhaled nitric oxide. *Acta Anaesthesiol Scand* 1998;**42**:391–8.

165 Buchser E, Leuenberger P, Chiolero R *et al.* Reduced pulmonary capillary blood volume as a long-term sequel of ARDS. *Chest* 1985;**87**:608–11.

166 Elliott CG, Morris AH, Cengiz M. Pulmonary function and exercise gas exchange in survivors of adult respiratory distress syndrome. *Am Rev Respir Dis* 1981;**123**:492–5.

167 Klein JJ, van Haeringen JR, Sluiter HJ *et al.* Pulmonary function after recovery from the adult respiratory distress syndrome. *Chest* 1976;**69**:350–5.

168 Desai SR, Wells AU, Rubens MB *et al.* Acute respiratory distress syndrome: CT abnormalities at long-term follow-up. *Radiology* 1999;**210**:29–35.

169 Alberts WM, Priest GR, Moser KM. The outlook for survivors of ARDS. *Chest* 1983;**84**:272–4.

170 Elliott CG. Pulmonary sequelae in survivors of the adult respiratory distress syndrome. *Clin Chest Med* 1990;**11**: 789–800.

171 Ghio AJ, Elliott CG, Crapo RO *et al.* Impairment after adult respiratory distress syndrome. An evaluation based on American Thoracic Society recommendations. *Am Rev Respir Dis* 1989;**139**:1158–62.

172 Peters JI, Bell RC, Prihoda TJ *et al.* Clinical determinants of abnormalities in pulmonary functions in survivors of the adult respiratory distress syndrome. *Am Rev Respir Dis* 1989;**139**:1163–8.

173 McHugh LG, Milberg JA, Whitcomb ME *et al.* Recovery of function in survivors of the acute respiratory distress syndrome. *Am J Respir Crit Care Med* 1994;**150**:90–4.

174 Davidson TA, Caldwell ES, Curtis JR *et al.* Reduced quality of life in survivors of acute respiratory distress syndrome compared with critically ill control patients. *JAMA* 1999;**281**:354–60.

175 Parsons PE. Mediators and mechanisms of acute lung injury. *Clin Chest Med* 2000;**21**:467–76.

176 Thickett DR, Armstrong L, Christie SJ *et al.* Vascular endothelial growth factor may contribute to increased vascular permeability in acute respiratory distress syndrome. *Am J Respir Crit Care Med* 2001;**164**:1601–5.

177 Pittet JF, Griffiths MJ, Geiser T et al. TGF-beta is a critical mediator of acute lung injury. *J Clin Invest* 2001;**107**:1537–44.

178 Roupie E. Incidence of ARDS. *Intensive Care Med* 2000;**26**:816–17.

179 Malik AB, Lo SK. Thrombin-endothelial interactions: role in lung vascular permeability. *Mol Aspects Med* 1985;**8**:515–54.

180 Hallgren R, Samuelsson T, Modig J. Complement activation and increased alveolar-capillary permeability after major surgery and in adult respiratory distress syndrome. *Crit Care Med* 1987;**15**:189–93.

181 Bernard GR, Brigham KL. Pulmonary edema. Pathophysiologic mechanisms and new approaches to therapy. *Chest* 1986;**89**:594–600.

182 Matthay MA, Eschenbacher WL, Goetzl EJ. Elevated concentrations of leukotriene D4 in pulmonary edema fluid of patients with the adult respiratory distress syndrome. *J Clin Immunol* 1984;**4**:479–83.

183 Miotla JM, Jeffery PK, Hellewell PG. Platelet-activating factor plays a pivotal role in the induction of experimental lung injury. *Am J Respir Cell Mol Biol* 1998;**18**:197–204.

184 Malik AB, Johnson A, Tahamont MV. Mechanisms of lung vascular injury after intravascular coagulation. *Ann NY Acad Sci* 1982;**384**:213–34.

185 Tate RM, Repine JE. Neutrophils and the adult respiratory distress syndrome. *Am Rev Respir Dis* 1983;**128**:552–9.

186 Strieter RM, Kunkel SL. Acute lung injury: the role of cytokines in the elicitation of neutrophils. *J Invest Med* 1994;**42**:640–51.

187 Worthen GS, Haslett C, Rees AJ et al. Neutrophil-mediated pulmonary vascular injury. Synergistic effect of trace amounts of lipopolysaccharide and neutrophil stimuli on vascular permeability and neutrophil sequestration in the lung. *Am Rev Respir Dis* 1987;**136**:19–28.

188 Zhao X, Alexander JS, Zhang S et al. Redox regulation of endothelial barrier integrity. *Am J Physiol Lung Cell Mol Physiol* 2001;**281**:L879–86.

189 Lum H, Roebuck KA. Oxidant stress and endothelial cell dysfunction. *Am J Physiol Cell Physiol* 2001;**280**:C719–41.

190 van Griensven M, Stalp M, Seekamp A. Ischemia-reperfusion directly increases pulmonary endothelial permeability in vitro. *Shock* 1999;**11**:259–63.

191 Fisher AB, Dodia C, Ayene I et al. Ischemia-reperfusion injury to the lung. *Ann N Y Acad Sci* 1994;**723**:197–207.

23

Pharmacological management of the pulmonary circulation in critically ill patients

JEAN-LOUIS VINCENT

INTRODUCTION

Pulmonary hypertension is very common on the intensive care unit (ICU), and is the result of various pathophysiological mechanisms that include:

- Hypoxic pulmonary vasoconstriction (HPV). HPV, the key regulator of local blood flow, effectively shunts blood away from hypoventilated areas to those alveoli that are being ventilated, preventing non-oxygenated blood from entering the pulmonary veins. During regional hypoxia, HPV thus improves ventilation/perfusion matching. However, severe HPV, as can occur in various forms of lung disease resulting in generalized alveolar hypoxia, such as pulmonary edema, atelectasis, extended pneumonitis, and airway obstruction, can contribute to the pulmonary hypertension often seen in such disease processes.
- Inflammatory mediators. Many mediators have been implicated in the pathogenesis of the pulmonary hypertension associated with inflammatory processes such as sepsis and acute respiratory distress syndrome (ARDS), including thromboxane, endothelin, and platelet activating factor (PAF).[1,2]
- Physical compression. When severe, lung edema that causes compression or distortion of blood vessels can cause pulmonary hypertension by increasing pulmonary resistance.

Regardless of the underlying mechanism, when pulmonary artery pressures increase, a point is reached when the right ventricle (RV) can no longer maintain adequate output and it starts to fail. The impact of pulmonary artery hypertension (PAH) on RV function will depend on its severity and its speed of onset.[3] In mild PAH, the increase in RV afterload is associated with a decline in RV ejection fraction (RVEF) and with RV dilatation; these compensatory mechanisms (defined by the Frank–Starling relation) allow for RV stroke volume to be maintained. However, in severe PAH, or when RV contractility is reduced by other contributing factors, such as sepsis,[4] compensatory mechanisms become inadequate and stroke volume falls. Accordingly, it is important to separate RV dysfunction (stroke volume maintained) from failure (stroke volume limited) (Figure 23.1). Importantly, the distinction between RV dysfunction and RV failure can be revealed by a short-term inhalation of nitric oxide (NO): NO will decrease pulmonary artery pressures and RV afterload, which in turn will be expected to increase the RVEF in all cases, but will increase stroke volume only if it is limited by the pulmonary hemodynamic alterations. At least two studies have shown that inhaled NO in patients with acute respiratory distress syndrome can increase RVEF but does not usually increase stroke volume.[5,6] However, Bhorade et al.[7] noted that inhaled NO did increase stroke volume and cardiac output in their study involving 26 patients with acute right ventricular dysfunction associated with shock and respiratory failure. The reasons for these differences are likely related to the greater severity of the right heart dysfunction in the latter study.[7]

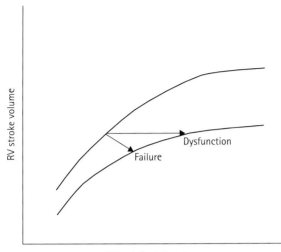

Figure 23.1 *Relationship between stroke volume and right ventricular (RV) end-diastolic volume in RV dysfunction (ventricular size increases but stroke volume is maintained so that only the ejection fraction falls) and in RV failure (both ejection fraction and stroke volume fall).*

Although RV failure is relatively rare, it is associated with high mortality. It is generally associated with conditions causing severe PAH, such as massive pulmonary embolism, or after cardiac surgery including heart transplant, mitral valve surgery, or repair of congenital heart disease. RV dysfunction is more common but less serious, and is most commonly due to inflammatory disease processes such as sepsis[8] and ARDS.

Treatment of PAH in the critically ill is essentially limited to those patients with associated RV failure. This chapter discusses the treatments currently available and the possibilities for future therapeutic strategies.

TREATMENT OF RV DYSFUNCTION/FAILURE

Various treatment strategies have been proposed for the treatment of RV failure in the setting of PAH. Most act to vasodilate the pulmonary circulation, thus reducing afterload to the right ventricle. However, the possibility of systemic vasodilation with resultant hypotension, particularly with agents used systemically, must be considered when using these drugs. The right ventricle is supplied by the right coronary artery, in which flow is dependent on the pressure gradient between the aorta and the right ventricle. Since RV pressures are generally lower than those in the left ventricle, RV perfusion takes place during both diastole and systole; as a consequence, even moderate degrees of arterial hypotension can be poorly tolerated. Thus, in some cases, the aortic pressure should be maintained at least at normal levels with

vasopressors to maintain hemodynamic stability and improve RV perfusion.[9]

The ideal agent is one that is selective for the pulmonary vasculature and reduces pulmonary artery pressure without affecting PaO_2. The available agents can be broadly divided into those that are administered systemically and those that can be given locally, i.e. by inhalation (see Chapter 13C).

Systemic agents

Several problems can arise with the administration of systemic vasodilators in the treatment of pulmonary hypertension, including arterial hypotension and alterations in gas exchange. The vasodilators used are typically non-selective and reduce vascular tone in all lung regions, including those that are poorly ventilated. As a result, all vasodilators can alter gas exchange. These effects can be counterbalanced in part by increases in cardiac output and mixed venous oxygen saturation (SvO_2). However, patients with compromised right ventricular function are likely to experience more severe side effects with systemic vasodilation.[10]

VASODILATORS

The principal vasodilating agents that can be administered systemically are as follows.

Nitrate compounds

Various nitrate compounds, including nitroglycerin, isosorbide dinitrate and sodium nitroprusside, have been used to treat pulmonary hypertension by vasodilating the pulmonary vasculature.[11–16] However, the degree of pulmonary vasodilation varies according to the agent used. Sodium nitroprusside is usually less effective than other nitrates because it decreases pulmonary vascular tone less and induces a proportionately greater decrease in aortic pressure.[13]

Prostacyclin (PGI_2) and prostaglandin (PG) E_1

These are very effective pulmonary vasodilators[17–19] that are, in part, metabolized in the lung vasculature,[20] so that their systemic effects are limited. These prostaglandins have additional properties that may be of benefit in patients with pulmonary hypertension, including their effects on platelet aggregation, leukocyte activation, and endothelin release.[21] However, they are more expensive than nitrates, so are usually reserved for patients who fail to respond adequately to nitrates.

PGE_1 is sometimes administered with vasopressor agents, such as norepinephrine, after cardiac surgery, to reduce RV afterload while maintaining RV perfusion.[22,23] In such cases, PGE_1 should be administered by the intravenous route and the vasopressor given through a left atrial catheter to increase the relative effects of the substances on their respective circuits. Prostacyclin has also been administered by inhalation with beneficial effects on pulmonary artery pressures (see below).

Hydralazine

Although hydralazine is no longer used for prolonged vasodilator therapy, the drug is very useful in acute conditions for two reasons: first, the increase in cardiac output is usually quite significant, as hydralazine can induce the release of norepinephrine from terminal nerves; and second, hydralazine alters gas exchange less than other vasodilators because the alterations in gas exchange in the lungs are compensated by a significant increase in SvO_2 secondary to the increase in cardiac output.[14] Hydralazine may also selectively increase renal blood flow.[24] The dose of hydralazine is 12.5–50 mg four to six times a day.

Calcium antagonists

Although calcium antagonists have been widely used in the prolonged treatment of chronic pulmonary hypertension, they are not commonly used in acute disease for several reasons.[25,26] First, they cause a significant reduction in arterial pressure. Second, their negative inotropic effects, although usually well tolerated, can be associated with complications in acute conditions. Third, they induce significant deterioration in gas exchange.

Angiotensin converting enzyme (ACE) inhibitors

ACE inhibitors are successful agents in the management of systemic hypertension and congestive cardiac failure. However, they are relatively ineffective in PAH,[27] and enalapril, the only commercially available intravenous preparation, induces significant systemic hypotension.

Adenosine

Adenosine is an endogenous nucleotide that plays an important physiological role in the maintenance of open vessels in the coronary circulation as well as in other regions. It has a short half-life of less than 10 seconds, as it is metabolized by adenosine deaminase. A key advantage of adenosine is that it is metabolized in the lungs, limiting its systemic effects. Adenosine reduces pulmonary artery pressure and pulmonary vascular resistance without increasing intrapulmonary shunt or reducing arterial PO_2.[28]

Other substances

Various other agents, including tolazoline,[29] urapidil,[30] serotonin antagonists[31] and potassium channel openers[21] have been used in the treatment of PAH, or are currently under investigation, as the search for the ideal pulmonary-specific vasodilator continues.

INOTROPIC AGENTS

As we have seen, an acute increase in pulmonary vascular resistance is often accompanied by a fall in cardiac output, and inotropes can be an important part of the management of these patients.

Isoproterenol and dobutamine

These agents can maintain cardiac output. β-Adrenergic stimulation can alter gas exchange by vasodilating effects on the pulmonary vasculature. Conversely, β-blocking agents increase PaO_2.[32] Dobutamine is usually preferred over isoproterenol as an inotropic agent, as it increases heart rate less, and therefore carries less risk of myocardial ischemia. However, isoproterenol can be a very useful drug in patients with relative bradycardia, typically after cardiac transplantation with cardiac denervation.

Phosphodiesterase (PDE) inhibitors

These agents combine vasodilating and inotropic properties, and have been called 'inodilating' agents. The most popular drugs in this group are milrinone and enoximone. Although the associated inotropic effects theoretically limit the hypotension, experience shows that this is not necessarily the case. A key limitation is the prolonged half-life of these drugs, making dose-titration difficult; if hypotension is induced, it may last for long periods. PDE inhibitors have been found to be particularly useful after cardiac surgery,[33,34] and enoximone has been used in combination with inhaled PGE_1 as prophylaxis against the development of right ventricular failure in children undergoing heart transplantation.[35]

Inhaled therapies

The use of inhaled agents can largely alleviate the two main shortcoming associated with systemic therapies:

- If the agent is delivered directly to the lungs and rapidly eliminated from there, the effects on systemic blood pressure will be negligible.
- If the agent is given by inhalation, it can reach only the open alveoli, and thus no alterations in gas exchange will occur.

Oxygen

Oxygen is at present the only selective pulmonary vasodilator available, and reduces pulmonary vascular resistance and increases cardiac index in patients with pulmonary hypertension.[36] Alveolar oxygen concentrations should thus be optimized in patients with pulmonary artery hypertension.

Inhaled nitric oxide (NO)

Inhaled NO is the most studied of these agents and has caused considerable excitement in this field. NO acts on vascular smooth muscle to cause vasodilation, and when given by inhalation it preferentially dilates the pulmonary vasculature and improves ventilation/perfusion matching.[37] Inhaled NO has been shown to reduce pulmonary artery pressures and improve oxygenation in various groups of patients, including those with ARDS, primary pulmonary hypertension, acute right heart syndrome, and post-cardiac surgery.[7,38–41] In addition, inhaled NO has been shown to improve RVEF,[5,6] although no consistent effects on cardiac output have been reported. In a study of 26 patients with acute right heart syndrome, Bhorade et al.[7] reported that inhaled NO, at a mean dose of 35 p.p.m., increased cardiac output, in contrast to many other studies where no effect on cardiac output has been noted.[5,6,42–45] These authors[7] suggested that these differences may have been due to their population of patients with demonstrated right ventricular failure, whereas other studies have included patients with lesser degrees of right ventricular dysfunction. However, while inhaled NO does appear to improve oxygenation and right ventricular function, it has not been shown to improve mortality,[46–48] and should be considered as a symptomatic treatment rather than a cure. In addition, the response to NO is very individual; only 50–60% of patients achieve an increase in PaO_2 following inhaled NO administration. Optimum dosing and timing schedules have also yet to be defined. Possible complications of inhaled NO therapy include the development of methemoglobinemia, which may be a problem in patients with reduced methemoglobin reductase activity,[49] nitrogen dioxide formation, and rebound hypoxemia or pulmonary hypertension, possibly related to altered endothelin levels,[50] if the drug is stopped abruptly.[51]

Aerosolized prostacyclin

Aerosolized prostacyclin causes selective pulmonary vasodilation; both prostacyclin and its analog, iloprost, have been shown to reduce mean pulmonary artery pressures and pulmonary vascular resistance in patients with PAH.[52–54] One study using sequential administrations of inhaled NO and iloprost in patients with primary pulmonary hypertension undergoing right heart catheterization has suggested that iloprost may be more effective than inhaled NO at acutely reducing pulmonary artery pressures and increasing cardiac output.[55]

KEY POINTS

- Pulmonary hypertension is common in the ICU, and treatment is not always necessary, being reserved for cases associated with right ventricular failure.
- Various drugs have been suggested and employed, but research continues to find the ideal agent that is selective for the pulmonary circulation, reducing pulmonary arterial pressures without reducing PaO_2.

- Inhaled therapies may be more effective than intravenous vasodilating therapy, but the systematic administration of these agents has not been shown to improve outcome.

REFERENCES

●1 Quinn JV, Slotman GJ. Platelet-activating factor and arachidonic acid metabolites mediate tumor necrosis factor and eicosanoid kinetics and cardiopulmonary dysfunction during bacteremic shock. Crit Care Med 1999;**27**:2485–94.

●2 Woolley DS, Puglisi RN, Quinn JV et al. Platelet activating factor mediates cardiopulmonary dysfunction during graded bacteremic shock. J Trauma 1996;**41**:291–6.

◆3 Chiche JD, Dhainaut JF. Inhaled nitric oxide for right ventricular dysfunction in chronic obstructive pulmonary disease patients: fall or rise of an idea? Crit Care Med 1999;**27**:2299–301.

◆4 Dhainaut JF, Lanore JJ, de Gournay JM et al. Right ventricular dysfunction in human septic shock. Prog Clin Biol Res 1988;**264**:343–8.

●5 Rossaint R, Slama K, Steudel W et al. Effects of inhaled nitric oxide on right ventricular function in severe acute respiratory distress syndrome. Intensive Care Med 1995;**21**:197–203.

●6 Fierobe L, Brunet F, Dhainaut JF et al. Effect of inhaled nitric oxide on right ventricular function in adult respiratory distress syndrome. Am J Respir Crit Care Med 1995;**151**:1414–19.

●7 Bhorade S, Christenson J, O'Connor M et al. Response to inhaled nitric oxide in patients with acute right heart syndrome. Am J Respir Crit Care Med 1999;**159**:571–9.

●8 Dhainaut JF, Pinsky MR, Nouria S et al. Right ventricular function in human sepsis: a thermodilution study. Chest 1997;**112**:1043–9.

◆9 Vincent JL. The measurement of right ventricular ejection fraction. Intensive Care World 1990;**7**:333–6.

●10 Weir EK, Rubin LJ, Ayres SM et al. The acute administration of vasodilators in primary pulmonary hypertension. Experience from the National Institutes of Health Registry on Primary Pulmonary Hypertension. Am Rev Respir Dis 1989;**140**:1623–30.

●11 Sibbald WJ, Short AI, Driedger AA et al. The immediate effects of isosorbide dinitrate on right ventricular function in patients with acute hypoxemic respiratory failure. A combined invasive and radionuclide study. Am Rev Respir Dis 1985;**131**:862–8.

●12 Pearl RG, Rosenthal MH, Schroeder JS et al. Acute hemodynamic effects of nitroglycerin in pulmonary hypertension. Ann Intern Med 1983;**99**:9–13.

●13 Pearl RG, Rosenthal MH, Ashton JP. Pulmonary vasodilator effects of nitroglycerin and sodium nitroprusside in canine oleic acid-induced pulmonary hypertension. Anesthesiology 1983;**58**:514–18.

●14 Brent BN, Berger HJ, Matthay RA et al. Contrasting acute effects of vasodilators (nitroglycerin, nitroprusside and hydralazine) on right ventricular performance in patients with chronic obstructive pulmonary disease and pulmonary hypertension: a combined radionuclide-hemodynamic study. Am J Cardiol 1983;**51**:1682–9.

◆15 Packer M, Halperin JL, Brooks KM et al. Nitroglycerin therapy in the management of pulmonary hypertensive disorders. Am J Med 1984;**76**:67–75.

●16 Rasch DK, Lancaster L. Successful use of nitroglycerin to treat postoperative pulmonary hypertension. Crit Care Med 1987;**15**:616–17.

◆17 Long WA, Rubin LJ. Prostacyclin and PGE1 treatment of pulmonary hypertension. Am Rev Respir Dis 1987;**136**:773–6.

●18 Prielipp RC, Rosenthal MH, Pearl RG. Hemodynamic profiles of prostaglandin E1, isoproterenol, prostacyclin, and nifedipine in vasoconstrictor pulmonary hypertension in sheep. Anesth Analg 1988;**67**:722–9.

●19 Prielipp RC, Rosenthal MH, Pearl RG. Vasodilator therapy in vasoconstrictor-induced pulmonary hypertension in sheep. Anesthesiology 1988;**68**:552–8.

◆20 Said SI. Pulmonary metabolism of prostaglandins and vasoactive peptides. Annu Rev Physiol 1982;**44**:257–68.

◆21 Strange JW, Wharton J, Phillips PG et al. Recent insights into the pathogenesis and therapeutics of pulmonary hypertension. Clin Sci (Lond) 2002;**102**:253–68.

●22 D'Ambra MN, LaRaia PJ, Philbin DM et al. Prostaglandin E1. A new therapy for refractory right heart failure and pulmonary hypertension after mitral valve replacement. J Thorac Cardiovasc Surg 1985;**89**:567–72.

●23 Vincent JL, Carlier E, Pinsky MR et al. Prostaglandin E1 infusion for right ventricular failure after cardiac transplantation. J Thorac Cardiovasc Surg 1992;**103**:33–9.

●24 Chelly JE, Doursout MF, Begaud B et al. Effects of hydralazine on regional blood flow in conscious dogs. J Pharmacol Exp Ther 1986;**238**:665–9.

◆25 Packer M. Therapeutic application of calcium-channel antagonists for pulmonary hypertension. Am J Cardiol 1985;**55**:196B–201B.

◆26 Neely CF, Stein R, Matot I et al. Calcium blockage in pulmonary hypertension and hypoxic vasoconstriction. New Horiz 1996;**4**:99–106.

●27 Zielinski J, Hawrylkiewicz I, Gorecka D et al. Captopril effects on pulmonary and systemic hemodynamics in chronic cor pulmonale. Chest 1986;**90**:562–5.

●28 Fullerton DA, Jones SD, Grover FL et al. Adenosine effectively controls pulmonary hypertension after cardiac operations. Ann Thorac Surg 1996;**61**:1118–23.

●29 Schranz D, Zepp F, Iversen S et al. Effects of tolazoline and prostacyclin on pulmonary hypertension in infants after cardiac surgery. Crit Care Med 1992;**20**:1243–9.

●30 Adnot S, Defouilloy C, Brun-Buisson C et al. Hemodynamic effects of urapidil in patients with pulmonary hypertension. A comparative study with hydralazine. Am Rev Respir Dis 1987;**135**:288–93.

●31 Domenighetti G, Leuenberger P, Feihl F. Haemodynamic effects of ketanserin either alone or with oxygen in COPD patients with secondary pulmonary hypertension. Monaldi Arch Chest Dis 1997;**52**:429–33.

◆32 Vincent JL, Berre J. Beta-blocking agents can increase PaO_2. Crit Care Med 1998;**26**:1613.

●33 Robinson BW, Gelband H, Mas MS. Selective pulmonary and systemic vasodilator effects of amrinone in children: new therapeutic implications. J Am Coll Cardiol 1993;**21**:1461–5.

●34 Feneck RO, Sherry KM, Withington PS et al. Comparison of the hemodynamic effects of milrinone with dobutamine in patients after cardiac surgery. J Cardiothorac Vasc Anesth 2001;**15**:306–15.

●35 Bauer J, Dapper F, Demirakca S et al. Perioperative management of pulmonary hypertension after heart transplantation in childhood. J Heart Lung Transplant 1997;**16**:1238–47.

●36 Roberts DH, Lepore JJ, Maroo A et al. Oxygen therapy improves cardiac index and pulmonary vascular resistance in patients with pulmonary hypertension. Chest 2001;**120**:1547–55.

◆37 Steudel W, Hurford WE, Zapol WM. Inhaled nitric oxide: basic biology and clinical applications. Anesthesiology 1999;**91**:1090–121.

●38 Pepke-Zaba J, Higenbottam TW, Dinh-Xuan AT et al. Inhaled nitric oxide as a cause of selective pulmonary vasodilatation in pulmonary hypertension. Lancet 1991;**338**:1173–4.

●39 Rossaint R, Falke KJ, Lopez F et al. Inhaled nitric oxide for the adult respiratory distress syndrome. N Engl J Med 1993;**328**:399–405.

●40 Sitbon O, Brenot F, Denjean A et al. Inhaled nitric oxide as a screening vasodilator agent in primary pulmonary hypertension. A dose-response study and comparison with prostacyclin. Am J Respir Crit Care Med 1995;**151**:384–9.

●41 Beck JR, Mongero LB, Kroslowitz RM et al. Inhaled nitric oxide improves hemodynamics in patients with acute pulmonary hypertension after high-risk cardiac surgery. Perfusion 1999;**14**:37–42.

●42 Lowson SM, Rich GF, McArdle PA et al. The response to varying concentrations of inhaled nitric oxide in patients with acute respiratory distress syndrome. Anesth Analg 1996;**82**:574–81.

●43 Bigatello LM, Hurford WE, Kacmarek RM et al. Prolonged inhalation of low concentrations of nitric oxide in patients with severe adult respiratory distress syndrome. Effects on pulmonary hemodynamics and oxygenation. Anesthesiology 1994;**80**:761–70.

●44 Walmrath D, Schneider T, Schermuly R et al. Direct comparison of inhaled nitric oxide and aerosolized prostacyclin in acute respiratory distress syndrome. Am J Respir Crit Care Med 1996;**153**:991–6.

●45 Rossaint R, Gerlach H, Schmidt Ruhnke H et al. Efficacy of inhaled nitric oxide in patients with severe ARDS. Chest 1995;**107**:1107–15.

●46 Dellinger RP, Zimmerman JL, Taylor RW et al. The Inhaled Nitric Oxide in ARDS Group. Effets of inhaled nitric oxide in patients with acute respiratory distress syndrome: results of a randomized phase II trial. Crit Care Med 1998;**26**:15–23.

●47 Lundin S, Mang H, Smithies M et al. Inhalation of nitric oxide in acute lung injury: results of a European multicentre study. The European Study Group of Inhaled Nitric Oxide. Intensive Care Med 1999;**25**:911–19.

◆48 Sokol J, Jacobs SE, Bohn D. Inhaled nitric oxide for acute hypoxemic respiratory failure in children and adults. Cochrane Database Syst Rev 2000;CD002787.

◆49 Jindal N, Dellinger RP. Inhalation of nitric oxide in acute respiratory distress syndrome. J Lab Clin Med 2000;**136**:21–8.

●50 Pearl JM, Nelson DP, Raake JL et al. Inhaled nitric oxide increases endothelin-1 levels: a potential cause of rebound pulmonary hypertension. Crit Care Med 2002;**30**:89–93.

●51 Lavoie A, Hall JB, Olson DM et al. Life-threatening effects of discontinuing inhaled nitric oxide in severe respiratory failure. Am J Respir Crit Care Med 1996;**153**:1985–7.

●52 Haraldsson A, Kieler-Jensen N, Ricksten SE. Inhaled prostacyclin for treatment of pulmonary hypertension after cardiac surgery or heart transplantation: a pharmacodynamic study. *J Cardiothorac Vasc Anesth* 1996;**10**:864–8.

●53 Olschewski H, Walmrath D, Schermuly R *et al.* Aerosolized prostacyclin and iloprost in severe pulmonary hypertension. *Ann Intern Med* 1996;**124**:820–4.

●54 Olschewski H, Ghofrani HA, Schmehl T *et al.* Inhaled iloprost to treat severe pulmonary hypertension. An uncontrolled trial. German PPH Study Group. *Ann Intern Med* 2000;**132**:435–43.

●55 Hoeper MM, Olschewski H, Ghofrani HA *et al.* A comparison of the acute hemodynamic effects of inhaled nitric oxide and aerosolized iloprost in primary pulmonary hypertension. German PPH study group. *J Am Coll Cardiol* 2000;**35**:176–82.

PART 8

Pulmonary circulation in special environments

24

High altitude, high-altitude pulmonary edema and the pulmonary circulation

MARCO MAGGIORINI AND PETER BÄRTSCH

INTRODUCTION

The physiological relevance of the Euler–Liljestrand reflex in healthy humans moving to altitude has not yet been fully understood. Mechanistically thinking, we could assume that moderately elevated pulmonary artery pressures (PAP) optimize oxygen delivery by recruiting ventilated but not blood-perfused lung areas. However, an excessive rise of PAP may harm and lead either to high-altitude pulmonary edema (HAPE),[1,2] an illness that can occur after rapid ascent without proper acclimatization, or within weeks or months to congestive right heart failure of high altitude, also named subacute mountain sickness.[3,4] This latter disease, which might more appropriately be termed 'cor pulmonale or acute right heart failure of high altitude', was first discovered in cattle in Colorado and named 'brisket disease'.[5] Brisket is the depending part of the neck where edema accumulates.

It is one of the most exciting and challenging goals to unravel the genetic basis of hypoxic pulmonary vasoconstriction (HPV) and its inter-individual variability. There is convincing evidence of a genetic basis in animals and humans. Excessive HPV and thus susceptibility to brisket disease has been bred out in Colorado cattle[6] and in Tibetans, the best-adapted human population to high altitude, HPV has virtually vanished.[7] Furthermore, in the Andes it was shown that susceptibility to HAPE runs in families.[8] This observation, if confirmed in a larger number, not only underlines the genetic basis of HPV but suggests also that hypoxic vasoconstriction of pulmonary arterioles may be a disadvantage when living at high altitude. In addition, it shows that HPV is not of vital importance since it appears to have vanished due to evolutionary adaptation to high altitude in Tibetans without deleterious consequences.

PULMONARY HYPERTENSION AT HIGH ALTITUDE

The physiological response of pulmonary circulation to hypobaric and normobaric hypoxia is to increase pulmonary arteriolar resistance. The magnitude of hypoxic pulmonary vasoconstriction is highly variable between humans. Sites of hypoxic pulmonary vasoconstriction are small pulmonary arterioles and veins of a diameter less than 900 μm, the veins accounting approximately for 20% of the total increase in pulmonary vascular resistance caused by hypoxia.[9,10] The structural differences at the site of hypoxic pulmonary vasoconstriction within humans appear to reflect a genetically determined and adaptive process.[7,11] This section discusses the different aspects of pulmonary circulation at altitude according to origin of the subjects.

Lowlanders

In healthy lowlanders at altitudes between 3800 and 4600 meters, invasively assessed resting mean PAP ranges between 15 and 35 mmHg (average 25 mmHg) and the

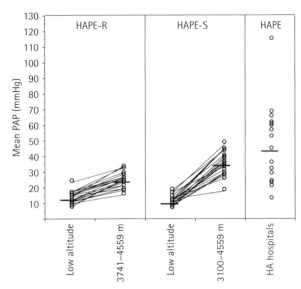

Figure 24.1 *The figure shows individual pulmonary artery pressure (PAP) values reported at low and approximately 24 hours after ascent at high altitude using a right heart catheter in high-altitude pulmonary edema resistant (HAPE-R)[12–14] and susceptible (HAPE-S) subjects[14,16] and mean PAP values reported in subjects with HAPE after hospital admission.[47,48,50,51] The figure illustrates that in 50% of the HAPE-susceptible subjects, mean PAP exceeds the 40 mmHg mark. The horizontal bars indicate median PAP value for each group of subjects.*

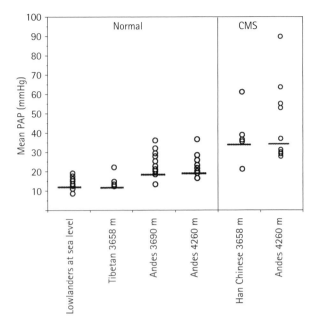

Figure 24.2 *The figure shows individual mean pulmonary artery pressure (PAP) values of sea-level residents and high-altitude residents (3500–4300 meters) in the Himalayas and in South America. The left panel shows the mean PAP values of healthy residents[7,18] and the right panel shows values of residents with chronic right heart failure of high altitude (CMS, chronic mountain sickness).[17,22] The horizontal bars indicate the median PAP value for each group of subjects.*

systolic PAP between 27 and 48 mmHg (average 37 mmHg)[12–14] (Figure 24.1). Mean PAP at altitudes above 5000 meters during exposure in a barochamber (Operation Everest II) in healthy and partially acclimatized volunteers was 24 mmHg at 6100 meters (barometric pressure 347 mmHg) and 34 mmHg at 7620 meters (282 mmHg). At both altitudes physical exercise significantly increased mean PAP to 41 and 54 mmHg, respectively.[15]

An abnormal increase in PAP is associated with life-threatening diseases in newcomers to high altitude. Individuals susceptible to HAPE had a mean PAP of 39 mmHg (range 22–47) at 3100 meters[16] and of 38 mmHg (31 and 51 mmHg) at an altitude of 4559 meters[14] (Figure 24.1). Indirect evidence of abnormally high PAP was reported after a prolonged stay at high altitude. Right heart failure associated with congestion has been described in infants of Han descent born at low altitude brought to reside in Lhasa[3] and Indian soldiers who failed to acclimatize at the extreme altitude of 5800–6700 meters.[4] This syndrome, which appears after an exposure of several weeks or months at high altitude, has been named infantile and adult subacute mountain sickness, respectively. Cases of severe pulmonary hypertension with chronic congestive right heart failure were described in immigrant Han populations after an average of 15 years of residence.[17]

High altitude populations

Mean resting PAP has been reported to be lowest in Tibetans compared to Han Chinese high-altitude residents and inhabitants of South and North America (Figure 24.2). At similar altitudes between 3658 and 3950 meters, mean PAP was on average 14 mmHg in Tibetans of Lhasa, 28 mmHg in Han Chinese residents of the Qinghai Province[7] and 20 mmHg among natives of South America.[18] In Leadville (CO, USA) mean PAP in 28 healthy men living at 3100 meters averaged 25 mmHg.[19] The absence of highly muscularized pulmonary arterioles in natives of Ladakh[20] and some, but not all, natives of the Andes[21] fits well with the data on PAP. All these findings indicate a genetic basis of hypoxic pulmonary vasoreactivity.

PAP may be increased in chronic mountain sickness (Figure 24.2). Pulmonary hemodynamic features of such patients were reported for a total of 16 natives of the Andes,[22] most of them examined at an altitude of 4300 meters, and five Han Chinese who developed the disease after having lived in Lhasa (3658 meters)[17] for a period between 11 and 36 years Mean PAP averaged 45 mmHg in South Americans and 40 mmHg in Han (Figure 24.2). Right atrial pressure, pulmonary artery occlusion pressure (wedge pressure) and cardiac output were within normal ranges in both groups of patients. Whether increased PAP is a cause or a consequence of the disease has not been established.

HIGH–ALTITUDE PULMONARY EDEMA

Epidemiology

There are two typical settings for HAPE, a condition that occurs within a few days of arrival at high altitude. The first setting involves high-altitude dwellers that return from a sojourn at low altitude[8,23,24] and the second involves unacclimatized lowlanders.[25] The first two publications suggesting that HAPE is a non-cardiogenic pulmonary edema were from Peru 1955 (re-entry HAPE) by Lizzarraga[23] and from the Rocky Mountains 1960 (unacclimatized lowlanders) by Houston.[25] Altitude, rate of ascent and, most importantly, individual susceptibility are the major determinants of HAPE in mountaineers and trekkers. The estimated incidence in visitors to ski resorts in the Rocky Mountains of Colorado is 0.01–0.1%.[26] The prevalence of HAPE is <0.2% in a general alpine mountaineering population when ascent occurs in three and more days to an altitude of 4559 meters.[27] When the same altitude is reached within 22 hours, the incidence increases to 7% in mountaineers without and to 62% in mountaineers with a history of radiographically documented HAPE.[28] The incidence of HAPE also increases from 2.5 to 15.5% when an altitude of 5500 m is reached by airlift[29] as opposed to trekking over 4–6 days.[30] Women may be less susceptible to HAPE than men.[27,31]

Signs and symptoms

HAPE presents within 2–5 days after arrival at high altitude.[29] It is rarely observed below altitudes of 2500–3000 meters and after 1 week of acclimatization at a particular altitude. In most cases, it is preceded by symptoms of acute mountain sickness (AMS). Early symptoms of HAPE include exertional dyspnea, cough and reduced exercise performance. As edema progresses, cough worsens and breathlessness at rest and sometimes orthopnea occur. Gurgling in the chest and pink frothy sputum indicate advanced cases.

Clinical examination reveals cyanosis, tachypnoea, tachycardia and elevated body temperature, which generally does not exceed 38.5°C. Crackles are discrete at the beginning, typically located over the middle lung fields. Often, there is a discrepancy between the minor findings at auscultation compared with the widespread disease on the chest radiograph. In advanced cases, signs of concomitant cerebral edema, such as ataxia and decreased levels of consciousness, are frequent findings.

Table 24.1 *Arterial blood gas analysis at an altitude of 4559 meters*

	PaO$_2$ (mmHg)	PaCO$_2$ (mmHg)	SaO$_2$ (%)
Controls (n = 22)	40 ± 5	30 ± 5	78 ± 7
HAPE (n = 4)	23 ± 3	28 ± 4	48 ± 8
P	<0.001	NS	<0.001

Mean values ± SD. PaCO$_2$/PaO$_2$, arterial partial pressure of CO_2/O_2; SaO$_2$, arterial oxygen saturation.

Laboratory evaluation

There are no characteristic findings in common laboratory examinations.[32] Abnormal results may be due to accompanying dehydration, stress and preceding exercise. Arterial blood gas measurements of four cases of advanced HAPE at 4559 meters demonstrate the severity of this illness[33] (Table 24.1). In early cases, values around 30 mmHg for PO$_2$ and 70% for SaO$_2$ are observed at this altitude. Chest radiographs and CT scans of early HAPE cases show a patchy, peripheral distribution of edema as shown in Figure 24.3.[34] The radiographic appearance of HAPE is more homogeneous and diffuse in advanced cases and during recovery.[35] Autopsies showed distended pulmonary arteries and diffuse pulmonary edema with bloody foamy fluid present in the airways but no evidence of left ventricular failure.[36]

Prevention

Slow ascent is the major measure of prevention that is effective even in susceptible individuals. Personal observations of nine ascents in seven mountaineers, who all developed HAPE more than once upon rapid ascent in the Alps, indicate that altitudes up to 7000 meters can be reached by these individuals without medical problems when the average daily ascent rate above 2000 meters does not exceed 350–400 m/day or with staged ascent. People should be advised not to ascend further with any symptoms of AMS or HAPE beginning and to avoid vigorous exercise during the first days of altitude exposure, since exercise-induced circulatory changes may enhance or cause pulmonary edema.[37] Furthermore, susceptibility to HAPE may be increased during and shortly after infection.[38]

Prophylaxis with nifedipine can be recommended for individuals with a history of unquestionable HAPE when slow ascent is not possible.[39] Sixty milligrams daily of a slow-release formulation should be given starting with the ascent and ending on the third or fourth day after arrival at the final altitude in the case of a prolonged stay or after returning to an altitude below 3000 meters, or to an altitude to which the individual is acclimatized. It should be emphasized that nifedipine helps to avoid HAPE and that it is not effective for preventing AMS.[40]

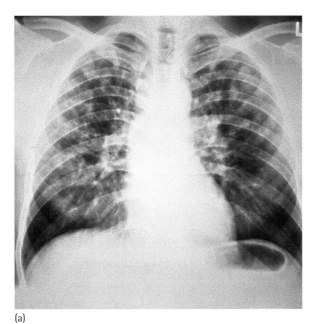

(a)

(b)

Figure 24.3 *(a) Radiograph of a female patient with high-altitude pulmonary edema (HAPE). Patchy infiltrates involve the right more than the left lung. (b) Computed tomography of the same patient shows the patchy distribution of the edema, which is predominantly located around the hilus of the right lung . (Illustrations by courtesy of Dr H Fischer, Regionalspital Visp, Switzerland.)*

Treatment

Immediate improvement of oxygenation is the treatment of choice. Specific recommendations on how to obtain this goal depend on where HAPE occurs. For the mountaineer in a remote area without medical care, descent has first priority, whereas the tourist with HAPE in a resort in the Rocky Mountains may stay at altitude if the arterial oxygen saturation can be kept above 90% with low-flow oxygen

(2–4 L/min) and monitoring by family or friends is guaranteed. Relief of symptoms is achieved within hours and complete clinical recovery usually occurs within 2–3 days. Although intermittent continuous positive end-expiratory airway pressure has been shown to improve SaO_2 in subjects with HAPE by 10–20%,[41,42] its use is not recommended because it may cause high-altitude cerebral edema (HACE) by decreasing venous return.[43]

When descent is impossible and supplemental oxygen is not available, portable hyperbaric chambers[44,45] and treatment with nifedipine (20 mg slow-release formulation every 6 hours) should be initiated until descent is possible. In mountaineers with HAPE at 4559 meters, persistent relief of symptoms, improvement of gas exchange and radiographical appearance were documented over 34 hours with 20 mg nifedipine every 6 hours.[46]

Pathophysiology of HAPE

PULMONARY ARTERY PRESSURE

Since the first hemodynamic measurements performed in patients with HAPE admitted to the hospital with HAPE, it has been shown that this condition is associated with elevated pulmonary artery pressure.[32,47–51] In a prospective hemodynamic evaluation of HAPE-susceptible subjects after rapid ascent to 4559 meters within 24 hours, it has been shown recently that mean PAP was elevated on average to 42 mmHg (range 36–51 mmHg) in those subjects who developed pulmonary edema during their stay at high altitude.[14] All these hemodynamic studies consistently show that in HAPE left atrial pressure, as assessed by occluded (or wedged) PAP, right atrial pressure and cardiac output are normal. Invasive hemodynamic evaluations at low and high altitude show that excessive reactivity of the pulmonary vessels is the mechanism leading to pulmonary hypertension of high altitude[12–14,16] (see Figure 24.1). In addition, the key role of elevated PAP in the pathogenesis of HAPE was demonstrated by the data showing that this condition is prevented or improved by the use of pulmonary vasodilators.[39,46,52]

The pathophysiological mechanism of high-altitude-associated pulmonary hypertension has been only incompletely understood. Inhibition of voltage-dependent potassium channels by PO_2 might be crucial.[53] However, other endothelium-based humoral mechanisms such as the synthesis of nitric oxide and endothelin may contribute to the mechanisms leading to excessive hypoxic pulmonary vasoconstriction.[54,55] The role of the autonomic nervous system in the initiation and progress of congestive heart failure in this particular setting remains to be determined.[56]

It should, however, be pointed out that not all subjects with high-altitude-associated pulmonary hypertension develop HAPE. About 40% of the HAPE-susceptible

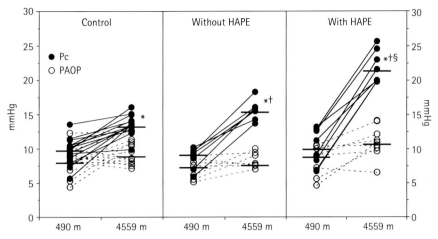

Figure 24.4 *Individual pulmonary capillary pressure (Pc, filled circles) and pulmonary artery occlusion pressure (PAOP, or wedge pressure, open circles), assessed using the arterial occlusion technique, in controls, high-altitude pulmonary edema (HAPE)-susceptible subjects without and with pulmonary edema.[14] The figure shows that in subjects who develop HAPE, Pc was higher than 19 mmHg, and that the increase in PAOP, though significant, is minimal.*

subjects do not redevelop HAPE after rapid ascent to 4559 meters.[57] Invasive hemodynamic measurements showed that PAP was on average lower in HAPE-susceptible subjects who did not develop HAPE than in those who did.[14] However, 10 young healthy adults with enhanced hypoxic pulmonary vasoreactivity following transient perinatal hypoxemia did not develop HAPE during an observation period of 72 hours after rapid ascent to 4559 meters despite an elevated systolic PAP pressure (62 mmHg; echocardiography).[58]

PULMONARY CAPILLARY PRESSURE

Using the arterial occlusion method, which is likely to measure pressures in vessels close to 100 μm in diameter,[59] it has been demonstrated recently that the pulmonary capillary pressure (Pc) is elevated in HAPE. Pc was, on average, 16 mmHg (range 14–18 mmHg) in HAPE-susceptible subjects without pulmonary edema and 22 mmHg (range 20–26 mmHg) in those who developed HAPE.[14] These results suggest that the Pc threshold value for edema formation in this setting is 20 mmHg (Figure 24.4). This is in keeping with previous experimental observations in dogs of a PO_2-independent critical capillary pressure of 17–24 mmHg, above which the lungs continuously gain weight.[60,61]

The question arises how increased arteriolar vasoconstriction causes an abnormal rise in capillary pressure in subjects susceptible to HAPE. The two most likely explanations are hypoxic constriction occurring at the level of the pulmonary veins[52] or inhomogeneous hypoxic vasoconstriction causing regional overperfusion of capillaries in areas with the least arterial vasoconstriction.[62] Since there is evidence that the small arterioles are the site of transvascular leakage in the presence of markedly

increased PAP in hypoxia[63] and that pulmonary veins contract in response to hypoxia,[64,65] increasing the resistance downstream of the region of fluid filtration,[66] inhomogeneous vasoconstriction is not mandatory to explain HAPE. Thus, alveolar flooding in subjects with HAPE is likely to result from elevated vascular pressures following excessive hypoxic constriction of the smallest pulmonary arterioles, veins or both. However, some element of regional heterogeneity of hypoxic pulmonary vasoconstriction (either at arterial and venous sites or both) is still necessary to explain the heterogeneity of regional edema, at least as we observe it on chest radiographs and CT scans.

There are data which suggest that in normoxia and hypoxia the increase in PAP during strenuous exercise is essentially related to the upstream transmission of increased left atrial pressure, with the increase in pulmonary vascular resistance being less important.[67,68] Furthermore, it has been reported that in HAPE-susceptible subjects PAP and PAOP increased more during exercise than in HAPE-resistant subjects.[37] This could be at least in part attributed to an impaired left ventricular filling, because of the dilation of the right ventricle and bulging of the septum to the left side.[69]

It has been suggested that pulmonary capillary hypertension may lead to increased hoop tension of the capillary wall, and hence stress failure of the blood/gas barrier.[70,71] However, the rapid regression of the leak after initiation of a vasodilator therapy[46] and the lack of an activation of the coagulation cascade in early HAPE[33] give some indirect evidence against this mechanisms in humans (Figure 24.5).

PERMEABILITY OF BLOOD/GAS BARRIER

Bronchoalveolar lavage (BAL) performed within a day after ascent to 4559 meters revealed elevated red blood cell

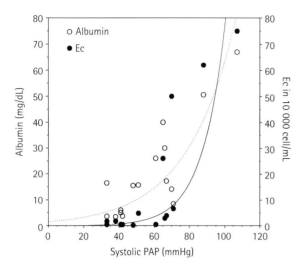

Figure 24.5 *Individual bronchoalveolar lavage (BAL) red blood cells (Ec) and albumin concentration plotted against systolic pulmonary artery pressure (PAP) at high altitude (4559 meters). The figure shows that the threshold systolic PAP for the appearance in the BAL fluid of albumin was 35 mmHg and the one for red blood cells >60 mmHg.[72]*

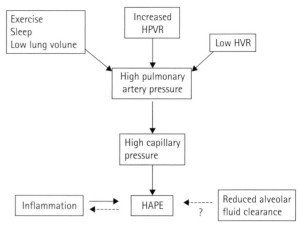

Figure 24.6 *The hallmark of the pathogenesis of high-altitude pulmonary edema (HAPE) is excessive hypoxic pulmonary vasoconstriction leading initially to an increased pulmonary capillary pressure. However, as shown in the figure, other factors may add to increase pulmonary capillary pressure or pulmonary capillary permeability. HPVR, hypoxic pulmonary vascular response; HVR, hypoxic ventilatory response.*

counts and serum derived protein concentration in their BAL fluid both in subjects with HAPE and in those who developed HAPE within the next 24 hours.[72] There was, however, no increase in alveolar macrophages and neutrophils, nor in the concentration of pro-inflammatory mediators [interleukin-1 (IL-1), tumor necrosis factor (TNF)-α, IL-8, thromboxane, prostaglandin E_2 and leukotriene B_4] at high altitude and there was no difference between HAPE-resistant and susceptible individuals. Interestingly, the albumin concentration and the number of red blood cells in the BAL fluid were significantly correlated with systolic PAP measured by echocardiography, the threshold for albumin being at a systolic PAP around 40 mmHg and for red blood cells around 60 mmHg (Figure 24.5). This fits well with the clinical observation of pink, frothy sputum in advanced HAPE.[29]

Analysis of BAL fluid of mountaineers with HAPE on Mount McKinley[73] and in hospitalized patients with HAPE[74] showed, however, in many but not all cases high concentrations of proteins, cytokines, leukotriene B_4 and increased granulocytes. Furthermore, urinary leukotriene E_4 excretion was increased in patients with HAPE reporting to clinics in the Rocky Mountains.[75] These observations suggest that in more advanced cases of HAPE, inflammation may occur and contribute to enhance the permeability of pulmonary capillaries.

In conclusion, all these recent results suggest that HAPE is initially a hydrostatic pulmonary edema, its pathophysiological mechanism being an excessive hypoxic pulmonary vasoconstriction of small arteries and veins, leading probably to an overdistension of the vessel wall, which opens intercellular junctions and possibly causes

stress failure of the alveolo-capillary membrane. Signs of inflammation found in the BAL fluid of patients with advanced HAPE are thus a secondary event, which may further add to increase the permeability of pulmonary capillaries, hence alveolar edema formation. Other non-hemodynamic factors that add to increase the risk for HAPE are discussed in the next section. The concept of the interaction of these various hemodynamic and non-hemodynamic elements is illustrated in Figure 24.6.

NON-HEMODYNAMIC RISK FACTORS

Behavioral and constitutional risk factors

Both a low hypoxic ventilatory drive, leading to increased pulmonary vasoconstriction,[76–78] and a smaller lung in relation to body size (decreased pulmonary vascular cross-sectional area)[79,80] are factors known to increase pulmonary artery pressure and hence susceptibility to HAPE. However, the considerable overlap for both factors between HAPE-susceptible and resistant individuals suggests that they are at best permissive but not compulsory regarding susceptibility to HAPE.

Congenital anomalies of the large pulmonary arteries[81,82] have been reported to be associated with an increased risk to develop HAPE at an altitude of about 2000 meters.

Increased permeability

It is conceivable that any process enhancing the permeability of the alveolar–capillary barrier would lower the pressure required for generating edema. Increased fluid accumulation during hypoxic exposure after priming by endotoxins or viruses in animals[83] and the association of preceding viral infections (predominantly of the upper

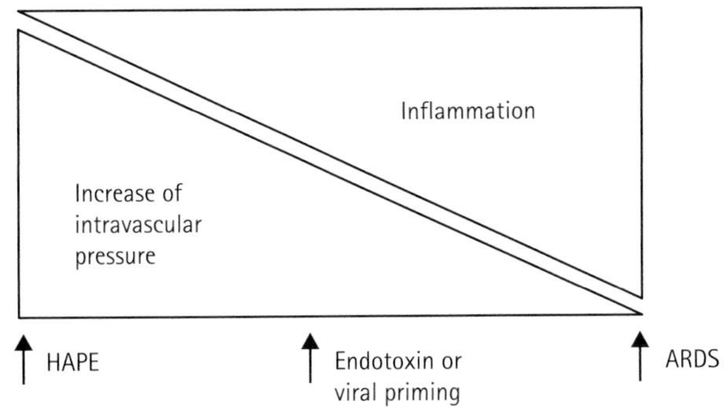

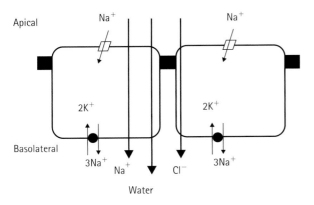

Figure 24.7 *Tentatively, the high pressure leak of pulmonary capillaries in high-altitude pulmonary edema (HAPE) contrasts with the inflammation-mediated low-pressure leak occurring in the acute respiratory distress syndrome (ARDS). It is conceivable that in some cases of HAPE, enhancement of capillary permeability by endotoxin or viral priming (systemic inflammation) lowers the pulmonary capillary pressure threshold for edema formation.*

Figure 24.8 *Alveolar epithelial apical and basolateral membrane ion channels and exchangers involved in active transepithelial sodium and water absorption. There is an active reabsorption of sodium; water and chloride follow passively. Acute hypoxia reduces alveolar fluid clearance by inhibition of apical sodium entry pathways and basolateral Na^+/K^+-ATPase activity. (Courtesy of H Mairbäurl.)*

respiratory tract) with HAPE in children visiting Colorado[38] support the concept shown in Figure 24.7. Under conditions of increased permeability, HAPE may also occur in individuals with normal hypoxic pulmonary vascular response.

Reduced fluid clearance from the alveolar space
Investigations obtained in cell cultures and animal models suggest that impairment of fluid clearance from the alveoli may be involved in the pathophysiology of HAPE. The water and sodium transport across type II pneumocytes is shown in Figure 24.8. Hypoxia decreases the transepithelial sodium transport[84] and accounts for decreased fluid clearance from the alveoli of hypoxic rats at an FIO_2 of

8%.[85] Mice partially deficient in the epithelial sodium channel show greater accumulation of lung water in hypoxia.[86] Transalveolar sodium transport can be stimulated by β_2-receptors.[85] Recently, it was reported that HAPE could be successfully prevented with the inhalation of salmeterol, a β_2-agonist.[87] Because of multiple actions of this drug, such as lowering pulmonary artery pressure, increasing ventilatory response to hypoxia and tightening cell-to-cell contacts, more specific drugs are needed for a precise evaluation of the role of alveolar fluid clearance from the alveoli for the pathophysiology of HAPE.

RIGHT HEART FAILURE OF HIGH ALTITUDE

Terminology

Carlos Monge and co-workers originally used the term 'subacute mountain sickness' to describe the persistence of headache, anorexia, nausea, dizziness and difficulty to sleep – usual symptoms of AMS – for weeks and months after arrival to high altitude.[88,89] Typically, in all these patients, mainly mining workers of the Peruvian Andes, physical findings suggesting elevated PAP, hence congestive right heart failure, were absent. Unfortunately, the name subacute mountain sickness was recently also used to describe the rapid development of congestive right heart failure which occurred within a few weeks or months after ascent to high altitude in Han infants and Indian soldiers.[3,4] In this chapter the name subacute mountains sickness is reserved for the description of the original syndrome published in 1937, and the term 'acute right heart failure of high altitude' is used to describe the syndrome described by Sui or Anand and co-workers. Accordingly, right heart failure in end-stage chronic mountain sickness disease has to be named 'chronic right heart failure of high altitude'. This chapter does not discuss the clinical aspects of Monge's disease, because pulmonary hypertension is only one key feature of this syndrome, excessive polycythemia, profound hypoxemia and mental deterioration being the others.

Epidemiology of acute right heart failure of high altitude

Acute right heart failure of high altitude occurred in 10–20% of Indian soldiers who were stationed at altitudes between 5800 and 6700 meters,[4] and was described in five infants and six children born in Leadville Colorado[90] and 15 infants in Lhasa.[3] The prevalence of acute right heart failure of high altitude in infants (age 3–16 months) and young children (age 4–6 years) is unknown. In Indian soldiers who acclimatized during 1 week at 3000 meters and 1–3 weeks at altitudes between 3000 and 4500 meters before arriving at their post at extreme altitude, symptoms of right heart failure developed between weeks 3 and 22, with an average of 11 weeks after arrival at high altitude. Symptoms disappeared at low altitude within a few weeks in all soldiers.

Clinical features of acute right heart failure of high altitude

Clinical features of pulmonary hypertension with acute right heart failure in infants, children and young adults were exertional dyspnea, orthopnea, cough, dependent edemas, even of the face, and oliguria. Additional symptoms were: effort angina in Indian soldiers and sleeplessness, irritability and cyanosis in infants in Lhasa. Clinical examination revealed tachypnea, tachycardia, stasis of the jugular veins, enlargement of the liver and ascites. All infants in Lhasa died. Autopsy revealed massive hypertrophy and dilatation of the right ventricle, dilatation of the pulmonary trunk, extreme medial hypertrophy of the muscular pulmonary arteries and muscularization of the pulmonary arterioles.[3]

In Indian soldiers, ECG showed right axis deviation and T-wave inversion V1 to V5–6. Signs of right ventricular hypertrophy were observed in 50% of the patients. Enlargement of the heart and prominent vascular pedicles but no pulmonary infiltrates were observed on chest radiographs. Echocardiography showed enlargement of the right ventricle and normal dimensions and ejection fraction of the left ventricle. Pericardial effusion was seen in 80% of the patients. There was no excessive polycythemia in these patients, who had a mean hemoglobin of 18 g/dL (range 14–23 g/dL) and a mean hematocrit of 61% (range 48–72%). At low altitude, symptoms of acute congestive right heart failure resolved completely without drugs within 12–16 weeks.[4]

Treatment of acute right heart failure of high altitude

There is no specific treatment for pulmonary hypertension of high altitude with or without congestive heart failure in addition to descent. The condition disappears after several weeks at sea level.[4] There are some data suggesting the use of pulmonary vasodilators. Acute testing of PAP reversibility at the altitude of La Paz was successful in 23 of 31 high-altitude residents with moderate to severe pulmonary hypertension without signs of right heart failure.[91] These results suggest that subjects with moderate to severe pulmonary hypertension of high altitude who respond to acute nifedipine testing could be candidates for long-term treatment with this vasodilator when return to low altitude is not possible. Whether this strategy affects outcome or improves symptoms related to pulmonary hypertension of high altitude remains to be determined.

Pathophysiology of acute right heart failure of high altitude

The pathophysiological mechanism of high-altitude-associated pulmonary hypertension leading to acute or chronic congestive heart failure in newcomers and residents of high altitude is incompletely understood. It is reasonable to assume that the initial stimulus leading to an excessive HPV may not differ from that associated with susceptibility to HAPE. The clinical findings of severe right heart failure, including ascites, and the considerable dilatation and hypertrophy of the right ventricle, without any evidence of left ventricular failure, clearly indicate that this condition is caused by an excessively elevated PAP at high altitude.[3,4] Pulmonary hemodynamics reported in Han Chinese who developed the condition after living in Lhasa for 11–36 years[17] strongly suggest that acute and chronic heart failure of high altitude share a common pathophysiological mechanism. Thus, it is conceivable that in an individual with abnormally increased hypoxic pulmonary vasoconstriction, rapid exposure to altitudes above 3500 meters may lead to HAPE, gradual ascent to and prolonged stay at extreme altitudes (>5000 meters) may lead to acute right heart failure and that residency between 3500 and 4000 meters for years leads to chronic right heart failure of high altitude. If the latter condition is associated with impaired mental function, excessive polycythemia (hematocrit >70%, hemoglobin >20 g/dL) and severe hypoxemia ($SaO_2 < 70\%$), the syndrome is named Monge's disease or chronic mountain sickness.[89]

Additional factors may also contribute to the development of right heart failure of high altitude. In Indian soldiers both with and without congestive heart failure, exposure to altitudes above 5800 meters increased total body water and sodium.[4,92] In the latter group, exposure to extreme altitude decreased the effective renal blood flow and increased plasma norepinephrine and aldosterone concentrations, while renin plasma activity did not change.[92] These findings suggest that activation of the neurohumoral system may contribute to edema and ascites formation in subjects susceptible to acute right heart failure of high altitude. Moreover, factors such as hypoventilation and impaired oxygen diffusion, because of subclinical pulmonary edema following elevated left ventricular endiastolic pressures (diastolic dysfunction), may also add to the pathogenesis of the disease. In Indian soldiers, polycythemia was moderate (average hemoglobin concentration <20 g/dL) and hence unlikely to be an important factor in this setting.

KEY POINTS

Pulmonary circulation at altitude

- Normal mean PAP in newcomers at altitudes between 3000 and 4500 meters ranges from 20 to 30 mmHg.
- Among high-altitude residents (altitudes between 3000 and 4000 meters), lowest mean PAP values were found in Tibetans (on average 14 mmHg) and highest values in Han Chinese in Tibet (on average 28 mmHg).
- Excessive hypoxic pulmonary vasoconstriction, leading to a mean PAP which mostly exceeds 40 mmHg, is the hallmark of maladaptation to high altitude in acute, prolonged and most likely also chronic exposure.

High-altitude pulmonary edema

- HAPE develops subjects within 2–5 days after acute exposure to high altitude. Typical symptoms and signs are: dyspnea at rest, incapacitating weakness, cough, tachycardia, hypoxemia and pulmonary crackles.
- A high recurrence rate in individuals with a history of HAPE indicates particular susceptibility of certain individuals for this disease.
- HAPE is caused by elevated pressures in leaky pulmonary arterioles ($\approx$100 μm) and capillaries as a consequence of an excessive hypoxic and presumably inhomogeneous constriction of small arteries or veins, or both.
- In early HAPE edema fluid is rich in albumin and contains red blood cells but there are no markers of an inflammatory response. Markers of inflammation are found in edema fluid of advanced HAPE, indicating that inflammation is a secondary event in more severe cases and is likely to enhance the leak.
- Additional factors such as exhaustive physical exercise, hypoxia-induced neurohumoral activation, impaired transepithelial sodium transport and viral infections may contribute to the development of HAPE.
- Pulmonary vasodilators, such as calcium channel blockers, are the drug of choice for prevention and treatment of HAPE.

Right heart failure of high altitude

- Right heart failure of high altitude following pulmonary hypertension develops either within weeks after acute exposure to altitudes >5800 meters, or after years of residency at high altitude.
- Clinical features are dependent edemas, stasis of the jugular veins and enlargement of the liver and ascites. Polycythemia, low oxygen saturation and mental dysfunction are the hallmarks of Monge's disease.
- Both acute and chronic right heart failure resolve completely once patients are brought to altitudes below 1000 meters.
- Treatments with pulmonary vasodilators have not been evaluated for treatment or prevention of congestive heart failure with prolonged exposure.

REFERENCES

◆1 Bärtsch P. High altitude pulmonary edema. *Med Sci Sports Exercise* 1999;**31**(Suppl 1):S23–7.
◆2 Schoene RB, Swenson ER, Hultgren HN. High altitude pulmonary edema. In: Hornbein TF, Schoene RB (eds), *High altitude – an exploration of human adaptation*. New York: Marcel Dekker, 2001;vol. 161:777–814.
●3 Sui GJ, Liu YH, Cheng XS *et al*. Subacute infantile mountain sickness. *J Pathol* 1988;**155**:161–70.
●4 Anand IS, Malhotra RM, Chandrashekhar Y *et al*. Adult subacute mountain sickness – a syndrome of congestive heart failure in man at very high altitude. *Lancet* 1990;**335**:561–5.
●5 Hecht HH, Kuida H, Lange RL *et al*. Brisket disease. *Am J Med* 1962;**32**:171–83.
6 Fagan KA, Weil JV. Potential genetic contributions to control of the pulmonary circulation and ventilation at high altitude. *High Alt Med Biol* 2001;**2**:165–71.
●7 Groves BM, Droma T, Sutton JR *et al*. Minimal hypoxic pulmonary hypertension in normal Tibetans at 3,658 m. *J Appl Physiol* 1993;**74**:312–18.
●8 Hultgren HN, Marticorena EA. High altitude pulmonary edema. Epidemiologic observations in Peru. *Chest* 1978;**74**:372–6.
9 Hakim TS, Michel RP, Minami H *et al*. Site of pulmonary hypoxic vasoconstriction studied with arterial and venous occlusion. *J Appl Physiol* 1983;**54**:1298–302.
10 Audi SH, Dawson CA, Rickaby DA *et al*. Localization of the sites of pulmonary vasomotion by use of arterial and venous occlusion. *J Appl Physiol* 1991;**70**:2126–36.
◆11 Moore LG. Human genetic adaptation to high altitude. *High Alt Med Biol* 2001;**2**:257–79.
●12 Kronenberg RG, Safar P, Wright F *et al*. Pulmonary artery pressure and alveolar gas exchange in men during acclimatization to 12,470 ft. *J Clin Invest* 1971;**50**:827–37.
13 Vogel JHK, Goss GE, Mori M *et al*. Pulmonary circulation in normal man with acute exposure to high altitude (14,260 feet). *Circulation* 1966;**43**(Suppl III):III-233.
●14 Maggiorini M, Mélot C, Pierre S *et al*. High altitude pulmonary edema is initially caused by an increase in capillary pressure. *Circulation* 2001;**103**:2078–83.

●15 Groves BM, Reeves JT, Sutton JR et al. Operation Everest II: elevated high altitude pulmonary resistance unresponsive to oxygen. J Appl Physiol 1987;63:521–30.

●16 Hultgren HN, Grover RF, Hartley LH. Abnormal circulatory responses to high altitude in subjects with a previous history of high-altitude pulmonary edema. Circulation 1971;44:759–70.

●17 Pei SX, Chen X J, Si Ren BZ et al. Chronic mountain sickness in Tibet. Q J Med 1989;71:555–74.

●18 Hultgren HN, Kelly J, Miller H. Pulmonary circulation in acclimatized mean at high altitude. J Appl Physiol 1965;20:233–8.

19 Vogel J, Weaver W, Rose R et al. Pulmonary hypetension on exertion in normal man living at 10,150 feet (Leadville Colorado). Med Thorac 1962;19:461–77.

●20 Gupta ML, Rao KS, Anand IS et al. Lack of smooth muscle in the small pulmonary arteries of the native Ladakhi. Is the Himalayan highlander adapted? Am Rev Respir Dis 1992;145:1201–4.

●21 Wagenvoort CA, Wagenvoort N. Hypoxic pulmonary vascular lesions in man at high altitude and in patients with chronic respiratory disease. Pathol Microbiol (Basel) 1973;39:276–82.

◆22 Hultgren H. Chronic mountain sickness. In: Hultgren H (ed.), High altitude medicine. San Francisco: Hultgren Publications, 1997;348–67.

●23 Lizzarraga L. Soroche agudo: edema agudo del pulmon. An Fac Med Univ Nac Mayor San Marcos de Lima Peru 1955;38:244–74.

24 Scoggin CH, Hyers TM, Reeves JT et al. High-altitude pulmonary edema in the children and young adults of Leadville, Colorado. N Engl J Med 1977;297:1269–72.

●25 Houston CS. Acute pulmonary edema of high altitude. N Engl J Med 1960;263:478–80.

26 Sophocles AM, Jr. High-altitude pulmonary edema in Vail, Colorado, 1975–1982. West J Med 1986;144:569–73.

27 Hochstrasser J, Nanzer A, Oelz O. Altitude edema in the Swiss Alps. Observations on the incidence and clinical course in 50 patients 1980–1984. Schweiz Med Wochenschr 1986;116:866–73.

28 Bartsch P, Maggiorini M, Mairbaurl H et al. Pulmonary extravascular fluid accumulation in climbers. Lancet 2002;360:571.

29 Singh I, Roy SB. High altitude pulmonary edema: clinical, hemodynamic, and pathologic studies. In: Command UARAD (ed.), Biomedicine of high terrestrial elevation problems. Washington DC: 1969;108–20.

●30 Hackett PH, Rennie D, Levine HD. The incidence, importance, and prophylaxis of acute mountain sickness. Lancet 1976;2:1149–54.

31 Hultgren HN, Honigman B, Theis K et al. High-altitude pulmonary edema at a ski resort. West J Med 1996;164:222–7.

●32 Kobayashi T, Koyama S, Kubo K et al. Clinical features of patients with high altitude pulmonary edema in Japan. Chest 1987;92:814–21.

33 Bartsch P, Waber U, Haeberli A et al. Enhanced fibrin formation in high-altitude pulmonary edema. J Appl Physiol 1987;63:752–7.

●34 Vock P, Fretz C, Franciolli M et al. High altitude pulmonary edema: findings at high altitude chest radiography and physical examination. Radiology 1989;170:661–6.

●35 Vock P, Brutsche MH, Nanzer A et al. Variable radiomorphologic data of high altitude pulmonary edema. Chest 1991;100:1306–11.

36 Nayak NC, Roy S, Narayanan TK. Pathologic features of altitude sickness. Am J Pathol 1964;45:381–91.

●37 Eldridge MW, Podolsky A, Richardson RS et al. Pulmonary hemodynamic response to exercise in subjects with prior high-altitude pulmonary edema. J Appl Physiol 1996;81:911–21.

38 Durmowicz AG, Noordeweir E, Nicholas R et al. Inflammatory processes may predispose children to high-altitude pulmonary edema. J Pediatr 1997;130:838–40.

*39 Bärtsch P, Maggiorini M, Ritter M et al. Prevention of high altitude pulmonary edema by nifedipine. N Engl J Med 1991;325:1284–9.

40 Hohenhaus E, Niroomand F, Görre S et al. Nifedipine does not prevent acute mountain sickness. Am J Respir Crit Care Med 1995;150:857–60.

41 Schoene RB, Roach RC, Hackett PH et al. High altitude pulmonary edema and exercise at 4,400 meters on Mount McKinley. Effect of expiratory positive airway pressure. Chest 1985;87:330–3.

42 Larson EB. Positive airway pressure for high-altitude pulmonary oedema. Lancet 1985;i:371–3.

43 Oelz O. High altitude cerebral oedema after positive airway pressure breathing at high altitude. Lancet 1983;ii:1148.

44 King JS, Greenlee RR. Successful use of the Gamow hyperbaric bag in the treatment of altitude illness at Mount Everest. J Wilderness Med 1990;i:193–202.

45 Taber RL. Protocols for the use of portable hyperbaric chamber for the treatment of high altitude disorders. J Wilderness Med 1990;1:181–92.

*46 Oelz O, Maggiorini M, Ritter M et al. Nifedipine for high altitude pulmonary oedema. Lancet 1989;ii:1241–4.

47 Antezana G, Leguia G, Guzman A. Hemodynamic study of high altitude pulmonary edema (12,000 ft). In: Brendel W, Zink R (eds), High altitude physiology and medicine. New York: Springer Verlag, 1982;232–41.

●48 Hultgren NH, Lopez CE, Lundberg E et al. Physiologic studies of pulmonary edema at high altitude. Circulation 1964;29:393–408.

49 Koitzumi T, Kawashima A, Kubo K et al. Radiographic and hemodynamic changes during recovery from high altitude pulmonary edema. Intern Med 1994;33:525–8.

50 Roy BS, Guleria JS, Khanna PK et al. Haemodynamic studies in high altitude pulmonary edema. Br Heart J 1969;31:52–8.

51 Penaloza D, Sime F. Circulatory dynamics during high altitude pulmonary edema. Am J Cardiol 1969;23:369–78.

52 Hackett PH, Roach RC, Hartig GS et al. The effect of vasodilators on pulmonary hemodynamics in high altitude pulmonary edema: a comparison. Int J Sports Med 1992;13(Suppl 1):S68–71.

●53 Weir EK, Archer SL. The mechanism of acute hypoxic pulmonary vasoconstriction: the tale of two channels. FASEB J 1995;9:183–9.

54 Duplain H, Sartori C, Lepori M et al. Exhaled nitric oxide in high-altitude pulmonary edema: role in the regulation of pulmonary vascular tone and evidence for a role against inflammation. Am J Respir Crit Care Med 2000;162:221–4.

55 Busch T, Bartsch P, Pappert D et al. Hypoxia decreases exhaled nitric oxide in mountaineers susceptible to

high-altitude pulmonary edema. *Am J Respir Crit Care Med* 2001;**163**:368–73.

56 Duplain H, Vollenweider L, Delabays A *et al.* Augmented sympathetic activation during short-term hypoxia and high-altitude exposure in subjects susceptible to high-altitude pulmonary edema. *Circulation* 1999;**99**:1713–18.

57 Bärtsch P, Vock P, Maggiorini M *et al.* Respiratory symptoms, radiographic and physiologic correlations at high altitude. In: Sutton JR, Coates G, Remmers JE (eds), *Hypoxia: the adaptation.* Philadelphia: BC Decker, 1990.

●58 Sartori C, Allemann Y, Trueb L *et al.* Augmented vasoreactivity in adult life associated with perinatal vascular insult. *Lancet* 1999;**353**:2205–7.

59 Hakim TS, Kelly S. Occlusion pressures vs. micropipette pressures in the pulmonary circulation. *J Appl Physiol* 1989;**67**:1277–85.

60 Homik LA, Bshouty Z, Light RB *et al.* Effect of alveolar hypoxia on pulmonary fluid filtration in *in situ* dog lungs. *J Appl Physiol* 1988;**65**:46–52.

61 Drake RE, Smith JH, Gabel JC. Estimation of the filtration coefficient in intact dog lungs. *Am J Physiol* 1980;**238**:H430–8.

62 Hultgren NH. High altitude pulmonary edema. In: Staub N (ed.), *Lung water and solute exchange.* New York: Marcel Dekker, 1978;437–64.

63 Whayne TF, Jr, Severinghaus JW. Experimental hypoxic pulmonary edema in the rat. *J Appl Physiol* 1968;**25**:729–32.

64 Raj JU, Chen P. Micropuncture measurement of microvascular pressures in isolated lamb lungs during hypoxia. *Circ Res* 1986;**59**:398–404.

65 Zhao Y, Packer CS, Rhoades RA. Pulmonary vein contracts in response to hypoxia. *Am J Physiol* 1993;**265**(1 Pt 1):L87–92.

●66 Mitzner W, Sylvester JT. Hypoxic vasoconstriction and fluid filtration in pig lungs. *J Appl Physiol* 1981;**51**:1065–71.

67 Naeije R, Mélot C, Niset G *et al.* Improved arterial oxygenation by a pharmacological increase in chemo-sensitivity during hypoxic exercise in normal subjects. *J Appl Physiol* 1993;**78**:1666–71.

68 Reeves JT, Dempsey JA, Grover RF. Pulmonary circulation during exercise. In: Weir EK, Reeves JT (eds), *Pulmonary vascular physiology and pathophysiology.* New York: Marcel Dekker, 1989;107–33.

69 Ritter M, Jenni R, Maggiorini M *et al.* Abnormal left ventricular diastolic filling patterns in acute hypoxic pulmonary hypertension at high altitude. *Am J Noninvas Cardiol* 1993;**7**:33–8.

●70 West JB, Tsukimoto K, Mathieu-Costello O *et al.* Stress failure in pulmonary capillaries. *J Appl Physiol* 1991;**70**:1731–42.

71 West J, Colice G, Lee Y *et al.* Pathogenesis of high-altitude pulmonary oedema: direct evidence of stress failure of pulmonary capillaries. *Eur Respir J* 1995;**8**:523–9.

●72 Swenson S, Maggiorini M, Mongovin S *et al.* High altitude pulmonary edema is a non-inflammatory high permeability leak of the alveolar-capillary barrier. *JAMA* 2002;**287**:2226–35.

●73 Schoene RB, Swenson ER, Pizzo CJ *et al.* The lung at high altitude: bronchoalveolar lavage in acute mountain sickness and pulmonary edema. *J Appl Physiol* 1988;**64**:2605–13.

●74 Kubo K, Hanaoka M, Yamaguchi S *et al.* Cytokines in bronchoalveolar lavage fluid in patients with high altitude

pulmonary edema at moderate altitude in Japan. *Thorax* 1996;**51**:739–42.

75 Kaminsky DA, Jones K, Schoene RB *et al.* Urinary leukotriene E4 levels in high-altitude pulmonary edema. A possible role for inflammation. *Chest* 1996;**110**:939–45.

●76 Hackett PH, Roach RC, Schoene RB *et al.* Abnormal control of ventilation in high-altitude pulmonary edema. *J Appl Physiol* 1988;**64**:1268–72.

●77 Matsuzawa Y, Fujimoto K, Kobayashi T *et al.* Blunted hypoxic ventilatory drive in subjects susceptible to high-altitude pulmonary edema. *J Appl Physiol* 1989;**66**:1152–7.

78 Hohenhaus E, Paul A, McCullough RE *et al.* Ventilatory and pulmonary vascular response to hypoxia and susceptibility to high altitude pulmonary oedema. *Eur Respir J* 1995;**8**:1825–33.

79 Viswanathan R, Jain SK, Subramanian S *et al.* Pulmonary edema of high altitude. II. Clinical, aerohemodynamic and biochemical studies in a group with history of pulmonary edema of high altitude. *Am Rev Respir Dis* 1969;**100**:334–49.

80 Podolsky A, Eldridge MW, Richardson RS *et al.* Exercise-induced VA/Q inequality in subjects with prior high-altitude pulmonary edema. *J Appl Physiol* 1996;**81**:922–32.

81 Fiorenzano G, Rastelli V, Greco V *et al.* Unilateral high-altitude pulmonary edema in a subject with right pulmonary artery hypoplasia. *Respiration* 1994;**61**:51–4.

●82 Hackett PH, Creagh CE, Grover RF *et al.* High altitude pulmonary edema in persons without the right pulmonary artery. *N Engl J Med* 1980;**302**:1070–3.

83 Carpenter TC, Reeves JT, Durmowicz AG. Viral respiratory infection increases susceptibility of young rats to hypoxia-induced pulmonary edema. *J Appl Physiol* 1998;**84**:1048–54.

84 Wodopia R, Ko HS, Billian J *et al.* Hypoxia decreases proteins involved in epithelial electrolyte transport in A549 cells and rat lung. *Am J Physiol Lung Cell Mol Physiol* 2000;**279**:L1110–19.

85 Vivona ML, Matthay M, Chabaud MB *et al.* Hypoxia reduces alveolar epithelial sodium and fluid transport in rats: reversal by beta-adrenergic agonist treatment. *Am J Respir Cell Mol Biol* 2001;**25**:554–61.

86 Scherrer U, Sartori C, Lepori M *et al.* High-altitude pulmonary edema: from exaggerated pulmonary hypertension to a defect in transepithelial sodium transport. *Adv Exp Med Biol* 1999;**474**:93–107.

●87 Sartori C, Allemann Y, Duplain H *et al.* Salmeterol for the prevention of high-altitude pulmonary edema. *N Engl J Med* 2002;**346**:1631–6.

88 Monge M, Monge C. Historical confirmation. In: *High altitude disease: mechanism and management.* Springfield, IL: CC Thomas, 1966.

●89 Monge C. High altitude disease. *Arch Intern Med* 1937;**59**:32–40.

90 Khoury GH, Hawes CR. Primary pulmonary hypertension in children living at high altitude. *J Pediatr* 1963;**62**:177–85.

∗91 Antezana AM, Antezana G, Aparicio O *et al.* Pulmonary hypertension in high-altitude chronic hypoxia: response to nifedipine. *Eur Respir J* 1998;**12**:1181–5.

92 Anand IS, Chandrashekhar Y, Rao SK *et al.* Body fluid compartments, renal blood flow, and hormones at 6,000 m in normal subjects. *J Appl Physiol* 1993;**74**:1234–9.

25

The pulmonary circulation in the underwater environment

STEPHEN J WATT

INTRODUCTION

During diving, the principal environmental change under water is a substantial increase in ambient pressure. This results in important physiological effects on ventilation, the handling of gases in tissues and the circulation. The distinction between disturbed physiology and a pathological result is blurred, but diving is associated with specific illnesses such as decompression sickness. The pulmonary circulation is important in enabling a return to normal environment after underwater exposure without pathological result protecting man from some adverse effects of pressure exposure. Knowledge of the role of the pulmonary circulation during diving is restricted by the difficulties of human investigation at pressure and we remain heavily dependent on animal data.

Diving techniques vary from the simple breath-hold diving at shallow depth, <30 msw (meters of seawater), carried out by snorkel divers or the pearl diving Ama of Korea, to deep saturation dives lasting several weeks now regularly conducted at depths of 350 msw.

Breath-hold diving is normally conducted from the surface but may be from a submerged air source such as the diving bell designed by Sir Edmund Halley in 1716. To remain under the water for more than a minute or two, a supply of breathing gas is necessary. This can be provided from the surface by hose or umbilical or from a cylinder containing compressed gas carried by the diver. The breathing apparatus may be a ventilated helmet, a demand valve system or a closed circuit rebreathing system. Whatever the technique, the diver is subject to the effects of pressure and the gas laws immediately on entering the water.

PHYSICAL PROPERTIES OF THE ENVIRONMENT

Under water, ambient hydrostatic pressure increases in a linear fashion by 1 atmosphere absolute (ATA) for every 10 meters increase in depth of seawater. Hence, in addition to being a measure of depth, meters of seawater (msw) may also be used as a unit of pressure. The scale of pressure change contrasts with changes on ascent to altitude, which are non-linear and where pressure reduces by only 0.5 ATA on ascent to 5500 meters.

The gas laws define the important physical concepts. Boyle's law states that 'for a fixed mass of gas at constant temperature the pressure is inversely proportional to the volume', i.e. a 1-liter balloon of gas at 1 ATA pressure (sea level) will contain 500 mL at 2 ATA, 250 mL at 4 ATA, etc. This has important implications for the gas-containing spaces within the body. Dalton's law states 'in a mixture of gases, the pressure exerted by one of the gases is the same as it would exert if it alone occupied the same volume'.

Hence the total pressure exerted by a gas mixture is the sum of the partial pressures of the constituents, e.g. in air at 1 ATA the pressure comprises the sum of partial pressures of approximately 0.79 ATA nitrogen and 0.21 ATA oxygen with minor contributions from other gases. Finally, Henry's law states that 'at constant temperature, the amount of gas which dissolves in a liquid, with which it is in contact, is proportional to the partial pressure of that gas'. A direct consequence is that the amount of nitrogen dissolved in body tissues at sea level relates to both the 0.79 ATA partial pressure of nitrogen in air and the solubility of nitrogen in body tissues. When a man breathing an air environment (79% nitrogen) is exposed to a change in pressure, the amount of nitrogen absorbed or released will relate to the change in total pressure.

Once under water, the pressure of gas in the lungs increases and more inert gas dissolves in body tissues. On ascent, pressure falls and this additional dissolved gas must be released gradually to prevent the formation of excessive gas bubbles, which place the diver at risk of decompression illness.

The important implications of diving for the pulmonary circulation relate to the following three main factors:

- hydrostatic pressure resulting from **immersion**;
- gas bubbles in tissue formed from dissolved gas which may result in **decompression illness**;
- exposure to high partial pressures of oxygen which may result in **pulmonary oxygen toxicity**.

IMMERSION

Immersion affects the circulation through three major mechanisms: hydrostatic pressure, temperature and the diving reflex. The effects of hydrostatic pressure have usually been studied in human subjects during immersion up to the neck (head out) in water. Immersed up to the neck in water, the pressure differential from neck to feet is approximately 150 cmH$_2$O in the upright position. This hydrostatic pressure forces blood from the lower extremities upwards and increases the intrathoracic blood volume and hence the pulmonary blood volume. During head-out immersion, Arborelius et al. observed rises in right atrial pressure and pulmonary arterial pressure of approximately 15 mmHg.[1] There was an associated 30% increase in cardiac output without any change in heart rate and calculated central blood volume increased by 700 mL.[1] Immersion reduces functional residual capacity and the engorgement of the pulmonary capillary circulation contributes to a reduction in lung volumes[2,3] and results in a degree of air trapping[4] demonstrated by an increase in closing volume. The increase in right atrial pressure results in diuresis. Immersion is frequently associated with cold and the resultant cutaneous vasoconstriction

also contributes to a shift of blood volume.[5] Cold, together with immersion, contribute to an acute rise in pulmonary blood volume which may result in acute pulmonary edema.[6] The cardiovascular effects of hydrostatic pressure and cold are modified by the diving reflex which is stimulated by immersion of the head or face in water[7] and is more marked in cold water.[7,8] It results in a bradycardia and some depression of myocardial contractility,[9] but the reflex is poorly developed in man compared with other diving mammals.

Ventilation/perfusion relationships are altered as the distribution of perfusion of the lung becomes more even during immersion.[1,10] However, gas exchange is impaired as a result of increased intrapulmonary shunt[11] and there is a reduction in diffusing capacity partly related to reduction in lung volume.[11]

The impact of these physiological effects on the free swimming diver is difficult to assess. The time course of effects on the pulmonary circulation is unclear as most studies have involved a stabilization period of 15–20 minutes of immersion and the immediate effects are variable.[1] The hydrostatic pressure differential between chest and legs varies as the diver may stand upright, swim horizontally or even head down, reversing the gradient. These rapid changes in differential hydrostatic pressure are likely to have marked effects on venous return and may be important in the pathogenesis of transient syncope under water as well as decompression illness.

PULMONARY EDEMA

Acute pulmonary edema may occur in divers[6,12] and is regarded as a rare but well recognized complication of diving. It frequently recurs with further dives and susceptible individuals are often hypertensive and may have an enhanced vasoconstrictor response to cold.[6] However, it may also occur in warm water or in divers using adequate thermal protection.[12] Pulmonary edema has also been reported in swimmers when working hard.[13]

Symptoms of cough, breathlessness and chest pain usually present during the dive and deteriorate until the dive ends, when hemoptysis may be observed. Since symptoms often lead to the dive being aborted and an unplanned or rapid ascent, the deterioration during ascent can readily be mistakenly attributed to decompression illness. Recovery after termination of the dive usually occurs over a short period but despite this, episodes are a serious threat to diver safety because symptoms of breathlessness are exacerbated by the use of breathing apparatus and increased gas density while in the water. Furthermore, if symptoms are attributed to pulmonary decompression illness, the problems of breathing apparatus and increased gas density may be imposed again during recompression treatment.

DECOMPRESSION ILLNESS

Decompression illness can be divided into two main types according to the pathological causation. Barotrauma is direct tissue injury associated with the change in volume of enclosed gas-containing spaces within or surrounding the body. The lungs represent an enclosed gas space when the mouth or glottis is closed or when a peripheral airway is obstructed; hence, in a breath-hold dive, the volume of the lung will reduce during descent and will increase again on ascent. A diver breathing a gas supply at ambient pressure maintains near-normal lung volumes. On ascent, gas within the lungs expands and must be exhaled or the lung may burst. Such episodes of pulmonary barotrauma may result from failure to breathe out on ascent or from a local pathological abnormality leading to gas trapping.[14,15] Air trapping resulting from increased pulmonary blood volume may be relevant to the pathogenesis of pulmonary barotrauma which has occasionally been reported after breath-hold dives.[16,17] Lung rupture occurs at alveolar level, and expanding extra-alveolar gas may track through the hilum to the mediastinum, rupture into the pleural cavity or burst into the pulmonary venous system. Both transpulmonary pressure gradient and differential pressure between the airways and the left atrium appear important factors in the development of air embolism.[18] In this situation, the pulmonary circulation provides a route for gas passing to the heart, resulting in cerebral air embolism.

Decompression sickness results in gas bubbles forming in body tissues from excess gas dissolved during prior exposure at higher pressure. The precise mechanisms causing the variety of clinical symptoms remain inadequately understood, but the pulmonary circulation is of considerable importance in one major mechanism.

The risk of decompression illness relates to the duration of exposure and depth (pressure) of the preceding dive or dives. Greater depth results in more inert gas dissolving in body tissues. Decompression procedures are based on dive depth and duration to take account of the inert gas load and are designed to provide a slow ascent in stages to permit excess gas to be expired. Originally these procedures were designed to avoid bubble formation, but the development of Doppler ultrasonic bubble detectors[19] has established that bubbles are formed during or after safe and symptom-free dives.[20–22] The amount of bubbles produced after a dive varies considerably both between and within individuals for reasons unknown but a bout of aerobic exercise before a dive has recently been shown to protect against both bubble formation and death from decompression illness in a rat model.[23] Many such factors may contribute to the unpredictable nature of decompression illness.

Bubbles form in many body tissues and may cause local pathology or pass through the peripheral venous system to the major veins and right heart.[24] Gas bubbles are not inert, the bubbles' surface is active and stimulates coagulation such that the bubble becomes a bubble/protein/platelet complex. As bubbles pass through the circulation, they have important effects on the endothelium which relate to the number of bubbles.[23] The number of bubble echoes seen increases with limited exertion such as a knee bend maneuver. Despite bubbles being readily detected in the right heart, very few are seen normally in the left heart or arterial circulation as the pulmonary circulation acts as a filter for bubble complexes and protects from arterial embolization. Clinical episodes of decompression sickness are associated with high bubble scores in the right heart[25] and with appearance of arterial or left heart bubbles.

The role of the pulmonary circulation in trapping venous gas emboli has been extensively studied in animal models. The pulmonary vasculature of dogs traps polystyrene microspheres injected into the pulmonary artery with increasing efficiency as the diameter increases, with only a small percentage of spheres greater than 8 μm reaching the arterial circulation. However, efficiency is affected by vasoactive drugs and by phase of respiration.[26] Bubbles formed during decompression of dogs have been found to range in size from 19 to 700 μm,[27] but, unlike microspheres, gas bubbles may deform in transit through vessels. Butler and Hills'[28] studies suggested that the threshold diameter for passage of bubbles through the lung must be less than 22 μm but also demonstrated that infused microbubbles of much larger diameter (up to 130 μm) would escape entrapment and appear in the systemic circulation following treatment with aminophylline. The same authors demonstrated a progressive elevation of pulmonary arterial pressure and pulmonary vascular resistance with continued air embolization and an apparent threshold effect for appearance of arterial bubbles at a pulmonary vascular pressure gradient of 34 mmHg.[29] This suggests that large volumes of gas bubbles can overload the circulation and open shunts for bubbles to access the systemic circulation. They also demonstrated that the appearance of arterial bubbles could be induced when pulmonary arterial pressure was elevated by diverting pulmonary blood flow from one lung to the other prior to air embolization.[30] However, in this case, the transit of bubbles may be related either to the pressure *per se* or to the increase in pulmonary blood volume in one lung.

These findings are consistent with the common clinical observation of transitory respiratory symptoms prior to the development of serious neurological decompression illness. Pulmonary decompression sickness, known as 'the chokes', is a rare but serious form of the disease associated with massive bubble formation which leads to cough, hemoptysis and dyspnea with clinical evidence of pulmonary edema. Such patients almost inevitably develop neurological abnormality and may progress to circulatory collapse.

The entrapment of bubbles within the pulmonary circulation may have long-term effects. Divers exposed to deep saturation dives have been shown to have abnormal lung function post-dive with reduced dynamic volumes and diffusing capacity.[31,32] These effects reverse slowly but some divers may sustain a permanent reduction in function. This has been attributed to both oxygen toxicity and to repeated episodes of microembolization during prolonged decompressions.[33] Significant reductions in diffusing capacity have been reported after single brief air dives,[34] but appear to be completely reversible.

Sustained experimental air embolism in sheep results in a large and sustained rise in pulmonary vascular resistance and pulmonary arterial pressure,[35] which is associated with increased vasoreactivity. Ultrastructural studies have shown that the air emboli attract clumps of neutrophils and damage the microvasculature by inducing gaps between endothelial cells with damage to the basement membrane and some associated edema.[36] This microvascular injury may be mediated by oxygen free radicals as it can be prevented by administration of catalase or superoxide dismutase.[37] One study has suggested that the abnormal lung function seen in saturation divers is a result of oxygen toxicity;[38] this does not explain all of the abnormality observed. In addition, in a recent deep dive, abnormal lung function appeared to be related to right heart bubble counts and the occurrence of decompression sickness.[39]

The recognition that cardiac shunts[40] and the presence of patent foramen ovale are a risk factor for neurological decompression sickness has cast further light on the role of the pulmonary circulation. Two studies[41,42] have demonstrated that the prevalence of patent foramen ovale is much greater in patients with neurological decompression sickness (approximately 65%) compared with the prevalence in the normal population or asymptomatic divers of 20–25%.[43–45] Patent foramen ovale can be demonstrated by contrast echocardiography using agitated normal saline to provide bubbles as contrast.[43] If passage of bubbles from right to left atrium cannot be seen after an initial injection, further injections following head-down tilt or Valsalva maneuver may provoke shunting across the foramen.[43] These maneuvers are frequently mimicked in diving by the changes in hydrostatic pressure and the need to equalize middle ear pressure on ascent.[46] The presence of patent foramen ovale may more than double a diver's risk of decompression illness.[47] The more widespread use of transesophageal echocardiography and also of transcranial Doppler examination of the cerebral arterial tree has expanded the understanding of this problem.[48] The appearance of contrast bubbles in the cerebral circulation after intravenous injection indicates the presence of right-to-left shunting. Echocardiography may confirm the presence of an intracardiac shunt, but where this is not detected, intrapulmonary shunt appears the likely explanation. This is consistent with Wilmshurst's investigation of explanatory factors for decompression illness in which abnormal lung function was commonly found in the absence of intracardiac shunt.[49] Investigation for the presence of right-to-left shunt is helpful in patients who have sustained neurological or cutaneous decompression illness to advise on the risk of future diving.

Factors that disturb the pulmonary circulation in a way that increases the risk of right to left intrapulmonary shunting are also likely to increase the risk of decompression illness. Asthma has previously been regarded as a significant potential risk factor for pulmonary barotrauma and hence a contraindication to diving. However, some asthmatics do dive and it has been difficult to prove this risk. One study[50] suggested that asthmatics do appear to have an increased risk of diving-related illness but not of barotrauma. This may reflect an increased risk of decompression sickness. Potential causes for venous bubbles reaching the arterial circulation in this situation include local disturbance of the pulmonary circulation with right-to-left shunt secondary to uneven ventilation, the possible distension of the pulmonary capillary bed secondary to increased negative transpulmonary pressure or the use of bronchodilators. Other pulmonary conditions may also carry an increased risk, for example, decompression sickness has been reported in association with a unilateral proximal occlusion of a pulmonary artery.[51] Smoking also appears to be a risk factor.[49]

OXYGEN TOXICITY

Diving normally involves exposure to breathing gas with an elevated partial pressure of oxygen. During a scuba dive to 50 msw breathing compressed air, the partial pressure of oxygen is 1.2 ATA. Short exposures at higher partial pressures occur during nitrox diving (up to 1.5 ATA), during decompression breathing oxygen (up to 2.5 ATA), and prolonged exposures at low pressure (0.4 ATA) occur during saturation diving. Oxygen exposure at relatively high dose (2–3 ATA) is part of the standard and effective therapy for decompression illness and is occasionally associated with minor symptoms of toxicity.

The pathogenesis of pulmonary oxygen toxicity has been extensively reviewed.[52] The pulmonary capillary endothelium appears the most sensitive tissue within the lung. This has been demonstrated both histologically[53,54] and by the use of biochemical markers of endothelial cell function in animal models.[55,56] Although there is some difference in species response to oxygen, histological studies from patients ventilated with high concentrations of oxygen suggest that the histological pattern of human oxygen toxicity is similar to that in animals.[57] Pulmonary oxygen toxicity has previously been assumed to have a threshold pressure for onset of 0.5 ATA,[58] but significant effects are observed below this pressure.[38,59] The pathological mechanism may not be the same at all pressures as animal data suggests that endothelial cell dysfunction may be less important at higher pressures.[60]

In the diving situation, acute pulmonary oxygen toxicity is characterized clinically by central chest discomfort and pain, cough and dyspnea. These symptoms reverse gradually over hours following exposure. Lung function tests have consistently demonstrated a reduction in vital capacity and of diffusing capacity.[52] Measurement of the pulmonary capillary blood volume and diffusing capacity of the alveolar membrane in volunteer studies[61] have indicated a reduction in pulmonary capillary blood volume, but more detailed information on the circulatory effects of developing oxygen toxicity is lacking.

The implications are perhaps most important because of the potential for interaction with other effects such as gas bubble injury to endothelium, water inhalation, pulmonary edema of immersion and the efficiency of the pulmonary vasculature to remove bubbles from the circulation.

CONCLUSIONS

During diving, the pulmonary circulation has an important role in preventing gas bubbles, produced in peripheral tissues, from gaining access to the arterial circulation, where they may generate the pathological sequence of decompression illness. Unfortunately, its ability to achieve this is readily compromised by other diving-induced insults such as the hydrostatic pressure of immersion, cold, oxygen exposure, water inhalation and transthoracic pressure. Knowledge of these effects and their interaction is valuable in the evaluation of diving casualties. Greater understanding of the formation of gas bubbles and the mechanisms that provide protection, principally the pulmonary circulation, might allow diving safety to be enhanced.

CASES

Patent foramen ovale

A 35-year-old diver conducted a single uneventful dive to 24 msw for 32 minutes. Five minutes after surfacing, she developed abdominal discomfort followed by paresthesiae of both legs distal to the thigh and both arms distal to the elbow. By the time of arrival at hospital, symptoms had improved spontaneously with only abdominal discomfort and tiredness persisting. All symptoms resolved during recompression therapy. Contrast echocardiography at a later date confirmed the presence of patent foramen ovale.

COMMENT

The early onset of neurological illness, which may be transient, after a non-provocative dive is strongly associated with right-to-left shunt.

Pulmonary edema

While diving to 23 msw, a diver noted inhalation of seawater spray from a leaking demand valve. During the ascent, chest tightness and breathlessness occurred. After surfacing, a pronounced cough with watery secretions persisted for almost 24 hours. A dive to 39 msw later the same day was uneventful until the ascent phase when breathlessness returned. Increasing distress with chest pain occurred during the staged ascent, ultimately necessitating assistance from the water. Cough recurred, with pink frothy sputum and hemoptysis. The patient was immediately taken to a recompression chamber where a diagnosis of pulmonary decompression illness was made. Recompression in a small chamber necessitated lying flat and breathing oxygen through a demand valve. This exacerbated symptoms, though some improvement occurred towards the end of the 5-hour treatment. On exit from the chamber, chest radiography in hospital confirmed bilateral alveolar edema, which resolved over the next 24 hours.

COMMENT

Seawater inhalation almost certainly induced significant alveolar injury and increased susceptibility to immersion-induced pulmonary edema. The rapid recovery despite ventilatory impediment is consistent with this diagnosis. Although inhalation injury might impair the pulmonary circulation's ability to filter bubbles, the absence of any other manifestations of decompression illness make this diagnosis unlikely.

KEY POINTS

- Under water, ambient hydrostatic pressure increases in a linear fashion by 1 atmosphere absolute (ATA) for every 10 meters increase in depth of seawater (msw).
- The important implications of diving for the pulmonary circulation relate to the following three main factors:
  - hydrostatic pressure resulting from **immersion**;
  - gas bubbles in tissue formed from dissolved gas, which may result in **decompression illness**;
  - exposure to high partial pressures of oxygen which may result in **pulmonary oxygen toxicity**.

- Immersion affects the circulation through three major mechanisms: hydrostatic pressure, temperature and the diving reflex.
- The prevalence of patent foramen ovale is much greater in patients with neurological decompression sickness (approximately 65%) compared with the prevalence in the normal population or asymptomatic divers of 20–25%.
- The pulmonary capillary endothelium appears the most sensitive tissue within the lung to oxygen toxicity.
- During diving, the pulmonary circulation has an important role in preventing gas bubbles, produced in peripheral tissues, from gaining access to the arterial circulation.

REFERENCES

1 Arborelius M, Balldin UI, Lilja B *et al.* Hemodynamic changes in man during immersion with the head above water. *Aerospace Med* 1972;**43**:592–8.

2 Prefaut C, Lupich E, Anthonisen NR. Human lung mechanics during water immersion. *J Appl Physiol* 1976;**40**:320–3.

3 Robertson CH, Engle CM, Bradley ME. Lung volumes in man immersed to the neck; dilution and plethysmographic techniques. *J Appl Physiol* 1978;**44**:679–82.

4 Lanphier EH, Rahn H. Alveolar gas exchange during breath-hold diving. *J Appl Physiol* 1963;**18**:471–7.

5 Glasser EM, Berridge FR. Effects of heat and cold on the distribution of blood within the human body. *Clin Sci* 1950;**9**:181–8.

6 Wilmshurst PT, Crowther A, Nuri M *et al.* Cold-induced pulmonary oedema in scuba divers and swimmers and subsequent development of hypertension. *Lancet* 1989;**i**:62–5.

7 Song SH, Lee WK, Chung YA *et al.* Mechanism of apneic bradycardia in man. *J Appl Physiol* 1969;**27**:323–7.

8 Sterba JA, Lundgren CEG. Diving bradycardia and breath-holding time in man. *Undersea Biomed Res* 1985;**12**:139–50.

9 Frey MAB, Kenney RA. Changes in left ventricular activity during apnoea and face immersion. *Undersea Biomed Res* 1977;**4**:27–37.

10 Lopez-Majano V, Data PG, Martignoni R *et al.* Pulmonary blood flow distribution in erect man in air and during breath-hold diving. *Aviat Space Environ Med* 1990;**61**:1107–15.

11 Lollgren H, Von Neiding G, Krekeler H *et al.* Respiratory gas exchange and lung perfusion in man during and after head-out water immersion. *Undersea Biomed Res* 1976;**3**:49–56.

12 Hampson NB, Dunford RG. Pulmonary oedema of scuba divers. *Undersea Hyperbaric Med* 1997;**24**:29–33.

13 Shupak A, Weiler R, Avell D *et al.* Pulmonary congestion induced by strenuous swimming: a field study. *Undersea Hyperbaric Med* 1998;**25**(Suppl):27.

14 Calder IM. Autopsy and experimental observations on factors leading to barotrauma in man. *Undersea Biomed Res* 1985;**12**:165–82.

15 Maklem H, Emhjellen S, Horgen O. Pulmonary barotrauma and arterial gas embolism caused by an emphysematous bulla in a scuba diver. *Aviat Space Environ Med* 1990;**61**:559–62.

16 Kol S, Weisz G, Melamed Y. Pulmonary barotrauma after a free dive – a possible mechanism. *Aviat Space Environ Med* 1993;**64**:236–7.

17 Bayne CG, Wurzbacher T. Can pulmonary barotrauma cause cerebral air embolism in a non-diver. *Chest* 1982;**81**:648–50.

18 Schaeffer KE, McNulty WP, Carey C *et al.* Mechanisms in development of interstitial emphysema and air embolism on decompression from depth. *J Appl Physiol* 1958;**13**:15–29.

•19 Smith KH, Spencer MP. Doppler indices of decompression sickness: their evaluation and use. *Aerospace Med* 1970;**41**:1396–400.

20 Masurel G, Gardette B, Comet M *et al.* Ultrasonic detection of circulating bubbles during Janus IV excursion dives at sea to 460 and 501 MSW. *Undersea Biomed Res* 1978;**5**(Suppl):29.

21 Brubakk AO, Petersen R, Grip A *et al.* Gas bubbles in the circulation of divers after ascending excursions from 300 to 250 MSW. *J Appl Physiol* 1986;**60**:45–51.

22 Spencer MP, Clarke HF. Precordial monitoring of pulmonary gas embolism and decompression bubbles. *Aerospace Med* 1972;**43**:762–7.

23 Nossum V, Koteng S, Brubakk AO. Endothelial damage by bubbles in the pulmonary artery of the pig. *Undersea Hyperbaric Med* 1999;**26**:1–8.

◆24 Nishi RY. Doppler and ultrasonic bubble detection. In: Bennett PB, Elliott DH (eds), *The physiology and medicine of diving*, 4th edn. London: WB Saunders, 1993;433–53.

25 Eatock BC. Correspondence between intravascular bubbles and symptoms of decompression sickness. *Undersea Biomed Res* 1984;**11**:326–9.

26 Ring GC, Blum AS, Kurbatov T *et al.* Size of microspheres passing through pulmonary circuit in the dog. *Am J Physiol* 1961;**200**:1191–6.

27 Hills BA, Butler BD. Size distribution of intravascular air emboli produced by decompression. *Undersea Biomed Res* 1981;**8**:163–70.

•28 Butler BD, Hills BA. The lung as a filter for microbubbles. *J Appl Physiol* 1979;**47**:537–43.

29 Butler BD, Hills BA. Transpulmonary passage of venous air emboli. *J Appl Physiol* 1985;**59**:543–7.

30 Butler BD, Katz J. Vascular pressures and passage of gas emboli through the pulmonary circulation. *Undersea Biomed Res* 1988;**15**:203–9.

31 Cotes JE, Davey IS, Reed JW *et al.* Respiratory effects of a single saturation dive to 300 meters. *Br J Ind Med* 1987;**44**:76–82.

32 Thorsen E, Hjelle J, Segedal K *et al.* Exercise tolerance and pulmonary gas exchange after deep saturation dives. *J Appl Physiol* 1990;**68**:1809–14.

33 Thorsen E, Segadal K, Myrseth E *et al.* Pulmonary mechanical function and diffusion capacity after deep saturation dives. *Br J Ind Med* 1990;**47**:242–7.

34 Dujic Z, Eterovic D, Denoble P *et al.* Effect of a single air dive on pulmonary diffusing capacity in professional divers. *J Appl Physiol* 1993;**74**:55–61.

35 Perkett EA, Brigham KL, Meyrick B. Continuous air embolization into sheep causes sustained pulmonary hypertension and increased pulmonary vasoactivity. *Am J Pathol* 1988;**132**:444–54.

36 Albertine KH, Weiner-Kronish JP, Koike K *et al.* Quantification of damage by air emboli to lung microvessels in anaesthetized sheep. *J Appl Physiol* 1984;**57**:1360–8.

37 Flick MR, Milligan SA, Hoeffel JM *et al.* Catalase prevents increased lung vascular permeability during air emboli in unanesthetized sheep. *J Appl Physiol* 1988;**64**:929–35.

38 Thorsen E, Segedal K, Reed J *et al. Effects of raised partial pressure of oxygen on pulmonary function in saturation diving.* Bergen: Norwegian Underwater Technology Centre, 1992.

39 Watt SJ, Ross JAS. Health and safety during Aurora 93. *Aurora 93 dive report.* Aberdeen: National Hyperbaric Centre Ltd, 1993.

40 Wilmshurst PT, Ellis BG, Jenkins BS. Paradoxical gas embolism in a scuba diver with an atrial septal defect. *Br Med J* 1986;**293**:1277.

•41 Moon RE, Camporesi EM, Kisslo JA. Patent foramen ovale and decompression sickness in divers. *Lancet* 1989;**i**:513–14.

•42 Wilmshurst PT, Byrne JC, Webb-Peploe MM. Relation between interatrial shunts and decompression sickness in divers. *Lancet* 1989;**2**:1302–6.

43 Lynch JJ, Schuchard GH, Gross CM *et al.* Prevalence of right-to left atrial shunting in a healthy population: detection by Valsalva maneuver contrast echocardiography. *Am J Cardiol* 1984;**53**:1478–80.

44 Hagen PT, Scholz DG, Edwards WD. Incidence and size of patent foramen ovale during the first 10 decades of life: an autopsy study of 965 normal hearts. *Mayo Clin Proc* 1984;**59**:17–20.

45 Cross SJ, Evans SA, Thomson LF *et al.* Safety of subaqua diving with a patent foramen ovale. *Br Med J* 1992;**304**:481–2.

46 Balestra C, Germonpre P, Marroni A. Intrathoracic pressure changes after Valsalva strain and other manoeuvres: implications for divers with patent foramen ovale. *Undersea Hyperbaric Med* 1998;**25**:171–4.

47 Bove AA. Risk of decompression sickness with patent foramen ovale. *Undersea Hyperbaric Med* 1998;**25**:175–8.

48 Glen S, Georgiadis D, Grosset DG *et al.* Transcranial doppler ultrasound in commercial air divers: a field study including cases with right to left shunting. *Undersea Hyperbaric Med* 1995;**22**:129–35.

49 Wilmshurst PT, Davidson C, O'Connell G *et al.* Role of cardiorespiratory abnormalities, smoking and dive characteristics in the manifestations of neurological decompression illness. *Clin Sci* 1994;**86**:297–303.

50 Corson KS, Dovenbarger JA, Moon RE *et al.* Risk assessment of asthma for decompression illness. *Undersea Biomed Res* 1991;**18**(Suppl):16–17.

51 Debatin JF, Moon RE, Spritzer CE *et al.* MRI of absent left pulmonary artery. *J Comput Assist Tomogr* 1992;**16**:641–5.

◆52 Clark JM. Oxygen toxicity. In: Bennett PB, Elliott DH (eds), *The physiology and medicine of diving*, 4th edn. London: WB Saunders, 1993;121–69.

53 Kistler GS, Caldwell PRB, Weibel ER. Development of fine ultra-structural damage to alveolar and capillary lung cells in oxygen poisoned rats. *J Cell Biol* 1967;**33**:605–28.

54 Crapo JD, Barry BE, Foscue HA *et al.* Structural and biochemical changes in rat lungs occurring during exposures to lethal and adaptive doses of oxygen. *Am Rev Respir Dis* 1980;**122**:123–43.

55 Block ER, Fisher AB. Depression of serotonin clearance by rat lungs during oxygen exposure. *J Appl Physiol* 1977;**42**:33–8.

56 Dobuler KJ, Catravas JD, Gillis NC. Early detection of oxygen-induced lung injury in conscious rabbits. *Am Rev Respir Dis* 1982;**126**:534–9.

57 Nash G, Blennerhasset JB, Pontoppidan H. Pulmonary lesions associated with oxygen therapy and artificial ventilation. *N Engl J Med* 1967;**279**:368–74.

◆58 Clark JM. Oxygen toxicity. In: Bennett PB, Elliott DH (eds), *The physiology and medicine of diving*, 3rd edn. London: Baillière Tindall, 1982;200–38.

59 Bruce Davis W, Rennard SI, Bitterman PB *et al.* Pulmonary oxygen toxicity – early reversible changes in human alveolar structures induced by hyperoxia. *N Engl J Med* 1983;**309**:878–83.

60 Allen MC, Watt SJ. Effect of hyperbaric and normobaric oxygen on pulmonary endothelial cell function. *Undersea Hyperbaric Med* 1993;**20**:39–48.

61 Puy RJM, Hyde RW, Fisher AB *et al.* Alterations in the pulmonary capillary bed during early oxygen toxicity in man. *J Appl Physiol* 1968;**24**:537–43.

26

The fetal pulmonary circulation

JOHN T REEVES, STEVEN H ABMAN AND KURT R STENMARK

INTRODUCTION

Remarkable recent advances in the embryology and physiology of the fetal circulation are of interest to physicians caring for newborns, children and/or adults. Regarding advances in embryology, it now appears that the assembly of the pulmonary arterial wall in the embryo requires the integration of the entire environment of the lung bud – the endothelium, mesenchyme and the airway epithelium, as well as extracellular matrix proteins and their corresponding integrin receptors. Moreover, for lung development to occur, fetal oxygen tension should be neither above nor below the usual fetal values. Importantly, for an understanding of postnatal pulmonary vascular disease, the processes responsible for assembling the arterial wall can become reactivated, perhaps in modified form, but still reactivated, by abnormal stimuli in the newborn or the adult. For example, after injury to an adult carotid artery, there is re-expression of an embryonic smooth muscle phenotype (Figure 26.1).[1] And in the lung circulation, matrix metalloproteinases, enzymes which are necessary to degrade matrix to allow for remodeling and growth of fetal blood vessels,[2] become activated by injury in the adult and may promote pathological vascular remodeling, in both pulmonary vascular and in coronary arterial diseases. Proteins in the basement membrane[3] and in the matrix have essential growth-promoting roles in the lung circulation before birth, and growth-inhibiting roles in normal vessels after birth, and the growth-promoting roles may be reactivated in postnatal vascular disease states.

Regarding advances in physiology, it appears that mechanisms (e.g. those involving ion channels, endothelial-dependent dilators and constrictors, and hormones), which are developed in the fetus for control of lung blood

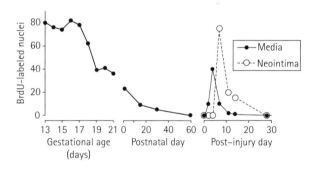

Figure 26.1 *In the embryonic rat, days 13 through 17 (left panel), high* in vivo *replication rates of carotid artery medial smooth muscle cells (filled circles) indicate about 80% of cells undergo cell division each 24 hours. In culture, these rapidly dividing cells grow autonomously, i.e. they are mitogen independent. At term (day 21 in the rat, left panel), replication has slowed. Cell growth slows further after birth (middle panel). (In culture, not shown, the late gestation and postnatal cells no longer exhibited autonomous growth, but required exogenous mitogens.) Following balloon injury to the endothelium in the adult rat,* in vivo *replication rates in the media and the neointima spiked to levels seen before birth (right panel). Cells cultured from the neointima showed autonomous growth, reminiscent of that in the embryo, suggesting that following injury cells could escape normal adult growth-suppressive activity. (Adapted from Weiser-Evans.[1])*

pressure and flow, are geared toward higher arterial tone than occurs after birth. But even in the adult, where control mechanisms are geared to a low resistance lung circulation, abnormal stimuli can reactivate some of the regulatory mechanisms which existed in the fetus, thereby promoting pulmonary hypertension. In addition, physicians increasingly recognize that fetal and neonatal disorders can cause adult disease. For example, pregnant women subjected to famine may give birth to infants who develop cardiovascular and obstructive airways disease as adults.[4] Intrauterine growth retardation impairs fetal airways growth, leading to impaired airflow after birth.[5] In addition, small doses of nicotine during pregnancy induces lung hypoplasia with abnormal accumulation of collagen around vessels.[6] Thus, the embryology and physiology of lung circulatory development may provide clues to adult disorders.

This chapter focuses on the recent advances (as we see them) in the embryology and physiology of the fetal circulation, where the concepts derived from the new work have implications for human disease.

PHILOSOPHICAL OVERVIEW

Historical aspects

In his classic description of the circulation of the blood published in 1628, Harvey did not ignore the fetal and newborn pulmonary circulation.[7] He recognized that *in utero* the two ventricles were 'nearly equal in all respects', and that after birth 'when the lungs are used', the right ventricle becomes less muscular than the left, because 'the right has only to drive blood through the lungs, whilst the left has to propel it through the whole body'. Historical details of the nearly four centuries after Harvey have been expertly reviewed.[8,9] In the 1930s and early 1940s, Sir Henry Barcroft, who may be considered the father of the fetal circulation, initiated a series of classical studies which showed by cineradiography the pattern of blood flow in the living fetal lamb, and suggested a lower lung blood flow before, than after, birth.[10] He realized that the fetus develops in a low oxygen environment and it was probably he who coined the term, 'Mt. Everest *in utero*'. In the 1950s, Geoffrey Dawes, applying the tools of physiology to the living exteriorized fetus, made many innovative, novel measurements, including the low pulmonary blood flow and high pressure in the fetus, and the several-fold increase in flow with the onset of breathing at birth. In the 1960s, Abraham Rudolph and colleagues developed the chronically instrumented, *in utero*, fetal lamb, which allowed measurement of vascular pressures, blood flows and blood gases under nearly ideal physiological conditions at various gestational ages. Application of this technique

greatly advanced the field and is the basis of much of our current physiological knowledge. Now the new tools of cellar biochemistry and genetics are opening entirely new vistas on our understanding of the fetal lung circulation.

Teleological aspects

The primary and sometimes difficult dilemma of the fetal lung circulation is to prepare itself for the moment of birth. Abruptly at birth, the newborn is deprived of oxygen from the placenta, and immediately must begin a life of independent existence, where oxygen is supplied by gas exchange between lung alveoli and the lung circulation. Remarkably, the *in utero* preparation for this drastic event occurs even though the lung is, in effect, a fluid-filled, non-essential organ. In the maturing fetus, the circulatory design seems directed at preserving blood flow, not to the lung, but to the placenta, which is the oxygen source and which receives some 60% of the output of the heart. Oddly, the heart appears to be pumping blood at near its maximal capacity. Therefore, and because all organs are perfused in parallel, if the placental flow is compromised, the fetus must rely upon a redistribution of the flow available. In such cases, there is preferential flow to the most essential organs such as placenta, brain and heart and away from less essential tissues such as the lung, which is, in effect, simply another systemic organ. Furthermore, because of this parallel perfusion of organs, even when fetal stress is absent there are constraints on increasing pulmonary blood flow. For example, a large, sustained vasodilation in the lung would shunt blood away from the placenta and be deleterious to fetal oxygenation. Therefore, the dilemma of the perinatal lung circulation is its disposition in fetal life toward a constricted state, versus the need for a sudden transition at birth to a state of sustained and profound vasodilation. To understand how the perinatal lung circulation solves the dilemma and what goes wrong when it does not, requires, in part, understanding the mechanisms of its formation.

EMBRYOLOGY

As has been known since the nineteenth century, the lung (like the liver) begins as an avascular bud from the primitive foregut. By the time of birth, this lung bud has developed into a complicated organ in which one arterial inflow, the bronchial artery, is destined to carry oxygenated blood, and another arterial inflow, the pulmonary artery, carries venous blood. Outflow from the organ is by a single venous system, and, unlike most other organs, the veins do not accompany the arteries. These observations have stood the tests of time.

The concept that has been in sway since the early 1800s,[11] and which is now being re-examined, is that the pulmonary arteries in mammals arise from a left aortic arch (the sixth arch in humans) and grow into the lung, following the airways. The idea was that the large arteries developed first, and subsequent vascular generations were formed from existing vessels, a process now designated as angiogenesis. Also by angiogenesis, the bronchial arteries budded out from the descending aorta and the pulmonary veins from the primitive cardiac sinus venosus. These views originated from histological examination where investigators could identify a vascular structure or a developed lumen, and there was no way that the histologists could know of the prior developmental events.

Application of the tools of molecular biology and genetics is beginning to question this classical sequence, and to suggest what some of these prior events might be. As a result, the views of the last two centuries, that lung blood vessels simply grow into the developing lung from pre-existing great vessels, is being questioned. Recent studies suggest that before light or electron microscopy can identify vascular structures, the lung bud is traversed by strands of primitive endothelial cells destined to form vessels (a process called vasculogenesis) and these strands can be identified by endothelial markers very early in gestation. A general sequence of events has been proposed.[12] Cells in the splanchnic mesoderm are assigned to an endothelial fate and become angioblasts, which then arrange themselves within an extracellular matrix to become cord-like structures. Possibly, this network of cords already anticipates the cardiovascular system with its heart, arteries, capillaries and veins. It has been suggested that even as the angioblast gives rise to the first-generation endothelial cells, the daughter cells are already assigned roles on the arterial or the venous side of the circulation.[13] Following the formation of the cord-like strands, there is the formation of vascular lumens, with large-caliber vessels forming through vascular fusion. There occurs recruitment of smooth muscle and pericytes to the endothelial tubes, resulting in the assembly of arterial walls.

But the endothelial cells, even before they have formed distinct blood vessels, may be responsible for organogenesis, itself. For example, neither the liver,[14] nor the pancreas[15] will develop as organs unless normal endothelial cell function is present. These recent results were interpreted to indicate that these cells provide the inductive signals for organ development, that is 'organs await blood vessels' go signal'.[16] If this is true for the lung, then endothelial cell formation and function will occur very early indeed in the developing embryo.

Such an embryological picture is quite different from that of the two prior centuries. If at their formation, the endothelial cord-like structures are already integrated into a network of arteries, capillaries and veins, the question of how they find each other to become connected, becomes less important than how they arrange themselves, and how each develops its different functions. Furthermore, the roles in development of matrix proteins, receptors, factors promoting differentiation and growth, and integrins begin to take center stage. The changing concept of how the pulmonary circulation is formed with emphasis on vasculogenesis, rather than only from ingrowth from pre-existing great arteries, not only provides a clearer picture of the embryology, but also it provides clues to the response of vessels to injury, as discussed below.

In the pulmonary circulation (and in other organs), a key early event occurs when primordial endothelial cells in the budding lung begin to express the receptor molecule, fetal liver kinase-1 (designated flk-1). When this receptor becomes activated by vascular endothelial growth factor (VEGF), cord-like endothelial cells begin to form tubes and enclose blood islands, resulting in the appearance of 'vascular lakes'.[17–21] In the human embryo, by about 50 days, and in the primitive mesenchyme distal to the budding airway, channelization (lumen development) begins within veins at the cardiac sinus venosus and approaches the capillary lakes. Beginning at about 10 weeks, when the 'lakes' have formed a primitive capillary network, and before airways have invaded the mesenchyme at the site, luminal connections develop between the network and the veins. Channelization then occurs in the pulmonary and bronchial arteries accompanying the airways, but it lags behind the developing lung buds. Within the developing lung, and as demonstrated by histological studies, channelization in vascular structures has a definite sequence: capillaries, pulmonary veins, the lumens of veins and capillaries become contiguous, and channelization of pulmonary and bronchial arteries which become contiguous to the capillary net. Finally, at about 19 weeks, the capillary network becomes a part of the alveolar wall, forming what will ultimately be the gas-exchanging surface.

In the lung bud, cross-talk between mesenchymal, epithelial and endothelial cells as well as the contribution from matrix proteins is essential for development. For example, if fetal lung mesenchyme is cultured in the absence of epithelial cells, it degenerates.[21] Grafting mesenchyme on to tracheal epithelium promotes branching morphogenesis.[22] The development of vessels depends on epithelium[23] and vice versa.[24] Extracellular matrix proteins are essential for development.[25] Also, apparently fetal development of the lung and its circulation requires the normal oxygen level found in the fetus (hypoxic by adult standards), where levels either above or below the healthy fetal values impair development (SA Gebb, personal communication). Thus, evolving concepts of vasculogenesis include the following:

- To a major extent the process is locally controlled.
- Signaling occurs among airway epithelial, vascular endothelial and mesodermal cells.

- Matrix proteins and their attachments to cells via integrin molecules are essential.
- There is a necessary and carefully controlled sequence of events.
- There is a balance between mechanisms facilitating new vessel formation and mechanisms which retard it.

(See also references 26–29.)

While these new developments are impressive, they raise fundamental questions. Where do the primitive endothelial cells come from, and how do they know where to go and what they are to do? What is the relationship between the branchial cleft arteries and the endothelial cells in the developing lung? Is it really true that the lung blood vessels arise initially by vasculogenesis, and what role does angiogenesis play? To obtain answers to these questions, investigators have plenty of work ahead.

FETAL PULMONARY CIRCULATORY DEVELOPMENT

Lung growth and the implications for the lung microcirculation

By the first third, and certainly by the first half of gestation, the primitive lung with its vessels and branching airways have been formed, but further differentiation and very substantial growth must subsequently occur. Although for the human fetus, little quantitative morphometric data are available on pulmonary capillary expansion for the last third of gestation, there are several reasons to believe the capillary bed is expanding rapidly during this period:

- From the 20th week until term, the fetus has its greatest absolute weight gain (Figure 26.2a).
- Both 'alveolar' surface area and lung volume are increasing rapidly, and accompany fetal weight gain (Figure 26.2b).

- 'Alveolar' surface area is closely related to lung volume implying regulation of parameters, which after birth, are necessary for gas exchange (Figure 26.2c).
- In nine human fetuses studied from the 18th week (i.e. when the capillaries actually 'break through' to the alveolar surface) to the 26th week of gestation capillary density and surface area increase exponentially.[18]
- Capillary network development accompanies 'alveolar' development.[17]
- Quantitative measurements in fetal lambs indicate the numbers of lung fifth and sixth generation arterioles increase 40-fold in the last 40% of gestation and the number of arteries per unit of lung volume increases 10-fold.[9,30]
- In fetal lambs, the increase in pulmonary vascularization with increasing gestation is accompanied by a fall in pulmonary vascular resistance.[31] Thus, it appears that while the conductive airways in the human fetus are all present by the 18th to 20th week of gestation, the expansion of respiratory surface area and pulmonary microcirculation which will be responsible for gas exchange, develops rapidly thereafter.

Fetal circulatory dynamics

As might be anticipated from the above, blood flows within the human fetus must be increasing rapidly after the 20th week of gestation. Indeed, the findings from ultrasound data in more than 200 normal human babies *in utero* indicate that the combined output for the two ventricles rises sharply after 20 weeks of gestation (Figure 26.3).[32] The right ventricular output increases with increasing gestational age. Throughout gestation, output from this chamber remains at about 60% of the combined ventricular output (Figure 26.3). By subtracting flow through the ductus arteriosus from the right ventricular output, the authors obtained an estimate of pulmonary

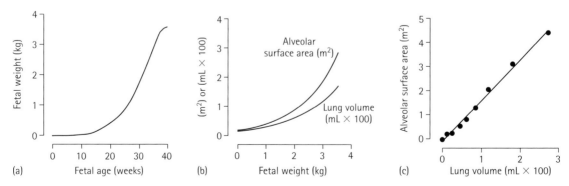

Figure 26.2 *Growth for humans of the fetus and fetal lung. (a) Approximate rate of fetal weight gain. (b) Increase in alveolar surface area and lung volume with fetal weight. (c) Strong relationship in the fetus of alveolar surface to lung volume. (Adapted from Langston et al.[70])*

blood flow (Figure 26.3), which increases with increasing age and remains at about 11% of the combined ventricular output until birth. From these non-invasive measurements, fetal lung blood flow was relatively higher in humans than in lambs, where values of about only 8% have been observed.

Although Mielke and Benda[32] did not report fetal weight, the rapid rise in total, right ventricular and pulmonary flow would correspond to the onset of the normal rapid weight gain as shown previously (Figure 26.2a). Assuming normal fetal weight gain, each of these three measures of flow would be directly proportional to weight. Because lung blood flow rises faster than pressure, vascular resistance falls. But even so, as term approaches, the increasing fetal 'alveolar' capillary surface area requires an increase in pulmonary arterial tone if pulmonary arterial pressure is to show the normal increase toward term.

Apparently, some of the fetal lung arterioles are particularly important in circulatory regulation late in fetal life. So called 'supernumerary' arterioles have been described in animals, and these arterioles have certain characteristics.[20,33,34] Supernumerary arterioles differ from the 'conventional' arteries which slavishly follow the airways, for they originate at right angles from the 'conventional' arteries. There are three to four times as many of them as 'conventional' arteries. In addition, they have a muscular 'baffle' valve at their origin and are more responsive than 'conventional' arteries to nitric oxide (NO), 5-hydroxytryptamine, and cyclic GMP (cGMP), but not more responsive to thromboxane. If existence and function of such supernumerary arteries are similar in the human fetus, then one might expect they play an important role in the regulation of the lung circulation, particularly in the late-stage fetus.

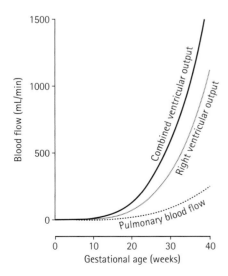

Figure 26.3 *Blood flows labeled for increasing gestional age as measured by ultrasound Doppler in human fetuses. (Adapted from Mielke and Benda.[32])*

Oxygen, NO and potassium ion channels in the vasoregulation of the fetal pulmonary circulation

The most obvious substance which might control the fetal lung circulation is oxygen tension. A role for oxygen in regulation is teleologically appealing, because low tension in the fetus would support the high arterial tone needed before birth, whereas after birth, the high oxygen tension which accompanies breathing would lower tone and promote an increase in lung blood flow. Hypoxic pulmonary vasoconstriction has been found in humans at 31–36 weeks of gestation.[35] In Rasanan's study,[35] when the mothers breathed a high oxygen mixture, the ultrasound measurements indicated that pulmonary blood flow increased in the fetus, while the right-to-left flow through the ductus arteriosus and the foramen ovale decreased – all of which was compatible with fetal pulmonary vasodilation. However, when the mothers breathed high oxygen at 20–26 weeks of gestation, these changes did not occur. The results in humans indicated that regulation of the fetal lung circulation by oxygen tension developed in the last half of gestation, as found in prior studies in fetal lambs.[36–39]

Fetal mechanisms for pulmonary vascular control, such as those involving potassium ion channels,[40] may be different from those in the adult. For example, in contrast to the normal adult, high oxygen tension in the fetal lung activates a calcium-sensitive potassium channel (K_{Ca}), allowing outflow of K ions from the vascular smooth muscle and inducing vasodilation.[41] Although the K_{Ca} channel may mediate, at least to some extent, the vasodilation in response both to NO and to oxygen, the former is presumably mediated by endothelium, while the latter involves smooth muscle. That a K_{Ca} channel is involved in the fetus is of interest, in that a voltage-dependent calcium channel (K_v) is involved in oxygen regulation of adult pulmonary arterial smooth muscle.

Surprisingly, oxygen, which is an important regulator of the lung circulation throughout all of life, causes only transient vasodilation in the fetal lamb near term. When the ewe breathes oxygen, the fetal pulmonary vascular flow promptly doubles (Figure 26.4) and resistance decreases approximately by half, but after 2 hours, the flow and resistance have returned toward the value observed before oxygen administration. Interestingly, whereas acetylcholine, a classic endothelium-dependent vasodilator, gives a transient dilation, an analog of cGMP, which acts directly on vascular smooth muscle gives a response which is sustained (Figure 26.4a). Not only acetylcholine, but other endothelial-dependent vasodilators, such as histamine, bradykinin, and tolazoline, all give transient vasodilation.[38] As discussed below, vasodilation in the fetus following partial compression of the ductus arteriosus, which increases mechanical shear stress on the endothelium, is also not sustained. Thus, while endothelial-dependent vasodilators cause a transient response, dilators which affect the smooth muscle cells directly, such as NO and 8-Br-GMP, give a sustained response. From all of the above, the implication is that oxygen acts via endothelium-dependent mechanisms in the fetus, and like other fetal endothelium-dependent vasodilators it causes a large, but transient dilation.

If in the fetus, oxygen-mediated vasodilation is largely mediated via the endothelium, NO release immediately comes to mind. Nitric oxide is among the most powerful vasodilators known. In endothelial cells, the enzyme nitric

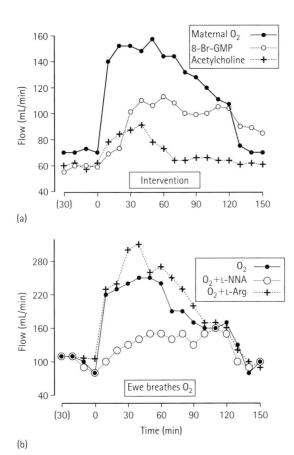

(a)

(b)

Figure 26.4 *Pulmonary blood flow in the mature fetal lamb before, during, and after each of three different 2-hour-long interventions. (a) The ewe breathes 100% oxygen (filled circles, unbroken line); with the ewe breathing air, infusion of the endothelial-independent vasodilator 8-bromo-guanosine monophosphate (8-Br-GMP) (unfilled circles, dotted line); and with the ewe breathing air, infusion of acetylcholine (plus signs, dashed line). (Adapted from Abman and Accurso.[71]) (b) The ewe breathes 100% oxygen without other interventions (filled circles, unbroken line), maternal oxygen plus the administration to the fetus of an inhibitor of nitric oxide synthase (eNOS), N-nitro-L-arginine (L-NNA) (unfilled circles, dotted line), and maternal oxygen plus supplemental L-arginine (L-Arg), an NO precursor (plus signs, dashed line). Data in (a) and (b) suggest endothelial-dependent vasodilation is transient, and much of the oxygen effect is endothelial-dependent. (Adapted from McQueston et al.[38])*

oxide synthase (eNOS) catalyses NO production by converting the amino acid, arginine, to citrulline. Once NO is produced by the endothelial cell, it easily crosses into the media and causes relaxation of vascular smooth muscle. That the mRNA for this enzyme appears in lung arteries of the lamb before the midpoint of gestation and persists is consistent with the concept that NO is important in fetal lung vasomotor control. In the lamb, the eNOS mRNA message, protein and activity all reach a peak by about 75% of gestation, and remain near that level through term.[42] Furthermore, when there is fetal growth retardation, the marked reduction in eNOS is thought to inhibit normal vascular development.[43] Isozymes NOS I and NOS II (potential sources of NO) have been identified in lung arterioles and appear to be important in the vasodilation that occurs on ventilation.[44,45] Thus, nitric oxide from several potential isozyme sources participates both in fetal lung vascular development and control.

In the fetal lamb, the oxygen-induced vasodilation was essentially blocked by the administration of an inhibitor of nitric oxide formation (Figure 26.4b),[37,38,46] suggesting that oxygen had acted by releasing nitric oxide from the endothelium. If so, then why is the endothelial-dependent vasodilation transient. One cannot invoke an inadequate supply of the circulating nitric oxide precursor, L-arginine, because increasing the supply does not prevent the transient nature of the oxygen effect (Figure 26.4b). Why there should be a transience of fetal pulmonary vasodilation from oxygen or other endothelial-dependent vasodilators remains an open question.

ENDOTHELIN

Endothelin-1 (ET-1) is a peptide which can induce either powerful vasoconstriction by activating endothelin A receptors (ET_A) or vasodilation by activating endothelin B receptors (ET_B). In fetal lambs, ET protein and ET_A and ET_B receptor mRNA expression were all found in the vasculature and maximal levels were seen as term approached, suggesting that the balance of these receptors could markedly influence fetal vascular tone.[47–49] Acute blockade of the ET_A receptor induced vasodilation, indicating that it normally functioned to mediate vasoconstriction in the fetal lung. Acute blockade of the ET_B receptor had no effect. These studies suggested that the balance of the endothelin system in the fetal lung was tipped toward vasoconstriction. However, the increase in ET_B receptor expression in late gestation and the finding of reduced ET_B expression in pulmonary hypertension suggested that chronic function of the ET_B receptor could be important. This proved to be the case. With blockade of the ET_B receptor in mature fetal lambs for 7 days, severe pulmonary hypertension resulted.[48] Furthermore, chronic blockade of the ET_B receptor markedly increased the levels of ET-1. The ET_B receptor appeared to function not only as a vasodilator, but also as a clearance receptor, serving to restrain the lung levels of ET-1. From studies such as these, it is clear that endothelin has important roles to play in the fetal lung circulation. Postnatally, chronic hypoxia induces upregulation of endothelin expression and activity, consistent with the concept of reactivation of fetal mechanisms of lung circulatory control.

ESTROGEN

The question naturally arises as to the effect of estrogen steroids on the fetal lung circulation. These steroids are well known vasodilators (acting at least in part, through stimulation of NO production), which, in pregnancy, are considered to induce the substantial arterial vasodilation and increased arterial diameter in the uterine circulation. Furthermore, estradiol levels are high in the mother, these hormones can cross the placenta, and fetal estrogen levels rise in late gestation. However, until recently, little was known of the hormonal effects in the fetus, much less on the fetal lung circulation. In a recent study, when estradiol was infused for 2–8 days in fetal lambs, there was a large and sustained pulmonary vasodilation, compatible with the concept that estrogen steroids are important in fetal pulmonary vascular control.[50] Oddly, while blockade of nitric oxide synthase inhibited the vasodilation, no alteration could be detected in expression of tissue nitric oxide synthase or the enzyme activity. Thus estradiol induced the vasodilation at least in part via nitric oxide, but the relationship between the steroid and nitric oxide production was obscure.

From the above, one might expect that chronic blockade of the estrogen receptors in the fetal lamb would induce fetal pulmonary vasoconstriction, but this did not occur.[51] Blockade of the estrogen receptor for 7 days did not alter fetal pulmonary hemodynamics. Neither did the blockade alter the pulmonary vasodilation in response to ventilation with gas containing high oxygen levels. Surprisingly, the main observed effect of blockade was to prevent the vasoconstriction in response to ventilation with gas containing low oxygen levels. The experimental results suggest that estrogen steroids do have a role in control of the perinatal lung circulation, but what that role is and its mechanisms require further study.

FETAL AND NEONATAL PULMONARY HYPERTENSION

Increased pulmonary arterial pressure

EXPERIMENTAL FETAL PULMONARY HYPERTENSION

An early and instructive animal model of fetal pulmonary hypertension has been to compress the ductus arteriosus

in the fetal lamb.[36] Normally, most of the right ventricular output flows from the main pulmonary artery through the ductus to the descending aorta and, as noted above, relatively little blood flows through the fetal lungs. However, when the ductus is partially compressed, more of the right ventricular output is forced through the lungs. Immediately on compression, pulmonary arterial pressure rises, flow increases and resistance falls, probably reflecting both active endothelial-dependent vasodilation in response to increased shear forces and passive vasodilation in response to the increased pressure. Remarkably, pulmonary vasoconstriction progressively occurs and over 2 hours, flow returns nearly to its pre-compression, control level (Figure 26.5a). During compression a fundamental change has occurred in pulmonary circulatory control. For example, after release of compression, oxygen administration to the ewe no longer causes pulmonary vasodilation (Figure 26.5b). Furthermore, repeat compression raises pressure, but no longer induces an initial pulmonary vasodilation (Figure 26.5a). If, as we suspect, the temporary, partial ductal compression has caused failure of endothelial-dependent vasodilation, then this endothelial function is at once seen as essential, but fragile.

When compression of the ductus was chronic, i.e. for 9–14 days, then oxygen administration to the mother had no vasodilating effect in the fetus (Figure 26.6a). Also, the normal vasodilation at birth did not occur (Figure 26.6b).[38] Hypoxemia was present despite ventilation with 100% oxygen. Thus, lambs born after several days of

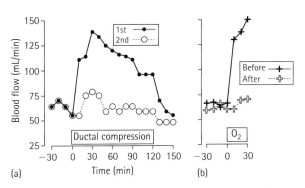

Figure 26.5 *Lung blood flow in the* in utero, *instrumented, mature lamb fetus. (a) Flow measurements before, during and after 2 hours of partial compression of the ductus arteriosus. With the initial compression (filled circles), flow increased sharply and then gradually fell toward the pre-compression value. When the partial compression was repeated (unfilled circles), there was little increase in flow. (b) An increase in lung blood flow occurred in the normal, instrumented, fetal lambs, when the ewe breathed 100% oxygen (O₂) (filled symbols). Following 2 hours of partial ductal compression, lung blood flow no longer increased when the ewe breathed oxygen. (Adapted from Abman and Accurso.[71])*

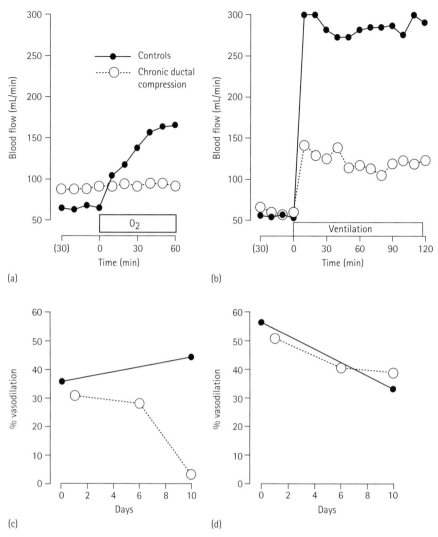

Figure 26.6 *Effects of chronic (≈ 10 days) partial compression of the ductus arteriosus in in utero, instrumented, mature lamb fetus. The figure suggests that ductal compression has impaired the ability of the endothelium to induce pulmonary vasodilation. (a) The normal fetus shows an increase in lung blood flow (filled circles), when the ewe breathes 100% oxygen (O_2), but the lamb with chronic ductal compression (unfilled circles), does not. (b) The normal fetus shows an increase in lung blood flow (filled circles), when the fetal lamb is ventilated, but the lamb with chronic ductal compression (unfilled circles), has a blunted increase in flow. (c) Acetylcholine (an endothelial-dependent vasodilator) infused into the normal fetal lamb induces pulmonary vasodilation (filled circles), on experimental day 0 and day 10, but the lamb with 10 days of chronic ductal compression (unfilled circles), failed to show vasodilation. (d) Atrial natriurietic peptide (an endothelial-independent vasodilator) caused vasodilation in both control lambs and those with chronic ductal compression. (Adapted from McQueston et al.[39])*

partial ductal compression *in utero* had pulmonary hypertension, low pulmonary blood flow and hypoxemia. Interestingly, infusing acetylcholine, an endothelial-dependent vasodilator, into the pulmonary circulation did not reduce the elevated pressure, resistance (Figure 26.6c), or hypoxemia, but infusing an endothelial-independent vasodilator (atrial natriuretic peptide, Figure 26.6d) or adding NO to the inspired air, both of which act directly on the pulmonary arterial vascular smooth muscle, resulted in vasodilation. These results suggested that the ductal compression had interfered with the vasodilating capacity of pulmonary endothelium, but not that of the vascular smooth muscle. Furthermore, while the results emphasized the important role of endothelium in the maintenance of normal fetal pulmonary vascular tone, they also implied that the endothelial vasodilating function might not be robust. Even in the early newborn period, endothelial-dependent relaxation can be impaired by a modest but chronic increase in pulmonary blood flow, findings compatible with a relatively vulnerable capacity of the endothelium for sustained vasodilation.[52,53]

PERSISTENT PULMONARY HYPERTENSION OF THE NEWBORN (PPHN)

When in humans the pulmonary arterial pressure and resistance do not fall at birth, or when the fall is not sustained, there results severe neonatal pulmonary hypertension, which is termed 'persistent pulmonary hypertension of the newborn', or PPHN. There are many potential causes, among which are pre- or postnatal hypoxia, prenatal ductal constriction, meconium aspiration, and/or prematurity. In the absence of treatment mortality is high. Inhalation of NO is increasingly replacing extracorporeal membrane oxygenation as treatment,[54] because it is less invasive, therapeutically effective, reduces hospital stay, and has fewer untoward effects, acutely and long term. Among the rationales for NO inhalation are that:

- NO is among the most potent known pulmonary vasodilators;
- being an inhaled small, water-soluble molecule, NO is delivered to alveoli where it easily diffuses directly into the arteriolar smooth muscle to reduce tone without requiring endothelial mediation;
- because it is rapidly removed by hemoglobin in the flowing blood, NO induces vasodilation of the constricted pulmonary arterial bed, without causing systemic hypotension;
- because low doses (<20 p.p.m.) of it are required, there is little risk of oxidant damage to tissues.

Following the effective use of inhaled NO in adults with primary pulmonary hypertension by Higgenbottam *et al.*,[55] Kinsella *et al.*[56] first showed that its use in PPHN could be followed by sustained improvement once the NO administration ceased.

Congenital diaphragmatic hernia (CDH)

The classical view of CDH is that one leaf of the diaphragm is incompletely formed or absent, with the result that abdominal contents enter the thoracic cavity and compress the lung during fetal development. This purely mechanical view may be incomplete. Possibly, a very early defect in the pleuroperitoneal fold within the developing embryo induces both the diaphragmatic defect and abnormal lung development.[57,58] In any event, underdevelopment of the pulmonary circulation results. The degree of underdevelopment, which may be severe in a hemithorax totally lacking a diaphragm, depends, at least in part, on the extent and timing of migration of the abdominal contents into the thorax. The opposite lung may also have an underdeveloped lung circulation. In the lungs, because the alveolar to arteriolar ratio is normal, the underdevelopment of the vascular system is considered to be appropriate for the underdevelopment of the airway structures. In addition to being underdeveloped,

the pulmonary arterioles have increased medial thickness. While mechanical compression of the lungs may be the dominant factor in the underdevelopment of pulmonary circulation, the cause of the medial hypertrophy is not clear.

Because during fetal life, fluid formed in the lung flows out the airways into the amniotic cavity, tracheal occlusion will, over time, distend the lung, and in experimental CDH, the external compression by the gut can be opposed. In fetal lambs, in which diaphragmatic hernia has been surgically created in early gestation and allowed to persist, 2 weeks of tracheal occlusion at about 75% of gestation prevents the arteriolar medial hypertrophy. Such experiments in CHD[59] emphasize the necessity of normal lung distension if the lung and its circulation are to develop normally.

There are likely additional factors. In the first place, it is not clear why medial hypertrophy of the pulmonary arterioles occurs in CDH. Furthermore, increased ET_A receptor activity, but not inadequate NO signaling, has been implicated in increasing pulmonary vascular tone in experimental congenital diaphragmatic hernia.[60] Understanding the factors causing the abnormal pulmonary vascular control is of clinical importance because decreasing pulmonary hypertension after birth in children with congenital diaphragmatic hernia is an important part of the therapy.

THE PULMONARY ARTERIAL WALL

Chronic thickening of the arterial wall is key to life-threatening pulmonary hypertension because it, *per se*, contributes to narrowing of the vascular lumen and obstruction of blood flow, and, in addition, medial hypertrophy and hyperplasia permit excessive vasoconstriction, and inhibit vasorelaxation. In the neonate, wall thickening often has its origins in some abnormal stimulus during fetal life. The risks of an abnormal pulmonary circulation after birth are not limited to the newborn, as physicians are now realizing that there are fetal and newborn origins of adult disease, including pulmonary hypertension and asthma.

Fetal pulmonary arterial wall

The cells which make up the fetal pulmonary arterial wall have several remarkable characteristics.

- Fetal cells have a greatly enhanced potential for replication. For example, adventitial fibroblasts from the main pulmonary artery of fetal calves at 40% gestation replicate much faster than do comparable cells from 8-day-old neonatal calves, and both replicate faster than those from adult cattle.[61] Furthermore, fibroblasts grow more slowly when taken from older than younger fetal calves, suggesting fibroblast growth rate diminished with advancing gestational age (M Das, unpublished). The enhanced replication rate appears to be due, at least in part, to the presence of specific isozymes of protein kinase C (PKC) that are present in the fetus, absent or diminished in the adult, and intermediate in the newborn. Smooth muscle cells and endothelial cells from fetal calves also exhibit faster growth than those from neonatal calves or adult cows.[62] Apparently then, mechanisms promoting rapid cellular eplication are diminished with advancing gestational age and after birth.

- Fetal pulmonary arterial smooth muscle and adventitial fibroblast cells show greater enhancement of replication in hypoxia than do adult cells.[62,63]
- Rapid replication of fetal vascular smooth muscle cells does not require exogenous mitogens (i.e. they exhibit autonomous growth) early in gestation, but such autonomous growth is absent near term and after birth.[64]
- Rates of apoptosis, i.e. programmed cell death, are high in the fetal vascular wall,[65] as vascular structures appear and disappear with great rapidity during development, and as the vessel walls are continually remodeled in later gestation.
- Fetal smooth muscle cells are 'plurifunctional'. Because in fetal life, circulatory control is developing at the same time the arterial wall is maturing, smooth muscle cells simultaneously replicate, secrete multiple matrix proteins, and maintain a contractile phenotype.[52,66] After birth, most vascular smooth muscle cells are considered to be well 'differentiated', implying that cells have prescribed functions and may replicate or secrete matrix proteins, but rarely do both simultaneously.
- Matrix proteins appear in a staged schedule, with those promoting cell growth, such as fibronectin and elastin, appearing early, and those with potential for retarding cell growth, such as perlecan, appearing later, coincidentally with slowing of vascular smooth muscle replication.

While growth of the fetus slows somewhat toward the end of gestation (Figure 26.2a), the newborn is still very active metabolically. The cells in the pulmonary arterial wall are also metabolically active at birth and retain the capacity for rapid proliferation, active matrix production, and vasoconstriction. Therefore, when an abnormal fetal lung circulation is carried into postnatal life, or when abnormal stimuli occur in the neonatal period, pulmonary arterial wall thickening occurs with extraordinary rapidity and remarkable magnitude. Indeed, life-threatening pulmonary hypertension is more common in the newborn period than at any other time of life.

Chronic hypoxic pulmonary hypertension in normal newborn calves

When a normal newborn calf at age 1–2 days is placed at high altitude to simulate the degree of hypoxemia which was present *in utero*, the normal transition of the pulmonary circulation is prevented, and severe pulmonary hypertension develops within a few days. Higher pressures develop more rapidly than in older cattle, and there is greater thickening in the walls of the pulmonary arterioles. The adventitial layer is particularly involved, because of proliferation of its resident fibroblast population and a marked increase in matrix proteins.

Given the multitude of subpopulations within a mixed population of fibroblasts, at any locus along the pulmonary arterial bed, fibroblasts have multifunctional capacities including rapid proliferation, migration, synthesis of connective tissue components, contractility, cytokine and mitogen production, and probably the capacity of transformation into other cell types.[65] Chronic hypoxia causes fibroblasts to reactivate fetal behaviors and mechanisms. For example, in the chronically hypoxic, pulmonary hypertensive neonatal calf, the normal pulmonary arterial regression of proteins related to fibronectin, elastin and collagen did not occur.[67] The persisting pattern of tropoelastin expression in these animals resembled that seen in fetal calves.[68] In addition, in this model of vascular injury and in other forms of injury to pulmonary and systemic arteries, fibroblasts are strongly suspected of being a source of cells in newly muscularized arteries and/or in arteries with increased medial thickness.

When muscular pulmonary arterial smooth muscle cells from hypertensive neonatal calves are cultured, they resemble fetal cells in more rapid rates of growth with and without serum present, and greater responsiveness to growth factors. Integrity of both the basement membrane[3] and the extracellular matrix[2] act to maintain the near quiescence of both fibroblasts and smooth muscle cells in the normal neonate. However, the lung arteries of the normal neonate retain fetal-like characteristics which can be re-expressed with chronic hypoxic injury. Furthermore, in adult models of vascular injury, there is also re-expression of fetal-like characteristics or genes in smooth muscle cells and fibroblasts.[65,69]

SUMMARY

We have focused on major advances in the embryology and physiology of the fetal lung circulation in recent years. No longer do we think that the lung arteries and veins invade the lung only by outgrowth from the great vessels by angiogenesis. While angiogenesis certainly occurs in the developing lung, preceding it are cords of primitive endothelial cells running through the early lung bud that may provide the template for the development of arteries, capillaries and veins, by the process of vasculogenesis. In the process of vasculogenesis, vessel wall assembly depends critically upon communication between the mesenchyme and the endothelium, airway and vessel, and a low (relative to that in the adult) arterial PO_2. It may be that these early endothelial cells are critical for the subsequent development of the organ itself. Although these concepts alter the conventional wisdom of nearly two centuries, their importance looks forward and not backward. On one hand, they provide a clearer understanding of how the lung circulation arises. On the other hand, because responses to injury often reactivate the mechanisms which existed during intrauterine development, these concepts are increasingly providing tantalizing insights into normal and abnormal repair in response to injury in the newborn and adult. For example, an injury to the endothelium calls upon responses which may involve the entire vessel wall, including not only its cells, but also its matrix and the basement membrane. Also for example, hypoxia may initially activate adventitial fibroblasts, the descendants of the primitive mesenchymal cells capable of performing many functions. The activated fibroblasts in turn, through production of cytokines, chemokines, growth factors, and extracellular matrix, likely influence other cells in the vessel wall and thus the overall function of the vessel. As in its embryological development, the structure of the neonatal and adult lung circulation and its response to injury depends upon interactions of cells, matrix, blood and tissue fluid, i.e. its entire environment.

The other major recent advance in understanding the fetal lung circulation has been in its function. Whilst we have long known that the fetal lung circulation is more reactive than that of the adult, we now begin to see how mechanisms of tone regulation (i.e. the K^+ channels employed, the fragility of endothelial-dependent vasodilation, the balance between endothelin constrictors and dilators, the roles of hormones) are used in the fetal lung circulation and how these can differ from those in the lung vessels of adults. Clues exist suggesting some of these regulatory functions *in utero* are reactivated in chronic pulmonary hypertension.

These advances in embryology are necessarily related to those in control mechanisms. Newer views on origins and assembly of lung arteries may relate to vascular function in fetal and neonatal pulmonary hypertension. For example, if abnormal stimuli activate the adventitial fibroblasts, which are descendants of the primitive mesenchyme, the fibroblasts not only reactivate patterns of fetal matrix synthesis, which leads to wall thickening, but

they also move into the media and toward the endothelium. They likely alter the compliance and contractility of the vessel. A more complete understanding of the fetal lung circulation, its formation, its function, and the relation of the two, will certainly lead to better modes of therapy in pulmonary hypertensive newborns and adults.

KEY POINTS

- Cords of primitive endothelial cells running through the early lung bud provide the template for the development of arteries, capillaries and veins, by the process of vasculogenesis.
- Vessel wall assembly depends critically upon a normal fetal arterial PO_2 as well as communication between the mesenchyme and the endothelium, airway and vessel.
- The presence of primitive endothelial cells is critical for the subsequent lung development.
- Postnatal responses to injury reactivate mechanisms which existed during fetal development.
- The control of the fetal lung circulation differs from that in the adult in, for example, the K^+ channels employed, the fragility of endothelial-dependent vasodilation, the balance between endothelin constrictors and dilators, and the roles of hormones.
- Adventitial fibroblasts are descendants of the primitive mesenchyme, and when activated not only do they reactivate patterns of fetal matrix synthesis, but also they move into the media and toward the endothelium, thereby altering compliance and contractility.

REFERENCES

1 Weiser-Evans MC, Quinn BE, Burkard MR *et al.* Transient reexpression of an embryonic autonomous growth phenotype by adult carotid artery smooth muscle cells after vascular injury. *Cell Physiol* 2000;**182**:12–23.

2 Rabinovitch M. Proteolytic modulation of the extracellular matrix. In: Weir EK, Archer SL, Reeves JT (eds), *The fetal and neonatal pulmonary circulations*. Armonk: Futura, 1999;117–30.

3 Belknap JK, Weiser-Evans MC, Grieshaber SS *et al.* Relationship between perlecan and tropoelastin gene expression and cell replication in the developing rat pulmonary vasculature. *Am J Respir Cell Mol Biol* 1999;**20**:24–34.

4 Lopuhaä CE, Rosenboom TJ, Osmond C *et al.* Atopy, lung function, and obstructive airways disease after prenatal exposure to famine. *Thorax* 2000;**55**:555–61.

5 Nikolajev K, Heinonen K, Hakulinen A *et al.* Effects of intrauterine growth retardation and prematurity on spirometric flow values and lung volumes at school age in twin pairs. *Pediatr Pulmonol* 1998;**25**:367–70.

6 Sekhon HS, Jia Y, Raab R *et al.* Prenatal nicotine increases pulmonary alpha 7 nicotinic receptor expression and alters fetal lung development in monkeys. *J Clin Invest* 1999;**103**:637–47.

◆7 Bowie A. *Harvey on the circulation of the blood.* London: George Bell & Sons, 1889 (A translation from the Latin of William Harvey's publication of 1628: *On the motion of the heart and Blood in Animals*).

◆8 Dawes GS. *Foetal and neonatal physiology.* Chicago: Year Book Publishers, 1968.

9 Rudolph AM. The development of concepts of the ontogeny of the pulmonary circulation. In: Weir EK, Archer SL, Reeves JT (eds), *The fetal and neonatal pulmonary circulations.* Armonk, NY: Futura, 1999.

10 Barclay AE, Franklin KJ, Pritchard MML. *The foetal circulation.* Springfield, IL: Charles C Thomas, 1945.

11 Rathke H. *Muller's Archiv*, p. 276. Referenced in Bremer JL. *Am J Anat* 1902;**1**:137–44.

12 Rupp PA, Little CD. Integrins in vascular development. *Circ Res* 2001;**89**:566–72.

13 Zhong TP, Rosenberg M, Mohideen MA *et al.* Protein gridlock, an HLH gene required for assembly of the aorta in zebrafish. *Science* 2000;**287**:1820–4.

14 Matsumoto K, Yoshitomi H, Rossant J *et al.* Liver organogenesis promoted by endothelial cells prior to vascular function. *Science* 2001;**294**:559–63.

15 Lammert E, Cleaver O, Melton D. Induction of pancreatic differentiation by signals from blood vessels. *Science* 2001;**294**:564–7.

16 Seydel C. Organs await blood vessel's go signal. *Science* 2001;**293**:2365.

17 Burri P. Fetal and postnatal development of the lung. *Am Rev Physiol* 1984;**46**:617–28.

18 DiMaio M, Gil J, Ciurea D *et al.* Structural maturation of the human fetal lung: a morphometric study of the development of the development of air-blood barriers. *Pediat Res* 1989;**26**:88–93.

19 deMello DE, Sawyer D, Galvin N *et al.* Early fetal development of lung vasculature. *Am J Respir Cell Mol Biol* 1997;**16**:568–81.

20 deMello DE, Reid LM. Embryonic and early fetal development of human lung vasculature and its functional implications. *Pediatr Dev Pathol* 2000;**3**:439–49.

•21 Gebb SA, Shannon JM. Tissue interactions mediate early events in pulmonary vasculogenesis. *Dev Dynamics* 2000;**217**:159–69.

22 Warburton D, Zhao J, Berberich MA *et al.* Molecular embryology of the lung: then, now, and in the future. *Am J Physiol Lung Cell Mol Physiol* 1999;**276**:L697–704.

23 Schwarz MA, Zhang F, Lane JE *et al.* Angiogenesis and morphogenesis of murine fetal distal lung in an allograft model. *Am J Physiol Lung Cell Mol Physiol* 2000;**278**:L1000–7.

24 Jakkula M, Le Cras TD, Gebb S *et al.* Inhibition of angiogenesis decreases alveolarization in the developing lung. *Am J Physiol Lung Cell Mol Physiol* 2000;**279**:L600–7.

25 Warburton D, Li DY, Faury G *et al.* Novel arterial pathology in mice and humans hemizygous for elastin. *J Clin Invest* 1998;**102**:1783–7.

26 Auerbach R, Auerbach W. Profound effects on vascular development caused by perturbations during organogenesis. *Am J Pathol* 1997;**151**:1183–6.

27 Hausladen JM, Davis EC, Pierce RA *et al.* Formation of the pulmonary vasculature: elastic fiber proteins as markers of cellular differentiation and vascular development. *Chest* 1998;**114**(Suppl 1):6S.

28 Morrell NW, Weiser MCM, Stenmark KR. Development of the pulmonary vasculature. In: Gaultier C, Bourbon JR, Post M (eds), *Lung development.* New York: Oxford University Press, 1999.

•29 Drake CJ, LaRue A, Ferrara N *et al.* VEGF regulates cell behavior during vasculogenesis. *Dev Biol* 2000;**224**:178–88.

30 Levin DL, Rudolph AM, Heyman MA *et al.* Morphological development of the pulmonary vascular bed in fetal lambs. *Circulation* 1976;**53**:144–51.

31 Lewis AB, Heyman MA, Rudolph AM. Gestational changes in pulmonary vascular responses in fetal lambs *in utero. Circ Res* 1976;**39**:536–41.

32 Mielke G, Benda N. Cardiac output and central distribution of blood flow in the human fetus. *Circulation* 2001;**103**:1662–8.

33 Bunton D, MacDonald A, Brown T *et al.* 5-Hydroxytryptamine and U46619-mediated vasoconstriction in bovine pulmonary conventional and supernumerary arteries: effect of endogenous nitric oxide. *Clin Sci* 2000;**98**:81–9.

34 Shaw AM, Bunton DC, Brown T *et al.* Regulation of sensitivity to 5-hydroxytryptamine in pulmonary supernumerary but not conventional arteries by a 5-HT(1D)-like receptor. *Eur J Pharmacol* 2000;**10**:69–82.

35 Rasanen J, Wood DC, Debbs RH *et al.* Reactivity of the human fetal pulmonary circulation to maternal hyperoxygenation increases during the second half of pregnancy. *Circulation* 1998;**97**:257–62.

•36 Abman SH, Accurso FJ. Acute effects of partial compression of the ductus arteriosus on the fetal pulmonary circulation. *Am J Physiol* 1989;**257**:H626–34.

◆37 Abman SH, Kinsella JP, Parker TA *et al.* Physiologic roles of nitric oxide in the perinatal circulation. In: Weir EK, Archer SL, Reeves JT (eds), *The fetal and neonatal pulmonary circulations.* Armonk, NY: Futura, 1999;239–60.

38 McQueston JA, Cornfield DN, McMurtry IF *et al.* Effects of oxygen and exogenous L-arginine on EDRF activity in the fetal pulmonary circulation. *Am J Physiol* 1993;**264**:H865–71.

39 McQueston JA, Kinsella JP, Ivy DD *et al.* Chronic pulmonary hypertension *in utero* impairs endothelium-dependent vasodilation. *Am J Physiol* 1995;**268**:H288–94.

◆40 Cornfield DN, Reeve HL, Weir EK. O_2-sensitive K^+ channel activity in the ovine pulmonary circulation shifts with maturation. In: Weir EK, Archer SL, Reeves JT (eds), *The fetal and neonatal pulmonary circulations.* Armonk, NY: Futura, 1999;303–17.

41 Cornfield DN, Reeve HL, Tolarova S *et al.* Oxygen causes fetal pulmonary vasodilation through activation of a calcium-dependent potassium channel. *Proc Natl Acad Sci USA* 1996;**93**:8089–94.

42 Parker TA, Le Cras TD, Kinsella JP *et al.* Developmental changes in endothelial nitric oxide synthase expression and activity in ovine fetal lung. *Am J Physiol Lung Cell Mol Physiol* 2000;**278**:L202–8.

43 Galan HL, Regnault TR, Le Cras TD *et al.* Cotyledon and binucleate cell nitric oxide synthase in an ovine model of fetal growth restriction. *J Appl Physiol* 2001;**90**:2420–6.

44 Rairigh RL, Parker TA, Ivy DD *et al.* Role of inducible nitric oxide synthase in the pulmonary vascular response to birth-related stimuli in the ovine fetus. *Circ Res* 2001;**88**:721–6.

45 Tzao C, Nickerson PA, Russell JA *et al.* Heterogeneous distribution of type I nitric oxide synthase in pulmonary vasculature of ovine fetus. *Histochem Cell Biol* 2000;**114**:421–30.

46 Shaul P. Regulation of endothelial nitric oxide synthase expression in the developing lung. In: Weir EK, Archer SL, Reeves JT (eds), *The fetal and neonatal pulmonary circulations.* Armonk: Futura, 1999;261–78.

47 Ivy DD, Abman SH. The role of endothelin in perinatal pulmonary vasoregulation. In: Weir EK, Archer SL, Reeves JT (eds), *The fetal and neonatal pulmonary circulations.* Armonk, NY: Futura, 1999;279–302.

48 Ivy DD, Parker TA, Abman SH. Prolonged endothelin B receptor blockade causes pulmonary hypertension in the ovine fetus. *Am J Physiol Lung Cell Mol Physiol* 2000;**278**:L758–65.

49 Ivy DD, Le Cras TD, Parker TA *et al.* Developmental changes in endothellin expression and activity in ovine fetal lung. *Am J Physiol Lung Cell Mol Physiol* 2000;**278**:L785–93.

50 Parker TA, Kinsella JP, Galan HL *et al.* Prolonged infusions of estradiol dilate the ovine fetal pulmonary circulation. *Pediatr Res* 2000;**47**:89–96.

51 Parker TA, Afshar S, Kinsella JP *et al.*Effects of chronic estrogen blockade on ovine pulmonary circulation. *Am J Physiol Heart Circ Physiol* 2001;**281**:H1005–14.

•52 Haworth SG. Development of the normal and abnormal pulmonary circulation. *Exp Physiol* 1995;**80**:843–53.

53 Reddy VM, Wong J, Liddicoat JR *et al.* Altered endothelium-dependent vasoactive responses in lambs with pulmonary hypertension and increased pulmonary blood flow. *Am J Physiol* 1996;**271**:H562–70.

◆54 Kinsella JP, Abman SH. Inhaled nitric oxide: current and future uses in neonates. *Semin Perinatol* 2000;**24**:387–95.

•55 Higenbottam TW, Pepke-Zaba J, Scott J *et al.* Inhaled 'endothelium-dependent relaxing factor' in primary pulmonary hypertension. *Am Rev Respir Dis* 1998;**137**:A107.

•56 Kinsella JP, Neish SR, Shaffer E *et al.* Low-dose inhalational nitric oxide in persistent pulmonary hypertension of the newborn. *Lancet* 1992;**340**:819–20.

57 Geer JJ, Allan DW, Babuik RP *et al.* State of the art review: recent advances toward and understanding of the pathogenesis of nitrofen-induced congenital diaphragmatic hernia. *Pediatr Pulmonol* 2000;**29**:394–9.

58 Jesudason EC, Connell MG, Fernig DG *et al.* Early malformations in congenital diaphragmatic hernia. *J Pediatr Surg* 2000;**35**:124–8.

59 Luks FI, Wild YK, Piasecki GJ *et al.* Short term tracheal occlusion corrects pulmonary vascular abnormalities in the fetal lamb with diaphragmatic hernia. *Surgery* 2000;**128**:266–72.

60 Thebaud B, de Lagausie P, Forgues D *et al.* ET(A)-receptor blockade and ET(B)-receptor stimulation in experimental congenital diaphragmatic hernia. *Am J Physiol Lung Cell Mol Physiol* 2000;**278**:L923–32.

61 Das M, Stenmark KR, Ruff LJ *et al.* Selected isozymes of PKC contribute to augmented growth of fetal and neonatal bovine adventitial fibroblasts. *Am J Cell Mol Physiol* 1997;**273**:L1276–84.

•62 Xu Y, Stenmark KR, Das M *et al.* Pulmonary artery smooth muscle cells from chronically hypoxic neonatal calves retain fetal-like and acquire new growth properties. *Am J Physiol* 1997;**273**:L234–45.

63 Das M, Bouchey DM, Moore MJ *et al.* Hypoxia-induced proliferative response of vascular adventitial fibroblasts is dependent on G-protein-mediated activation of mitogen-activated protein kinases. *J Biol Chem* 2001;**276**:15631–40.

64 Cook CL, Weiser MC, Schwartz PE *et al.* Developmentally timed expression of an embryonic growth phenotype in vascular smooth muscle cells. *Circ Res* 1994;**74**:189–96.

◆65 Stenmark KR, Das M, Bouchey D *et al.* Contribution of the adventitial fibroblast to pulmonary vascular disease. In: Weir EK, Archer SL, Reeves JT (eds), *The fetal and neonatal pulmonary circulations.* Armonk: Futura, 1999;67–86.

66 Wohrley JD, Frid MG, Moiseeva EP *et al.* Hypoxia selectively induces proliferation in a specific subpopulation of smooth muscle cells in the bovine neonatal pulmonary arterial media. *J Clin Invest* 1995;**96**:273–81.

67 Durmowicz AJ, Parks WC, Hyde DM *et al.* Persistent, re-expression, and induction of pulmonary arterial fibronectin, tropoelastin, and type I procollagen mRNA expression in neonatal hypoxic pulmonary hypertension. *Am J Pathol* 1994;**145**:1411–20.

68 Stenmark KR, Durmowicz AJ, Roby JD *et al.* Persistence of the fetal pattern of tropoelastin gene expression in severe neonatal bovine pulmonary hypertension. *J Clin Invest* 1994;**93**:1234–42.

69 Weiser-Evans MC, Schwartz PE, Grieshaber NA *et al.* Novel embryonic genes are preferentially expressed by autonomously replicating rat embryonic and neointimal smooth muscle cells. *Circ Res* 2000;**87**:608–15.

70 Langston C, Kida K, Reed M *et al.* Human lung growth in late gestation and in the neonate. *Am Rev Respir Dis* 1984;**129**:607–13.

71 Abman SH, Accurso FJ. Sustained fetal pulmonary vasodilation with prolonged atrial natriuretic factor and GMP infusions. *Am J Physiol* 1991;**260**:H183–92.

PART 9

Disorders causing intrapulmonary shunt

27

Hepatopulmonary syndrome

MICHAEL J KROWKA

INTRODUCTION

In an 1884 German publication, Dr M Fluckiger described a 37-year-old woman with profound cyanosis and digital clubbing who died following an episode of hematemesis and probable hepatic coma. A postmortem examination conducted by Professor v. Recklinghausen demonstrated cirrhosis, enlarged twisted veins around the esophagus and abnormally **dilated pulmonary vessels**.[1] Approximately 75 years later, in 1959, a case report describing the death of a 17-year-old male with severe hypoxemia and juvenile cirrhosis, Rydell and Hoffbauer emphasized the dramatic clinical relationship between hypoxemia and hepatic dysfunction. Their post-mortem study described both precapillary dilatations and direct arteriovenous communications as demonstrated by vascular injections of the pulmonary arteries with a plastic vinyl acetate solution.[2] Berthelot and colleagues from England confirmed these pulmonary vascular observations in their 1969 autopsy study of 12 patients with microscopic 'lung spiders' that complicated advanced liver disease.[3] The entity of hypoxemia due to such pulmonary vascular abnormalities in the setting of liver disease was later termed 'hepatopulmonary syndrome' by Knudsen and Kennedy in 1979.[4] Over the last 20 years the international importance of and intrigue surrounding the hepatopulmonary syndrome (HPS) has steadily unfolded as a consequence of the clinical experiences during pre- and post-liver transplant evaluations.

A continuum of pulmonary vascular pathology can occur in the setting of chronic liver disease (Figure 27.1).

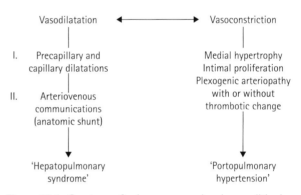

Figure 27.1 *Spectrum of pulmonary vascular abnormalities in advanced liver disease.*

It is hypothesized that the pulmonary arterial and capillary beds experience the 'downstream' effects of circulating vascular mediators that exist due to hepatic dysfunction. This chapter focuses on the concept of **pulmonary vascular dilatation** that causes arterial hypoxemia in the setting of liver and portal circulation dysfunction.[5,6] HPS is distinct from portopulmonary hypertension, the other major insult to the pulmonary circulation associated with liver disease (discussed in Chapter 13F).

DIAGNOSTIC CRITERIA

The **triad** of hepatic dysfunction, pulmonary vascular dilatation and arterial hypoxemia characterizes HPS.[5,6] Specific diagnostic criteria currently followed by most clinical investigators are summarized in Table 27.1.

Hepatic dysfunction

Pediatric and adult patients with HPS most commonly have chronic liver disease (cirrhosis) with portal hypertension. However, HPS has been reported in the setting of non-cirrhotic portal hypertension.[6,7] In addition, pulmonary vascular dilatations have been demonstrated at autopsy in the setting of fulminant hepatic failure.[8] Severity of liver disease characterized by the Child–Pugh classification (ascites, encephalopathy, bilirubin, albumin and prothrombin time) correlates poorly with the severity of hypoxemia.[9]

Pulmonary vascular dilatation

Non-invasive diagnosis of pulmonary vascular dilatations rests upon detecting the abnormal passage of microbubbles (Figure 27.2) or technetium-radiolabeled macroaggregated albumin ([99mTcMAA], Figure 27.3) through

Table 27.1 *Hepatopulmonary syndrome diagnostic criteria*

Liver disease
- Cirrhosis with portal hypertension (any cause)
- Noncirrhotic portal hypertension

Hypoxemia
- $PaO_2 < 70$ mmHg; or
- Alveolar−arterial (A−a) oxygen gradient >20 mmHg

Pulmonary vascular dilatation
- 'Positive' contrast-enhanced echocardiogram showing microbubble opacification in the left atrium >3 cardiac cycles after right ventricular opacification; or
- [99mTcMAA] brain uptake >5% following lung perfusion scanning

PaO_2, arterial partial pressure of O_2; [99mTcMAA], technetium-radiolabeled macro-aggregated albumin.

dilated capillary beds or discrete arteriovenous communications.[10,11] Normally, microbubbles (>10 μm) or [99mTcMAA] (20–60 μm) are absorbed or trapped, respectively, and do not pass through capillaries (<8 μm in diameter). [99mTcMAA] lung scanning offers the advantage of quantifying the degree of pulmonary vascular dilatation by measuring brain versus lung uptake.[11,12] Neither method, however, can distinguish between diffuse vascular dilatations and discrete arteriovenous communications.

Pulmonary angiography has demonstrated at least two types of vascular abnormality that characterize HPS (Figure 27.4). The common type I pattern is characterized by a normal to diffuse spongy/blush appearance during the arterial phase of imaging.[6,13,14] The rare type II lesions are seen as discrete arteriovenous communications (which may be amenable to coil embolotherapy to improve oxygenation and reduce the risk of brain embolic events). It is not uncommon for the angiogram images to be reported as 'normal', suggesting only rapid venous filling.[2,9] HPS patients with $PaO_2 > 300$ mmHg breathing 100% oxygen are unlikely to have clinically significant lesions demonstrated by pulmonary angiography.[9] This invasive procedure should be conducted in a select group of HPS patients and only if coil embolotherapy is to be considered.

Unlike portopulmonary hypertension associated with vasoconstriction, the pulmonary vascular dilatations in HPS are characterized by normal or reduced pulmonary vascular resistance measured during right heart catheterization.[5] Cardiac outputs may be quite high due to the hyperdynamic circulatory state created by hepatic dysfunction. Pulmonary artery pressures may be slightly increased in HPS due to the high-flow state through the pulmonary vascular bed.

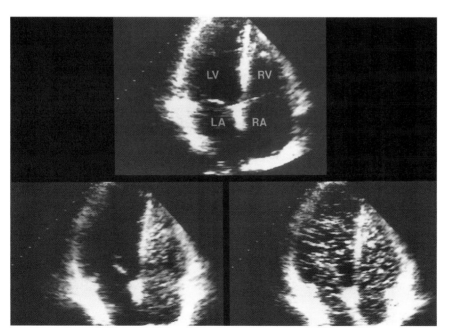

Figure 27.2 *Transthoracic echocardiogram demonstrating: (top) normal four-chamber view; RA, right atrium; RV, right ventricle; LA, left atrium; LV, left ventricle; (bottom left) normal right heart chamber opacification following peripheral vein injection of agitated saline; (bottom right) left heart chamber opacification four to six cardiac cycles later due to abnormal intrapulmonary passage of microbubbles through dilated precapillary and capillary vessels. Reproduced with permission from Krowka MJ, Cartese DA. Hepatopulmonary syndrome: Current concepts in diagnostic and therapeutic considerations.* Chest *1994;5:1528–37.*

Arterial hypoxemia

A schematic that demonstrates precapillary/capillary dilatation and anatomic shunt pathophysiology associated with

HPS is shown in Figure 27.5.[2,3] Such pathology causes arterial hypoxemia from three mechanisms:[15–19]

- low ventilation/perfusion ($\dot{V}/\dot{Q}$) ratio due to excess perfusion ($\dot{Q}$) to a given area of ventilation ($\dot{V}$);

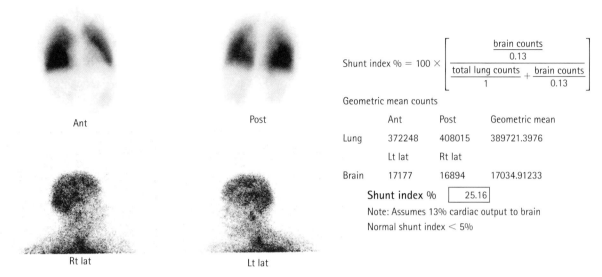

$$\text{Shunt index \%} = 100 \times \left[\frac{\dfrac{\text{brain counts}}{0.13}}{\dfrac{\text{total lung counts}}{1} + \dfrac{\text{brain counts}}{0.13}} \right]$$

Geometric mean counts

	Ant	Post	Geometric mean
Lung	372248	408015	389721.3976
	Lt lat	Rt lat	
Brain	17177	16894	17034.91233

Shunt index % $\boxed{25.16}$

Note: Assumes 13% cardiac output to brain
Normal shunt index $< 5\%$

Figure 27.3 *Technetium-radiolabeled macro-aggregated albumin brain and lung perfusion scan demonstrating a 25% brain uptake in a patient with nodular regenerative hyperplasia, portal hypertension and severe hepatopulmonary syndrome. Reproduced with permission from Ref 9.*

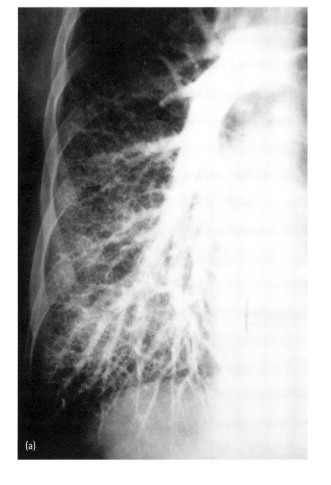

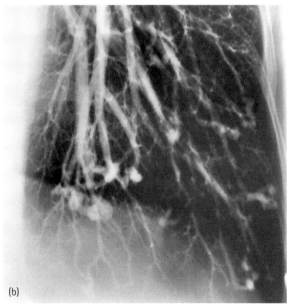

Figure 27.4 *Pulmonary angiograms demonstrating (a) diffuse, spongy arterial pattern and (b) discrete arteriovenous communications.*

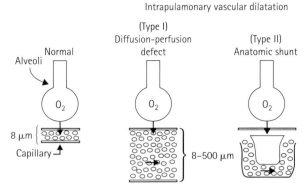

Intrapulamonary vascular dilatation

Figure 27.5 *The schematic of abnormal physiology associated with dilated precapillary/capillary vessels and direct arteriovenous communications.*

- impaired diffusion of oxygen molecules through dilated perialveolar vessels (a diffusion-perfusion defect);
- true anatomic (intrapulmonary) right-to-left shunt.

The multiple inert gas elimination technique (MIGET) has been the gold standard in studying the physiology of hypoxemia in the presence of pulmonary vascular dilatations.[15,17] Following a venous infusion of inert gases with varying solubilities, exhalation and arterial concentrations allow numerical approximations of pulmonary ventilation/perfusion relationships.[15] The dramatic response to 100% inspired oxygen in the setting of severe hypoxemia breathing room air argues against the existence of a clinically significant right-to-left anatomic shunt in most patients with HPS.[9] The accuracy and interpretation of MIGET in the setting of severe hypoxemia due to diffuse vascular dilatation (not distinct arteriovenous communications) has been questioned.[20]

Clinically, many patients with HPS have near normal PaO_2 (>500 mmHg) when breathing 100% oxygen.[9] High concentrations of alveolar O_2 are able to completely penetrate dilated capillary channels and thus PaO_2 improves. For this reason it is unlikely that most cases of HPS involve true 'shunt'. Worsening of arterial oxygenation when moving from the supine to standing position (orthodeoxia) has been documented in HPS.[3,9] Orthodeoxia has been attributed to the predominance of vascular dilatations in the lung bases, effects of gravity on blood flow and reduced cardiac output when standing.

The severity of arterial hypoxemia breathing room air correlates modestly with 100% inspired oxygen and [99m]TcMAA lung scanning (Figure 27.6). These studies may have varying prognostic importance. Indeed, multiple reasons for hypoxemia (lung atelectasis caused by hepatic hydrothorax, effects of massive ascites upon the diaphragms, chronic obstructive lung disease and interstitial lung disease) may exist in approximately 20–30% of patients with pulmonary vascular dilatations.[9,21]

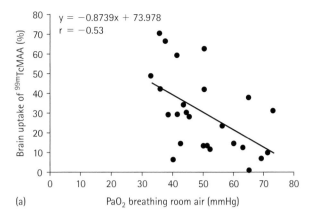

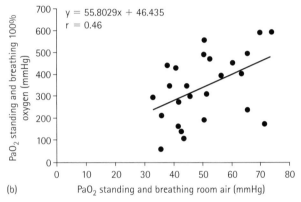

Figure 27.6 *Relationships between arterial partial pressure of O_2 (PaO_2) breathing room air and (a) technetium-radiolabeled macro-aggregated albumin ([99m]TcMAA) lung scans with brain uptake per cent; (b) PaO_2 breathing 100% oxygen using a two-way valve, sealed mouth piece with nose clips (all studies done in the standing position). Reproduced with permission from Ref 9.*

SCREENING AND DIAGNOSTIC ALGORITHM

Screening for hypoxemia

Oxyhemoglobin saturation (SaO_2) measured by pulse oximetry, arterial partial pressure of oxygen (PaO_2) and the alveolar–arterial (A–a) oxygen gradient characterize the degree of hypoxemia in patients with liver disease.[22] The obvious advantage of pulse oximetry is that the measurement is non-invasive. However, this method has been reported to overestimate oxyhemoglobin saturations obtained via arterial puncture and blood gas analysis by approximately 4%.[23] Pulse oximetry ($SpO_2 < 94\%$) detected all subjects with a $PaO_2 < 60$ mmHg in the same study.[23]

Indeed, PaO_2 and A–a oxygen gradient determinations require arterial puncture, but this method can be safely accomplished by experienced individuals even in the setting of thrombocytopenia and coagulopathy due to liver disease. Owing to hyperventilation which accompanies liver disease, most investigators concur that PaO_2

Algorithm for HPS screening and diagnosis

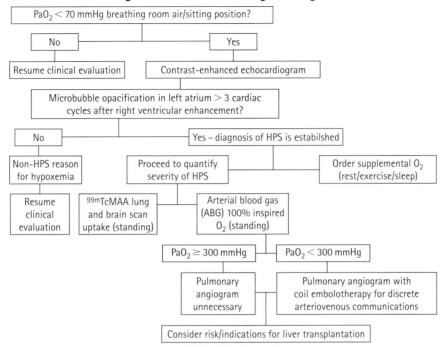

Figure 27.7 *Hepatopulmonary syndrome (HPS) screening and diagnostic algorithm currently followed at the Mayo Clinic.* [99m]*TcMAA, technetium-labeled macro-aggregated albumin; PaO₂, arterial partial pressure of O₂.*

values <70 mmHg should be considered abnormal.[5,6,12] Determination of the (A−a) oxygen gradient, which takes into consideration not only the PaO_2, but also the $PaCO_2$ effect on oxygenation, provides the most sensitive assessment of abnormal arterial oxygenation. Normal (A−a) oxygen gradient is age dependent, but usually considered abnormal if greater than 20 mmHg.[17] The measurement of the (A−a) oxygen gradient, however, must take into consideration the daily barometric pressure in calculating the alveolar partial pressure of oxygen. Although hypoxemia is common in liver disease and not necessarily due to HPS, patients with severe hypoxemia (PaO_2 <50 mmHg) should be considered to have hepatopulmonary syndrome **until proven otherwise**.

Screening for pulmonary vascular dilatations

Most centers screen for pulmonary vascular dilatation using transthoracic, contrast-enhanced echocardiography.[10] If necessary, contrast transesophageal echocardiography can distinguish between intracardiac shunts and intrapulmonary vascular dilatations by direct imaging of the intra-atrial septum and pulmonary veins, respectively. [99m]TcMAA lung scanning should be accomplished if the screening PaO_2 (and contrast echocardiogram) suggest HPS.

The HPS screening and diagnostic algorithm followed at the Mayo Clinic is shown in Figure 27.7.

INCIDENCE

The frequency of transthoracic echo-detected pulmonary vascular dilatation associated with liver disease has ranged from 7 to 47% (Table 27.2). Hypoxemia was reported in 32–65% of those with 'positive' contrast-enhanced echocardiograms and in 5–17% of all patients screened.[10,24–30] A subclinical or *forme fruste* aspect of HPS may exist which, over time, results in progressive hypoxemia.[10,11]

PATHOPHYSIOLOGY

Circulating mediators that result in diffuse vascular dilatations, discrete arteriovenous communications, and possible angiogenesis, have not been identified in humans.[2,3] Increased levels of exhaled nitric oxide have been documented in HPS with resolution of such findings and hypoxemia following successful orthotopic liver transplantation (OLT).[31–33] Recently, animal models have provided links between hepatic dysfunction and the pulmonary endothelium.[34–36] A bile duct ligation rat model of cirrhosis and portal hypertension has focused on the role of circulating endothelin-1.[35] Increased levels of endothelin-1 (originating from the liver) may affect endothelin A and endothelin B receptors in the pulmonary

Table 27.2 *Frequency of positive transthoracic contrast-enhanced echocardiograms and hypoxemia when screening for hepatopulmonary syndrome*

Study	No. of patients	Positive echo	Hypoxemia[*,†]
1985 Park *et al.*[24]	73	4 (5%)	not done
1990 Krowka *et al.*[10]	40	5 (13%)	2 (5%)[*]
1992 Hopkins *et al.*[26]	53	25 (47%)	8 (15%)[*]
1994 Jensen *et al.*[27]	47	11 (23%)	6 (13%)[*]
1996 Donovan *et al.*[25]	125	39 (31%)	not done
1997 Vedrinne *et al.*[28]	37	12 (33%)	not done
1998 Mimidis *et al.*[29]	56	8 (14%)	normal PaO_2
2001 Anand *et al.*[30]	88	17 (27%)	11 (17%)[†]

[*]PaO_2, arterial partial pressure of O_2 <70 mmHg
[†]Alveolar-arterial oxygen gradient >20 mmHg

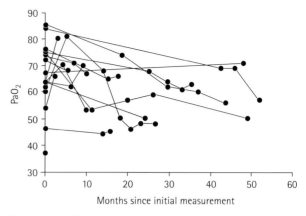

Figure 27.8 *'Natural history' of arterial partial pressure of O_2 (PaO_2) change documented in patients with hepatopulmonary syndrome (HPS) awaiting liver transplantation.*

vascular bed . These receptors normally cause vasodilation (endothelin B receptors on the luminal side of the endothelium) and vasoconstriction (endothelin A and B receptors on smooth muscle which surround the vessels). Genetic predisposition and the effects of endothelin receptor expression/distribution in liver disease require further study.[35,36] Finally, angiogenesis and the role of vascular endothelial growth factor (VEGF) remain unproved hypotheses in the evolution of HPS. Autopsy descriptions reported by Berthelot *et al.*[3] documented an apparent increase in the number of perialveolar vessels compared to controls.

CLINICAL PRESENTATION AND NATURAL HISTORY

The natural history of HPS is poorly defined.[37] HPS appears to develop slowly over months to years after the onset of hepatic dysfunction. Young children, as well as adults, may have profound presentations of cyanosis due to HPS. Clubbing, cyanosis and spider angiomas of the skin in the setting of liver disease strongly suggest the existence of pulmonary vascular dilatations. Correlation with the stage of liver disease (as documented by the Child–Pugh classification or with the existence of esophageal varices) is poor.[9,11,12] The chest radiograph is frequently unremarkable; patterns consistent with lower lung field 'interstitial lung disease' may be reported, but subsequent chest CT scanning reveals peripheral, diffusely dilated vessels.[14]

Once the diagnosis of HPS is established, progressive worsening of hypoxemia over months to years has been reported with an approximate mortality of 41% at 2.5 years from diagnosis.[37] Patients with HPS awaiting liver transplantation tend to have a progressive, symptomatic deterioration in PaO_2, which occurs over many months (Figure 27.8).

TREATMENT OPTIONS

By definition, HPS patients are hypoxemic at rest. This may worsen with exercise and sleep.[4] Therefore, one of the fundamental interventions to improve the symptoms of dyspnea and fatigue associated with HPS should be the provision of supplemental oxygen. Most patients respond well to low-flow oxygen (1–5 L/min) via nasal cannula. As HPS advances, additional oxygen can be provided by face masks or face tents during the waiting time for liver transplantation.

The definitive treatment of HPS remains OLT.[5,6] Nonsurgical approaches have been attempted, providing some improvement in hypoxemia, but none has provided resolution of hypoxemia due to HPS. Rarely, spontaneous resolution of HPS has occurred with improvement in liver disease.[6]

Pharmacological

Medication approaches have been disappointing in providing a consistent and reproducible improvement in the hypoxemia associated with HPS. Small series have involved the open-label use of vascular mediators such as almitrine bismesylate,[37] somatostatin analog[16,38] and garlic preparation;[39] except for garlic, significant improvement in PaO_2 could not be consistently demonstrated in these studies. Case reports have advocated anti-inflammatory approaches utilizing oral and intravenous indomethacin and high-dose aspirin (2 g/day in children with portal vein thrombosis).[40] Attempts to improve oxygenation in HPS with β-blockers, estrogen inhibitors, and plasma exchange have been unsuccessful;[6] cytoxan and prednisone have been reported to reverse HPS.[41]

As a means to block the vasodilatory effects of nitric oxide, intravenous methylene blue was administered to seven hospitalized patients with severe HPS (PaO_2

<60 mmHg) in an open-label trial. Improvements in hypoxemia and the hyperdynamic circulatory state were reported after 5 hours following the administration of methylene blue (3 mg/kg over 15 minutes).[42]

Interventional radiology

The placement of TIPS (transjugular intrahepatic portosystemic shunting) to improve hypoxemia due to HPS remains controversial and cannot be advised at this time without further prospective study.[43,44] Coil embolotherapy to occlude discrete arteriovenous communications in patients with severe hypoxemia and type II HPS lesions has resulted in significant increases in PaO_2 in two adults.[45]

Orthotopic liver transplantation

The existence of HPS has evolved from an 'absolute' or 'relative' contraindication to 'indication' for liver transplantation in highly selected patients.[46–48] Complete resolution of hepatopulmonary syndrome, even in the setting of severe hypoxemia ($PaO_2 < 50$ mmHg), has been well documented.[6,48,49] In a retrospective review of 81 patients with HPS who underwent OLT, normalization of the pretransplant abnormal oxygenation was documented at 3–15 months post-OLT in both children and adults.[48] Prolonged intubation and mechanical ventilation occurred in 22% of HPS patients surviving the liver transplant procedure. Mortality following OLT in patients with HPS has been related to the severity of pretransplant PaO_2 and the degree of intrapulmonary vascular dilatation as measured by ^{99m}TcMAA lung perfusion scanning. Patients with a pre-OLT $PaO_2 < 50$ mmHg had a 30% mortality within 90 days of liver transplantation; no intraoperative deaths were reported. Brain uptake >20% following ^{99m}TcMAA lung scanning has been associated with higher mortality.[48–50] Significant mortality (38%) within 1 year of living related OLT in pediatric patients has been reported.[49] Key clinical observations in HPS patients who have undergone OLT are summarized in Table 27.3.

Other surgical options

Cavoplasty in Budd–Chiari syndrome and surgical ligation of portosystemic shunts have been reported to correct hypoxemia in highly selected HPS cases.[7]

FUTURE DIRECTIONS

Identification of the circulating vascular mediators and genetic predispositions associated with the pulmonary vascular remodeling associated with HPS remain high priorities for clinical investigation.

Table 27.3 *Outcomes following orthotopic liver transplantation (OLT) in hepatopulmonary syndrome (HPS)*

- An *indication* for OLT per Pediatric and Adult UNOS criteria*
- Resolution of the syndrome in 62–82% (3–15 months)[48,49]
- Mortality ranges from 16–38% within 1 year post-transplant[48,49]
- Pretransplant risk factors for increased mortality within 90 days of transplant
  - $PaO_2 < 50$ mmHg[48]
  - ^{99m}TcMAA brain uptake > 20%[49,51]
- Prolonged intubation/mechanical ventilation (4–77 days) in 22%[48]
- Recurrence of HPS following OLT extremely rare

PaO_2, arterial partial pressure of O_2; ^{99m}TcMAA, technetium-labeled macro-aggregated albumin; UNOS, United Network for Organ Sharing (6/28/01).

KEY POINTS

- The clinical triad of hepatic dysfunction, pulmonary vascular dilatations and arterial hypoxemia characterizes hepatopulmonary syndrome (HPS).
- Pulmonary vascular pathology documented in HPS includes diffuse precapillary/capillary dilatations, discrete arteriovenous communications and possible angiogenesis.
- Arterial hypoxemia may be severe and is caused by excess perfusion to ventilation ratios, diffusion-perfusion impairment and anatomic right-to-left shunts.
- Hypoxemia associated with HPS is usually progressive and correlates poorly with severity of chronic liver disease with a median survival of approximately 3 years.
- Liver transplantation may result in complete resolution of arterial hypoxemia caused by HPS; however, post-transplant mortality and time until syndrome resolution is strongly correlated to the severity of pretransplant PaO_2.

REFERENCES

1 Fluckiger M. Vorkommen von trommelschlagelformigen fingerendphalangen ohne chronische veriinderungen an den lungen oder am herzen. *Wien Med Wochenschr* 1884;**49**:1457–8.

●2 Rydell R, Hoffbauer FW. Multiple pulmonary arteriovenous fistulae in juvenile cirrhosis. *Am J Med* 1956;**21**:450–9.

3 Berthelot P, Walker JG, Sherlock S *et al.* Arterial changes in the lungs in cirrhosis of the liver: lung spider nevi. *N Engl J Med* 1966;**274**:291–8.

4 Kennedy TC, Knudsen RJ. Exercise-aggravated hypoxemia and orthodeoxia in cirrhosis. *Chest* 1977;**72**:305–9.

◆5 Krowka MJ. Leading article: Hepatopulmonary syndromes. *Gut* 2000;**46**:1–4.

◆6 Herve P, Lebrec D, Brenot F *et al*. Pulmonary vascular disorders in portal hypertension. *Eur Respir J* 1998;**11**:1153–66.

7 Krowka MJ. Hepatopulmonary syndrome and extrahepatic vascular abnormalities. *Liver Transpl* 2001;**7**:656–7.

8 Williams A, Trewby P, Williams R *et al*. Structural alterations to the pulmonary circulation in fulminant hepatic failure. *Thorax* 1979;**34**:447–53.

*9 Krowka MJ, Wiseman GA, Burnett OL *et al*. Hepatopulmonary syndrome: a prospective study of relationships between severity of liver disease, PaO_2 response to 100% oxygen, and brain uptake after ^{99m}TcMAA lung scanning. *Chest* 2000;**118**:815–24.

●10 Krowka MJ, Tajik AJ, Dickson ER *et al*. Intrapulmonary vascular dilatations (IPVD) in liver transplant candidates. *Chest* 1990;**97**:1165–70.

●11 Abrams GA, Nanda NC, Dubovsky EV *et al*. Use of macroaggregated lung perfusion scan to diagnose hepatopulmonary syndrome: a new approach. *Gastroenterology* 1998;**114**:305–10.

12 Whyte MKB, Hughes JMB, Peters AM *et al*. Analysis of intrapulmonary right to left shunt in hepatopulmonary syndrome. *J Hepatol* 1998;**29**:85–93.

13 McAdams HP, Erasmus J, Crockett R *et al*. The hepato-pulmonary syndrome: radiologic findings in 10 patients. *AJR Am J Roentgenol* 1996;**166**:1379–85.

14 Lee KN, Lee HJ, Shin WW *et al*. Hypoxemia and liver cirrhosis (hepatopulmonary syndrome) in eight patients: comparison of the central and peripheral pulmonary vasculature. *Radiology* 1999;**211**:549–53.

15 Edell ES, Cortese DA, Krowka MJ *et al*. Severe hypoxemia and liver disease. *Am Rev Respir Dis* 1989;**140**:1631–5.

16 Soderman C, Juhlin-Dannfelt A, Lagerstrand B *et al*. Ventilation-perfusion relationships and central hemodynamics in patients with cirrhosis; effects of somatostatin. *J Hepatol* 1994;**21**:52–7.

17 Agusti AGN, Roca J, Bosch J *et al*. The lung in patients with cirrhosis. *J Hepatol* 1990;**10**:251–7.

18 Melot C, Naeije R, Dechamps P *et al*. Pulmonary and extra-pulmonary contributors to hypoxemia in liver cirrhosis. *Am Rev Respir Dis* 1989;**139**:632–40.

19 Crawford ABH, Regnis J, Laks L *et al*. Pulmonary vascular dilatation and diffusion-dependent impairment of gas exchange in liver cirrhosis. *Eur Respir J* 1995;**8**:2015–21.

20 Thorens JB, Junod AF. Hypoxemia and liver cirrhosis: a new argument in favor of a 'diffusion-perfusion' defect. *Eur Respir J* 1992;**5**:754–6.

●21 Martinez G, Barbaera JA, Navasa M *et al*. Hepatopulmonary syndrome associated with cardiorespiratory disease. *J Hepatol* 1999;**30**:882–9.

*22 Abrams GA, Sanders MK, Fallon MB. Utility of pulse oximetry in the detection of arterial hypoxemia in liver transplant patients. *Liver Transpl* 2002;**8**:391–6.

23 Krowka MJ, Dickson ER, Cortese DA. Hepatopulmonary syndrome: clinical observations and lack of therapeutic response to somatostatin analogue. *Chest* 1993;**104**:515–21.

24 Park SC, Beerman LB, Gartner JC *et al*. Echocardiographic findings before and after liver transplantation. *Am J Cardiol* 1985;**55**:1373–8.

25 Donovan CL, Marcovitz, Punch JD *et al*. Two-dimensional and dobutamine stress echocardiography in the preoperative assessment of patients with end-stage liver disease prior to orthotopic liver transplantation. *Transplantation* 1996;**61**:1180–8.

26 Hopkins WE, Waggoner AD, Barzilai B. frequency and significance of intrapulmonary right-to-left shunt in end-stage hepatic disease. *Am J Cardiol* 1992;**70**:516–19.

27 Jensen DM, Pothamsetty S, Ganger D *et al*. Clinical manifestations of cirrhotic patients with intrapulmonary shunts. [Abstract] *Gastroenterology* 1994;**106**:A912.

28 Vedrinne JM, Duperret S, Bizollon T *et al*. Comparison of transesophageal and transthoracic contrast echocardiography for the detection of intrapulmonary shunt in liver disease. *Chest* 1997;**111**:1236–40.

29 Mimidis KP, Vassilakos PI, Mastoakou AN *et al*. Evaluation of contrast echocardiography and lung perfusion scan in detecting intrapulmonary vascular dilatation in normoxemic patients with early liver cirrhosis. *Hepatogastroenterology* 1998;**45**:2303–7.

30 Anand AC, Mukherjee D, Rao KS *et al*. Hepatopulmonary syndrome: prevalence and clinical profile. *Indian J Gastroenterol* 2001;**20**:24–7.

31 Rolla G, Brussino L, Colagrande P *et al*. Exhaled nitric oxide and oxygenation abnormalities in hepatic cirrhosis. *Hepatology* 1997;**27**:842–7.

32 Sogni P, Garnier P, Gadano A *et al*. Endogenous pulmonary nitric oxide production measured from exhaled air is increased in patients with severe cirrhosis. *J Hepatol* 1995;**23**:471–3.

●33 Cremona G, Higenbottam TW, Mayoral V *et al*. Elevated exhaled nitric oxide in patients with hepatopulmonary syndrome. *Eur Respir J* 1995;**8**:1883–5.

34 Nunes H, Lebrec D, Mazmanian M *et al*. Role of nitric oxide in hepatopulmonary syndrome in cirrhotic rats. *Am J Respir Crit Care Med* 2001;**164**:9879–85.

●35 Fallon MB, Abrams GA. Pulmonary dysfunction in chronic liver disease. *Hepatology* 2000;**32**:859–65.

36 Eddahibi S, Adnot S. Endothelins and pulmonary hypertension, what directions for the near future? *Eur Respir J* 2001;**18**:1–4.

37 Krowka MJ, Dickson ER, Cortese DA. Hepatopulmonary syndrome: clinical observations and lack of therapeutic response to somatostatin analogue. *Chest* 1993;**104**:515–21.

38 Krowka MJ, Cortese DA. Severe hypoxemia associated with liver disease: Mayo Clinic experience and the experimental use of almitrine bismesylate. *Mayo Clin Proc* 1987;**62**:164–73.

39 Abrams GA, Krowka MJ, Crapo RO *et al*. Treatment of hepatopulmonary syndrome with allium sativum (garlic). *J Clin Gastroenterol* 1998;**27**:232–5.

40 Song JY, Choi JY, Ko JT *et al*. Long term aspirin therapy for hepatopulmonary syndrome. *Pediatrics* 1996;**97**:917–20.

41 Cadranel JL, Milleron BJ, Cadrenal JF *et al*. Severe hypoxemia-associated intrapulmonary shunt in chronic liver disease improvement after medical treatment. *Am Rev Respir Dis* 1992;**146**:526–7.

42 Schenk P, Madl C, Rezaie-Majd S *et al*. Methylene blue improves hepatopulmonary syndrome. *Ann Intern Med* 2000;**133**:701–6.

43 Riegler JL, Lang KA, Johnson SP *et al.* Transjugular intrahepatic portosystemic shunt improves oxygenation in hepatopulmonary syndrome. *Gastroenterology* 1995;**109**:978–83.

44 Corley DA, Scharschmidt B, Bass N *et al.* Lack of efficacy of TIPS for hepatopulmonary syndrome. *Gastroenterology* 1997;**113**:728–31.

*45 Poterucha JJ, Krowka MJ, Dickson E *et al.* Failure of hepato-pulmonary syndrome to resolve after liver transplantation and successful treatment with embolotherapy. *Hepatology* 1995;**21**:96–100.

46 Van Thiel DH, Schade RR, Gavaler JS *et al.* Medical aspects of liver transplantation. *Hepatology* 1984;**4**(Suppl 1):79S–83S.

47 Maddrey WC, Van Theil DH. Liver transplantation: an overview. *Hepatology* 1988;**8**:948–59.

◆*48 Krowka MJ, Porayko MK, Plevak DJ *et al.* Hepatopulmonary syndrome with progressive hypoxemia as an indication for liver transplantation: case reports and literature review. *Mayo Clin Proc* 1996;**72**:44–53.

49 Egawa H, Hasahara M, Inomata Y *et al.* Long-term outcome of living related liver transplantation for patients with intrapulmonary shunting and strategy for complications. *Transplantation* 1999;**67**:712–17.

*50 Abrams GA, Krowka MJ, Fallon MB. Prospective evaluation of outcomes and predictors of mortality in patients undergoing liver transplantation for hepatopulmonary syndrome. *Hepatology* 2001;**34**(Pt 2):184A.

28

Pulmonary arteriovenous malformations

CLAIRE L SHOVLIN AND JAMES E JACKSON

INTRODUCTION

Historical overview

Pulmonary arteriovenous malformations (PAVMs) are abnormal vascular structures that provide a direct capillary-free communication between the pulmonary and systemic circulations. First described at postmortem,[1] affected individuals were subsequently recognized exhibiting the physiological consequences of a massive right-to-left shunt (dyspnea, cyanosis, clubbing and polycythemia). Some also demonstrated the consequences of paradoxical emboli through the shunts with the development of brain abscess.[2]

Soon after PAVMs were first described during life, a link with the inherited condition hereditary hemorrhagic telangiectasia (HHT, Osler–Weber–Rendu syndrome) was appreciated.[3] More than 90% of PAVMs are now known to be due to HHT, although sporadic cases undoubtedly also occur. With the introduction of surgical treatments for cyanotic congenital heart disease in the 1960s, a further type of PAVM became apparent, as PAVMs developed in the lung not receiving inferior caval blood via surgically generated cavopulmonary or atriopulmonary shunts.[4] The associations of PAVMs with the two disease processes HHT and cavopulmonary shunts have led to important breakthroughs in our understanding of their pathogenesis.

The clinical picture of PAVMs

It is often assumed that all patients with clinically significant PAVMs will have prominent respiratory symptoms. Unexplained and frequently profound hypoxemia is the hallmark of large PAVMs, but the majority of PAVM patients are asymptomatic (Table 28.1). In such patients, PAVMs are not benign, since the individuals remain at high risk of paradoxical embolism. Catastrophic embolic cerebral events (cerebral abscess and embolic stroke),

Table 28.1 *Clinical features of pulmonary arteriovenous malformations (PAVMs) on presentation (published series*)*

	Mean (%)	Range	No. of patients
Respiratory			
Asymptomatic	49	25–58	260
Dyspnea	49	27–71	483
Chest pain	14	6–18	198
Hemoptysis	11	4–18	479
Hemothorax	<1	0–2	192
Cyanosis	30	9–73	275
Clubbing	32	6–68	267
Bruit	49	25–58	263
Embolic phenomenon			
Cerebral abscess	9	0–25	368
CVA or TIA	27	11–55	401

*Series described in references 9 and 10. CVA, cerebrovascular accident; TIA, transient ischemic attack.

and transient ischemic attacks occur in patients regardless of the degree of respiratory symptoms,[5,6] and still carry significant morbidity and mortality.[7,8]

These complications can be limited if the condition is recognized and treated. Treatment of the asymptomatic patient was advocated as early as 1950,[11] but the benefits of intervention were mitigated by the significant morbidity associated with surgical resection. With the advent of embolization therapy in the late 1970s,[12] a parenchymal-sparing treatment regimen became available for patients. In experienced centers, there are proven long-term physiological benefits and excellent safety profiles of embolization. This has supported the trend towards earlier treatment of the asymptomatic patient, accompanied by clinical screening of high-risk groups.

Significant clinical concerns remain, however. First, many PAVM patients remain under regular follow-up in respiratory units without consideration of intervention. Second, published and anecdotal data suggest higher rates of complications in inexperienced hands. These include peri-procedural events and long-term development of systemic arterial feeders to the sac, resulting in catastrophic hemorrhage,[13] but are not widely recognized. Finally, modern detection methods reveal more disease than is treatable with today's technologies and much of current management lies in the long-term prevention of cerebral embolic events in patients with residual disease following maximal embolotherapy.

varying according to the relative vascular resistances of the shunt and normal lung. Where PAVMs are present in dependent portions of the lung, gravitational forces will increase flow through these shunts, a phenomenon first noted by auscultation, and more recently quantitated. As the majority of PAVMs are at the lung bases, orthodeoxia (desaturation on standing) is frequent.[22]

In chronically adapted patients, there is a reduced total pulmonary vascular resistance (PVR), low-normal mean pulmonary arterial pressure (PAP) and increased cardiac output ($\dot{Q}$).[23] In our recent study of 66 patients with a mean shunt of 12.8 ± 1%, the mean pulmonary artery pressure prior to embolization was 15.3 mmHg (range 8–36) with mean systolic and diastolic pressures of 26 and 8.8 mmHg, respectively.[10] In canine models, increased cardiac output is directly proportional to the increased flow through the shunt accompanied by an increase in stroke volume (presumably reflecting the increased left ventricular end diastolic pressure), with no effect on heart rate.[24] Effects of exercise on shunt flow have been contradictory,[23,25] probably reflecting variation in the size and compliance of feeding arteries to PAVMs with consequently variable capacity for further dilatation in response to increased cardiac output.

The true anatomic shunts of PAVMs are usually distinguished from the diffusion-perfusion defects that arise in patients with intrapulmonary vascular dilatations secondary to the hepatopulmonary syndrome

DEFINITIONS

Pulmonary arteriovenous malformations are abnormal vessels replacing the pulmonary capillary bed between the pulmonary arterial and venous circulations. They range in size from communications within the microvasculature (telangiectases[14]), to large complex structures consisting of a bulbous aneurysmal sac between dilated feeding arteries and draining veins[15] (Figure 28.1). Approximately 70% of PAVMs are basally situated.[5,16–20] Dilated feeding arteries and dilated veins are characterized by walls of varying degrees of thickness even over relatively short segments, with disorganized adventitia. Medial thinning is observed, but also prominent are areas of focal thickening with abundant elastin tissue and a varying contribution of smooth muscle cells.[14,21]

PAVMs result in a right-to-left shunt because they allow blood to flow directly from the right to left side of the circulation. In normal individuals, the anatomic shunt is less than 2% of the cardiac output, ascribed to the post-pulmonary drainage of bronchial veins into the pulmonary vein and thebesian vessels into the left atrium. PAVMs provide a low-resistance shunt pathway, with the fraction of the cardiac output flowing through the fistula

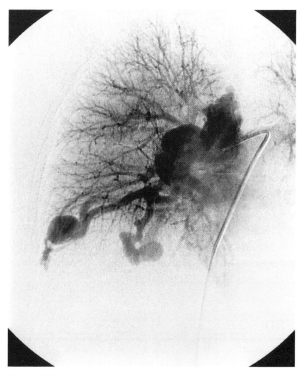

Figure 28.1 *Selective right pulmonary angiogram demonstrating two large basal pulmonary arteriovenous malformations (PAVMs).*

(HPS) in which the anatomic basis appears to be due to smaller vessels than usually discussed as representing PAVMs, and a physiological not anatomic shunt is produced (see Chapter 27).

INCIDENCE/EPIDEMIOLOGY

There have been no studies to assess the incidence of PAVMs in the general population, but due to the association with other diseases, an estimate may be made.

Careful family and personal histories and examination reveals that the majority of PAVMs occur in individuals affected by the inherited vascular disorder hereditary hemorrhagic telangiectasia (HHT, Osler–Weber–Rendu syndrome, discussed in the subsequent section). PAVMs affect more than 25% of HHT patients.[26,27] Since 1984, 242 PAVM patients have been reviewed at the Hammersmith hospital: for 223, records are available and of these, features of HHT were present in 203 (91%). The final proportion may be even higher given the late onset penetrance of the disorder. Recent careful epidemiological surveys suggest HHT incidences far in excess of previously quoted figures, including greater than 1 in 2500 in the Jura Valley in France[28] and the Dutch Antilles,[29] 1 in 6400 in Denmark[30] and 1 in 5000–8000 in Japan.[31] Assuming a conservative HHT prevalence of 1 in 8000 for the UK population of 60 million, there will be approximately 2000–2500 HHT-associated PAVM cases, and for the US population of 300 million, more than 10 000 cases. The majority of these will be undiagnosed. Further cases occur as a result of surgical treatments of several forms of complex cyanotic congenital heart disease, and these two etiological processes point towards pathogenic mechanisms (see below).

PAVMs only occasionally appear to develop in the prenatal or perinatal period,[32,33] and in these there is a 2:1 male:female predominence, in contrast to the female preponderance of approximately 1.6:1 seen in teenagers and adults.[5,6,10] Screening of individuals over a period of years shows that PAVMs can develop in adult life in radiologically and/or physiologically normal vessels,[34,35] although it is likely that functional changes at a cellular or microscopic level predate the development of the macroscopic lesions. Once present, PAVMs tend to increase in size,[36] particularly during puberty, and in female patients during pregnancy.[34]

ETIOLOGY

Macroscopic PAVMs may develop idiopathically, posttrauma (when they are more correctly termed arteriovenous fistulae), in association with hereditary hemorrhagic telangiectasia (HHT, accounting for the majority of PAVMs), and following surgery for congenital heart disease. They have also been described more rarely in association with other vascular conditions. In the absence of any previous trauma or cardiac surgery, a very careful search for HHT in the patient and their family is warranted, due to the importance of presymptomatic screening and treatment for other family members.

Hereditary hemorrhagic telangiectasia (HHT; Osler–Weber–Rendu syndrome) and PAVMs

HHT is usually recognized by physicians because of the consequences of abnormal dilated vessels developing in the systemic circulation, leading to epistaxes, mucocutaneous telangiectasia and iron deficiency anemia secondary to chronic nasal and/or gastrointestinal hemorrhage. In addition to PAVMs, large arteriovenous malformations (AVMs) also occur in several systemic vascular beds such as the cerebral, spinal, and hepatic circulations (Table 28.2). In contrast to cerebral AVMs that are thought to develop perinatally, the overwhelming majority of abnormal vessels in HHT, including PAVMs, develop postnatally. As a result, HHT exhibits age-dependent penetrance, with most index patients presenting in early to midadulthood. Manifestations are often progressive, with mucocutaneous and gastrointestinal telangiectasia in particular continuing to develop with time. PAVMs occur in at least 25% of HHT patients,[26,37] when they are often multiple. However, the diagnosis of HHT is frequently missed by physicians managing PAVM patients and made by us at the time of review.

MOLECULAR BASIS OF HHT

HHT is inherited as an autosomal dominant trait, and essentially indistinguishable forms of HHT arise from mutations in at least three genes: *endoglin* on chromosome 9,[38] *ALK1* encoding activin receptor-like kinase I, on chromosome 12,[39] and a third as yet unassigned gene.[35] Intriguingly, PAVMs occur most commonly in HHT patients with *endoglin* mutations, but PAVMs also occur in *ALK1*[40] and non-*endoglin*, non-*ALK1*[35] families.

Numerous different *endoglin* and *ALK1* mutations have been described to date in HHT (Figure 28.2). The prevailing view is that the mutations generate null alleles and that the molecular mechanism of HHT development is via haploinsufficiency. For *endoglin*, evidence includes the mutations resulting in absent mRNA[41] or unstable/ improperly processed proteins,[42,43] half-normal expression of endoglin on the endothelial cell surface,[21] and the fact that the human HHT phenotype can be recapitulated in endoglin$^\pm$ heterozygous mice.[44] Furthermore, there is no detectable clinical difference in phenotype between HHT patients with null (absent mRNA) mutations,

Table 28.2 *Important clinical features of hereditary hemorrhagic telangiectasia (HHT) patients and age-related penetrance*

Feature	Overall frequency (%)	Approximate penetrance at age (years)				
		0	15	25	45	90
Epistaxes (nose bleeds) (%)	>90	0	40	60	90	97
Mucocutaneous telangiectasia (%)	75	0	11	30	50	75
Chronic GI hemorrhage (%)	25	0	<1	1.5	12	25
Pulmonary AVMs (PAVMs) (%)	30					
Hepatic AVMs* (%)	20					
Cerebral AVMs (CAVMs) (%)	10					
Spinal AVMs (%)	<2					

*Data on age-related penetrance adapted from 324 patients reviewed in reference 90. Note that hepatic arteriovenous malformations (AVMs) are usually silent. GI, gastrointestinal.

endoglin mutations in HHT

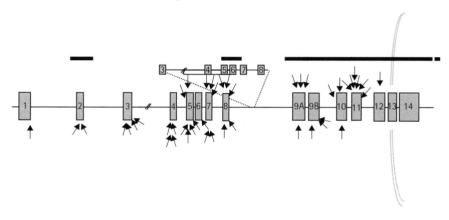

ALK1 mutations in HHT

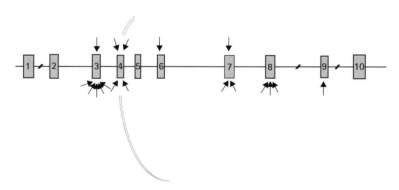

Figure 28.2 *A selection of hereditary hemorrhagic telangiectasia (HHT)-associated mutations.*

in-frame or out-of-frame deletions.[41] In all HHT cases resulting from *ALK1* mutations that have been characterized at the level of the endothelial cell, ALK1 surface expression is also half that of normal.[45] Debate continues whether there may be occasional examples of *endoglin* mutations acting in a dominant negative manner,[43,46] but since the most severe HHT phenotypes are seen in patients with proven null mutations,[41] any dominant negative mutants would be unlikely to contribute to a significant proportion of HHT cases.

The mechanisms whereby endoglin or ALK1 haploinsufficiency leads to the vascular anomalies seen in HHT have not been clarified, though the importance of endoglin and ALK1 in the development and maintenance of the vasculature has been demonstrated repeatedly by null mouse models (see for example references 44 and 47). Endoglin and *ALK1* encode transmembrane proteins expressed on vascular endothelial cells. These proteins modulate signaling by TGF-β family members, establishing a role of the TGF-β superfamily in mediating this disorder of the pulmonary circulation several years before the association with primary pulmonary hypertension (PPH). The TGF-β superfamily, including TGF-βs, activins, bone morphogenetic proteins (BMPs), growth/differentiation factors (GDFs) and inhibins, signal through heteromeric complexes composed of type I and type II cell surface receptor serine-threonine kinases.[48–51] These ligands, their receptors and downstream signaling moieties regulate a diverse series of fundamental pathways in development and pathophysiology. There is significant crosstalk with other signaling pathways, and interaction with additional proteins may support the potential diversity within the signaling system. Endoglin is a co-receptor for several members of the TGF-β superfamily,[52] whereas ALK1 is a type I receptor serine-threonine kinase. Each is known to influence at least TGF-β_1 signaling,[47,53] and there is likely to be a direct physical interaction between endoglin and ALK1.[45]

TRIGGERS FOR VASCULAR DEFECTS IN HHT

As in other vascular malformation syndromes, in any one individual with HHT, the majority of vascular beds develop normally with macroscopic malformations developing in only a small fraction. Similar to many other autosomal dominant diseases, different family members with the same underlying mutation have highly disparate phenotypes, which in the case of HHT may range from life-threatening events in childhood to non-penetrance.

Physiological factors, including changes in hemodynamics and hormones, are likely to play a role in generating this phenotypic diversity. Pulmonary AVMs are more common in women than in men with HHT, and have been shown to enlarge during pregnancy, with increased risk of pulmonary hemorrhage and death.[34] However, the heterozygous *endoglin* mouse emphasizes the importance of modifier genes and other potential factors such as plasma TGF-β_1 concentrations on disease expression.[54]

THE OVERLAP BETWEEN PPH AND HHT

The recent identification of the fundamental role of BMPR2 in pulmonary hypertension has indicated a further critical role of TGF-β superfamily signaling in pulmonary vascular responses.[55,56] The differences between these two diseases generating dilated pulmonary AVMs and the obstructive PPH lesions, at first sight appear overwhelming. A recent study, however, has demonstrated that PPH indistinguishable to that seen in classical PPH families with *BMPR2* mutations is observed in a proportion of HHT patients with *ALK1* mutations, but normal *BMPR2* sequence.[57] Intriguingly, PAVMs are less common in *ALK1* than *endoglin* HHT families.[58] This suggests that dysregulation of the vascular signaling pathways which produce the vascular dilations characteristic of HHT may also lead to the abnormalities resulting in PPH.

Cavopulmonary shunts

Surgical treatments of several forms of complex cyanotic congenital heart disease, particularly tetralogy of Fallot, rely on the establishment of anastomoses between the vena cavae and pulmonary arteries. Classic Glenn anastomoses result in PAVMs in the pulmonary artery not receiving the caval flow[4] – these PAVMs are macroscopically indistinguishable from sporadic and HHT-associated macroscopic PAVMs. It has been suggested that following superior bidirectional cavopulmonary anastomosis (BCPA), the development of functional intrapulmonary shunts [detectable by perfusion scans using technetium-99m (^{99m}Tc)-labelled albumin macroaggregates, see below] may be universal.[59] The key pathogenic feature appears to be the route taken by hepatic venous effluent, since PAVMs are found in the lung which receives no or minimal hepatic venous return.[60] This suggests that normal hepatic venous effluent protects the pulmonary circulation from development of PAVMs, though the exact mechanism remains the subject of experimental study.

CLINICAL PRESENTATION OF PAVMs

Untreated macroscopic PAVMs carry significant risks. The abnormal vessels may hemorrhage into a bronchus or the pleural cavity, sometimes with a fatal outcome.[34,61] However, it is the functional consequences of capillary-free communications between pulmonary and systemic circulations that most commonly cause problems (see Table 28.1). Pulmonary arterial blood passing through such right-to-left shunts escapes oxygenation, leading to hypoxemia. Furthermore, the absence of a filtering capillary bed allows paradoxical embolism of particulate matter which can reach the systemic arteries, causing clinical sequelae, particularly in the cerebral circulation. In historical series, mortality rates in untreated patients ranged from 4 to 40%, brain abscess occurred in up to 25%, and up to 80% of patients had MRI evidence of previous embolic CVAs (reviewed in reference 9). While these data probably overestimate the risks in patients managed with modern medical therapies, comparable data in series spanning more recent years are unlikely to become available as the majority of identified patients are offered treatment.

In spite of the significant hazards of untreated PAVMs, approximately 50% of patients have no respiratory symptoms at the time of presentation, even with physical signs such as cyanosis, clubbing, or a vascular bruit, or abnormal chest radiographs (see Table 28.1 and reference 10). The commonest symptom is dyspnea, but this may not be appreciated until after the condition has been treated. (PAVM patients even tolerate worsening hypoxemia on exercise well, reflecting their low pulmonary

Table 28.3 *Comparison of screening regimens*

	Study time (min)	Effective radiation dose	Availability	Other considerations
CXR PA and lateral	15	0.08 mSv	General	
Oxygen saturations	25	Nil	General	
Arterial blood gases	5	Nil	General	Arterial sample
100% O_2 study	30	Nil	General but local validation needed	Arterial samples (x2) Quantifies R–L shunt
Tc scan	30	<1 mSv[63]	Expertise limited	Quantifies R–L shunt
Spiral CT scan	30	4 mSv*	General	
Echocardiography	20	Nil	Expertise limited	

CT, computed tomography; CXR, chest x-ray; PA, posterior-anterior.

*Calculated for a 120 kVp, 5 mm slice, 24 cm scan, 1.0 s rotation (D McRobbie, personal communication).

vascular resistance and ability to generate a supranormal cardiac output which may increase further on exercise.[23]) Pleuritic chest pain of uncertain etiology occurs in up to 10% of patients. A similar percentage experience hemoptysis which may be due to accompanying endobronchial telangiectasia.

It is particularly important to recognize patients with paroxysmal neurological symptoms that may be attributable to transient ischemic attacks secondary to paradoxical emboli. These are not necessarily the more severely affected, as judged by respiratory symptoms or signs – many patients have no respiratory symptoms when presenting with the neurological complications, particularly transient ischemic attacks, stroke or cerebral abscess.

INVESTIGATIONS FOR PAVMs

The majority of PAVM patients are at risk of developing further lesions and therefore serial investigations are likely to be necessary. In an ideal setting therefore, PAVMs would be diagnosed at minimum cost and radiation dose. Many patients are diagnosed as a result of radiological investigations following clinical presentation with respiratory symptoms or signs. An abnormal plain chest radiograph is a classical mode of presentation, and optimal thoracic CT scans should identify all PAVMs suitable for embolization therapy.[62] Ideally, non-invasive diagnostic strategies should be employed, in particular to quantify the right-to-left shunt, both to assist the initial diagnosis where it is in doubt, and to provide a means to monitor both the response to treatment, and the development of any new lesions.

Different institutions have developed and optimized different regimens according to locally available expertise and the published results in any particular institution should not be extrapolated to another. No single test or group of tests is perfect, and there are no specific recommendations as to the precise type of diagnostic tests

which should be undertaken (Table 28.3). However, local expertise leads to within-center consistencies.

Specific investigations

STRUCTURAL INVESTIGATIONS

Chest radiographs

The radiographic appearances of PAVMs range from apparent normality (paticularly if diffuse small telangiectasia are present, or lower lobe lesions are obscured by a hemidiaphragm on the PA projection), through prominent bronchovascular markings, to the classical rounded mass with visible feeding or draining vessels. The sensitivity of plain radiographs varies widely according to the size and distribution of PAVMs.

Thoracic CT scanning

Compared to conventional axial CT scanning, helical scans (from apices to bases) are preferable both to increase sensitivity and to reduce the radiation burden for patients at risk of recurrent disease. Small lesions are less likely to be missed between the contiguous axial sections obtained by reconstructing the 'spiral' of information, because the sections are genuinely contiguous, unaffected by respiration as images are acquired in a single breath-hold. Sensitivity is further enhanced by reducing slice thickness and reconstructing the acquired data with a 50% overlap. Contrast is not required. Three-dimensional reconstructions provide impressive images,[62] although these are not required for diagnosis. Where there are difficulties with interpreting the circulatory origin of dilated apparently vascular structures, confirmation of right-to-left shunting is helpful.

METHODS TO DETECT AND QUANTIFY THE RIGHT-TO-LEFT SHUNTS

Flow-through anatomic intrapulmonary shunts can be detected by impaired oxygenation, or by tracing the passage of particles which should impact in the pulmonary capillaries, but can pass through shunt vessels. The first two methods described also provide the means for accurate quantification of the shunt.

Impaired oxygenation on room air

The simplest method for detecting a right-to-left shunt is the demonstration of hypoxemia breathing room air, but the differential diagnosis of hypoxemia is wide, and additional investigations are required to suggest that this is due to PAVMs rather than other etiologies. Further desaturation on assuming the upright posture, orthodeoxia, may be useful supporting evidence as the majority of PAVMs are in the lower lobes. The detection of hypoxemia alone, either by age-defined PaO_2, or SaO_2 from pulse oximetry is insufficiently sensitive to be used as a single diagnostic test.[26] Although in one study, SaO_2 in the erect posture, measured by pulse oximetry, was associated with sensitivity of 100% if $SaO_2 \le 97\%$,[64] our more recent data indicate that significant PAVMs diagnosed by thoracic CT scanning have been present with $SaO_2 \ge 98\%$ on room air.[7]

Impaired oxygenation following 100% O_2 rebreathing

One hundred per cent inspired oxygen rebreathing (to wash out alveolar nitrogen and eliminate ventilation/ perfusion mismatching) has been considered the gold standard for non-invasive methods of measuring the shunt as a fraction of the cardiac output.

$$\frac{Qs}{Qt} = \frac{(CcO_2 - CaO_2)}{(CcO_2 - C\bar{v}O_2)}$$

where CcO_2 represents the oxygen content of end-capillary blood, estimated from alveolar PO_2 (P_AO_2) obtained from the alveolar gas equation as it is assumed that $PcO_2 = P_AO_2$. $C\bar{v}O_2$ represents the oxygen content of mixed venous blood, estimated (since right heart catheterization is not performed) by assuming a normal arteriovenous oxygen content difference ($Ca - C\bar{v}$) of 5 mL/100 mL.

There are several practical problems with this method which depends upon good patient technique, two sets of arterial blood gas sampling without contamination by air bubbles, and calibration of the oxygen electrode with blood tonometry or commercially available sealed buffer solutions at high PaO_2. In addition, recent data highlight that the ($Ca - C\bar{v}$) estimate of 5 mL/100 mL is too high for the majority of HHT patients (mean value 4.4 mL/100 mL), resulting in an underestimate of the size of the shunt by approximately 10%.[65] The lower than normal ($Ca - C\bar{v}$) probably reflects the higher than normal cardiac output, and presence of systemic left-to-right shunts in patients with telangiectasia or larger AVMs due to HHT.[65] At best, the sensitivity of this test approaches 90%, though this depends upon local expertise.

Radionuclide scanning

Following intravenous injection of technetium-99m (^{99m}Tc)-labelled albumin microspheres (7–25 μm) or macroaggregates (10–80 μm), the right-to-left shunt can be assessed by calculating the quantity of tracer reaching the systemic circulation compared to the total quantity received.[66] Ideally, renal flow should be measured directly using a second tracer,[65] although often the calculation assumes that the right kidney receives 10% of the cardiac output. Recent data from our institution which has extensive experience with this method indicated that a shunt measurement >3.5% had 87% sensitivity and 61% specificity for the presence of PAVMs.[64]

Right-to-left shunt measurements obtained by ^{99m}Tc-scanning methods correlated well with 100% inspired oxygen methods in two centers, with correlation coefficients of at least 0.77.[65,66] However, the methods cannot be used interchangeably in follow-up of shunt size in a particular patient[65] as the measurements include subtly different parameters. For example, in contrast to Tc scanning, 100% oxygen methods will underestimate the shunt (even if $Ca - C\bar{v}$ is measured rather than assumed) if microsopic AVMs are participating in gas exchange. Conversely, 100% oxygen methods (but not radionuclide scanning) will include the normal anatomic shunt due to venous admixture which may total up to 2% of the cardiac output.

Contrast echocardiography

This method traces the circulatory transit of microbubbles generated by intravenously injected echocontrast. In contrast to intracardiac shunts (in which contrast passes immediately from the right to the left ventricle), right-to-left shunting through PAVMs results in a delayed appearance of microbubbles in the left ventricle and systemic arteries (within 5–10 cardiac cycles). The shunt currently cannot be quantified by this method.

Contrast echocardiography is widely advocated as the most sensitive method of detecting right-to-left shunting, and is widely used in the congenital heart disease population, particularly for detection of microscopic disease.[59,60] Initial reports in the adult HHT population suggested 100% sensitivity,[27] but these figures are being revised downwards with further data suggesting a false-negative rate of at least 10%.[67] Two studies have compared the sensitivity of contrast echocardiography with the 100% oxygen rebreathing method: in one, they were similar,[27] whereas in a second, contrast echocardiography was more sensitive (93% compared to 66%) though the sensitivity of the oxygen shunt method was less than reported in other series.[67] Further refinement of these methods, including the use of spectral Doppler techniques and quantification of contrast echocardiography signals, is under development.[68]

However, the correlation of contrast echocardiography and direct measurement of pulmonary venous SaO_2 or angiographically visible vessels during cardiac catheterization is poor. Although more than 90% of lungs with pulmonary venous desaturation were correctly detected by

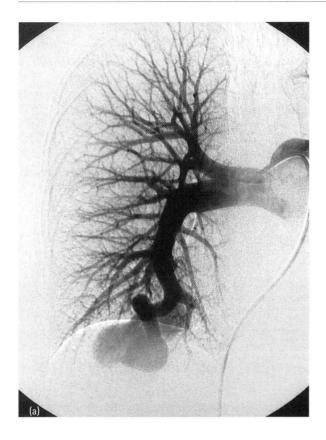

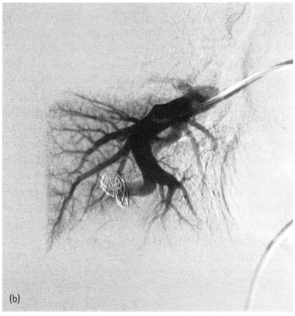

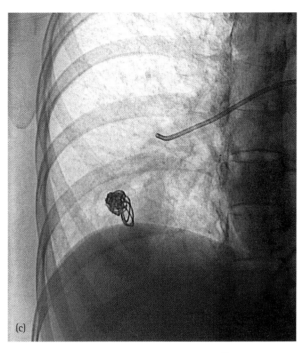

Figure 28.3 *(a) Pre- and (b) post-embolization angiograms, and (c) post-embolization chest radiographs of a patient with pulmonary arteriovenous malformations (PAVMs).*

contrast echocardiography in a recent study,[69] in 6 out of 11 cases with strongly positive echocardiography as assessed by two blinded observers, no clinically relevant shunt was present.

Magnetic resonance imaging

MR scanning has been less effective than CT or pulmonary angiography as small PAVMs with rapid blood flow are not visualized.[70] Methodology is improving, however,[71,72] and since this modality provides no radiation burden, we expect that the frequency of its use will increase.

TREATMENT/MANAGEMENT

Expectant management is indicated only when physician and patient are fully informed of the risks of leaving PAVMs untreated – PAVMs are not benign lesions that can be safely ignored.

Management modalities

EMBOLIZATION, THE MAINSTAY OF TREATMENT

Embolization techniques, described in detail elsewhere,[73] lead to occlusion of the feeding vessels to PAVMs with thrombus which organizes either on thrombogenic fibers associated with carefully positioned metallic coils or secondary to the stasis of blood by an occluding balloon, or, more rarely, other devices[74] (Figure 28.3). Embolization series published to date provide clear evidence for regression of the PAVM sac,[62] in addition to reduction in the right-to-left shunt and improvement in hypoxemia (Table 28.4). While physiological measurements related to the shunt consistently demonstrate more dramatic

Table 28.4 *Outcomes in pulmonary arteriovenous malformation (PAVM) treatment series*

Center/reference	No. of patients	R–L shunt*		PaO$_2$/SaO$_2^\dagger$		Residual shunt present (%)
		Pre	Post	Pre	Post	
Baltimore/Yale						
pre 1983[75]	10	44%	24%	43 mmHg (sitting)	64 mmHg (sitting)	100
1978–1987[19]	76	?	?	47 mmHg	68 mmHg	?
1978–1995[76]	45	?	?	56.6 mmHg	84.1 mmHg	?
Hammersmith						
1984–1990[77]	16	28%	13%	87.5% (supine)	92.4% (supine)	100
1987–1994[20]	53	23%	9%	83%	93%	60
1994–1999[10]	66	12.8%	5.9%	93%	96%	72
San Francisco						
1986–1991[25]	8	25%	13%	55 mmHg (seated)	77 mmHg (seated)	?
Netherlands						
1990–1995[78]	32	16.6%	7.4%	9.6 kPa (sem-rec‡)	11.5 kPa (sem-rec‡)	63
Denmark						
1994–1998[79]	12	21^{TP}	13^{TP}	266 mmHg (100% FiO$_2$)	439 mmHg (100% FiO$_2$)	73

* Per cent shunt quantitation by 100% FiO$_2$ rebreathing,[25,78] Tc scanning,[20] or contrast echocardiography;[79] R–L, right–left.
$\dagger$ Erect posture except where stated, as erect SaO$_2$ (arterial oxygen saturation) best predictor of shunt size.[64]
$\ddagger$ Sem-rec, semi-recumbent.
^{TP} Calculated from PaO$_2$ (arterial partial pressure of O$_2$).

improvements than exercise capacity, we have recently demonstrated a small but significant difference between the pre- and post-embolization workload measurements in patients who have been maximally treated.[10]

SURGERY

Embolization has generally supplanted surgical procedures, due to reduced periprocedural risks, parenchymal sparing in patients at risk of recurrent disease, and the documented physiological benefits. Although no surgical series describes physiological outcomes in any detail, procedural morbidity has been reduced since the historical mortality data were obtained, particularly with the use of video-assisted thoracoscopic techniques.[80] There may therefore be situations in which limited surgical resection is more appropriate than embolization. However, the likelihood of recurrent disease in non-resected lobes of PAVM patients (especially when there is underlying HHT) remains. Ideally, surgery should only be undertaken after full consideration of the best available embolization outcome, if necessary involving assessment by other units with expertise in embolization – a recent suggestion that surgery should be favored over embolization,[81] arose from poor embolization results at a single center.[76]

MEDICAL MANAGEMENT

Although formal treatment of PAVMs either by angiographic embolization techniques or by surgery is required to radically alter the long-term prognosis,

several medical maneuvers are recommended in patients suspected of having PAVMs. Antibiotic prophylaxis is recommended prior to dental and surgical interventions – our medical alert card for patients has been approved by The British Society for Antimicrobial Chemotherapy and Dental Formulary Subcommittee. Female patients should be advised to defer pregnancy pending formal assessment and treatment in view of the risks of PAVM growth and rupture during pregnancy.[34] There are no data on additional maneuvers to reduce thromboembolic risks, but based on the high frequency of cerebral thromboembolic complications in these patients,[82] options such as cessation of hormonal therapy or possible benefits of antiplatelet therapy may be considered on a case-by-case basis for patients experiencing transient ischemic attacks, even if there is underlying HHT.

Importance of regular follow-up with shunt assessments

Following initially complete embolization or surgical resection, residual macroscopic disease may develop several months after treatment, following a period of vascular remodeling. It is well recognized that removal of a low-resistance shunt can unmask or provoke the development of additional PAVMs elsewhere in the pulmonary circulation, and occasionally, new pulmonary artery feeder vessels to the treated lesion. As a result, review of all patients and right-to-left shunt measurement after several months is generally recommended, and a series of treatments may be needed.

Table 28.5 *Pulmonary artery (PA) pressures in patient with coexisting pulmonary hypertension pre- and post-embolization**

	PA pressures (mmHg)			SaO$_2$ (%)	
	Systolic	Diastolic	Mean	Supine	Erect
Pre-embolization	60	30	40	94	95
Post-embolization	40	15	27	97	96

SaO$_2$, arterial oxygen saturation.

*Pulmonary hypertension ascribed to coexistent ischaemic heart disease.

Special circumstances

MANAGEMENT STRATEGY FOR PREGNANT PATIENTS

Since our initial description of pregnancy-induced PAVM growth,[34] we have witnessed a consistent and near-predictable deterioration in PAVM status post-pregnancy, with evidence of some spontaneous improvement postpartum. There have also been patients who have embarked on pregnancy after maximal embolotherapy and have had life-threatening hemoptysis in late pregnancy. We recommend pre-pregnancy screening and maximal treatment, and in addition, alert patients and their medical practitioners to this possibility of hemoptysis which would require urgent admission and management. Embolization in the second and third trimesters is feasible and safe.[83]

MANAGEMENT IN PRESENCE OF PRE-EXISTING PULMONARY HYPERTENSION

Occasionally, it may be deemed inappropriate to treat PAVMs. This may be the case in rare patients in whom pulmonary hypertension and PAVMs coexist, as removal of a low-resistance shunt would be expected to aggravate the pulmonary hypertension.[25,78] Even in these cases, in our experience, there may be unpredictable beneficial responses to embolization, probably reflecting a greater proportional fall in cardiac output than rise in pulmonary vascular resistance (Table 28.5). Test occlusion with measurement of PA pressures may be warranted.

SEVERE DIFFUSE DISEASE: A ROLE FOR LUNG TRANSPLANTATION?

Lung transplantation has been undertaken in a few patients with severe hypoxemia secondary to diffuse disease (see, for example, reference 84). However, the long-term complications of PAVMs are likely in most cases to be less than transplantation-associated morbidity. Three PAVM patients in our clinic (one male, two female) who elected not to proceed with transplantation after discussion of the risks at two different UK transplant centers have since remained stable over 8, 9 and 13 years, and one has had three successful pregnancies. In a retrospective series of 16 cyanosed patients with diffuse PAVMs (mean PaO$_2$ 47 mmHg) for whom follow-up data were available for between 0.3 and 17 years, the 2-year survival rate was 91%, and over a mean follow-up period of 6 years, 11 of the original 16 were working or studying full time.[85]

Which PAVMs are safe to leave untreated?

SMALL PAVMs (≤3 mm FEEDING ARTERY)

Technical issues limit the size of feeding arteries which can be embolized. In addition, there is a widely held belief that it is the larger PAVMs that are predominantly responsible for embolic events based on suggestions that a feeding artery size of greater than 3 mm can be used to predict the likelihood of certain neurological sequelae.[82] A 3 mm 'rule' has become established in conventional practice, and is now being used to define PAVMs of importance for screening purposes.[71,72,86] Physiological considerations suggest that pathological thromboemboli could pass through vessels of much smaller caliber. Many centers routinely treat PAVMs with feeding vessels between 2 and 3 mm in diameter,[10,87] and we recommend medical PAVM treatment for all patients with residual shunts, irrespective of the size of the feeding vessels, as smaller feeding vessels have been associated with cerebral abscess.[7] We now classify our post embolization patients into three groups:

- group I in whom complete occlusion of all angiographically visible PAVMs is achieved;
- group II in whom complete occlusion of all PAVMs with feeding vessels ≥3 mm diameter is achieved;
- group III in which further embolizations are planned.

N.B.: In many centers, groups I and II would be considered 'complete' treatment. In our latest series of 58 patients in whom all vessels down to 2 mm in diameter had been embolized, 40 (69%) had residual disease, in keeping with the three other major series since 1990 (60–73%, Table 28.4). We suspect that an indication by a center that suggests they have little or no residual disease post-treatment reflects insensitive methods of detecting residual disease, unless they are focusing purely on the small percentage of PAVM patients who have single PAVMs and do not have HHT.

MICROSCOPIC DISEASE OR FALSE-POSITIVE RESULTS?

With the introduction of non-invasive screening tests for PAVMs it has become evident that in some cases, angiography does not detect shunts previously identified by non-invasive methods, and which cannot be attributed to intracardiac lesions. Ten of the 25 patients with positive contrast echocardiogram studies in one series,[27] 20% in a second[67] and 6 of 11 patients in a third[69] did not have lesions detected by subsequent angiography or pulmonary venous oxygen saturation measurements.

Are these apparent shunts 'false positives' or do they represent lesions too small for detection by the previously accepted gold standard of pulmonary angiography? There is a paucity of data in normal adult controls, and there is limited further information on the echopositive angio-negative HHT patients such as KCO measurements or long-term neurological sequelae. It is therefore possible that a significant proportion of these and possibly other screening modality 'false positives' reflect normal variation, rather than microscopic PAVM disease. There are, however, considerable data indicating that microscopic PAVMs may be present in HHT patients with macroscopic PAVMs. In some angiographic sessions, a continuum in lesion sizes from grossly dilated sacs to vessels associated with rapid shunt flow though macroscopically normal may be observed. Furthermore, CO transfer coefficient (KCO) may be reduced, suggesting the presence of microvascular disease.[10,20] As the primary goal should be to detect all lesions which carry potential clinical sequelae, we believe it is safer to assume that 'false positives' represent microscopic PAVM disease, with attendant requirements for medical follow-up.

Hammersmith screening protocols

Our assessments for patients with possible PAVMs routinely include posteroanterior and lateral chest radiographs and SaO_2 in erect and supine postures, accompanied by spirometry and assessment of gas transfer (KCO). Patients are then directed to thoracic CT scans to visualize the size and structure of putative PAVMs, and ^{99m}Tc-radionucleide shunt studies. Contrast echocardiography is performed as part of research protocols only (see following section and Figure 28.4).

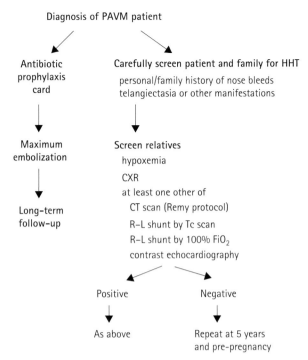

Figure 28.4 *Algorithm for investigation of a pulmonary arteriovenous malformation (PAVM) patient. CT, computed tomography; CXR, chest x-ray; FiO$_2$, fraction of inspired oxygen; HHT, hereditary hemorrhagic telangiectasia; R–L, right–left.*

Detection of underlying HHT and family screening of PAVM patients

Diagnosis and treatment of any PAVM is only one part of the management of a PAVM patient. It is crucial that the physician is alert to the possibility of HHT in the patient and therefore other family members. PAVMs may be the first sign of HHT in the presenting patient, and may be the only feature of HHT evident in patients through their 30s, 40s, 50s and beyond. (The mean penetrance of HHT reaches 95% by 40 years of age, but is only 62% by 16 years,[88–90] Table 28.2.) Mucocutaneous telangiectasia are often subtle. Furthermore, the majority of patients will not volunteer a personal or family history of nosebleeds unless specifically asked, and allowed time to check with relatives, at least 80% of PAVM patients will have underlying HHT, a diagnosis that should be sought in all cases (see algorithm, Figure 28.4). All patients with PAVMs should be alerted to the possibility of HHT in their family.

Current clinical diagnostic criteria for a definitive diagnosis of HHT require the presence of three out of four key features, namely:

- spontaneous recurrent epistaxis,
- telangiectases at characteristic sites,
- a visceral manifestation and
- an affected first-degree relative[91] (Table 28.2).

Table 28.6 *Complications of treatment in pulmonary arteriovenous malformation (PAVM) treatment series*

	Center	No. of patients	No. of PAVM	Complications expressed as % of patients				
				Angina	Pleurisy	Parenchymal infarction	Paradoxical embolus	Balloon deflation
Expectant management								
Hammersmith 1995–99[10]	1	66	225				54%	
Interventional series								
Baltimore/Yale pre-1983[75]	2	10	58	10%	20%		several	
Baltimore/Yale 1978–87[19]	2	76	276	5%	10%	1.3%	2.6%	
France pre-1991[87]	3	19	58	–	26%	31%	2%	
Baltimore-Yale[94]	2		96	4%	5%		2–3%*	10%*4/96
Netherlands[78]	4	32	92	–	9%	–	4.5%	3%
Hammersmith[20]	1	53	200	3%	9%	–	2%	
Baltimore/Yale 1978–95[76] large PAVM 8 mm diam	2	45	–	2%	31%			
Denmark 1994–98[79]	5	12	20	0	36%			
Japan, pre- 1998[13]	6	7	14					57%†
Hammersmith 1995–99[10]	1	66	225	5%	5%	3%	1.5%†	

* 1/96 PAVMs.
† Early in series: has not recurred since introduction of detachable coils.
† 50% of these had systemic arterial feeder.

Detailed management of the non-pulmonary aspects of HHT is beyond the scope of this text and the reader is referred to several recent reviews.[9,92,93] Families can be provided with information about HHT patient self-help groups, HHT Foundation International (http://www.hht.org) and the UK Telangiectasia Self Help group (http://www.telangiectasia.cwc.net).

PAVM screening programs in patients with HHT deserve consideration, as these involve large numbers of individuals (PAVM screening cannot be limited to individuals with particular genotypes as previously suggested). Not every asymptomatic offspring of an HHT-affected patient can pass through the entire repertoire of screening methods. For rapid exclusion of PAVMs, readily available, low-cost, simple screening tests with sensitivities approaching 100% are required. Based on published data of sensitivities of over 85%, different units use oximetry ($SaO_2 \geq 98\%$), arterial blood gases, 100% oxygen breathing, contrast echocardiography, thoracic CT scanning or a combination of methods, but there is no consensus. The optimal screening intervals are unknown. Current recommendations are to screen every 5–10 years or if the patient is approaching a period known to be associated with PAVM enlargement and rupture, such as puberty or pregnancy. Given the development of lesions over a 2- to 3-year period, even these rarely instituted regimens may be insufficient. It is particularly important to screen prior to, or if necessary during pregnancy, in view of the maternal risks of PAVMs[34,61] and the opportunity for safe embolization

procedures even in the third trimester. (It should be noted that desaturation due to right-to-left shunting may be masked by physiological factors during pregnancy.)[34]

COMPLICATIONS OF PAVM TREATMENT

Embolization has been widely introduced, but it is important to note that treatment outcomes are not equivalent at all centers. Published series show varying efficacy and consistent within-center improvements with operator experience and/or technical developments. The severity and frequency of reported procedural complications also varies (Table 28.6). For example, the most common symptom developing post-procedure is self-limiting pleurisy, the frequency varying from 9 to 36% of patients according to the series. Transient angina or arrhythmias have been reported in between zero and 29% of patients. In addition, inappropriate placement of coils or balloons by less experienced operators may lead to significant difficulties in subsequent management of PAVMs.[13] These data highlight the importance of embolization being undertaken in centers with sufficient experience and a proven track record.

Coil or balloon displacement

Paradoxical emboli could result in tissue infarction, potentially most severe in cerebral and coronary circulations.

This has been a well recognized risk of pulmonary angiography, and great care is taken to avoid this possibility. It is instructive therefore, to compare the low rates in PAVM treatment series (Table 28.6) to the 35% incidence of pulmonary emboli of cyanoacrylate or platinum coils following embolization of cerebral AVMs.[95] For PAVMs, in addition to embolization of coils or balloons, the thrombotic mass in the embolized sac has the potential to embolize prior to organization, and there are some data to suggest this may be the case, particularly when there is a persistent feeder, as in one individual treated by an experienced center.[96] Avoidance of strenuous exercise in the week following embolization, as suggested by the Dutch group,[96] may be appropriate.

Recanalization with systemic feeding artery

Recanalization by further pulmonary arterial feeders may result in requirements for further embolization, but it is the risk of recanalization by systemic arterial feeders that poses the greater potential risk to patients. This has been described in as many of 50% of cases from smaller series (4/8 PAVMs[13]). Although it may be considered that this may pose less of a problem than the original right-to-left shunt,[97] the risk of systemic arterial pressures in the dilated PAVMs cannot be underestimated. We are aware of a number of cases where massive hemoptysis has occurred attributable to systemic arterial feeders to PAVMs developing post-embolization.

Precipitation of right ventricular failure if coexistent pulmonary hypertension

As discussed above, in rare patients in whom pulmonary hypertension and PAVMs coexist, removal of a low-resistance shunt may aggrevate the pulmonary hypertension.[25,78] As there may be unpredictable beneficial responses to embolization, measurement of pulmonary artery pressures following temporary inflation of an occlusion balloon may be warranted (see Table 28.5).

FUTURE DIRECTIONS OF THERAPY

We suspect that in expert hands, transcatheter embolization techniques may have reached potential technical limits: it is doubtful that advances will permit routine embolization of feeding vessels of less than 2 mm in diameter. We would suggest that new medical therapeutic modalities developed from a clear understanding of the pathogenic basis of PAVMs are likely to provide the next significant advance. The importance of such maneuvers will depend on elucidation of the true natural history of the smaller shunt vessels.

KEY POINTS

- Fifty per cent of patients with PAVMs are asymptomatic. However, all patients with PAVMs are at risk of stroke and cerebral abscess due to paradoxical emboli through the right-to-left shunt. PAVMs can be readily detected by non-invasive methods, and safely treated.
- Treatment should be considered for all patients to limit complications from PAVMs. Embolization is the treatment of choice, and can be repeated. Surgery should be only rarely undertaken because of the likelihood of extensive or recurrent disease. All patients with PAVMs should receive antibiotic prophylaxis for dental or surgical procedures.
- Ninety per cent of PAVM patients will have hereditary hemorrhagic telangiectasia and an 'at-risk' family. All PAVM patients with HHT need long-term follow-up to assess for growth of new PAVMs. No relatives of patients with PAVMs should be allowed to present with catastrophic consequences of a cerebral abscess.

REFERENCES

1 Churton TL. Multiple aneurysm of pulmonary artery. *Br Med J* 1897;**1**:1223.
2 Reading B. A case of congenital telangiectasia of the lung complicated by brain abscess. *Texas State J Med* 1932;**23**:462.
3 Rundles RW. Hemorrhagic telangiectasia with pulmonary artery aneurysm: case report. *Am J Med Sci* 1945; **210**:76–81.
●4 Kopf G, Laks H, Stansel H *et al.* Thirty-year follow-up of superior vena cava-pulmonary artery (Glenn) shunts. *J Thorac Cardiovasc Surg* 1990;**100**:662–71.
●5 Dines DE, Arms RA, Bernatz PE *et al.* Pulmonary arteriovenous fistulas. *Mayo Clin Proc* 1974;**49**:460–5.
●6 Dines DE, Steward JB, Bernatz PE. Pulmonary arteriovenous fistulas. *Mayo Clin Proc* 1983;**58**:176–81.
7 Benjamin A, Jackson JE, Shovlin CL. Cerebral abscess in patients with pulmonary arteriovenous malformations (abstract). *Am J Respir Crit Care Med* 2002;**165**:A330.
8 Easey A, Wallace GMF, Hughes JMB *et al.* Should asymptomatic patients with hereditary haemorrhagic telangiectasia (HHT) be screened for cerebral malformations? Data from 22,061 years of patient life. *J Neurol Neurosurg Psychiatry* 2002;**74**:743–8.
◆9 Shovlin CL, Letarte M. Hereditary haemorrhagic telangiectasia and pulmonary arteriovenous malformations: issues in clinical management and review of pathogenic mechanisms. *Thorax* 1999;**54**:714–29.
●10 Gupta P, Mordin C, Curtiss J *et al.* PAVMs: effect of embolization on right-to-left shunt, hypoxemia and exercise

tolerance in 66 patients. *AJR Am J Roentgenol* 2002;**179**:347–55.

11 Lindskog G, Liebow A, Kausel H *et al.* Pulmonary arteriovenous aneurysm. *Ann Surg* 1950;**132**:591–610.

•12 Postmann W. Therapeutic embolization of arteriovenous pulmonary fistulas by catheter technique. In: Kelop O (ed.), *Current concepts in pediatric radiology.* Berlin: Springer, 1977;23–31.

13 Sagara K, Miyazono N, Inoue H *et al.* Recanalization after coil embolotherapy of pulmonary arteriovenous malformations: study of long term outcome and mechanism for recanalization. *Am J Roentgenol* 1998;**170**:727–30.

14 Hales M. Multiple small arteriovenous fistulas of the lungs. *Am J Pathol* 1956;**32**:927–37.

15 Anabtawi IA, Ellison RG, Ellison LT. Pulmonary arteriovenous aneurysms and fistulas. *Ann Thorac Surg* 1965;**1**:277–85.

16 Stringer C, Stanley A, Bates R *et al.* Pulmonary arteriovenous fistula. *Am J Surg* 1955;**89**:1054–80.

17 Bosher L, Blake A, Byrd B. An analysis of the pathologic anatomy of pulmonary arteriovenous aneurysms with particular reference to the applicability of local excision. *Surgery* 1959;**45**:91–104.

•18 Shumacker H, Waldhausen J. Pulmonary arteriovenous fistulas in children. *Ann Surg* 1963;**158**:713–20.

•19 White RI, Lynch-Nyhan A, Terry P *et al.* Pulmonary arteriovenous malformations: techniques and long-term outcomes of embolotherapy. *Radiology* 1988;**169**:663–9.

•20 Dutton JAE, Jackson JE, Hughes JMB *et al.* Pulmonary arteriovenous malformations: results of treatment with coil embolization in 53 patients. *Am J Roentgenol* 1995;**165**:1119–25.

21 Bourdeau A, Cymerman U, Paquet M-E *et al.* Endoglin expression is reduced on normal vessels but still detectable in arteriovenous malformations of patients with hereditary hemorrhagic telangiectasia type I. *Am J Pathol* 2000;**156**:911–23.

•22 Ueki T, Hughes JMB, Peters AM *et al.* Oxygen and ^{99m}Tc-MAA shunt estimations in patients with pulmonary arteriovenous malformations: effects of changes in posture and lung volume. *Thorax* 1994;**49**:327–31.

•23 Whyte MKB, Hughes JMB, Jackson JE *et al.* Cardiopulmonary response to exercise in patients with intrapulmonary vascular shunts. *J Appl Physiol* 1993;**75**:321–8.

24 Waldhausen J, Abel F. The circulatory effects of pulmonary arteriovenous fistulas. *Surgery* 1966;**59**:76–80.

•25 Pennington D, Gold W, Gordon R *et al.* Treatment of pulmonary arteriovenous malformations by therapeutic embolization. *Am Rev Respir Dis* 1992;**145**:1047–51.

•26 Haitjema T, Disch F, Overtoom TTC *et al.* Screening family members of patients with hereditary hemorrhagic telangiectasia. *Am J Med* 1995;**99**:519–24.

•27 Kjeldsen AD, Oxhøj H, Andersen PE *et al.* Pulmonary arteriovenous malformations: Screening procedures and pulmonary angiography in patients with hereditary hemorrhagic telangiectasia. *Chest* 1999;**116**:432–9.

28 Bideau A, Brunet G, Heyer E *et al.* An abnormal concentration of cases of Rendu-Osler disease in the Valserine valley of the French Jura: a geneological and demographic study. *Ann Hum Biol* 1992;**19**:233–47.

29 Jessuron GA, Kamphuis DJ, Zande FH *et al.* Cerebral arteriovenous malfomations in the Netherlands Antilles. High prevalence of hereditary hemorrhagic telangiectasia-related single and multiple cerebral arteriovenous malformations. *Clin Neurol Neurosurg* 1993;**95**:193–8.

30 Kjeldsen AD, Vase P, Green A. Hereditary hemorrhagic telangiectasia (HHT): a population-based study of prevalence and mortality in Danish HHT patients. *J Intern Med* 1999;**245**:31–9.

31 Dakeishi M, Shioya T, Wada Y *et al.* Genetic epidemiology of hereditary hemorrhagic telangiectasia in a local community in the northern part of Japan. *Hum Mutat* 2002;**19**:140–8.

32 Higgins C, Wexler L. Clinical and angiographic features of pulmonary arteriovenous fistulas in children. *Radiology* 1976;**119**:171–5.

33 Olgunturk R, Oguz D, Tunaoglu S *et al.* Pulmonary arteriovenous malformation in the newborn. *Turkish J Pediatr* 2001;**43**:332–7.

•34 Shovlin CL, Winstock AR, Peters AM *et al.* Medical complications of pregnancy in hereditary haemorrhagic telangiectasia. *Q J Med* 1995;**88**:879–87.

35 Wallace GMF, Shovlin CL. A hereditary haemorrhagic telangiectasia family with pulmonary involvement is unlinked to the known HHT genes, endoglin and ALK-1. *Thorax* 2000;**55**:685–90.

36 Shovlin CL, Jackson JE. Pulmonary arteriovenous malformations and aneurysms. In: Gibson J, Geddes D, Costabel U *et al.* (eds), *Respiratory medicine*, 3rd edn. London: Harcourt, 2002.

37 Kjeldsen A, Oxhoj H, Andersen P *et al.* Prevalence of pulmonary arteriovenous malformations (PAVMs) and occurrence of neurological symptoms in patients with hereditary haemorrhagic telangiectasia. *J Int Med* 2000;**248**:255–62.

•38 McAllister KA, Grogg KM, Johnson DW *et al.* Endoglin, a TGF-β binding protein of endothelial cells, is the gene for hereditary haemorrhagic telangiectasia type 1. *Nat Genet* 1994;**8**:345–51.

•39 Johnson DW, Berg JN, Baldwin MA *et al.* Mutations in the activin receptor-like kinase 1 gene in hereditary haemorrhagic telangiectasia type 2. *Nat Genet* 1996;**13**:189–95.

40 McDonald J, Miller FJ, Hallam SE *et al.* Clinical manifestations in a large hereditary hemorrhagic telangiectasia (HHT) type 2 kindred. *Am J Med Genet* 2000;**93**:320–7.

41 Shovlin CL, Hughes JMB, Scott J *et al.* Characterization of endoglin and identification of novel mutations in hereditary hemorrhagic telangiectasia. *Am J Hum Genet* 1997;**61**:68–79.

•42 Pece N, Vera S, Cymerman U *et al.* Mutant endoglin in hereditary hemorrhagic telangiectasia type I is transiently expressed intracellularly and is not a dominant negative. *J Clin Invest* 1997;**100**:2568–79.

43 Paquet M-E, Pece-Barbara N, Vera S *et al.* Analysis of several endoglin mutants reveals no endogenous mature or secreted protein capable of interfering with normal endoglin function. *Hum Mol Genet* 2001;**10**:1347–57.

•44 Bourdeau A, Dumont DJ, Letarte M. A murine model of hereditary hemorrhagic telangiectasia. *J Clin Invest* 1999;**104**:1343–51.

45 Abdalla S, Pece-Barbara N, Vera S *et al.* Analysis of ALK-1 and endoglin in newborns from families with hereditary hemorrhagic telangiectasia type 2. *Hum Mol Genet* 2000;**9**:1227–37.

46 Lux A, Gallione C, Marchuk D. Expression analysis of endoglin missense and truncation mutations: insights into protein structure and disease mechanisms. *Hum Mol Genet* 2000;**9**:745–55.

47 Oh S, Seki T, Goss K *et al.* Activin receptor-like kinase 1 modulates transforming growth factor-β1 signaling in the regulation of angiogenesis. *Proc Natl Acad Sci USA* 2000;**97**:2626–31.

48 Wrana JL, Attisano L, Wieser R *et al.* Mechanism of activation of the TGF-b receptor. *Nature* 1994;**370**:341–7.

◆49 Heldin C-H, Miyazono K, ten Dijke P. TGF-β signalling from cell membrane to nucleus through SMAD proteins. *Nature* 1997;**390**:465–71.

◆50 Massague J, Chen Y-G. Controlling TGF-β signalling. *Genes Dev* 2000;**14**:627–44.

◆51 Miyazono K, Kusanagi K, Inoue H. Divergence and convergence of TGF-β/BMP signaling. *J Cell Physiol* 2001;**187**:265–76.

•52 Pece Barbara N, Wrana JL, Letarte M. Endoglin is an accessory protein that interacts with the signaling receptor complex of multiple members of the transforming growth factor-β superfamily. *J Biol Chem* 1999;**274**:584–94.

•53 Lastres P, Letamendia A, Zhang H *et al.* Endoglin modulates cellular responses to TGF-β1. *J Cell Biol* 1996;**133**:1109–21.

54 Bourdeau A, Faughnan M, McDonald M-L *et al.* Potential role of modifier genes influencing transforming growth factor-beta1 levels in the development of vascular defects in endoglin heterozygous mice with hereditary hemorrhagic telangiectasia. *Am J Pathol* 2001;**158**:2011–20.

•55 Deng Z, Morse J, Slager S *et al.* Familial primary pulmonary hypertension (gene *PPH1*) is caused by mutations in the bone morphogenetic protein receptor-II gene. *Am J Hum Genet* 2000;**67**:737–44.

•56 Lane K, Machado R, Pauciulo M *et al.* Heterozygous germline mutations in BMPR2, encoding a TGF-β receptor, cause familial primary pulmonary hypertension. *Nat Genet* 2000;**26**:81–4.

•57 Trembath R, Thomson J, Machado R *et al.* Clinical and molecular features of pulmonary hypertension in hereditary hemorrhagic telangiectasia. *N Engl J Med* 2001;**345**:325–34.

58 Berg JN, Guttmacher AE, Marchuk DA *et al.* Clinical heterogeneity in hereditary haemorrhagic telangiectasia – are pulmonary arteriovenous malformations more common in families linked to endoglin? *J Med Genet* 1996;**33**:256–7.

59 Vettukattil J, Slavik Z, Monro J *et al.* Intrapulmonary arteriovenous shunting may be a universal phenomenon in patients with the superior cavopulmonary anastomosis. *Heart* 2000;**83**:425–8.

60 Larsson E, Solymar L, Eriksson B *et al.* Bubble contrast echocardiography in detecting pulmonary arteriovenous malformations after modified Fontan operations. *Cardiol Young* 2001;**11**:505–11.

61 Ference BA, Shannon TM, White RI *et al.* Life threatening pulmonary hemorrhage with pulmonary arteriovenous malformations and hereditary hemorrhagic telangiectasia. *Chest* 1994;**106**:1387–92.

62 Remy J, Remy-Jardin M, Wattinne L *et al.* Pulmonary arteriovenous malformations: Evaluation with CT of the chest before and after treatment. *Radiology* 1992;**182**:809–16.

63 Administration of Radioactive Substances Advisory Committee (ARSAC). Notes for guidance on the administration of radioactive substances to persons for diagnosis, treatment or research. Oxford: ARSAC, 1998.

•64 Thompson RD, Jackson JE, Peters AM *et al.* Sensitivity and specificity of radioisotope right-left shunt measurements and pulse oximetry for the early detection of pulmonary arteriovenous malformations. *Chest* 1999;**115**:109–13.

•65 Mager J, Zanen P, Verzijbergen F *et al.* Quantification of right to left shunt with ⁹⁹mTc labeled albumin macroaggregates and 100% oxygen in patients with hereditary haemorrhagic telangiectasia. *Clin Sci* 2002;**102**:127–34.

•66 Chilvers ER, Peters AM, George P *et al.* Quantification of right to left shunt through pulmonary arteriovenous malformations using ⁹⁹Tcᵐ albumin microspheres. *Clin Radiol* 1989;**39**:611–14.

•67 Nanthakumar K, Graham A, Robinson T *et al.* Contrast echocardiography for detection of pulmonary arteriovenous malformations. *Am Heart J* 2001;**141**:243–6.

68 Blomley M, Harvey C, Hughes J *et al.* Can relative signal changes in the intensity of systemic spectral doppler signals after bolus injections of microbubbles measure pulmonary AV shunting noninvasively. *Radiology* 1999;**213**:1145.

69 Feinstein J, Moore P, Rosenthal D *et al.* Comparison of contrast echocardiography versus cardiac catheterization for detection of pulmonary arteriovenous malformations. *Am J Cardiol* 2002;**89**:281–5.

70 Gutierrez F, Glazer H, Levitt R *et al.* NMR imaging of pulmonary arteriovenous fistulae. *J Comput Assist Tomogr* 1984;**8**:750–2.

71 Maki D, Siegelman E, Roberts S *et al.* Pulmonary arteriovenous malformations: three dimensional gadolinium-enhanced MR-angiography – initial experience. *Radiology* 2001;**219**:243–6.

72 Ohno Y, Hatabu H, Takenaka D *et al.* Contrast-enhanced MR perfusion imaging and MR angiography: utility for management of pulmonary arteriovenous malformations for embolotherapy. *Eur J Radiol* 2002;**41**:136–46.

73 Coley S, Jackson J. Pulmonary arteriovenous malformations. *Clin Radiol* 1998;**53**:396–404.

74 Apostolopoulos S, Kelekis N, Papiannis J *et al.* Transcatheter occlusion of a large pulmonary arteriovenous malformation with use of a cardioseal device. *J Vasc Intervent Radiol* 2001;**12**:767–9.

•75 Terry P, White R, Barth K *et al.* Pulmonary arteriovenous malformations: physiologic observations and results of balloon embolization. *N Engl J Med* 1983;**308**:1197–200.

•76 Lee D, White R, Egglin T *et al.* Embolotherapy of large pulmonary arteriovenous malformation: long term results. *Ann Thorac Surg* 1997;**64**:930–40.

•77 Jackson J, Whyte M, Allison D *et al.* Coil embolization of pulmonary arteriovenous malformations. *Cor Vasa* 1990;**32**:191–6.

•78 Haitjema T, Overtoom T, Westermann CJJ *et al.* Embolization of pulmonary arteriovenous malformations: results and follow-up in 32 patients. *Thorax* 1995;**50**:719–23.

•79 Andersen P, Kjeldsen A, Oxhoj H et al. Embolotherapy for pulmonary arteriovenous malformations in patients with hereditary haemorrhagic telangiectasia. Acta Radiol 1998;**39**:723–6.

80 Watanabe N, Munakata Y, Ogiwara M et al. A case of pulmonary arteriovenous malformation in a patient with brain abscess successfully treated with video-assisted thoracoscopic resection. Chest 1995;**108**:1724–7.

81 Puskas J, Allen M, Moncure A et al. Pulmonary arteriovenous malformations: therapeutic options. Ann Thorac Surg 1993;**56**:253–8.

*82 Moussouttas M, Fayad P, Rosenblatt M et al. Pulmonary arteriovenous malformations. Cerebral ischemia and neurologic manifestations. Neurology 2000;**55**:959–64.

83 Gershon A, Faughnan M, Chon K et al. Transcatheter embolotherapy of maternal pulmonary arteriovenous malformations during pregnancy. Chest 2001;**119**:470–7.

84 Reynaud-Gaubert M, Thomas P, Gaubert J-Y et al. Pulmonary arteriovenous malformations: lung transplantation as a therapeutic option. Eur Respir J 1999;**14**:1425–8.

85 Faughnan M, Lui Y, Wirth J et al. Diffuse pulmonary arteriovenous malformations. Characteristics and prognosis. Chest 2000;**117**:31–8.

86 Khalil A, Farres M-T, Mangiapan G et al. Pulmonary arteriovenous malformations: diagnosis by contrast-enhanced magnetic resonance angiography. Chest 2000;**117**:1399–403.

87 Remy-Jardin M, Wattine L, Remy J. Transcatheter occlusion of pulmonary arterial circulation and collateral supply: failures, incidents, and complications. Radiology 1991;**180**:699–705.

88 Porteous MEM, Burn J, Proctor SJ. Hereditary haemorrhagic telangiectasia: a clinical analysis. J Med Genet 1992;**29**:527–30.

89 Shovlin CL, Hughes JMB, Tuddenham EGD et al. A gene for hereditary haemorrhagic telangiectasia maps to chromosome 9q3. Nat Genet 1994;**6**:205–9.

90 Plauchu H, de Chadarévian J-P, Bideau A et al. Age-related profile of hereditary hemorrhagic telangiectasia in an epidemiologically recruited population. Am J Med Genet 1989;**32**:291–7.

*91 Shovlin CL, Guttmacher AE, Buscarini E et al. Diagnostic criteria for hereditary hemorrhagic telangiectasia (Rendu-Osler-Weber syndrome). Am J Med Genet 2000;**91**:66–7.

◆92 Guttmacher AE, Marchuk DA, White RI. Hereditary hemorrhagic telangiectasia. N Engl J Med 1995; **333**:918–24.

◆93 Haitjema T, Westermann CJJ, Overtoom TTC et al. Hereditary haemorrhagic telangiectasia (Osler-Weber-Rendu syndrome) – new insights in pathogenesis, complications, and treatment. Arch Intern Med 1996;**156**:714–19.

94 Pollak J, Egglin T, Rosenblatt M et al. Clinical results of transvenous systemic embolotherapy with a neuroradiologic detachable balloon. Radiology 1994;**191**:477–82.

95 Kjellin I, Boechat MI, Vinuela F et al. Pulmonary emboli following therapeutic embolization of cerebral arteriovenous malformations in children. Pediatr Radiol 2000;**30**:279–83.

96 Mager J, Overtoom T, Mauser H et al. Early cerebral infarction after embolotherapy of a pulmonary arteriovenous malformation. J Vasc Intervent Radiol 2001;**12**:122–3.

97 Clark J, Pugash R. Recanalization after coil embolization of pulmonary arteriovenous malformations. Am J Roentgenol 1998;**171**:1426.

Index